BIOMEDICAL TECHNOLOGY and DEVICES HANDBOOK

The Mechanical Engineering Handbook Series

Series Editor
Frank Kreith
Consulting Engineer

Published Titles

Air Pollution Control Technology Handbook
Karl B. Schnelle, Jr. and Charles A. Brown
Computational Intelligence in Manufacturing Handbook
Jun Wang and Andrew Kusiak
Fuel Cell Technology Handbook
Gregor Hoogers
Handbook of Heating, Ventilation, and Air Conditioning
Jan F. Kreider
Hazardous and Radioactive Waste Treatment Technologies Handbook
Chang Ho Oh
Inverse Engineering Handbook
Keith A. Woodbury
Opto-Mechatronic Systems Handbook: Techniques and Applications
Hyungsuck Cho
The CRC Handbook of Mechanical Engineering
Frank Kreith
The CRC Handbook of Thermal Engineering
Frank Kreith
The Handbook of Fluid Dynamics
Richard W. Johnson
The MEMS Handbook
Mohamed Gad-el-Hak
Biomedical Technology and Devices Handbook
James Moore and George Zouridakis

Forthcoming Titles

Handbook of Mechanical Engineering, Second Edition
Frank Kreith and Yogi Goswani
Multi-Phase Flow Handbook
Clayton T. Crowe
Shock and Vibration Handbook
Clarence W. de Silva

BIOMEDICAL TECHNOLOGY and DEVICES HANDBOOK

Edited by

James Moore
George Zouridakis

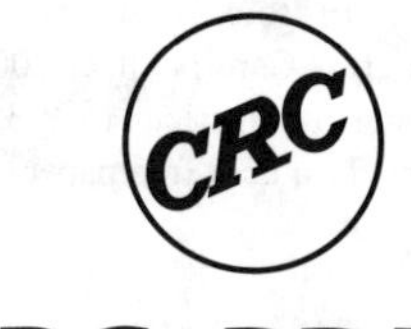

CRC PRESS

Boca Raton London New York Washington, D.C.

Library of Congress Cataloging-in-Publication Data

Biomedical technology and devices handbook / edited by James Moore and George Zouridakis.
p. cm. -- (The mechanical engineering handbook series)
Includes bibliographical references and index.
ISBN 0-8493-1140-3 (alk. paper)
1. Biomedical engineering--Handbooks, manuals, etc. 2. Medical instruments and apparatus--Handbooks, manuals, etc. I. Moore, James E., Jr., 1964- II. Zouridakis, George. III. Series.

R856.15.B565 2003
610′.28--dc21 2003046278

Direct all inquiries to CRC Press LLC, 2000 N.W. Corporate Blvd., Boca Raton, Florida 33431.

Visit the CRC Press Web site at www.crcpress.com

International Standard Book Number 0-8493-1140-3
Library of Congress Card Number 2003046278
Printed in the United States of America 1 2 3 4 5 6 7 8 9 0
Printed on acid-free paper

Preface

In an attempt to summarize the field of medical technology, a natural tendency is to begin to list the areas of medicine in which technology is being applied. If, on the other hand, one tries to name an area of medicine in which it is not being applied, it becomes clear that technology is a dominant factor in modern healthcare delivery. The domain of biomedical technology has evolved through the interaction of physicians, scientists, and engineers who have combined their skills to develop better methods for diagnosing and treating disease. Recent advances in the fields of molecular biology, biomaterials, tissue engineering, and imaging have given clinicians exciting new tools. The ever-increasing significance of computational sciences, bioinformatics, visualization, telecommunications, and robotics gives promise of new clinical devices and procedures that will revolutionize medical practice.

The majority of clinicians are fascinated by, and very receptive to, new technological advances. However, the degree to which novel technologies are included in the everyday practice depends on many factors. In the free-market environment of the U.S., financial considerations such as potential market share, intellectual property protection, regulatory approval, and insurance reimbursement often determine the fate of an emerging technology. On the other hand, if the market demands that a new technology become available, it will find its way into clinical practice.

The rapidly evolving nature of biomedical technology development makes it difficult to define exactly the field itself, much less attempt to describe its entirety in a single volume. Thanks to the expertise and special effort of the contributing authors, this handbook represents our attempt at preparing a current and, as much as possible, comprehensive professional reference source, as well as a textbook for undergraduate and graduate students in biomedical engineering programs. Yet, it should at best be considered a still photo of a swiftly moving, constantly reshaping cloud.

Preface

Acknowledgments

A volume with such diversity in topics could not have come together without enthusiastic contributions from scientists with diverse interests. Included here are contributions from 61 authors, representing 28 universities and hospitals, in 10 countries around the world — Canada, Denmark, Germany, Italy, Israel, Japan, Taiwan, Turkey, U.K., and the U.S. This handbook is a testament to their extraordinary effort and belief in the purpose of its existence.

We would also like to acknowledge the hard work and endless support of the CRC Press staff, particularly Cindy Carelli, Helena Redshaw, Elizabeth Spangenberger, and Naomi Lynch. Dr. Moore also acknowledges the support of the Engineering College at Florida International University, where he was on faculty for much of the preparation of this handbook.

The effort behind this handbook would not have been possible without the support and understanding of our families. From James Moore, much heartfelt love and appreciation to Peggy Moore and their wonderful children Gerald, James III, and Jacquelyne. From George Zouridakis, lots of love and gratitude to his wife Maria Kataki, M.D., and their princess, Antonia.

Editors-in-Chief

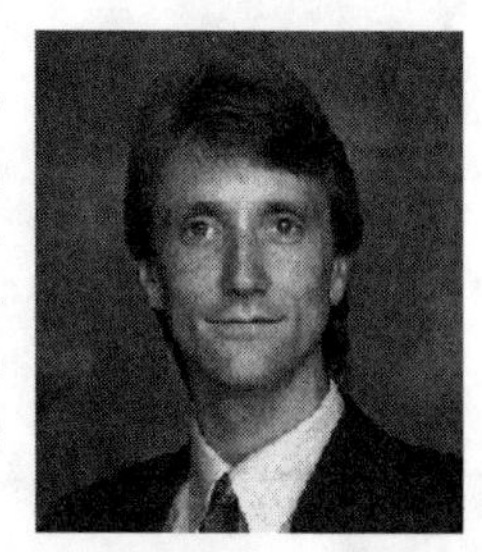

James E. Moore, Jr., Ph.D., was born in Toccoa, GA to James and Joyce Moore. He received his bachelor's degree in mechanical engineering with highest honor from the Georgia Institute of Technology, followed by an M.S. and Ph.D. from the same school and institute. After a postdoctoral fellowship at the Swiss Institute of Technology in Lausanne, he accepted a faculty position at Florida International University. His research focuses on the role of mechanical factors in cardiovascular disease development and treatment. His personal interests include music and ultimate frisbee.

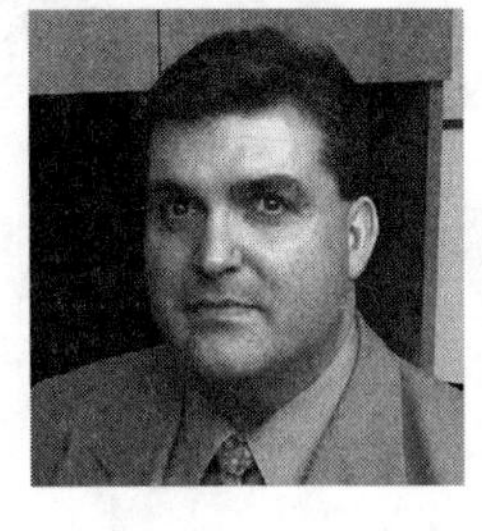

George Zouridakis, Ph.D., was born in Chania, Greece. He received a Dr. Ing. degree in electronics engineering from the University of Rome La Sapienza in Italy, followed by an M.S. and Ph.D. in biomedical and electrical engineering, respectively, from the University of Houston. He then joined the Department of Neurosurgery at the University of Texas–Houston Medical School as an assistant professor, where his clinical activities included intraoperative monitoring, functional brain mapping, and deep brain stimulation. Recently, he joined the Department of Computer Science at the University of Houston as an associate professor, and is currently the director of the Biomedical Imaging Lab. His research interests are in the areas of biomedical imaging, computational biomedicine, and functional brain mapping. He has authored a book, *A Concise Guide to Intraoperative Monitoring* (CRC Press, 2001), and is an associate editor of the *IEEE Transactions on Biomedical Engineering.*

Contributors

Stelios T. Andreadis
Department of Chemical Engineering
State University of New York at Buffalo
Amherst, New York

Nurullah Arslan
Department of Industrial Engineering
Fatih University
Istanbul, Turkey

Kyriacos A. Athanasiou
Department of Bioengineering
Rice University
Houston, Texas

Hisham S. Bassiouny
Department of Surgery
University of Chicago
Chicago, Illinois

Daniel S. Beasley
The University of Memphis
Memphis, Tennessee

Timothy Bill
Department of Plastic Surgery
University of Virginia
Charlottesville, Virginia

A.G. Brown
Department of Histopathology and Morbid Anatomy
Barts & The London School of Medicine & Dentistry, Queen Mary
Univeristy of London
London, U.K.

Kristine S. Calderon
Department of Health Promotion, Education, and Behavior
University of South Carolina
Columbia, South Carolina

Rajiv Chopra
Sunnybrook and Women's College Health Sciences Centre
Toronto, Ontario, Canada

Kevin Cleary
Imaging Science and Information Systems (ISIS) Center
Department of Radiology
Georgetown University Medical Center
Washington, D.C.

Eric Crumpler
Biomedical Engineering Institute
Florida International University
Miami, Florida

Michael A. Curi
Department of Surgery
University of Chicago
Chicago, Illinois

Eric M. Darling
Department of Bioengineering
Rice University
Houston, Texas

Maria de la Cova
Hialeah Hospital
Hialeah, Florida

Dario Farina
Laboratory for Neuromuscular System Engineering
Department of Electronics
Politecnico di Torino
Torino, Italy

Yuriy Fofanov
Department of Computer Science
University of Houston
Houston, Texas

Juan Franquiz
Biomedical Engineering Institute
Florida International University
Miami, Florida

Stephen L. Gaffin
Thermal and Mountain Medicine Division
U.S. Army Research Institute of Environmental Medicine
Natick, Massachusetts

Thomas J. Gampper
Department of Plastic Surgery
University of Virginia
Charlottesville, Virginia

Roman Joel Garcia
Department of Biological Sciences
Florida International University
Miami, Florida

Icel Gonzalez
Herbert Jay Gould, School of Audiology and Speech-Language Pathology
University of Memphis
Memphis, Tennessee

Herbert Jay Gould
The University of Memphis
Memphis, Tennessee

S.E. Greenwald
Department of Histopathology and Morbid Anatomy
Barts & The London School of Medicine & Dentistry, Queen Mary
Univeristy of London
London, U.K.

Mark A. Grevious
Department of Surgery
University of Illinois at Chicago
Chicago, Illinois

Craig J. Hartley
Baylor College of Medicine
Houston, Texas

Carla S. Hatten
Premier Neurodiagnostic Services
Sugarland, Texas

Hermann Hinrichs
Department of Neurology II
University of Magdeburg
Germany

Clark T. Hung
Cellular Engineering Laboratory
Department of Biomedical Engineering
Columbia University
New York, New York

Noriko Iida
Department of Physiology
School of Medicine
University of Hiroshima
Hiroshima, Japan

Darshan Iyer
Biomedical Imaging Lab
Department of Computer Science
University of Houston
Houston, Texas

Marc Jalisi
Biomedical Engineering Institute
Florida International University
Miami, Florida

Steven A. Jones
Department of Biomedical Engineering
Louisiana Tech University
Ruston, Louisiana

Eiji Kawasaki
Unit of Metabolism/Diabetes and Clinical Nutrition
Nagasaki University School of Medicine
Nagasaki, Japan

Spencer Kee
Critical Care and Anesthesiology
M.D. Anderson Cancer Center
Houston, Texas

Elisa E. Konofagou
Department of Radiology–MRI Research
Brigham and Women's Hospital
Harvard Medical School
Boston, Massachusetts

Lidia Kos
Department of Biological Sciences
Florida International University
Miami, Florida

Tong-Bin Li
Department of Computer Science
University of Houston
Houston, Texas

Robert S. Litman
College of Pharmacy
Nova Southeastern University
Fort Lauderdale, Florida

Eduardo Lopez
Miami, Florida

Francis Loth
Department of Mechanical and Industrial Engineering
Department of Bioengineering
University of Illinois at Chicago
Chicago, Illinois

Christopher K. Macgowan
Department of Medical Imaging
University of Toronto
Toronto, Canada

Robert L. Mauck
Cellular Engineering Laboratory
Department of Biomedical Engineering
Columbia University
New York, New York

Anthony J. McGoron
Biomedical Engineering Institute
Florida International University
Miami, Florida

Liran Mendel
Heller Institute of Medical Research
Military Physiology Unit
Sheba Medical Center
Tel Hashomer, Israel

Roberto Merletti
Laboratory for Neuromuscular System Engineering
Department of Electronics
Politecnico di Torino
Torino, Italy

James E. Moore, Jr.
Biomedical Engineering Institute
Florida International University
Miami, Florida

Daniel S. Moran
Heller Institute of Medical Research
Military Physiology Unit
Sheba Medical Center
Tel Hashomer, Israel

Michael R. Moreno
Biomedical Engineering Institute
Florida International University
Miami, Florida

Charles C. Nguyen
School of Engineering
Catholic University of America
Washington, D.C.

B. Montgomery Pettitt
Department of Computer Science
University of Houston
Houston, Texas

Carl A. Pinkert
Department of Pathology and Laboratory Medicine
University of Rochester Medical Center
Rochester, New York

Dejan B. Popović
Center for Sensory Motor Interaction
Aalborg University
Aalborg, Denmark

Marco Pozzo
Laboratory for Neuromuscular System Engineering
Department of Electronics
Politecnico di Torino
Torino, Italy

Timothy P.L. Roberts
Department of Medical Imaging
University of Toronto
Toronto, Canada

Lewis B. Schwartz
Department of Surgery
University of Chicago
Chicago, Illinois

C. Corey Scott
Department of Bioengineering
Rice University
Houston, Texas

Reza Tabrizchi
Division of Basic Medical Sciences
Faculty of Medicine
Memorial University of Newfoundland
St John's, Newfoundland, Canada

George Triadafilopoulos
Division of Gastroenterology
School of Medicine
Stanford University
Stanford, California

Pei-Shan Tsai
College of Nursing
Taipei Medical University
Taipei, Taiwan

Arnold Vainrub
Department of Chemistry
University of Houston
Houston, Texas

Thomas D. Wang
Division of Gastroenterology
School of Medicine
Stanford University
Stanford, California

Tonja Weed
Department of Plastic Surgery
University of Virginia
Charlottesville, Virginia

Michael D. Weil
Sirius Medicine, LLC
Fort Collins, Colorado

Carolyn B. Yucha
College of Nursing
University of Florida
Gainesville, Florida

George Zouridakis
Biomedical Imaging Lab
Department of Computer Science
University of Houston
Houston, Texas

Contents

I Basic Clinical Measurements

II Imaging Techniques

III Biological Assays

IV Genetic and Tissue Engineering

V Interventional Disease Treatment

VI Ambulatory Adaptations

VII Recovery

VIII Alternative and Emerging Techniques

I

Basic Clinical Measurements

Introduction: Technology as a Tool for Aiding Initial Diagnosis

From the moment we enter a doctor's office or hospital, we are confronted with equipment designed to improve the diagnosis and treatment of disease. Most of the initial clinical evaluation is aided by seemingly simple devices. However, the fact that these devices have become commonplace does not detract from the elegance of their technological development.

The widespread use of basic clinical technologies has greatly benefited patient care; body temperature, heart activity, blood pressure, and brain activity can be measured much faster and more accurately than ever before. Moreover, certain patterns in the data gathered by these relatively simple devices can often be used to provide an accurate diagnosis, as in the case of cardiac arrhythmia.

In this section, the underlying technology of devices used at the front lines of clinical medicine is presented, along with basic information on their use and the potential risks they may pose to patients. Continued advances in this area will enhance the ability of primary care physicians to identify and treat disease accurately and efficiently.

This section includes the following chapters:

1. Measuring Body Temperature
2. Ultrasonic Blood Flow and Velocity Measurement
3. Electromagnetic Blood Flow Measurements
4. Electromyography: Detection, Processing, and Applications
5. Evoked Potentials
6. Electroencephalography
7. Hearing and Audiologic Assessment

1

Measuring Body Temperature

Daniel S. Moran
Heller Institute of Medical Research

Stephen L. Gaffin
U.S. Army Research Institute for Environmental Medicine

Liran Mendel
Heller Institute of Medical Research

CONTENTS

1.1 Introduction

Knowledge of body temperature is required for a wide range of physiological and clinical studies. However, body temperature is not uniform throughout, neither in distribution within the body nor over time, and decisions must be made as to where to measure temperature, and by what means. The choice of an appropriate temperature measurement site and method requires some knowledge of how the human body responds to environmental factors and is described below.

Several mathematical models have been developed to describe the distribution of body temperature in humans in various environments, and under widely ranging physiological conditions.[1] A theoretical concept of a warm "core" surrounded by a cooler "shell" is widely used to describe the body's central region of temperature that is defended by a variety of physiological mechanisms.[2] This core is a roughly cylindrical region along the axis of the trunk and includes the inner regions of the neck and head. While there are small differences in temperature from place to place within the core that depend on local blood supply, metabolic rate and the temperature of neighboring tissue, a single temperature is used as a reasonable approximation of core temperature (T_c).[3]

Under neutral environmental conditions of an ambient temperature of 28 to 30°C and 40 to 60% relative humidity, T_c is approximately 37°C in a resting, healthy nude subject.[4] The skin temperatures of the forehead, trunk, fingers and toes are progressively cooler. In a cold environment, skin temperatures of these areas could be much lower and, if sufficiently cold, the skin may freeze even though the temperature of the core may have fallen only a degree or two. The wearing of clothes, by providing insulation, could substantially raise those peripheral skin temperatures and defend against hypothermia.

In order to properly interpret temperature measurements at any given site, some knowledge is required of the physical and physiological factors that create that temperature, and how changes in those factors

0-8493-1140-3/04/$0.00+$1.50

may alter temperature. Skin temperature of a nude resting human is largely determined by the environmental temperature, relative humidity, wind speed, intensity of solar radiation, atmospheric pressure, metabolic rate and skin blood flow.[5] This blood flow varies over a wide range depending on the body's requirements at the time. During exercise at room temperature, as body temperature rises, the flow of warm blood from the core to the extremities substantially increases, raising the temperature of the skin to dissipate this heat by radiation, conduction, convection and the evaporation of sweat.[6] The relative contribution of each heat dissipation mechanism varies with physiological status and environmental conditions. At cold ambient temperatures at rest, blood flow to the skin is reduced to minimize heat loss from the core, and skin temperature falls.[5]

Even at rest and under constant environmental conditions, body temperature rises and falls about 0.5°C from a mean of approximately 37.0°C in a circadian cycle, lowest in the morning and highest in the late afternoon, but varying somewhat from person to person. Where, then, is the best place to measure the temperature-skin or core? It really depends on the nature of what is intended; is this a clinical study of fever, or a physiological study of heat loss to the environment? For most purposes, the best measure of abnormal health and altered physiological status is the measurement of T_c. Those measurements can be made sequentially during the course of an experiment lasting minutes to hours or illness or, if periodically over days, at the same time each day to account for the circadian variation.

Body temperature is a result of the steady state between the rates of metabolic heat production plus absorption from the environment and the rate of heat dissipation. When the absorption of heat from high environmental temperature and/or high metabolic rate from exercise is greater than the body's ability to dissipate it, temperature rises and the condition of hyperthermia results. Fever, on the other hand, results when an infection or absorbed substance causes a release of cytokines from various body tissues that circulate to the brain, act on the thermoregulatory center and raise the "set point" temperature from 37°C. Under such a condition, a 37°C body temperature is "considered" by the hypothalamus to be a hypothermic state. The body defends this new set point temperature and elevates T_c by means of an increased metabolic rate through shivering and by reduced dissipation of heat through vasoconstriction, two classic homeostatic mechanisms of hypothermia.

Hypothermia results when heat is dissipated from the body faster than it is produced. It usually occurs because of a cold environmental temperature or an increased conduction of heat by water because of water immersion. In addition, hypothermia may result from the wearing of wet clothes in cold weather, or from a reduction of metabolic heat rate due to severe illness. Regardless of the mechanisms, hyperthermia, fever and hypothermia can be fatal.

1.1.1 History of the Thermometer

Illness has long been known to lead to fever.[7] It is written in Deuteronomy, "The Lord shall smite thee with a consumption, with a fever, and with an inflammation...," said God to Moses, threatening him to uphold the commandments.[8]

The first quantitative instruments for measuring temperature were devised by 17th century Florentine glassblowers. In some of these instruments, carefully weighted hollow glass balls were suspended in a liquid medium whose density depended on its temperature. The balls would float or sink depending on the local density of the medium that varied slightly with the temperature. The temperature of liquid depended on the ambient temperature surrounding the instrument, its distance from the outer surface of the liquid and the convective movement of the liquid. This system was not very accurate because the temperature indicated by the glass balls depended not only on ambient temperature, density and location, but also on the shape of the containers, as this influenced convection currents.

The first pioneer in the history of the thermometer was Galileo, who prepared a "thermoscope" from a thin glass tube with one end inserted into a sealed bulb containing liquid.[7] As temperature rose and fell, the liquid volume expanded and contracted causing the level of the liquid in the tube to rise and fall. However, because one end of the tube was open to the air, the height of the liquid was influenced by atmospheric pressure as well as by temperature. This was clear to the astronomer

Olaus Roemer in 1702, who recognized the importance of sealing the open end of the tube as well as the bulb. Roemer also developed a temperature scale based on two fixed points, the boiling point of water defined as 60° and the temperature of melting ice set at 7.5°.[9] In 1720, Daniel Gabriel Fahrenheit added what he considered a more "rational" scale to his thermometer assigning a value of 0° to the freezing point of a saturated solution of salt and water, and setting the upper point by "placing the bulb of the thermometer in the mouth or armpit of a healthy male."[9] Eventually, this scale was modified so that it could be conveniently calibrated by defining the freezing and boiling points of distilled water as 32 and 212°F, respectively. Today, the most widely used scale is the centigrade scale, suggested by Celsius in 1742. Celsius originally set the boiling point of water as 0° and the freezing of ice at 100°, but these points were reset into its present format by the Danish botanist Linnaeus in 1750.[7]

In 1868 Carl Wunderlich published *Fever in Disease*, which summarized his observations of thousands of temperature measurements in patients with various diseases.[10] He found that fevers rarely exceeded 105°F and that a practical thermometer for clinical use required the measurement of only the limited temperature range of 95 to 105°F. For convenience, he added a small kink in the tube to prevent the mercury from returning to the bulb when the thermometer was removed from the fevered patient. His views that temperature should be measured in all patients met considerable resistance from the conservative medical community, and years passed before temperature determinations became routine in medical practice.

In a different approach to temperature measurements, 19th century chemists found that esters of cholesterol formed loose structures — today called liquid crystals — that changed color as their temperature changed. These were first introduced by Lehmann in 1877 as a means of measuring skin temperature (T_{sk}), but they were not employed by others for a century. Initially, the crystals were mixed with black pigments, and adhered to a flat surface that was placed on the skin. Because surface veins provided local warm regions, they could be readily identified on the liquid crystal surface by their color, which was different from that of the rest of the cooler skin. Nevertheless, this method was not suitable for widespread physiological or medical use, had a narrow temperature range and a long response time, was uncomfortable to patients and was limited to a specialized laboratory environment. Furthermore, it could be used only once and then was thrown away.

This changed with the advent of microencapsulation technology. Simplified devices containing microencapsulated liquid crystals embedded onto flexible surfaces were developed. These had improved contact areas created by using inflated airbags with transparent windows to press them against uneven and curved skin surfaces. Advances in chemistry led to the development of reusable liquid crystal devices, each responding to small temperature changes, and which could be produced in physiologically relevant ranges of temperatures. Such systems have been used to diagnose pathological conditions in the breast, lower back and veins.[11,12] However, the liquid crystal technique was only useful when a pathology led to alterations in skin temperature, but not to changes in core temperature alone.

The most widely used instruments for measuring core temperature are the mercury and alcohol thermometers. However, in recent years the use of mercury thermometers has been declining, and they have been banned from some government laboratories because of increasing concern over mercury toxicity to the environment and, for mercury spills, the imposition of substantial penalties by the U.S. Environmental Protection Agency. Exceptions to this prohibition may be extended if investigators can show that alcohol-based thermometers cannot be used.

Infrared thermometers inserted into the ears are increasingly being used in hospital and home-care environments because of their convenience, economic benefit and environmental safety.

A relatively new method for measuring core temperature is the "temperature pill." This is a small sealed sensor containing a miniaturized transmitter whose frequency depends upon temperature. A nearby receiver translates the frequency into temperature and records the results over time.

We will review here different devices and methods to measure T_c as a diagnostic tool for illnesses and infectious diseases, with a view to their practical incorporation to prevent heat or cold injuries during commercial activities, sporting events, military training and combat.

An ideal thermometer must satisfy several conditions:[13]

- It must be accurate to at least 0.1° in order to monitor temperatures associated with fever, as well as the normal circadian variation in temperature.
- It must provide a true local temperature and not be influenced by changes in temperature of distant areas of the body such as in the limbs and skin, or by the environmental temperature.
- It must be stable long enough so that, after calibration, its accuracy is maintained.
- It must be small enough and of a shape appropriate to where it can be used in the body (mouth, rectum, esophagus).
- The area of use should not influence the temperature being measured. For instance, heavy breathing usually cools a mouth thermometer.
- It must be simple to operate.

Errors preventing true measurements of the body core temperature include noncompliance with the measuring protocol, e.g., inserting a rectal thermometer to an incorrect depth, an insufficient measuring time, and possible chemical incompatibility between the sensor and the surrounding medium.[13]

1.2 Noninvasive Sites for T_c Measurements

1.2.1 Oral

The method of inserting a thermometer into the sublingual pocket (i.e., under the tongue) is the most widely used method for measuring body temperature in the home environment, in the clinic and often in clinical research because of the convenience of easy accessibility of the mouth. The temperature in this region is usually, but not always, close to core temperature because of the large regional arterial blood flow from a branch of the carotid artery. Furthermore, this thermometer responds rapidly with changes in T_c. Nevertheless, this measurement may be substantially affected by the following factors:

- The skin on the head or face being cooler than the rest of the body
- Exposure to cold air
- Rapid or irregular mouth breathing patterns, especially in athletes or crying children, that may increase local evaporation thus lowering the temperature
- Ingestion of hot or cold beverages
- Recent smoking
- Neurological compromise making compliance difficult, e.g., by heat illness
- Differences in the temperature in different parts of the mouth cavity

1.2.2 Axilla

Measuring temperature at the axilla ("armpit") is slower than oral temperature measurement, as it takes longer to reach equilibrium. In addition, this method is less accurate than measurements in the rectum, mouth or ear.[14] This temperature is usually appreciably lower than the T_c, especially in athletes. Due to its inherent inaccuracy, it is not recommended for clinical use.

1.2.3 Tympanic Membrane

The tympanic membrane receives blood from branches of the internal carotid artery that also supply blood to the thermoregulatory center in the hypothalamic region of the brain, and is close to core temperature. A thermometer was developed to measure the temperature in this site, in part because of the easy access of the ear canal. However, many studies show that this method of measurement is unreliable, especially during physical effort in the heat, due to errors in measurements introduced by dirt, and inaccurate placement of the thermometer by an unskilled person.[13-17]

1.2.4 Body Surface

Skin temperature is normally measured by thermistors placed on the skin, covered by a layer of insulation and secured in place by tape. Because skin temperature varies from region to region, an integrated skin temperature is normally taken by averaging recorded temperatures on the skin in a dozen or more different places, unless a temperature is required at a specific site. This body surface temperature does not reflect T_c, but only the temperature of the skin.

1.3 Invasive Sites for T_c Measurements

1.3.1 Rectal

The rectum contains a high density of blood vessels with a large blood flow from the core, and is an accurate and convenient location for measuring core temperature. Temperatures obtained from the rectum are usually slightly higher than those taken from other regions, especially during leg exercise, since there is a warming effect of blood returning to the core from the metabolically active leg muscles. On the other hand, in severe pathological conditions such as the hypodynamic state of shock, in which metabolic rate may fall, then the rectal temperature (T_{re}) may be lower than T_c.

In particular, the rectum is the most widely used location for physiological and clinical studies of heat illnesses and for diagnostic tests, especially in babies and children. For accuracy, the thermometer must be inserted a consistent distance into the rectum. Furthermore, the response time for determining rectal temperatures is somewhat slower than those of other locations such as the esophagus. This slow response time is a disadvantage when rapid changes in core temperature are being studied. This method also has the disadvantage of requiring a hardwire connection to a recording device, thus limiting physical activities. However, in a side-by-side comparison between rectal, aural and axillary temperatures, it was concluded that rectal temperature monitoring offered the greatest combination of accuracy and precision.[14]

1.3.2 Esophagus

A small thermistor or thermocouple attached to a thin insulated wire can be swallowed so that it remains in place within the esophagus, above the entry to the stomach. This deep body location is close to the heart and aorta. Measurements at this location respond rapidly to changes in core temperature.

The main reason it is not more widely used is the difficulty of insertion. The esophageal thermistor is threaded through the nasal passages and down into the esophagus. This process may be uncomfortable and may irritate the nasal passages, and not all persons can tolerate the procedure.[18] Among other problems with this method is assurance that it is located correctly in the esophagus, and that the subject has not recently consumed any hot or cold beverages. This temperature measurement, although less accurate than pulmonary artery measurements, is appropriate for use in physiological research, but has relatively little use in clinical practice.

1.3.3 Pulmonary Artery

The pulmonary artery is a large vessel containing blood with low oxygen content extending from the right ventricle to the lungs where the blood is then reoxygenated. To reach this location, an invasive procedure carrying significant medical risk is required. A long, flexible catheter (narrow tube) containing a tiny thermistor is inserted into a large vein in the neck, leg or arm, threaded toward the heart, through the vena cava into the right heart chamber, down through the atrium and ventricle and then floated up into the pulmonary artery. The large blood flow through the pulmonary artery from the core and surroundings makes this location very accurate for measuring T_c. Obviously, its use is severely limited to special situations where such an invasive procedure is justified.[19]

1.3.4 Urinary Bladder

This discontinued older method was based on the belief that the temperature of the urine was closely related to the temperature of the body, and involved measuring the temperature of fresh urine. However, it was found that the temperature of urine did not accurately reflect core temperature, and depended on the rate of urination. As a result, this method is rarely used.

1.4 Methods and Instruments for T_c Measurement

Temperature is a measure of the average kinetic energy of the particles in a system. When heat is added to a system the kinetic energy of all the atoms is increased, their electrons become more energetic and their temperature rises. The operation of thermistors and thermocouples described below is based on this principle.

1.4.1 Digital Electronic Thermometers

Digital electronic thermometers contain one of two types of temperature-sensing elements — thermistors or thermocouples. They are connected by long, narrow flexible cables to an electronic "black box" where temperature is displayed digitally, usually to 0.1°C. These thermometers can be used for measuring rectal, oral or axillary temperatures, and are convenient for use in research, in the clinic and in the home environment. Their use increased when mercury thermometers were banned in a number of countries for environmental protection and safety reasons. Both the thermistor- and thermocouple-based digital thermometers are stable, accurate and respond rapidly to changes in temperature. They are smaller than the other types of temperature probes because the temperature sensing elements of both types of temperature transducers are tiny ($<50\ \mu m^2$).

1.4.1.1 Thermistors

Thermistors contain an alloy of heavy metals of the types used as semiconductors, and their atoms form microscopic crystal lattices. When this alloy is placed in an electric circuit at a constant ambient temperature, a stable voltage is maintained.[20] Electrons in semiconducting metals are easily released by only a small increase in thermal energy, i.e., by an increase in temperature. When the electronic circuit is made, at a given voltage, freed electrons cross the semiconductor lattice.[21] The number of thermal electrons released by the alloy increases exponentially with temperature and, by Ohm's law, the electrical resistance of the lattice falls exponentially. A rise in temperature, therefore, leads to a reduced voltage and, by precalibration, this voltage measurement is converted to and displayed as temperature.[13]

1.4.1.2 Thermocouples

A thermocouple contains a junction of two wires composed of different metals welded together. When placed in an electric circuit, a current will flow when the two metals are at different temperatures.[15,16] The physical basis for current flow across the junction is as follows:

In any given metal, some of the electrons present can move freely, almost as if they were in a gas. If one end of a wire is heated, more electrons will be freed in the warmer region. With its higher energy, these electrons carrying negative charges will undergo a net diffusion toward the cooler region. When two different metals of intrinsically different physical and chemical properties are welded together, inevitably, the number of electrons "freed" by each metal at a given temperature, their rate of migration down a thermal gradient, and their rates of heat flow are different on the two sides of the weld. As a result of those differences, heat and electrons will flow across one side of the junction and be absorbed into the other. In open circuit, the flow of electrons across the junction continues until the net negative charge created by the movement of negatively charged electrons on one side of the junction produces a negative electromotive force (emf) that counterbalances the flow. In addition to this thermally produced emf at the junction, there is a small chemical effect due to the difference in chemical potential between the two metals.

In an open circuit, at the junction, the two metals produce an emf proportional to the difference in temperature between the two sides of the junction, and for most pairs of metals this emf is in the order of microvolts per °C difference. In practice, two separate thermocouples are run simultaneously in a differential mode, with one maintained at a constant reference temperature and the other used as the temperature probe. When placed on or into warm tissue, heat transfers across the wall of this probe and its temperature approaches the local body temperature. The voltage generated by the difference in temperature between the two probes is converted to temperature, by precalibration.

1.4.1.3 Response Time of Temperature Measurements

The time required for an accurate measurement can be seconds or minutes, depending on which of the two possible modes of operation are employed by the thermal probes. In the steady-state mode, requiring several minutes, the final temperature is displayed only after the sensor has reached thermal equilibrium. In the predictive mode, the initial rate of change of temperature is measured for a few seconds and a mathematically calculated final temperature is predicted. The prediction of the final temperature depends upon when, exactly, the probe is first in contact with the body. While this method is faster, it is obviously not as reliable since it is an extrapolation. Moreover, this method is particularly technician-dependent since the probe must be accurately placed and the thermometer must be activated with precision.

1.4.2 Infrared Radiation Detectors

A new and popular method for measuring body temperature at home and in many clinics is the aural thermometer that measures temperature from the tympanic membrane or tympanic canal. A branch of the internal carotid artery supplies blood to the thermoregulatory center in the hypothalamus region of the brain, while another branch supplies the tympanic membrane. Because a high proportion of blood flow from the heart goes to the brain, the temperature of the brain is close to the temperature of the heart and core.

Within the ear, infrared (IR) radiation is emitted from all surfaces, at frequencies dependent on local temperature. An IR probe can be placed inside the ear canal to measure inner ear temperature. This measurement is rapid, cost-effective, noninvasive and, especially, convenient compared to other methods. However, despite its use in certain sports activities the aural thermometer is usually not considered accurate enough for most research.[22,23] For instance, in one study, aural temperatures were approximately 3°F lower than rectal temperatures taken at the same time.[24]

In use, a disposable otoscope probe is placed into the patient's ear. This probe consists of a flaring cylinder with a highly polished interior surface. It collects IR radiation from the direction in which it is aimed, and only that radiation strikes the transducer. The field of view "seen" by the transducer depends on both its distance from the target surface and viewing angle. Conventional wave-guides in commercial use have conical fields of view of 45° around their axes. The radius of the field of view for such a wave-guide is equal to its distance from the target.

IR thermometers operate very rapidly, typically in less than 5 sec, because they simply record radiation; they do not have to absorb heat from a tissue that requires time for adequate heat transfer to the transducer.

1.4.2.1 Tympanic Temperature

The tympanic membrane is both well supplied with arterial blood and convenient to access and could be an important site for measuring T_c. A disadvantage of this site, however, is the need to maneuver the probe to obtain input from the tympanic membrane, exclusively, and not from any other local tissues, so that the measurement is accurate and reproducible.

1.4.2.2 Ear Canal

The temperature within the ear canal is not uniform. It is usually warmest close to the inner ear and coolest near the ear lobe, and is influenced by ambient temperature.[24] Algorithms have been designed to utilize the ear canal temperatures to provide a temperature close to the core temperature. Using this site has the advantages that no special maneuvers of the IR probe are required, and it is simple and very convenient to access. However, a correction factor must be applied to the data to better account for the cooler temperature of the ear canal due to heat lost to the environment.

1.4.2.3 Shortcomings of IR Measurements

Despite the apparent ease of this method, numerous studies have reported difficulties in obtaining true tympanic temperatures.[15-17]

These thermometers typically have a viewing angle that is too wide, resulting in a field of view that is too large to measure exclusively temperature of the tympanic membrane. In fact, the probes from these devices may not even "see" the membrane at all because of poor user technique, or because of atypical anatomy of a particular ear canal. Research has shown that even when the thermometer is placed correctly, the temperature recorded from the tympanic membrane includes a component from an averaged temperature of the ear canal wall. As a result, temperature readings are generally lower than the actual temperature of the tympanic membrane and lower than T_c.[15-17] In order to compensate for these lower readings, some instruments contain an offset system for compensation. The system is calibrated from previously obtained data and shows computerized and updated temperatures from other locations (e.g., oral, rectal, axilla). One method for overcoming these difficulties is scanning, in which a series of measurements of the tympanic membrane are taken. The maximal temperature measured is considered the temperature of the tympanic membrane.

There are several scientific reports on the accuracy of the aural thermometer.[13-17] For example, when the measurement technique of the medical staff is inconsistent, inaccurate measurements are recorded. The lack of standardization stemming from the use of different types of thermometers results in a wide range of readings. Cerumen (earwax) buildup on the thermometer speculum causes an inaccurate measurement when a disposable probe is not used or the top is broken from improper use of the instrument. Additional factors that can cause a false result in the accuracy of the measurement include an abnormally high temperature gradient between the interior and exterior parts of the ear canal due to wind, inadequate depth of insertion of the thermometer inside the ear canal, and external conditions such as environmental temperature.

In summary, because of the complexity of the system and the many sources of error such as environmental factors and the anatomy of the ear, aural temperature is not reliable for establishing either fever or hypothermia. Hooker and Houston[17] summarized in 1996 a study that dealt with comparing temperature measurement in the ear as opposed to the oral cavity in the emergency room: "Tympanic thermometers are convenient and well accepted and do not require contact with mucous membranes. However, most authors have shown that the tympanic thermometer is very insensitive to fever and current research indicates that its sensitivity is not as good as that of oral electronic thermometers in the detection of fever." On the basis of other reports and on our own experience, we caution against relying on these thermometers in screening for fever in the emergency rooms.

1.4.3 Temperature Pill

Advances in microcircuitry technology have led to the development of a sophisticated "temperature pill" (T_{pill}). This large vitamin pill-sized device is sealed with biocompatible epoxy and/or silicone, and contains both a battery and an FM transmitter whose frequency depends upon the local temperature. A small receiver nearby ($6 \times 2.5 \times 12$ cm) picks up the signal, amplifies it, converts frequency to temperature after appropriate calibration, and can display the temperature and record it for later retrieval. The temperature pill is manufactured in a form smaller than 0.5 in. diameter $\times$ 1 in. and is swallowed. As the pill traverses the alimentary tract the local temperature is recorded on a receiver attached to the subject's belt. Other sensors and additional FM circuits can be included within the pill to simultaneously measure blood pressure, heart rate, pH and local chemistry. The temperature pill system has been found to be accurate, reliable and comfortable compared to esophageal and rectal temperature measurements and, importantly, has been certified by the FDA. The measurements were found to be valid not only during the steady state, but also during rising and falling body temperatures.[25] The pill temperature and response time tended to be intermediate between T_{re} and T_{es}.[25] Because of the few limitations to its use, T_{pill} is increasingly used in physiological research[26] and even in unusual clinical situations such as in monitoring core temperatures of saturation divers in the North Sea, so that they might avoid developing hypothermia.[27]

Not only can the pill be swallowed for short (approximately 1 to 2 days) application, but it can be manufactured small enough (9 mm diameter × 35 mm) to pass through a 10-mm endoscopic tube for long-term implantation, and has been used to monitor intrauterine temperature and pressure for up to 10 months.[28]

This device (pill and receiver) provides considerable advantages over previous techniques in experimental physiology because: (1) it does not require limiting the physical activity of the subject since no wire is required between the temperature sensor and the recorder; (2) it is not limited to the laboratory or hospital environment, but can be used in field settings; and (3) it may be used experimentally as well as clinically.

Disadvantages of the temperature pill include: (1) discomfort in swallowing for some individuals; (2) as the pill progresses down the gastrointestinal tract, local temperatures vary from place to place, and are subject to different influences on its local temperature; (3) high cost of the receiver (approximately $2000, and each pill costs approximately $40 for a one-time use); (4) impractical or not cost-effective for most clinical uses and (5) inappropriate for the home environment.

1.5 Summary

Until as recently as 1987, the esophageal temperature was considered the optimal method for measuring core temperature in the research setting; since then, it has been rectal temperature.[19] If that could not be measured, then at that time oral temperature was considered the best alternative. Nevertheless, measuring temperature with a mercury thermometer under the tongue still remains the most popular and accepted method in the world. In many instances, where it is not possible to measure temperature orally, and when measurement of body core temperature is needed, the measurement takes place in the rectum.

In recent years, a great deal of effort has been expended in advancing sophisticated new techniques in medicine such as magnetic resonance technology and biotechnology leading to improved diagnostic capability and new approaches to therapy. At the same time old, familiar methods are being replaced. Nevertheless, despite the favorable climate for developing new technology, and the need of medical staff and sportsmen for a simple, user-friendly, noninvasive and comfortable device for measuring core temperature, that instrument has not yet been developed. Measuring temperature in the brain or the pulmonary artery would be the "gold standard" for temperature measurements, but it is rarely possible to do so. This review summarized the alternative methods.

References

1. Havenith, G., Human surface to mass ratio and body core temperature in exercise heat stress — a concept revisited, *J. Therm. Biol.*, 26, 387–393, 2001.
2. Elizondo, R., Regulation of body temperature, in *Human Physiology*, Rhodes, R.A and Pflanzer, R.G., Eds., Saunders College Publishing, Philadelphia, 1989, pp. 823–840.
3. Wenger, C.B., Human adaptation to hot environments, in *Medical Aspects of Harsh Environments*, Pandolf, K.B. and Burr, R.E., Eds., Borden Institute, Walter Reed Army Medical Center, Washington, D.C., 2002, pp. 51–86.
4. Bligh, J. and Johnson, K.G., Glossary of terms for thermal physiology, *J. Appl. Physiol.*, 35, 941–961, 1973.
5. Pozos, R.S. and Danzl, D.F., Human physiological responses to cold stress and hypothermia, in *Medical Aspects of Harsh Environments*, Pandolf, K.B. and Burr, R.E., Eds., Borden Institute, Walter Reed Army Medical Center, Washington, D.C., 2001, pp. 351–382.

6. Sawka, M.N. and Wenger, C.B., Physiological responses to acute exercise heat stress, in *Human Performance Physiology and Environmental Medicine at Terrestrial Extremes*, Pandolf, K.B., Sawka, M.N., and Gonzalez, R.R., Eds., Benchmark Press, Indianapolis, 1988, pp. 97–151.
7. Ring, E.F.J., Progress in the measurement of human body temperature, *IEEE Eng. Med. Biol. Mag.*, 17, 19–24, 1998.
8. The Bible, Deuteronomy 28:22.
9. Gough, J.B., Fahrenheit's thermometer, in A *History of the Thermometer and Its Uses in Meteorology*, Johns Hopkins Press, Baltimore, 1996.
10. Wunderlich, C., *On the Temperature in Disease: A Manual of Medical Thermometry*, Transl., New Sydenham Society, London, 1871.
11. Sterns, E.E., Zee, B., SenGupta, S., and Saunders, F.W., Thermography. Its relation to pathologic characteristics, vascularity, proliferation rate, and survival of patients with invasive ductal carcinoma of the breast. *Cancer*, 77, 1324–1328, 1996.
12. Yang, W.J. and Yang, P.P., Literature survey on biomedical applications of thermography, *Biomed. Mater. Eng.*, 2, 7–18, 1992.
13. Cetas, T.C., Thermometers, in *Fever: Basic Mechanisms and Management*, Mackowiak, P.A., Ed., Lippincott-Raven Publ, Philadelphia, 1997, pp. 11–34.
14. Cattenaeo, C.G., Frank, S.M., Hesel, T.W., El Rahmany, H.K., Kim, L.J., and Tran, K.M., The accuracy and precision of body temperature monitoring methods during regional and general anesthesia, *Anesth. Analg.*, 90, 938–945, 2000.
15. Amoateng-Adjepong, Y., Del Mundo, J., and Manthous, C.A., Accuracy of an infrared tympanic thermometer, *Chest*, 115, 1002–1005, 1999.
16. Briner, W.W., Jr., Tympanic membrane vs rectal temperature measurement in marathon runners, *JAMA*, 276, 194, 1996.
17. Hooker, E.A. and Houston, H., Screening for fever in an adult emergency department: oral vs tympanic thermometry, *South. Med. J.*, 89, 230–234, 1996.
18. Stuart, M.C., Lee, S.M.C., and Williams, W.J., Core temperature measurement during supine exercise: esophageal, rectal and intestinal temperature, *Aviat. Space Environ. Med.*, 71, 939–945, 2000.
19. Brengelmann, G.L., Dilemma of body temperature measurement, in *Man in Stressful Environments: Thermal and Work Physiology*, Shiraki, K. and Yousef, M.K., Eds., Thomas, Springfield, 1987, pp. 5–22.
20. Childs, P.R.N., Greenwood, J.R., and Long, C.A., Review of temperature measurement, *Rev. Sci. Instrum.*, 71, 2959–2978, 2000.
21. Bloomfield, L.A., Thermometers and thermostats, in *How Things Work. The Physics of Everyday Life*, John Wiley & Sons, Indianapolis, 2001.
22. Armstrong, L.E., Maresh, C.M., Crago, A.E., Adams, R., and Roberts, W.O., Interpretation of aural temperatures during exercise, hyperthermia, and cooling therapy, *Med. Exerc. Nutr. Health*, 3, 9–16, 1994.
23. Armstrong, L.E., Crago, A.E., Adams, R., Senk, J.M., and Maresh, C.M., Use of the infrared temperature scanner during triage of hyperthermic runners, *Sports Med. Training Rehab.*, 5, 1–3, 1994.
24. Ash, C.J., Cooke, J.R., McMurry, T.A., and Auner, C.R., The use of rectal temperature to monitor heat stroke. *Missouri Med.*, May, 288, 1992.
25. O'Brien, C., Hoyt, R.W., Buller, M.J., Castellani, J.W., and Young, A.J., Telemetry pill measurement of core temperature in humans during active heating and cooling, *Med. Sci. Sports Exerc.*, 30, 468–472, 1998.
26. Coyne, M.D., Kesick, C.M., Doherty, T.J., Kolka, M.A., and Stephenson, L.A., Circadian rhythm changes in core temperature over the menstrual cycle: method for noninvasive monitoring, *Am. J. Physiol. Regul. Integr. Comp. Physiol.*, 279, R1316–R1320, 2000.

27. Mekjavic, I.B., Golden, F.S., Eglin, M., and Tipton, M.J., Thermal status of saturation divers during operational dives in the North Sea, *Undersea Hyperb. Med.*, 28, 149–155, 2001.
28. NASA, Implantable Biotelemetry System for Preterm Labor and Fetal Monitoring, http://technology.arc.nasa.gov/techopps/biotelemetry.html, 2002.

2

Ultrasonic Blood Flow and Velocity Measurement

Craig J. Hartley
Baylor College of Medicine

CONTENTS

2.1 Introduction

During the last 50 years, ultrasound has developed into a widely used research and clinical modality with its most widespread and familiar applications in noninvasive two-dimensional and color Doppler imaging.[1–4] From its earliest days, ultrasound has also found nonimaging medical applications using noninvasive as well as invasive, intraoperative, implantable, and intravascular transducers and sensors to measure dimensions, displacement, velocity, and flow. We will concentrate here on the ultrasonic measurement of blood flow and velocity.

2.2 Ultrasound Physics

Ultrasound is usually defined as a mechanical vibration with a frequency above the range of human hearing. The frequencies (f) usually employed in medical applications are in the range between 500 kHz and 100 MHz. Acoustic signals at these frequencies can be directed and coupled into body tissues where they propagate at the speed of sound. While traveling through the various tissues, the sound waves undergo absorption, refraction, reflection, and scattering, which depend on the acoustic properties of

0-8493-1140-3/04/$0.00+$1.50

the tissues (density, speed of sound, absorption coefficient, and homogeneity) and the changes in these properties at the tissue interfaces.[5,6] Thus, sound, which is transmitted into body tissues, undergoes a very complex series of interactions in which it can be partially passed, redirected, reflected, and/or weakened by each tissue and interface through which it passes. The reflections at the interfaces returning to the sending transducer produce the images with which we are familiar.

The speed of sound (c) in water, blood, and most body tissues is approximately 1500 ± 100 m/sec or 1.5 mm/μsec, so that at frequencies from 500 kHz to 100 MHz, the wavelength ($\lambda = c/f$) is between 0.015 and 3.0 mm.[7] The higher frequencies have shorter wavelengths and give higher resolutions, but are also attenuated to a greater extent and do not penetrate as far into the tissue without unacceptable loss of signal.[6] Thus, low frequencies (1 to 5 MHz) are used where greater penetration is required (noninvasive imaging and Doppler), and higher frequencies (5 to 50 MHz) are used where high resolution is required (invasive and intravascular imaging and velocimetry). Frequencies used for blood flow and velocity measurements from extravascular cuff type transit-time and Doppler probes are between 450 kHz and 20 MHz.

2.3 Ultrasonic Transducers

An important part of any ultrasound instrument is the transducer, which converts electrical energy to mechanical vibration and vice versa and defines the direction, frequency, and geometry of the sound beam. The active element is usually a piezoelectric material that ranges from single crystal quartz, which has a high sensitivity and narrow bandwidth, to polymers which have lower sensitivity but wider bandwidth.[8–10] The choice of material depends on the application; one of the more common materials used in medical ultrasound is piezoelectric ceramic such as lead-zirconate-titanate (LZT or PZT).[11] Ceramics have properties that are intermediate between crystals and polymers, provide a good compromise between sensitivity and bandwidth, and are available from several suppliers in sheets with metallic electrodes (silver, gold, or nickel) plated to each face.[12] The ceramic is generally fabricated in "thickness mode" where the thickness (1/2 wavelength) determines the resonant frequency which can range from a few hundred kilohertz to over 100 MHz.[13] When properly polarized during manufacture, the piezoelectric material thins or thickens when a voltage is applied, and conversely develops an electrical potential between its electrodes when subjected to a mechanical force. It can thus act as both a transmitter and a receiver of ultrasound. The sheets are cut into discs, squares, or strips for fabrication into a complete transducer consisting of the piezoelectric element or elements; acoustic matching layers; acoustic backing; acoustic focusing or diverging lenses; a holder or body consisting of metal, plastic, silicone rubber, or epoxy; lead wires; and an electrical connector. The word "transducer" is often used to refer to the piezoelectric element or to the completed device which is also referred to as a "scan head," "array," "probe," "sensor," or "crystal" depending on its configuration, shape, and application.[9] Imaging transducers are relatively complex because the sound beam must be electrically steered or mechanically directed to scan an area of interest. However, ultrasound can also be used in nonimaging applications to measure dimensions, velocity, flow, and displacement of tissues and fluids utilizing the principles outlined below. Compared to imaging, these methodologies use fairly simple transducers and signal processing, and many can produce outputs compatible with standard physiologic recorders and data acquisition systems.

2.4 Transit-Time Dimension

One of the first applications of ultrasound in medicine was to measure dimensions using the transit-time principle.[14–16] If a pulse of sound transmitted by one transducer is received by a second transducer or is reflected by a target back to the same transducer, the pulse arrival time (t) is related to the distance (d) between the transducers or to the reflector by the speed of sound (c) as shown in Figure 2.1A and 2.1B. The equations for the one-way (t_{1way}) and two-way (t_{2way}) transit times are shown in Figure 2.1 and below.

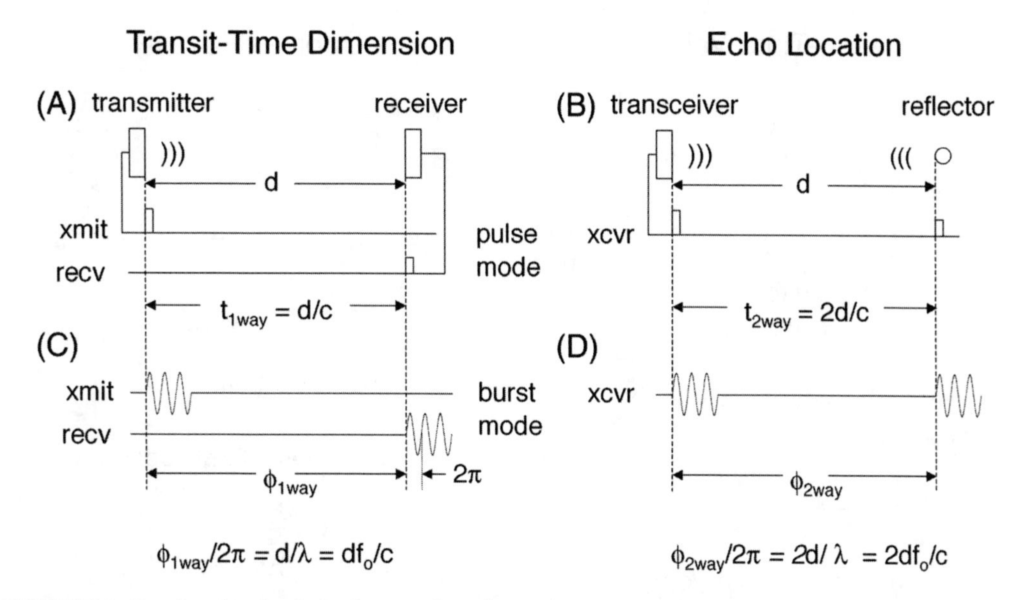

FIGURE 2.1 Drawing showing how ultrasound can be used to measure distance via transit-time (A,C) or pulse echo (B,D) methods for pulse (A,B) or burst (C,D) excitation of the transmitter. Equations are shown relating one-way (1way) and two-way (2way) transit-time (t) and phase (ϕ) to the distance (d) between the crystals or from the crystal to a reflector, where c is the speed of sound (~1500 m/sec or 1.5 mm/μsec), λ is the wavelength, and f_o is the ultrasonic frequency.

$$t_{1way} = d/c \tag{2.1}$$

$$t_{2way} = 2d/c \tag{2.2}$$

If a flip/flop is set at transmission of the pulse and reset upon receipt of the pulse, the width provides a simple measure of the distance between the transducers updated at a typical pulse repetition frequency (PRF) of 1 to 10 kHz. Compared to imaging, the signal processing is very simple. This method requires that the transducers be inserted into or attached to the tissue of interest and is commonly used to measure ventricular diameters,[14,16] myocardial segment length[15,17] and wall thickness,[18,19] and arterial diameter.[20,21] With proper synchronization, several dimensions can be measured simultaneously.[14,15,22] Although the accuracy is limited by the wavelength (typically 0.3 mm at 5 MHz), the sensitivity to motion or change in dimension is on the order of 1 μm.

If a tone burst is transmitted instead of a single-cycle pulse, the phase (ϕ) of the received burst measured in radians with respect to the transmitted burst could also be used as a measure of distance as shown in Figure 2.1C and 2.1D. The equations for one-way and two-way phase are also shown below in terms of the wavelength (λ) and the transmitted burst frequency (f_o).

$$\phi_{1way}/2\pi = d/\lambda = df_o/c \tag{2.3}$$

$$\phi_{2way}/2\pi = 2d/\lambda = 2df_o/c \tag{2.4}$$

In general, pulse mode is used to measure distance with two transducers,[14,18,22] and burst mode is used to measure change in position or displacement of tissues with a single echo transducer.[23–27]

If the fluid and/or the target are moving, the velocity (V) affects the arrival time, the phase, and the frequency of the received signals as shown in Figure 2.2. In pulse mode, the moving fluid speeds up the arrival of a pulse moving with the flow (t_{2-1}) and retards the arrival of a pulse moving against the flow (t_{1-2}). If we alternately transmit from each crystal, receive on the other, and subtract the arrival times, the difference in arrival times (Δt) divided by the average arrival time (t_{avg}) is directly proportional to the velocity as shown in the equation below provided that $V \ll c$.

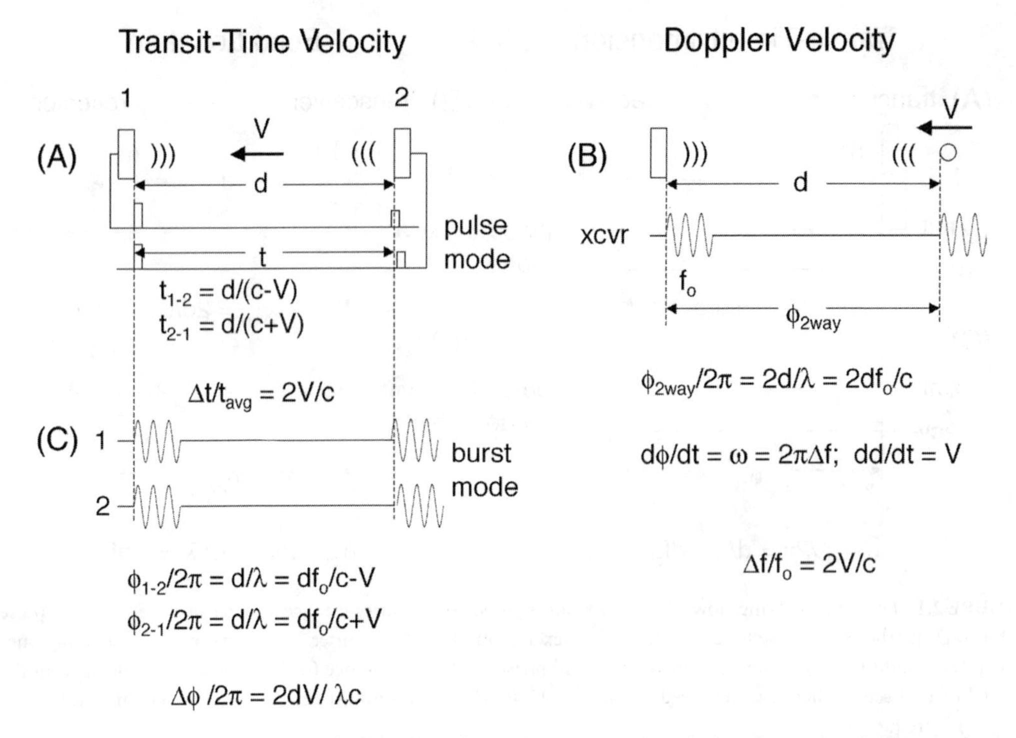

FIGURE 2.2 Drawing showing how ultrasound can be used to measure the velocity of a moving fluid or a reflecting target via transit-time (A,C) or Doppler (B) methods. The fluid velocity (V) adds or subtracts from the speed of sound (c) to change the arrival time (t) or phase (ϕ) of pulses traveling with (2–1) or against (1–2) the flow. The difference in transit-times (Δt) or phase ($\Delta\phi$) is proportional to the velocity. Since the phase of an echo (ϕ_{2way}) is proportional to distance (d), the derivative of phase (Doppler frequency, Δf) is proportional to the derivative of distance (reflector velocity, V). The equations hold only when $V \ll c$ and the velocity is in the direction of sound propagation.

$$\Delta t/t_{avg} = 2V/c \tag{2.5}$$

In burst mode, the relative phase of the received bursts ($\Delta\phi$) is also proportional to velocity.

$$\Delta\phi/2\pi = 2dV/\lambda c \tag{2.6}$$

In echo mode, the phase of the echo changes with each successive burst as the target moves with respect to the transducer. If we differentiate both sides of Equation 2.4 noting that the derivative of phase is angular frequency ($\omega = 2\pi f$) and the derivative of distance is velocity, we get an equation relating the Doppler shift frequency (Δf) to the velocity (V) of the reflector.[28]

$$\Delta f/f_o = 2V/c \tag{2.7}$$

Thus, ultrasound can be used to measure either distance or velocity depending on the conditions, the transducer, and the signal processing applied.

2.5 Transit-Time Velocity and Flow

The differential transit-time principle was first applied to the measurement of biologic flows in the 1950's[29,30] and is now in wide use in both industrial and medical applications. This method can operate with catheter-mounted transducers immersed in the fluid,[31] or with extravascular or cuff-type probes[30,32] as shown in Figure 2.3. The simplest approach is to place the transducers diagonally on opposite sides of the vessel (Figure 2.3A). This requires modification to Equations 2.5 and 2.6 to account for the angle

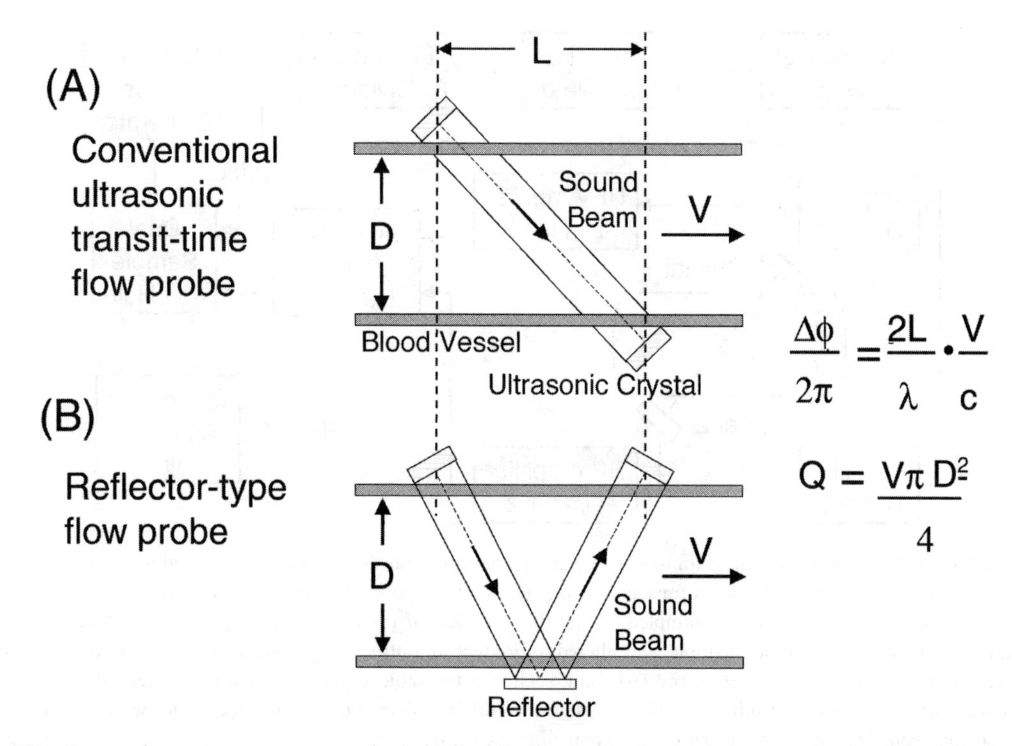

FIGURE 2.3 Ultrasonic transit-time methods for measuring blood flow through an exposed vessel using a conventional probe (A) or a reflector probe (B). The governing equation relating the difference in phase between upstream and downstream transits (Δϕ) to the average velocity (V) along the sound path is shown. In theory if the crystals are wider than the vessel, flow anywhere in the lumen contributes equally to the average velocity. Flow (Q) is then determined by multiplying velocity by the cross-sectional area. Because of the angle, the sensitivity is proportional to the length (L) along the vessel between the crystals rather than to the crystal spacing.

between the sound beam and the direction of flow, but with the constant angle, the difference between upstream and downstream transit-times (or phase shift) is still proportional to the average velocity along the sound path as shown by the equations in Figure 2.3 and below.

$$\Delta\phi/2\pi = 2LV/\lambda c \tag{2.8}$$

Volume flow (Q) is calculated by multiplying the average velocity across the lumen by the cross-sectional area of the vessel.

$$Q = V\pi D^2/4 \tag{2.9}$$

To be sensitive to volume flow and independent of vessel diameter and velocity profile, the sound beam must cover the entire vessel uniformly.[33] To achieve this, the piezoelectric crystals must be at least as long as the vessel diameter. In addition, the sensitivity to flow increases with the length of the probe (L) and the ultrasonic frequency ($f_o = c/\lambda$). These requirements and the need for stable and rigid geometries and insensitivity to variations in vessel angle have led to some innovative probe configurations. The reflector probe shown in Figure 2.3B allows the two transducers to be mounted in a rigid frame, and the dual path minimizes the sensitivity to angle variations.[34] Implantable transit-time probes based on the reflector design are available from Transonic Systems, Ithaca, NY in sizes to fit vessels from under 1 mm up to several centimeters.[35]

A simplified block diagram of a transit-time flowmeter is shown in Figure 2.4.[36] It uses the burst mode illustrated in Figure 2.2C with both crystals driven simultaneously. After the short transit-time, the bursts are received at the same time, and their phases are compared and sampled. After amplifying and filtering

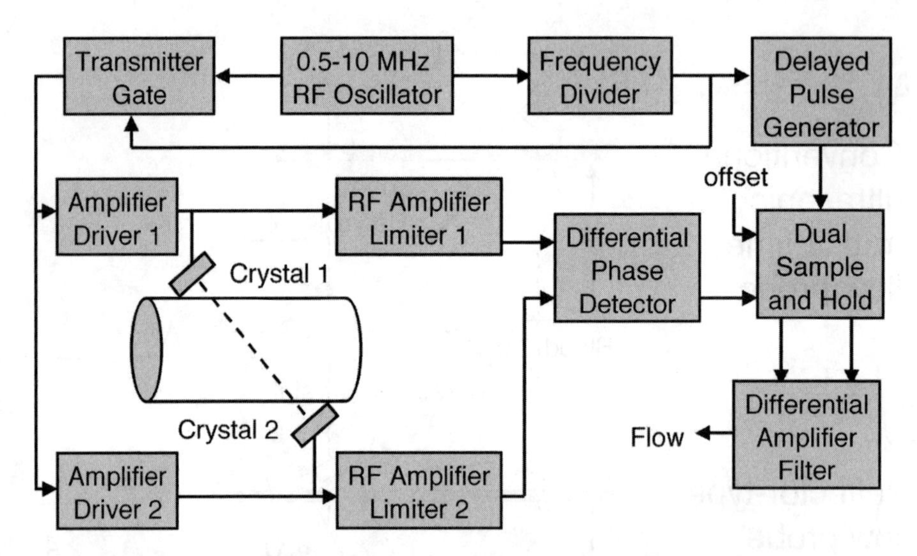

FIGURE 2.4 Simplified block diagram of one implementation of a transit-time flowmeter based on measuring the differential phase of ultrasonic bursts traveling simultaneously in opposite directions between two crystals as illustrated in Figure 2.2C. The phase is sampled during the reception of the burst by a delayed pulse following each transmission, held until the next sample, and filtered to produce an output proportional to flow. Other designs use alternate pulsing of the two crystals and switching such that the same signal path is used for each direction of measurement. This cancels or minimizes the effects of small differences in component values which would otherwise cause unacceptable offsets in measuring the very small phase shifts.

to remove the pulse repetition frequency (PRF), the flow signal can be displayed and recorded. Notice that an offset must usually be added to compensate for any differences in components or transducers in the signal path. In a more practical implementation, electronic switches are included to alternately reverse the crystal connections and/or the inputs to the phase detector in an attempt to cancel any differences in the crystals or in the signal paths. That, and the careful matching of load impedances during transmission and reception, and improved transducer designs have minimized zero-drift and made the ultrasonic transit-time flowmeter a practical and widely used device.[34]

2.6 Doppler Velocity

Another method to measure blood flow with ultrasound is Doppler velocimetry.[28,37,38] As indicated in Equation 2.7, the velocity of a target can be estimated by measuring difference in frequency between the transmitted wave and the signal reflected from the target. The difference frequency is known as the Doppler frequency and is directly proportional to the component of velocity along the sound beam. When applied to blood flow measurement, the situation is complicated by several factors as shown in Figure 2.5: (1) the direction of blood flow is not generally in the direction of the sound beam, (2) the blood cells that reflect the sound are very small and are poor reflectors,[39–42] (3) many cells are in the sound beam or sample volume (SV) at the same time, and (4) the cells don't necessarily move at the same velocity or direction. The signals from each blood cell or reflector add together with each blood cell, contributing a signal whose amplitude and frequency vary according to its velocity, direction, and position within the sample volume. The practical implications of these complicating factors will be explained below.

2.7 Continuous Wave Doppler

The first Doppler velocimeters utilized continuous wave (CW) ultrasound with one transducer acting as a constant transmitter and another simultaneously as a receiver.[37,38] The transducers can be placed on a catheter inside the vessel[43–46] or more commonly on a probe or cuff outside the vessel as shown in Figure

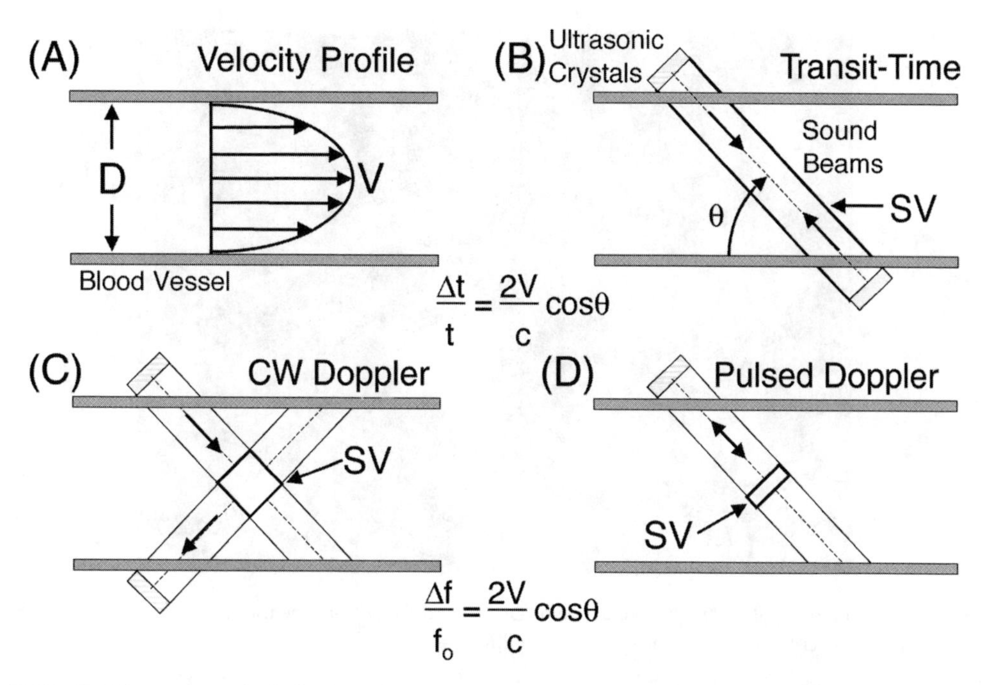

FIGURE 2.5 Ultrasonic methods for measuring blood flow in an exposed vessel: (A) an idealized velocity profile for laminar flow, (B) transit-time, (C) continuous wave (CW) Doppler, and (D) pulsed Doppler. The transit-time method (B) requires two crystals on opposite sides of the vessel, its sample volume (SV) includes the entire sound path between the crystals, and no reflectors are required in the fluid for operation. The CW Doppler method (c) also uses two crystals which can be on the same or opposite sides of the vessel. Its SV is the region where the transmitting and receiving sound beams cross, and its operation requires reflectors (blood cells) in the fluid. The pulsed Doppler method (D) uses a single crystal, and its sample volume can be controlled electronically in both length and position along the sound beam. In addition, the pulsed Doppler method can measure velocity from several SV's along the sound beam simultaneously. Normalized equations governing transit-time and Doppler methods are very similar in form. In each case the measured parameter (differential transit-time or Doppler frequency shift) varies in proportion to the average velocity (V) in the sample volume.

2.5C.[38,47] From outside the vessel, the angle between each transducer and the direction of flow (θ) must be considered as shown by the equation below.

$$\Delta f/f_o = 2(V/c)\cos\theta \tag{2.10}$$

The volume from which signals originate is often referred to as the sample volume (SV). In the transit-time flowmeter, the sample volume consists of the area between the crystals as shown in Figure 2.5B, and velocity is thus averaged across the entire lumen. In CW Doppler, signals are generated by any reflector in the area where the transmitting and receiving beams cross, as shown in Figure 2.5C. Because of absorption and attenuation, reflections from close targets will have higher signals than distant targets, and reflections from targets near the edges of the beams are weaker than from those near the center. Thus, the sample volume has an amplitude as well as a geometry, and the summing of the signals within the sample volume produces a weighted average due to these nonuniformities. Although the shape of the sample volume can be varied by controlling the beam shapes and crossing zone through sizing, angling, and focusing of the transducers, the control is limited, and the size and shape of the sample volume in CW Dopplers is often ill-defined.

2.8 Pulsed Doppler Velocity

Pulsed Doppler systems allow better control of the sample volume by transmitting and receiving short pulses from the same transducer at different times as shown in Figure 2.5D.[28,48,49] The axial length of the

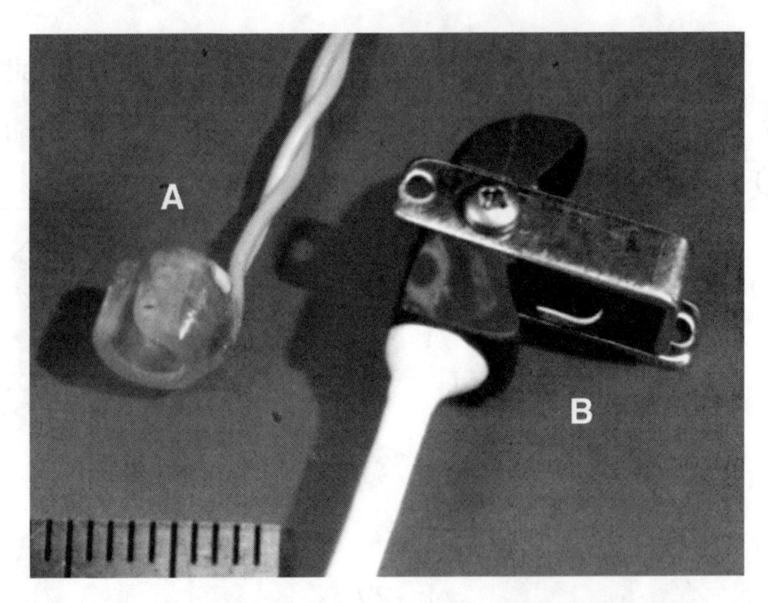

FIGURE 2.6 Photo of a pulsed Doppler cuff-type probe (A) and a reflector type transit-time probe (B) each sized to fit a 4-mm-diameter blood vessel. The scale is in millimeters.

sample volume is determined primarily by the lengths of the transmit and receive pulses, and its position along the sound beam is controlled by the time delay between transmission and reception. By controlling the beam width through focusing and sizing, the dimensions and shape of the sample volume can be controlled much more accurately in pulsed vs. CW Doppler systems.

Also shown in Figure 2.5A is the velocity profile across the vessel which may be parabolic as shown or much more complex. The way the sample volume intersects the velocity profile is extremely important in interpreting the signals from any of the ultrasonic velocimeters. Ideally, if volume flow is to be sensed, the sample volume should cover the entire vessel uniformly to average the entire lumen (best done with transit time but also possible with CW and pulsed Doppler methods); and if local velocity is to be sensed, the sample volume should be as small as possible (best done with the pulsed Doppler method). Figure 2.6 shows a photograph of a 20-MHz pulsed Doppler cuff (A) and a transit-time probe with a stainless steel reflector (B). Both are sized to fit around a 4-mm-diameter vessel.

2.9 Doppler Signal Processing

The final Doppler signal is a summation of the signals from each reflector in the sample volume with the frequency determined by the reflector velocity and angle, and the amplitude determined by its position in the sample volume. The result is a wideband signal with its spectral content related to the velocity distribution within the sample volume. The task of the Doppler signal processor is to extract the information contained in the signal and to present it in a meaningful way. The available options include audio only for listening,[37] frequency-to-voltage conversion for a recorder output,[38,50] and spectral analysis and display.[47] An additional concern is whether nondirectional or directional demodulation is needed.[51,52]

A block diagram of a directional 20-MHz pulsed Doppler velocimeter with frequency-voltage conversion is shown in Figure 2.7. A 20-MHz oscillator provides all of the timing and phase reference signals via frequency division and phase shifting. The transducer is energized at a PRF of 62.5 kHz by an 8-cycle tone burst similar to that shown in Figure 2.2B. The returning echoes are amplified and compared in-phase to two reference signals in quadrature (90° out-of-phase). The two-phase signals are sampled after a variable delay (which defines the location of the sample volume) and filtered to produce in-phase (I) and quadrature (Q) Doppler signals. These I and Q signals, when plotted on an X-Y display, show in polar coordinates the amplitude and phase of the Doppler vector which rotates at the Doppler frequency

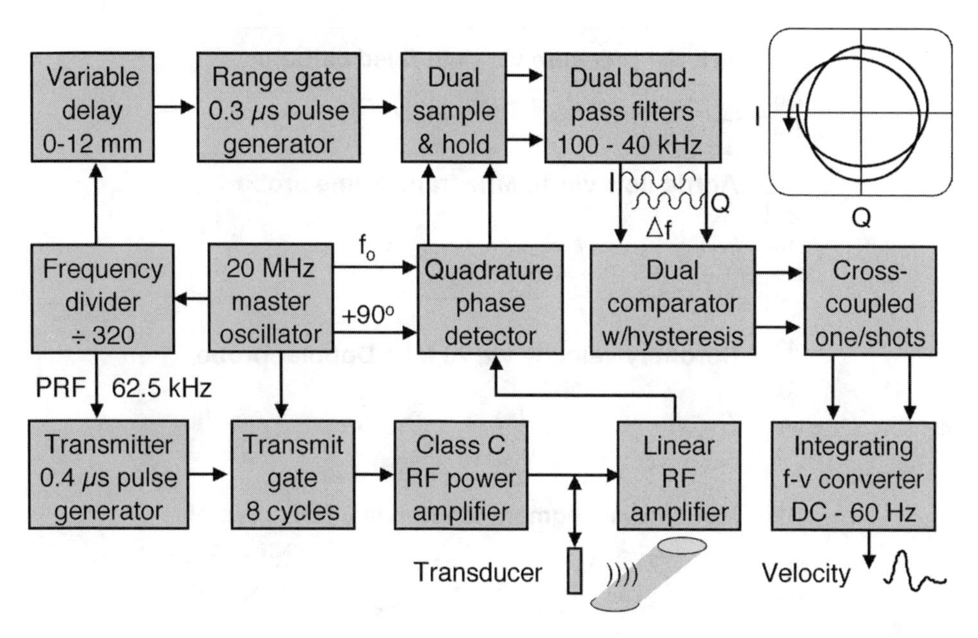

FIGURE 2.7 Block diagram of a 20-MHz pulsed Doppler velocimeter using quadrature phase detection and range-gating. After sampling and filtering, the in-phase (I) and quadrature (Q) Doppler signals can be viewed as the X and Y components of a phase vector which rotates at the Doppler frequency in a direction determined by the direction of flow. The Doppler signals can be further processed to produce a directional waveform proportional to the average frequency as shown, or they can be connected to a spectrum analyzer.

in a direction determined by the direction of flow. The signal processor must measure the frequency of rotation or angular velocity of the vector, the direction of rotation, and generate a suitable output (instantaneous, mean, peak, average, or spectrum). In complex flow regimes, there may be motion in several directions at once producing a very complex signal. The processor shown counts all X and Y axis (zero) crossings of the Doppler vector using the sign of the other signal to determine the direction and produces a directional display of the average frequency.[49,51]

The simple CW Doppler devices introduced in the early 1960s used nondirectional demodulation (producing only the X or Y component of the vector) and often contained only an audio output that was interpreted by listening to the signal. When used in research applications, a recordable and quantifiable output was required, and several methods were developed to generate a voltage proportional to the average frequency of the signal. The simplest of these is the zero-crossing counter (ZCC) that operates by counting the number of times the audio signal passes through zero in a given interval.[38,53] With a slight increase in complexity, the ZCC method can work with quadrature inputs to provide a direction-sensitive output[45,51,54] as shown in Figure 2.7. The ZCC method is simple, reliable, provides an accurate output for single frequency or narrow band signals with good signal-to-noise ratios, and is incorporated into many commercially available CW and pulsed Doppler devices.[22,49] As an example, Figure 2.8 shows simultaneously measured arterial pressure, 10-MHz transit-time aortic flow, 20-MHz Doppler coronary flow, and 5-MHz transit-time myocardial dimension signals from a dog with implantable ultrasonic sensors. The transit-time flow probe is configured as in Figure 2.4 with burst excitation and phase detection, the segment length crystals are configured as in Figure 2.1A with pulse excitation, and the Doppler velocity signal is derived from a 20-MHz pulsed Doppler probe as in Figure 2.6A with the sample volume centered in the vessel where the velocity gradient is small and the spectrum tends to be narrow. However, the performance of a ZCC degrades with wideband signals and with low or marginal signal/noise ratios often encountered in noninvasive applications,[53] and a better signal processor is required.

From the first applications of Doppler ultrasound, it was recognized that there was valuable information in the shape of the spectrum that could be appreciated by listening to the sounds, but that was difficult to

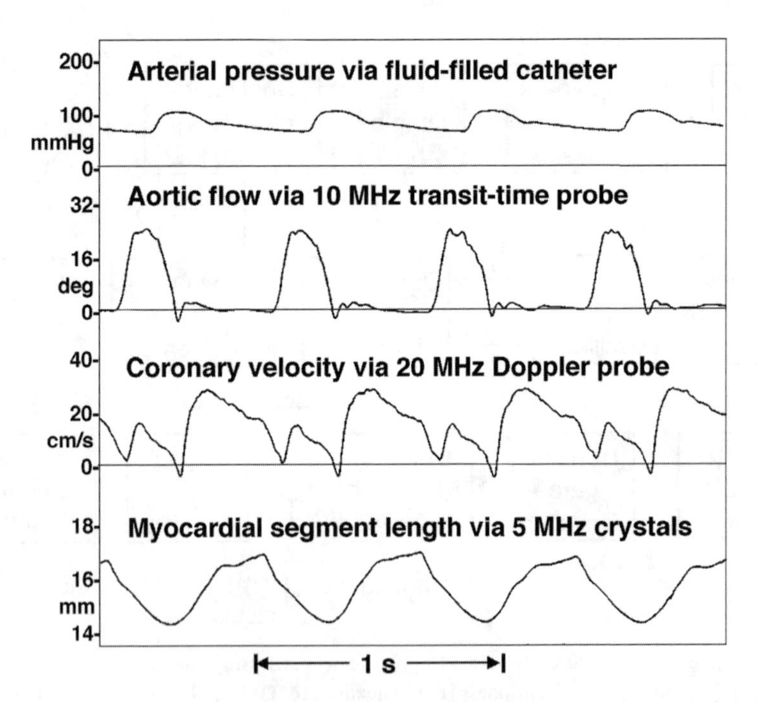

FIGURE 2.8 Multiple physiologic signals from an instrumented dog. Pressure was measured with a fluid-filled catheter placed in the descending aorta and connected to an external pressure transducer, aortic flow was measured with a 10-MHz transit-time probe on the ascending aorta, coronary flow was measured with a 20-MHz pulsed Doppler probe on the left anterior descending coronary artery, and LV myocardial segment length was measured with a pair of 5-MHz transit-time crystals (sonomicrometry) imbedded into the myocardium.

quantify or display. Early attempts at spectral analysis used swept filters,[55] banks of filters,[56] phase-locked loops,[57–59] or zero-crossing-interval histograms (ZCIH)[60] to produce various forms of time-frequency displays using analog signal processing. The advent of digital signal processing in the 1970s enabled a wide range of additional methods for spectral analysis which continue to be improved upon.[4] The most common spectral analyzer in use today is the fast Fourier transform (FFT) which is used in various forms in most clinical Doppler devices.[59] Other methods have included autoregressive (AR),[61] time-frequency distribution,[62,63] and others too numerous to include. The FFT algorithm acquires a series of short (64 to 1024 point) samples of the Doppler signal upon which a spectrum is calculated and displayed. Then, after a short time delay, a new set of samples is acquired and a new spectrum is calculated either in real-time or from previously sampled data. Depending on the time resolution required, the time delay may or may not exceed the total number of samples in the FFT resulting in either overlap or complete separation of adjacent spectra. Figure 2.9 shows FFT (A) and ZCC (B) displays of the Doppler signal taken from the author's common carotid artery using a 10-MHz pulsed Doppler probe held against the neck. The velocity scale on the right is calculated from the Doppler shift on the left using Equation 2.10 with a 45° angle. The dark line on the FFT display shows the peak of the spectrum and corresponds to the maximum velocity in the sample volume. The ZCC signal approximates the average velocity in the sample volume. Note that the peaks of the spectral velocity signal are more uniform than the peaks of the ZCC signal. We and others have found that the maximum velocity derived from the spectrum is a more robust signal that is less affected by vessel wall motion, probe motion, signal strength, noise, or slight misalignment of the probe.[62,64–66]

2.10 Multigate and Color Doppler

Pulsed Doppler devices are often used to measure the velocity distribution across a vessel, valve, or chamber during the cardiac cycle. Multiple range-gating allows velocity to be sensed at several locations

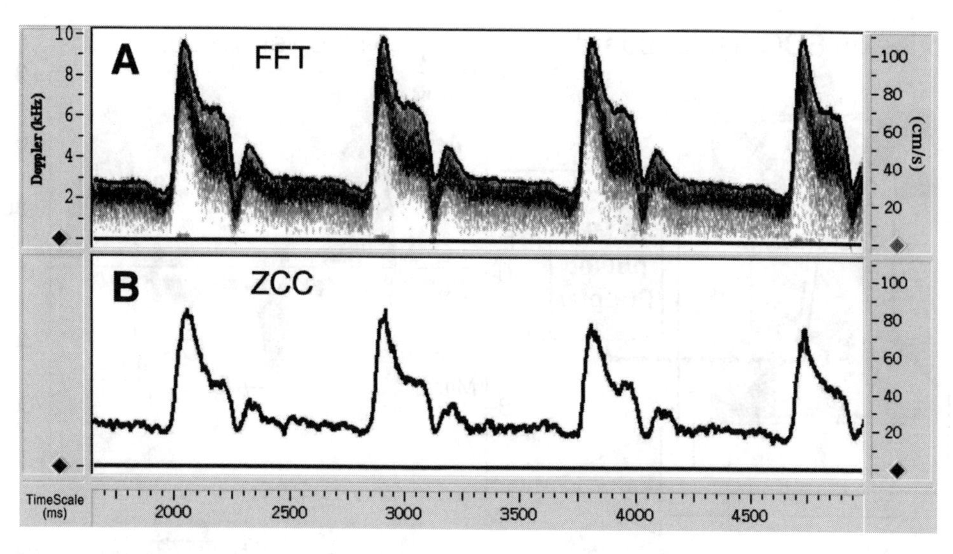

FIGURE 2.9 FFT display (above) and average zero-crossing frequency signal (below) from a common carotid artery made with a 10-MHz pulsed Doppler transducer applied to the neck. The solid line over the FFT display shows the maximum frequency calculated from the spectrum.

or sample volumes along the sound beam at the same time.[28] The simplest method uses several analog processors operating in parallel to produce quadrature audio signals from each gate or depth. The complexity of parallel processing limits the number of gates typically from 8 to 80.[67–70]

Digital processing can also be used with no practical limits on the number of range gates.[69,71,72] This approach is used in color Doppler imaging devices to sense velocity over a two-dimensional region in the image.[4,73] Color Doppler instruments allow visual interpretation of velocity patterns and distributions, but quantification is difficult because the number of samples from each measurement site is limited by the need to maintain a high frame rate for the image and because of the way frequencies are mapped into colors.

2.11 Feature Extraction

The Doppler signal contains potentially valuable information about the flow field within the sample volume, and spectral processing is the best way to extract the maximum number of parameters. The underlying assumption is that frequency components in the Doppler spectrum are directly related to velocity components within the sample volume. As an example, Figure 2.10 shows intracardiac velocity signals taken noninvasively from an anesthetized mouse using a 10-MHz probe applied just below the sternum and pointed toward the heart with the sample volume placed in the left ventricle at a depth of 7 to 8 mm. Using the envelope or maximum value of the spectrum, several useful parameters relating to cardiac function can be extracted as shown. From the aortic outflow wave, these include heart rate and period, systolic time intervals, peak ejection velocity, mean velocity, rise time, peak acceleration, and area under the ejection curve (stroke distance). From the mitral filling wave, we can measure filling times, peak early filling velocity, peak late filling velocity, and areas and slopes of the waves. Thus, with proper signal processing, Doppler velocimetry can provide useful indexes of left ventricular systolic and diastolic function[74] as well as peak and mean filling and ejection velocities.[64]

It is also possible to measure flow and velocity in peripheral arteries of animals as small as mice using transit-time and pulsed Doppler ultrasound.[35,65] Figure 2.11 shows Doppler velocity signals (D) taken noninvasively from nine sites (C) in an anesthetized mouse (A) using a 20-MHz Doppler probe (B). The shape of the velocity wave in a given vessel is a function of the vascular impedance of the arteries distal to the measurement site and is often used to estimate the severity of vascular disease and stenoses.[4,75,76]

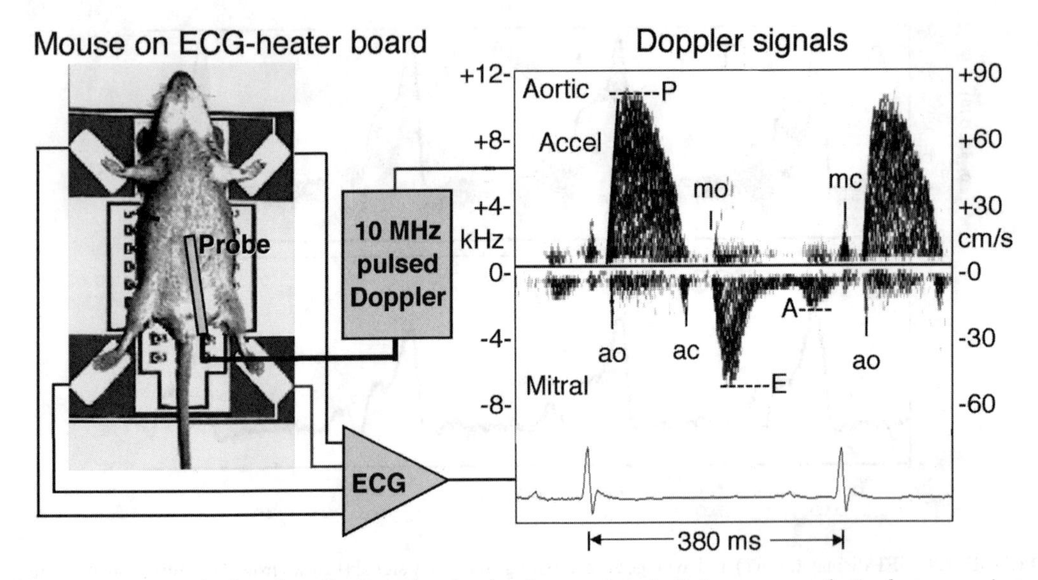

FIGURE 2.10 FFT display of cardiac Doppler signals taken noninvasively from an anesthetized mouse using a 10-MHz probe placed just below the sternum and pointed toward the heart. With the sample volume in the left ventricle, both inflow and outflow signals can be obtained. Labels show the opening (o) and closing (c) of the aortic (a) and mitral (m) valves, peak ejection velocity (P) and acceleration (Accel), and peak early (E) and late (A) filling velocities. From these signals, it is possible to obtain accurate timing of cardiac events such as pre-ejection time, filling and ejection times, and isovolumic contraction and relaxation times as indexes or systolic and diastolic ventricular function.

It can be seen in Figure 2.11 that the upstroke of the velocity wave at each site with respect to the ECG increases with distance from the heart. By measuring the difference in arrival times and the distance between measurement sites, the pulse-wave velocity of the arteries between the sites can be calculated.[77] Pulse-wave velocity is a function of arterial stiffness and is known to increase with age, hypertension, and other conditions[78,79] and has been proposed as an independent risk factor for cardiovascular disease.[80] Pulse-wave velocity can be measured noninvasively with Doppler ultrasound.

2.12 Converting Velocity to Volume Flow

In general, the measurement of volume flow requires knowledge of the average luminal velocity and the cross-sectional area of the vessel at the site where velocity is measured. There are several possible ways to accomplish this using ultrasound. Transit-time velocimetry can be converted to volume flow if the sound beam covers the entire vessel uniformly.[33,34] This turns out to be fairly easy to accomplish in practice, and most of the commercially available transit-time flowmeters utilize this principle.[35] Continuous wave Doppler could also be sensitive to volume flow if the sound beam covered the entire vessel uniformly, the cross-sectional area was known, and the output was related to the average frequency or first moment of the spectrum.[47,81–83] Although numerous attempts have been made, it has proven difficult to obtain uniform insonation together with an accurate measure of vessel diameter. In theory, pulsed Doppler can be used to measure the flux of blood through a surface which intersects the vessel.[84,85] This method is known as the *attenuation compensated flowmeter* and should sense volume flow independent of vessel size, orientation, or velocity profile. The method utilizes two sound beams: a broad beam which covers the entire vessel; and a smaller one that is centered in the vessel and used to estimate the attenuation along the signal path. Although the method has been proven to work in the laboratory, it has been difficult to implement practically due to problems in obtaining uniform insonation of one and only one vessel.

Pulsed Doppler can also be used to measure the velocity profile using a movable range-gate or multiple range-gates.[28] The point velocity measurements could then be combined with an area estimate to calculate

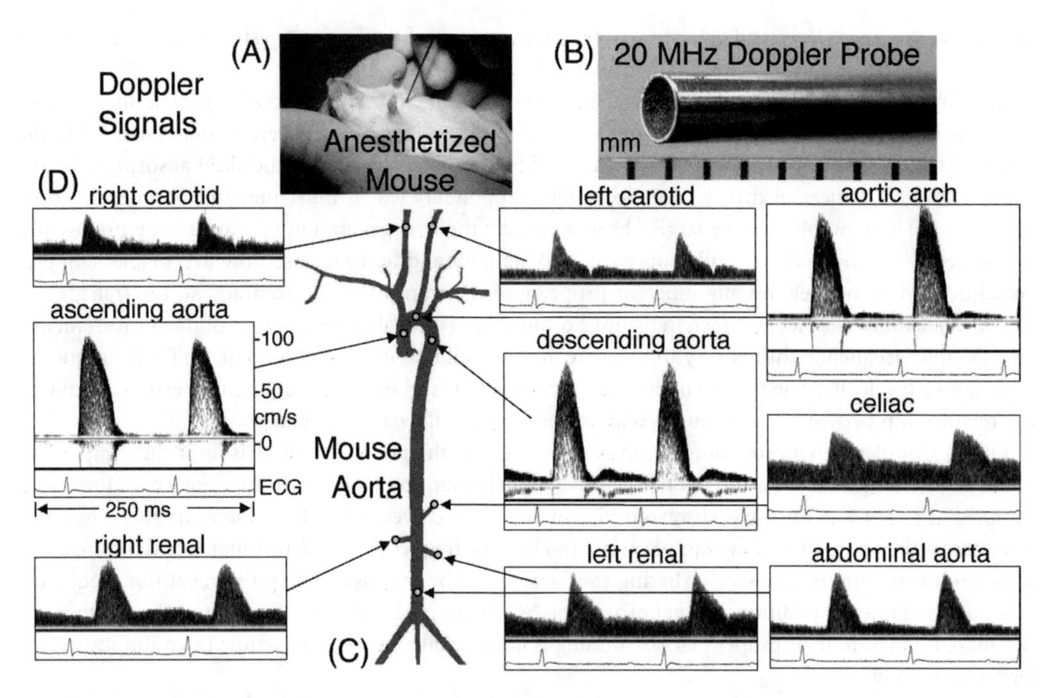

FIGURE 2.11 Doppler signals (D) from several peripheral vessels (C) in an anesthetized mouse (A) taken with the 2-mm-diameter 20-MHz probe (B). All signals were taken with the mouse supine except for the renal signals which were obtained with the mouse prone and the probe placed lateral to the spine.

the volume flow.[32,67,68,86] Still another approach is to measure the centerline velocity using a Doppler crystal mounted at a known angle in a rigid cuff of known diameter (Figure 2.6A), assume a parabolic velocity profile where the centerline velocity is twice the average (Figure 2.5A), and calculate volume flow based on the assumptions (Equation 2.9). It has been shown that, despite the obvious shortcomings, this method works fairly well in practice[87] and is much simpler than the algorithms using multiple range-gates.

2.13 Other Applications of Doppler Velocimetry

In addition to the applications mentioned above, noninvasive Doppler ultrasound is used to estimate the degree of stenosis in peripheral vessels such as carotid and femoral arteries by alterations to the Doppler spectrum and blood flow waveforms.[4,55,76] Flow disturbances including turbulence and vorticity can also be detected and evaluated.[65,88–90] Doppler catheters can be used to assess deeper vessels such as coronary arteries to estimate the effects of stenoses on coronary blood flow and vascular reserve.[91–94] Doppler is also used to detect and quantify valvular heart disease including insufficiency and stenosis by estimating regurgitant fraction and pressure drop.[95,96]

2.14 Artifacts and Limitations

There are numerous potential sources of error when using ultrasound to sense blood velocity or flow. Doppler and transit-time instruments measure only the component of velocity along the sound beam and provide no information about the other components of the velocity vector. Thus, some assumptions regarding the true direction of flow are required to estimate actual velocity or flow. Usually it is assumed that velocity is parallel to the vessel walls and that the Doppler device measures a component of this velocity according to the angle between the sound beam and the vessel axis (Figure 2.5). However, branching, curvature, tortuosity, stenosis, pulsatility, turbulence, etc. can invalidate this assumption and produce errors in the estimation of velocity. These errors are minimal with transit-time methods because the sample volume is large and velocity is averaged over most of the lumen to estimate volume flow, but the errors can be significant with Doppler methods.

Stability and accuracy are concerns with both transit-time and Doppler methods. The first transit-time flowmeters had unacceptable drift and zero stability,[30] and it was this severe problem that led to the development of Doppler methods.[38] Drift is caused by geometric instability and fluid absorption by the probe and by the thermal drift in the electronic components which must measure nanosecond time differences. These problems have largely been solved by the new generation of transit-time probes and instruments, and both short- and long-term zero stability and accuracy are now acceptable. Doppler velocimetry does not rely on any inherent property of the transducer for accuracy, so the transducers can be made much simpler as shown in Figure 2.6 and are not critical to the accuracy of the measurements. The Doppler frequency shift is easy to measure and to calibrate in the instrument, and zero frequency is always zero velocity. The probe either works or it doesn't, and most of the potential errors are due to the relationship between the measured velocity and volume flow as described above.

Pulsed Doppler signal processing involves sampling and the possibility of aliasing if the sample rate is not high enough.[97–99] In a directional Doppler velocimeter, the Doppler vector (Figure 2.7) must be sampled at least twice during each revolution for the sampled version to have the same frequency and direction as the true vector. If the sample rate is too low, the frequency is underestimated and the apparent direction of rotation is reversed.[98] Aliasing can be resolved by increasing the pulse repetition frequency and sampling rate, by additional signal processing,[97,98] or simply by shifting the spectral display to place the aliased signals in their proper place.[98] Aliasing is not a problem with transit-time or continuous-wave Doppler methods.

A related problem is range ambiguity resulting from having multiple pulses in flight at the same time. This is caused by high PRF and low absorption such that the echoes from one pulse are still being received when the next pulse is transmitted. Since the echoes from the two pulses overlap, the range-gate samples from two (or more) locations at the same time. This often occurs in commercial ultrasound systems when used in "high PRF mode" to avoid aliasing at high velocities. The solution is to lower the PRF if possible.

It is often desired in fluid mechanical studies to make point velocity measurements at several locations to determine the shape of the velocity profile[100,101] or to detect the presence, location, and duration of flow disturbances.[65] The pulsed Doppler method can provide this. The sample volume in a pulsed Doppler system has dimensions determined by the diameter, wavelength, and focusing of the transducer, by the burst length, gate length, gate delay, and filtering within the instrument, and by the acoustic properties of the scattering medium. The result is a complex four-dimensional surface (x, y, z, and amplitude) over which the signals are averaged. Assuming that each red cell generates a spectral component proportional to its velocity, the spectral distribution should represent the weighted velocity distribution within the sample volume. However other factors contribute to further broadening of the spectrum. These include transit-time and geometric broadening[102] which are due to the limited bandwidth of the short burst, the limited time each scatterer spends in the sample volume, and the geometry of the beam and transducer. The result is a Doppler spectrum that is always broader than the velocity distribution would predict.

In sensing volume flow with Doppler, it is assumed that the average frequency of the Doppler spectrum represents the average velocity in the sample volume (Figure 2.8). The presence of flow disturbances, turbulence, and/or vorticity can seriously affect the accuracy of this assumption by generating variable nonaxial velocity components in the sample volume. The spectral width and dynamics can be used to detect these effects,[88,89] but under those conditions the average frequency does not relate well to the average axial velocity.

The nature of the Doppler spectrum defies rigorous analysis by conventional means because it is dynamic and nonstationary.[4] For instance, FFT analyzers work best on long samples with stationary spectra. Frequency resolution improves with longer samples but at the expense of temporal resolution. To be useful for Doppler signals, compromises must be made. Typically, short (1 to 20 msec) samples are used, and a stationary condition is assumed over this short interval. But this condition is violated especially during rapid acceleration. Despite its well-known limitations, the FFT remains the standard for Doppler signal analysis.

2.15 Summary

Over the last 20 years, transit-time ultrasound has supplanted the electromagnetic flowmeter as the "gold standard" for measuring blood flow in animals and in man from extracorporeal probes placed on exposed arteries. At the same time, pulsed Doppler ultrasound has become the method of choice for high-resolution and noninvasive measurements of blood velocity and for the detection of flow disturbances secondary to cardiovascular disease. Both methods are capable of sensing flow in vessels from <0.2 mm and up in animals ranging from mice to man and larger.

References

1. Wells, P.N.T., *Biomedical Ultrasonics*, Academic Press, New York, 1977.
2. Altobelli, S.A., Voyles, W.F., and Greene, E.R., *Cardiovascular Ultrasonic Flowmetry*, Elsevier, New York, 1985.
3. Kremkau, F.W., *Doppler Ultrasound: Principles and Instruments*, W.B. Saunders, Philadelphia, 1990.
4. Evans, D.H. et al., Doppler Ultrasound: Physics, Instrumentation, and Clinical Applications, John Wiley & Sons, New York, 1989.
5. Morse, P.M. and Ingard, K.U., *Theoretical Acoustics*, McGraw-Hill, New York, 1968.
6. Christensen, D.A., *Ultrasonic Bioinstrumentation*, John Wiley & Sons, New York, 1988.
7. Goldman, D.E. and Hueter, T.F., Tabular data of the velocity and absorption of high-frequency sound in mammalian tissues, *J. Acoust. Soc. Am.*, 28, 35, 1956.
8. Snook, K.A. et al., Design, fabrication, and evaluation of high frequency, single-element transducers incorporating different materials, *IEEE Trans. Ultrason. Ferroelect. Freq. Contr.*, 49, 169, 2002.
9. Shung, K.K. and Zipparo, M.J., Ultrasonic transducers and arrays, *IEEE Eng. Med. Biol.*, 15, 20, 1996.
10. Ritter, T.A. et al., A 30-MHz piezo-composite ultrasound array for medical imaging applications, *IEEE Trans. Ultrason. Ferroelect. Freq. Contr.*, 49, 217, 2002.
11. Kossoff, G., The effects of backing and matching on the performance of piezoelectric ceramic transducers, *IEEE Trans. Sonics Ultrason.*, SU-13, 20, 1966.
12. Desilets, C.S., Fraser, J.D., and Kino, G.S., The design of efficient broad-band piezoelectric transducers, *IEEE Trans. Sonics Ultrason,*. SU-25, 115, 1978.
13. Zipparo, M.J., Shung, K.K., and Shrout, T.R., Piezoceramics for high-frequency (20–100 MHz) single-element imaging transducers, *IEEE Trans. Ultrason. Ferroelect. Freq. Contr.*, 44, 1038, 1997.
14. Rushmer, R.F., Franklin, D.L., and Ellis, R.M., Left ventricular dimensions recorded by sonocardiometry, *Circ. Res.*, 4, 684, 1956.
15. Theroux, P. et al., Regional myocardial function during acute coronary artery occlusion and its modification by pharmacologic agents in the dog, *Circ. Res.*, 35, 896, 1974.
16. Stegall, H.F. et al., A portable simple sonomicrometer, *J. Appl. Physiol.*, 23, 289, 1967.
17. Hill, R.C. et al., Perioperative assessment of segmental left ventricular function in man, *Arch. Surg.*, 115, 609, 1980.
18. Sasayama, S. et al., Dynamic changes in left ventricular wall thickness and their use in analyzing cardiac function in the conscious dog, *Am. J. Cardiol.*, 38, 870, 1976.
19. Gallagher, K.P. et al., Significance of regional wall thickening abnormalities relative to transmural myocardial perfusion in anesthetized dogs, *Circulation*, 62, 1266, 1980.
20. Pagani, M. et al., Measurements of multiple simultaneous small dimensions and study of arterial pressure dimension relations in conscious animals, *Am. J. Physiol. Heart Circ. Physiol.*, 235, H610, 1978.
21. Bertram, C.D., Ultrasonic transit-time system for arterial diameter measurement, *Med. Biol. Eng. Comput.*, 15, 489, 1977.
22. Hartley, C.J. et al., Synchronized pulsed Doppler blood flow and ultrasonic dimension measurement in conscious dogs, *Ultrasound Med. Biol.*, 4, 99, 1978.

23. Baker, D.W. and Simmons, V.E., Phase track techniques for detecting arterial blood vessel wall motion, *Proc. 21st ACEMB*, 8.6, 1968. (Abstract)
24. Hokanson, D.E. et al., A phase-locked echo tracking system for recording arterial diameter changes in vivo, *J. Appl. Physiol.*, 32, 728, 1972.
25. Hartley, C.J. et al., Doppler measurement of myocardial thickening with a single epicardial transducer, *Am. J. Physiol. Heart Circ. Physiol.*, 245, H1066, 1983.
26. Zhu, W. et al., Validation of a single crystal for the measurement of transmural and epicardial thickening, *Am. J. Physiol. Heart. Circ. Physiol.*, 251, H1045, 1986.
27. Hartley, C.J. et al., An ultrasonic method for measuring tissue displacement: technical details and validation for measuring myocardial thickening, *IEEE Trans. Biomed. Eng.*, 38, 735, 1991.
28. Baker, D.W., Pulsed ultrasonic Doppler blood flow sensing, *IEEE Trans. Sonics Ultrason.*, SU-17, 170, 1970.
29. Kalmus, H.P., Electronic flowmeter system, *Rev. Sci. Instrum.*, 25, 201, 1954.
30. Franklin, D.L., Baker, D.W., and Ellis, R.M., A pulsed ultrasonic flowmeter, *IRE Trans. Med. Electron.*, 6, 204, 1959.
31. Plass, K.G., A new ultrasonic flowmeter for intravascular application, *IEEE Trans. Biomed. Eng.*, BME-11, 154, 1964.
32. Keller, H.M. et al., Non-invasive measurement of velocity profiles and blood flow in the common carotid artery by pulsed Doppler ultrasound, *Stroke*, 7, 370, 1976.
33. Rader, R.D., A diameter-independent blood flow measurement technique, *Med. Instrum.*, 10, 185, 1976.
34. Drost, C.J., Vessel diameter-independent volume flow measurements using ultrasound, *Proc. 17th San Diego Biomed.Symp.*, 299–302, 1978. (Abstract)
35. D'Almeida, M.S., Gaudin, C., and Lebrec, D., Validation of 1 and 2 mm transit-time ultrasound flow probes on mesenteric artery and aorta of rats, *Am. J. Physiol. Heart Circ. Physiol.*, 268, H1368, 1995.
36. Hartley, C.J., A phase detecting ultrasonic flowmeter, *Proc 25th ACEMB*, 331972. (Abstract)
37. Satomura, S., Ultrasonic Doppler method for the inspection of cardiac functions, *J. Acoust. Soc. Am.*, 29, 1181, 1957.
38. Franklin, D.L., Schlegal, W., and Rushmer, R.F., Blood flow measured by Doppler frequency shift of back-scattered ultrasound, *Science*, 134, 564, 1961.
39. Carstensen, E.L., Li, K., and Schwan, H.P., Determination of the acoustic properties of blood and its components, *J. Acoust. Soc. Am.*, 25, 286, 1953.
40. Shung, K.K., Sigelmann, R.A., and Reid, J.M., Scattering of ultrasound by blood, *IEEE Trans. Biomed. Eng.*, BME-23, 460, 1976.
41. Angelsen, B.A.J., A theoretical study of the scattering of ultrasound from blood, *IEEE Trans. Biomed. Eng.*, 27, 61, 1980.
42. Shung, K.K., Physics of blood echogenicity, *J. Cardiovasc. Ultrasonography*, 2, 401, 1983.
43. Stegall, H.F., Stone, H.L., and Bishop, V.S., A catheter-tip pressure and velocity sensor, *Proc. 20th Annual Conf. on Engineering in Medicine and Biology*, 27.4, 1967. (Abstract)
44. Benchimol, A. et al., Aortic flow velocity in man during cardiac arrythmias measured with the Doppler catheter-flowmeter system, *Am. Heart J.*, 78, 649, 1969.
45. Kalmanson, D. et al., Retrograde catheterization of left heart cavities in dogs by means of an orientable directional Doppler catheter-tip flowmeter: a preliminary report, *Cardiovasc. Res.*, 6, 309, 1972.
46. Reid, J.M. et al., A new Doppler flowmeter system and its operation with catheter mounted transducers, *Cardiovascular Applications of Ultrasound*, Reneman, R.S., Ed., Elsevier, New York, 1974, pp. 183–197.
47. Brody, W.R. and Meindl, J.D., Theoretical analysis of the CW Doppler ultrasonic flowmeter, *IEEE Trans. Biomed. Eng.*, 21, 183, 1974.

48. Peronneau, P.A. et al., Theoretical and practical aspects of pulsed Doppler flowmetry: real-time application to the measurement of instantaneous velocity profiles *in vitro* and *in vivo*, *Cardiovascular Applications of Ultrasound*, Reneman, R.S., Ed., Amsterdam, North-Holland, 1974, pp. 66–84.
49. Hartley, C.J. and Cole, J.S., An ultrasonic pulsed doppler system for measuring blood flow in small vessels, *J. Appl. Physiol.*, 37, 626, 1974.
50. Satomura, S., Study of the flow patterns in peripheral arteries by ultrasonics, *J. Acoust. Soc. Jpn*, 15, 151, 1959.
51. McLeod, F.D., A directional Doppler flowmeter, *Proc. 7th ICMBE*, 14, 1967. (Abstract)
52. Coghlan, B.A. and Taylor, M.G., Directional Doppler techniques for detection of blood flow velocities, *Ultrasound Med. Biol.*, 2, 181, 1976.
53. Lunt, M.J., Accuracy and limitations of the ultrasonic Doppler blood velocimeter and zero-crossing detector, *Ultrasound Med. Biol.*, 2, 1, 1975.
54. Hartley, C.J. and Cole, J.S., A single crystal ultrasonic catheter tip velocity probe, *Med. Instrum.*, 8, 241, 1974.
55. Felix, W.R. et al., Pulsed Doppler ultrasound detection of flow disturbances in arteriosclerosis, *J. Clin. Ultrasound*, 4, 275, 1976.
56. Cross, G. and Light, L.H., Direction-resolving Doppler instrument with improved rejection of tissue artifacts for transcutaneous aortovelography, *Physiol. Soc.*, 5P, 1971.
57. Giddens, D.P. and Khalifa, A.M., Turbulence measurements with pulsed Doppler ultrasound employing a frequency tracking method, *Ultrasound Med. Biol.*, 8, 427, 1982.
58. Sainz, A.J., Roberts, V.C., and Pinardi, G., Phased-locked loop techniques applied to ultrasonic Doppler signal processing (blood flow measurements), *Ultrasonics*, 14, 128, 1976.
59. Brigham, E.O., *The Fast Fourier Transform*, Englewood Cliffs, NJ, Prentice-Hall, 1974.
60. Daigle, R.E. and Baker, D.W., A readout for pulsed Doppler velocity meters, *ISA Trans.*, 16, 41, 1977.
61. Kitney, R.I. and Giddens, D.P., Analysis of blood velocity waveforms by phase shift averaging and autoregressive spectral estimation, *J. Biomech. Eng.*, 105, 398, 1983.
62. Evans, D.H., Doppler signal processing, *Cardiovascular Ultrasonic Flowmetry*, Altobelli, S.A., Voyles, W.F., and Greene, E.R., Eds., Elsevier, New York, 1985, pp. 239–261.
63. Cohen, L., Time-frequency distributions — a review, *Proc IEEE*, 77, 941, 1995.
64. Hartley, C.J., Michael, L.H., and Entman, M.L., Noninvasive measurement of ascending aortic blood velocity in mice, *Am. J. Physiol. Heart Circ. Physiol.*, 268, H499, 1995.
65. Hartley, C.J. et al., Noninvasive cardiovascular phenotyping in mice, *ILAR J.*, 43, 147, 2002.
66. Sudhir, K. et al., Measurement of volumetric coronary blood flow with a Doppler catheter: validation in an animal model, *Am. Heart J.*, 124, 870, 1992.
67. Casty, M. and Giddens, D.P., 25+1 channel pulsed ultrasound doppler velocity meter for quantitative flow measurements and turbulence analysis, *Ultrasound Med. Biol.*, 10, 161, 1984.
68. Stacey-Clear, A. and Fish, P.J., Repeatability of blood flow measurement using multichannel pulsed Doppler ultrasound, *Br. J. Radiol.*, 57, 419, 1984.
69. Hoeks, A.P.G., Reneman, R.S., and Peronneau, P.A., A multigate pulsed Doppler system with serial data processing, *IEEE Trans. Sonics Ultrason.*, 28, 242, 1981.
70. Kajiya, F. et al., Evaluation of human coronary blood flow with an 80-channel 20 MHz pulsed Doppler velocitometer and zero-cross and Fourier transform methods during cardiac surgery, *Circulation*, Suppl. III, 53, 1986.
71. Brandestini, M.A., A digital 128-channel transcutaneous blood-flowmeter, *Biomed. Tech.*, 21, 291, 1976.
72. Nowicki, A. and Reid, J.M., An infinite gate pulse Doppler, *Ultrasound Med. Biol.*, 7, 41, 1981.
73. Merritt, C.R., Doppler color flow imaging, *J. Clin. Ultrasound*, 15, 591, 1987.
74. Taffet, G.E. et al., Noninvasive indexes of cardiac systolic and diastolic function in hyperthyroid and senescent mouse, *Am. J. Physiol. Heart Circ. Physiol.*, 270, H2204, 1996.
75. Hartley, C.J. et al., Hemodynamic changes in apolipoprotein E-knockout mice, *Am. J. Physiol. Heart Circ. Physiol.*, 279, H2326, 2000.

76. Skidmore, R., Woodcock, J.P., and Wells, P.N.T., Physiological interpretation of Doppler-shift waveforms, *Ultrasound Med. Biol.*, 6, 7–10, 219–225, 227, 1980.
77. Hartley, C.J. et al., Noninvasive determination of pulse-wave velocity in mice, *Am. J. Physiol. Heart Circ. Physiol.*, 273, H494, 1997.
78. Avolio, A.P. et al., Effects of aging on arterial distensibility in populations with high and low prevalence of hypertension: comparison between urban and rural communities in China, *Circulation*, 71, 202, 1985.
79. Nichols, W.W. and O'Rourke, M.F., *McDonald's Blood Flow in Arteries: Theoretical, Experimental, and Clinical Principles*, Edward Arnold, London, 1998.
80. Arnett, D.K., Evans, G.W., and Riley, W.A., Arterial stiffness: A new cardiovascular risk factor? *Am. J. Epidem.*, 140, 669, 1994.
81. Arts, M.G.J. and Roevros, J.M.G.J., On the instantaneous measurement of blood flow by ultrasonic means, *Med. Biol Eng.*, 10, 23, 1972.
82. Gerzberg, L. and Meindl, J.D., Mean frequency estimator with applications in ultrasonic Doppler flowmeters, *Ultrasound in Medicine*, White, D.N. and Brown, R.E., Eds., Plenum, New York, 1977, pp. 1173–1175.
83. Gill, R.W., Performance of the mean frequency Doppler demodulator, *Ultrasound Med. Biol.*, 5, 237, 1979.
84. Hottinger, C.F., Blood flow measurement using the attenuation-compensated volume flowmeter, *Ultrasonic Imaging*, 1, 1, 1979.
85. Hottinger, C.F. and Meindl, J.D., Unambiguous measurement of volume flow using ultrasound, *IEEE*, 63, 984, 1975.
86. Marquis, C. et al., Femoral blood flow determination with a multichannel digital pulsed Doppler; an experimental study on anaesthetized dogs, *Vasc. Surg.*, 17, 95, 1983.
87. Ishida, T. et al., Comparison of hepatic extraction of insulin and glucagon in conscious and anesthetized dogs, *J. Endocrinol.*, 112, 1098, 1983.
88. Cloutier, G., Chen, D., and Durand, L.G., Performance of time-frequency representation techniques to measure blood flow turbulence with pulsed-wave Doppler ultrasound, *Ultrasound Med. Biol.*, 27, 535, 2001.
89. Cloutier, G., Allard, M.F., and Durand, L.G., Characterization of blood flow turbulence with pulsed-wave and power Doppler ultrasound imaging, *J. Biomech. Eng.*, 118, 318, 1996.
90. Wang, Y. and Fish, P.J., Comparison of Doppler signal analysis techniques for velocity waveform, turbulence, and vortex measurement: a simluation study, *Ultrasound Med. Biol.*, 22, 635, 1996.
91. Cole, J.S. and Hartley, C.J., The pulsed Doppler coronary artery catheter: Preliminary report of a new technique for measuring rapid changes in coronary artery flow velocity in man, *Circulation*, 56, 18, 1977.
92. Wilson, R.F. et al., Transluminal, subselective measurement of coronary artery blood flow velocity and vasodilator reserve in man, *Circulation*, 72, 82, 1985.
93. Sibley, D.H. et al., Subselective measurement of coronary blood flow velocity using a steerable Doppler catheter, *J. Am. Coll. Cardiol.*, 8, 1332, 1986.
94. Hartley, C.J., Review of intracoronary Doppler catheters, *Int. J. Cardiac Imaging*, 4, 159, 1989.
95. Hatle, L., Non-invasive assessment and differentiation of left ventricular outflow obstruction with Doppler ultrasound, *Circulation*, 64, 381, 1981.
96. Hatle, L. et al., Noninvasive assessment of pressure drop in mitral stenosis by Doppler ultrasound, *Br. Heart J.*, 40, 131, 1978.
97. Tortoli, P., Valgimigli, F., and Guidi, G., Clinical evaluation of a new anti-aliasing technique for ultrasound pulsed Doppler analysis, *Ultrasound Med. Biol.*, 15, 749, 1989.
98. Hartley, C.J., Resolution of frequency aliases in pulsed Doppler velocimeters, *IEEE Trans. Sonics Ultrasonics*, SU-28, 69, 1981.
99. Bom, N., De Boo, J., and Rijsterborgh, H., On the aliasing problem in pulsed Doppler cardiac studies, *J. Clin. Ultrasound*, 12, 559, 1984.

100. Rabinovitz, R.S. et al., Fluid dynamics of the left main coronary bifurcation, *Proc. 40th ACEMB,* 154, 1987. (Abstract)
101. Vieli, A., Jenni, R., and Anliker, M. Spatial velocity distributions in the ascending aorta of healthy humans and cardiac patients, *IEEE Trans. Biomed. Eng.*, 33, 28, 1986.
102. Newhouse, V.L. et al., The dependence of ultrasound Doppler bandwidth on beam geometry, *IEEE Trans. Sonics Ultrason.*, SU-27, 50, 1980.

3

Electromagnetic Blood Flow Measurements

Reza Tabrizchi
Memorial University of Newfoundland

Noriko Iida
University of Hiroshima

CONTENTS

3.1 Introduction

The formula that defines Ohm's law perhaps best illustrates the dynamics of blood flow through blood vessels. Essentially, Ohm's law states that potential difference (δP) between two points is equal to the products of current (flow of electrons) (I) and resistance to flow (R). So the flow of electrons (i.e., current) is determined by two factors, the potential difference between two points of flow, and the resistance to flow, as given by Equation 3.1.

$$\delta P = I \times R \text{ and } I = \delta P/R \tag{3.1}$$

Thus, by comparison, flow of fluids (F) through a pipe (blood vessel) is determined by two factors: the pressure difference (gradient) (δP) between the two points in the vessels, which is the force that pushes the fluid through the pipe, and the resistance (R) to that flow, as defined by Equation 3.2.

$$F = \delta P/R \tag{3.2}$$

In defining blood flow through a vessel, it must be noted that it is the pressure difference between the two ends of the vessels and not the absolute pressure that determines the rate of blood flow. Quantitative definition of blood flow is a quantity of blood that passes a specific point in circulation by a specified period of time.[1] Units ascribed to blood flow can be liters per minute, or milliliters per minute. In an average 70-kg man, the blood flow in circulation is 5 l/min, and this is referred to as cardiac output.

The first person to give a value to blood flow in circulation was William Harvey (1628). He estimated the cardiac output (~3 l/min) from post-mortem measurements of left ventricular diastolic volume. Subsequently, Stephen Hales (1733), in assessing circulatory dynamics, calculated circulation rates by measuring the velocity of the blood as it traveled along veins, arteries, and capillaries. Hales also measured cardiac output based on the same technique as Harvey's and introduced the term of peripheral resistance as it applies in the arterial circulation.[2]

0-8493-1140-3/04/$0.00+$1.50

The actual method for the measurement of cardiac output in living humans and animals was not achieved until the physiologist Adolph Fick (1870) introduced his principle. Interestingly, Fick never used the principle that he formulated to measure cardiac output; that task was left to Grehart and Quinquardt (1886). Essentially, *Fick's principle* stated that the amount of a substance taken up by an organ is the product of blood flow to the organ and the concentration difference of the substance between the arterial and venous systems. Grehart and Quinquardt used Fick's method to measure cardiac output in dogs.[2]

One popular substance that has been used to measure cardiac output using Fick's method is oxygen. Calculation of cardiac output (pulmonary blood flow) can be obtained based on Fick's principle using the following formula:

$$\text{PBF} = [\text{Oxygen usage ml/min}]/[(\text{A} - \text{V}) \text{ oxygen difference ml/100 ml}] \times 100 \qquad (3.3)$$

where PBF is pulmonary blood flow, A is arterial blood oxygen amount (ml/100 ml), and V is venous blood oxygen amount (ml/100 ml).[3]

Perhaps since the introduction of Fick's principle, the other most notable event in the history of blood flow measurements was the use of electromagnetic flowmeters. Fabre[4] in France was the first person to use the concept of electromagnetic induction for the measurement of blood flow noninvasively. Kolin[5,6] in the United States and Wetterer[7] in Germany were the first individuals independently to use electromagnetic flowmeters in the measurement of absolute blood flow in blood vessels invasively. It was soon recognized that the simple advantages of the electromagnetic flowmeter were linearity and accuracy over flow ranges in unopened blood vessels. In addition, this type of meter was capable of measuring not only forward flow but also backward flow. Moreover, more recent modern development has yielded probes that allow for measurement of blood flow in vessels without exposing them. However, the most important advantage of electromagnetic flow probes is that it allows for the recording of changes in flow less than 0.01 sec, and for the recording of pulsatile changes in flow, as well as steady flow.

3.2 Methodology and Instrumentation

3.2.1 Basic Principle

The basis for electromagnetic blood flow probes is Faraday's law and induction of electromagnetic force (EMF).[8,9] Faraday's law states that when a current is passed through a magnetic field, a force termed EMF is generated and can be measured as a voltage. Equation 3.4 defines Faraday's law:

$$E = -d\Phi/dt \qquad (3.4)$$

Here, E is the EMF (volts, V), Φ is magnetic flux (weber, Wb), and t is time (sec). Simply, $d\Phi/dt$ defines change in flux with respect to time. EMF and $d\Phi/dt$ always have opposite potentials.

When conductive fluid flows between the force of a magnetic field, an electromagnetic force is generated in the fluid (i.e., blood or saline) which is perpendicular to the direction of the magnetic field and the direction of the motion of the fluid. For example, if a conductive particle (Q) is in a fluid and has a velocity (v), and is then placed in a magnetic field, the charged particle (Q) will experience a force (F). The expression that describes such a scenario is given by Equation 3.5:

$$F = Q \times v \times B \qquad (3.5)$$

Here, F is force (Newtons, N), Q is electrical charge (coulombs, C), v is velocity (m/sec), and B is flux density of magnetic field (Wb/m^2).

However, put another way, when charged particles in a fluid such as blood pass in a perpendicular manner through a magnetic field, a voltage is generated. This voltage can subsequently be detected by electrodes placed perpendicular to the direction of flow. The voltage generated is directly proportional to the rate of flow; the expression that describes such an event is given by Equation 3.6:

$$E = B \times d \times v \tag{3.6}$$

where E is electromagnetic force (V), B is flux density of magnetic field (Wb/m^2), d is the distance between the two detecting electrodes (m), and v (m/sec) is mean flow velocity of the conductive fluid in the vessel.

With the assumption of uniform flow by the fluid, the relationship between flow and velocity of flow in a cylinder (i.e., blood vessel) is given by Equation 3.7:

$$V = v \times A \tag{3.7}$$

where V is rate of flow in the cylinder (m^3/sec), v is velocity of fluid (m/sec), and A is the cross-sectional area of the cylinder (m^2). The area of a circle is πr^2 where r is the radius (m); it can also be written as $\pi d^2/4$ where d is the diameter of the cylinder. From here, we will use $\pi d^2/4$ as the area for the cylinder, where d is the distance between the two electrodes for the detection of the voltage that is generated. Thus, Equation 3.7 can be rewritten as:

$$v = 4 \times V/\pi d^2 \tag{3.8}$$

Substituting $4 \times V/\pi d^2$ in Equation 3.6 for velocity and rearranging the equation to obtain flow (Equation 3.9),

$$V = [E \times \pi d]/4B \tag{3.9}$$

Equations 3.7 through 3.9 relate rate of flow of fluids to the voltage generated due to flow, diameter of the cylindrical vessel and flux density imposed on the conductive fluid. It essentially indicates that the rate of flow in a cylinder is directly proportional to the product of the voltage generated and the diameter of the cylinder in which the fluid is flowing, and is inversely proportional to flux density of the magnetic field. Equation 3.9 can be written in centimetre-gramme-second (CGS) electromagnetic units:

$$V = [E \times \pi d]/[4B] \times 10^8 \tag{3.10}$$

where V is flow (cm^3/sec), E is electromagnetic force (V), d is the distance between the two detecting electrodes (cm) (assumed to be lumen diameter), and B is magnetic flux density (gauss, G).

Equation 3.6 describes the voltage generated in a flowmeter due to flow of a conductive fluid written in CGS electromagnetic units:

$$E = [d \times B \times v] \times 10^{-8} \tag{3.11}$$

where E is voltage generated (V), d is distance between two detecting electrodes (cm), B is magnetic flux density (G), and v is velocity of conductive fluid (cm/sec).

Depicted in Table 3.1 are typical voltages generated by electromagnetic flow probes (using Equation 3.11) for blood flows in aorta of groups of four different species. Here, the assumption is that the distance between the two detecting electrodes is the lumen diameter of the blood vessels, and the magnetic flux density generated by the probe is 300 G.

3.2.2 Electromagnetic Flow Probes (Perivascular)

The probes that are utilized for measurement of blood flow each consist of an electromagnet, a coil that generates the magnetic flux with appropriate current, and two electrodes that are present to detect the flow signal (Figure 3.1). For example, a coil consisting of 100 turns of wire in four layers will generate a magnetic flux density of approximately 70 G with a current of 250 mA.[10] A probe with such characteristics

TABLE 3.1 Typical Values of Voltage Signal Generated by Blood Flow in Aorta of Five Species[a]

Species	Mean Velocity; Ascending Aorta (cm/sec)[b]	Size of Diameter of Aorta (cm)[b]	Signal Generated (μV)
Human	16	3.0	144
Dog	22	1.56	103
Rabbit	32	0.46	44
Rat	22	0.26	17

[a] Values obtained using Equation 3.11 and assuming a magnetic flux density of 300 G.
[b] Values from Milnor, W. R., *Hemodynamics,* 2nd Ed., Williams & Wilkins, Baltimore, 1989, chap. 5 and 6.

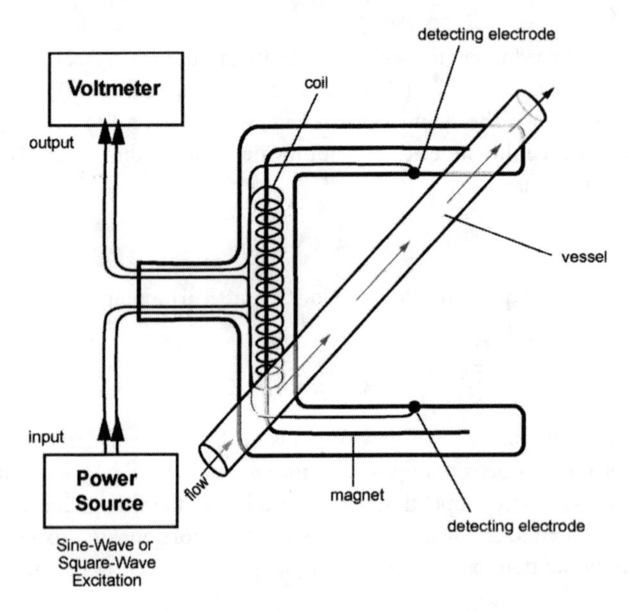

FIGURE 3.1 Schematic of electromagnetic flow probe consisting of an electromagnet, a coil, and detecting electrodes, as well as input and output systems.

will generate little heat, which is important for detecting electrodes as the thermic effects contribute to baseline drift. The detecting electrodes can be platinum wires. Usually, these components are encapsulated into varying sizes so that they can be used on various blood vessels with varying diameters. Probes are also specifically designed to be used either acutely (Figure 3.2) or chronically (Figure 3.3). In addition, special designs such as the forceps probe can be used for acute flow measurements (Figure 3.4). Obviously, different numbers of turns and different currents can be used to create a greater quantity of magnetic flux density as defined by Equation 3.12. The probe is subsequently connected to an appropriate recorder that has either digital or dial readout. In addition, permanent recordings are made using a pen-driven polygraph or stored on diskettes via a computer using the appropriate software.

The magnetic flux density for an electromagnetic probe can be obtained using Equation 3.12:

$$B = [\mu \times N \times I]/L \tag{3.12}$$

Here, B is magnetic flux density (Wb/m^2), μ is the permeability of free space, $4\pi \times 10^{-7}$ (Wb/A/m), N is the number of turns of wire for assembly of the coil, I is the current (A), and L is the length in meters of the wire used to make the coil (Figure 3.1). In practical terms, the field generated can be increased by placement of ferromagnetic material as part of the coil. Thus, Equation 3.12 is modified by the insertion of μ_r, the relative permeability of ferromagnetic material used (e.g., value for iron is 5000), and is written as:

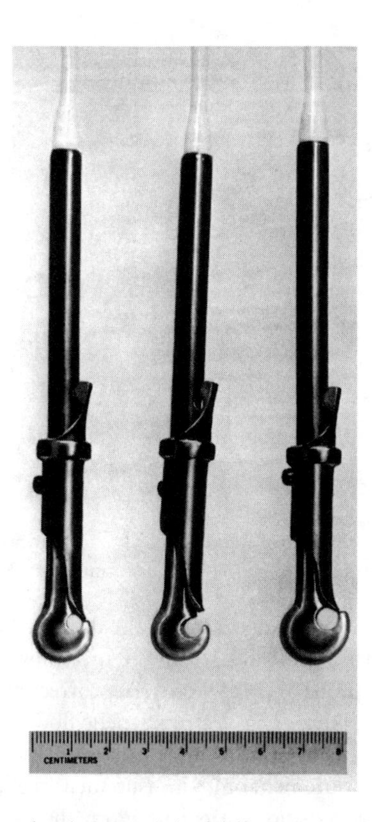

FIGURE 3.2 Electromagnetic flow probes (400H series) of different internal diameters for acute measurement of blood flow. (Reproduced with permission from Carolina Medical Electronics Inc., King, NC.)

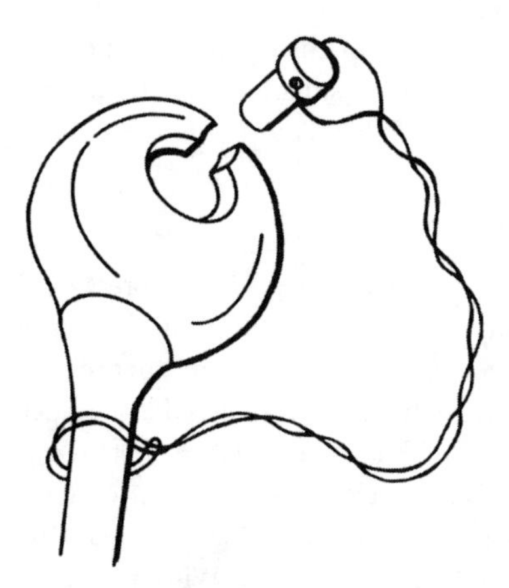

FIGURE 3.3 Electromagnetic flow probe (Dowel) with slot closure for chronic use of blood flow measurements. (Reproduced with permission from Carolina Medical Electronics Inc., King, NC.)

$$B = [\mu_r \times \mu \times N \times I]/L \tag{3.13}$$

Different types of currents can be used in excitation to generate the electromagnetic field. The electrical waveform can be square-wave, sine-wave, or trapezoidal-wave in nature.[11,12] Typical carrier signal for different types of currents are 400, 250, and 1000 cps for sine-wave, square-wave, and trapezoidal-wave, respectively.

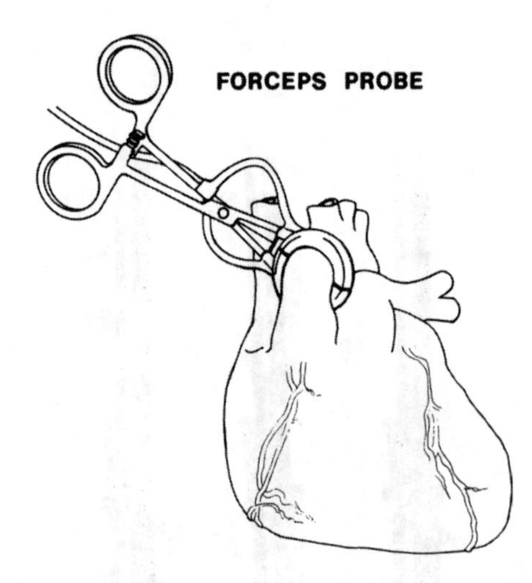

FIGURE 3.4 Forceps electromagnetic flow probe (200 series) for acute measurement of blood flow in arteries or veins. (Reproduced with permission from Carolina Medical Electronics Inc., King, NC.)

Careful selection of probe size is quite important, as the distance between the electrodes defines the lumen diameter. This obviously has a great impact on the measurement of blood flow. It is important to have good contact between the probe and the vessel. The correct placement of the probe around the blood vessel is also of critical importance. The electromagnetic flow probe must be perpendicular to the long axis of the vessels in which the blood flow is to be measured. Incorrect placement of the probes on the vessel will result in incorrect measurement or no measurement at all. The electromagnetic flow probes can be placed on the vessel in two positions. Depending on the position, the polarity can either be negative or positive on the recorder.

In acute implantation of electromagnetic flowmeters, it is advisable to have a snug fit, and up to 20% occlusion is recommended. This will provide good vessel-to-electrode contact without significant impediment on total blood flow or the pulse wave. For chronic implantation, the probe should be 10 to 20% larger than the vessel lumen. A snug fit in chronic situations will result in necrosis of the vessel wall (due to interruption in vaso vasorum blood flow). This is most important for larger blood vessels such as the aorta.

3.2.3 Practical Consideration

Recording of cardiovascular events in a laboratory (blood pressure, blood flow, electrocardiogram) is usually a time-varying periodic function.[2] Furthermore, it is not surprising that each variable has its own characteristic waveform that changes repetitiously over time. In order to accurately measure such variables over time, its waveform characteristics have to be analyzed and understood. Ultimately, the main goals of recording any physiological event within the circulatory system is to obtain an accurate recording of the event that is reproducible. To this end, a clear understanding of the errors associated with the recording of the events must first be understood. Errors can arise from many sources, including the operator, the environment, and the recording modules/instruments. Within the recording system, errors can arise and be associated with components such as amplifiers, processors, recorders, transducers, catheters, and so on. Simply put, a thorough understanding of the entire setup is absolutely necessary for meaningful and accurate recordings of any cardiovascular parameter.

It must be recognized that recording blood flow or, for that matter, any cardiovascular parameter requires appropriate amplification, processing, storing, and analysis of the signal. It then follows that certain minimum criteria must be met by the recording instrument (electromagnetic flowmeters are no exception) if meaningful blood flow measurements are to be made accurately and be reproducible under a variety of conditions. These pertinent factors are phase/amplitude linearity and adequate frequency response of the recording modules and apparatus.

3.2.3.1 Phase Linearity

This is a reference to the capability of the recording module to provide a signal (i.e., rate of flow) that is as close as the measurement of the event that is being presented to it. Deviation from linearity of input and output will result in phase distortion. This will manifest itself in complex displacement of the output signal in the time axis, and thus result in erroneous measurement of blood flow.

3.2.3.2 Amplitude Response

The recording module is required to have a frequency response great enough to measure the highest harmonic of the flow variable that is being measured. There appears to be no evidence to indicate that there are significant propagated waves in terms of blood flow that exist above 30 Hz, and it seems that those above 20 Hz are fairly small.[2] For example, Patel and associates[13] have reported that there is little information beyond the 11th harmonic component (~30 Hz), and Bergel and Gessner[14] seem to suggest that the limit is about the 8th harmonics in pulmonary artery and aortic flow pulses. It is reasonable to assume that a flowmeter that has a frequency response of >60 Hz will be capable of measuring blood flow in most species.

3.2.3.3 Amplitude Linearity

This aspect of the recording system is a little more complex and it has to do with various factors, namely, drift, noise, hysteresis, and calibration of the flowmeters. In general, the term amplitude linearity refers to the ability of the recording system to produce an output signal that is directly proportional in magnitude to the input signal amplitude. Clearly, this should apply not only to above zero baseline values but also to below the zero line, and must also include the entire range of the measurements. This is an important criterion in measuring blood flow using an electromagnetic flow probe. Therefore, it is imperative that before choosing a flowmeter the approximate range of the variable to be assessed must be known. Obviously, such values can be obtained from reference to the literature. Currently, commercially available flowmeters are capable of measuring blood flow in ranges of 5 ml/min to 20 l/min.

3.2.3.3.1 Drift

Drift associated with an electromagnetic flowmeter will affect accurate measurements of blood flow. In cases where there is drift of the baseline without actual changes to slope (i.e., sensitivity), measurement of blood flow will be out of phase by the amount of change associated with the baseline. This, of course, may be either negative or positive from the zero baseline. However, when there is drift associated with the slope or actual calibration of the flowmeter, it will lead to alteration of the sensitivity curve. When using an electromagnetic flowmeter for measurement of blood flow over a period of time, no matter how well the system is calibrated, changes in zero baseline or calibration can occur, and this will result in erroneous measurement of blood flow. Certainly, physiochemical changes in blood vessels can contribute to drifting, which can ultimately have an effect on zero line stability and actual flow measurements. It is recognized that zero line stability can be greatly enhanced with good contact between electrode-to-blood vessel wall. It seems that heat production in the probe is also another source of zero line instability, especially in smaller blood vessels. It has been reported that interelectrode voltages are altered if the temperature at one electrode is changed in relation to the other.[15] In smaller blood vessels, thermic effects may be considerable and may produce substantive drift. Therefore, appropriate precautions need to be taken in order to avoid drift, and care must be taken in calibration of the instrument. In addition, frequent checks of zero baseline as well as calibration of sensitivity are imperative. Simply, periodic checking and readjustments are necessary for accurate and reproducible measurement of blood flow when using an electromagnetic flowmeter. Moreover, it seems that electronic zero obtained by switching off the magnet does not always coincide with the mechanical zero. Therefore, it is advisable that whenever possible, an occlusive cuff or snare placed on the artery beyond the probe be used to obtain mechanical zero. Zero can be obtained naturally when recordings are being carried out in the ascending aorta or pulmonary artery as zero occurs during the latter portion of diastole.

3.2.3.3.2 Noise

Clearly, a potential problem in recording any signal is unwanted noise. The signal-to-noise ratio can have a significant impact on the accuracy of the instrument, and the noise is most likely seen in the low-frequency recordings. This becomes an important factor especially when measuring low velocity flow. Obviously, since the velocity of flow is a function of frequency in experiments using a flowmeter, the signal-to-noise ratio becomes smaller at higher frequencies.

In general, noise is part of the output of an instrument, and it can be generated by the instrument, caused by external interference, or both. It is useful to distinguish the noise from the actual signal being measured. This can be done by assessing signal-to-noise ratio. Essentially, in order to determine the value that signifies the noise that is either generated or is associated with an instrument, the signal-to-noise ratio at the input is divided by the signal-to-noise ratio at the output. Needless to say, the ideal ratio is unity. When noise exists, it is desirable to identify its source and eliminate it completely or reduce it as much as possible. Most often, elimination or reduction in noise levels can be achieved by proper grounding. In addition, high frequency noise may be dealt with by the introduction of low-frequency band electronic filters provided that the filter does not eliminate or reduce the signal that is being measured. In practical terms, a flowmeter with a magnetic field of about 100 G that generates a mean signal of ~5 μV should have a noise level of no more than 0.1 μV. This translates into a signal-to-noise ratio of ~50, which is acceptable.

3.2.3.3.3 Hysteresis

An important source of error that can have a direct impact on systems linearity is hysteresis. A definition of the term means a "lag of effect." In terms of measurements, this defines the ability of the instrument to produce an output that follows the input independently. In electromagnetic flowmeters, there are several sources of error that may be ascribed to hysteresis, for example, the nonuniformity of the magnetic field. The magnetic field produced by the magnets of the probe only covers a small length of the vessel. This essentially results in the magnetic field not being uniform along the vessel axis, and more importantly, it is not uniform across the lumen of the vessel. This can result in reduction in sensitivity by as much as 20 to 50%.[14] However, this reduction is constant for a given probe and will be contained in the calibration factor. Another source may be polarization effects. Polarization effects at the recording electrodes alter contact impedance between the electrode and vessel wall. These effects may not follow similar patterns at the two recording electrodes. Under such conditions, the voltage observed is less than the one that can be calculated theoretically by the given equation. Other sources include shunting by conductive vessel walls and surrounding conductive fluids, which will be discussed and dealt with in detail later on in the chapter.

3.2.3.3.4 Calibration

Clearly, calibration of the flowmeter has to be carried out over the range of input amplitude that must be measured by the meter. In essence, the increase in flow and the resulting output signals need to be measured. A plot of the input vs. output values should result in a linear calibration relationship. The frequency characteristics can be obtained by pumping a conductive fluid (preferably blood) through a blood vessel with the flow probe placed on the vessel. The obvious limitation of such a procedure is that it is difficult to produce flows of sufficient amplitude at frequencies that are higher than 20 Hz.

Hydraulic calibration. Sinusoidal flow oscillation can be generated by a crank-driven piston pump for this form of calibration. The piston displacement should generate the sinusoidal function such that there is negligible second harmonic content. A fresh blood vessel should be used for this calibration, and it should be cannulated and stretched appropriately and held in a rigid position. The flowmeter should be placed around the vessel and held in a steady state, and pressure should be applied to the fluid to keep the vessel in contact with the probe. The necessary pressure is about 100 mmHg, but should be increased if needed during the calibration procedure to insure that the vessel is pressed against the probe at all times. Obviously, a loss of contact between blood vessel and the two electrodes of the probe will result in electrode imbalance and drift. This will most likely result in disappearance of the output signal, and should be easy to detect. Such a setup can be used for calibration of a flowmeter and in determination of frequency response of the probe. Saline can be used for this procedure, and frequency of up to 20 Hz can be employed.[11]

Electrical calibration. Electrical circuitry of a flowmeter can also be tested using electrical calibration. This can be achieved by applying a signal to its input terminal so that a voltage can be detected by the flow probes electrodes. This is the carrier signal which can be a square-wave or sine-wave. A sine-wave carrier signal can be obtained from the magnet driven circuit in the flowmeter, and the flow signal may be generated by the output from a low-frequency oscillator (1 to 40 cps). Modulation can be performed by an electronic multiplier, and the generated waveform can be fed into the flowmeter input at the appropriate voltage range (~100 μV). Both outputs can be recorded at various frequencies.[11]

Dynamic calibration of an electromagnetic flowmeter (for both sine-wave and square-wave) using a simple transistor circuit has also been described by Hill.[16] In this technique, the magnetic current is modulated using a square frequency wave at 1 Hz in order to provide a suitable input to the flowmeter. Subsequently, both the input square wave as well as the square wave from the flowmeter are sampled using a computer. The Fourier analysis transforms the two waves at different frequencies (up to 50 Hz) and can be utilized to yield a calibration of amplitude and phase lag for the flowmeter.[16]

Both hydraulic and electrical calibrations can be used to assess the accuracy expected from a flowmeter. It seems that no significant differences exist between the two methods of calibration but, as mentioned already, there is a limitation on frequency that can be employed using the hydraulic method.[11] It should be noted that signal-to-noise ratio has an impact on the accuracy of the instrument, and the noise is most often problematic in the low-frequency recordings.

The amplitude frequencies of commercially available flowmeters (Biotronex BL 613 sine-wave flowmeter) determined experimentally has been noted to be flat ±5% between 45 and 54% of the given value for the instrument, with relatively good phase linearity >60 Hz.[2] However, it has also been reported that probes with square-wave excitation can have a reduction of output of 10% at 7 cps, and where the output lagged the input by 4.5°/cps.[11] In contrast, meters with gate sine-wave excitation have reductions of 10% at 24 cps and a lag time of 2.2°/cps.[11]

In commercially available flowmeters, the amplitude/frequency responses of the probe are usually given as ±3 dB. This essentially means that the frequency at which the amplitude is decreased by approximately 30% is considered to be at 3-dB frequency. It is advisable that the dynamics of frequency characteristics of the probes be determined individually by the investigator. However, typically it may be assumed that flowmeters have a usable frequency response that is 50% of the theoretical limit and 25% of the practical limit of the carrier frequencies ascribed to them.

3.2.3.4 Impact of Vessel Wall

There are two types of errors that can be associated with the placement of a flowmeter cuff on blood vessels. The first source of these errors directly relates to the conductivity of the blood vessel wall, and the second error can be attributed to the serous fluid between the blood vessel and the flowmeter cuff.[17]

Consideration has to be given to error arising from the conductivity of blood vessels and relates to two main factors assuming that conductivity of blood is larger than 10^{-7} (ohm meter)$^{-1}$. These two factors are: (1) ratio of inside to outside diameter of the vessels and (2) the conductivity of blood to blood vessel wall which has been determined to be of the order of 4.0 (i.e., blood is four times more conductive than the vessel wall).[18] Based on the fact that the typical conductivity ratio of blood to blood vessel wall is a constant, then the error arising from this can specifically be ascribed to the ratio of inside and outside diameter of the vessel in question where flow is being measured. The relationship between reduction in signal (i.e., voltage as described in Equation 3.11) and ratio of the inside and outside diameter of the blood vessel is relatively linear. For example, in vessels where the ratio of inside to outside diameter is 0.7, 0.8, and 0.9, the error is approximately 11, 9, and 5%, respectively.[17] These are values by which the voltage will deviate from the theoretical value, the actual impact being that a lower voltage will be detected by the recording electrodes, which is attributed to electrical shunting. It is apparent that as the vessel wall becomes thinner and the ratio of inside diameter to outside diameter reaches unity, the error is substantially reduced. Thus, typical errors here are of the order of –5 to –10% deviation from the actual true signal generated by flow. It should also be mentioned that the theoretical calculation for this error is based on Equation 3.11, which assumes the mean velocity for flow in a given cylinder, and more importantly the fact that flow is rotationally symmetrical.[17] Clearly, blood flow in blood vessels is not always rotationally symmetrical (see Section 3.2.3.5).

Error associated with serous fluid between the blood vessel and the detecting electrodes of the flowmeter can occur due to polarization and electrical shunting. Any tissue fluid or blood lying between the vessel and the flowmeter cuff can provide an additional electric shunt, which will ultimately manifest itself as a reduction in the voltage detected by the electrodes. For example, for a vessel where the ratio of inside to outside diameter is 0.8, a conductive film of a thickness of between 2 and 4% of the outside radius of the vessel will result in error greater than 10% but less than 20%. For a vessel in which the ratio of inside diameter to outside is 0.9, a conductive film of thickness between 2 and 4% of the outside radius of the vessels will result in an error of 5 to 10%.[17] Again, as with the error associated with vessels conductivity, with the vessel wall becoming thinner and the ratio of inside diameter to outside diameter reaching unity, the actual error occurring as a result of electric shunting due to conductive fluids between the electrode and vessel wall will decline.[17] To effectively reduce error due to electric shunting, the flowmeter should be cuffed tightly around the blood vessel. It is obvious that a typical thickness of film of conductive fluid is hard to predict, and error attributed to this factor has to be estimated for individual vessels and each flowmeter cuff.

Experimentally, it has been found that meticulous preparation of a blood vessel for *in vivo* recording of blood flow in small blood vessels in animals such as rats and rabbits improves zero-line stability.[19] Essentially, careful dissection and cleaning of blood vessels allows for a mechanically good electrode-to-wall contact. There has been marked improvement in stability in blood flow measurement after removal of the adventitial tissue. In addition, removal of the adventitial layer may remove serous fluid and thus reduce the thickness of the conductive fluid outside the vessel which would be in contact with the recording electrodes of the probe. Moreover, nonstatic serous fluid can also cause problems with zero-line stability due to polarization of the charge around the recording electrode. Certainly, the removal of adventitial tissue will allow for much better contact of the probe with the blood vessel, pulling the ratio of inside vessel diameter to outside diameter closer to unity as well. As already mentioned, the film of conductive fluid outside the vessel and in contact with electrodes provides for electric shunting, thus reducing the actual voltage recorded by the flowmeter.[17] However, a smaller ratio between the inside and outside diameter of blood the vessel will diminish the impact of this source of error, as well as that associated with conductivity of the vessel. A foreseen problem associated with stripping the adventitial tissue is the occurrence of spasm. In fact, spasm may occur and has been observed both proximal and distal to the prepared area.[19] Thus, careful cleaning and dissection of the vessel on which the probe is to be placed is quite important, perhaps critical for accurate and reproducible blood flow measurements.

Clearly, changes in vessel wall thickness displace the ratio between probe diameter and inner vessel diameter. This physical factor appears to be of considerable importance when dealing with small probes and vessels even with constant electrode-to-wall contact. This also emphasizes the critical importance of selection of the probe diameter for accurate measurements of blood flow using an electromagnetic flowmeter.

3.2.3.5 Impact of Blood Cells and Flow Rate

It would appear that both hematocrit and flow rate can have an impact on blood flow measurements using electromagnetic flow probes. It would also appear that sensitivity of flow measurements by an electromagnetic flow probe is reduced with an increase in flow rate and/or hematocrit.[20]

A critical assumption that is made when using an electromagnetic flowmeter for the measurement of blood flow in a blood vessel is that the velocity of the fluid in a circular vessel is dependent only on the distance from the center of the vessel. This assumption is compromised in any measurement of blood flow in a vessel where there is asymmetrical flow. Theoretical analysis indicates that radial asymmetry has a considerable effect on the voltage output of an electromagnetic flowmeter. Within the cardiovascular tree, asymmetrical flow can arise near heart valves, large arterial branches, and where there is partial obstruction in blood vessels (e.g., plaque). It is also recognized that the presence of a bend in a circular flow pipe causes radial asymmetry of velocity profile under either turbulent or laminar conditions. In addition, asymmetric regurgitation or eddying within a vessel may also give rise to radial asymmetry in circulation. Experimentally, it has been reported that asymmetry may cause the instrument to indicate incorrect discharge rate, and errors in measurements as great as 2:1 have been observed.[21]

However, reports on the impact of hematocrit on blood flow measurement using electromagnetic flowmeters are conflicting. While some investigators have found that the instrument is less sensitive when using blood instead of saline,[10] others have reported no differences.[22] The presence of a cell-free zone has been used to explain the non-Newtonian behavior of blood flow in blood vessels. This phenomenon has been used as a basis for explaining the impact of blood cells on differential flow measurement by electromagnetic flowmeters. However, an alternative to this view is the idea of the existence of finite unsheared laminae in the liquid and radially distributed cells resulting in a nonlaminar flow of blood. In general, the erythrocytes flow with their main surface aligned parallel to the direction of flow. If this is the case, the electrical resistance of blood would be greater in diametral as opposed to circumferential directions. During a laminar flow of blood, symmetrical circulating currents are set up across the section of the vessel. These currents are partially directed along the vessel and partially circumferential. The possible differences in the resistivity in these directions could affect the potential difference between the detecting electrodes of the electromagnetic flow probe. This could account for changes in sensitivity due to flow and changes in the concentration of hematocrit. Taken together, it seems that altered sensitivity in the ability of electromagnetic flowmeters to measure blood flow may be explained by the anisotropic conductivity of blood as a consequence of differences in conductivity of radial and circumferential direction of flow which also could be accompanied by the nonuniform radial distribution of cells.[20]

3.2.4 Implantation of Perivascular Electromagnetic Flowmeters in Experimental Animals

The most commonly used term for electromagnetic flowmeter is *probe.* It generally consists of an electromagnet to generate a magnetic field and two electrodes to sense the voltage, and is encapsulated in an inert hard plastic casing that permits it to be placed around a blood vessel. The lumen or inner diameter of the holder slightly deforms the vessel so that its cross-section area is fixed. In this way, the transducer can be used to measure the flow rate. It is advisable to cover the outside of the probe and cord with medical silicon to reduce an alien feeling in the body of the animal. The length of cord (lead wire to the plug from the probe) must be selected by body size of the animal. A probe for chronic implantation is specially ordered to fit the animal's size. The probe should be placed on a straight portion of the vessel and as far as possible from junctions and branches. This is to avoid the turbulent flow in the region where the probe is implanted. Normally, stain on electrodes of probes removed from vessels should be wiped out by soft gauze carefully so as that the electrodes are not damaged. The probe should then be washed with water and subsequently the probe's head should be immersed in physiological saline (>30 min) in order to stabilize the electrode status. The probe should be kept in a clean condition after natural drying. It is recommended that the entire probe, with the exception of part of the connector, be sterilized by ethylene oxide gas or formalin gas.

3.2.4.1 Probe Implantation in Conscious Rat

Probes can be implanted on superior mesenteric artery, renal artery, or terminal aorta from a retroperitoneally position by left flank incision in an anesthetized (thiamylal sodium; 50 mg/kg, i.p.) animal.[23,24] A probe with an internal diameters of 1, 1.5, and 2.0 mm can be used for the renal artery, superior mesenteric artery, and terminal aorta, respectively. The lead wire to the plug from the probes is then tunneled subcutaneously to the back of the neck, exteriorized and secured. The outer end of the wire needs to be secured to the neck muscle. A polyethylene catheter can be inserted into the femoral artery for measurement of arterial blood pressure, and into either a jugular vein or the femoral vein for the administration of drugs. These catheters are then tunneled subcutaneously to the back of the neck,

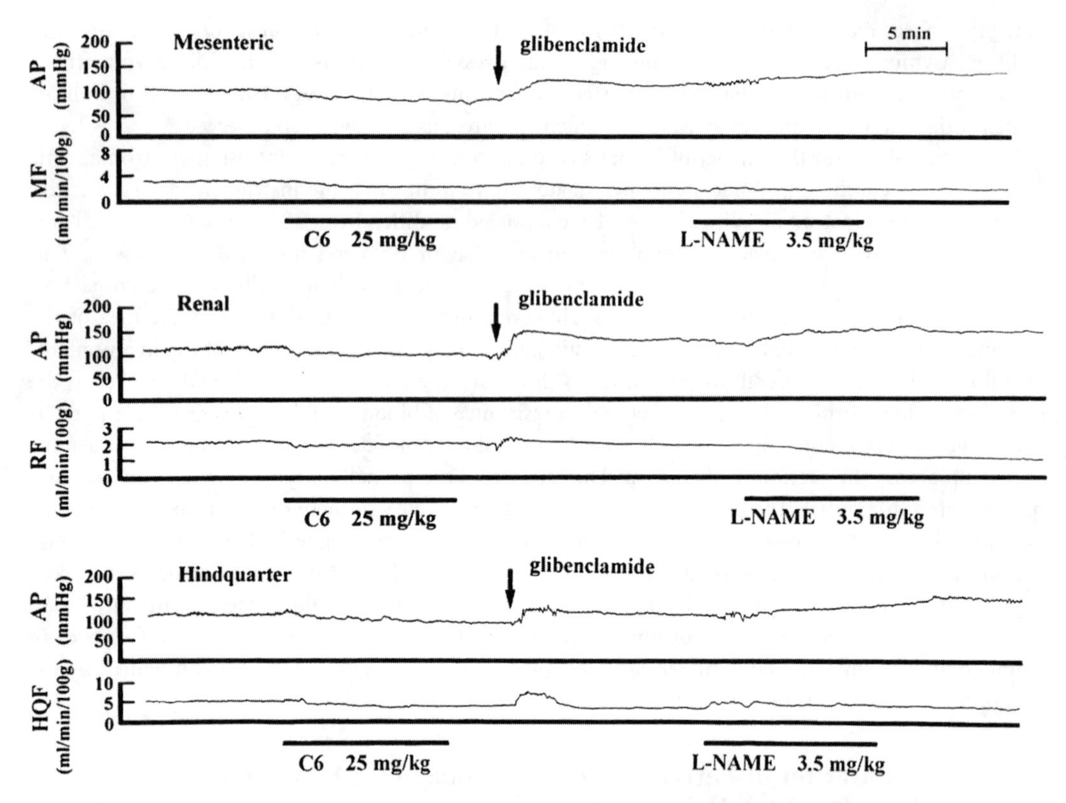

FIGURE 3.5 Original tracing of arterial pressure and blood flow measurements in conscious rats. Blood flow measurements were made with electromagnetic flow probes implanted on superior mesenteric artery (MF), renal artery (RF), and hindquarter (HQF).

exteriorized and secured. Each animal will then be allowed to recover and is placed in a polyethylene cage, with access to food and water ad libitum. Three or four days post-surgery, the exteriorized plug from the probe can be connected to an external cable from the flowmeter circuit, and flow can be monitored. In addition, a blood pressure catheter will be connected to a pressure transducer via appropriate tubing for simultaneous measurement of flow and pressure from the conscious animal. In Figure 3.5, arterial pressure (mmHg) and regional vascular flows (mesenteric, renal, and hindquarter; ml/min × 100 g body wt) measured in conscious rats after administration of hexamethonium bromide (C6), glibenclamide (0.67 mg/kg i.v.), and N^{ω}-nitro-L-arginine methyl ester (L-NAME) is shown. Flow measurements were made in separate animals using a Type FI, Nihon Koden: 1-, 1.5-, or 2-mm ID probe and flowmeter circuit (Nihon Koden MFV-3100). In Table 3.2., a comparison of total basal regional blood flow values of terminal aorta, renal artery, superior mesenteric artery, celiac artery, and carotid artery in conscious, normotensive, and spontaneously hypertensive rats are shown as measured by electromagnetic flow probes.[24,25]

3.2.5 Electromagnetic Transducer (Intravascular)

Mills[26] was the first to design and utilize catheters with an electromagnetic flow probe mounted at the tip for intravascular measurement of blood velocity. This type of probe uses the same principle as the external electromagnetic flow probes.[27] However, the magnetic field is external to the probe, so that voltages are generated by the blood flowing around it rather than through it. The Mills catheter-tipped flowmeter has been used to measure blood velocity in venous[28] as well as arterial[29] circulation in humans.

The intravascular flowmeter can also be used to measure blood velocity at various sites in the circulatory system of dogs.[30,31] Moreover, comparisons between blood velocity measurements at various sites

TABLE 3.2 Basal Regional Blood Flow Values Measured using Electromagnetic Flow Probes in Conscious Normotensive or Spontaneously Hypertensive Rats

Regions	Spontaneously Hypertensive Rats	Normotensive Rats
Terminal aorta (T)[25]	4.56 ± 1.68 (13)	5.84 ± 1.31 (11)
Renal artery (R)[25]	1.69 ± 0.67 (8)	1.72 ± 0.34 (8)
S. Mesenteric artery (M)[25]	4.78 ± 1.54 (7)	4.36 ± 0.66 (8)
Celiac artery (Ce)[23]	2.25 ± 0.44 (15)	2.07 ± 0.44 (15)
Carotid artery (C)[25]	2.03 ± 0.48 (7)	1.64 ± 0.21 (8)
2 (R + C) + T + M + Ce	19.00	19.00

Note: Values are from Iriuchijima[25] and Iida.[23] The values are mean ± SD, (n).

in the circulatory system in dogs by intravascular probes has yielded values comparable to measurements using external flow probes (e.g., ascending, descending, and abdominal aorta).[31]

An important difference between the perivascular vs. intravascular probe/sensor is that the perivascular probe measures blood velocity/flow across the entire cross-sectional area of the vessels. In contrast, the intravascular sensor measures only the velocity of blood flowing in the region around the sensor. This difference means that with an intravascular sensor, the velocity measured is dependent on the profile of the velocity of blood flowing close to the sensor, and this may not necessarily be reflective of mean velocity of flow within that vessel. Thus, in order to assess the mean velocity within a given vessel using such sensors one needs to record the velocity of blood at different points over the cross-sectional area of that vessel.[31]

To determine the rate of blood flow (volume of flow per unit of time) using the intravascular flow probes, the cross-sectional area of the vessel in which the flow is being measured needs to be known. Otherwise, the velocity of flow needs to be calibrated in milliliters per minute or liters per minute by reference to cardiac output as measured by another technique.[32,33] It has been recognized that small errors may be introduced into calculations of rate of blood flow if the average diameter of blood vessels are used. For example, in man it has been reported that the cross-sectional areas of the ascending aorta and the main pulmonary artery diameter change by a total of 11% (–5 to +5%) and 18% (–9 to +9%), respectively, between the end-diastole and end-systole cycles.[34,35] Thus, such factors may need to be taken into account when estimating rate of blood flow by intravascular methods. However, it has also been suggested by Nichols et al.[32] that changes in cross-sectional areas of vessels during cardiac cycles may be affected by a number of conditions, namely, site of measurement and experimental conditions and techniques. For example, there appear to be minimal changes in the cross-sectional diameter of the aorta at the upper border of the sinus of Valsalva,[32] which perhaps makes it an ideal site for assessment of blood flow using an intravascular sensor. In addition, another potential problem that may arise when using an intravascular flow sensor in the pulmonary artery is introduction of motion artifacts. This could result in signal artifacts that in turn could result in the underestimation of systolic blood velocity. The basis for this artifact has been attributed to right ventricular contraction which may cause catheter movement in the direction of axial flow within the pulmonary artery. To circumvent this problem, use of fairly rigid catheters may result in reduction in longitudinal motion.[32]

Precautions may also need to be taken when using intravascular electromagnetic flowmeters, as there is a possibility of current leakage. This becomes quite important close to, or within, the hearts in humans. Obviously, such leakage could cause electrical disturbances in the myocardium, precipitating cardiac arrhythmias. Furthermore, a high current density may produce thermic effects at the tip of the catheter, and this may cause the development of small blood clots. These issues have been considered by Jones and Wyatt[36] and Buchanan and Shabetai,[37] who have concluded that Mills-type probes are fairly safe for human use. In addition, it has been reported that Carolina probes also meet electric and thermal safety specifications that are required for *in vivo* use in human subjects.[38] Nonetheless, care must be taken when using such catheters in humans, and careful monitoring of the insulation for electric and thermal safety is highly recommended prior to their use in human subjects.

3.2.6 Noninvasive Electromagnetic Flowmetry

Noninvasive electromagnetic flowmetry has been used to measure blood flow in humans. Lee and associates[39] first described this technique in detail in humans. In particular, reports of blood flow measurement made by noninvasive and invasive methods were found to show similar waveform contour.[39] Boccalon and associates[40] have also described the technique of measuring limb blood flow in humans using noninvasive electromagnetic flowmetry. In general, the technique uses the same principle as the magnetic flow probes. Here, the limb is placed in a magnetic field and the blood flow induces electromagnetic force that can be detected by skin surface electrocardiograph electrodes. The technique has been reported to provide reliable and reproducible data and appears to be quite easy to use.[41,42] The noninvasive electromagnetic flowmetry has been used to assess global pulsatile arterial blood flow in the lower limbs of humans.[43,44]

Technical evaluation of this technique by Boccalon and associates[45] has revealed that blood chemical composition (e.g., $[Na^+]$ and $[K^+]$) within the limits of the normal physiological range does not have an impact on flow signal detected by the surface electrodes. However, it seems that reduction in hematocrit from 45 to 29% results in a variation within 10% of the invasive technique. In final analysis, measurement of blood flow by a noninvasive electromagnetic flowmetry method using skin surface electrodes requires the background subtraction of ballistocardiographic signal (due to the vibration of electrode wires in magnetic field), and the electrocardiograph signal. In addition, it may be necessary to also filter out random noise which may in part be generated by nonsynchronous signals such as muscle twitching and tension. Furthermore, low-frequency drift due to changes in the position of the electrodes, perspiration and/or drying of electrode electrolytes may also occur. This essentially will result in electrode polarization and lead to reduction in voltage detected by the skin surface electrodes.[45] Therefore, investigators planning to measure blood flow using this technique need to be aware of these factors.

One important factor that also needs special consideration when measuring arterial blood flow by a noninvasive electromagnetic flowmetry technique is venous flow. A critical feature of the noninvasive electromagnetic flowmetry is that only the pulsatile components of the flow are measured. Therefore, in a case where flow in a limb is being measured far from the heart, the venous flow by virtue of being continuous will not have an impact on the signal that is being recorded (i.e., arterial flow). Likewise, where the pulsatile venous flow is due to respiration, its influence can be circumvented and nullified by a waveform averaging technique. Furthermore, in a case where venous pulsatile flow is synchronized with the heart rate, it only appears to affect the diastolic part of the waveform below zero line.[45] The latter is not of critical importance in assessment of arterial blood flow.

3.3 Discussion

A method capable of directly measuring beat-to-beat blood flow (i.e., cardiac output and/or regional flow) is most desirable. Furthermore, it is also important if the instrument employed is able to measure the quantity of blood that passes a specific point. Obviously, electromagnetic flow probes are instruments that are capable of measuring beat-to-beat blood flow, as well as volume of blood flow in a unit of time. In fact, it is well recognized that electromagnetic flow probes, when used properly for measurement of blood flow, can provide investigators with one of the most accurate methods of flow (volume of blood in unit time or velocity rate per unit time) measurements *in vivo*. Of course, it is mandatory that an ideal flowmeter have certain special attributes if blood flow is to be measured accurately in a reproducible manner. Clearly, the most important properties associated with an ideal flowmeter are that it must: (1) be nonobstructive to flow, (2) not interfere with the profile of flow, (3) provide linear response for both forward and backward flow, (4) have an adequate frequency response range, and (5) possess a stable zero baseline over the duration of the time period of flow measurements.

Here, in the case of the electromagnetic flow probes, the principle of electromagnetic flux has been exploited based on Faraday's law to produce an instrument that is capable of measuring blood flow invasively and noninvasively with very good accuracy and precision. For the purpose of noninvasive flow measurements, probes have been refined to measure blood flow and velocity locally or globally in a region, while in the case of the invasive technique, flowmeters have been modified for measurement of local or extracorporeal flow via perivascular or intravascular modules in large as well as small blood vessels.

In general, blood flow measurements are made under a variety of conditions and for many different reasons. For example, electromagnetic flow probes have been used in experimental animals to assess the impact of altered physiological conditions or the effect of chemicals on regional blood flow (e.g., blood flow to kidney, mesentery, hindlimb, liver, etc.) and cardiac output. In addition, measurement of blood flow in the various regions of the body in pathophysiological conditions (such as hypertension, congestive heart failure, diabetes) have provided useful information as to the changes that occur in the rate, and to the profile of flow. Moreover, in humans an understanding of changes in the rate and the profile of blood flow has been used to assess and define pathophysiology. In addition, blood flow measurements have been employed to determine the impact of drugs in the circulatory system in humans.

Electromagnetic flow probes now set the bench mark for accurate and precise measurement of blood flow in both experimental and clinical conditions. In fact, it is accurate to say that electromagnetic flow probes are considered "gold standard" for measurement of cardiac output and regional blood flow in both animals and humans. In addition, they are routinely used to calibrate flow modules, as well as to gauge the accuracy and precision of other instruments such as Doppler flowmeters. Moreover, electromagnetic flow probes have been utilized as internal calibration modules with nuclear magnetic resonance techniques for assessment of blood flow in humans. Kerr et al.[46] devised a method of integrating a nuclear magnetic resonance instrument with an electromagnetic flow sensor as a secondary standard for measurement of blood flow in the lower extremities in human subjects. Volumetric calibration of the instrument indicated precise and accurate measurement of flow over a range of 0 to 100 ml/min. An assessment of the calibration module and the electromagnetic sensor was found to be linear for a rate of flow between 5 to 100 ml/min with a regression coefficient of 0.99. It was reported that the assessment of blood flow in the extremities using such an apparatus would enable one to distinguish limb ischemia and claudication without allowing the operator to make a distinction between the two.[46] Evidently, such an instrument appears to allow for direct measurement of pulsatile blood flow in a noninvasive manner but it also has its limitation. Of note is the fact that only pulsatile flow can be measured; lack of ability to measure flow lower than 5 ml/min and the inability to measure flow in most distal portions of the arterial tree (i.e., toes and fingers) are the other limitations associated with this technique.[46]

Perivascular electromagnetic flow probes have been employed to measure regional blood flow in many species either anesthetized or conscious. For example, blood flow to mesenteric, renal, and limbs have been recorded and reported in the literature from anesthetized canines,[47] felines,[48] rats,[49] porcines,[50,51] and primates.[52,53] In addition, flow to the same regions have been recorded and are available in the literature in conscious canines,[54] felines,[55] and rats.[23,24] Hepatic blood flow (hepatic artery and portal vein) measurements have also been reported by use of electromagnetic flow probes.[56,57] Blood flow measurements in carotid, hepatic, and portal veins in canine have also been reported.[58] Blood flow has also been reported in the vena cava (45 ml/min/kg), coccygeomesenteric vein (8.3 ml/min/kg), mesenteric vein (6.7 ml/min/kg), and hepatic portal vein (15 ml/min/kg) of chickens using electromagnetic flow probes.[59]

Electromagnetic flowmetry has also been effectively used in the measurement of coronary blood flow in both animals and humans. In anesthetized and conscious dogs, blood flow through the left circumflex coronary artery has been reported to range between 18 and 33 ml/min,[60,61] and 24 and 60 ml/min,[62] respectively. In addition, coronary blood flow measurement in primates appears to indicate that flow in the left descending coronary artery can range between 12 and 26 ml/min.[63] Moreover, Folts and associates[64] have reported phasic changes in human right coronary blood flow before and after repair of aortic insufficiency using electromagnetic flowmetry during surgery. Flows reported in the right coronary artery prior to aortic valve replacement ranged between 79 and 153 ml/min, while flow increased post-valve replacement was reported to range between 140 and 220 ml/min.[64]

Comparing aortic flow characteristics in monkeys using electromagnetic (invasive) and Doppler (non-invasive) flowmetry indicates that there is good correlation and no significant differences between the two systems in values gathered for peak flow, cardiac output, stroke volume and maximal rate of change of flow velocity.[65] In addition, frequency domain analysis (magnitude and phase) of flow waveform revealed very modest differences between the two methods. However, significant differences were noted in time to peak flow, and time to maximal rate of changes of flow velocity between the two methods. Essentially, these events appeared to occur significantly earlier in the Doppler than with the electromagnetic flow characteristics. The reasons for this observation remain unresolved and may relate to several factors. There was a real possibility that the Doppler signal may have been contaminated by the motion of the opening of the aortic valve leaflets during early systole. Equally conceivable was the possibility that the setting of the frequency-response of an electromagnetic flowmeter may have been inadequate for recording the rapidly changing flow rate in early systole.[65]

Heerdt et al.,[66] comparing the method of thermodilution vs. electromagnetic flowmetry in a clinical setting, have also reported good correlation (r = 0.92) between the two techniques. However, they also revealed wide variation in cardiac output measurements using thermodilution in some patients with tricuspid regurgitation, thus suggesting that underlying pathophysiology may have a significant impact on the capability of the technique that is used for measuring flow.[66] Therefore, it is imperative to understand the limitations of the techniques used for measurement of blood flow. It is also recognized that inaccuracies in estimating volume of flow using probes occurs more often as the result of inaccuracies in the measurement of aortic cross-sectional areas than the evaluation of blood flow velocity. For example, a comparison in estimating blood flow in the ascending aorta in man revealed that there is a greater similarity in measurement of flow between electromagnetic and Doppler flowmetry when compared to thermodilution. In essence, the underestimation (by >10%) of cardiac output measurements appear to be due to error in the measurement of the cross-sectional area of the ascending aorta.[67]

In Table 3.3, values presented for cardiac output using electromagnetic flow probes and dye/thermodilutions have been reported in a number of species including rats,[68-72] dogs,[66,73-75] rabbits,[76-79] and porcines[80-84] both in anesthetized and conscious states. Overall, comparison of cardiac output measurements between the two techniques reveals that similar values are obtained for electromagnetic vs. dye/thermodilution methods. Cardiac output measurements using electromagnetic flowmetry have also been made in other species such as felines[85,86] and primates.[87] Furthermore, it is evident that a comparison between cardiac output measurements using electromagnetic flow probes vs. microspheres techniques in rats,[88-90] rabbits,[76] and porcines[91,92] also seems to show fairly comparable results (Table 3.3). There are obviously some modest discrepancies between cardiac output values obtained with different techniques in some species (e.g., conscious porcine; microsphere vs. electromagnetic flowmetry), but such differences are most likely related to experimental conditions. In human subjects, an assessment of cardiac output using electromagnetic flowmetry[32,93] vs. dye/thermodilution[32,66] techniques indicates that comparable values are obtained (Table 3.3) even though assessment of cardiac output by the method of thermodilution under certain circumstances has been suggested to yield higher values for cardiac output than electromagnetic flowmetry.

TABLE 3.3 Cardiac Index (ml/min per kg) or Output (ml/min) Measurements by Different Techniques in Different Species

Species	Electromagnetic Probes	Microspheres	Dye/Thermodilutions
Rat (A)	180– 250[a] [68]	291–343[a] [88,90]	186–274[a] [71]
Rat (C)	230–350[a] [68-70]	270–311[a] [88]	387–421[a] [72]
Dog (A)	1200–4800[b] [66]	—	3100–5490[b] [75]
Dog (C)	1990–2300[b] [73]	—	1900–3520[b] [74]
Rabbit (A)	83–131[a] [75]	90–131[a] [76]	85–143[a] [78]
Rabbit (C)	174–192[a] [77]	151–213[a] [76]	214–286[a] [79]
Porcine (A)	62–91[a] [80]	172–212[a] [92]	64–85[a] [81,83]
Porcine (C)	190–223[a] [81]	121–221[a] [91]	166–278[a] [84]
Human (A)	2315–6300[b] [93]	—	3500–8500[b] [66]
Human (C)	5100–8300[b] [32]	—	6100–8800[b] [32]

Note: A = anesthetized; C = conscious. [a]ml/min per kg; [b]ml/min.

Clearly, among the many advantages offered by the technique of electromagnetic flowmetry in assessing cardiac output, when compared to either microsphere or dye/thermodilution techniques in either experimental and/or clinical conditions, is the fact that electromagnetic flowmetry offers the opportunity of measurement of beat-to-beat flow rate. In addition, use of electromagnetic flowmetry will allow for an assessment of such things as peak flow within a given vessel. Nonetheless, measurement of blood flow/cardiac output using electromagnetic flowmetry has its limitations, and investigators who wish to use this technique to assess flow rates must be aware of them.

References

1. Tabrizchi, R. and Pugsley, M.K., Methods of blood flow measurements in the arterial circulatory system, *J. Pharmacol. Methods,* 44, 375, 2000.
2. Nichols, W.W., O'Rourke, M.F. and Hartley, C., *McDonald's Blood Flow in Arteries, Theoretical, Experimental and Clinical Principles*, 4th ed., Edward Arnold, London, 1998, chaps. 6 and 10.
3. Keele, C.A. and Neil, E., *Samson Wright's Applied Physiology,* 12th ed., Oxford University Press, London, 1971, p. 107.
4. Fabre, P., Utilisation des forces electromotrices d'induction pour l'enregistrement des variations de vitesse des liquides conducteurs: un nouvel hemodromograph sans palette dans le sang, *C.R. Acad. Sci. Paris,* 194, 1097, 1932.
5. Kolin, A., An electromagnetic flowmeter: principle of the method and its application to blood flow measurements, *Proc. Soc. Exp. Biol. Med.,* 35, 53, 1936.
6. Kolin, A., An electromagnetic recording flowmeter, *Am. J. Physiol.,* 119, 355, 1937.
7. Wetterer, E., Eine neue Methode zur Registrieung der Blutstromunggsgeschwindkiet am unerоffneter Egass, *Z. Biol.,* 98, 26, 1937.
8. Bevir, M.K., The theory of induced voltage electromagnetic flowmeters, *J. Fluid Mech,*. 43, 577, 1970.
9. Scott, E.A. and Sandler, G.A., Electromagnetic blood flowmeters and flow probes: theoretic and practical considerations, *Am. J. Vet. Res.,* 39, 1567, 1978.
10. Khouri, E.M. and Gregg, D.E., Miniature electromagnetic flowmeter applicable to coronary arteries, *J. Appl. Physiol.,* 18, 224, 1963.
11. Gessner, U. and Bergel, D.H., Frequency response of electromagnetic flowmeters, *J. Appl. Physiol.,* 19, 1209, 1964.
12. Yanof, H.M., A trapezoidal-wave electromagnetic blood flowmeter. *J. Appl. Physiol.,* 16, 566, 1961.
13. Patel, D.J., deFreitas, F.M. and Fry, D.L., Hydraulic input impedance to aorta and pulmonary artery in dogs, *J. Appl. Physiol.,* 18, 134, 1963.
14. Bergel, D.H. and Gessner, U., III, The electromagnetic flowmeter, *Meth. Med. Res.,* 11, 70, 1966.
15. Wyatt, D.G., Problems in the measurements of blood flow by magnetic induction, *Phys. Med. Biol. J.,* 289, 1961.
16. Hill, R.D., A rapid technique for dynamic calibration of electromagnetic flowmeters, *J. Appl. Physiol.,* 53, 294, 1982.
17. Gessner, U., Effects of the vessel wall on electromagnetic flow measurements, *Biophysics,* 1, 627, 1961.
18. Schwan, H.P. and Kay, C.F., Specific resistance of body tissue, *Circ. Res.,* 4, 664, 1956.
19. Nornes, H., Electromagnetic blood flowmetry in small vessel surgery, *Scand. J. Thor. Cardiovasc.,* 10, 144, 1976.
20. Dennis, J. and Wyatt, D.G., Effect of hematocrit value upon electromagnetic flowmeter sensitivity, *Circ. Res.,* 24, 875, 1969.
21. Goldman, S.C., Marple, N.B. and Scolink, W.L., Effects of flow profile on electromagnetic flowmeter accuracy, *J. Appl. Physiol.,* 18, 652, 1963.
22. Westersten, A., Herrold, G. and Assali, N.S., Gated sine wave blood flowmeter, *J. Appl. Physiol.,* 15, 533, 1960.

23. Iida, N., Different flow regulation mechanisms between celiac and mesenteric vascular beds in conscious rats, *Hypertension,* 25, 260, 1995.
24. Iida, N., Nitric oxide mediates sympathetic vasoconstriction at supraspinal, spinal, and synaptic levels, *Am. J. Physiol.*, 276, H918, 1999.
25. Iriuchijima, J., Regional blood flow in conscious spontaneously hypertensive rats, *Jpn. J. Physiol.*, 33, 41, 1983.
26. Mills, C.J., A catheter-tip electromagnetic velocity probe, *Phys. Med. Biol.*, 11, 323, 1966.
27. Mills, C.J., Measurement of pulsatile flow and flow velocity, in *Cardiovascular Fluid Dynamics,* Vol. 1, Bergel, D.H., Ed., Academic Press, New York, 1972, p. 51.
28. Wexler, L. et al., Velocity of blood flow in normal human venae cavae, *Circ. Res.*, 23, 349, 1968.
29. Gabe, I.T. et al., Measurement of instantaneous blood flow velocity and pressure in conscious man with a catheter-tip velocity probe, *Circulation,* 40, 603, 1969.
30. Bond, R.F. and Barefoot, C.A., Evaluation of an electromagnetic catheter tip velocity sensitive blood flow probe, *J. Appl. Physiol.*, 23, 403, 1967.
31. Warbasse, J. R. et al., Physiologic evaluation of a catheter-tip electromagnetic velocity probe, *Am. J. Cardiol.*, 23, 424, 1969.
32. Nichols, W.W. et al., Evaluation of a new catheter-mounted electromagnetic velocity sensor during cardiac catheterization, *Cathet. Cardiovasc. Diag.,* 6, 97, 1980.
33. Nichols, W.W. et al., Experimental evaluation of a multisensor velocity-pressure catheter, *Med. Biol. Eng. Comput.*, 23, 79, 1985.
34. Greenfield, J.C., Jr. and Patel, D.J., Relation between pressure and diameter in the ascending aorta in man, *Circ. Res.*, 10, 778, 1962.
35. Greenfield, J.C., Jr. and Griggs, D.M., Jr., The relation between pressure and diameter in the main pulmonary artery of man, *J. Appl. Physiol.*, 18, 557, 1963.
36. Jones, M.A.S. and Wyatt, D.G., The surface temperature of electromagnetic velocity probes, *Cardiovasc. Res.*, 4, 338, 1970.
37. Buchanan, J. W. and Shabetai, R., True power dissipation of catheter tip velocity probes, *Cardiovasc. Res.*, 6, 211, 1972.
38. Peterson, K.L. et al., Assessment of left ventricular performance in man: instantaneous tension-velocity-length relations obtained with the aid of an electromagnetic velocity catheter in the ascending aorta, *Circulation,* 47, 924, 1973.
39. Lee, B.Y. et al., A clinical evaluation of a noninvasive electromagnetic flowmeter, *Angiology,* 26, 317, 1975.
40. Boccalon, H.J. et al., Non-invasive electromagnetic measurement of the peripheral pulsatile blood flow: experimental study and clinical applications, *Cardiovasc. Res.*, 12, 66, 1978.
41. Lee, B.Y. et al., Noninvasive flowmetry in vascular surgery: use of a noninvasive electromagnetic flowmeter, *Jpn. J. Surg*,. 11, 219, 1981.
42. Cunningham, L.N. et al., A noninvasive electromagnetic flowmeter, *Med. Instrum.*, 17, 237, 1983.
43. Boccalon, H., Critical study of the measurement of pulsatile flow in artheritis patients, value of non-invasive electromagnetic flowmetry, *J. Mal. Vasc.*, 10(Suppl. A), 20, 1985.
44. Boccalon, H., Flowmeter monitoring following lumbar sympathectomy, *J. Mal. Vasc.* 10(Suppl. A), 88, 1985.
45. Boccalon, H. et al., Noninvasive electromagnetic blood flowmeter: theoretical aspects and technical evaluation, *Med. Biol. Eng. Comput.*, 20, 671, 1982.
46. Kerr, T.M. et al., Measurement of blood flow rates in the lower extremities with use of nuclear magnetic resonance based instrument, *J. Vasc. Surg.*, 14, 649, 1991.
47. De Backer, D. et al., Regional effects of dobutamine in endotoxic shock, *J. Surg. Res.*, 65, 93, 1996.
48. Mraovitch, S., Kumada, M., and Reis, D.J., Role of the nucleus parabrachialis in cardiovascular regulation in cat, *Brain Res.*, 232, 57, 1982.
49. Pete, G. et al., Insulin-like growth factor-I decreases mean blood pressure and selectively increases regional blood flow in normal rats, *Proc. Soc. Exp. Biol.*, 213, 187, 1996.

50. Vacca, G. et al., The effect of distension of the stomach on peripheral blood flow in anesthetized pigs, *Exp. Physiol.*, 81, 385, 1996.
51. Molinari, C. et al., Effect of progesterone on peripheral blood flow in prepubertal female anesthetized pigs, *J. Vasc. Res.*, 38, 569, 2001.
52. Udelsman, R. et al., Hemodynamic effects of corticotropin releasing hormone in the anesthetized cynomolgus monkey, *Peptides*, 7, 465, 1986.
53. Spelman, F.A., Oberg, P.A. and Astley, C., Localized neural control of blood flow in the renal cortex on the anesthetized baboon, *Acta Physiol. Scand.*, 127, 437, 1986.
54. Vanter, S.F. and McRitchie, R. J., Reflex limb dilatation following norepinephrine and angiotensin II in conscious dogs, *Am. J. Physiol.*, 230, 557, 1976.
55. Baccelli, G. et al., Cardiovascular changes during spontaneous micturition in conscious cats, *Am. J. Physiol.*, 237, H213, 1979.
56. Matuschak, G.M., Pinsky, M.R. and Rogers, R.M., Effects of positive end-expiratory pressure on hepatic blood flow and performance, *J. Appl. Physiol.*, 62, 1377, 1987.
57. Alexander, B., Blumgart, L.H. and Mathie, R.T., The effect of propranolol on the hyperaemic response of the hepatic artery to portal venous occlusion in the dog, *Br. J. Pharmacol.*, 96, 356, 1989.
58. Hallberg, D. and Pernow, B., Effect of substance P on various vascular beds in the dog, *Acta Physiol. Scand.*, 93, 277, 1975.
59. Sturkie, P.D. and Abati, A., Blood flow in mesenteric, hepatic portal and renal portal veins on chickens, *Pflügers Arch.*, 359, 127, 1975.
60. Cevese, A. et al., The effect of distension of the urinary bladder on coronary blood flow in anesthetized dogs, *Exp. Physiol.*, 76, 409, 1991.
61. Martin, U., Dorge, L. and Fischer, S., Comparison of desulfatohirudin (REVASC) and heparin as adjuncts to thrombolytic therapy with reteplase in a canine model of coronary thrombosis, *Br. J. Pharmacol.*, 118, 271, 1996.
62. Dulas, D., Homans, D.C. and Bache, R. J., Effects of urapidil on coronary blood flow during graded treadmill exercise, *J. Cardiovasc. Pharmacol.*, 24, 1004, 1994.
63. Taira, N. et al., Sustained coronary constriction and its antagonism by calcium-blocking agents in monkeys and baboons, *Circ. Res.*, 52, I40, 1983.
64. Folts, J.D. et al., Phasic changes in human right coronary blood flow before and after repair of aortic insufficiency, *Am. Heart J.*, 97, 211, 1979.
65. Spencer, K.T. et al., Doppler and electromagnetic comparisons of instantaneous aortic flow characteristics in primates, *Circ. Res.*, 68, 1369, 1991.
66. Heerdt, P.M. et al., Comparison of cardiac output measured by intrapulmonary artery Doppler, themodilution, and electromagnetometry, *Ann. Thorac. Surg.*, 54, 959, 1992.
67. Coats, A.J. et al., Validation of the beat-to-beat measurement of blood velocity in the human ascending aorta by a new high temporal resolution Doppler ultrasound spectral analyzer, *Br. Heart J.*, 68, 223, 1992.
68. Kawaue, Y. and Iriuchijima, J., Changes in cardiac output and peripheral flows on pentobarbital anesthesia in the rat, *Jpn. J. Physiol.*, 34, 283, 1984.
69. Sardella, G.L. and Ou, L.C., Chronically instrumented rat model for hemodynamic studies of both pulmonary and systemic circulation, *J. Appl. Physiol.*, 74, 849, 1993.
70. Hinojosa-Laborde, C., Forhlich, B.H. and Cowley, A.W., Jr., Contribution of regional vascular responses to whole body autoregulation in conscious areflexic rats, *Hypertension*, 17, 1078, 1991.
71. Sweet, C.S. et al., Measurement of cardiac output in anesthetized rats by dye dilution using a fiberoptic catheter, *J. Pharmacol. Methods*, 17, 189, 1987.
72. Siren, A.L. et al., Mechanisms of central hemodynamic and sympathetic regulation by mu opioid receptors: effects of dermorphin in the conscious rat, *J. Pharmacol. Exp. Ther.*, 248, 596, 1989.
73. Puybasset, L. et al., Hemodynamic effects of sub-chronic NO synthase inhibition in conscious dogs: role of EDRF/NO in muscular exertion, *Arch. Mal. Coeur. Vaiss.*, 88, 121, 1995.

74. Laks, M., Callis, G. and Swan, H. J., Hemodynamic effects of low doses of norepinephrine in the conscious dog, *Am. J. Physiol.*, 220, 171, 1971.
75. French, W.J. et al., Ejection fraction derived using dye dilution and angiographic methods, *Am. Heart J.*, 104, 104, 1982.
76. Saxena, P.R. et al., Regional and systemic haemodynamic changes evoked by 5-hydroxytryptamine in awake and anaesthetized rabbits, *Eur. J. Pharmacol.*, 50, 61, 1978.
77. Saxena, P.R. et al., Electromagnetic flow-probe implantation for cardiac output measurements in rabbit, *J. Pharmacol. Methods*, 3, 125, 1980.
78. Bhattacharya, S., Glucksberg, M.R. and Bhattacharya, J., Measurement of lung microvascular pressure in the intact anesthetized rabbit by the micropuncture technique, *Circ. Res.*, 64, 167, 1989.
79. Beilin, L.J. and Bhattachyarya, J., The effect of prostaglandin synthesis inhibitors on renal blood flow distribution in conscious rabbits, *J. Physiol.*, 269, 395, 1977.
80. Gelman, S., Rabbani, S. and Bradley, E.L., Jr., Inferior and superior vena cava blood flows during cross-clamping of the thoracic aorta in pigs, *J. Thorac. Cardiovasc. Surg.*, 96, 387, 1988.
81. Fiser, W.P. et al., Cardiovascular effects of protamine sulfate are dependent on the presence and type of circulating heparin, *J. Thorac. Cardiovasc. Surg.*, 89, 63, 1985.
82. Stuesse, D.C. et al., Hemodynamic effects of S-nitrosocyteine, an intravenous regional vasodilator, *J. Thorac. Cardiovasc. Surg.*, 122, 371, 2001.
83. Asher, A.S. et al., Effect of increasing inspired oxygen concentration on hemodynamics and regional blood flows, *Crit. Care Med.*, 16, 1235, 1988.
84. Law, W.R. et al., Pentoxifylline treatment of sepsis in conscious Yucatan minipigs, *Circ. Shock*, 37, 291, 1992.
85. Francis, G.R. and Whiting, R.L., On-line computation of peripheral resistance and stroke volume in the conscious cat obtained by the use of chronically-implanted electromagnetic flow transducer, *Br. J. Pharmacol.*, 312P, 60, 1977.
86. Dreteler, G.H. et al., Systemic and regional hemodynamic effects of the putative 5-HT_{1A} receptor agonist flesinoxan in the cat, *J. Cardiovasc. Pharmacol.*, 14, 770, 1989.
87. Chimoskey, J.E. et al., Effects of ketamine on ventricular dynamics of unanesthetized baboons, *Cardiovasc. Res. Cent. Bull.*, 14, 53, 1975.
88. Tabrizchi, R. and Pang, C.C.Y., Influence of intravenous infusion on regional blood flow in conscious rats, *J. Pharm. Pharmacol.*, 45, 151, 1993.
89. Dutta, P., Ryan, D.E. and Tabrizchi, R., The influence of phosphodiesterase inhibitor, rolipram, on hemodynamics in lipopolysaccharide-treated rats, *Jpn. J. Pharmacol.*, 85, 241, 2001.
90. Tabrizchi, R., The influence of tumor necrosis factor-α on the cardiovascular system of anaesthetized rats, *Naunyn-Schmiedeberg's Arch. Pharmacol.*, 363, 307, 2001.
91. Manohar, M. and Parks, C.M., Porcine brain and myocardial perfusion during enflurane anesthesia without and with nitrous oxide, *J. Cardiovasc. Pharmacol.*, 6, 1092, 1984.
92. Manohar, M., Impact of 70% nitrous oxide administration on regional distribution of brain blood flow in unmedicated healthy swine, *J. Cardiovasc. Pharmacol.*, 7, 463, 1985.
93. Lewis, G.J. et al., Use of electromagnetic flow probes to assess myocardial performance in man, *Eur. J. Cardiol.*, 7, 283, 1978.

4

Electromyography: Detection, Processing, and Applications

Marco Pozzo
Politecnico di Torino, Italy

Dario Farina
Politecnico di Torino, Italy

Roberto Merletti
Politecnico di Torino, Italy

CONTENTS

4.1 Introduction

An essential characteristic of animals is their ability to move in the surrounding environment. The actuators of movement are the muscles whose contractions generate forces on the skeletal segments to which they are connected. Functional properties of muscles, that is, their contractile properties, cannot easily be investigated *in vivo*, both because of the difficulty of inserting force sensors in series with the tendons and because, in normal conditions, different muscles act on the same skeletal segment. Besides mechanical properties, the activity of skeletal muscles is also associated with the generation of electric signals that can be recorded by electrodes inserted in the muscle (*intramuscular recordings*) or fixed over the skin (*surface recordings*). The electric signals generated by the muscles during their activity are referred to as *electromyographic* (*EMG*) signals.

Although muscles have been subject of study for centuries, only recently has the importance of their electrical activity been acknowledged for the study of their properties. Galvani (1737–1789) showed that muscle contractions can be induced by electrical stimulation. Duchenne (1949) first used electrical stimulation to investigate the contractile muscle properties. In 1929 Adrian and Bronk measured muscle electrical activity by needle electrodes, the so-called concentric needle, with the possibility of detecting potentials of single motor units.

0-8493-1140-3/04/$0.00+$1.50

The first recording of surface electromyographic signals was performed by Raymond in 1849 with a primitive type of galvanometer. In 1922 Gasser and Erlanger presented for the first time the myoelectric signal on an oscillograph and in 1944 Inmann and co-workers first reported data on the activity of different muscles of the shoulder investigated by the analysis of surface EMG signals.

In the last 10 to 20 years the methods for EMG signal detection and processing have been largely refined and the quantity and quality of information that can be extracted from these recordings is now important for research and clinical applications in a number of fields, including rehabilitation medicine, ergonomics, sport and space medicine, and neurophysiology. This chapter focuses on the methods for EMG signal detection and processing and on the current and potential future applications of these techniques.

4.2 EMG Signal Generation and Detection

4.2.1 Basic Physiology of EMG Signal Generation

4.2.1.1 The Motor Unit

Skeletal muscles are comprised by nearly parallel cells, the *muscle fibers*, that constitute the contractile structural units. In humans, muscle fibers have a variable length from a few millimeters to several centimeters and a diameter in the range from approximately tens to one hundred micrometers (Dubowitz and Brooke, 1973). Each fiber is able, if excited, to shorten its rest length. The contraction of the fibers is due to biochemical processes whose description is beyond the scope of this chapter.

Muscle fibers are activated by the central nervous system through electric signals transmitted by motoneurons. A motoneuron innervates a group of muscle fibers which thus constitute the smallest functional unit of the muscle. The motoneuron and the fibers it innervates are called a *motor unit*, a term introduced by Sherrington in 1929 (Figure 4.1). The number of muscle fibers innervated by the same motoneuron (and thus constituting a motor unit) is termed *innervation ratio* and can considerably vary for different muscles. The smallest innervation ratio (lower than 10) has been observed in the eye muscles and the greatest (larger than 2000) in the leg muscles. The innervation ratio is variable also in the same muscle where large motor units can have a number of fibers ten times larger than small motor units (Brandstater and Lambert, 1973; Burke and Tsairis, 1973).

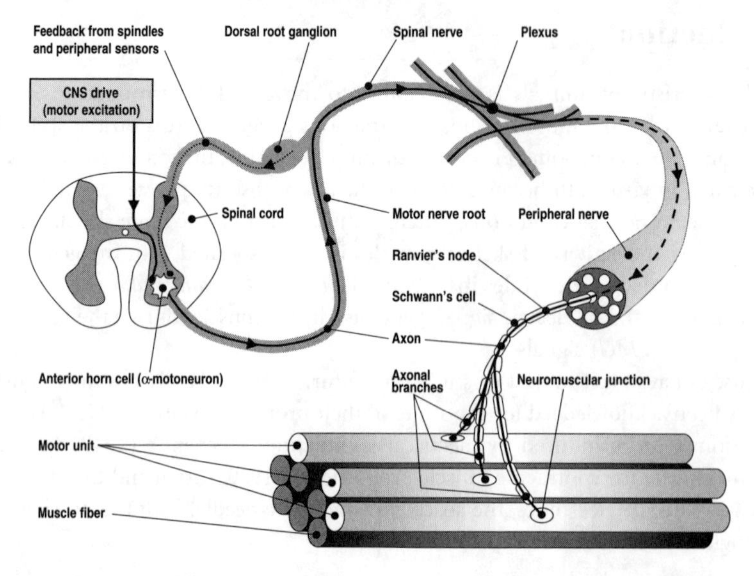

FIGURE 4.1 Motor unit structure. The motoneuron innervates a certain number of muscle fibers by the neuromuscular junctions.

Muscle fibers have different properties that allow their classification in at least two categories. On the basis of biomechanical characteristics, muscle fibers are divided into *type I* fibers (*slow*) and *type II* fibers (*fast*) (Saltin and Gollnick, 1983). Type I fibers have a mechanical response (*single twitch*) longer than type II fibers, and they are oxidative and fatigue resistant. Usually, type I fibers are smaller than type II fibers and are innervated from axons with smaller diameter. Type II fibers are glycolytic, easily fatiguing and innervated from axons with a larger diameter than type I fibers. In the same motor unit all the fibers are of the same type (Henneman, 1980), thus the classification in type I and type II fibers can be extended to motor units. The proportion of type I and type II motor units depends on the muscle and, in the same muscle, on the subject (Le Bozec and Maton, 1987).

Muscle fibers of a motor unit are randomly distributed in a territory approximately circular (Buchthal et al., 1957). The density of muscle fibers in a motor unit is much smaller than the density of muscle fibers in the muscle, thus the geometrical territory of a motor unit collects fibers of different units (McMillan and Hannam, 1991). Although the data in the literature are rather controversial, there are indications for a slight predominance of type I fibers in surface layers of certain muscles (Lexell et al., 1984, 1986).

Each axon reaches the innervated fibers at their neuromuscular junctions, which are usually located in the central part of the fibers (Masuda et al., 1983b).

4.2.1.2 The Action Potential

If a microelectrode is inserted in a muscle cell, a rest potential of 70 to 90 mV, negative inside the cell with respect to the extracellular environment, is measured. The generation of this potential depends on the balance of ions passing through the membrane (Dumitru, 1995). The electric impulse that is propagated along the motorneuron arrives at the neuromuscular junction and determines the excitation of the muscle fiber membrane. In this case, a potential distribution located in a part of the membrane is generated (Figure 4.2). A charge density (*depolarization zone*) corresponds to this potential distribution.

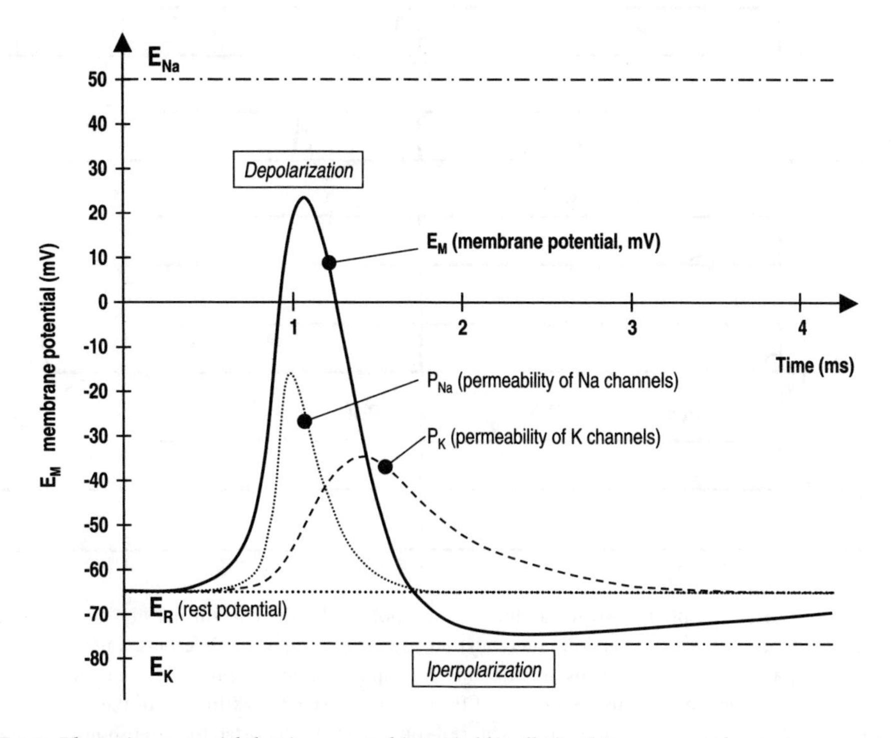

FIGURE 4.2 The action potential that is generated in excitable cells (in this case a squid axon is represented). The permeabilities to sodium and potassium ions are qualitatively presented as functions of time. The dynamics of membrane permeabilities to different ionic species determines the shape of the action potential.

If the *line source model* (Johannsen, 1986) is assumed, the transmembrane current that is generated is the second spatial derivative of the potential.

The depolarization zones propagate along the muscle fibers from the neuromuscular junctions to the tendons' endings. The velocity with which the action potential propagates depends on the fiber diameter and type and is referred to as *conduction velocity.* At the neuromuscular junction and tendons the intracellular action potentials are generated and extinguished, respectively. Although the physical description of these phenomena is controversial (Dimitrova, 1974; Dimitrov and Dimitrova, 1998; Gootzen et al., 1991; Griep et al., 1982; Gydikov et al., 1986; Kleinpenning et al., 1990; McGill and Huynh, 1988; Merletti et al., 1999; Plonsey, 1977), generally it is assumed that the total current density along the entire muscle fiber is zero at each time instant (Dimitrov and Dimitrova, 1998; Gootzen et al., 1991).

The action potential can be analytically represented in the space domain; Rosenfalck (1969) proposed, for example, the following function:

$$V_m(z) = \begin{cases} Az^3 e^{-\lambda_z} + B & z > 0 \\ 0 & z \leq 0 \end{cases} \tag{4.1}$$

with $\lambda = 1$ mm^{-1}, $A = 96$ mV · mm^{-3}, and $B = -90$ mV. Later, other analytical descriptions derived from Equation 4.1 (Dimitrov, 1987) have been proposed. Figure 4.3 reports the schematic representation of

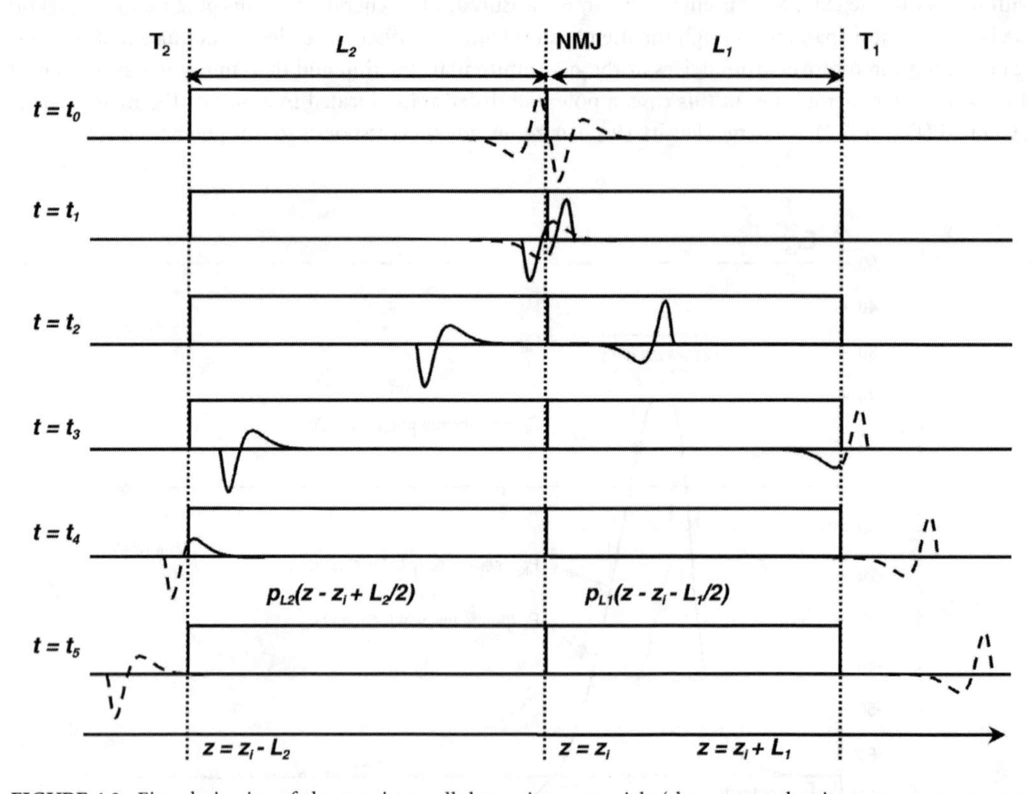

FIGURE 4.3 First derivative of the two intracellular action potentials (the current density sources are proportional to the second derivative of the action potentials) propagating in opposite directions along the muscle fiber as a function of space for six different instants of time corresponding to the pre-generation situation (t_0), the generation (t_1), the propagation (t_2), the extinction of the first source (t_3), the extinction of the second source (t_4) and the final instant (t_5). Dotted lines do not represent real sources but are reported to better show the propagation phenomena. T_1 and T_2 represent the tendons, z_i is the position of the neuromuscular junction, L_1 and L_2 the lengths of the fiber from the neuromuscular junction to tendon T_1 and T_2, respectively. (From Farina, D. and Merletti, R., *IEEE Trans. Biomed. Eng.*, 48, 637–645, 2001. With permission.)

the action potential first derivative generation, propagation, and extinction along a muscle fiber, assuming the analytical description of Equation 4.1 for the intracellular action potential.

The summation of the single fiber action potentials determines the motor unit action potential that propagates at the conduction velocity of 3 to 5 m/s.

4.2.1.3 Motor Unit Control Properties

The central nervous system controls the activation of motor units to optimize the interaction between our body and the surrounding environment. Muscle force is regulated by two mechanisms: motor unit recruitment (*recruitment*) and firing frequency modulation (*rate coding*) (Basmajian and De Luca, 1985). These two mechanisms are present in different proportions for different muscles.

In general, smaller muscles (e.g., hand muscles) recruit all their motor units within 0 to 50% MVC and rely mainly on firing rate modulation, with peaks in the firing rate as high as 60 firings per second, to reach higher force levels (Milner-Brown et al., 1973). On the contrary, larger limb muscles rely mainly on recruitment for force modulation, with recruitment up to 90% MVC and beyond and a reduced firing rate range, peaking at about 35 to 40 firings per second.

4.2.1.3.1 The Size Principle

The recruitment order is not random but it is related to the motor unit properties (Henneman, 1980). The recruitment proceeds from motor units with lower innervation ratio and smaller exerted force toward motor units with more fibers and which produce higher forces. This phenomenon, observed for the first time by Henneman (1965), is known as *size principle* and has been extensively experimentally validated. The Henneman principle is an efficient strategy of the CNS: at low force levels, only small, low-force motor units are active, resulting in an higher precision in the modulation of the force and low fatigue, as required in skilled tasks.

Conduction velocity of action potentials is linked to the fiber contractile properties and follows, in general, the size principle, with motor units with lower conduction velocity recruited before motor units with higher conduction velocity (Andreassen and Arendt-Nielsen, 1987). Recruitment strategies can vary because of peripheral conditions' changes of the neuromuscular system.

4.2.1.3.2 The Common Drive

The muscle is incapable of generating purely constant-force contractions; fluctuations in force, at a dominant oscillation frequency of about 1 to 2 Hz, are observable as a consequence of the mechanical transfer function of the muscle-nerve system.

The central control is not independent for all the motor units; cross-correlation among mean firing rates of different motor units shows that their oscillations are correlated. This phenomenon, described by De Luca and Erim (1994) in more than 300 contractions and in many muscles (Kamen and De Luca, 1992), indicates that the control comes from a single source (*common drive*). A common drive can determine different recruitment patterns because the motoneurons present different degrees of excitability (*Henneman principle*). Selective recruitment of motor units at different force levels then depends on the sensitivity of motoneurons to be activated (De Luca and Erim, 1994) and on the interconnections of neural nets at the spinal level.

4.2.1.4 EMG Signals Generated in Voluntary and Electrically Elicited Contractions

When the motor units are activated by the central nervous system, they produce an action potential and, thus, repetitive activation generates motor unit action potential trains. The potential trains of the active motor units add together to generate the *interference EMG signal*. The single motor unit action potential train is the convolution of the motor unit action potential and the Delta function train describing the firing pattern. The analytical model is a bank of filters whose impulse responses are the action potentials and whose outputs are summed. The inputs are the Delta function trains describing the motor unit activations (Basmajian and De Luca, 1985) (Figure 4.4a).

The muscles can also be activated without the input command from the central nervous system, using externally generated currents (e.g., by means of electrical muscle stimulators) which excite the terminal nerve branches. In this case all the motor units are activated at approximately the same time instants

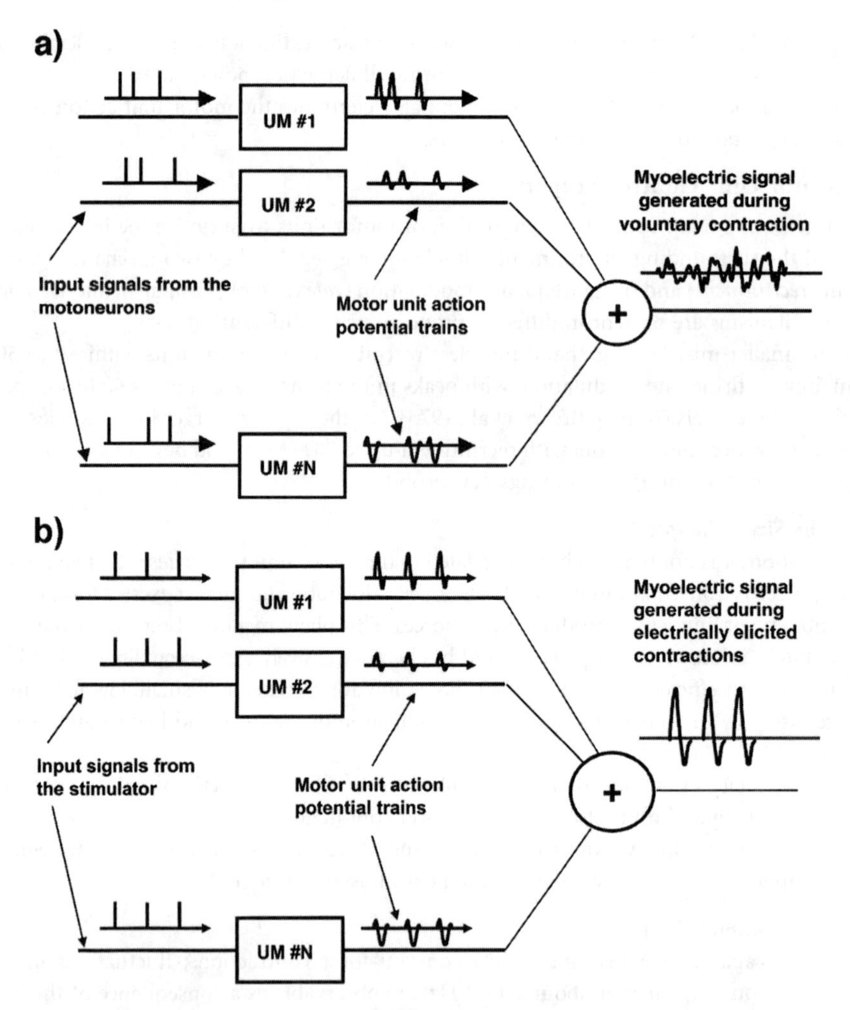

FIGURE 4.4 Models of generation of EMG signals from voluntary (a) and electrically elicited (b) contractions. The inputs to the filter bank are Delta trains which reflect the central nervous system activation strategy (a) or the frequency of the stimulation current induced by an external device (b). The impulse responses are the motor unit action potentials and depend on the conduction velocity, recording system, motor unit location, etc. (see text). (From Basmajian, V.J. and De Luca, C.J., *Muscle Alive*, Williams & Wilkins, Baltimore, 1985. With permission.)

and their activation frequency is equal to the stimulation frequency. The generated signal is called *M-wave* and is the synchronous summation of the potentials of the stimulated motor units. The model of signal generation is in this case similar to that described for the voluntary contractions but the inputs are synchronized Delta trains (Figure 4.4b).

4.2.2 The Volume Conductor

4.2.2.1 Effect of the Tissues between Sources and Recording Electrodes

The generation of the intracellular action potential determines an electric field in any point of the surrounding space. The potential generated by a motor unit can thus be detected also in locations relatively far from the source. The biological tissues separating the sources and the detecting electrodes are referred to as *volume conductors* and their characteristics strongly affect the detected signal.

Under the static hypothesis, in a volume conductor, the current density, the electric field, and the potential satisfy the following relationships (Plonsey, 1977):

$$\nabla \cdot J = I \quad J = \overline{\overline{\sigma}} E \quad E = -\nabla \varphi \tag{4.2}$$

where J is the current density in the volume conductor ($A \cdot m^{-2}$), I the current density of the source ($A \cdot m^{-3}$), E the electric field ($V \cdot m^{-1}$), and φ the potential (V).

From Equations 4.2, the Poisson equation is obtained:

$$-\frac{\partial}{\partial x}\left(\sigma_x \frac{\partial \varphi}{\partial x}\right) - \frac{\partial}{\partial y}\left(\sigma_y \frac{\partial \varphi}{\partial y}\right) - \frac{\partial}{\partial z}\left(\sigma_z \frac{\partial \varphi}{\partial z}\right) = I \tag{4.3}$$

which is the general relation between the potential and the current density in a non-homogenous and anisotropic medium in Cartesian coordinates.

If the medium is homogenous, the conductivities do not depend on the point and the following equation is obtained:

$$-\sigma_x \frac{\partial^2 \varphi}{\partial x^2} - \sigma_y \frac{\partial^2 \varphi}{\partial y^2} - \sigma_z \frac{\partial^2 \varphi}{\partial z^2} = I \tag{4.4}$$

The solution of Equation 4.4 provides, theoretically, the potential in any point in space when the characteristics of the source and the medium are known. The transmembrane current can be approximated by simple functions, but the analytical solution of Equation 4.4 can be obtained only in cases in which the boundary conditions can be described in particularly simple coordinate systems. This problem has been investigated by many researchers, with different degrees of simplification. The simplest assumption for the solution of Equation 4.4 is to deal with a homogeneous, isotropic, infinite volume conductor. In this case, assuming a source distributed on a line, the potential distribution in the volume conductor is given by the following relationship:

$$\varphi(r,z) = \frac{1}{2\sigma} \int_{-\infty}^{+\infty} \frac{I(s)}{\sqrt{r^2 + (z-s)^2}} ds \tag{4.5}$$

where $I(z)$ is the current density source and σ is the conductivity of the medium. In case of anisotropic medium, with $\sigma_x = \sigma_y = \sigma_r \neq \sigma_z$, Equation 4.5 becomes:

$$\varphi(r,z) = \frac{1}{2\sigma_r} \int_{-\infty}^{+\infty} \frac{I(s)}{\sqrt{r^2 \frac{\sigma_z}{\sigma_r} + (z-s)^2}} ds \tag{4.6}$$

where σ_z and σ_r are the conductivities of the medium in the direction of the line source and in the radial direction, respectively. This is the case of the muscle tissue.

More complex descriptions of the volume conductor have been proposed and include finite limb dimensions, non-homogeneous media, and tissues with properties dependent on the temporal frequency (characterized by impedances rather than by resistances) (Stegeman et al., 2000; Farina and Merletti, 2001). In all the cases, the volume conductor has a low-pass filter characteristic whose cutoff frequency depends on the distance of the source from the detection point, i.e., the more distant the source, the more selective the equivalent low-pass filter of the volume conductor (Figure 4.5).

4.2.2.2 Effect of the Volume Conductor on the Detected Potentials

Depending on the recording modality, the volume conductor may have a negligible or important effect on the acquired EMG signals. In case of intramuscular recordings, the detection system is located very close to the sources and thus the detected potentials are only slightly altered by the

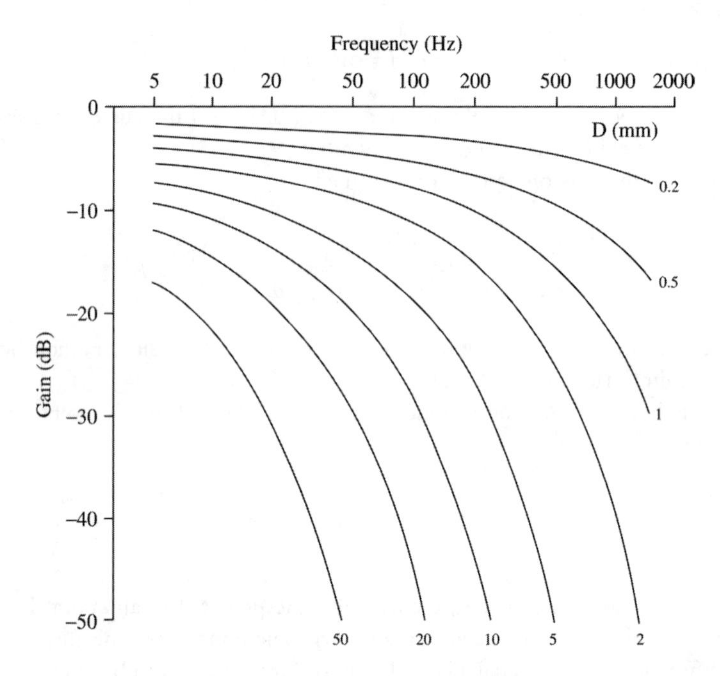

FIGURE 4.5 Spatial transfer function of a homogeneous volume conductor for different distances between the source and the detection point. (From Lindström, L. and Magnusson, R., *Proc. IEEE*, 65, 653–662, 1977. With permission.)

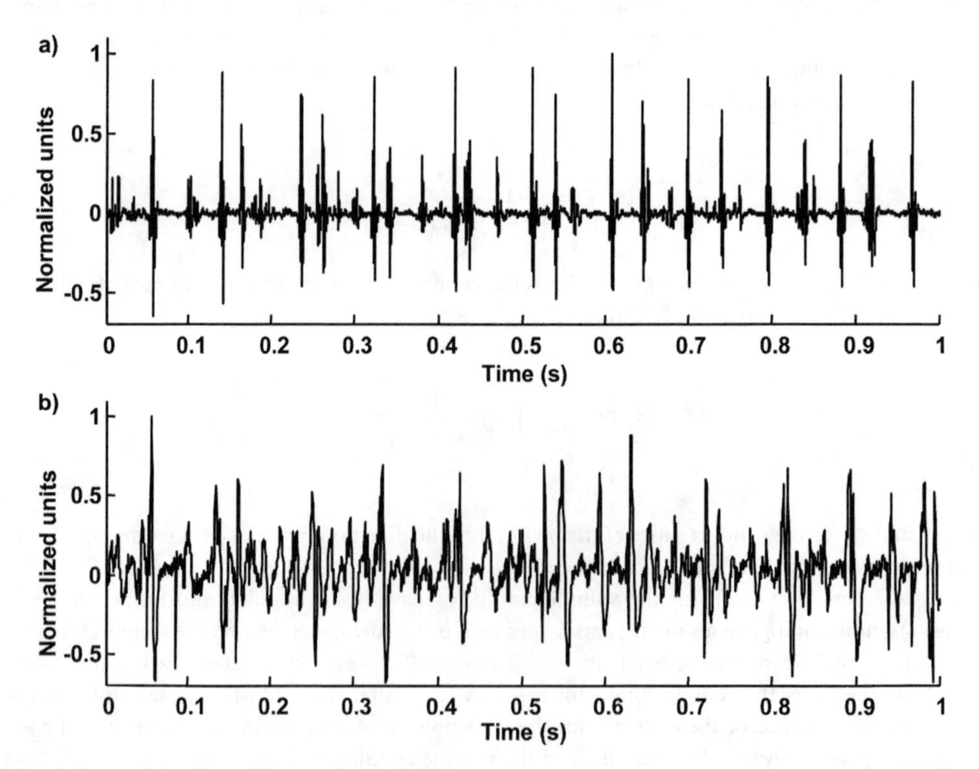

FIGURE 4.6 (a) Signals recorded monopolarly with intramuscular wires during a contraction at 10% MVC of the tibialis anterior muscle. (b) Surface EMG signals recorded over the skin with a single differential system (interelectrode distance 5 mm). Signals in (a) and (b) were collected at the same time during the same muscle contraction. (From Farina, D., Advances in Myoelectric Signal Detection, Processing and Interpretation in Motor Control Studies, Ph.D. thesis, Politecnico di Torino and Ecole Centrale de Nantes, 2001.)

tissues separating sources and electrodes. In this case the signal bandwidth is up to 1 to 5 KHz. If EMG signals are recorded over the skin surface, the volume conductor plays a major role in determining signal features. The low-pass effect of the tissues results in a signal with frequency content below 300 to 400 Hz. Figure 4.6 shows EMG signals recorded at the same time from the tibialis anterior muscle by invasive and surface recording systems. The different spectral content and degree of potential overlapping are evident.

The distance of the source from the recording system in case of surface methods implies poor spatial selectivity, i.e., the contribution of a source is not confined in a narrow region of space. For muscles that are close to each other, it may happen that signals generated by one muscle are also detected over other muscles due to the conduction of the signal by the volume conductor. The signal detected on a non-active muscle and generated by another active muscle is referred as *crosstalk* and represents an important problem for proper surface EMG signal interpretation. Figure 4.7 shows an example of signals generated by electrical stimulation of one muscle (selective activation) and recording on other muscles to assess the amount of crosstalk in this muscle group. Some considerations on crosstalk, important from the practical point of view, can be drawn directly from Figure 4.7:

1. Crosstalk signals detected by multichannel recordings are non-propagating, synchronous potentials.
2. Crosstalk signals appear at the end of propagation of the signals generated by the active muscle.
3. The amount of crosstalk between two muscles does not only depend of the distance between them.

These considerations are interpreted by the observation that the most contribution to crosstalk is due to the end-of-fiber potentials, generated by the extinction of the motor unit action potentials at the tendons. End-of-fiber potentials can be reduced by particular spatial filters, although clear criteria of filter design for the reduction of end-of-fiber potentials, and thus for the reduction of crosstalk, are still not known.

The effect of the volume conductor on the detected potentials determines the differences between intramuscular and surface recordings. Surface recordings present poor spatial selectivity and provide a global information about the muscle activity. On the contrary, intramuscular recordings are extremely selective and give localized information on muscle activity (often limited to four to five motor units). The features of the two types of EMG recordings (invasive and non-invasive) determine their specific fields of application. Invasively recorded signals have been largely used in diagnosis and in motor control studies, particularly when it is necessary to reliably identify the motor unit firing instants. However, the invasive recordings do not directly allow estimation of some motor unit physiological properties, such as conduction velocity. Surface EMG signals allow peripheral property investigation but from these signals it is difficult to separate the single motor unit action potentials. Given the different features of EMG signals detected intramuscularly or at the skin surface, the methods for the detection and processing and the applications of invasive and non-invasive electromyography are very different.

4.2.3 Equipment, Detection, and Recording Techniques

4.2.3.1 Intramuscular Electrodes

In the following text, the term *electrode* will refer to the passive electrical interface between the patient and the equipment, whose active electronic circuitry will be referred to as the *input stage* or the *front end* of the EMG amplifier. Usually, part of the front end is directly attached to the electrode, with the aim of improving interference immunity (Hageman et al., 1985). This part of the conditioning circuitry is usually named as *active probe* or, more simply, *probe.*

Since 1929 when Adrian and Bronk proposed the concentric needle electrode, a number of systems for the detection of intramuscular EMG signals have been developed. The concentric needle electrode detects signals in monopolar configuration through a wire insulated in the cannula of the needle. Other needle electrodes have been proposed in more recent times and have been adapted to the specific algorithms for information extraction. Buchthal et al. (1957) extended the idea of the concentric needle

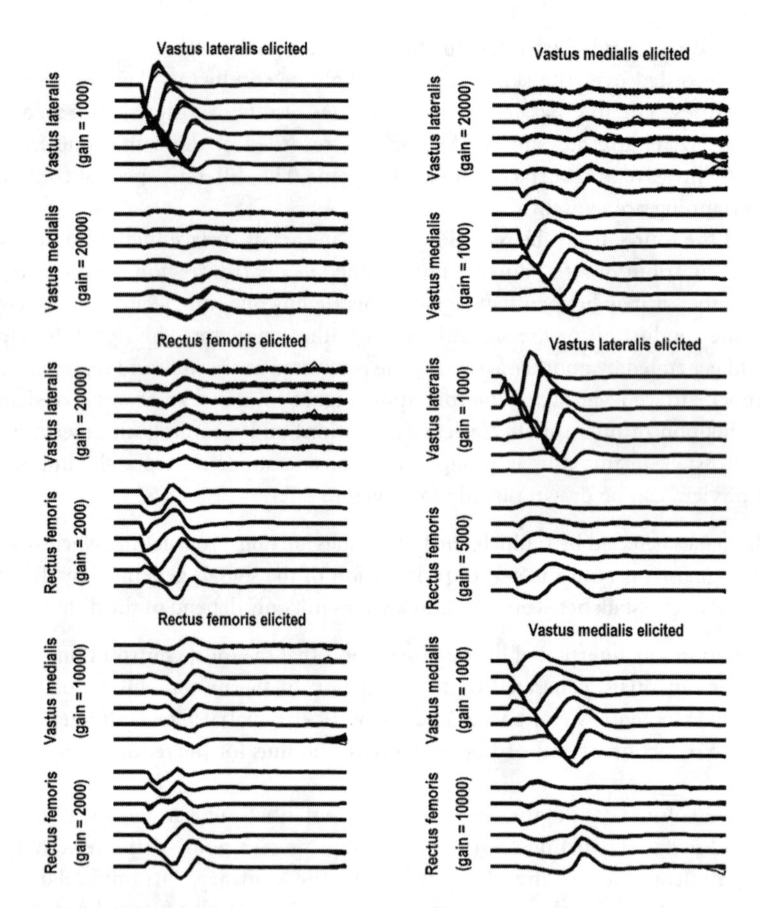

FIGURE 4.7 Signals recorded from the vastus lateralis (VL), vastus medialis (VM), and rectus femoris (RF) muscles in six conditions of selective stimulation (2 Hz stimulation frequency) of one muscle and recording from a muscle pair (one stimulated and one not stimulated). In each case, the responses to 20 stimuli are reported. In this subject, the distances between the arrays (center to center) are 77 mm for the pair VL-RF, 43 mm for the pair VM-RF, and 39 mm for the pair VL-VM. Note the different gains used for the active and non-active muscles. For this subject the ratio between average ARV values (along the array) is, for the six muscle pairs, 2.8% (VL-VM), 2.5% (VM-VL), 6.5% (RF-VL), 6.6% (VL-RF), 15.6% (RF-VM), and 7.0% (VM-RF). The signals detected from a pair of muscles are normalized with respect to a common factor (apart from the different gain), thus are comparable in amplitude, while the signals detected from different muscle pairs are normalized with respect to different factors. (From Farina, D., Merletti, R., Indino, B., Nazzaro, M., and Pozzo, M., *Muscle Nerve*, 26, 681–695, 2002. With permission.)

by placing 12 insulated wires in the cannula of a needle. With this system it was possible to record the motor unit electrical activity from many points in the muscle, thus analyzing the decrease of signal amplitude with the distance and investigating the motor unit territory. In 1972 De Luca and Forrest described the quadripolar needle, consisting of four detecting surfaces arranged in order to detect the motor unit action potentials from different locations in space. This recording system provides four representations of the same motor unit activity, thus adding information for the automatic decomposition of the EMG signal into the constituent motor unit action potential trains (see also Section 4.3.1.1, "Decomposition of Intramuscular EMG Signals into Motor Unit Action Potential Trains"). Figure 4.8 reports some examples of needle electrodes for the detection of EMG signals.

In 1960, Basmajian et al. proposed wire electrodes for the detection of intramuscular EMG signals. Wire electrodes may be made from any small diameter, non-oxidizing, stiff wire with insulation. They can be inserted in the cannula of a needle and bent at the tip; the needle is inserted in the muscle and

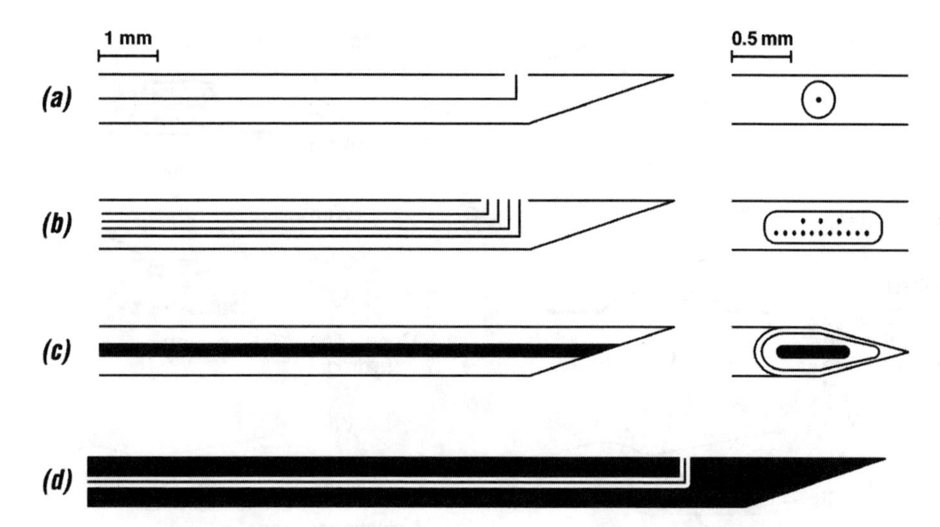

FIGURE 4.8 Various types of intramuscular electrodes. (a) Single fiber electrode with one detection surface; (b) multipolar electrode; (c) concentric needle electrode; (d) macro EMG electrode. (Redrawn from Stålberg, E., *J. Neurol. Neurosurg. Psychiatry*, 43, 475–483,1980. With permission.)

then removed, with the wires left in the muscle. The advantages with respect to needle electrodes is that the wires can be hardly felt when the needle is removed, thus allowing strong contractions without discomfort or pain. However, their position cannot be adjusted after the needle removal, while a needle can be moved in the muscle to search for the optimal position. Usually, wire electrodes are preferred in studies in which the EMG activity is recorded over long periods and under movement, since they are more stable than needle electrodes.

Gydikov et al. (1986) proposed more recently subcutaneous *branched electrodes*, which consisted of two isolated parallel wires connected together to prevent relative displacement between the wires. The isolation of one of the wires is removed at one point and the isolation of the other wire at two points spaced by 1 to 2 mm. The point of removal of the isolation forms the leading-off area. The signals recorded by the first wire are subtracted to the signals detected by the second wire (the two un-insulated points of the second wire detect a signal which is the average of the potentials in the two points). These wires are inserted subcutaneously by means of a needle and were proven to detect EMG signals with enough selectivity for single motor unit analysis.

4.2.3.2 Surface Electrodes

A surface electrode consists of a conductive medium with defined dimensions and shape, which is electrically connected to the skin of the patient, and kept in place by means of an appropriate fixation method: single- or double-sided adhesive tape, strap, etc.

Commonly used materials in electrode manufacturing are solid silver or gold (Ko and Hynecek, 1974), sintered silver and silver chloride, carbon, and sponge saturated with electrolyte gel or conductive hydrogel; the former are also referred to as *dry* electrodes since they do not make use of conductive gel. Several electrodes are available with a pre-gelled adhesive surface; they can advantageously be used where the stability of the contact during movement is needed, e.g., in gait analysis. An overview of different types of surface electrodes is shown in Figure 4.9.

Electrodes can be used in a monopolar configuration (with an additional reference electrode, placed on an electrically inactive area) or in pairs, especially in applications where simple muscle activation needs to be detected (e.g., in biofeedback applications). In this case, disposable adhesive or recessed electrodes are preferred, usually with a surface area up to 2 cm^2 in order to keep a stable contact and provide a large pickup area and a low contact impedance. Among recessed types, Gereonic (USA) electrodes and equivalents are extensively used in clinical applications, due to the intrinsically better performance of their constitution, as will be discussed later.

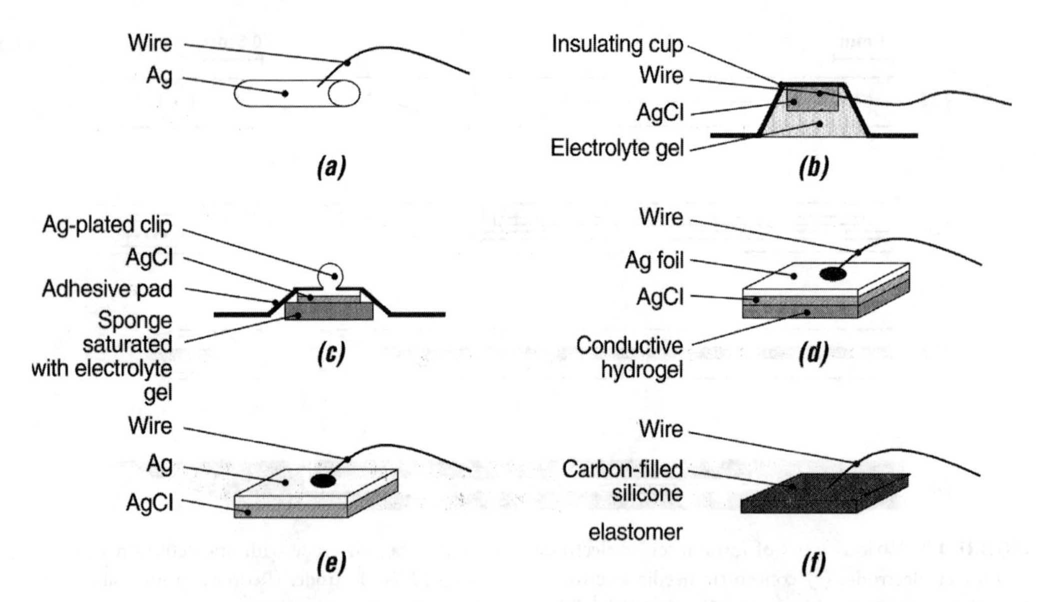

FIGURE 4.9 Overview of different surface electrodes. (a) Ag or AgCl bar electrode; (b) recessed electrode; (c) disposable electrode with electrolyte-saturated sponge; (d) disposable hydrogel electrode; (e) silver-silver chloride electrode; (f) carbon-filled elastomer dry electrode. (Redrawn and adapted from Bronzino, J.D., *The Biomedical Engineering Handbook*, CRC Press, Boca Raton, FL, 1995, p. 750, Fig. 50.4. With permission.)

Besides dry and gelled electrodes, capacitively coupled electrodes exist; here, the detection surface is coated with a thin layer of dielectric substance and the skin-electrode junction behaves like a capacitor. Although they do not require a conductive medium, they have a higher inherent noise and a low reliability over time (Potter and Menke, 1970) and for these reasons they are not used in electromyography.

In advanced EMG applications and for research purposes, surface electrodes can be combined in mono- and bidimensional arrays (also referred as *arrays, matrixes,* or *grids*) to provide multichannel information and to implement spatial filtering for improving the selectivity of the recording (Figure 4.10; see also Section 4.2.3.3, "Surface EMG Spatial Filtering").

Arrays and matrixes usually use silver-silver chloride bars or pins, and are not suitable for long-term recordings or in non-isometric conditions. Recently, a novel type of semidisposable adhesive arrays that overcome these drawbacks has become available from Spes Medica (Italy). With respect to "dry" electrode arrays, they feature a lower and more stable contact impedance and a reduced generation of motion artifact (see later in the text).

4.2.3.2.1 Electrode Technology

The process of detecting a biological signal involves the transduction of the ionic current, flowing through the body, into electrical current (electron flow) into the equipment input circuits. This process is carried out by reduction-oxidation reactions that occur at the interface between the electrodes and the aqueous ionic solutions of the body. Note that, in practical situations, a certain degree of ionic exchange always takes place even with dry silver electrodes, e.g., due to ions contained in the natural moisture or sweat of the skin. The current flowing through the input amplifier is due both to the non-infinite input impedance of the input stage and also to the unavoidable non-zero DC bias currents drawn by the amplifier.

A current flowing through an electrode has the effect of removing electrons from the surface and oxidizing superficial atoms that go into solution as positive ions; thus, the potential of the electrode surface changes with respect to the bulk of the electrode. This voltage, known as the *half-cell* potential, is generated whenever a metal comes in contact with an ionic solution. In a general (and simplified) case, when two ionic solutions of different activity are separated by a ion-selective semipermeable membrane, an electrical potential E is generated between the two solutions, as described by the *Nernst equation* (Weast, 1974):

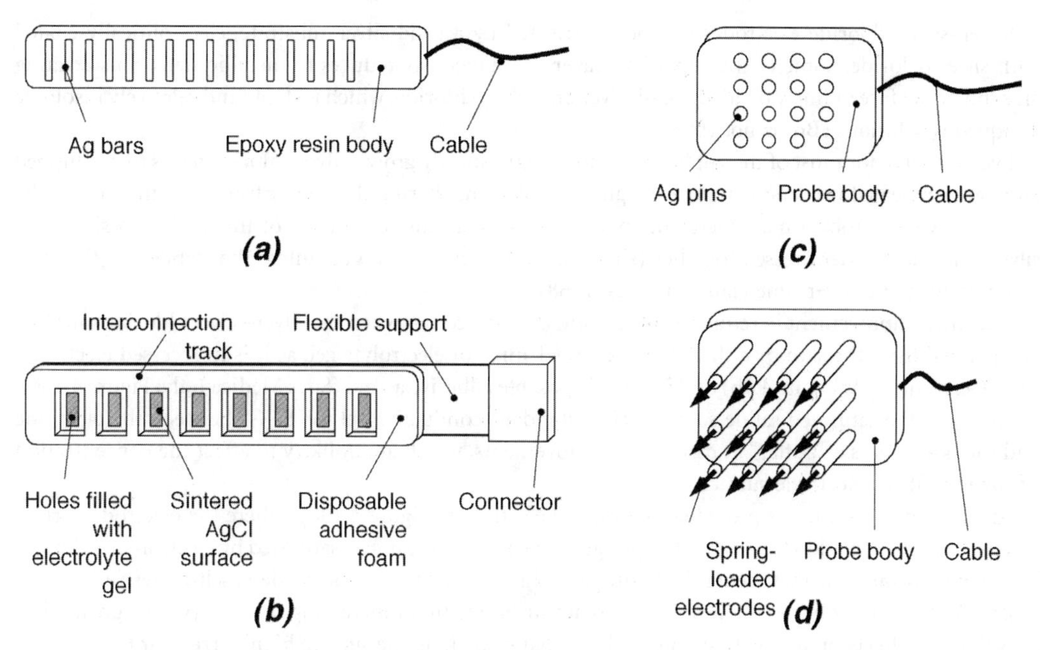

FIGURE 4.10 Examples of mono- and bidimensional surface electrode arrays. (a) Dry silver bar electrode array; (b) Spes Medica (Italy) semi-disposable adhesive electrode array; (c) silver pins electrode grid; (d) spring-loaded electrode grid with sharp tips.

$$E = \frac{RT}{nF} \ln\left(\frac{a_1}{a_2}\right) \tag{4.7}$$

where R is the universal gas constant, T is the absolute temperature, n is the valence of the ion, and a_1 and a_2 are the activities (which are functions of concentration and mobility) of the ion on the two sides of the membrane.

From an electrochemical point of view, electrodes can be divided into two main categories: *polarizable* and *non-polarizable*, the definition of polarizability being a change of the half-cell potential due to current passing through the membrane. This voltage variation, which is referred to as *overvoltage*, is the result of changes in charge distribution in the solution in contact with the electrode and has three main components; namely, the *ohmic* component, the *concentration* component, and the *activation over potentials* component (Webster, 1992).

Perfectly polarizable electrodes (i.e., electrodes made from noble metals, such as platinum) exhibit a capacitive behavior and allow a current flow between the electrode and the electrolyte solution by changing the charge distribution in the solution. Polarizability is a concern in surface EMG electrodes, especially when movement is present. If the electrode moves with respect to the electrolyte solution, the charge distribution at the interface will change, thus inducing a voltage change at the skin-electrode contact that will appear as a *motion artifact*, i.e., a slow variation of the sensed voltage, with a spectral range that extends usually from DC up to 20 Hz. Furthermore, changes in charge distribution will reflect on the skin-electrode contact impedance, whose variations (especially unbalance with respect to the reference electrode) may adversely affect the quality of the signal.

Non-polarizable electrodes exhibit a more ohmic behavior and a better performance in surface EMG recording, and are by far the preferred type. Among them, silver–silver chloride electrodes are those that more closely approximate the ideal behavior; moreover, they have less electrical noise than equivalent polarizable electrodes, especially at the lower frequencies of the surface EMG band, and are recommended for measurements at low signal levels.

Silver–silver chloride electrodes can be constituted by a solid silver substrate, electrolitically coated with silver chloride. Some of the superficial layer spontaneously reduces to metallic state, thus creating an exposed surface of finely divided metal silver and silver chloride, which is stable and relatively insoluble in aqueous solutions (Bronzino, 1995).

Even if usable for most of the applications, the electrolitically grown silver chloride tends to be chipped away after repeated use, and can possibly go into solution, altering the concentration of the ions at the interface. A more robust manufacturing method is to use a sintered surface of finely divided silver and silver chloride powder pressed together (sintered electrodes), which guarantees the stability of the electrode performance over time (Janz and Ives, 1968).

A further improvement in reduction of motion artifacts comes when the silver–silver chloride interface is separated from the skin by a thick layer (about 1 mm) of electrolyte gel, as it is in recessed electrodes (e.g., Gereonic USA; Figure 4.9b) and in semidisposable adhesive arrays (Spes Medica Italy; Figure 4.10b). In this case, the saturated saline solution (i.e., standard conductive gel for ECG) between the electrode and the skin acts as a "buffer" in case of fluid movements, which are unlikely to affect the concentration of the ions at the electrode surface.

An alternative solution is provided by *hydrogel* electrodes (Figure 4.10d), where the electrode surface is separated from the skin by a layer of a sponge with microscopic pores, saturated by electrolytic solution. The main advantage is that, being the hydrogel foil is very sticky, the electrode is self-adhesive.

An effective solution for increasing the contact surface without increasing the area (with a greater low pass filtering effects on the surface potentials) is that of making the surface highly irregular by means of grooves on the surface (Blok et al., 1997).

4.2.3.2.2 Electrode Impedance

Although a large number of papers and even complete books on the topic exist (Geddes, 1972), the concepts behind a complete description of the skin-electrode interface are generally poorly understood, mainly due to the highly non-linear and non-repetitive nature of the phenomena and the large number of secondary aspects involved.

Controversial results about skin-electrode contact impedance and proper skin treatment exist in literature. A detailed analysis of these crucial topics goes beyond the goals of this chapter; nevertheless, a basic overview of the main concepts is appropriate.

The skin-electrode interface can be considered a boundary between two media: a multilayer, non-homogeneous, and anisotropic conductive media (skin, subcutaneous tissue, and muscle) that contains the sources of the electrical field, and an isotropic media (the electrode itself) (Grimnes, 1982).

The skin-electrode interface can be represented by an electrical network of impedances modeling the various tissues, plus one or more batteries representing the half cell potentials that are created at the different interfaces.

As shown in Figure 4.11a, an electrical model of the skin-electrode contact can be as sophisticated as desired, e.g., taking into account the effects of sweat ducts. A simplified, although effective, version of this model is commonly used and is represented in Figure 4.11b.

The main problem in finding a satisfactory representation resides in a correct numerical evaluation of the model parameters. Unfortunately they strongly depend on many factors among which the electrode type, the electrode area, and the skin treatment play a major role.

An additional complication resides in the highly non-linear behavior of the skin-electrode interface. This implies that for a correct evaluation of the skin-electrode impedance, the measurements should recreate the same experimental conditions in which the electrode will operate during EMG acquisition.

Of particular concern must be the choice of the test frequency, which should lie in the same range of surface EMG bandwidth (10 to 400 Hz), and particularly the test current, which should match the situation during EMG detection, where the current is virtually zero (except for the DC bias currents of the input amplifiers, in the pA to nA range). Such an experimental condition is difficult to obtain but can be extrapolated by several measurements at progressively decreasing current

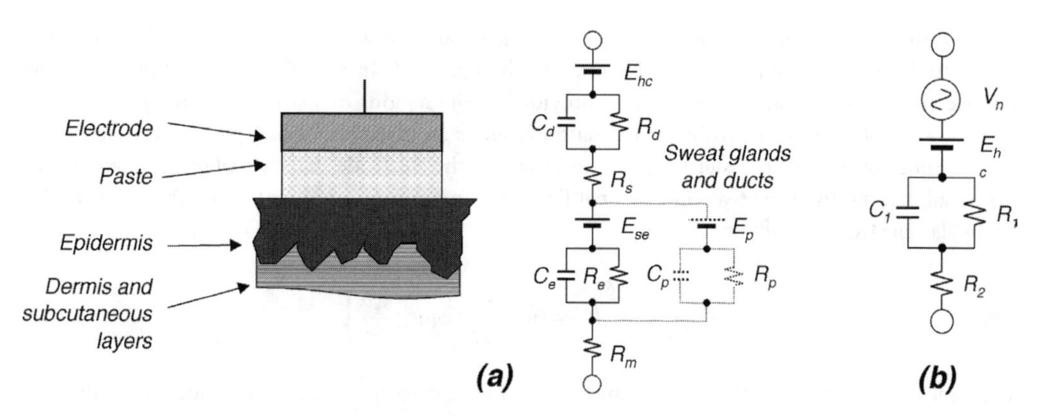

FIGURE 4.11 Electrical models of the skin-electrode interface. (a) The model proposed by Neuman; (b) a simplified electrical model that takes into account also the noise produced at the interface. (From Neuman, M.R., *Medical Instrumentation*, Webster, J.G., Ed., Houghton Mifflin, Boston, 1978, 215–272.)

densities (Bottin, 2002). As shown later, the impedance value extrapolated at zero current can be much higher than expected.

4.2.3.3 Surface EMG Spatial Filtering

The detection of EMG signals with electrodes placed over the skin always implies a filtering of the signal in the spatial domain. The spatial filtering effects are due to the electrode size and shape and to the particular combination of the signals recorded by different electrodes. In both cases, spatial filtering can be effectively used for better extracting information from the signal. In particular, the most common use of spatial filtering techniques is the enhancement of the spatial selectivity of the surface recordings by means of high-pass transfer function design (Reucher et al., 1987a, 1987b). One of the most crucial limitations of the conventional surface EMG techniques is indeed their poor spatial resolution. This means that it is difficult to distinguish, from surface signals, sources that are closely placed in the muscle. As a consequence, surface EMG methods allow, at medium to high contraction levels, only a statement about the compound activity of a large number of motor units (e.g., amplitude or global spectral parameters).

4.2.3.3.1 Spatial Filtering of Electrodes with Physical Dimensions

Consider a potential $\phi(x,z)$ generated over the skin by a muscle fiber, where x and z are the spatial coordinates transversal and parallel to the fiber, respectively, and suppose that the potential is moving along the fiber direction. The potential detected in space over the skin, in case of point detection electrodes, is a section of $\phi(x,z)$ for $x = x_0$:

$$\varphi(z) = \phi(x_0, z) \tag{4.8}$$

where x_0 is the transversal distance of the point electrode from the fiber in the skin plane. In the case of electrodes with physical dimensions, as a first approximation, at each detection location the potential is integrated under the electrode area (Helal and Bouissou, 1992). This integration can be mathematically described as the two-dimensional convolution of the potential distribution over the skin with a function that depends on the electrode shape and size (Farina and Merletti, 2001). This function assumes a constant value, equal to the inverse of the electrode area, in the region of space corresponding to the electrode area and zero outside:

$$h_{size}(x,z) = \begin{cases} \dfrac{1}{S} & f(-x,-z) \le 0 \\ 0 & f(-x,-z) > 0 \end{cases} \tag{4.9}$$

where S is the electrode area and $f(x,z) < 0$ the mathematical expression that defines the electrode shape. The electrode is thus included in the area described by $f(x,z) < 0$. In Equation 4.9 the impulse response of an electrode with physical dimensions is provided in the regions of space described by $f(-x, -z) < 0$ and $f(-x, -z) > 0$ since the convolution operation requires an inversion of the spatial coordinates.

From Equation 4.9, the transfer function equivalent to the electrode shape is obtained (analytically or numerically) computing the two-dimensional Fourier transform $H_{size}(k_x,k_z)$ of $h_{size}(x,z)$. In the case of a rectangular electrode we obtain:

$$H_{size}(k_x,k_z) = \mathrm{sinc}\left(\frac{k_x a}{2\pi}\right)\mathrm{sinc}\left(\frac{k_z b}{2\pi}\right) \tag{4.10}$$

where $\mathrm{sinc}(s) = \sin(\pi s)/(\pi s)$ if $s \neq 0$ and $\mathrm{sinc}(0) = 1$. In the case of a circular electrode with radius r:

$$H_{size}(k_x,k_z) = \begin{cases} 2\dfrac{J_1(r\sqrt{k_x^2+k_z^2})}{r\sqrt{k_x^2+k_z^2}} & (k_x,k_z) \neq (0,0) \\ 1 & (k_x,k_z) = (0,0) \end{cases} \tag{4.11}$$

where $J_1(k)$ is the first-order Bessel function of the first kind (Zwillinger, 1996).

From Equations 4.10 and 4.11, the spatial transfer function of electrodes with physical dimensions represents a low-pass filter whose cut-off frequency depends on the electrode area; the larger the area, the more selective the filter (i.e., high frequencies are more attenuated). Figure 4.12a represents the two-dimensional transfer function of a circular electrode and Figure 4.12b the two-dimensional Fourier transform of the surface potential that would be detected with that electrode.

4.2.3.3.2 *Linear Combinations of Signals Detected by Point Electrodes*

The spatial filtering operation described above occurs with any type of surface electrodes and depends on the contact area. Acquiring monopolar signals, the spatial filtering due to electrode size is the only filtering operation performed by the detection system. In practical applications, monopolar signals are rarely recorded; rather, the signals acquired are the linear combination of those recorded from different electrodes placed over the muscle under study. The simplest of these recording systems is the longitudinal single differential which detects the difference between signals detected by two electrodes

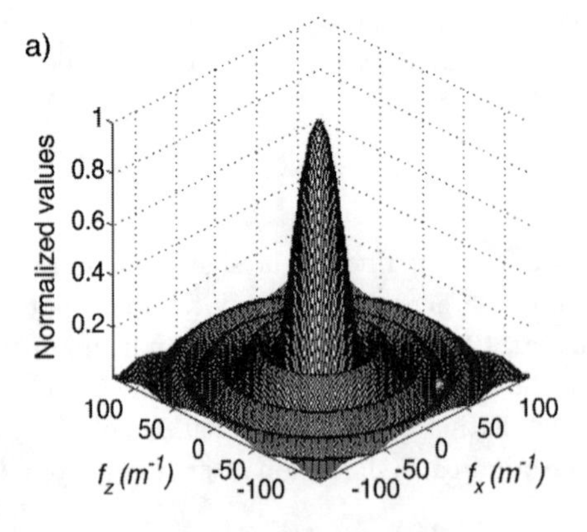

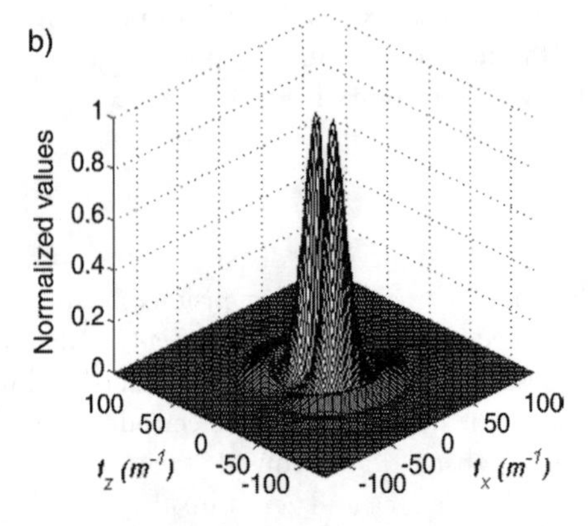

FIGURE 4.12 Magnitude of the transfer function of a large (for demonstrative purposes) circular electrode with radius equal to 15 mm (a) and absolute value of the two-dimensional Fourier transform of the potential detected over the skin with such a system and generated by an intramuscular action potential approximated with Rosenfalck's analytical expression at a depth of 2 mm in the muscle (b). The functions are normalized with respect to their absolute maximum value. (From Farina, D. and Merletti, R., *IEEE Trans. Biomed. Eng.*, 48, 637–645, 2001. With permission.)

located along the muscle fiber direction. This operation is equivalent to a spatial filtering operation which attenuates low spatial frequencies. The usefulness of this filtering operation is based on the properties of the volume conductor.

As discussed previously, deep motor units generate surface potentials with narrower bandwidth with respect to those generated by more superficial motor units. In the spatial domain this implies that deeper motor units present surface potentials with slower variations with respect to superficial units. This effect is due to the low-pass filtering of the tissues separating the sources from the recording electrodes (Figure 4.5). The application of spatial filters obtained by linear combinations of surface EMG signals is based on these characteristics of the sources and aims at the selective attenuation of the contributions to the surface EMG signal of far sources. The considerations drawn for the single differential system can be extended to more complex one-dimensional electrode configurations or to the two spatial directions.

Given a general two-dimensional arrangements of electrode whose signals are summed together in a linear combination with a set of weights, the impulse response of the spatial filter is (Reucher et al., 1987a; 1987b):

$$h(x,z) = \sum_{i=0}^{M} a_i \delta(x + x_i)\delta(z + z_i) \tag{4.12}$$

where x and z are the spatial coordinates in the transversal and longitudinal directions, respectively, x_i and z_i are the coordinates of the location of the electrode i, $M+1$ is the number of electrodes, and a_i $(i = 0,\ldots, M)$ are the weights given to the linear combination.

The two-dimensional Fourier Transform of the impulse response (12) provides the transfer function:

$$H(f_x, f_z) = \sum_{i=0}^{M} a_i e^{j2\pi f_x x_i} e^{j2\pi f_z z_i} \tag{4.13}$$

where f_x and f_z are the spatial frequencies in the transversal and longitudinal direction, respectively.

Selecting the weights a_i, it is possible to design transfer functions with particular characteristics. Usually the spatial filters are designed in order to meet the basic condition:

$$H(0,0) = \sum_{i=0}^{M} a_i = 0 \tag{4.14}$$

which implies the rejection of the DC components in the two spatial directions. This assures the absence of common mode signals. Given condition (4.14) and given the geometry of the electrode configuration, M degrees of freedom remain for the design of the spatial filter transfer function.

4.2.3.3.3 Spatial Filter Design

Indications about filter design in one or two dimensions can be partly derived from the field of image processing. The aim in the design of spatial filters is to enhance high spatial frequencies and, thus, to increase spatial selectivity. A class of spatial high-pass filters, called *Laplace filters*, performs the second spatial derivative and has been applied for surface EMG detection by many researchers. The one-dimensional longitudinal double differential system belongs to this filter category and approximates the second spatial derivative in the direction of propagation of the action potentials. With respect to the single differential system, the double differential allows better rejection of spatial common mode components, such as the end-of-fiber potentials (Figure 4.7). The double differential system is realized with three electrodes in a row, the central electrode weighted with the factor –2 and the others with +1. If the electrodes are arranged transversal with respect to the muscle fibres rather than parallel, a *TDD* (*transversal double differential*) results.

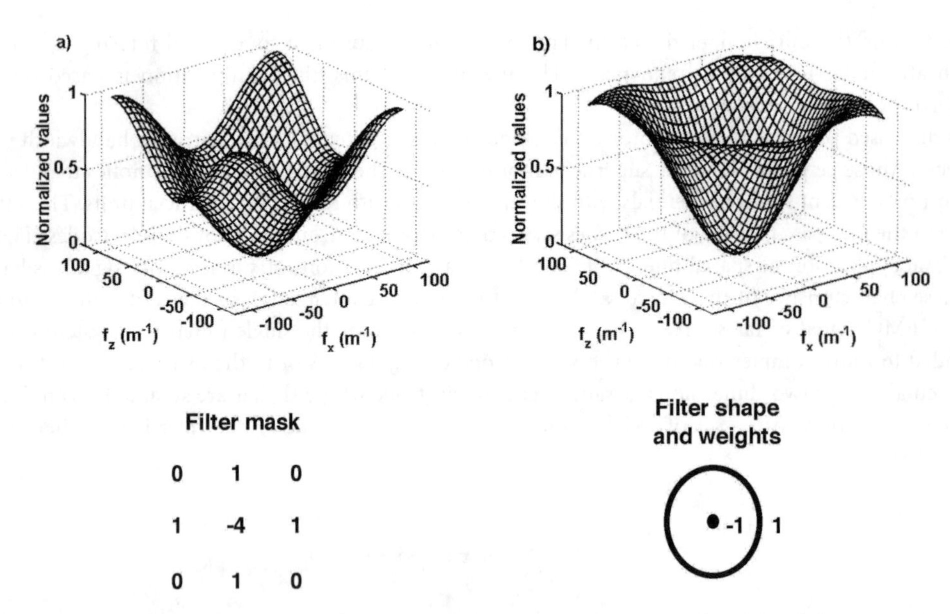

FIGURE 4.13 Magnitude of the two-dimensional transfer function of the NDD-filter (a) and the concentric single ring system (b). The filter masks are also shown. The interelectrode distance is 5 mm in (a); the radius is 5 mm in (b). (Adapted from Disselhorst-Klug et al., 1997 and Farina and Cescon, 2001.)

The same concepts can be applied to two-dimensional electrode configurations. Reucher et al. (1987a, 1987b) have shown that a two-dimensional Laplace filter, the *NDD* (*normal double differentiating*) filter, allows very high spatial selectivity with the possibility of separating single motor unit activities even at maximum voluntary contractions. The weighting factors of each lead of the NDD-filter can be determined from an approximation of the Laplace operator by a Taylor series (Jähne, 1989). The NDD-filter can be represented by the so called *filter mask*:

$$M_{NDD} = \begin{bmatrix} 0 & 1 & 0 \\ 1 & -4 & 1 \\ 0 & 1 & 0 \end{bmatrix} \tag{4.15}$$

Rows and columns of the filter mask represent the position of the recording electrodes and the entries the respective weighting factors. Thus, an NDD-filter can be realized by five cross-wisely arranged electrodes whereby the central electrode is weighted with the factor –4 and the surrounding electrodes with the factor +1. In contrast to the LDD-filter, the NDD-filter performs a spatial double differentiation in two orthogonal directions and builds in this way a two-dimensional spatial high-pass filter.

The impulse response of the NDD-filter and other two-dimensional filter arrangements can be obtained by applying Equation 4.13. Figure 4.13 shows the two-dimensional transfer function of the NDD-filter. Figure 4.14 shows a matrix-based spatial filtering device.

Other spatial filter arrangements consisting of more than five electrodes have been developed and used for detection of single motor units (Disselhorst-Klug et al., 1997).

4.2.3.3.4 Linear Combinations of Signals Detected by Electrodes with Physical Dimensions

Using electrode systems that perform the linear combination of signals detected by non-point electrodes, the surface EMG signal is spatially filtered by the equivalent transfer functions describing the electrode shape and size and the spatial arrangement of the weights associated to each electrode (i.e., the two spatial filtering operations described above are applied to the detected signal). In this way it is possible to design spatial filters whose transfer functions have properties that are not achievable with matrixes of point electrodes. Examples of these systems are those comprised of ring electrodes. Farina and Cescon (2001)

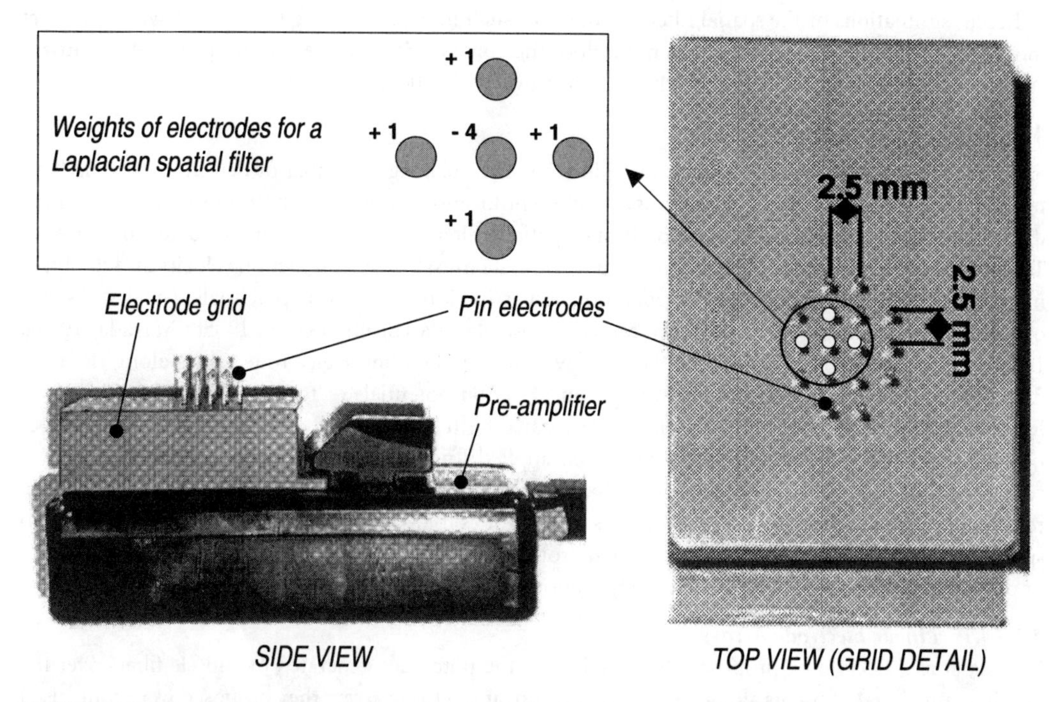

FIGURE 4.14 Matrix of electrodes for detection of spatially filtered EMG signals. The weights given to five electrodes to obtain a signal filtered by the Laplacian filter are shown. (Modified from Disselhorst-Klug et al., *Eur. J. Appl. Physiol.*, 83, 144–150, 2000. With permission.)

recently analyzed the transfer function of these systems and compared them with the matrixes of point electrodes. They demonstrated that, by assuming rings with negligible thickness and a central point electrode, an approximation of the equivalent transfer function of the system comprised by a point electrode and a concentric ring is given by:

$$H_{Mappr}(k_y) = 1 - J_0(rk_y) \tag{4.16}$$

where $J_0(z)$ is the zero-order Bessel function of the first kind. These concepts can be extended to configurations of more than one ring as well, forming a class of isotropic concentric ring detection systems. Figure 4.13 shows the transfer function in Equation 4.16.

4.2.3.3.5 Crosstalk and Spatial Selectivity

Spatial high-pass filters enhance the signals of motor units located close to the recording electrodes and suppress the contributions of more distantly located traveling sources. For this reason spatial filters have been considered for reducing cross talk in applications of surface EMG in which the detection of the muscular coordination pattern is of interest (Koh and Grabiner, 1993; Winter et al., 1994). Different kinds and different orders of spatial filters have been applied for crosstalk reduction. However, the experimental results have shown that cross talk is not reduced by spatial high-pass filtering (van Vugt and van Dijk, 2001).

This apparent discrepancy between theory and practice becomes clearer when the simplifications adopted for the development of the spatial filter theory are considered in greater detail. In particular, the derivation of the spatial filter transfer functions is based on the assumptions that only traveling signals are detected by the electrodes, while the non-traveling components shown, for example, in Figure 4.7 are not considered. Since these components are the major contributions to cross talk, the reduction of cross talk cannot be predicted by the spatial filter theory reported above.

Recent simulations of the spatial filter responses to such non-propagating potentials have shown that most of the spatial high-pass filters do not reduce the contributions of the non-propagating potentials, and in some cases they even enhance them (Dimitrova et al., 2002; Farina et al., 2002).

4.2.3.4 Spatial Sampling

Sampling the surface EMG signal over the skin consists in placing a number of detection systems (that might perform spatial filtering operations) in different locations over the skin. In this case the potential distribution is sampled in particular points and spatially filtered in each point by the detection systems. The availability of many channels may be used to estimate muscle fiber conduction velocity and to obtain more information on the processes of generation and extinction of the action potentials. The first systems of this type were proposed by De Luca, Merletti, and Masuda (Broman et al., 1985b; Masuda, 1983a, 1983b, 1985a, 1985b; Merletti and De Luca, 1989), who applied linear electrode arrays along the fiber direction to estimate the velocity of propagation of action potentials or to identify innervation zones. Recently, more complex systems with electrodes located both longitudinally and in the transversal direction with respect to the muscle fibers have been applied for the estimation of motor unit anatomical properties (Kleine et al., 1999, 2001; Prutchi, 1995; Roeleveld et al., 1997a, 1997b). Currently, some research groups are using systems of hundreds of electrodes for sampling the surface potential in the two spatial directions. The information extracted from this type of signals was shown to be extremely important both for research and clinical applications (Drost et al., 2001; Kleine et al., 2001).

4.2.3.4.1 Linear Electrode Arrays

Masuda et al. (1983a) first proposed the sampling of the potentials generated by muscle fibers over the skin in many different points along the muscle. The linear electrode arrays they proposed were comprised of point electrodes from which single or double differential signals could be extracted. These systems were shown to provide information about single motor unit anatomical properties, such as the location of the innervation zones and the length of the muscle fibers. Later, linear electrode arrays were applied and further developed by other research groups (Merletti et al., 1999; Roy et al., 1986b). Figure 4.15 shows signals detected from the biceps brachii muscle by a linear electrode array. The generation of the action potentials at the motor end plate can be observed from the surface signals as the point from which the potentials start the propagation in the two directions (toward the tendon regions). It is possible to follow the action potentials from the generation at the neuromuscular junction to the extinction at the

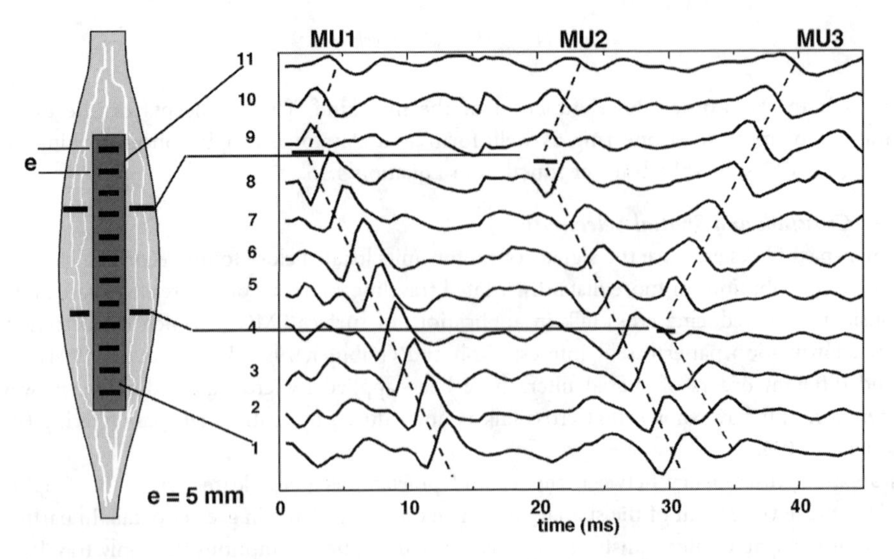

FIGURE 4.15 Detection of surface EMG signals by a linear electrode array of 16 electrodes (interelectrode distance 10 mm) from the biceps brachii muscle during a voluntary low force level contraction. The action potentials of three motor units with different locations of the innervation zone are shown. (Modified from Merletti et al., 1999.)

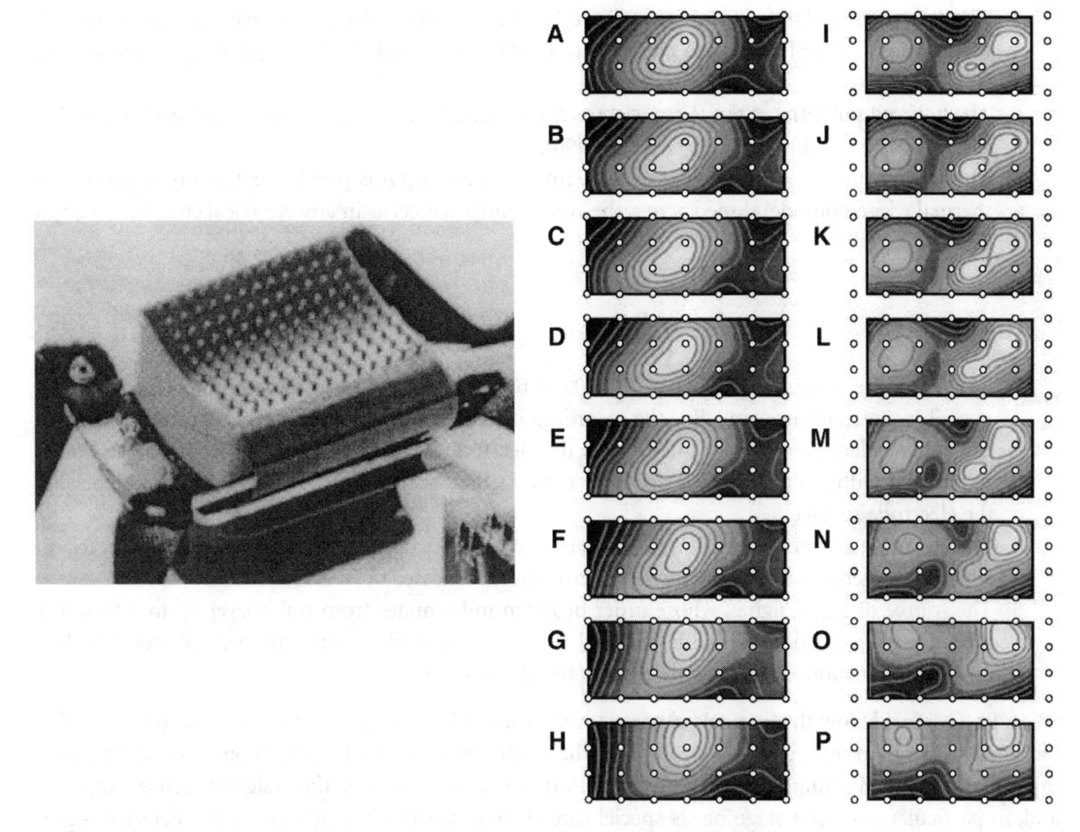

FIGURE 4.16 High density surface matrix of electrodes (left) and topographical maps of the root mean square value for monopolarly detected signals (A–H) and single differential signals (I–P) (right), at increasing force levels (5, 10, 15, 20, 35, 50, and 100% MVC, A–G and I–O) and at the end of a fatiguing exercise at 50% MVC (H, P). The maps are computed from recordings with a two-dimensional system similar to that shown on the left from the upper trapezius muscle. (Modified from Kleine et al., 2000b.)

tendons. The pattern corresponding to the propagation of the signals in both directions is typical of single motor unit action potentials and can be used to identify the contributions of the single motor units in the interference signals. In the example shown, three motor units can clearly be distinguished.

4.2.3.4.2 Bidimensional Arrays

The systems for signal detection can be placed in either direction over the muscle. The placement of electrodes in the transversal direction can be used to analyze the rate of decrease of the potential with increasing transversal distance from the source. This decrease depends on the depth of the motor unit, which thus can be estimated from this type of recordings. Roeleveld et al. (1997a) first proposed such recording techniques.

Systems of about 100 electrodes (Figure 4.16) have been developed (Zwillinger, 1996) and are being used in advanced studies on muscle functions. In particular, from these systems it is possible to compute maps of potential amplitude and to investigate the distribution of muscle electrical activity in different tasks. Figure 4.16 shows examples of these amplitude maps in case of upper trapezius muscle assessment.

4.2.3.5 Amplifier Design

4.2.3.5.1 The Input Stage: Overview

In the previous sections we examined the electrical behavior of intramuscular and surface electrodes, and we pointed out that the tissue-electrode assembly, although involving many complex interactions, can be well represented by a simplified electrical model that takes into account:

1. The contact impedance, comprised of a resistive and a capacitive component, usually in the 10-kΩ to 1-MΩ range (Basmajian and De Luca, 1985; Blok et al., 1997), depending on the type of electrode.
2. The half-cell potential at the tissue-electrode interface, that can be as high as 200 mV and higher in practical cases (Ragheb and Geddes, 1990).
3. The intrinsic noise of the tissue-electrode interface. Its origin is purely electric and is due to the thermal white noise developed across the contact impedance, as in any electrical circuit; it is given by:

$$E_{thermal,RMS} = \sqrt{4kTRB} \tag{4.17}$$

   where k is the Boltzmann constant (1.3805×10^{-23} J/K), T is the absolute temperature, R is the overall input resistance, and B is the recording bandwidth. In intramuscular detection this noise can be considered a given parameter once the electrode type has been selected. This noise can be minimized with proper surface electrode manufacturing and skin treatment, and by increasing the electrode surface.
4. The electrode contact noise, due to the ionic exchanges occurring at the skin-electrode interface, which is, in general, higher than the intrinsic thermal noise.
5. The source of EMG signal, whose order of magnitude ranges from noise level up to 5 to 6 mV for surface signals detected with standard electrodes, and whose maximum amplitude in intramuscular detection is strongly affected by the electrode used.

An EMG signal below the intrinsic electrode noise cannot be distinguished from noise; thus, it is this parameter (which, in turn, depends strongly on the electrode) that sets the lower boundary of the useful input range of an EMG amplifier. The above specifications clearly show that the design of such an amplifier and, in particular, its input stage needs special care since it sets the final quality of the detected signal (Silverman and Jenden, 1971; van der Locht and van der Straaten, 1980).

Regardless of the type of recording (intramuscular or surface), the input stage of an EMG amplifier is composed by an *instrumentation amplifier* (*IA*) that performs the difference between a signal detected within the volume conductor, with respect to a remote reference placed in an electrically inactive area (*monopolar* detection) or to another electrode placed in the same volume conductor (*bipolar* or *differential* detection).

A realistic electrical model of the input stage comprises:

1. The finite input impedance of the amplifier, composed by a resistive and a capacitive component, usually a resistor of 10^7 to 10^{12} Ω in parallel to a 5- to 10-pF capacitor.
2. The input bias current, in the nA to pA range, depending on the input transistors (BJT or FET) and whether the amplifier includes an internal compensation.
3. The input voltage noise, which can be considered white in the EMG bandwidth, with additional flicker (*1/f*) noise below 10 Hz, and expressed by:

$$E_{in,noise} = e_n \cdot \sqrt{B} \tag{4.18}$$

   where e_n is the voltage noise spectral density of the amplifier and B is the bandwidth over which the noise is detected; this value is usually slightly lower in BJT input stages, and is approximately proportional to the bias current. Typical values for the noise spectral density with BJT amplifiers range between 20 and 40 nV/√Hz at 1 kHz (Metting van Rijn, 1993; Metting van Rijn et al., 1991b).
4. The input current noise, expressed by:

$$I_{in,noise} = i_n \cdot \sqrt{B} \tag{4.19}$$

where i_n is the current noise spectral density and B is the bandwidth. This value is much lower in BJT input stages with respect to FET input stages, and is approximately inversely proportional to the bias current. Typical values in BJT amplifiers range from 1 to 60 fA/√Hz at 1 KHz, depending on the bias current.

5. The finite *Common Mode Rejection Ratio* (*CMRR*), which is the ability of the amplifier to reject common mode signals (i.e., the same signal applied at both inputs), defined as Ad/Ac and, in dB, as:

$$CMRR_{dB} = 20\log(Ad / Ac) \tag{4.20}$$

where $Ad = V_{out}/Vd$ is the differential gain (with Vd being the differential voltage across the two inputs) and $Ac = V_{out}/Vc$ is the common mode gain (when the common mode voltage Vc is applied at both inputs).

Other issues of amplifier design, such as the limited gain-bandwith product or *GBW* (i.e., the maximum value of the product $B \cdot Ad$), are usually not a concern in EMG applications. A complete model of the system comprised of tissue, electrode, and amplifier input stage is represented in Figure 4.17.

The intrinsic noise of the input amplifier is given by the joint effect of the two statistically independent sources of noise, the input voltage noise and the input current noise. The overall input noise of the amplifier is then given by:

$$V_{noise,amp} = \sqrt{E_{in,noise}^{\ 2} + (Z_s \cdot I_{in,noise})^2} \tag{4.21}$$

with the notation of Figure 4.17 and $E_{in,noise}$ and $I_{in,noise}$ expressed as in Equations 4.18 and 4.19.

As an example of design of a surface EMG amplifier (bandwidth 20 to 500 Hz), we may consider the use of a commercially available instrumentation amplifier for biomedical use (Texas Instruments INA121), featuring a typical voltage noise density of 20 nV/√Hz and a current voltage noise density of 1 fA/√Hz. Considering an unlucky but not uncommon source impedance of 100 kΩ, the voltage and

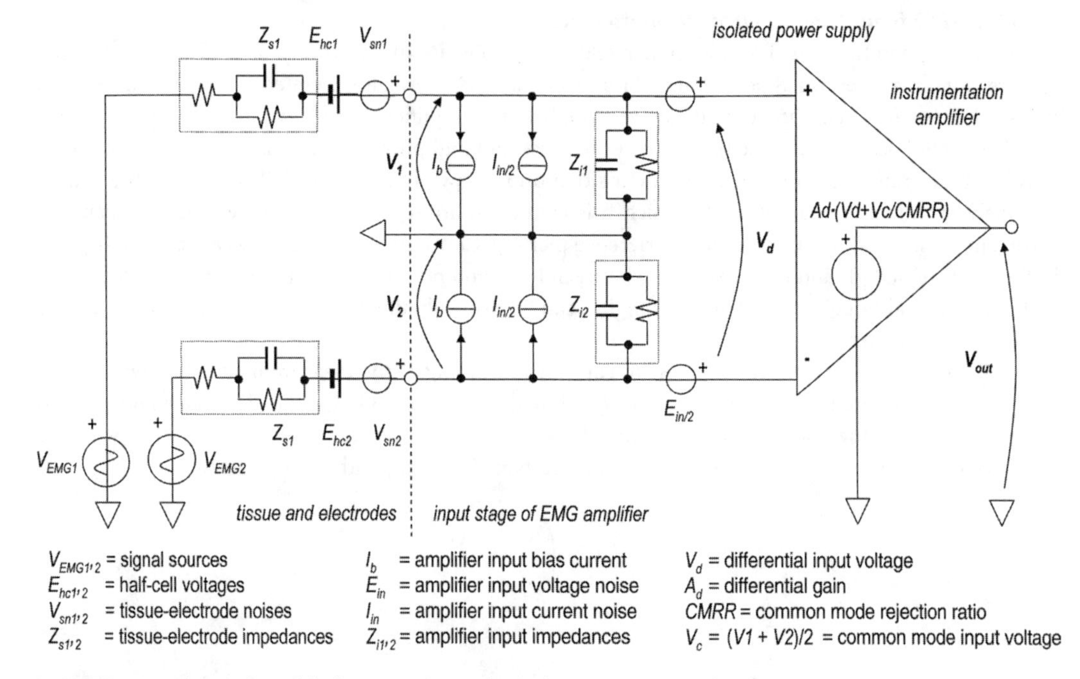

FIGURE 4.17 Electrical model of an EMG tissue-electrode system connected to the input stage of an EMG amplifier; the figure represents the main sources of non-idealities, such as non-zero source impedance, source noise, finite amplifier input impedance, input noise.

current noise contributions will be, respectively, $E_{in} = 0.44\ \mu V_{RMS}$ and a negligible $Z_s \cdot I_n = 2.2\ nV_{RMS}$. The overall input noise of the amplifier will be about $V_{noise,amp} = 0.44\ \mu V_{RMS}$.

If we consider the overall electrode noise (thermal plus contact), we may be surprised that in general this is much higher than the above calculated input noise; in this case, it is this factor that sets the performance limit of the system, and further efforts to improve the noise introduced by the amplifier will not result in increased performance. As a rule of thumb, a good amplifier should have an input noise that is not exceeding half of the intrinsic electrode noise. For a good surface electrode, this noise is 1 to 5 μV_{RMS}.

Note that, when performing spectral analysis on acquired signals, it is important to know not only the overall noise of the system but also its spectral density over the bandwidth, which sets the limit in the frequency domain. This is given by:

$$E_{noise,RMS,total} = \sqrt{V_{noise,amp}^2 + E_{thermal,RMS}^2} \tag{4.22a}$$

$$e_{noise,RMS,total} = E_{noise,RMS,total} / \sqrt{B} \tag{4.22b}$$

When choosing the gain of the first stage (Ad), design considerations will suggest to attain the highest possible gain so that the noise contributions of subsequent stages will not be an issue, and expensive low-noise amplifiers will be needed only in the first stage.

Special care, however, must be taken in order to avoid saturation caused by the half-cell potential of the electrodes, which are DC coupled to the inputs. A high-pass filter usually follows the input stage in order to remove such DC components (Figures 4.19 and 4.21); in typical cases, with half-cell potentials as high as 200 mV and beyond, a differential gain of 20 to 50 is usually selected.

If the gain of the instrumentation amplifier is selected by an external resistor, it is possible to place a capacitor in series with it, so that the differential gain will be lower in DC (i.e., unity gain) than in the EMG band; this, however, can create unwanted transients in case of electrically elicited EMG signals, which require additional circuitry to reduce artifact amplitude (Knaflitz and Merletti, 1988).

4.2.3.5.2 The Input Stage: Sources of Interference

In practical applications, an EMG amplifier seldom operates in an electrically noise-free environment; sources of interference such as power line cables, externally and internally generated magnetic and electrical fields, HF interference and ripples in the power supply of the amplifier can greatly impair the quality of the signal. A careful design must take these sources into account and provide solutions to reduce their effect.

A block diagram of a typical measurement situation is shown in Figure 4.18. The body of the patient and the instrumentation amplifier to which it is connected are represented together with the parasitic capacitances that play a major role in interference pick-up. Common values of body capacitance (C_b) are in the range of 300 pF, and the capacitance between body and power (C_p) is in the pF range (Huhta and Webster, 1973), although values ten times higher can be easily obtained. The resulting current, i_p, can be as high as 0.5 to 5 µA.

A primary source of interference is due to capacitive coupling of the measurement cables with power lines (C_{c1}, C_{c2}); the induced currents (i_{c1} and i_{c2}) flow through the body via the electrodes and close to earth by means of the body-earth capacitance (C_b) and the isolation capacity (C_{iso}) in series with the reference contact impedance (Z_r). The differential voltage due to C_{c1} and C_{c2} is given by:

$$Vd = i_c \cdot Z_s \cdot \left(\frac{\Delta Z_s}{Z_s} + \frac{\Delta i_c}{i_c} \right)$$

where

$$i_c \equiv \frac{i_{c1} + i_{c2}}{2} \quad \text{and} \quad Z_s \equiv \frac{Z_{s1} + Z_{s2}}{2} \tag{4.23}$$

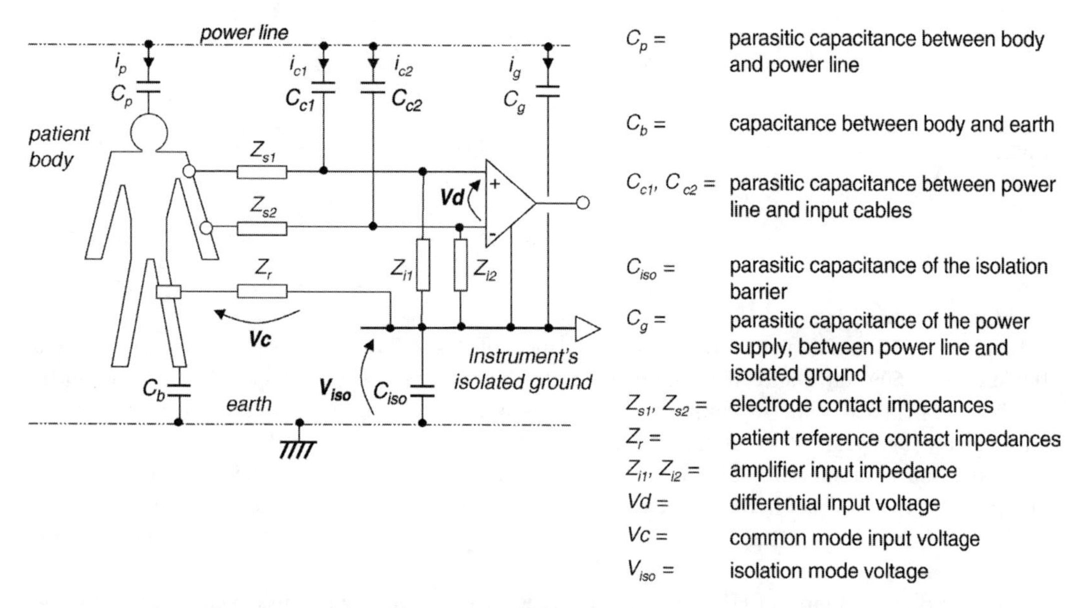

FIGURE 4.18 Typical working environment of an EMG amplifier; the body of the patient and the instrumentation itself are connected to power line cables and earth through parasitic capacitances. (Reproduced from Metting van Rjin, A.C., Peper, A., and Grimbergen, C., *Med. Biol. Eng. Comp.*, 28, 389–397, 1990. With permission.)

Since the induced voltage is differential, it is by no means attenuated by the CMRR; on the contrary, it is amplified together with the EMG signal.

The only effective way to reduce its effect is by keeping the parasitic capacitances C_{c1} and C_{c2} as low as possible. This can be done by making the connection tracks between the electrodes and the front-end as short as possible (i.e., placing the amplification circuitry very close to the electrodes); otherwise, the use of shielded cables with *active guarding* (i.e., driving the shield with a buffer whose input is connected to the common mode voltage) is an effective countermeasure.

Placing the front-end close to the electrodes has the further advantage of reducing the magnetically induced interference, whose amplitude is proportional to the area of the loop formed by the measurement cables. Twisting the cables to reduce this area is only partially effective if the area of the loop that includes the reference path is not negligible.

Another important source of interference is due to common mode voltage (Vc in Figure 4.18) generated by the capacitances between the body and the power lines (C_p in Figure 4.18). Connecting both the patient and the isolated ground to an electrically "clean" earth (thus shunting C_b and C_{iso}) is not a viable solution, because it infringes the safety requirements of biomedical instrumentation.

Considering the body and the electrode contact impedances negligible with respect to that of the parasitic capacitors, and introducing some other simplifications, basic calculations using realistic values of $C_p = 3$ pF, $C_b = 300$ pF, $C_g = C_{iso} = 10$ pF, and $Z_r = 100$ kΩ give a common mode voltage of 63 mV_{RMS}, which is enough to create an equivalent input interference of 1.9 μV_{RMS} (2.8 μV_{PP})* when using a commercially available instrumentation amplifier with a typical CMRR of 90 dB.

A major role in interference generation is played by the so-called *potential divider effect* (Huhta and Webster, 1973), caused by non-equal electrode impedances and unbalanced input impedances of the amplifier. This generates a differential voltage that is related to the common mode voltage by:

* In the case of sinusoidal interference, as in this case, the relationship between RMS and peak-to-peak value is: $V_{PP} = \sqrt{2} \cdot V_{RMS}$, while in the case of white noise, the relationship is approximately $V_{pp} \approx 6 \cdot V_{RMS}$.

$$Vd = Vc\frac{Z_s}{Z_i}\left(\frac{\Delta Z_s}{Z_s} + \frac{\Delta Z_i}{Z_i}\right)$$

where

$$Z_s \equiv \frac{Z_{s1} + Z_{s2}}{2} \text{ and } Z_i \equiv \frac{Z_{i1} + Z_{i2}}{2} \tag{4.24}$$

with the notation of Figure 4.18.

In a practical situation, with equal input impedances of $Zi = 1$ GΩ and a mean contact impedance of 100 kΩ with a 50% unbalance, the multiplying factor between Vc and Vd will be $50 \cdot 10^{-6}$; in case of the previously calculated value of common mode voltage, the resulting input interference will have an unacceptably high value of about 3.2 μV_{RMS}.

Another source of interference comes from high-frequency (*HF*) emissions of neighboring equipment. The effects of the HF itself in the signal are the same as in the case of power line interference, although with a greatly reduced CMRR. The presence of a low-pass filter in the signal conditioning, however, solves this problem.

A less predictable source of HF-induced interference comes from the intrinsic rectifying effect of the input stage, which behaves like a primitive AM/FM demodulator generating signal components within the EMG bandwidth. An effective solution is to place small HF ceramic disc capacitors (unaffecting the performance in the EMG band) between each input and the reference (Metting van Rjin et al., 1990).

Finally, special care must be taken in circuit board design: the use of large ground tracks connected in a "star" configuration is mandatory to reduce crosstalk between different parts of the circuit (especially in multichannel amplifiers), which could even turn into auto-oscillations.

4.2.3.5.3 DRL Circuits and Power Line Removal

The ultimate performance limit is set by the intrinsic electrode noise (whose RMS value is usually in the microvolt range); keeping the other sources of noise and interference below or within this limit ensures that the maximum possible performance of the equipment is obtained.

The previous examples showed that, in practical situations, interferences can seriously degrade the performance of an EMG amplifier. Since the designer has little or no control over electrode impedance unbalance and parasitic capacitances, the most effective way to reduce such interferences is to reduce the amplitude of the common mode itself.

This is normally done by the use of a *DRL* (*Driven Right Leg*) circuit, named following its extensive use in ECG amplifiers, where the reference is connected to the patient's right leg. It is basically composed by a circuit that senses the patient's common mode voltage, and reapplies it on the reference electrode with amplification and reversed phase.

Using a DRL circuit the common mode voltage will be greatly reduced, with an increase in the equivalent CMRR of tens of decibels (Pallas-Areny, 1988; Winter and Webster, 1983). However, because the DRL is a feedback system, special design care is needed to avoid instability. Further details on DRL circuit design can be found in texts on ECG equipment. Design of a DRL for multichannel acquisition system can be found in Metting van Rjin et al. (1990).

An additional advantage of the DRL circuit is the increased patient safety, since the resistor always connected in series to this output limits the maximum current flowing into the body in case of system malfunction. The common mode voltage needed by the DRL circuit can be also used for guarding the shields of the input cables.

In surface EMG amplifiers, analog *notch filters* (i.e., filters whose transfer function has a dip centered at a specific frequency) have been sometimes used to reduce the common-mode interference coming from power lines. These filters introduce a phase reversal in the spectral components above the notch frequency, with a substantial change in the shape of the motor unit action potentials (although the total power of the signal is only slightly affected). This is usually not a good practice, except in cases where only the amplitude and not the shape of EMG signal is of interest (e.g., in biofeedback applications).

More effective ways of reducing line interference make use of digital adaptive filters located after signal sampling and A/D conversion. They lock on a predetermined waveform, estimate its amplitude and phase, and remove it by subtraction (Mortara, 1977).

4.2.3.5.4 Filtering and Amplification

In an EMG amplifier, the input stage is followed by a *band-pass filter* (i.e., a filter that rejects all the frequencies below and above preset values). The high-pass filtering is needed to remove the unwanted DC offset generated by the half-cell potential of the electrodes, which is DC-coupled in the input stage and, in lower percentage, by the offset voltage of the input amplifier itself. This offset, if amplified together with the EMG signals by the next amplification stages, could reduce the useful dynamic range of the signal or even saturate the last stages.

High-pass filtering has the additional advantage of removing signals below 10 to 20 Hz in surface recordings and below 50 to 100 Hz in intramuscular recordings. This frequency region contains motion artifacts that, in intramuscular recording, are due to movements of the lead wires while in surface EMG can be generated during non-isometric contractions (e.g., in gait analysis).

Low-pass filtering is needed mainly to remove unwanted noise beyond the bandwidth of interest that could lead to a degradation of the *signal-to-noise ratio* (i.e., the ratio between the amplitude of the signal and the background noise). The signal-to-noise ratio is defined as:

$$SNR_{dB} = 20\log\left(\frac{S}{N}\right) \tag{4.25}$$

where S is the amplitude of the signal and N of the noise. In case of white noise, it is expressed by:

$$N = n \cdot \sqrt{B} \tag{4.26}$$

where n is the total noise spectral density and B is the bandwidth. In case of cascaded amplification stages the equivalent input noise must be evaluated stage by stage and the different contributions must be summed quadratically, their effects being statistically independent.

A well-designed EMG acquisition system should use a sampling frequency high enough to acquire the highest spectral components of interest in the signal; in this case, filtering will avoid aliasing of the wideband background noise. A summary of the recommended high and low cut-off frequencies for EMG amplifiers (Basmajian and De Luca, 1985; Hermens et al., 1999) is reported in Table 4.1.

TABLE 4.1 Recommended Bandwidth for EMG Amplifiers

Electrode Type and Application	Recommended High-Pass Filter (Hz)	Recommended Low-Pass Filter (Hz)
Surface electrode		
for EMG spectral analysis	< 10	500
for movement analysis	10–20	500
for special wideband applications	10–20	1.000
Wire electrode		
for general applications	20	1.000
for signal decomposition	1.000	10.000
Monopolar and bipolar needle electrode		
for general applications	20	1.000
for signal decomposition	1.000	10.000
Single fiber electrode	20	10.000
Macroelectrode	20	10.000

Except for applications where the shape of the motor unit action potentials is not of interest (e.g., in biofeedback), not only a proper choice of the bandwidth is an issue, but also its phase linearity. Filters with Butterworth or Chebychev response (Franco, 1988) show a steeper *roll-off* (i.e., the slope at the cut-off frequency), but also exhibit a non-linear phase response; this will delay the various spectral components by different amounts, thus introducing a change in the shape of the motor unit action potential. What is worse, because this effect is frequency dependent, the shape of the motor unit action potential can change as a consequence of motor unit action potential scaling (e.g., due to fatigue-induced changes in the conduction velocity). Filters with Bessel response are usually better suited in EMG applications due to their linear phase response. Once again, the use of notch filters should be avoided in all applications where the shape of the EMG signal is of interest.

The choice of the proper gain is simply related to the input range of the A/D conversion system; a correct gain should be suitable to bring the signal into its full input range, thus maximizing the signal resolution. As an example, to acquire an EMG signal with a maximum amplitude of 5 mV using an A/D converter system with an input range of –5 to 5V, the maximal resolution will be reached with a total gain of about 2000.

4.2.3.5.5 Galvanic Isolation

Safety regulations in medical care require that the patient be isolated from external, non-biomedical equipment (such as oscilloscopes, computers, etc.) that can be connected to an EMG amplifier. They also prescribe maximum leakage currents in case the patient touches the case of an ungrounded instrument during a bioelectric recording.

This degree of safety can be obtained by *galvanic isolation* (i.e., no resistive conductive path should exist) between the EMG amplifier and any external equipment that can be connected to it. A typical way to obtain this condition is by optical coupling the circuits connected to the patient (also called the *patient circuit*), while supplying the power by means of a medical grade, transformer-isolated power supply *(DC/DC converter)* or a battery (Figure 4.19).

A coupling capacitance C_{iso} less than 300 pF is suggested, since it will not alter the electrical situation of the patient, C_b, also within this range. It also ensures a maximum leakage current of 20 μA_{RMS} in the worst case, which is considerably lower than the value prescribed by safety requirements.[†]

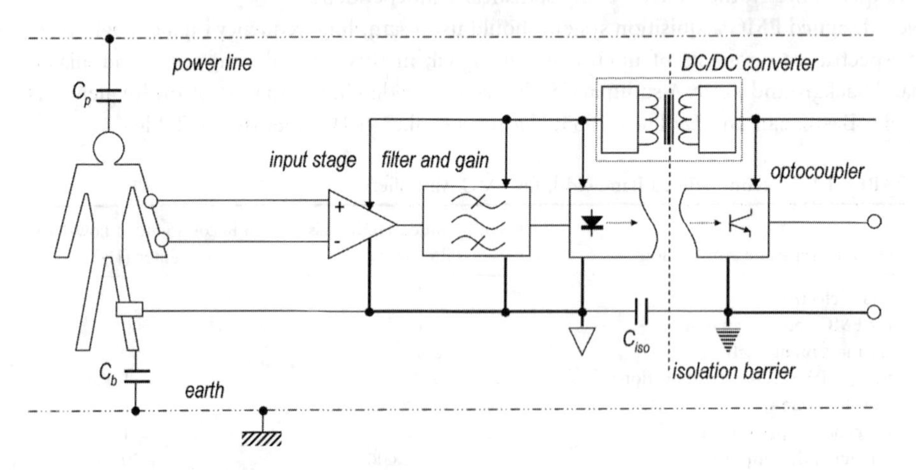

FIGURE 4.19 Block diagram of an EMG amplifier, showing the power supply rails, the galvanic isolation circuitry, and its parasitic isolation capacitance, $C_{iso.}$

[†] The maximum accepted value of the leakage current can vary from country to country. In Europe, type BF biomedical equipment should have a maximum leakage current of 100 μA_{RMS} during normal working.

The optical coupling can be either analog or digital. In the first case, the optocoupler being intrinsically noisy, it should be placed at the end of the amplification chain. Digital coupling can be implemented after A/D conversion, and generally allows better performance both in terms of noise and lower value of the isolation capacitance. A low value of isolation capacitance is needed not only as a safety requirement, but also because it is a potential source of interference on the input signal.

Technical specifications of an optocoupler or isolation amplifier are: the maximum isolation voltage, the isolation capacitance, and the *Isolation Mode Rejection Ratio* (*IMRR*), which depends on the isolation capacitance and defines the ability of the optocoupler to suppress feed-through of interferences across the isolation barrier (Metting van Rijn et al., 1991a). In a well-designed EMG amplifier, an IMRR value of 150 dB or above is usually needed. An effective but often impractical way of greatly increasing the IMRR, with positive effects on interference reduction, is using battery-powered front-end stages.

4.2.3.5.6 Sampling and A/D Conversion

After proper conditioning and, in most cases, optoisolation, the EMG signal is usually sent to an acquisition system for data recording and/or online display.

The acquisition system can be a bank of A/D (*analog-to-digital*) converters, residing internally to the equipment (e.g., in portable EMG acquisition system, such as EMG *dataloggers*) or an external PC acquisition board. In any case, the interface between the "analog world" and the display/acquisition system is always composed by one or more A/D converters; thus, the concepts expressed in this section are of general use.

When an analog signal is fed into and A/D converter, it undergoes two different effects — *sampling* and *quantization*. Sampling is the process of acquiring the values of the signal at equally spaced time intervals, which define the *sampling frequency* of the system (Figure 4.20a). From a spectral point of view, this has the effect of creating *aliases* of the spectrum of the signal, spaced by twice the sampling frequency

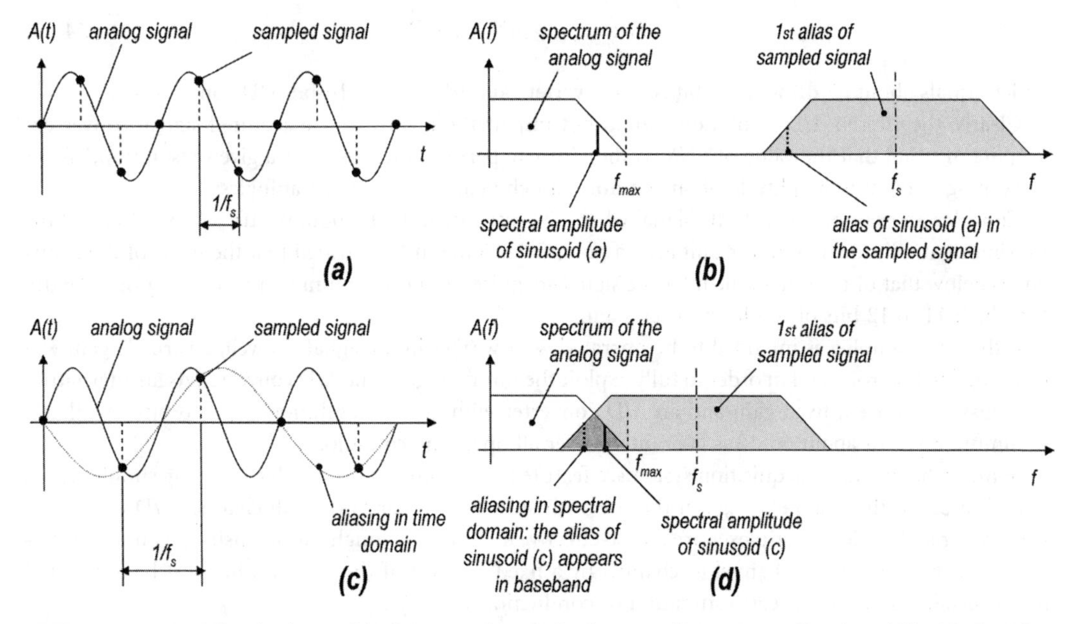

FIGURE 4.20 Sampling in time and in frequency domain in the case of correct sampling (a and b) with $f_s > 2f_{max}$, and in the case of incorrect sampling (c and d) with $f_s < 2f_{max}$. In the latter case, the first alias of the sampled signal partially overlaps the original spectrum of the signal, impairing a correct reconstruction of the signal. The effect is known as aliasing and the reconstructed waveform differs in frequency and phase from the original one. In case of violation of the Nyquist theorem, an aliased frequency component would appear in baseband with a frequency of $f_a = f_s - f$, where f was its original frequency and f_s is the sampling frequency.

(Figure 4.20b). The well-known Nyquist theorem states that the original signal can be fully reconstructed from its samples if the sampling frequency is at least twice the maximum frequency of interest:

$$fs \geq 2 \cdot f_{\max} \tag{4.27}$$

Thus, sampling is a loss-less process, and a correct choice of the sampling frequency will not introduce any distortion or loss of information in the reconstructed signal.

The quantization of a sampled signal consists in expressing the analog value of the samples in terms of digital words, or steps, that have limited resolution. The amplitude of each step is referred to as *least significant bit*, or *LSB*. Differently from sampling, the quantization introduces an approximation in the reconstructed signal, since all the numerical values between two subsequent steps will be represented by the same digital value. This can be modeled as an additive noise that is added to the signal in order to obtain its digitized representation. The maximum peak-to-peak amplitude of this so-called *quantization noise* is then 1 LSB.

The effect of A/D conversion of an analog signal is then to limit its signal-to-noise ratio to a value that, in the optimal case (when the full input range of the A/D converter is exploited), equals the *quantization signal-to-noise ratio* that, for signals with uniform amplitude distribution, equals:

$$SNR_q = \frac{S_{\max}}{V_{LSB}} \leq \frac{2^N}{1} \tag{4.28}$$

where $S_{\max}$ is the maximum amplitude of the signal fed into the A/D, V_{LSB} is the value of its LSB in volts and N is the number of bits.

The maximum achievable value of SNR_q (i.e., when the full input range of the A/D is exploited) for signals with gaussian amplitude distribution, as an EMG signal can be considered, is:

$$SNR_{q,dB,\max} \approx (6N - 4.8)dB \tag{4.29}$$

which equals about 67 dB with 12-bit A/D converters and 91 dB with 16-bit A/D converters.

Clearly, the chosen A/D resolution should not impair the quality of the acquired signal; conversely, keeping in mind that the value of SNR_q is the ultimate performance limit for a given resolution, efforts in keeping maximum amplitude of analog noise much below 1 LSB are meaningless.

Consider an example of an EMG signal where the intrinsic noise is about 0.5 μV_{RMS} (3 μV_{PP}) and the maximum amplitude of a motor unit action potential is 5 to 6 mV. Provided that the noise of the front-end is below that of the signal, the intrinsic signal-to-noise ratio is then limited to a maximum of 66 dB, for which 11 to 12 bits of resolution is enough.

If the EMG amplier is intended to be operated with weaker input signals as well, a variable gain will be needed in the front-end in order to fully exploit the input range of the A/D converter. As an alternative, it is possible to use a fixed gain and an A/D converter with greater resolution (e.g., 16 bits), so that a minimum SNR_q of about 66 dB is guaranteed over all operating conditions.

In multichannel EMG acquisition systems, a feature that is sometimes desirable is having simultaneous sampling on all the channels (e.g., in the use with surface EMG arrays). Multichannel A/D converters with integrated analog multiplexer are a cost-effective solution, although the acquisition is not simultaneous but is shifted from channel to channel by a fixed amount of time. This shift must be accounted for in certain applications (e.g., estimation of conduction velocity).

If a very tight temporal relationship between channels is required (e.g., in conduction velocity calculation), the time shift between samples must be compensated either on-line with the use of *digital signal processors* (*DSP*) or off-line. As previously discussed, a correct sampling frequency ensures that the entire signal can be completely reconstructed from its samples; then, a time shifting of less than one sampling time can be performed in the spectral domain, where this operation is equal to a multiplication by a complex exponential.

One important issue to stress is that the design of the low-pass (*anti-aliasing*) filter and the choice of sampling frequency are strongly correlated. Since real filters exhibit a finite roll-off above the cutoff frequency, a portion of the aliased spectrum, although attenuated, comes into the baseband spectrum.

The designer should then select the order of the filter and sampling frequency in a manner to ensure the amplitude of the aliased spectrum in the bandwidth of interest is less than the A/D resolution of 1 LSB.

When evaluating the required filter order for a given sampling frequency and A/D resolution, if the sampling frequency is not much higher than the Nyquist frequency of $2 \cdot f_{max}$, unrealistic filter orders would be required if only the filter mask is taken into account. Fortunately, in practical cases the acquired signal has limited bandwidth and decreased spectral amplitude toward its upper spectrum boundary. Thus, the joint effects of low-pass filtering and limited bandwidth with decreased amplitude at higher frequencies allow the design of more reasonable filter orders.

Numerical evaluations of the filter order as a function of the sampling frequency and resolution require a knowledge of the mean spectrum of the EMG signal, or a reliable mathematical model of it (Shwedik et al., 1977).

4.2.3.6 EMG Equipment

This section is devoted to the description of EMG equipment that is currently used in clinical applications, in sport and occupational medicine, and in basic and applied research. These biomedical devices include electromyographs, gait analysis systems, and biofeedback modules. An additional application of EMG for the control of motorized prostheses will also be described.

4.2.3.6.1 Electromyographs

An electromyograph for clinical use (either for intramuscular or surface EMG) usually consists of a multichannel EMG amplifier, an embedded or external acquisition board, and a PC equipped with a software for signal visualization, acquisition, off-line review, and sometimes processing. An optional stimulation board may also be included for the acquisition of electrically elicited EMG activity. The latter may be useful, among other applications, for the measurement of the motor nerve conduction (*MNC*) velocity by applying an electrical stimulus on a motor nerve and measuring the delay of the elicited EMG response detected on the surface of the stimulated muscle. The compatibility of the EMG front-end with the electrical stimulation board is ensured by an additional *blanking* circuitry, synchronized with the stimulator ouput, whose aim is to reduce the amplitude of stimulation artifact on the electrically elicited EMG signal (Knaflitz and Merletti, 1988; Merletti et al., 1992). Figure 4.21 depicts a general block diagram of the system.

The analog front-end is comprised of a set of instrumentation amplifiers that allow, by means of a network of configuration switches, the detection of EMG signal in monopolar, single differential and sometimes double differential mode. The amplification and, in some cases, the low and high cutoff frequencies are user selectable.

All the circuitry in electrical contact with the patient (the so-called *patient circuit*) is isolated from the rest of the equipment by means of an optical and galvanic isolation barrier that guarantees the required high degree of safety for the patient even in case of system malfunctioning (Figure 4.21).

4.2.3.6.2 EMG Dataloggers

Several applications, such as sport or occupational medicine, sometimes require long-term EMG measurements in the field. In these cases, a portable, battery-powered EMG acquisition system is required. This kind of equipment, usually known as a *datalogger*, consists of a number of surface EMG probes and a wearable multichannel acquisition unit, equipped with a removable storage media (sometimes a standard PCMCIA memory card) and/or with a PC interface for off-line downloading the acquired EMG signals on an external computer.

The acquisition unit is usually equipped with a user interface (display and keys) that, by means of an embedded microprocessor, microcontroller or DSP, allows the setting of the various acquisition options such as the number of channels, sampling frequency, etc. (Figure 4.22).

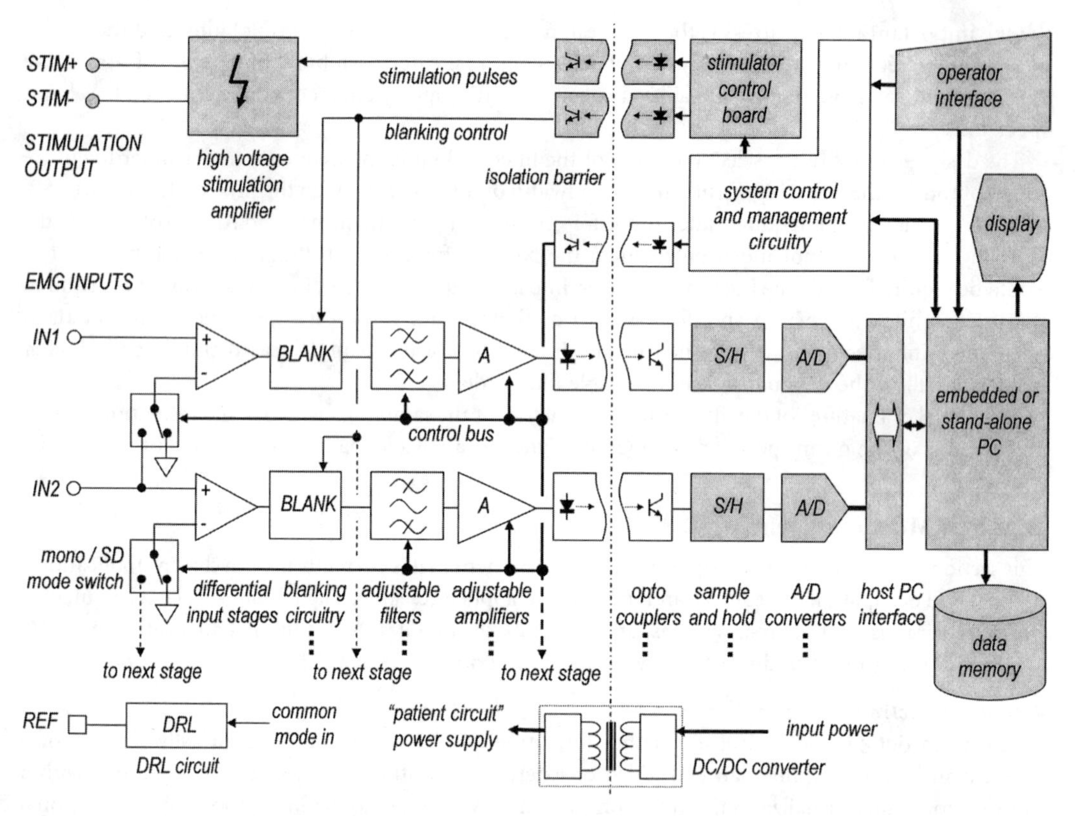

FIGURE 4.21 Block diagram of a multichannel electromyograph, comprised of analog EMG front-end, isolation circuits, A/D acquisition board, PC with screen and user interface, and optional electrical stimulation board. The acquisition board and the PC (shaded in gray) may be embedded in the same enclosure of the electromyograph, which acts as stand-alone equipment, or may be external and a standard PC may be used instead. An optional stimulation board may also be included; in this case, the analog front-end is equipped with an additional circuitry for the reduction of stimulation artifacts.

To improve the immunity to external interference and to distribute the overall weight, the analog EMG front-end is usually embedded into the probes, and the conditioned and amplified signals are fed into the acquisition unit by means of thin and wearable cables.

EMG dataloggers feature only a limited number of functions with respect to electromyographs (e.g., the detection method, gain and high and low cutoff frequency are fixed), they do not include a stimulation board, usually do not allow the real-time visualization of the EMG signal and generally have a limited number of channels.

4.2.3.6.3 Gait Analysis Systems

Gait and movement analysis is one of the most common applications of surface EMG. Basically, it is the detection of muscle activation by means of bipolar surface electrodes during normal movement (such as gait), with the aim of studying the activation patterns of the various muscles involved and their degree of synchronization.

In gait analysis foot switches and/or goniometers are used to provide the correlation between EMG and the various phases of gait (swing and stance). Complex and expensive camera systems are sometimes also used to track and reconstruct the movements in a three-dimensional space. Additional details on gait analysis can be found in Section 4.4, "Applications of EMG in Basic Research and Clinical Routine."

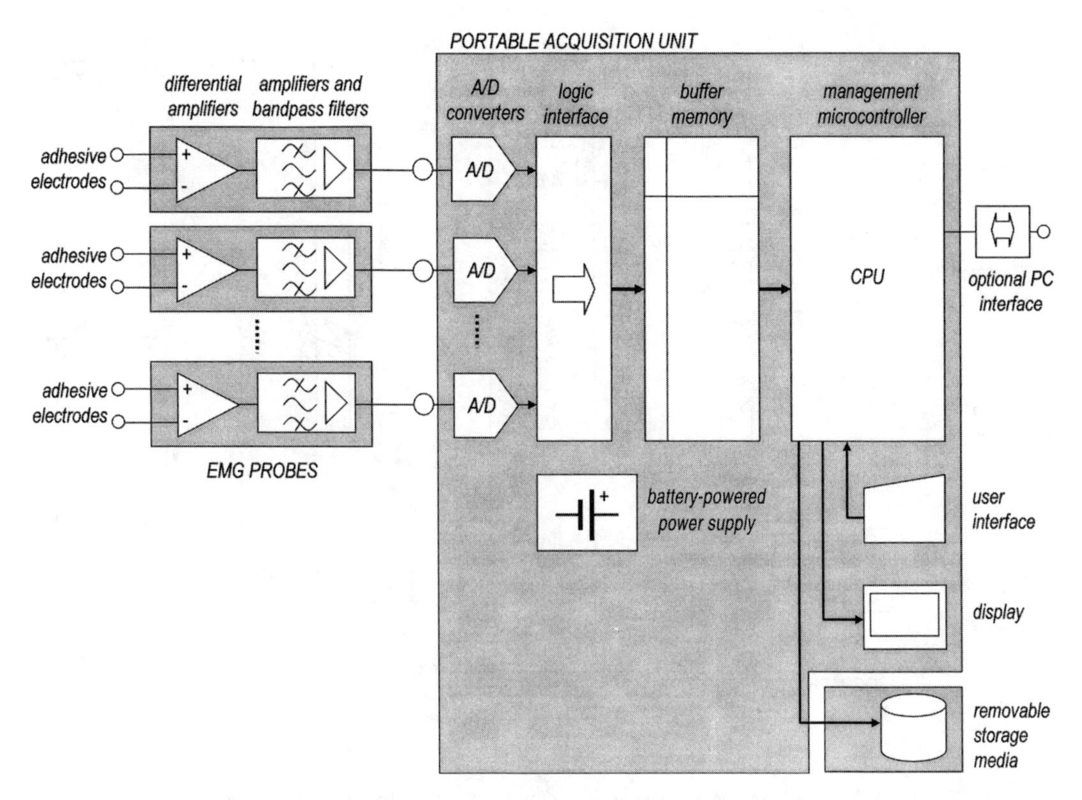

FIGURE 4.22 Block diagram of an EMG datalogger. When compared with a standard electromyograph, a datalogger shows a more simplified EMG front-end, which is usually embedded directly into the probes rather than into the main unit. Acquired data are stored on a high capacity non-volatile memory, that in some cases can be removed and plugged into an external PC for off-line data review and processing. Some types of dataloggers do not use a removable memory, but are equipped with a host PC interface for the downloading of the data. The equipment is battery powered and all the internal circuitry is designed for a low power consumption for an extended battery life.

The equipment usually consists of a set of bipolar surface EMG probes that collect a single channel of EMG data for each muscle by means of special, low-artifact surface electrodes.

The signals are fed into a wearable acquisition unit, usually fixed to the patient by means of a belt. The acquisition unit includes a bank of A/D converters, a multiplexer that converts the parallel samples into a stream of serial data and a trasmitting circuitry. On the other side, a receiver de-serializes the data that are fed into a PC for signal acquisition, review, and processing (Figure 4.23).

To guarantee the requested degree of safety and patient isolation, the transmitter and the receiver are coupled by means of an electrically isolated link, such as fiber optic, optical isolated copper cable or point-to-point radio transmission.

Low-cost systems usually do not comprise the A/D converters, and the analog signals are optically isolated and fed directly into a general purpose PC analog acquisition board by means of a multipolar cable.

4.2.3.6.4 Biofeedback

Several studies in occupational medicine demonstrate the incidence of insufficient muscle relaxation in the occurrence of musculoskeletal disorders. It has also been experimentally demonstrated that mental stress can contribute to involuntary muscle activation, especially in the neck-shoulder region, which in turn may lead to chronic muscle pain.

In these and in other cases, *biofeedback* (which provides the patient a real-time indication of his/her muscle activity) proves to be a useful method for training the patient in relaxing the muscle where an excessive activation exists or in increasing an insufficient activation level. The hardware usually consists

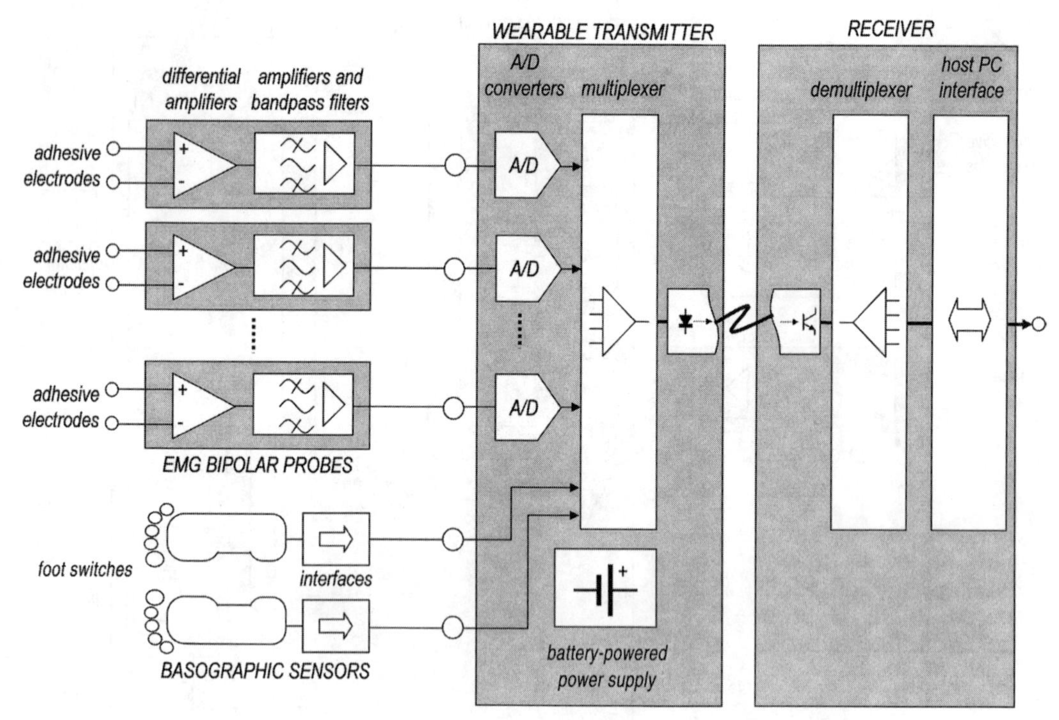

FIGURE 4.23 Block diagram of an EMG gait analysis system. The wearable transmission unit collects the EMG signals of the various muscles from the bipolar probes, converts and serializes the data into a serial stream which is transmitted to the receiver by means of an electrically isolated link (fiber optic, optocoupled cable, or radio). The receiver de-serializes the data and feeds it into the host PC for signal review, acquisition, or processing. Dedicated input channels are available for the connection of additional sensors such as goniometers, footswitches, or foot pressure sensors.

of a miniaturized, single-channel EMG amplifier with surface electrodes connected to a suitable muscle that can provide the patient with a real-time feedback of the muscle activation in a visual or acoustic way.

Classical biofeedback equipment usually includes a presettable threshold, so that it can raise a warning to the user when the muscle activity crosses a preset threshold (Figure 4.24).

Recent studies (Hägg, 1991) formulated the so-called *Cynderella theory*, which hypothesizes that there are low-threshold motor units that are always recruited as soon as the muscle is activated, and stay active until total muscle relaxation; clearly, these motor units are more prone to overload that may lead to degenerative processes. Although areas of debate on this theory still exists (Westgaard and De Luca, 2001), this hypothesis has in general been acknowledged by the research community.

In this paradigm a continuous, low voluntary effort muscle activity under the safety threshold could also lead to muscular disorders. A biofeedback system based on the Cynderella hypothesis would rather provide indications about the presence of *gaps* (i.e., short periods of EMG inactivity) in the activation pattern instead of giving a feedback solely based on amplitude.

The hardware consists of an EMG analog front-end, an A/D converter, and a DSP or microcontroller unit that is a detector of gaps. A non-volatile memory is usually also included, together with a PC interface for the downloading of the measurements. The warning of insufficient muscle relaxation may be given to the user with an optical or acoustic alarm or, in a more private way, by means of a wearable vibrating device (Figure 4.25).

Biofeedback can also be used for the treatment of incontinence, as a tool for training the patients in increasing control of the muscles of the pelvic floor suffering from excessive relaxation.

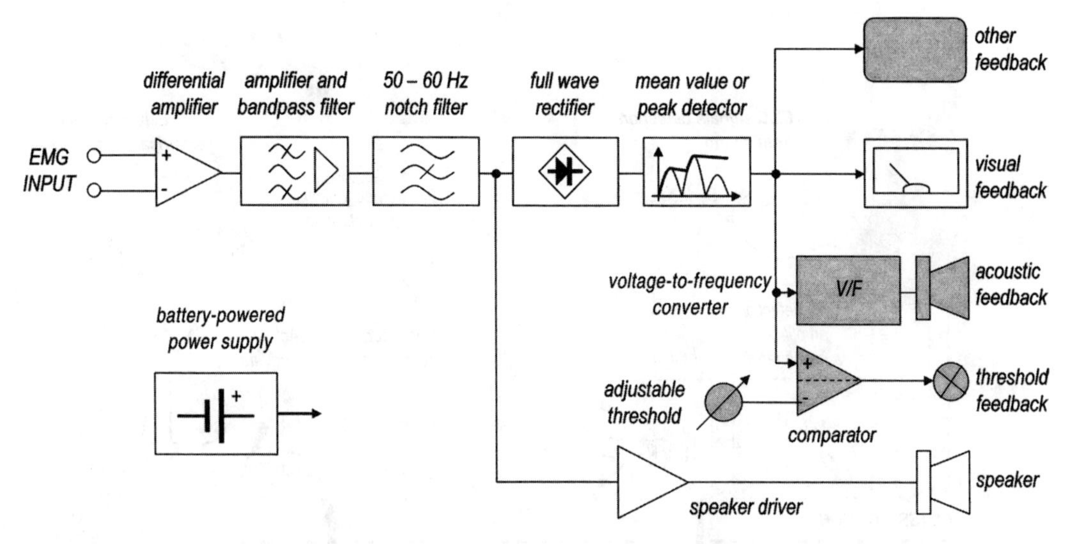

FIGURE 4.24 Block diagram of a "classic" biofeedback, comprised of analog EMG front-end, full wave rectifier, peak detector, and activity level indicator (usually consisting of a bar of visual indicators). An optional alarm with presettable threshold can also be included, as well as a storage memory. Note that in this case only the amplitude, and not the shape of the signal, is of interest. The use of a notch filter is then possible to reduce the amount of power line interference, even if this introduces a distortion in the shape of the signal.

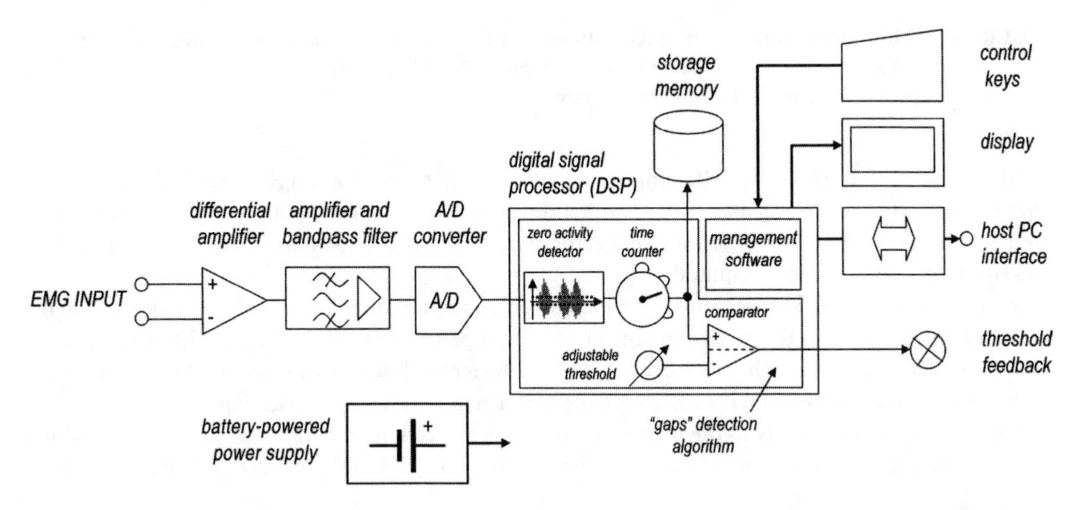

FIGURE 4.25 Block diagram of a biofeedback based on the Cynderella theory. Here the EMG signal, properly conditioned, amplified, and converted into digital data, is fed into a Digital Signal Processor (DSP) that contains an algorithm for the detection and evaluation of gaps in the EMG activity. A storage memory is usually also included that allows to download off-line the measurements by means of host PC interface.

4.2.3.6.5 EMG-Controlled Prostheses

In some commercially available limb prostheses such as artificial elbows, wrists, and hands, the motors may be controlled by means of EMG signals detected from muscles above the level of amputation (Figure 4.26). An embedded processor evaluates the electrical activity from nerves (ENG), from residual stump muscles (EMG), or from other muscles, and by means of appropriate algorithms decides which prosthesis function to activate in order to satisfy the intent of the central nervous system. Depending on the algorithm used, EMG processors can be classified as either *multistate* or *pattern based.*

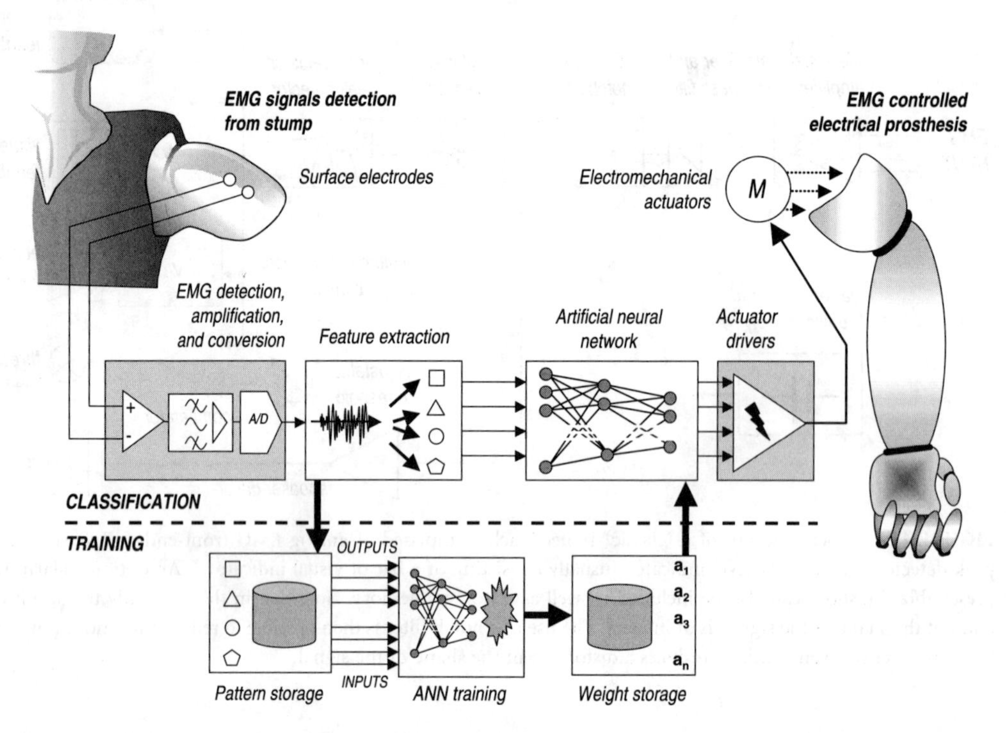

FIGURE 4.26 Block diagram of a surface EMG controlled prosthesis. From the surface signals detected from muscles under the control of the subject, a feature set is extracted. An Artificial Neural Network (ANN) classifies the feature patterns and drives the electronics for prosthesis control.

In *multistate controllers*, the EMG amplitude range (or its rectified average value) is divided into a number of levels or *states*, each associated with a different prosthesis function. The number of states is limited to two or three to avoid performance error due to the excessive demand on the operator's ability to generate the proper EMG amplitude.

An increased number of functions may be obtained by the use of *EMG pattern controllers* (Hudgins et al., 1994), based on EMG signals present in activation patterns of agonist/antagonist muscles. With proper selection of patterns that are repeatable and sufficiently different with respect to each other, up to five functions can be obtained with acceptable performance in function selection.

Other recent developments in the field have been in the direction of *artificial neural networks*, which proved to be successful in pattern classification because of their trainability, adaptability, and robustness.

4.3 EMG Signal Processing

4.3.1 Intramuscular EMG Processing

Intramuscular and surface EMG signals present different characteristics, mainly due to the influence of the volume conductor on the detected potentials. This implies that the techniques used for their processing are based on different approaches and that the information that can be extracted from the signals are rather different. Intramuscular EMG signals historically have been used to get information at the single motor unit level since, from the invasively detected signals, the separation of the motor unit action potential trains is feasible even at relatively high force contraction levels. On the contrary, from surface EMG signals, a global analysis of the muscle properties is usually performed, since in this case the separation of the contributions to the signal is extremely difficult. Moreover, peripheral properties of the

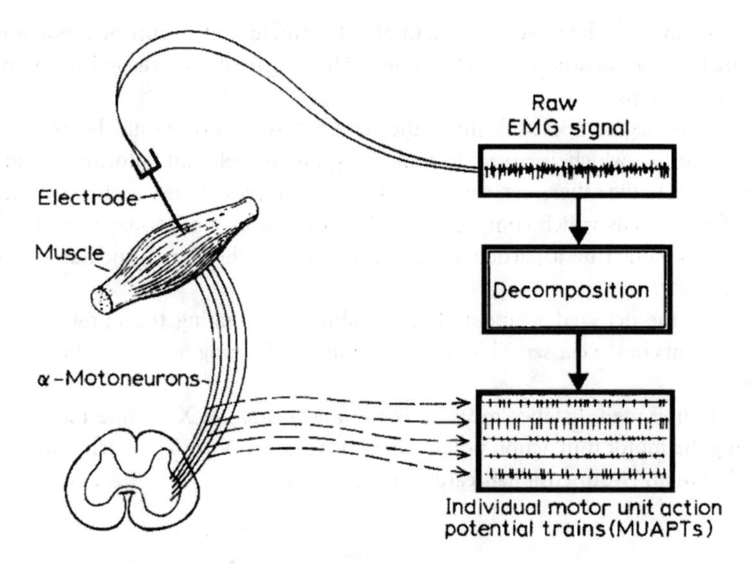

FIGURE 4.27 Schematic representation of the detection and decomposition of intramuscular EMG signals. The signals are detected by electrodes inserted in the muscle. An interference signal, constituted by the activity of a number of motor units, is then obtained. The aim of the EMG signal decomposition algorithms is to identify the times of occurrence of all the active MUs that consistently contribute to the interference signal. (From Basmajian, J.V. and De Luca, C.J., *Muscles Alive: Their Functions Revealed by Electromyography*, 5th ed., Williams & Wilkins, Baltimore, 1985. With permission.)

neuromuscular system are usually investigated by surface EMG while mainly control properties are addressed in the case of intramuscular signals. The joint use of intramuscular and surface systems allows extraction of more information than that obtained by the use of only one of the two methods.

4.3.1.1 Decomposition of Intramuscular EMG Signals into Motor Unit Action Potential Trains

The decomposition of an intramuscular EMG signal into its constituent motor unit action potential trains requires the ability to detect the discharges of the motor units significantly contributing to the signal and to correctly associate each detected motor unit action potential with the motor unit that generated it. EMG signal decomposition therefore involves the two basic steps of detecting motor unit action potentials and recognizing detected motor unit action potentials. The schematic representation of the process of intramuscular EMG signal decomposition is shown in Figure 4.27.

To identify the occurrences of motor unit action potentials within a signal or to segment the signal into portions that contain motor unit action potentials, common characteristics of motor unit action potential shapes, which differentiate them from background signal noise, are used. To classify detected motor unit action potentials, the motor unit action potentials produced by the same motor unit should be more similar in shape than motor unit action potentials produced by different motor units, and the differences in motor unit action potential shapes should be quantified and characterized. Intramuscular EMG signal decomposition can thus involve the following steps (Stashuk, 1999):

1. Signal segmentation
2. Motor unit action potential representation
3. Motor unit action potential clustering
4. Supervised motor unit action potential classification
5. Resolution of superimposed motor unit action potentials

The motor unit action potential detection is usually based on a threshold applied to the raw or filtered signals, or to the derivative, etc. The threshold can be selected either manually by the user or automatically on the basis of a portion of the signal where only noise and no activity is present. The detected segments can be isolated action potentials of a single motor unit or a portion of an action potential or more than one action potential or noise. The nature of the detected segment is established by further processing steps.

For the subsequent segment classification, the detected segments should be represented by their features. The feature set, which is a vector containing all the relevant information to distinguish a waveform with respect to the others, can simply contain the samples of the waveform in the time domain, characteristics of the signals which compactly provide indications on its shape (peak value, duration, etc.), or the values obtained by a particular transformation of the signal, such as Fourier transform, wavelet coefficients, etc.

The clustering of the detected segments has the aim of estimating the number of classes and of classifying the segments in the classes. This is usually done by defining measures of distance between the feature vectors.

The most commonly used distance measure is the Euclidean. Let $\mathbf{X}_i$ denote the *i*th N-dimensional pattern describing the motor unit action potential: $\mathbf{X}_i = (x_{i1}, x_{i2}, \ldots, x_{iN})^T$. The Euclidean distance between two objects (X_i, X_k) in an N-dimensional feature space is then:

$$d(\mathbf{X}_i, \mathbf{X}_k) = \sqrt{(\mathbf{X}_i - \mathbf{X}_k)^T (\mathbf{X}_i - \mathbf{X}_k)} = \sqrt{\sum_{j=1}^{N} \left(x_{ij} - x_{kj}\right)^2} \tag{4.30}$$

Most algorithms for intramuscular EMG decomposition are limited to the segmentation and clustering part. Some others include an additional step based on supervised classification to assign objects by a clustering based on a training set of objects correctly classified in the training phase.

In the segmentation phase, the detected segments may represent superimposition of more than one motor unit action potential. Superimposed motor unit action potentials are usually not classified in the previous classification steps. The degree of superimposition depends on the distance between the time of occurrences of the waveforms involved and on the waveform shapes. In particular cases, it is possible to obtain an almost zero energy signal by the superimposition of different waveforms (destructive superimposition). The resolution of superimposed waveforms is the most difficult task of a decomposition algorithm and currently there are no general fast solutions. Some algorithms skip the resolution of superimpositions and are limited to the classification of non-overlapping waveforms in the signal. In this way, incomplete firing patterns are obtained.

4.3.1.2 Spike-Triggered Averaging of the Force Signal

Stein et al. (1972) proposed a method to estimate single motor unit contractile properties recording intramuscular EMG signals and joint torque. The method is based on the averaging of the joint torque signal using the detected single motor unit firing instants as triggers. It is well known, indeed, that the averaging of a deterministic signal appearing always in the same way after a stimulus allows reduction of the background noise (in this case mainly the twitches of the other motor units) and extraction of the response to the stimulus. This technique can be applied only at very low firing rates since the force twitches of the motor units have durations of the order of hundreds of milliseconds and are fused for frequencies above 8 to 10 Hz. If the twitches are fused there is no possibility of separating them. For this reason, techniques based on the averaging of a subset of the detected firing instants have been proposed; in this case only the most distant firing instants are used for the averaging.

Due to its limitations, spike-triggered averaging technique is usually applied during non-physiological contractions with the subject using particular feedback techniques to maintain a constant firing rate of the investigated motor unit. Even in these ideal conditions, the technique of twitch averaging has some drawbacks and it is not yet clear how much it is affected by motor unit synchronization, non-linear force summation or jitter in the latency between the electrical and mechanical response (Calancie and Bawa, 1986). All the previous factors are neglected in the averaging theory, which assumes the deterministic signal to be independent from the background noise.

Despite these limitations, the spike triggered averaging technique has been applied extensively to investigate basic relationships among motor unit twitch, recruitment threshold, and firing rate and has provided important results on neuromuscular physiology.

4.3.1.3 Macro EMG

The selective needle or wire electrodes only pick up potentials from the few muscle fibers of a specific motor unit, lying within the uptake radius of the electrode. This motor unit action potential does not represent the real motor unit action potential, which allows the interpretation of motor unit properties, such as motor unit size.

The number of fibers participating in the motor unit action potential detected by the selective electrode are dependent on the area and geometry of the recording electrode, the fiber density of the motor unit, and the position of the electrode in relation to the center and periphery of the motor unit territory in the muscle. Ideally, to describe the motor unit properties, a compound signal should be recorded that contains the summed action potentials from the majority of fibers in the motor unit. To obtain such a standardized signal, Stålberg (1980) introduced the averaging of macrointramuscular signals. The technique was based on the concomitant detection of intramuscular EMG signals by a selective electrode and a large electrode 15 mm long. The signal detected by the large intramuscular electrode is spike-trigger averaged using the decomposition of the selective fiber recording as trigger. *Macro motor unit action potentials* are obtained in this way. The size parameters of the macro motor unit action potentials, such as the peak-to-peak voltage or area, are related to the overall size of the contributing motor unit. With respect to the averaging of surface EMG signals, the macro motor unit action potential has the advantage that fewer discharges are needed to obtain a clean averaged potential and can be used also in muscles that are not easily accessible with surface electrodes.

4.3.1.4 Estimation of Motor Unit Conduction Velocity from Invasive Recordings

Buchthal et al. (1955) first proposed an invasive method for single motor unit conduction velocity estimation. Their technique was based on the detection of intramuscular EMG signals at two locations at a known distance and on the estimation of the delay between the two detected potentials. In this way, conduction velocity could be estimated during either voluntary or electrically elicited contractions. The technique is time-consuming and suffers from some methodological limitations, the most important being the difficulty of obtaining potentials of similar shape from two extremely selective detection systems. High selectivity indeed implies large changes of the detected waveform shapes as a consequence of small electrode movements. If the two signal shapes are slightly different, the delay can be defined on the basis of different criteria, such as the distance between zero crossings or peaks (the criteria will lead to different results in case of different shape). If the shape of the two signals is consistently different, the delay becomes meaningless.

Troni et al. (1983) proposed a simpler method based on the estimation of the delay in the detection of action potentials elicited by intramuscular electrical stimulation. A pair of electrodes served for direct stimulation of a small muscle portion, and another invasive electrode served to detect the elicited muscle fiber action potentials.

4.3.2 Surface EMG: Single Channel Processing

Most of the techniques used for surface EMG signal analysis consider signal epochs of hundreds of milliseconds and provide information related to a large number of active motor units. The most commonly used techniques are amplitude and spectral estimation. They provide indications about muscle activity and fatigue. In this case, the surface EMG signal is modeled as a colored stochastic process. Single channel processing techniques generally do not attempt to analyze at the single motor unit level.

4.3.2.1 Amplitude Estimation

If the EMG is modeled as a stochastic process and EMG amplitude is defined as its time-varying standard deviation, then EMG amplitude estimation can be described mathematically as the task of best estimating

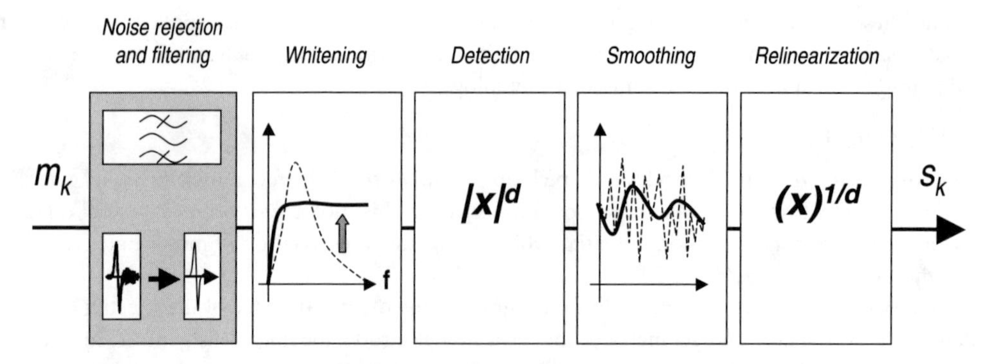

FIGURE 4.28 Block diagram of a single channel estimator of signal amplitude, including interference noise reduction and whitening of the signal. In the detection and relinearization phase d = 1 for ARV and d = 2 for RMS.

the standard deviation (RMS) of a colored random process in additive noise. This estimation problem has been studied for several years, with continuous improvement in amplitude estimation techniques. Historically, Inman et al. (1944) are credited with the first continuous EMG amplitude estimator. They implemented a full-wave rectifier followed by a resistor-capacitor low-pass filter.‡ Subsequent investigators studied the type of non-linear detector that should be applied to the waveform.

To improve amplitude estimation, especially in relation to estimation variance, a standard cascade of sequential processing stages can be used (Figure 4.28), which are (Clancy et al., 1994, 1999a, 1999b, 2000, 2002):

1. Noise and interference attenuation
2. Whitening
3. Demodulation
4. Smoothing
5. Relinearization

Noise and interference attenuation attempt to limit the adverse effects of motion artifacts, power line interference, etc. The correlation between neighboring EMG samples is a consequence of the limited signal bandwidth due to the low-pass filtering effects of the tissues as the signal field diffuses from its source to the measurement apparatus. Decorrelation, that is whitening, makes the samples statistically uncorrelated, increases the "statistical bandwidth," and reduces the variance of amplitude estimation. Demodulation rectifies the whitened EMG and then raises the result to a power (either 1 for *averaged rectified value* [*ARV*] or 2 for RMS). Smoothing filters the signal, increasing the signal-to-noise ratio, albeit at the expense of adding bias error to the estimate and time lag in the case of causal processors. Finally, relinearization inverts the power law applied during the demodulation stage, returning the signal to units of EMG amplitude.

Clinically, EMG amplitude is used to study muscle coordination and activation intervals. For example, EMG amplitude is used in gait analysis to determine when various muscles are active throughout the gait cycle. Various abnormalities (e.g., stroke, sport injuries) can cause alterations in muscular coordination.

4.3.2.2 Estimation of Muscle Activation Intervals

The estimation of on-off timing of human skeletal muscles during movement has important clinical applications (Craik and Oatis, 1994). The surface EMG signal is a useful means in this respect. In ideal cases of absence of noise and cross talk, the detection of the intervals of time during which the muscle is active would be a trivial task, based on a near zero threshold. In practical cases, the EMG signal recorded over a muscle contains additive noise. In non-stationary cases, such as during movement, the signal-to-noise ratio can considerably change in time since the muscle activity is changing while the noise remains

‡ They termed their processor an "integrator" — a misnomer they acknowledged in their original work. This incorrect term is still frequently used.

almost constant. As a consequence, the most crucial signal part is the beginning of the contraction, when the signal amplitude is low and the signal-to-noise ratio extremely poor. In these conditions the discrimination of EMG activity in noise is a complex signal processing task. In addition, crosstalk between nearby muscles may affect the indications on muscle activation intervals, since crosstalk can be misunderstood as co-activation. The problem of crosstalk reduction or identification is not yet solved, as already stated, thus the only possible solution to verify the presence or absence of crosstalk is to perform, prior to the measurement, voluntary selective contractions (if possible) of the muscles investigated and to check the absence of crosstalk in the signals recorded on the closely located muscles.

The problem of identification of muscle activity in noise has been addressed in the past in many different ways. The techniques, referred to as *single threshold methods*, are based on the comparison of the rectified raw signals and an amplitude threshold whose value depends on the mean power of the background noise. Other methods compare a low-pass filtered version of rectified data (the *signal envelope*) with a threshold based on the noise-related envelope. For this purpose, different types of filters have been proposed, leading to results difficult to compare. Methods based on the envelope time evolution, rather than on its instantaneous value, have been proposed. With these techniques, onset is detected when a weighted average of N consecutive samples overcomes a given threshold.

A more advanced approach has recently been proposed in Bonato et al. (1998), where two thresholds are applied on whitened data with the possibility of setting the probabilities of false-positive and of correct detection. This approach led to a bias on onset estimate lower than 10 ms with a standard deviation lower than 15 ms on phenomenologically simulated data with 8 dB SNR. Maximum likelihood methods such as cumulative sum, approximated generalized likelihood ratio, and approximated cumulative sum focus on abrupt changes of the variance of the whitened process by using no windowing, a sliding window, and two contiguous sliding windows, respectively. None of these methods can separate coactivation from cross talk; they provide indications about the presence of an EMG signal, as recognized in background noise. Figure 4.29 shows an example of detection of muscle activation intervals from surface EMG traces with two different algorithms (Merlo et al., 2003).

4.3.2.3 Spectral Analysis

4.3.2.3.1 Voluntary Contractions

The spectral analysis of the surface EMG signal has been applied to the study of muscle fatigue and of motor unit recruitment strategies. Piper (1912) first reported changes in the EMG power spectrum during maximal force contractions. Later, the changes in the spectral content of EMG signals were quantified by the centroid frequency, the median frequency, the ratio between the power of the signal in the low and high frequency bands (defined by a fixed threshold) (Stulen and De Luca, 1981) or different percentile frequencies.

The theoretical bases for the interpretation of the changes of EMG spectral content in light of the underlying physiological processes were provided by De Luca (1981), Lago and Jones (1977), and Lindström (1970). Lindström and Magnusson (1977) described the effect of the detection system on the spectrum of the recorded signal. Their theoretical predictions were later experimentally validated in many studies. Stulen and De Luca (1981) derived the theoretical relationships between the surface EMG power spectral density and the mean motor unit conduction velocity, indicating in this way the potential role of surface EMG spectral analysis in the objective quantification of muscle fatigue. The work by Lago and Jones (1977) clarified the effect of motor unit firing rate on the spectrum of the signal detected over the skin, and observed that different control strategies may influence the EMG spectrum.

After these pioneering works, many studies focused on the application of surface EMG spectral analysis for the investigation of muscle fatigue and motor control strategies. The experimental evidence provided by Arendt-Nielsen and Mills (1985) and Merletti et al. (1989, 1992) indicated that surface EMG spectral analysis provides reliable indications on muscle fatigue. The relevance of this application was demonstrated by the development of instruments (*fatigue monitors*) for real-time computation of spectral variables (Stulen and De Luca, 1982). Other studies showed the potential usefulness of spectral variables for the identification of recruitment modalities or for the estimation of the proportion between different types of muscle fibers (Sadoyama et al., 1988).

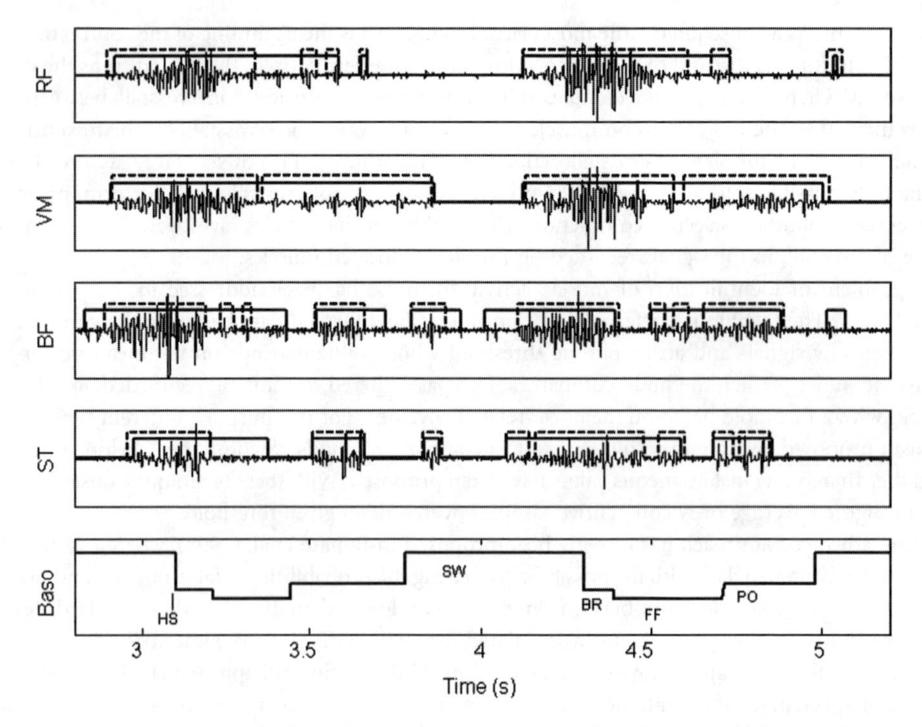

FIGURE 4.29 Surface EMG signals detected during the gait of a healthy subject from the rectus femoris, vastus medialis, biceps femoris, and semitendinosus muscles. A four-level coded basography (FF = Foot-Flat, PO = Push-Off, SW = SWing, BR = BRake, HS = Heel Strike), indicating the phases of the gait, is also shown (bottom trace). The activation intervals of the four muscles have been estimated by two algorithms. Solid line indicates the result of the algorithm developed by Merlo et al. (2003); dotted lines indicate those obtained with the algorithm developed by Bonato et al., 1998. Note how big the difference in the estimation can be when different algorithms are used. (From Merlo et al., 2003. With permission.)

The most commonly used method for the estimation of EMG power spectrum is the periodogram, defined by the square of the magnitude of the Fourier transform of the signal (Kay and Marple, 1981). If the signal is quasi-stationary, i.e., if the signal spectrum changes slowly with time, it is divided in epochs (which can overlap) and the spectrum is computed for each epoch with a short-time Fourier transform (*STFT*) (Cohen, 1989). If we consider a contraction of 60 s and we assume that the signal is approximately stationary within time intervals shorter than 1 s, it is sufficient to divide it into 60 epochs of 1 s each and compute for each of them the power spectrum. In this way, information localized in time and frequency are obtained. Of course, decreasing the window length determines an increase in spectral estimation variance and bias and a decrease of frequency resolution, thus it is not possible to indefinitely decrease the window length for improving the time resolution.

The spectral estimation from the signal epochs can also be performed by parametric methods (*autoregressive moving average*, or *ARMA*), based on the identification of a finite number of parameters. In this case, the signal is modeled as generated by filtering white noise with a filter with transfer function defined as the ratio between polynomial functions (thus it depends on a finite number of coefficients, given the degrees of the polynomials) (Kay and Marple, 1981). Among the parametric methods, the autoregressive techniques (*AR*) have been widely applied for surface EMG analysis with a model order in the range of 5 to 10. By windowing non-stationary signals and estimating an AR model in each window, a time varying AR (*TVAR*) analysis is obtained. For fatigue assessment, STFT and TVAR have been proven to be similarly sensitive to the window length and type and to provide similar information on the spectral changes assessed by mean and median frequencies. Figure 4.30 shows examples of spectrum estimation by different approaches.

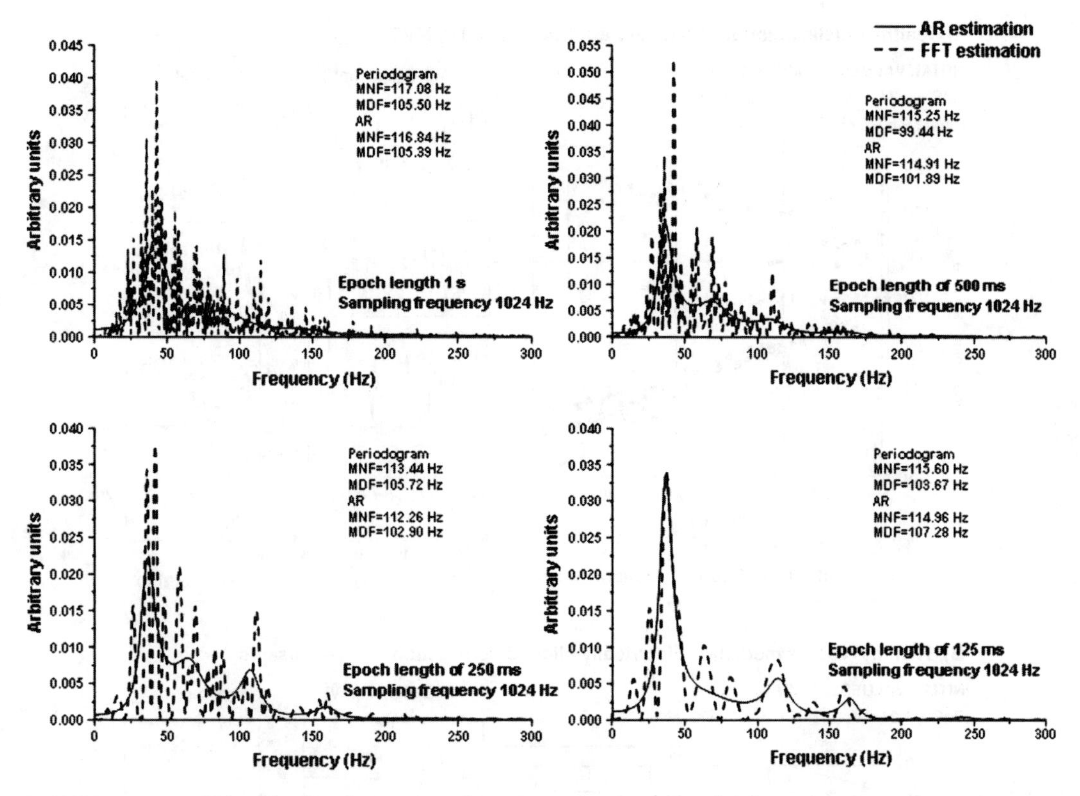

FIGURE 4.30 Examples of spectral estimation from EMG signal epochs of different lengths with periodogram-based and AR approaches. Note the difference in the estimation obtained by the two techniques but the very limited effect on characteristic frequencies. (From Farina, D. and Merletti, R., *J. Electromyogr. Kinesiol.*, 10, 327–336, 2000. With permission.)

The information provided by the power spectral density can be synthesized by a few variables. Among these, the most commonly used are the mean (*MNF*) and median (*MDF*) spectral frequencies, defined as the first-order spectral moment and as the frequency dividing the spectrum in two parts of equal power, respectively. Other spectral descriptors have been proposed, such as the percentile frequencies or an average of many percentile frequencies, spectral moments of higher order, etc.

4.3.2.3.2 Electrically Elicited Contractions

Electrically evoked signals may be considered deterministic and quasi-periodic signals with period determined by the stimulation frequency imposed by the stimulator. Each M-wave is a finite energy, finite duration signal whose frequency content can be described by the energy spectral density. During a sustained stimulated contraction the motor unit action potential properties change with time, in particular their conduction velocity (CV) decreases, determining changes in the M-wave. If only one value of conduction velocity was present (i.e., all the motor unit action potentials had the same conduction velocity and conduction velocity changes with time), then the M-wave would only change its scale with changing conduction velocity. Due to the distribution of conduction velocities among the motor units, the M-wave is not simply scaling with time but rather it is changing both shape and scale. However, usually changes of scale are monitored with the approximation of minor shape changes. The scale changes can be computed, as in the voluntary contraction case, by characteristic spectral frequencies. Figure 4.31 shows fatigue analyses during voluntary and electrically elicited contractions.

Since the EMG spectrum during electrically elicited contractions is used mainly for monitoring scale changes, other approaches to estimate a scale factor between deterministic signals provide similar indi-

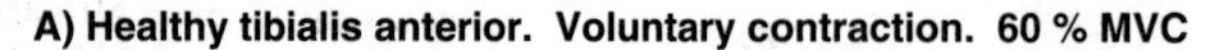

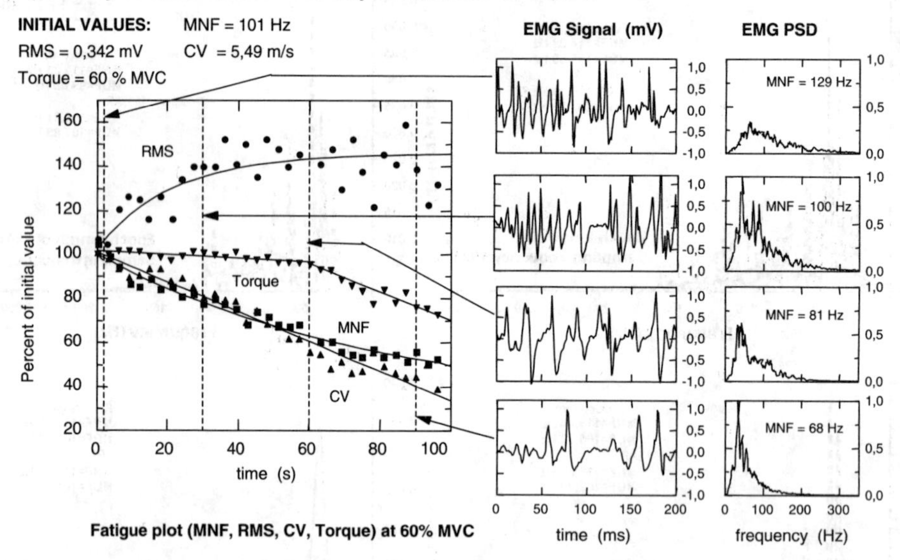

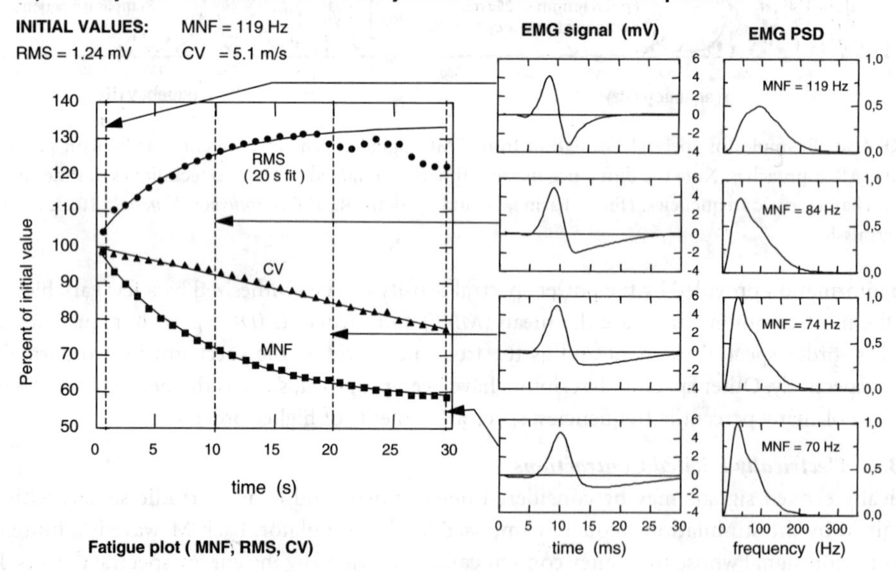

FIGURE 4.31 Example of spectral compression during a voluntary (a) and an electrically elicited contraction (b). Some signal epochs are shown together with the spectral estimations (with periodogram-based approach). All variables are normalized to their initial value to obtain the fatigue plot. Note the myoelectric manifestation of muscle fatigue, with a decrease in MNF and conduction velocity and an increase in RMS even at constant force level (PSD = power spectral density, RMS = root mean square value, MNF = mean frequency, CV = conduction velocity). (From Merletti, R. and Lo Conte, L.R., *J. Electromyogr. Kinesiol.*, 7, 241–250, 1997. With permission.)

cations. Among them, the distribution function method, the expansion in Hermite-Rodriguez functions, pseudo-joint delay-scale estimators, and maximum likelihood estimators of the scale factor have been proposed. In most cases, alternative approaches, based on the time domain analysis of the signal, have the advantage with respect to spectral analysis of being less sensitive to truncations of the M-waves due to high stimulation rates when the M-wave duration is larger than the stimulation period.

4.3.3 Surface EMG: Multichannel Processing

4.3.3.1 Estimation of Muscle Fiber Conduction Velocity

4.3.3.1.1 Two Channel-Based Methods for Conduction Velocity Estimation

Conduction velocity of the potentials propagating along the muscle fibers can be estimated non-invasively by computing the "average" delay between surface EMG signals detected at two different points along the fiber direction. A global estimation of conduction velocity is obtained if signal epochs are considered, as it is usually the case with surface recordings. Considering that there is a distribution of conduction velocities and thus a distribution of delays, the definition of a unique delay to characterize the detected signals is critical. Indeed, from a mathematical point of view we cannot strictly refer to delayed signals if they are not exactly the same and shifted in time. Thus, the delay between two EMG signals must be defined.

The most commonly used definition of delay between EMG signals is the time shift which, when applied to one of the two signals, minimizes the mean square error between the two. The cost function to be minimized is:

$$e_t(\hat{\theta}) = \sum_{n=1}^{N} \left[x_2(n+\hat{\theta}) - x_1(n) \right]^2 \tag{4.31}$$

where x_1 and x_2 are the two sampled signals from which the delay has to be estimated.

This definition corresponds to the maximum likelihood delay estimation between two signals with additive white gaussian noise (Farina et al., 2001b). This definition coincides with the delay of the maximum of the cross-correlation function often estimated using *spectral matching* (McGill and Dorfman, 1984; Merletti and Lo Conte, 1995), described below.

In the frequency domain, the mean square error (Equation 4.31) can be written as:

$$e_f(\hat{\theta}) = \frac{2}{N} \sum_{k=1}^{N/2} \left| X_2(k) e^{j2\pi k\hat{\theta}/N} - X_1(k) \right|^2 \tag{4.32}$$

where N is the number of samples in the signal epoch, and $X_1(k)$, $X_2(k)$ are the Fourier transforms of the two signals. As a consequence of the Parseval's theorem, it follows that $e_t(\hat{\theta}) = e_f(\hat{\theta})$, thus, Equations 4.31 and 4.32 are equivalent. However, using Equation 4.32, $\hat{\theta}$ is not limited to be a multiple of the sampling interval but rather can be selected as any real value. The temporal resolution is, thus, in principle not limited if Equation 4.32 is used instead of Equation 4.31. The problem is solved by finding the minimum of $e_f(\hat{\theta})$ with an iterative algorithm which converges to the optimal point in a few iterations by finding the zero of its first derivative using a gradient method, that is starting from a coarse estimation of the delay and updating this estimate moving along the gradient direction (McGill and Dorfman, 1984).

The normalized cross-correlation function of the two signals from which the delay is estimated is given by:

$$\rho_{1,2}(\tau) = \frac{\sum_{n=1}^{N} x_2(n+\tau) x_1(n)}{\sqrt{\sum_{n=1}^{N} x_1^2(n) \sum_{n=1}^{N} x_2^2(n)}} = \frac{R_{1,2}(\tau)}{\sigma_1 \sigma_2} = \frac{1}{2\sigma_1\sigma_2} \left[\sigma_1^2 + \sigma_2^2 - e_t(\tau) \right] \tag{4.33}$$

where e_t is given by Equation 4.31. Thus, the minimum of the mean square error (in time or frequency domain) corresponds to the maximum of the cross-correlation function.

Other approaches have been proposed to estimate the delay between two surface EMG signals, among them the *phase method* and the *distribution function method*.

4.3.3.1.2 Multichannel-Based Methods for Conduction Velocity Estimation

If more than two signals detected along the fiber direction are available, new delay estimators can be defined on the basis of the alignment of all the available signals. Assuming that the systems used to detect the EMG signals are placed between the innervation zone and tendon region, then, ideally, all the detected signals are equal in shape but delayed. If the electrodes are equally spaced, in ideal conditions of pure propagation without shape changes, the delay between adjacent signals is constant and its maximum likelihood estimation is the minimization of the sum of the mean square errors between each signal assumed as the reference and the other signals aligned (Farina et al., 2001b):

$$e_{MLE} = \sum_{k=1}^{K} \sum_{n=1}^{N} \left[x_k(n) - \frac{1}{K} \sum_{m=1}^{K} x_m(n + (m-k)\theta) \right]^2 \quad (4.34)$$

where N is the number of samples in the signal epoch considered. Equation 4.34 is the generalization of Equation 4.31 to the case of any number of channels. Again, the mean square error can be minimized in the frequency domain with iterative algorithms. Figure 4.32 shows the comparison between two- and multichannel estimators of conduction velocity.

Other methods for multichannel conduction velocity estimation are based on beamforming technique (i.e., the best alignment corresponds to the minimum mean square error between the aligned waveforms and a reference waveform) or on the assumption of possible changes between the delay along the detecting array.

4.3.3.2 Estimation of Motor Unit Conduction Velocity Distribution

The methods previously described for the estimation of muscle fiber conduction velocity from surface EMG signals imply the assessment of the mean value of conduction velocity of the active motor units. The estimation of the distribution of conduction velocities of the active motor units is certainly preferred but implies the separation, in the interference surface EMG signal, of the contributions of the different motor units and the estimation of the velocity of propagation of each of them. Techniques based on deconvolution approaches have been proposed (Davies and Parker, 1987). However, these methods still have many limitations in practical applications. Other methods, based on the identification of each motor unit action potential in the signal, have been proposed (Farina et al., 2000b) and applied in basic physiological investigations. These methods have the great disadvantage of being limited by the superposition of the waveforms, i.e., the detection of the motor unit action potential is limited to the highest energy waveforms which thus bias the distribution estimation. The application of spatial sampling and filtering methods provides in this case a powerful detection method for improving source separation and thus limit the problem of waveform superimposition.

4.3.3.3 Decomposition of Multichannel Surface EMG Signals

Techniques for the decomposition of the surface EMG signals into its constituent motor unit action potential trains are being developed and preliminary applications have been shown (Gazzoni et al., 2001; Kleine et al., 1999, 2001). The approaches followed are usually similar to those used for intramuscular EMG signal decomposition and are based on a segmentation and a classification phase. However, in case of surface EMG signals, the number of superimpositions is much higher than in the case of intramuscular signals due to the low spatial resolution of the technique. Thus, complete firing patterns cannot be obtained from surface EMG decomposition by simple segmentation/classification schemes. It is clear that the detection technique is in these cases of primary importance for successful decomposition. Spatial filters allow the reduction of the number of contributions detected. The use of spatial sampling, on the other hand, increases the information for the classification of the contributions by providing different views, from many points in space, of the same potentials. Information, such as motor unit activation instants and recruitment, can be extracted by these methods in particular conditions and can be used for non-invasively obtaining information about single motor unit control properties (Figure 4.33). More advanced approaches are currently under development with the aim of overcoming the problem of potential overlapping.

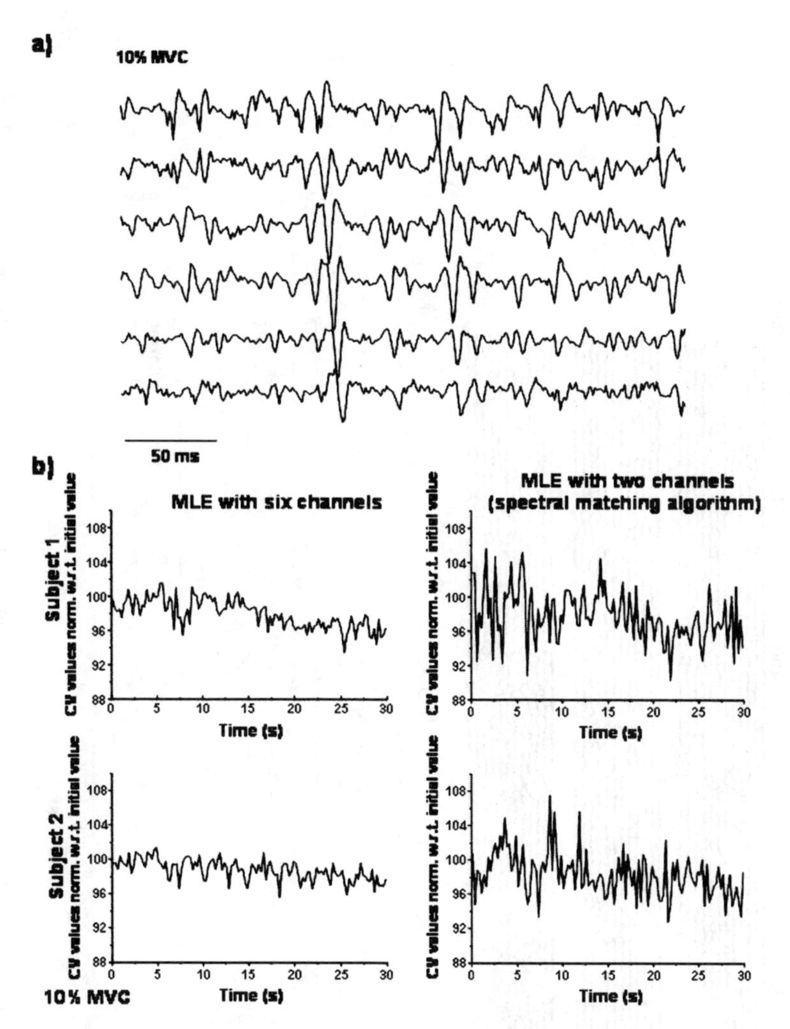

FIGURE 4.32 (a) Example of a multichannel EMG signal detected from the biceps brachii muscle at 10% MVC. (b) Estimations of mean muscle fiber conduction velocity from two subjects during a contraction of the same type of that shown in (a). The estimations obtained using two and six surface EMG channels are shown. Note the reduction in estimation variance by increasing the number of channels. Estimates are normalized with respect to the initial values. (From Farina, D., Muhammad, W., Fortunato, E., Meste, O., Merletti, R., and Rix, H., *Med. Biol. Eng. Comput.*, 39, 225–236, 2001b. With permission.)

4.3.4 Surface EMG for the Control of Powered Prostheses

The use of the surface EMG signal as the input signal to control powered prostheses has found applications for individuals with amputations or congenitally deficient upper limbs. The idea is to control the prosthesis by the activity of a muscle that can be controlled by the subject (see Section 4.2.3.6.5).

The simplest processing algorithms for the control of prostheses are based on the estimation of the EMG signal amplitude. A function of the prosthesis is in this case associated to a set of amplitude levels. The performance will depend on the number of levels and on the type of estimator used for amplitude calculation. Methods to reduce the variance of amplitude estimation have been described in Section 4.3.2.1 and in this type of application play a very important role. Moreover, increasing the number of EMG channels, i.e., locating more than one electrode pair over the muscle, variance of amplitude estimation is further reduced.

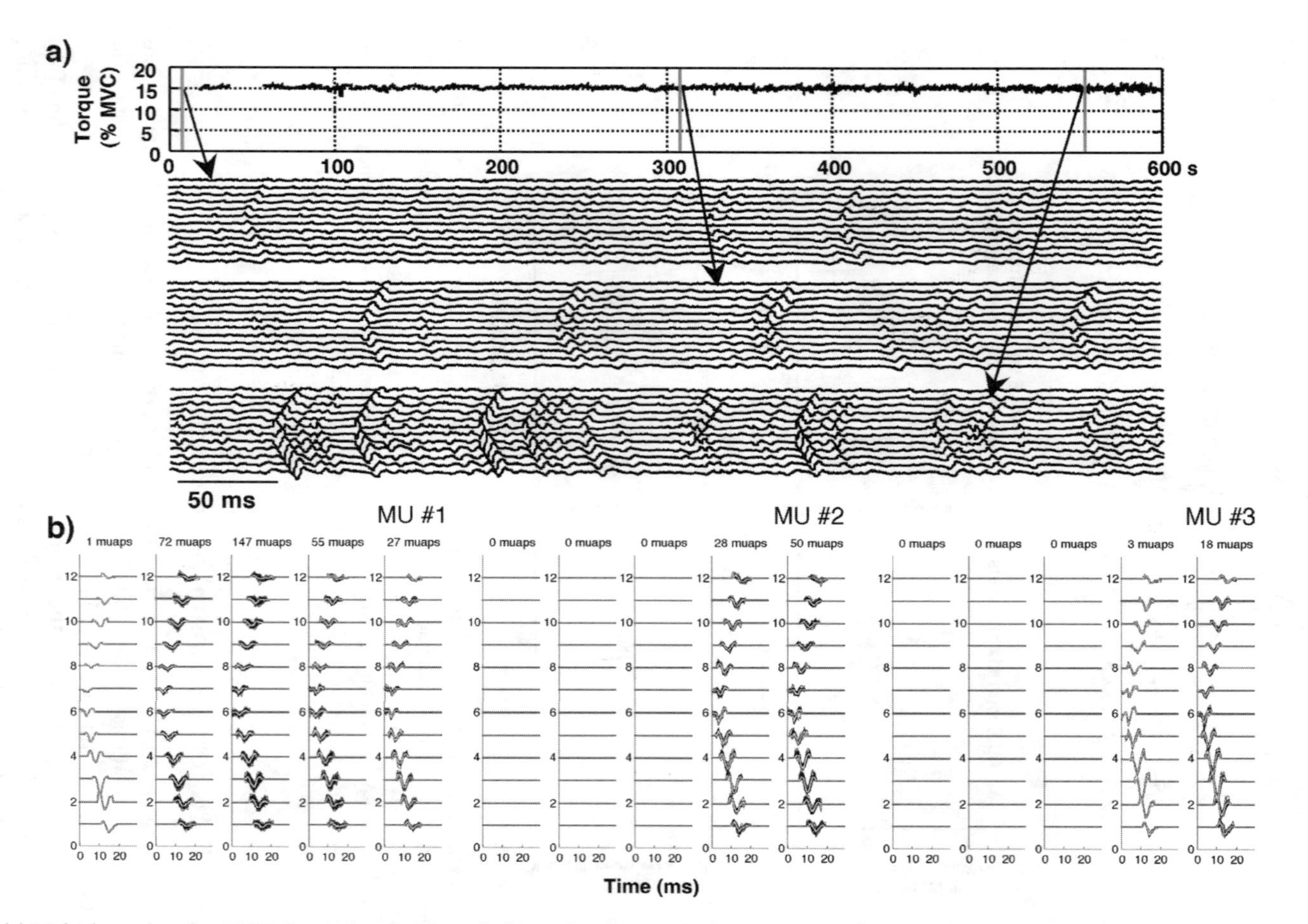

FIGURE 4.33 (a) Multichannel surface EMG signals detected from the biceps brachii muscle during a 10-min-long contraction at 15% MVC. (b) Decomposition and classification of motor unit action potentials from three motor units, extracted from the signals shown in (a). All the firings of the same motor units are superimposed in five 2-min epochs. It can be observed that motor unit #1 is active from the beginning of the contraction, while motor units #2 and #3 are recruited at the end of the contraction. (From Gazzoni, M., Farina, D., and Merletti, R., *Acta Physiol. Pharmacol. Bulg.*, 26(1–2), 67–71, 2001. With permission.)

More complex algorithms are based on the recognition of a pattern in the surface EMG signal rather than on the estimation of the level of muscle activity. The identification of patterns is based on the building of feature sets that are able to distinguish between different types of muscle activation. Commonly used feature sets are based on the coefficient of ARMA models which can be computed from a single or multi-channel EMG recording.

4.3.5 Joint Intramuscular and Surface Recordings

4.3.5.1 Control and Conduction Properties of Single Motor Units

As appears from the brief review provided on the methods for information extraction from EMG signals, it is possible to extract from intramuscular signals control properties of single motor units, while from surface recordings it is feasible to estimate the peripheral properties of the neuromuscular system. The two techniques thus provide different information about the muscle contraction. The control and peripheral properties of the neuromuscular system are, however, strictly related and techniques for their joint analysis are certainly useful in many applications.

One possible approach is to record both intramuscular and surface EMG signals using the intramuscularly detected potentials as triggers to obtain single motor unit action potentials, at the surface, from which to estimate the conduction velocity. Techniques of this type have been applied and proposed in the past. Recently, Farina et al. (2002d) combined advanced methods for intramuscular signal detection (multichannel wire detection) and surface EMG detection (multichannel arrays) with reliable methods for conduction velocity estimation, providing a joint technique for reliable assessment of motor unit conduction and control properties. Figure 4.34 reports single motor unit control and conduction property analysis from joint intramuscular and surface recordings.

4.3.5.2 Estimation of Motor Unit Depth and Size

With the use of multichannel surface EMG recordings triggered by the intramuscularly detected motor unit action potentials it is possible to estimate motor unit size (Roeleveld, 1997a) (with results similar to those obtained by macro EMG) and depth (Roeleveld, 1997b). These methods are based on the distribution of the electric potential over the skin in the direction perpendicular to the muscle fibers, rather than longitudinal. The transversal decrease of signal amplitude is related to the depth of the motor unit which can thus be estimated (within large approximations) and motor unit action potential amplitude can be compensated by the estimated depth in order to reflect only the motor unit size.

4.4. Applications of EMG in Basic Research and Clinical Routine

4.4.1 Fundamentals of Clinical EMG

4.4.1.1 Intramuscular Electrode Placement

Characterization of the distribution of the shapes of the motor unit action potentials of each active motor unit is required in order to recognize detected motor unit action potentials. This consequently requires that motor unit action potentials of each motor unit are individually detected (i.e., not in superposition with the motor unit action potentials of any other motor units) several times. This places constraints on methods and protocols for detecting decomposable EMG signals. Thus, the peak level of force is often below 50% of maximal voluntary contraction (MVC). However, signal complexity at a certain %MVC level of contraction is related to a number of physiological factors such as the number of motor units in the muscle, the muscle fiber diameter, the density of motor unit muscle fibers, the motor unit recruitment thresholds, and the motor unit rate coding strategies. When compared with larger muscles such as the biceps brachii, smaller muscles such as the first dorsal interosseous have fewer motor units, tend to have a narrower range of recruitment thresholds, and use large amounts of rate coding. Therefore, for comparable %MVC contractions, smaller muscles will on average generate more complex signals than signals

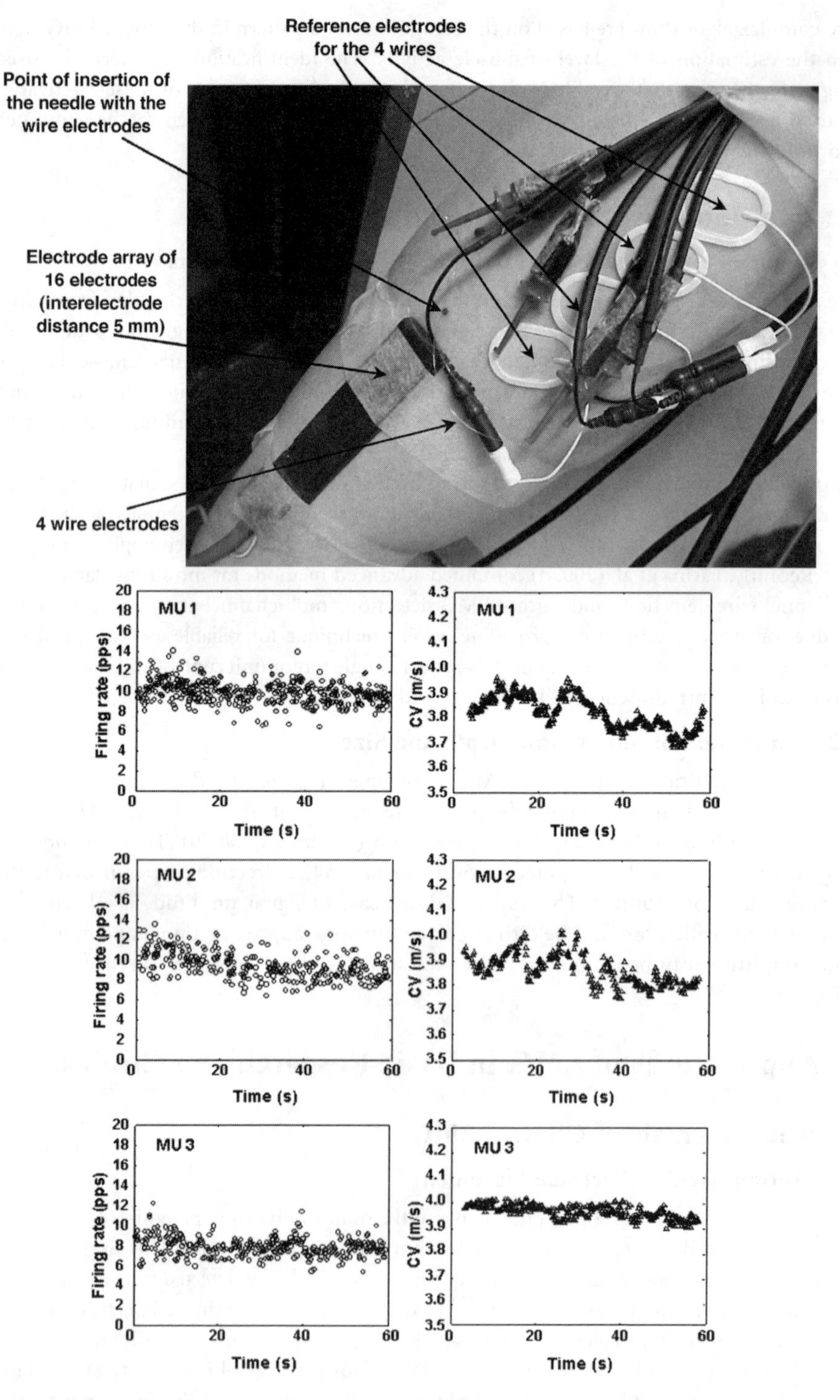

FIGURE 4.34 (a) Joint detection of intramuscular and multichannel surface EMG signals from the tibialis anterior muscle. (b) Estimation of instantaneous firing rate and conduction velocity from three motor units whose activity was detected during a voluntary contraction of the tibialis anterior muscle at 25% MVC with intramuscular and surface recordings (firing rate estimated from intramuscular recordings and conduction velocity from the surface recordings). (Adapted from Farina, D., Arendt-Nielsen, L., Merletti, R., and Graven-Nielsen, T., *J. Neurosci. Meth.*, 115, 1–12, 2002. With permission.)

detected in larger muscles. In addition, the need to minimize needle movement usually requires that the rate of change of force be less than 10% MVC/sec.

In the case of wire recordings, the problems due to the movement of the muscle when contracting are less important than with needle detection. However, it is usually more difficult to correctly place the electrodes since it is not possible to monitor the signals while the electrodes are moved in the muscle. For this reason it is highly recommended, when wire detection is used, to insert more than one wire per needle. This will enhance the likelihood of detecting at least one signal from which the desired characteristics can be obtained.

4.4.1.2 Fundamentals of Clinical Practice in Surface EMG

The massive use of intramuscular EMG techniques in past years has led to a well established clinical practice. Unfortunately, this is not true in surface EMG, where common fallacies, especially about electrode placement issues, still exist (Hermens et al., 1999).

4.4.1.2.1 Electrode Placement

In Section 4.2.3.2 some characteristics of the skin-electrode contact for proper EMG recording have been highlighted. They are: a repeatable, stable over time, and as low as possible contact impedance, a stable value of the half-cell potential (little motion artifacts) and the lowest possible intrinsic noise of the equipment, lower than that generated by the electrode-skin interface.

The above features can be obtained by a correct selection of the electrode type and a proper treatment of the skin prior to the application of the electrode. Additional constraints should be taken into account when evaluating the proper size and interelectrode distance (in case of bipolar or multichannel recordings), since geometrical factors greatly affect the features of the acquired signals by introducing filtering effects. Finally, provisions for a correct location on the muscle must be considered in order to attain a proper recording of surface motor unit action potentials. A summary of the issues that must be taken into account for proper EMG recording is reported in Table 4.2.

In clinical applications with bipolar electrodes, it is somewhat common practice to apply the electrodes over the muscle belly or on the endplate, in order to maximize the signal amplitude. This, however, is a fallacy, as this position is highly sensitive to shifts of the innervation zone, which can produce dips in the amplitude of the signals and strong alterations of the shape of the motor unit action potentials and their spectral content (Farina et al., 2001a). Locating the electrodes in between the endplate and the tendon is recommended.

TABLE 4.2 Issues That Play a Major Role in a Correct Acquisition of Surface EMG Signal

Aspects of Electrode Selection and Placing	Desired Function or Parameters to Take into Account
Manufacturing technology	Low contact impedance
	Low motion artifacts
	Low contact noise
	Good mechanical adherence to the skin
Skin treatment	Low value of contact impedance
	Stability of impedance over time
Electrode dimensions	Usability on the selected muscle
	Filtering effect of the electrode (spatial filtering)
Detection technique	Selectivity
	Insensitivity to external interferences
	Insensitivity to crosstalk
	Filtering effect of the detection technique (spatial sampling)
Electrode placement	Minimal sensitivity w.r.t. muscle geometry (i.e., innervation zone)
	Minimal alteration of motor unit action potentials due to movement
	Maximum amplitude of the signal
Signal acquisition	Selection of correct bandpass and gain
	Selection of correct sampling frequency

TABLE 4.3 Summary Table of SENIAM Recommendations

Parameter	Recommended Value or Condition
Electrodes (bipolar montage)	
Electrode size	Diameter < 10 mm
Interelectrode distance (IED)	< 20 mm or < 1/4 the muscle length, whichever is smaller
Electrode location	Between the most distal innervation zone and the distal tendon or between the most proximal innervation zone and the proximal tendon; not over an innervation zone
Reference electrode location	Wrist, ankle, processus spinosus of C7, or other electrically inactive area
Amplifier	
High-pass filter (low frequency cut-off)	
for EMG spectral analysis	< 10 Hz
for movement analysis only	10–20 Hz
Low-pass filter (high frequency cut-off)	
for general applications	~ 500 Hz (sampling frequency > 1000 samples/s)
for special wide band applications	~ 1000 Hz (sampling frequency > 2000 samples/s)
Input referred voltage noise level	< 1 μV_{RMS} (in the 10–500 Hz bandwidth)
Input referred current noise level	< 10 pA_{RMS} (in the 10–500 Hz bandwidth)
Input impedance	> 100 MΩ (for conventional electrodes) > 1000 MΩ (for pasteless "dry" pin electrodes)
Gain	suitable to bring the signal into the input range of the A/D converter with desired input resolution
Sampler and A/D converter	
Sampling frequency	> 1000 samples/s (general applications) > 2000 samples/s (wide band applications)
Number of bits of A/D	12 (requires amplifier with variable gain) 16 (fixed gain amplifiers may be used)

Despite the large number of scientific papers on the topic, the issue of a correct EMG detection that takes into account all the above issues is still poorly understood. Considerable effort came from the European Community within the European Concerted Action SENIAM (Hermens et al., 1999), whose aim was to deliver recommendations for a correct clinical procedure in surface EMG assessment. A summary of these recommendations is reported in Table 4.3.

4.4.1.2.2 Crosstalk

When the issue of electrode placement is considered, cross talk should also be taken into account. As already stated, the issue of cross talk in surface EMG signal detection is far from being completely understood and only a few studies can be found in the literature with the aim of investigating cross talk. Almost no studies are present on the problem of cross talk in relation to electrode placement, even if it is common experience, for large muscles, to identify electrode locations that lead to smaller crosstalk signals than others. To assess cross talk in cases where more sophisticated detection techniques are lacking, it is recommended, after electrode placement, to ask the subject to perform selective voluntary movements (or at least movements in which mainly one muscle is involved) and to record from different muscles to qualitatively validate the absence of cross talk. If crosstalk results are not at acceptable levels, it is recommended to change electrode location, when possible.

4.4.1.2.3 Skin Treatment

Once the electrode type has been selected, a proper skin treatment can greatly enhance the quality of the recording. Although common practice in clinical routines, cleaning the surface with alcohol does not provide substantial improvement of the skin-electrode contact, at least with silver–silver chloride recessed-type electrodes. A light abrasion with standard ECG abrasive paste, or "stripping" the skin with

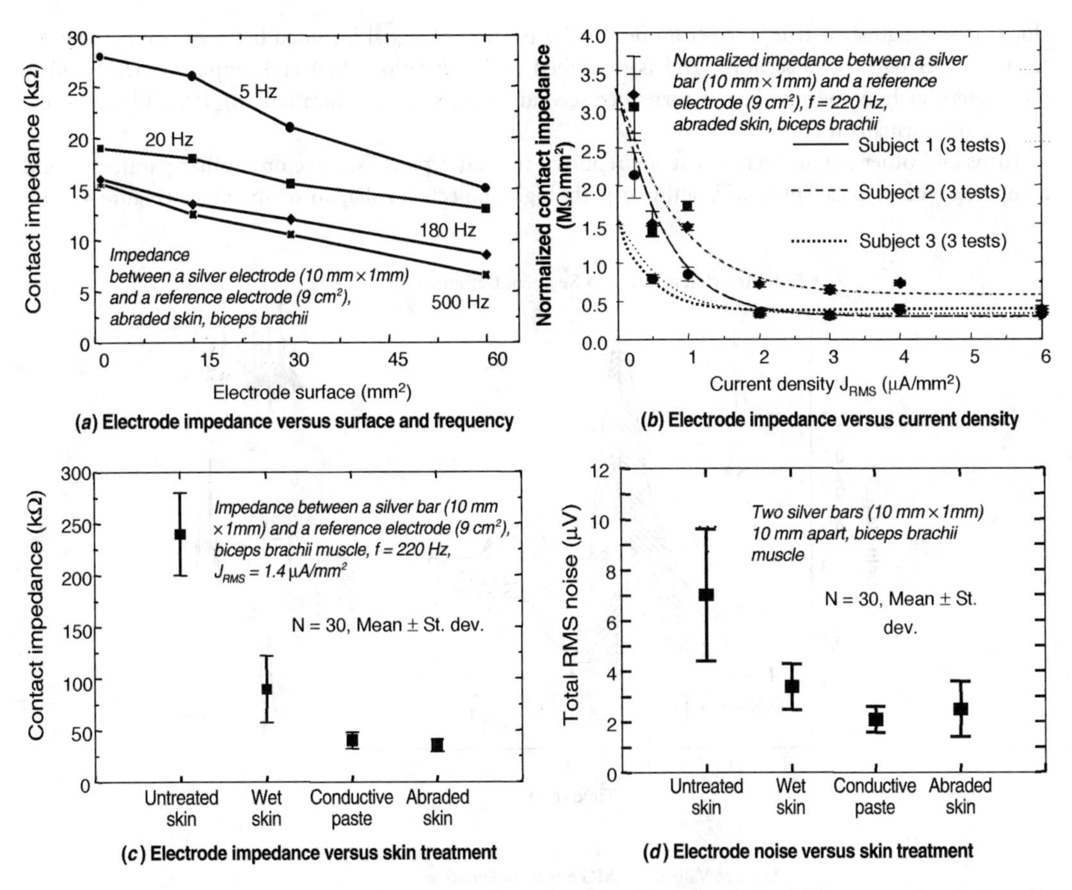

FIGURE 4.35 Evaluations of skin-electrode impedance (magnitude) and noise in different experimental conditions with silver electrodes. (a) Impedance as a function of surface and frequency; (b) impedance as a function of current density; (c and d) impedance and noise with different skin treatments. (Data kindly provided by Bottin, A., Politecnico di Torino, Torino, Italy.)

adhesive tape helps to remove the most superficial layer of dead cells, with advantages both in terms of impedance and noise (Figure 4.35c and 4.35d).

4.4.2 Basic and Clinical Applications of EMG

Many methods for information extraction from both intramuscular and surface EMG signals have been developed in the last decades, some of which found wide application in the clinical field, while others remain confined in research laboratories. However, applications of EMG (and, in particular, surface EMG, whose non-invasivity is particularly attractive) are finding growing interest in clinical routine, sport and occupational medicine, mainly due to improvements undergone by the equipment and the signal processing techniques in the last years. This section will give a very short overview of the main analysis methods used in basic research and in clinical applications. The interested reader can refer to the references provided for more details.

4.4.2.1 Intramuscular EMG

4.4.2.1.1 Turns and Amplitude

The *turns and amplitude* (T&A) method has been extensively used, with some refinements, during the past 20 years for the analysis of intramuscular EMG (Fuglsang-Frederiksen, 1981). A *turn* in the EMG signal is defined by a change in the slope, with some special features (e.g., the maximum and minimum slope) to distinguish a "true" turn from noise. The portion of signal included between two subsequent turns is referred to as a *segment*, and is described by its duration (*SD*) and amplitude (*SA*). Other parameters such as the number of turns per second, mean segment duration (*MSD*), and amplitude (*MSA*) are normally used.

Turns and other parameters are usually reported in scatter plots vs. force or another parameter, and compared with "typical" plots of healthy or pathologic subjects for diagnostic inference (Figure 4.36).

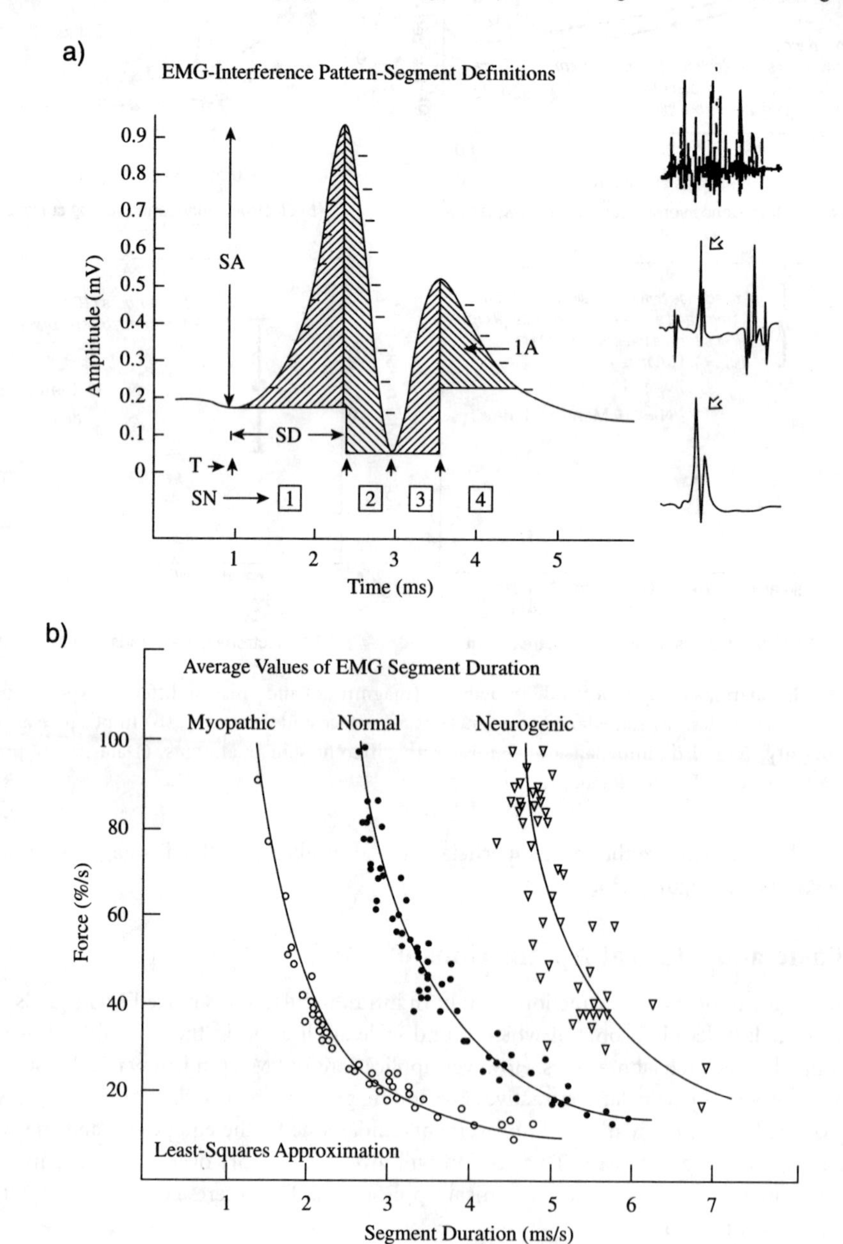

FIGURE 4.36 Turns and amplitude method. (a) Definition of parameters for turns. In the insets on the right, short epochs of EMG signals are shown. A turn (T) is defined as a polarity reversal. Turns identify the beginning and end of a segment, of duration SD, amplitude SA, and integrated area IA. Each of these parameters can be computed as a mean value per unit of time. (b) Plot of mean segment duration (on the abscissa) versus rate of force increase in healthy and pathological subjects. (From Gilai, A.N., Analysis of turns and amplitude in EMG, in *Computer-Aided Electromyography and Expert Systems*, Desmedt, J.E., Ed., Elsevier, New York, 1989. With permission.)

4.4.2.1.2 Macro EMG and Scanning EMG

As already indicated in Section 4.3.1.3, the *macro EMG* technique (Stålberg, 1980) consists of the use of a modified single fiber EMG (*SFEMG*) needle, where the body of the needle is exposed and acts as a macro electrode, its acquisition triggered by the SFEMG signal (Figure 4.8).

Clinical routine usually requires recordings of at least 20 *macro motor unit action potentials*, obtained at different depths and with 2–5 different needle insertions, while the muscle is activated at 30% or less of its maximal force. Peak-to-peak and area of the macro motor unit action potential are then evaluated and compared against reference values of healthy subjects, reported for different muscles and ages (Stålberg and Fawcett, 1982).

Another technique that relies on the triggering technique is *scanning EMG*, which provides an electrophysiological cross-section of a motor unit (Stålberg and Antoni, 1980). The recording method makes use of two intramuscular electrodes: a single fiber electrode for triggering and a concentric electrode for acquisition, inserted at least 2 cm away and in the direction of the fibers. The muscle is voluntarily activated at 30% MVC force or less.

The concentric electrode is then connected to a mechanic linear actuator, controlled by the acquisition system; after triggered recording and averaging of some potentials at each site, the concentric electrode is pulled in steps of 50 μm or multiples, so that a corridor of about 20 mm of length is investigated.

Analysis of the scanning EMG consists of visual interpretation of the graphics obtained, where the averaged motor unit action potentials are plotted with respect to their spatial distribution.

4.4.2.1.3 Intramuscular EMG Decomposition

Decomposition of the intramuscular EMG signals is a very powerful technique for in-depth studies down to motor unit level, allowing the evaluation of motor unit recruitment strategy and firing rate; for this reason it is extensively used in basic physiological studies. This technique gives consistent results in case of moderate interference pattern, i.e., at low force level, while it may take considerable processing time or even fail in highly interferent EMG signals.

In clinical practice the decomposition of intramuscular signals has still limited applications, due to the difficulties in electrode placement and the long processing time.

4.4.2.1.4 Compound Muscle Action Potential (CMAP) and Motor Nerve Conduction (MNC)

An approach for the assessment of peripheral nerve pathologies is the electrical stimulation of the motor nerves while detecting the electrically elicited surface EMG response of the muscle; the resulting signal is the M-wave or *compound muscle action potential* (*CMAP*), composed by the synchronized summation of all the innervated and recruited motor units (Desmedt, 1989).

CMAP amplitude is also used for the diagnosis of diseases like myastenia gravis and Lambert-Eaton myastenic syndrome, where both axons and muscle fibers are normal, but impulse transmission at the neuromuscular junctions may fail. In myastenia gravis, repeated electrical stimulation results in abnormal CMAP amplitude decrease, while in Lambert-Eaton's myastenic syndrome (*LEMS*) patients the effect is an increased amplitude after repeated stimulation.

An important diagnostic parameter is the *motor nerve conduction* (*MNC*) velocity, calculated by the ratio of distance between the stimulation and detection electrodes and time shift between stimulation and elicited response. Abnormally low values of this parameter may reveal axonal damage or nerve demyelination. The measurement is usually performed by stimulation of two points along the nerve path and dividing their distance by the difference between the two delays. This approach eliminates the delay due to neuromuscular junction and muscle conduction velocity.

4.4.2.1.5 Fourier Analysis

The Fourier analysis of EMG signal consists of the evaluation of its global spectral parameters usually during fatiguing isometric contractions at a constant-force level.

Of particular interest are the initial value of the median (*MDF*) and mean (*MNF* or *MPF*) frequencies of the power spectrum, and their slope (rate of decrease with respect to time), since they have been demonstrated to be related to conduction velocity and, in turn, fiber type composition, both in experimental studies and with mathematical models (see, for example, Lindström [1970]).

The result of an EMG Fourier analysis is the so-called *fatigue plot* or *muscle fatigue pattern* (Figure 4.31), where the relative change of conduction velocity, amplitude, and spectral parameters vs. time is represented.

This type of examination can then be advantageously used in the assessment of muscle diseases which is reflected in an abnormal fiber type composition (abnormal predominance of type II fibers, high muscle fatiguability) or congenital myopathy (abnormal predominance of type I fibers). Despite its numerous advantages, however, its use is still not completely accepted in diagnostic routine.

Studies by Roy et al. (1989) demonstrated a correlation between back pain and higher initial values of MNF and steeper slope, suggesting the application of this technique to the study of musculoskeletal disorders. In the last years, surface electromyography has been extensively used in ergonomics and occupational medicine for the assessment of work-related pathologies deriving, for example, from repetitive monotonous work.

EMG spectral analysis also finds applications in sports medicine, as a tool for providing fatigue indexes and rough indications about fiber type composition. Thus, it can advantageously be used for the validation of specific trainings that privilege the strengthening of a specific type of fibers (e.g., type I, fatigue-resistance fibers in endurance runners and type II, fast-twitch fibers in sprinters and weight lifters) (Felici et al., 2001; Sadoyama et al., 1988). The technique is expected to be of help in the evaluation of musculoskeletal disorders related to fiber types.

4.4.2.1.6 Multichannel Surface EMG and Measurements of Conduction Velocity

A typical example of multichannel surface EMG signals (SD detection) acquired from a healthy subject is shown in Figure 4.37a; it is possible to note the typical V-shaped patterns, reflecting the phenomena of motor unit action potential generation at the endplate and propagation toward the tendons.

The estimation of the width of the innervation zone is indeed a useful clinical tool to reveal pathologies such as primary myopathies, where the spread of motor endplates tends to an abnormally extended endplate region.

Also, multichannel surface EMG allows the high accuracy measurement of muscle conduction velocity (Farina et al., 2000b), a powerful diagnostic tool for basic physiological studies (as this parameter is related to fiber type) and in clinical applications. Patients with lower motoneuron disease, Duchenne dystrophy, and congenital myopathies show an abnormal range of conduction velocity values when compared to that of healthy subjects (Figure 4.37b and c) (Desmedt, 1989). Figure 4.38a and c show a multichannel recording from the biceps brachii of a myotonic subject attempting to hold a constant contraction level. Muscle performance deteriorates rapidly and force decreases (not shown in Figure 4.38) because muscle fiber conduction properties change. As shown in Figure 4.38a, action potentials propagate for a progressively shorter distance, the contractile mechanisms are no longer excited and force decreases despite the recruitment of new motor units. Figure 4.38c is a zoom of Figure 4.38a. If a healthy subject is asked to mimic the same force pattern, the decrement of force is obtained through de-recruitment of motor units and reduced firing rate, as indicated in Figure 4.38b and d. Figure 4.38d is a zoom of Figure 4.38b (Drost et al., 2001).

A growing interest in the use of multichannel surface EMG has been observed in the last years. The method is non-invasive, and gives information about global muscle physiology and, with some limitations, on single motor unit properties. On the other hand, it can only be applied to superficial muscles having parallel fibers.

Besides arrays, other electrode montages such as bi-dimentional grids have been developed in the last years and are finding applications in the assessment of muscle pathologies.

4.4.2.1.7 Surface EMG Decomposition

Decomposition of surface EMG signals is indeed a very challenging issue for the limited selectivity of the detection method with respect to intramuscular EMG. Besides non-invasivity, application of decomposition to multichannel surface EMG has the great advantage of allowing estimation of single motor unit conduction velocity, which permits in-depth investigations of recruitment strategies in relationship

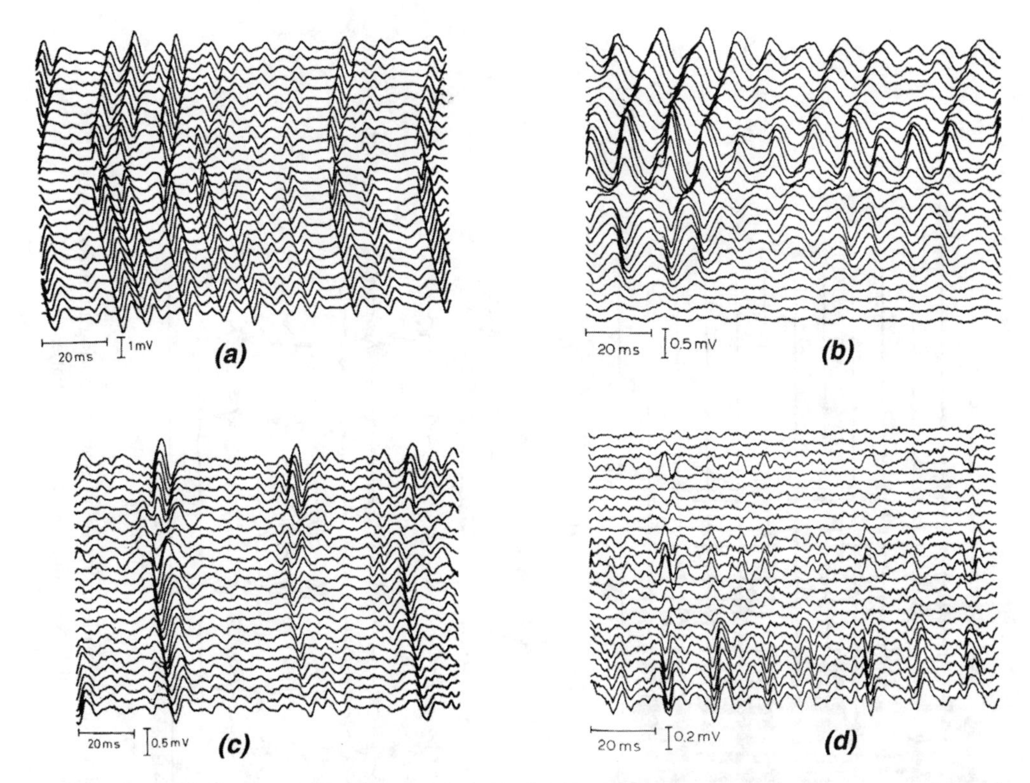

FIGURE 4.37 Multichannel surface EMG signal acquired with 2.5-mm interelectrode distance array from biceps brachii muscle during voluntary contraction. (a) Healthy subject; (b) patient affected by Duchenne dystrophy: the motor unit action potentials appear to be wider and slower in propagation; (c) patient affected by lower motoneuron disease: the conduction velocity of the motor unit action potentials is higher than in control subjects; (d) patient affected by progressive muscular dystrophy (limb girdle type): no propagating patterns can be observed. (From Meyer, M., Hilfiker, P., and Gygi, A., Surface EMG for diagnosis of neuromuscular diseases, in *Computer-Aided Electromyography and Expert Systems*, Desmedt, J.E., Ed., Elsevier, New York, 1989. With permission.)

to peripheral physiological features (i.e., fiber type and size) (Kleine et al., 2000). Although this technique needs further improvements and validation, it is certainly promising for clinical applications.

4.4.2.1.8 Movement and Gait Analysis

In kinesiologic applications a global indication of activity of different muscles is of greater interest than a detailed insight into a single muscle. Bipolar surface EMG detection is by far the preferred technique because it is non-invasive, less sensitive to movement than intramuscular detection, and gives a more global indication of the muscle activity, more directly correlated to the mechanical outcome.

Electrode pairs are placed on each muscle in an active area between tendon and the innervation zone (which can shift under the skin with movement [Farina et al., 2001a]). During the electrode placement phase, a preliminary evaluation of muscle geometry, using of a surface EMG array, can be of great help in finding the best position.

The issue of crosstalk is of special concern in this application, and the operator should be aware of methods for proper electrode placement that reduce this adverse effect.

Electromyographic data is then used to provide muscle activation times and intensity, usually by means of the "envelope" of the EMG signal. One example of application is the evaluation of pathological co-contraction of antagonist muscles, resulting in joint stiffness, observed in pathological (e.g., spastic) subjects during gait (Figure 4.39).

This information is often integrated with kinematic and dynamic quantities coming from additional sensors, such as joint angle sensors, soles for measurements of ground reaction forces and pressure

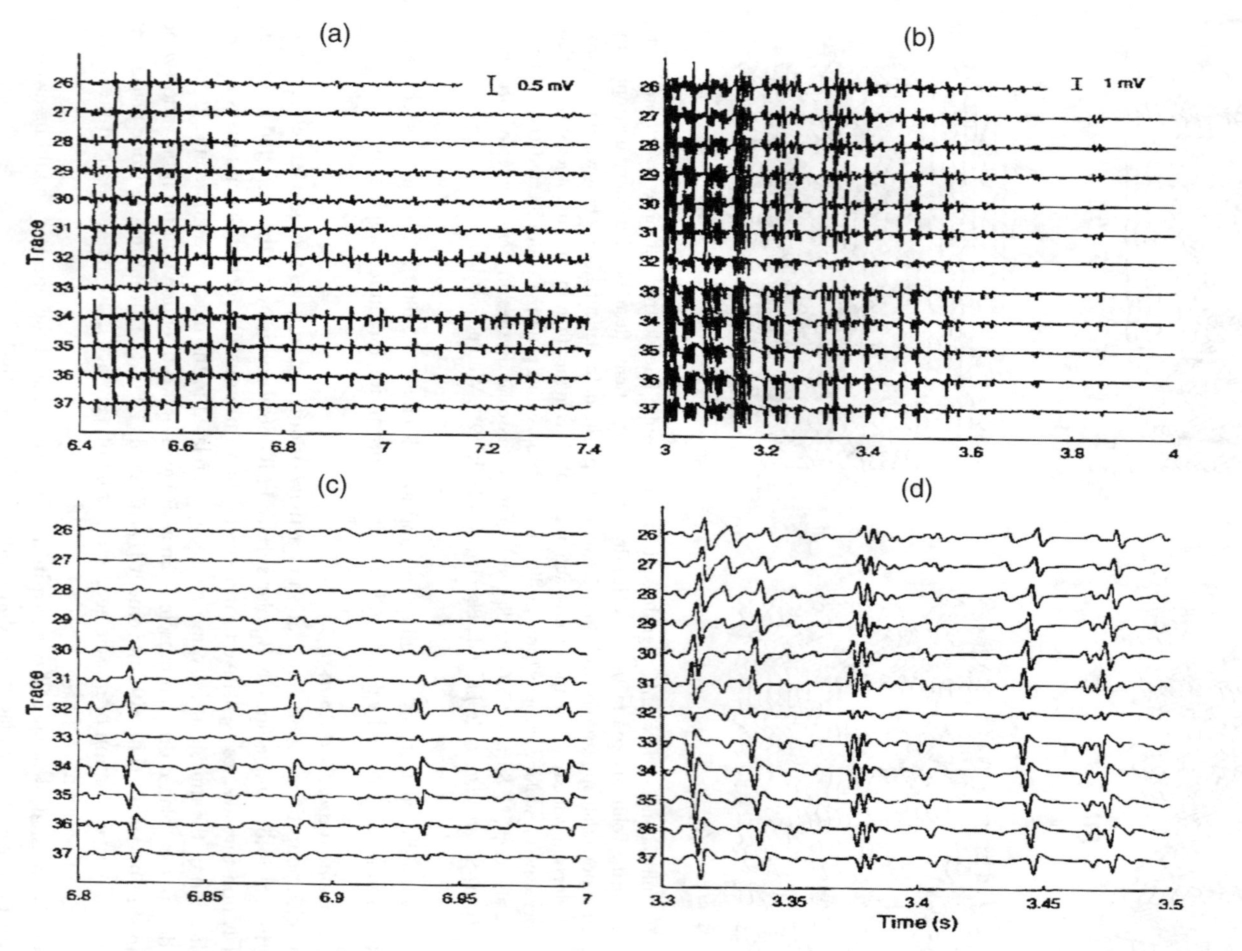

FIGURE 4.38 Multichannel surface EMG signals detected from the biceps brachii muscle of a patient affected by myotonia during a transient paresis (a and c), and a healthy subject (b and d) performing a decreasing force contraction. Note the conduction blocking in the patient. (From Drost, G., Blok, J.H., Stegeman, D.F., van Dijk, J.P., van Engelen, B.G., and Zwarts, M.J., *Brain*, 124, 352–360, 2001. With permission.)

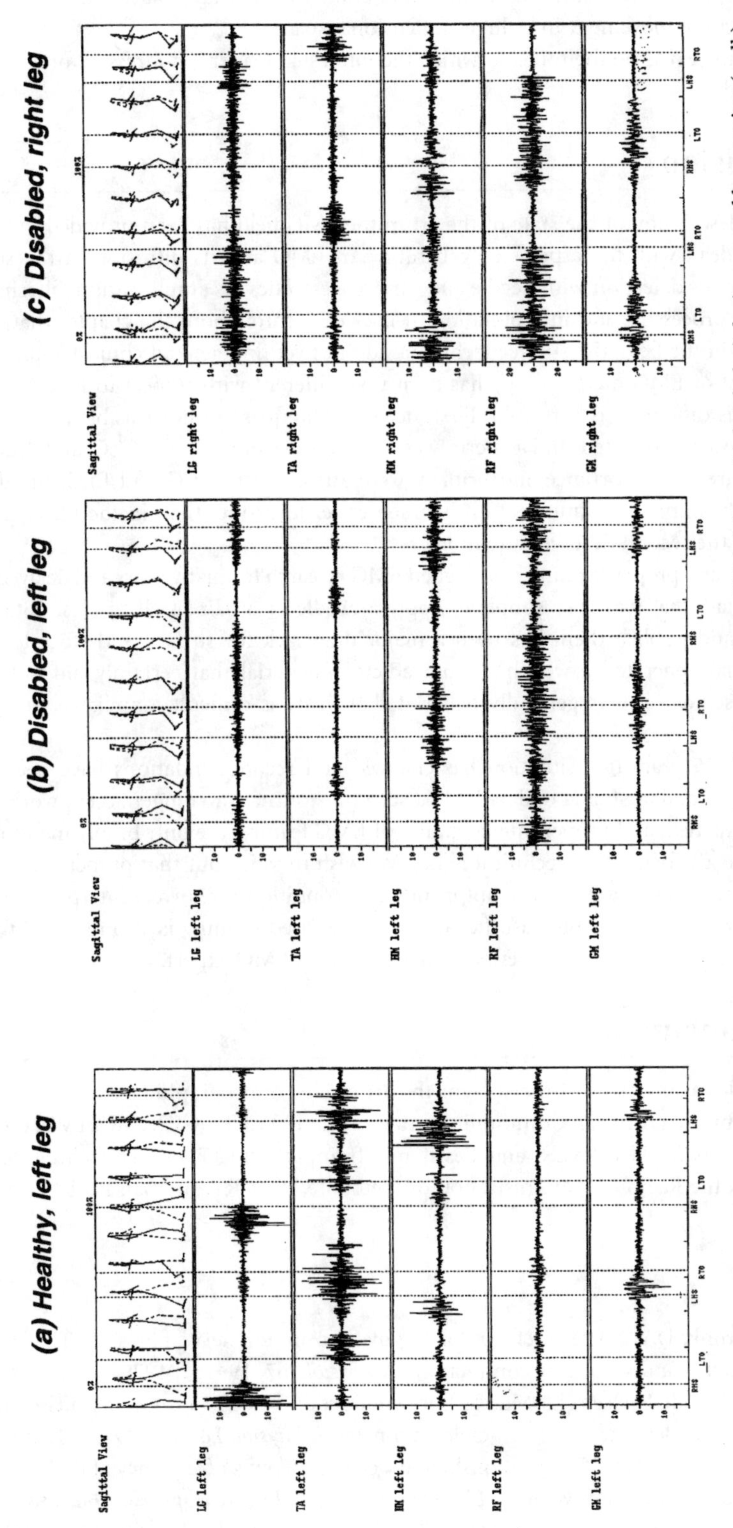

FIGURE 4.39. Example of gait analysis on normal (a) and spastic-type diplegic cerebral palsy subject ([b] left leg and [c] right leg) during normal locomotion (walk); a high degree of co-contraction of muscles and lack of temporal sequencing in the disabled subject is evident when compared to the healthy pattern. (From Craik and Oatis, 1994.)

distribution, or footswitches for evaluation of gait events and phases (the so-called *basographic* data). PC-based camera systems can also be used, in conjunction with markers placed at the limb joints, in order to reconstruct the movement in a three-dimensional space.

Extended literature exists on the topic, to which the interested reader is addressed for a more detailed view of the methods.

4.5 Conclusion

A comprehensive description of the state of the art in the EMG field has been provided in this chapter. Different sections dealt with the aspects of generation of EMG and its diffusion in the surrounding conductive medium, its detection with needle and surface electrodes, its amplification, filtering, and A/D conversion, and its processing and interpretation. It is evident throughout the chapter that, despite the extensive literature in the field, the surface techniques do not yet find general clinical application.

The development of EMG methodology has been very different with respect to ECG and EEG. The basic reason for this difference is threefold. First, needle techniques are not feasible in ECG and EEG. Second, standards were proposed and experts were trained as soon as the ECG and EEG methods developed. Third, greater importance and priority were attributed to ECG and EEG. In addition, the ECG signal is much simpler and information is much easier to extract than in the EMG case. Among these three reasons the second deserves attention.

Lack of standards and proper training has plagued EMG research for many years and delayed its clinical development. The fact that it is very simple to apply a needle or a pair of electrodes, obtain a signal, draw conclusions, and publish them has been a major drawback for surface and (to a lesser degree) needle EMG and has generated a wealth of contradictory material that certainly did not attract the clinician. As a consequence, it is generally believed that EMG is difficult, unreliable, and of limited diagnostic value.

In the last 10 to 15 years this situation has changed and recommendations have been published (Hermens et al., 1999) and are being updated. Most scientific journals no longer accept works with poor methodology. Clinical tests and proper interpretation of EMG features are only briefly mentioned in this chapter which is mostly focused on technical issues. We wish to point out that proper methodology, so often missing in past works, is a necessary but insufficient condition for correct interpretation of EMG. Studying this chapter is necessary but insufficient, and supervised training is also required to reach the level of knowledge, competence, and experience that qualify an EMG expert.

Acknowledgments

This chapter provides a summary of the state of the art of electromyographic techniques and of EMG research sponsored by the European Community (projects SENIAM, PROCID, and NEW), the European Space Agency (projects MESM, EXER, and Resistance Training Using Flywheel Technology for Crew Stationed in Space), the Regional Administration of Piemonte, the CRT, and San Paolo Foundations in Torino, Italy.

References

Adrian, E.D. and Bronk, D.W., The discharge of impulses in motor nerve fibres. II. The frequency of discharge in reflex and voluntary contractions, *J. Physiol.*, 67, 19–151, 1929.

Andreassen, S. and Arendt-Nielsen, L., Muscle fibre conduction velocity in motor units of the human anterior tibial muscle; a new size principle parameter, *J. Physiol. London*, 391, 561, 1987.

Arendt-Nielsen, L. and Mills, K.R., The relationship between mean power frequency of the EMG spectrum and muscle fibre conduction velocity, *Electroencephalogr. Clin. Neurophysiol.*, 60, 130–134, 1985.

Basmajian, J.V. and De Luca, C.J., *Muscles Alive: Their Functions Revealed by Electromyography*, 5th ed., William & Wilkins, Baltimore, 1985.

Blok, J., van Asselt, S., van Dijk, J., and Stegeman, D., On an optimal pastless electrode to skin interface in surface EMG, in SENIAM 5: The State of the Art on Sensors and Sensor Placement Procedures for Surface ElectroMyoGraphy: A Proposal for Sensor Placement Procedures, Hermens, H.J. and Freriks, B., Eds., Roessingh Research and Development, The Netherlands, 1997.

Bonato, P., D'Alessio, T., and Knaflitz, M., A statistical method for the measurement of muscle activation intervals from surface myoelectric signal during gait, *IEEE Trans. Biomed. Eng.*, 45, 287–299, 1998.

Bottin, A., Impedance and noise of the skin-electrode interface in surface EMG recordings, Proc. XIVth ISEK Congress, Wien, 2002.

Brandstater, M.E. and Lambert, E.H., Motor unit anatomy. Type and spatial arrangement of muscle fibres, in *New Developments in Electromyography and Clinical Neurophysiology*, Desmedt, J.E., Ed., S. Karger, Basel, 1973.

Broman, H., De Luca, C.J., and Mambrito, B., Motor unit recruitment and firing rates interaction in control of human muscles, *Brain Res.*, 337, 311–319, 1985.

Broman, H., Bilotto, G., and De Luca, C.J., Myoelectric signal conduction velocity and spectral parameters: influence of force and time, *J. Appl. Physiol.*, 58, 1428–1437, 1985.

Bronzino, J.D., *The Biomedical Engineering Handbook*, CRC Press, Boca Raton, FL, 1995.

Buchthal, F., Guld, P., and Rosenfalck, P., Propagation velocity in electrically activated muscle fibers in man, *Acta Physiol. Scand.*, 34, 75–89, 1955.

Buchthal F., Guld, C., and Rosenfalck, P., Multielectrode study of the territory of a motor unit, *Acta Physiol. Scand.*, 39, 83–104, 1957.

Buchthal, F., Guld, C., and Rosenfalck, P., Volume conduction of the motor unit action potential investigated with a new type of multielectrode, *Acta Physiol. Scand.*, 38, 331–354, 1958.

Burke, R.E. and Tsairis, P., Anatomy and innervation ratios in motor units of cat gastrocnemius, *J. Physiol.*, 234, 749–765, 1973.

Calancie, B. and Bawa, P., Limitations of the spike-triggered averaging technique, *Muscle Nerve*, 9, 78–83, 1986.

Clancy, E.A., Electromyogram amplitude estimation with adaptive smoothing window length, *IEEE Trans. Biomed. Eng.*, 46, 717–729, 1999a.

Clancy, E.A. and Farry, K.A., Adaptive whitening of the electromyogram to improve amplitude estimation, *IEEE Trans. Biomed. Eng.*, 47, 709–719, 2000.

Clancy, E.A. and Hogan, N., Single site electromyograph amplitude estimation, *IEEE Trans. Biomed. Eng.*, 41, 159–167, 1994.

Clancy, E.A. and Hogan, N., Probability density of the surface electromyogram and its relation to amplitude detectors, *IEEE Trans. Biomed. Eng.*, 46, 730–739, 1999b.

Clancy, E.A., Morin, E.L., and Merletti, R., Sampling, noise reduction and amplitude estimation issues in surface electromyography, *J. Electromyogr. Kinesiol.*, 12, 1–16, 2002.

Cohen, L., Time-frequency distributions: a review, *Proc. IEEE*, 77, 941–981, 1989.

Cooper, R., Osselton, J.W., and Shaw, J.C., *EEG Technology*, Butterworth, London, 1969, pp. 14–22.

Craik, R.L. and Oatis, C.A., *Gait Analysis Theory and Applications*, C.V. Mosby, St. Louis, MO, 1994.

Davies, S. and Parker, P., Estimation of myoelectric conduction velocity distribution, *IEEE Trans. Biomed. Eng.*, 34, 98–105, 1987.

De Luca, C.J. and Erim, Z., Common drive of motor units in regulation of muscle force, *Trends Neurosci.*, 17, 299–305, 1994.

De Luca, C.J. and Forrest, W.J., An electrode for recording single motor unit activity during strong muscle contractions, *IEEE Trans. Biomed. Eng.*, 19, 367–372, 1972.

Desmedt, J.E., *Computer-Aided Electromyography and Expert Systems*, Elsevier, New York, 1989.

Dimitrov, G.V., Changes in the extracellular potentials produced by unmyelinated nerve fibre resulting from alterations in the propagation velocity or the duration of the action potential, *Electromyogr. Clin. Neurophysiol.*, 27, 243–249, 1987.

Dimitrov, G.V. and Dimitrova, N.A., Precise and fast calculation of the motor unit potentials detected by a point and rectangular plate electrode, *Med. Eng. Physics*, 20, 374–381, 1998.

Dimitrova, N.A., Model of the extracellular potential field of a single striated muscle fiber, *Electromyogr. Clin. Neurophysiol.*, 14, 53–66, 1974.

Dimitrova, N.A., Dimitrov, G.V., and Nikitin, O.A., Neither high-pass filtering nor mathematical differentiation of the EMG signals can considerably reduce crosstalk, *J. Electromyogr. Kinesiol.*, 12, 235–246, 2002.

Disselhorst-Klug, C., Silny, J., and Rau, G., Improvement of spatial resolution in surface-EMG: a theoretical and experimental comparison of different spatial filters, *IEEE Trans. Biomed. Eng.*, 44, 567–574, 1997.

Disselhorst-Klug, C., Bahm, J., Ramaekers, V., Trachterna, A., and Rau, G., Non-invasive approach of motor unit recording during muscle contractions in humans, *Eur. J. Applied Physiol.*, 83, 144–150, 2000.

Drost G., Blok, J.H., Stegeman, D.F., van Dijk, J.P., van Engelen, B.G., and Zwarts, M.J., Propagation disturbance of motor unit action potentials during transient paresis in generalized myotonia: a high-density surface EMG study, *Brain*, 124, 352–360, 2001.

Dubowitz, V. and Brooke, M.H., *Muscle Biopsy: A Modern Approach*, Vol. 2, W.B. Saunders, London, 1973, p. 475.

Duchenne, G.B.A., *Physiologie des Movements* (transl. by E.B. Kaplan), W.B. Saunders, Philadelphia, 1949.

Dumitru, D., *Electrodiagnostic Medicine*, Hanley & Belfus, Philadephia, 1995.

Farina, D., Advances in Myoelectric Signal Detection, Processing and Interpretation in Motor Control Studies, Ph.D. thesis, Politecnico di Torino and Ecole Centrale de Nantes, 2001.

Farina, D. and Cescon, C., Concentric ring electrode systems for non-invasive detection of single motor unit activity, *IEEE Trans. Biomed. Eng.*, 48, 1326–1334, 2001.

Farina, D. and Merletti, R., Comparison of algorithms for estimation of the EMG variables during voluntary isometric contractions, *J. Electromyogr. Kinesiol.*, 10, 327–336, 2000.

Farina, D. and Merletti, R., A novel approach for precise simulation of the EMG signal detected by surface electrodes, *IEEE Trans. Biomed. Eng.*, 48, 637–645, 2001.

Farina, D., Fortunato, E., and Merletti, R., Non-invasive estimation of motor unit conduction velocity distribution using linear electrode arrays, *IEEE Trans. Biomed. Eng.*, 41, 380–388, 2000.

Farina, D., Merletti, R., Nazzaro, R., and Caruso, I., Effect of joint angle on surface EMG variables for the muscles of the leg and thigh, *IEEE Eng. Med. Biol. Mag.*, 20, 62–71, 2001a.

Farina, D., Muhammad, W., Fortunato, E., Meste, O., Merletti, R., and Rix H., Estimation of single motor unit conduction velocity from the surface EMG signal detected with linear electrode arrays, *Med. Biol. Eng. Comput.*, 39, 225–236, 2001b.

Farina, D., Merletti, R., Indino, B., Nazzaro, M., and Pozzo, M., Surface EMG crosstalk between knee extensor muscles: experimental and model results, *Muscle Nerve*, 26, 681–695, 2002.

Farina, D., Arendt-Nielsen, L., Merletti, R., and Graven-Nielsen, T., Assessment of single motor unit conduction velocity during sustained contractions of the tibialis anterior muscle with advanced spike triggered averaging, *J. Neurosci. Meth.*, 115, 1–12, 2002.

Felici, F., Rosponi, A., Sbriccioli, P., Filligoi, G.C., Fattorini, L., and Marchetti, M., Linear and non-linear analysis of surface electromyograms in weightlifters, *Eur. J. Appl. Physiol.*, 84, 337–342, 2001.

Franco, S., *Design with Operational Amplifiers and Analog Integrated Circuits*, McGraw-Hill, New York, 1988.

Fuglsang-Frederiksen, A., Electrical activity and force during voluntary contraction of normal and diseased muscle, *Acta Neurol. Scand.*, 63 (Suppl. 83), 1–60, 1981.

Gazzoni, M., Farina, D., and Merletti, R., Motor unit recruitment during constant low force and long duration muscle contractions investigated with surface electromyography, *Acta Physiol. Pharmacol. Bulg.*, 26(1–2), 67–71, 2001.

Geddes, L.A., *Electrodes and the Measurement of Bioeletric Events*, Wiley, New York, 1972.

Gilai, A.N., Analysis of turns and amplitude in EMG, in *Computer-Aided Electromyography and Expert Systems*, Desmedt, J.E., Ed., Elsevier, New York, 1989.

Gootzen, T.H., Stegeman, D.F., and Van Oosterom, A., Finite limb dimensions and finite muscle length in a model for the generation of electromyographic signals, *Electroencephalogr. Clin. Neurophysiol.*, 81, 152–162, 1991.

Griep, P., Gielen, F., Boon, K., Hoogstraten, L., Pool, C., and Wallinga de Jonge, W., Calculation and registration of the same motor unit action potential, *Electroencephalogr. Clin. Neurophysiol.*, 53, 388–404, 1982.

Grimnes, S., Psychogalvanic reflex and changes in electrical parameters of the skin, *Med. Biol. Eng. Comp.*, 20, 734–740, 1982.

Gydikov, A., Gerilovski, L., Radicheva, N., and Troyanova, N., Influence of the muscle fiber end geometry on the extracellular potentials, *Biol. Cybern.*, 54, 1–8, 1986.

Hageman, B., Luhede, G., and Luczak, H., Improved active electrodes for recording bioelectric signals in work physiology, *Eur. J. Appl. Physiol.*, 54, 95–98, 1985.

Hägg, G.M., Static work load and occupational myalgia – a new explanation model, in *Electromyographical Kinesiology*, Anderson, P., Hobart, D., and Danoff, J., Eds., Elsevier Science, Amsterdam, 1991, pp. 141–144.

Helal, J.N. and Bouissou, P., The spatial integration effect of surface electrode detecting myoelectric signal, *IEEE Trans. Biomed. Eng.*, 39, 1161–1167, 1992.

Henneman, E., Somjem, G., and Carpenter, D.O., Functional significance of cell size in spinal motoneurons, *J. Neurophysiol.*, 28, 560, 1965.

Henneman, E., Skeletal muscle: the servant of the nervous system, in *Medical Physiology,* Mountcastle, V.B., Ed., 1980.

Hermens, H., Freriks, B., Merletti, R., Stegeman, D., Blok, J., Rau, G., Disselhorst-Klug, C., and Hägg, G., European recommendations for surface electromyography, Roessingh Research and Development, Enschede, The Netherlands, 1999.

Hudgins, B., Parker, P., and Scott, R., Control of artificial limbs using myoelectric pattern recognition, *Med. Life Sci.*, 12, 21–38, 1994.

Huhta, J.C. and Webster, J.G., 60-Hz interference in electro-cardiography, *IEEE Trans. Biomed. Eng.*, 20, 657–658, 1973.

Inman, V.T., Saunders, J.B., and Abbott, L.C., Observations on the function of the shoulder joint, *J. Bone Jt. Surg.*, 26, 1–30, 1944.

Jähne, B., *Digitale Bildverarbeitung*, Springer-Verlag, Heidelberg, 1989, ch. 5, pp. 88–128.

Janz, G.J. and Ives, D.J.G., Silver–silver chloride electrodes, *Ann. N.Y. Acad. Sci.*, 148, 210, 1968.

Johannsen, G., Line source models for active fibers, *Biol. Cybern.*, 54, 151–158, 1986.

Kamen, G. and De Luca, C.J., Firing rate interactions among human orbicularis oris motor units, *Int. J. Neurosci.*, 64, 167–175, 1992.

Kay, S.M. and Marple, L.M., Spectrum analysis — a modern perspective, *Proc. IEEE*, 69, 1380–1413, 1981.

Kleine, B.U., Praamsta, P., Blok, J.H., and Stegeman, D.F., Single motor unit discharge patterns recorded with multi-channel sEMG, Proc. Symp. Muscular Disorders in Computer Users, Copenhagen, 1999, pp. 175–179.

Kleine, B.U., Blok, J.H., Oostenveld, R., Praamstra, P., and Stegeman, D.F., Magnetic stimulation-induced modulations of motor unit firings extracted from multi-channel surface EMG, *Muscle Nerve*, 23(7), 1005–1015, 2000.

Kleine, B.U., Schumann, N.P., Stegeman, D.F., and Scholle, H.C., Surface EMG mapping of the human upper trapezius muscle: the typography of monopolar and bipolar surface EMG amplitude and spectrum parameters at varied forces and fatigue, *Clin. Neurophysiol.*, 111, 686–693, 2000b.

Kleine, B.U., Praamstra, P., Stegeman, D.F., and Zwarts, M.J., Impaired motor cortical inhibition in Parkinson's disease: motor unit responses to transcranial magnetic stimulation, *Exp. Brain Res.*, 138, 477–483, 2001.

Kleinpenning, P., Gootzen, T., Van Oosterom, A., and Stegeman, D.F., The equivalent source description representing the extinction of an action potential at a muscle fiber ending, *Math. Biosci.*, 101, 41–61, 1990.

Knaflitz, M. and Merletti, R., Suppression of stimulation artifacts from myoelectric evoked potential recordings, *IEEE Trans. Biomed. Eng.*, 35, 758–763, 1988.

Ko, W.H. and Hynecek, J., Dry electrodes and electrode amplifiers, *Biomedical Electrode Technology*, Academic Press, New York, 1974, pp. 169–181.

Koh, T.J. and Grabiner, M.D., Evaluation of methods to minimize crosstalk in surface electromyography, *J. Biomech.*, 26, 151–157, 1993.

Lago, P.J. and Jones, N.B., Effect of motor unit firing time statistics on E.M.G. spectra, *Med. Biol. Eng. Comput.*, 5, 648–655, 1977.

Le Bozec, S. and Maton, B., Differences between motor unit firing rate, twitch characteristics and fibre type composition in an agonistic muscle group in man, *Eur. J. Appl. Physiol.*, 56, 350–355, 1987.

Lexell, J., Downham, D., and Sjostrom, M., Distribution of different fibre type in human skeletal muscles — a statistical and computational study of the fibre type arrangement in m. vastus lateralis of young, healthy males, *J. Neurol. Sci.*, 65, 353–365, 1984.

Lexell, J., Downham, D., and Sjostrom, M., Distribution of different fibre type in human skeletal muscles — a statistical and computational study of the fibre type arrangement in m. vastus lateralis from three groups of healthy men between 15 and 83 years, *J. Neurol. Sci.*, 72, 211–222, 1986.

Lindström, L., On the Frequency Spectrum of the EMG Signals, Thesis, Chalmers University of Technology, Göteborg, 1970.

Lindström, L. and Magnusson, R., Interpretation of myoelectric power spectra: a model and its applications, *Proc. IEEE*, 65, 653–662, 1977.

Masuda, T., Miyano, H., and Sadoyama, T., The propagation of motor unit action potential and the location of neuromuscular junction investigated by surface electrode arrays, *Electroencephal. Clin. Neurophysiol.*, 56, 507–603, 1983.

Masuda, T., Miyano, H., and Sadoyama, T., The distribution of myoneural junctions in the biceps brachii investigated by surface electromyography, *Electroencephal. Clin. Neurophysiol.*, 56, 597–603, 1983b.

Masuda, T., Miyano, H., and Sadoyama, T., A surface electrode array for detecting action potential trains of single motor units, *Electroencephal. Clin. Neurophysiol.*, 60, 435–443, 1985.

Masuda, T., Miyano, H., and Sadoyama, T., The position of innervation zones in the biceps brachii investigated by surface electromyography, *IEEE Trans. Biomed. Eng.*, 32, 36–42, 1985b.

McGill, K.C. and Dorfman, L.J., High resolution alignment of sampled waveforms, *IEEE Trans. Biomed. Eng.*, 31, 462–470, 1984.

McGill, K. and Huynh, A., A model of the surface recorded motor unit action potential, *Proc. 10th Annu. Int. IEEE Conf. Eng. Med. Biol.*, pp. 1697–1699, 1988.

McMillan, A.S. and Hannam, A.G., Motor-unit territory in the human masseter muscle, *Arch. Oral Biol.*, 36, 435–441, 1991.

Merletti, R. and De Luca, C.J., New techniques in surface electromyography, in *Computer Aided Electromyography and Expert Systems*, Desmedt, J.E., Ed., Elsevier Science, Amsterdam, 1989.

Merletti, R. and Lo Conte, L., Advances in processing of surface myoelectric signals. I, *Med. Biol. Eng. Comp.*, 33, 362–372, 1995.

Merletti, R. and Lo Conte, L.R., Surface EMG signal processing during isometric contractions, *J. Electromyogr. Kinesiol.*, 7, 241–250, 1997.

Merletti, R. and Parker, P., Eds., *Electromyography Physiology, Engineering and Non Invasive Applications*, Wiley/IEEE Press Publication, in press.

Merletti, R., Knaflitz, M., and De Luca, C.J., Electrically evoked myoelectric signals, *Crit. Rev. Biomed. Eng.*, 19, 293–340, 1992.

Merletti, R., Lo Conte, L., Avignone, E., and Guglielminotti, P., Modelling of surface EMG signals. I. Model implementation, *IEEE Trans. Biomed. Eng.*, 46, 810–820, 1999.

Merlo, A., Farina, D., and Merletti, R., A fast and reliable technique for muscle activity detection from surface EMG signals, *IEEE Trans. Biomed. Eng.*, 50(3), 316–323, March 2003.

Metting van Rijn, A.C., The Modelling of Biopotential Recordings and Its Implications for Instrumentation Design, Proefschrift ter verkrijging van der graad van doctor aan de Technische Universitiet Delft, Delft, Technische Universiteit Delft, 1993.

Metting van Rjin, A.C., Peper, A., and Grimbergen, C., High quality recordings of bioelectric events. I. Interference reduction theory and practice, *Med. Biol. Eng. Comp.*, 28, 389–397, 1990.

Metting van Rijn, A.C., Peper, A., and Grimbergen, C., The isolation mode rejection ratio in bioelectric amplifiers, *IEEE Trans. Biomed. Eng.*, 38, 1154–1157, 1991.

Metting van Rjin, A.C., Peper, A., and Grimbergen, C., High quality recordings of bioelectric events. II. Low noise, low power multichannel amplifier design, *Med. Biol. Eng. Comp.*, 29, 433–440, 1991.

Meyer, M., Hilfiker, P., and Gygi, A., Surface EMG for diagnosis of neuromuscular diseases, in *Computer-Aided Electromyography and Expert Systems*, Desmedt, J.E., Ed., Elsevier, New York, 1989.

Milner-Brown, H.S., Stein, R.B., and Yemm, R., Changes in firing rate of human motor units during linearly changing voluntary contractions, *J. Physiol.*, 230, 371–390, 1973.

Mortara, D.W., Digital filters of ECG signals, *Computers in Cardiology*, IEEE Press, New York, 1977, pp. 511–514.

Neuman, M.R., Biopotential electrodes, in *Medical Instrumentation*, Webster, J.G., Ed., Houghton Mifflin, Boston, 1978, 215–272.

Pallas-Areny, R., Interference-rejection characteristics of biopotential amplifiers: a comparative analysis, *IEEE Trans. Biomed. Eng.*, 35, 953–959, 1988.

Piper, H., *Electrophysiologic Menschlicher Muskeln*, Springer-Verlag, Berlin, 1912.

Plonsey, R., Action potential sources and their volume conductor fileds, *IEEE Trans. Biomed. Eng.*, 56, 601–611, 1977.

Potter, A. and Menke, L., Capacitive type of biomedical electrode, *IEEE Trans. Biomed. Eng.*, 17, 350, 1970.

Prutchi, D., A high resolution large array (HRLA) surface EMG system, *Med. Eng. Phys.*, 17, 442–454, 1995.

Ragheb, T. and Geddes, L.A., Electrical properties of metallic electrodes, *Med. Biol. Eng. Comp.*, 28, 182–186, 1990.

Reucher, H., Rau, G., and Silny, J., Spatial filtering of noninvasive multielectrode EMG. I. Introduction to measuring technique and applications, *IEEE Trans. Biomed. Eng.*, 34, 98–105, 1987a.

Reucher, H., Rau, G., and Silny, J., Spatial filtering of noninvasive multielectrode EMG. II. Filter performance in theory and modelling, *IEEE Trans. Biomed. Eng.*, 34, 106–113, 1987b.

Roeleveld, K., Stegeman, D.F., Falck, B., and Stalberg, E.V., Motor unit size estimation: confrontation of surface EMG with macro EMG, *Electroencephal. Clin. Neurophysiol.*, 105, 181–188, 1997a.

Roeleveld, K., Stegeman, D.F., Vingerhoets, H.M., and Van Oosterom, A., The motor unit potential distribution over the skin surface and its use in estimating the motor unit location, *Acta Physiol. Scand.*, 161, 465–472, 1997b.

Rosenfalck, P., Intra and extracellular fields of active nerve and muscle fibers. A physico-mathematical analysis of different models, *Acta Physiol. Scand.*, 321, 1–49, 1969.

Roy, S.H., De Luca, C.J., and Casavant, D.A., Lumbar muscle fatigue and chronic lower back pain, *Spine*, 14, 992–1001, 1989.

Sadoyama, T., Masuda, T., Miyata, H., and Katsuta, S., Fibre conduction velocity and fibre composition in human vastus lateralis, *Eur. J. Appl. Physiol.*, 56, 767, 1988.

Saltin, B. and Gollnick, P.D., Skeletal muscle adaptability: significance for metabolism and performance, in *Handbook of Physiology: Skeletal Muscle*, Peachey, L.D., Adrian, R.H., and Geider, S.G., Eds., Williams & Wilkins, Baltimore, 1983.

Shwedik, E., Balasubramanian, R., and Scott, R., A nonstationary model for the electromyogram, *IEEE Trans. Biomed. Eng.*, 24, 417–424, 1977.

Silverman, R. and Jenden, D., A novel high performance preamplifier for biological applications, *IEEE Trans. Biomed. Eng.*, 430, 1971.

Stålberg, E., Macro EMG, a new recording technique, *J. Neurol. Neurosurg. Psychiatry*, 43, 475–483, 1980.

Stålberg, E. and Antoni, L., Electrophysiological cross section of the motor unit, *J. Neurol. Neurosurg. Psychiatry*, 43, 469–474, 1980.

Stålberg, E. and Fawcett, P.R.W., Macro EMG in healthy subjects of different ages, *J. Neurol. Neurosurg. Psychiatry*, 45, 870, 1982.

Stashuk, D. and De Luca, C.J., Decomposition of surface detected myoelectric signals, *Proc. VIII Conf. IEEE Eng. Med Biol*, 1, 547–550, 1986.

Stashuk, D.W., Decomposition and quantitative analysis of clinical electromyographic signals, *Med. Eng. Phys.*, 21, 389–404, 1999.

Stegeman, D.F., Blok, H.J., Hermens, J.H., and Roeleveld, K., Surface EMG models: properties and applications, *J. Electromyogr. Kinesiol.*, 10, 313–326, 2000.

Stein, R.B., French, A.S., and Yemm, R., New methods for analysing motor function in man and animals, *Brain Res.*, 40, 187–192, 1972.

Stulen, F.B. and De Luca, C.J., Frequency parameters of the myoelectric signal as a measure of muscle conduction velocity, *IEEE Trans. Biomed. Eng.*, 28, 512–522, 1981.

Stulen, F.B. and De Luca, C.J., Muscle fatigue monitor: a non invasive device for observing localized muscular fatigue, *IEEE Trans. Biomed. Eng.*, 29, 760–769, 1982.

Troni, W., Cantello, R., and Rainero, I., Conduction velocity along human muscle fibers *in situ*, *Neurology*, 33, 1453–1459, 1983.

van der Locht, H.M. and van der Straaten, J.H., Hybrid amplifier-electrode module for measuring surface electromyographic potentials, *Med. Biol. Eng. Comp.*, 18, 119–122, 1980.

van Vugt J.P. and van Dijk, J.G., A convenient method to reduce crosstalk in surface EMG, *Clin. Neurophysiol.*, 112, 583–592, 2001.

Weast, R.C., *Handbook of Chemistry and Physics*, 55th ed., CRC Press, Boca Raton, FL, 1974.

Webster, J.G., *Medical Instrumentation: Application and Design*, Houghton Mifflin, Boston, 1992.

Westgaard, R. and De Luca, C.J., Motor control of low-threshold motor units in the human trapezius muscle, *J. Neurophysiol.*, 85, 1777–1781, 2001.

Winter, B.B. and Webster, J.G., Reduction of interference due to common mode voltage in biopotential amplifiers, *IEEE Trans. Biomed. Eng.*, 30, 58–65, 1983.

Winter, D.A., Fuglevand, A.J., and Archer, S.E., Crosstalk in surface electromyography: theoretical and practical estimates, *J. Electromyogr. Kinesiol.*, 4, 15–26, 1994.

Zwillinger, D., *Standard Mathematical Tables and Formulae*, CRC Press, Boca Raton, FL, 1996.

5

Evoked Potentials

CONTENTS

Hermann Hinrichs
University of Magdeburg

5.1 Basic Operational Mechanisms

The ongoing background electroencephalogram (EEG) is discussed in Chapter 6 of this book. In this chapter we discuss techniques for extracting from the ongoing EEG measures of the brain's specific reaction to peripheral sensory stimulation, which are known as *evoked potentials* (EPs). A comprehensive description of the underlying physiological mechanisms may be found in Kandel et al. (2000). Techniques for measuring EPs can also be used to measure sensory nerve potentials that occur before the effects of peripheral stimulation are apparent in the brain. A brief overview of the main technical components necessary to record an EP is provided in Figure 5.1.

EPs can be extracted from the background EEG if subjects are exposed to repeated brief sensory stimuli. For standard neurological applications, *auditory*, *somatosensory*, and *visual* stimuli are the most important. The corresponding specific EPs are called AEPs, SEPs, and VEPs, respectively. The most common methods of stimulation are (1) presenting auditory clicks via earphones (AEP), (2) presenting brief electrical pulses to peripheral sensory nerves such as the *median* or the *tibial nerve*, and (3) presenting inverting checkerboard patterns on a computer screen (VEP). Further modalities, involving olfactory or thermal stimuli, for example, will not be discussed here. Different subtypes of AEP and SEP can be observed with different latencies after stimulus onset. In this chapter we focus on the earliest responses known as the *brainstem AEP* (BAEP) and the *early SEP.* There are later AEP and SEP components, but these reflect higher processing stages and have gained less importance in everyday neurological examination. The required frequency of repeated stimulus presentation strongly varies with modality and ranges from about 1 Hz for VEPs to 2 to 3 Hz for SEPs, up to 10 to 20 Hz for BAEPs.

In contrast to the more-or-less random background EEG, EPs are to a large extent reproducible when peripheral stimuli are repeatedly presented. This is the reason why they can be measured, despite the fact that their amplitude is much lower than that of the background EEG. The basic technique needed to extract these small signals is to *average* (Epstein and Boor, 1988) the voltages measured in short EEG epochs that are synchronized with the stimulus presentation. Assuming a stable EP pattern and a background EEG that

0-8493-1140-3/04/$0.00+$1.50

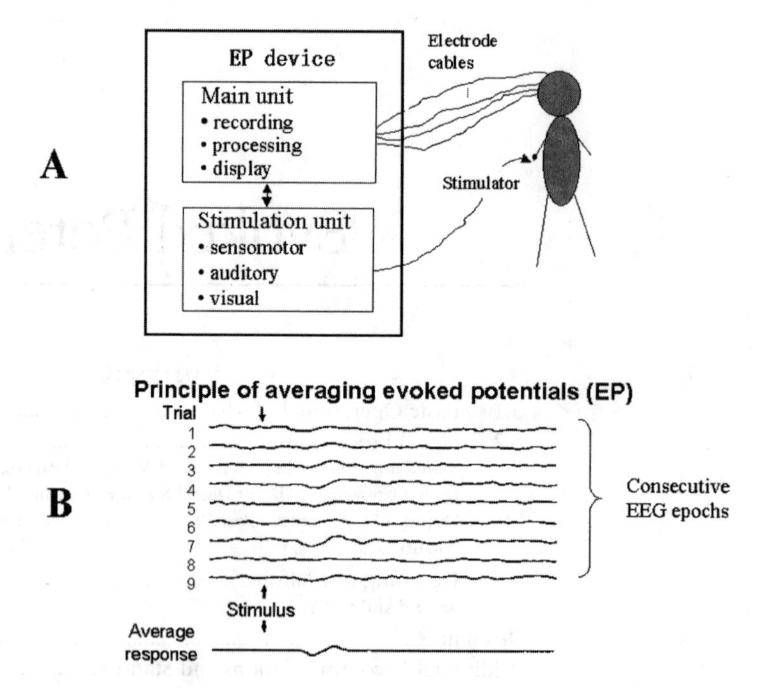

FIGURE 5.1 (A) Basic components of an EP recorder; (B) principle to extract an EP from an ongoing EEG (for details see Figure 5.11).

is random with respect to the stimulation timing, such averaging will attenuate the background EEG amplitude by $1/\sqrt{n}$, where n is the number of averaged epochs. Because the EP fraction of the signal remains constant, the EP emerges from the background more and more clearly with a growing number of averaged epochs. In principle, the EP can be determined with arbitrary precision by adding sufficient epochs. However, practically there are limits (1) because of limited examination time, and (2) because EP morphology is not perfectly stable due to physiological noise, habituation, and other effects. Also, as discussed below, minor signal distortions due to artifacts often cannot be fully controlled and therefore degrade EP quality and reproducibility. The number of repeated stimuli needed for a reliable EP measurement significantly depends on the modality, ranging from about 50 (VEP) up to more than 1000 (BAEP).

The EP reflects specific neurophysiological functions, in contrast to the background EEG, which provides an overview of global brain function. A normal EP indicates that both the specific sensory pathways as well as the corresponding brain areas are intact. In contrast, pathological EPs permit — to varying extents, depending on the modality — diagnostic conclusions about the origin and type of the underlying malfunction. Due to the considerable intra-individual variability of the EP, it is good practice in terms of quality control to derive at least two consecutive EP measurements and check if they are similar. In special applications, like function monitoring in the intensive care unit, or during operations, EPs may be repeatedly acquired according to fixed or random schedules in order to monitor brain functions continuously over hours, days, or even weeks.

In contrast to the background EEG, the EP is usually recorded from only a few (typically two) electrodes placed over the specific brain areas. In addition, one or two additional electrodes are sometimes placed on the neck to record cervical SEPs. Thus, only two to four EP channels are generally recorded. The electrical activity is measured against electrodes placed somewhere else on the skull where activity related to the EP is negligible. In accordance with the organization of the relevant sensory nerve pathways, the brain responses are mainly ipsilateral (BAEP) or contralateral (VEP, SEP) to the side of stimulation. For a comprehensive examination, therefore, EP recordings with alternating sides of stimulation are needed. Alternatively, in certain situations bilateral stimulation may be useful. Appropriate electrode sites for recording the various EP types are as follows, labeled according to the internationally

10-20 electrode positioning system

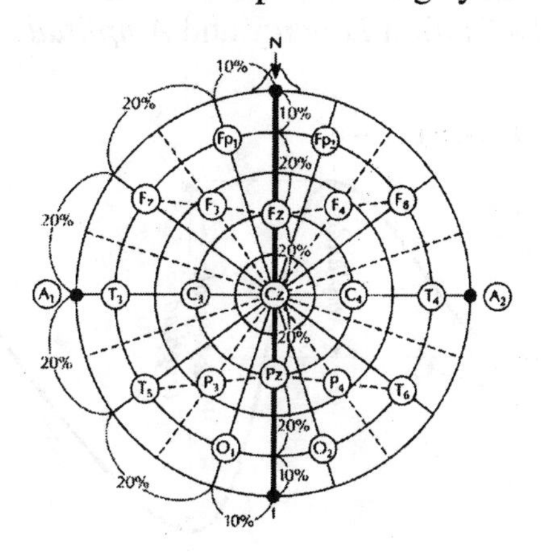

Usual electrode positions for EP recording

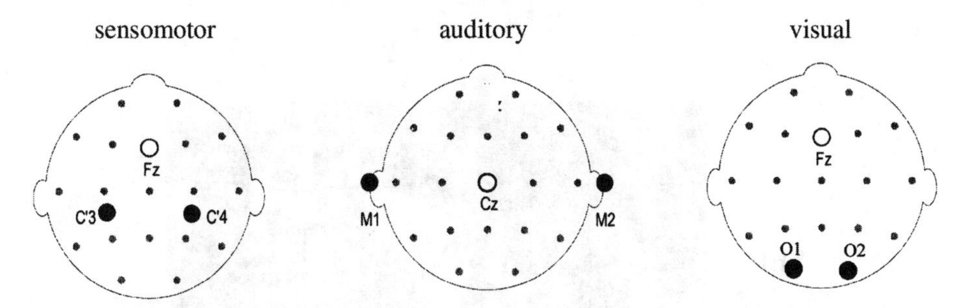

FIGURE 5.2 (Upper) The international 10-20 system (Jasper, 1958) for electrode placement and labeling. (Lower) Scalp locations (according to the 10-20 system) used for different EP modalities. M1 and M2 indicate the left and right mastoids located close to the ears.

standardized 10-20 positioning system (Jasper, 1958) (see Figure 5.2): (1) VEP: O1 (left) and O2 (right) vs. Fz; (2) BAEP: left and right mastoid vs. Cz; (3) SEP: left and right sensory cortex vs. Fz. For instance, for the median nerve, the appropriate positions are C3′ and C4′, which are slightly more posterior than C3 and C4. Cervical potentials may be acquired from the C2 position (not shown in Figure 5.2) on the neck, again using Fz as reference electrode.

Details regarding the various stimulation techniques are explained below. EP recorders are usually embedded in general neurophysiological devices capable of recording and analyzing electromyographic (EMG) activity, neurographic measures (nerve velocity, etc.), and EP. All these methods share the same amplifiers, stimulation units (where applicable), and computer environment. Alternatively, there are some EEG recorders on the market capable of recording and analyzing EPs as an additional tool.

As shown symbolically in Figure 5.3 the EP elicited by the stimulus exhibits a sequence of one or more positive and negative deflections (also called *peaks* or *components*) arising from the noise floor which are usually characterized by their *latency* (i.e., the delay between stimulus onset and the peak of the deflection) and *amplitude.* The surface EP typically covers an amplitude range of 5 to 10 μV (VEP, SEP) or 0.5 μV (BAEP). The first clear and stable VEP component (a positive deflection, see Figure 5.4) occurs at about 100 msec (called P100 or P1) after stimulus onset, frequently preceded by a small negative deflection at 75 msec (N75), and followed by another negative deflection at about 145 msec (N145), all reflecting visual cortex activity. The latencies of the earliest cortically recorded SEP components are around 10 msec, depending on the site of stimulation. In principle, the more proximal the stimulation is, the shorter the latency. In clinical examinations, it is most usual to stimulate the median nerve. The corresponding

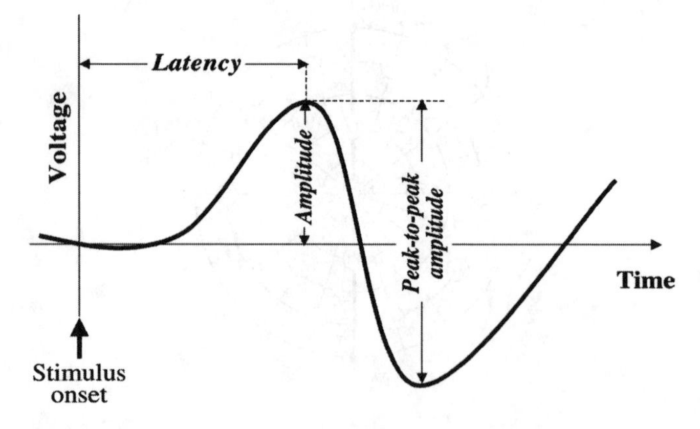

FIGURE 5.3 Definition of parameters used for EP quantification.

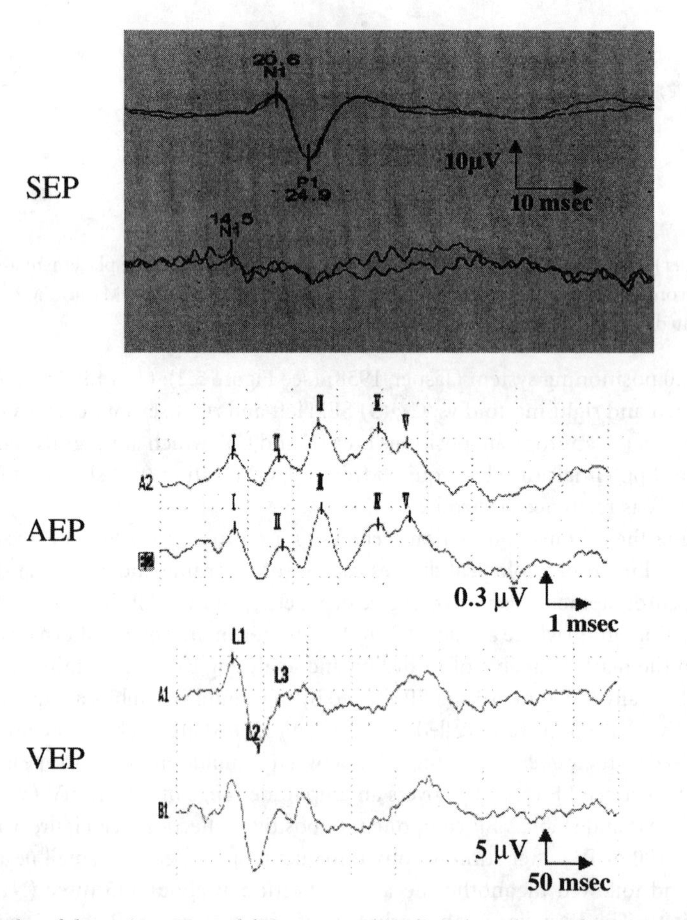

FIGURE 5.4 Examples of the various EP-modalities. As usual in clinical routine, each EP is recorded and displayed twice in order to control its reproducability. Note the different scaling of time and amplitude.

SEP shows a pronounced negative peak in the scalp recording at about 20 ms (N20) post-stimulus, followed by a positive deflection at around 25 msec (P25). In addition, under favorable conditions (i.e., low noise), an early negative wave may be observed at 13 msec (N13). This component coincides with a strong negative peak obtained in recordings from the neck (C2 electrode site). Both peaks, therefore, represent the same neurophysiological entity arising as a post-synaptic potential in the spinal cord. Similar temporal relations can be observed with SEPs derived when stimulating arbitrary sensory nerves. BAEPs recorded at the scalp start with an early peak at around 2 msec after stimulus onset and extend up to approximately 6 msec. Five principal signal deflections can be distinguished, which are labeled I to V, in order of their occurrence. Components I and II are attributed to the *acoustic nerve*, whereas the three later peaks (III, IV, V) originate in the brainstem. Two additional peaks may be found in the latency range of 6 to 10 msec. However, these components have not gained clinical importance.

The main SEP and VEP components (N20, P25, P100) are generated in close vicinity to the relevant scalp electrode. In contrast, the early cortical SEP component N13 as well as all BAEP components originate in regions located far away from the electrodes. They can nevertheless be measured due to volume conduction in the brain. In order to distinguish between these two mechanisms, the terms *near field* and *far field potentials* have been introduced.

Because of the strongly differing temporal structures of the different EPs, the amplifier frequency band best suited to record them varies significantly. Reasonable bandpass settings are approximately 1 to 100 Hz (VEP), 5 to 1000 Hz (SEP), and 100 to 3000 Hz (BAEP). These settings are somewhat arbitrary and depend on individual laboratory standards rather than official recommendations. The number of epochs needed to extract an EP mainly depends on its amplitude. Typical values are 64 to 128 (VEP), 128 to 256 (SEP), and 1024 to 2048 (BAEP).

With respect to EP evaluation, the most important characteristics are the latencies of certain components and — to a lesser extent due to large inherent variability — their amplitudes. In addition, sometimes latency or amplitude differences between consecutive peaks may carry further diagnostic information.

The differential amplifiers used for EP recording are very much similar to EEG amplifiers, except for the larger bandwidth needed for BAEP acquisition. The same holds for considerations regarding the main physical properties of the electrodes providing the appropriate low impedance contact between skin and amplifier input. However, the requirements to be able to transmit very low frequencies approaching direct current (DC) is less restrictive with EPs, because this frequency range is less important here. Therefore, the selection of electrode types is less critical with EPs than with EEG.

As in the case of EEG recording, external signal components often overlay the original EP and thus corrupt the measured signal, even after averaging. There are both technical and biological sources of these so-called *artifacts*. Among the biological artifacts picked up by the amplifiers are residual electrocardiogram (ECG), electromyogram (EMG) generated by muscles in the vicinity of the electrode, electrooculogram (EOG) resulting from eye movements, and slowly fluctuating electrode voltages induced by transpiration, which influences the electrode's electrochemical conditions. Some examples are demonstrated in Figure 5.5. Technical artifacts have a variety of causes, including inductive nonsymmetric coupling of the 50/60 Hz line (mains) frequency, which usually occurs when electrode impedances are excessively large, fluctuating electrode voltages caused by electrode movement, distortions of the ambient electrostatic field due to movement of the patient or the technician, unstable electrical contact between the electrode and the amplifier input, and bad or poorly cleaned electrode material.

The significance of these artifacts differs depending on the type of EP. For example, low frequency disturbances caused by EOG or transpiration hardly influence BAEPs, whereas VEPs may be severely distorted by these artifacts. By contrast, under favorable conditions a VEP may not be significantly degraded by EMG, which would, however, severely affect BAEP quality. A general rule for EP recording, therefore, is to exclude artefactual epochs as much as possible from the averaging process. Under difficult conditions, as, for instance, in intensive care units, 50- or 60-Hz line (mains) frequency artifacts sometimes cannot be avoided. Notch filters are capable of selectively suppressing these frequencies. However, these filters, although available on most devices, must be applied with great caution in the case of SEPs, because they may suppress parts of the real EP signal as well. Thus the usage of notch filters is still debated

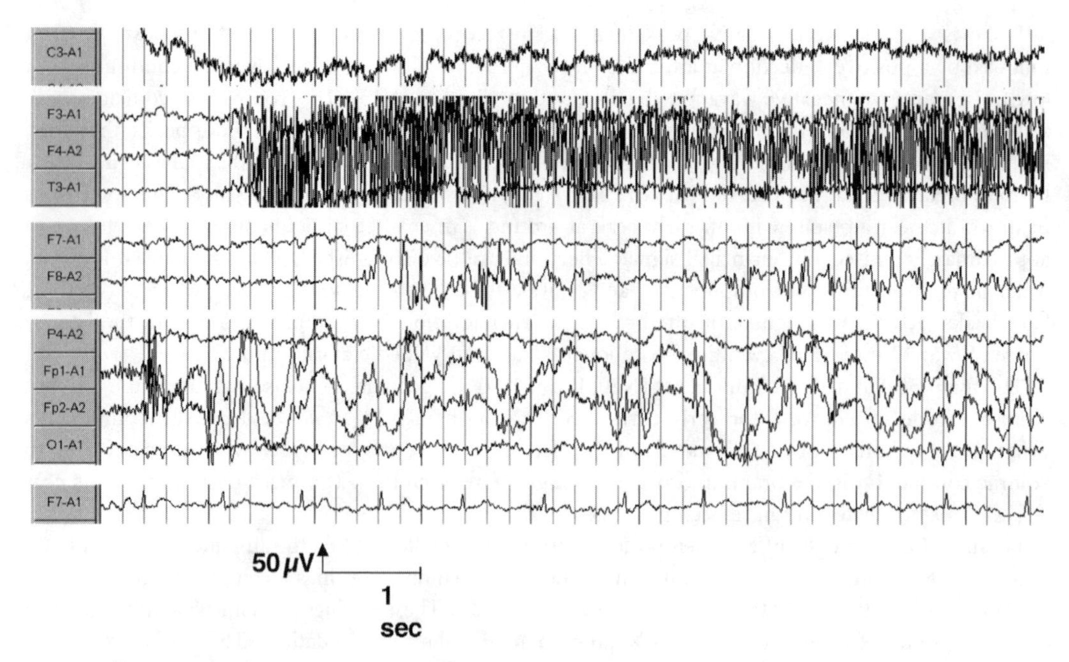

FIGURE 5.5 Examples of different types of EEG-artifacts (shown only selected channels per artifact) that may affect the quality of the EP extracted from these signals: line (mains) artifact, i.e., 50 Hz activity; electromyogram (EMG) acitivity generated by scalp-muscles if the subject is not sufficiently relaxed; movement of electrodes on the skin; eye movements: the moving eye — as an electrical dipole — generates slowly varying electrical potentials which are picked up by the EEG electrodes; electrocardiographic (ECG) activity embedded in the ongoing EEG.

with respect to SEP. Even with VEPs, notch filters must be applied very carefully because they may cause latency shifts.

Traditionally, during EP acquisition the actual digitally recorded epoch as well as the emerging average potential were displayed on an analog cathode ray tube (CRT). Once acquired, the EP was written as a hard copy to photosensitive paper strips. The evaluation was completed by interactive amplitude and latency measurement, either using the hard copy or done directly on the screen, sometimes supported by cursors. Modern EP systems are supported by digital post-processing aides including automatic peak detection. Also, signal display now greatly benefits from modern digital displays offering better quality and larger flexibility (e.g., easy rescaling, color marking of selected signal epochs). The graphical resolution of these screens is much better than is actually required if one takes into account the signal-to-noise ratio of the EPs. In addition to the ability to produce additional hard copy documentation, modern EP devices offer the possibility of storing the data on digital media such as magnetic disks, and so forth. Details regarding these issues are discussed in the next section.

There are now a large variety of digital post-processing methods, such as source analysis to localize the intracerebral neural generators of individual EP components from multichannel recordings, decomposition by principal component analysis, sophisticated peak detection techniques, and so forth. However, routine EP interpretation still relies almost exclusively on inspection of peak latencies and amplitudes. Only for special applications such as monitoring of long-term cerebral function are automated procedures routinely applied.

5.2 Signal Processing

In this section, the main elements of a modern fully digital EP recorder will be described. An excellent overview of EP techniques is found in a book edited by Deuschl and Eisen (1999) comprising separate

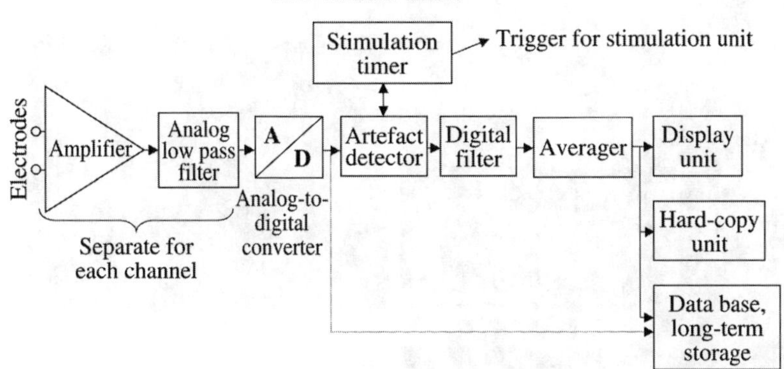

FIGURE 5.6 Technical block diagram of an EP recorder. The digital filters allow for filtering of the signal with a variable bandwidth according to the actual needs. In some designs this feature may be replaced by switchable analog filters. Yet another solution might be to filter the averaged rather than the raw data. There is still no canonical technical concept. For later evaluation, arbitrary sets of averaged EPs can be fetched from the archive.

chapters (written by different groups of authors) for the various EP modalities. As shown in Figure 5.6, an EP recording may be subdivided into the following stages:

- Stimulators
- Electrodes
- Analog preamplifier; safety considerations
- Analog-to-digital conversion
- Digital signal processing; filtering, averaging, and scaling
- Signal display on screen and on paper
- Long-term data storage and retrieval

5.2.1 Stimulators (see Figure 5.7)

5.2.1.1 SEP

The basic stimulation unit consists of an electronic circuit capable of applying short electrical impulses (50 to 200 μsec) of predefined yet scalable constant currents or voltages to the skin. A pair of electrodes (metal plates of a few millimeters diameter) provides the necessary low resistance electrical contact between the poles of the stimulator and the skin. Usually the cathode is placed a few centimeters proximal to the anode, both with an orientation parallel to the sensory nerve fiber under consideration. The selection of electrode material is not critical (e.g., refined steel or silver are suitable). In order to enhance the electrical contact, an electrolytic paste or saline solution is brought into the gap between electrode surface and skin by various methods. Today most stimulators feed constant currents through the closed loop during the stimulation period. Constant voltage stimuli may be used as well, although they lead to less reliable stimulation in the case of nonoptimal electrical contacts.

For the adjustment of stimulus strength the following procedure is performed before recording. Starting from a low value, the current is usually increased until a motor response is observed. For the subsequent repeated stimulation this current intensity is maintained or even slightly increased. In the case of pathological SEPs, it is often helpful to record the SEP also from the contralateral hemisphere. This SEP may serve as a reference for the interpretation. Due to the electrical stimulation a large amplitude artefact is seen in the averaged EP at zero latency. However, due to the short pulse duration and the short time constant of the filter settings (see below), this artefact does not interfere with the EP components under consideration. Typical stimulators allow the stimulation frequency to be varied over a wide range (typical values are 0.5 to 10 Hz). For safety reasons the application unit (providing the stimuli) is electrically insulated from the other electronic circuits of the recording unit.

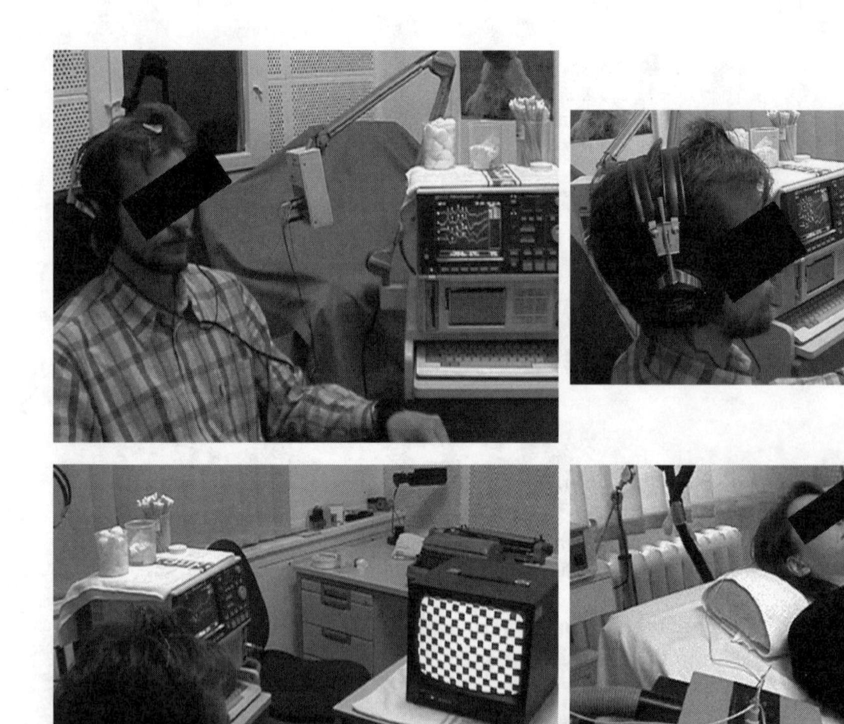

FIGURE 5.7 Recording an EP. (Upper) AEP; auditory stimulation is accomplished by a headset. (Lower left) VEP; note the monitor in front of the subject providing the flickering checkerboard pattern used for stimulation. (Lower right) SEP; note the electrode pair applied at the subjects's wrist for electrical stimulation of the median nerve. For EP recordings of other nerves the electrodes have to be placed accordingly.

5.2.1.2 BAEP

Simple rectangular auditory pulses (clicks) of 100-μsec duration are presented to the subject over ordinary high-quality headphones. Typical pulse generators provide both rarefaction and compression pulses, including alternating sequences. A sound pressure level of around 70 dB above sensory level (SL) is required to acquire stable BAEP, with the precise value varying between laboratories. The SL is the minimal sound pressure that is detected by the subject with a probability larger than chance. It must be determined individually for each subject before the EP acquisition starts. BAEPs are usually recorded separately for each ear. In order to prevent interference from ambient noise, the opposite ear is usually "neutralized" by applying white noise at a sound pressure level of approximately 30 dB below the click intensity. Typical auditory stimulators allow the stimulation frequency to be adjusted over a range of around 1 to 50 Hz, and the intensity to be adjusted up to 100 dB or louder.

5.2.1.3 VEP

Sequentially inverting black and white checkerboards presented on a regular computer screen is currently the most popular method of visual stimulation. A reasonable value for the total field of view of the stimulation pattern, in terms of degrees of visual angle, is in the range of 15° by 12°, with about eight squared checks per row. The pattern should be presented at the largest possible contrast ratio and with good luminance. These parameters must be carefully controlled and kept constant because the VEP latency and amplitude varies with these physical features. Normative VEP parameter values are useful only if the the luminance and contrast values are specified. Typical values for the luminance and contrast ratio are 35 to 50 cd/m^2 and 50 to 95%, respectively (Altenmüller et al., 1989; Celesia and Brigell, 1999), as measured by a photometer device. The checkerboard is typically inverted at a rate of about 1 Hz. Again, the stimulators provide a large range of possible frequency values as well as different settings of the checkerboard (number of checks per row and per column, half-field stimulation, etc.). For the stimulation of unconscious patients, there is a variant of this type of stimulator in which grids of light-emitting diodes (LEDs) are placed in a pair of goggles. Groups of these LEDs are switched on and off alternately. This stimulation can be applied even with the eyes closed. Yet another stimulation device involves repeatedly flashing bulbs, but is used only rarely. Usually each eye is stimulated separately in separate sessions, with the opposite eye being hidden by a shield. Some laboratories append a third session with binocular stimulation.

5.2.2 Recording Electrodes (see Figure 5.8)

Measuring the EP requires the setting up of a closed loop passing the current from its neuronal source through the various layers of tissue to the electronic amplifier, and back again through the head tissue to the neuronal source. Within this circuit, the coupling between skin surface and amplifier input plays a critical role: in contrast to the brain tissue, the skin itself usually exhibits a high resistance and therefore the electrode must be combined with a wet electrolyte in order to bridge this junction. The number of electrodes needed for EP recording is less than with EEG. Therefore, the standard method of electrode fixation is to use a special electrolytic paste that softly glues the electrode, and at the same time provides a good electrical contact. For special cases like long-term monitoring, the fixation of the electrodes is enhanced by the application of a collodium-acetone solution.

Among the metals used for electrodes are silver, gold, platinum, tin, and refined steel. Electrodes may consist of a plate covering an area of a few square millimeters, but thin needles of refined steel are also

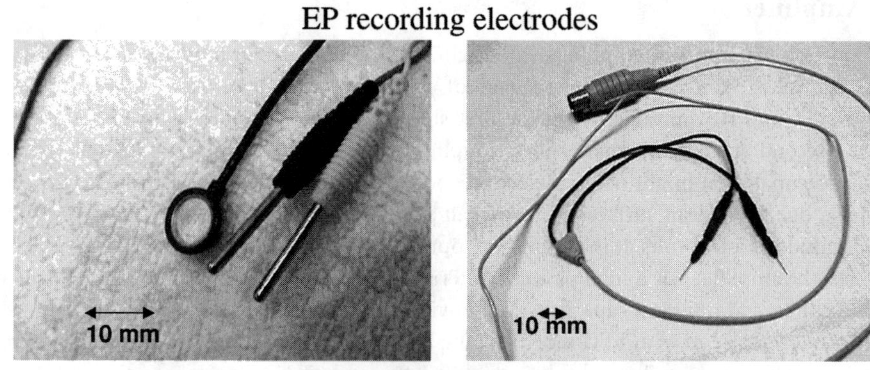

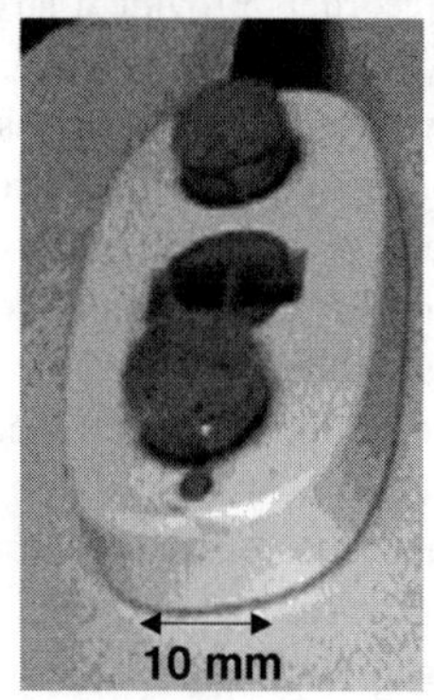

FIGURE 5.8 Examples of electrodes used for EP recording and stimulation. (Upper) Recording electrodes. (Lower) Pair of electrodes arranged in a fixed frame to apply electrical stimuli for somatosensory stimulation.

frequently used. The polarization observed with pure noble metal (see Chapter 6 for details) does not play a role here, because low frequency components — which would be suppressed by polarizing electrodes — do not significantly contribute to the EP waveform. If EPs are to be recorded cortically (e.g., for presurgical evaluation, or even during operations) grids or strips with a fixed geometrical arrangement of a large number of electrodes are available that allow for a multichannel recording to achieve a high spatial resolution. However, this topic is beyond the scope of this chapter. Recently, *graphite* electrodes have been introduced which have special advantages for EEG recordings during magnetic resonance tomography (MRI).

The electrolyte-electrode unit is, physically speaking, an electrochemical element similar to a battery, generating a DC voltage that is uniquely defined by the sort of metal used for the electrode. This voltage is several magnitudes larger than the EEG and EP voltage. Given identical electrode types for all recording sites, the voltage cancels out if differential amplifiers are used. Cancellation of this voltage is a prerequisite for being able to amplify the EEG by a factor of approximately 10,000 (or even more in some available devices) without blocking the amplifiers. If different electrode metals are used simultaneously, resulting in different electrode potentials, amplifier overload may result in clipped signals. Mixing of electrode types should therefore be avoided.

For a good quality recording the impedance of the electrode-skin junction should be kept below 5 kΩ. In contrast to the EEG, this value can well be achieved under almost any conditions, given the small number of electrodes needed for EP recording. Abrading the skin may help to reach this value, as well as slightly moving the electrode. Keeping impedances as low as possible keeps electrical noise low and reduces the risk of picking up the 50- or 60-Hz line (mains) frequency. The measurement of electrode impedance is usually a special function included in the EP recorder, using the same measurement method as in EEG recorders. Details can be found in Chapter 6.

5.2.3 Amplifier

Standard low noise operational amplifiers with high input impedance (in most cases >10 MΩ) are used to amplify the voltage differences between pairs of electrodes (i.e., *diffential amplifiers* are used). The amplifier is split into two modules, with the first stage providing a modest gain of about 10. Before entering the second stage, the signals pass a coupling capacitor that removes potential residual high voltage DC potentials that might occur if electrode potentials are not perfectly equal over the electrodes involved (e.g., due to unclean surfaces). The overall gain in most EP systems is at least 10,000 yielding a signal amplitude of a few volts at the amplifier's output. Due to the DC blocking capacitor between its two modules, the amplifier has a high pass characteristic with a low frequency cut-off that is defined by the capacitor. If several different capacitors are provided, a switch allows several cut-off frequencies to be selected. Traditionally, as with EEG recorders, the *time constant* of this circuit is specified in addition to the lower cut-off frequency. Typical values are 1, 0.3, 0.1, and 0.03 sec, corresponding to 0.16, 0.5, 1.6, and 5 Hz, respectively. Modern digitized EP recorders provide a larger flexibility than older ones with respect to these settings. This flexibility is accomplished by providing just one high capacity coupling capacitor in the amplifier and defining the final cut-off frequency using a digital filter (see below). The same approach is usually used to filter out higher frequencies, according to the demands of the various EP modalities: The amplifier transmits the signal with an upper cut-off frequency meeting the demands of all EP modalities. Then the signal is converted from the analog to the digital domain, with the final bandwidth being defined afterwards using digital filters.

Because of the large amplitude range covered by the various EP modalities, as well as the superimposed EEG, it is desirable to have different amplifier gain factors (also known as sensitivity, specified in terms of microvolts per unit). The average EEG amplitudes observed during BAEP recording are well below the values observed during VEP recording, due to the fact that the background EEG is almost perfectly suppressed by the high-pass filter applied during BAEP acquisition. On the other hand, BAEP average waveforms exhibit much smaller amplitudes compared to the VEP. Variable amplifier gain therefore helps to adjust the actual signal amplitude range to the input range of the analog-to-digital converter (ADC;

see below), thereby keeping digitization noise low. Another solution to this problem, which is easier to realize with modern digital components, is to extend the ADC input range by increasing the number of bits per sample, thereby extending the input range without increasing digitization noise.

Besides providing adequate signal transmission, the amplifiers must be designed to match the safety demands of the relevant *IEC 601* norm. The main goal is to rule out the possibility that the current flowing from the amplifier backward through the tissue exceeds 100 μV, even in the case of a technical failure of the electronics. This can be achieved by placing appropriate resistors between the electrode cable and the amplifier input pins. In addition, modern EP amplifiers usually use optical transmitters to provide full electrical insulation between the front-end preamplifier and subsequent electronics, in order to prevent high voltages entering into the front end. This isolation is known as *floating input,* because there is no stable relationship between the absolute signal potentials within the preamplifier and the ground potential of the subsequent amplification stages.

One important characteristic of the differential amplifier is its *common mode rejection* (CMR) characteristic, which is defined by the ratio g1/g2, where g1 is the gain applied to the difference between the voltages at the two inputs, and g2 is the gain applied to the voltage that is common to the two inputs. A large CMR is a prerequisite for efficient suppression of unwanted signal components that are common to the inputs. Modern EP amplifiers achieve a CMR of 80 dB or even better, thereby reducing common signal components by at least 1:10,000.

The intrinsic amplifier noise level significantly depends on the bandwidth. Given a setting of 1 to 100 Hz, as would be appropriate for VEP recording, the resulting noise will be about 0.5 μV_{eff} before amplification, whereas this level may go up to 3 μV_{eff} if the bandwidth is extended to approximately 3000 Hz, as in the case of BAEP recordings. The total noise is slightly larger because the thermal noise originating at the electrodes adds to this noise.

5.2.4 Analog-to-Digital Converter (ADC)

Going from analog to digital signal representation (see Figure 5.9A) requires constraints to be placed on (1) the spectral bandwidth, (2) the amplitude resolution, and (3) the amplitude range. The sampling rate and the number of bits per sample (sometimes called *resolution*) then need to be adapted appropriately.

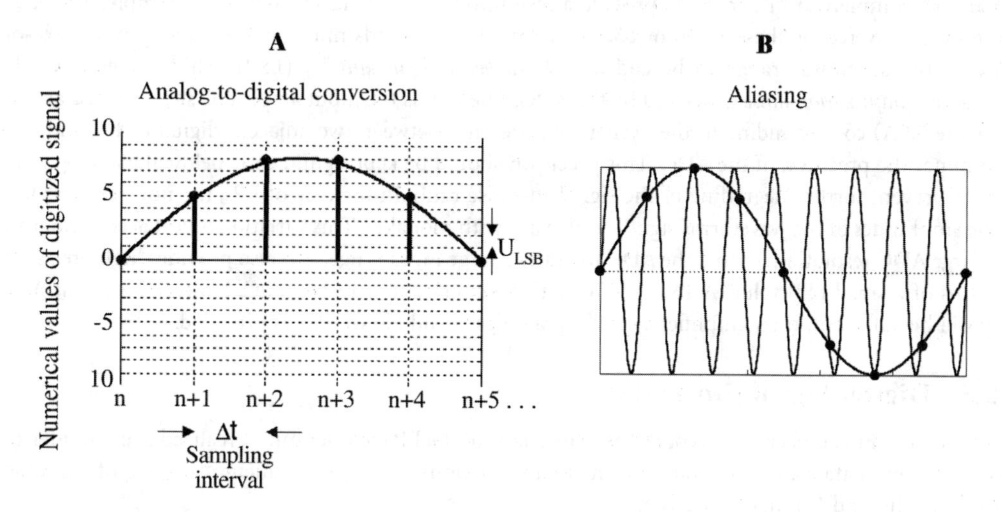

FIGURE 5.9 (A) Principle of analog to digital conversion. The continuous analog signal is converted into a sequence of numbers (indicated on the y-axis) representing the signal amplitudes at discrete points in time with a limited number of different amplitude values. The resulting temporal and amplitude resolution are labeled as Δt and U_{LSB} in the figure. The sampling rate thus is 1/Δt. (B) Aliasing: A high frequency component (thin line) mimics a low frequency component (bold line) if sampled with a too low rate.

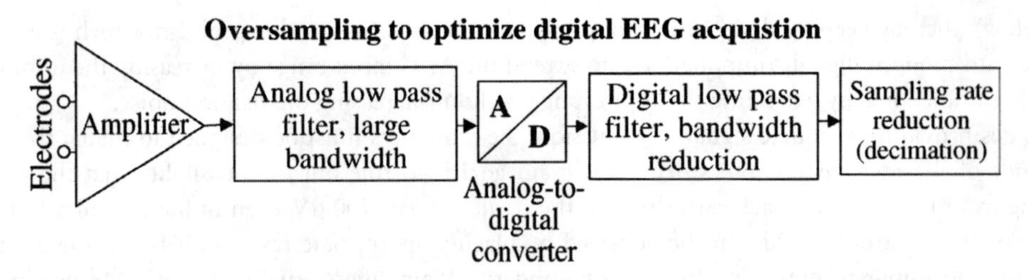

FIGURE 5.10 After passing an analog filter of large bandwidth the signals are digitally sampled with a correspondingly high rate. A subsequent digital filter substantially reduces the bandwidth. Finally, the digital data rate is reduced accordingly. Usual reduction ratios (the *decimation factor*) are 1:4 or 1:16.

According to the *Shannon Nyquist theorem*, the minimum sampling rate *fs* for adequate digital representation of analog signals is 2*fn, where fn is the highest frequency occurring in the signal. If this rule is violated (i.e., fs< 2*fn), a component at frequency f > fn will result in a spurious frequency component of a lower frequency after digitization, with the frequency of the spurious component being given by fn-(f-fn). This effect is known as *aliasing* (see Figure 5.9B). To prevent such distortion, analog low-pass filters (*anti-aliasing filters*) with an appropriate cut-off frequency are used to suppress high frequencies before digitization. Due to the limited steepness of the roll-off characteristic of the filter, the sampling rate should be slightly higher than twice the cut-off frequency fc. Given the largest EP bandwidth of 3 kHz, reasonable minimum values for fc and fs are 3 and 10 kHz, respectively. Better performance, in terms of phase linearity within the passband (i.e., below 3 kHz), can be achieved by increasing fc to, for instance, 6 kHz, and fs to 20 kHz. In technical terms, this corresponds to mild oversampling (see Figure 5.10). The advantage of this approach is that the final 3 kHz cut-off frequency can be realized using digital filters (see below). Such filters provide superior performance and better control of the overall filter characteristics, especially with respect to phase linearity, which is important because of potential EP latency shifts that might arise from different phase shifts. In case of SEPs and VEPs, the bandwidth can be adapted by changing the parameters of the digital filter accordingly.

Current commercial EP recorders provide a resolution of either 12 or 16 bits per sample. The ADC input range covered by these 4,096 or 65,536 different code words must be determined by a trade-off between the amplitude range to be coded and the *least significant bit* (LSB), which determines the additional *quantization noise* generated by the ADC. The LSB is the input amplitude step (labeled as U_{LSB} in Figure 5.9A) corresponding to the numerical difference between two adjacent digital codes, and thus determines the precision of the ADC. This precision should be kept significantly below the analog noise level to prevent further degrading of the signal-to-noise ratio. In the case of EPs, the noise level as well as the amplitudes of the waveforms significantly vary with modality. This variation is best accommodated by a large ADC resolution, so that the ADC tolerates a large input range, and also provides high precision, in terms of a small LSB value. A 16-bit ADC is thus superior to a 12-bit ADC. However, a 12-bit ADC may still be sufficient, if an amplifier with adaptable gain and bandwidth is provided.

5.2.5 Digital Signal Processing

Once the EEG/EP has been digitized, all basic functions of the EP recorder can be realized using numerical algorithms and data transfer operations. The main functions are: (1) subsequent *averaging* of stimulus-related epochs, and (2) digital filtering.

5.2.5.1 Averaging

The stimulation unit sends a trigger signal to the recorder each time a stimulus is presented. Let us assume the set of indices $\{t_j, j=1, 2, \ldots nt\}$, denoting the temporal stimulation sequence. Averaging of an EP for one channel can then be formally described as:

$$EP_i = \frac{1}{nt}\sum_{j=1}^{nt} EEG_{t_j+i}$$

where EEG_{t_j+i} is the i-th sample of the t_j-th epoch and EP_i is the ith sample of the averaged EP. During the recording process nt is continuously increased until the predefined number of epochs is reached. This process is schematically shown in Figure 5.11.

With respect to signal quality, most EP recorders automatically detect and reject gross artifacts before averaging. These simple pattern recognition algorithms mainly check the signal for unusually large amplitudes or amplitude gradients, so that minor artifacts may remain undetected. However, due to the averaging procedure, these minor artifacts will not significantly degrade the final EP waveform, with the exception of continuous small amplitude EMG artifacts, which may significantly corrupt the EP and should be avoided.

5.2.5.2 Digital Filtering

With respect to EP recording, filtering means suppression of selected frequency ranges either toward the upper or lower frequencies (*low-pass* or *high-pass* filtering). In addition, a dedicated filter is usually provided for the selective suppression of one fixed frequency component (*notch filter*), with the aim of rejecting 50- or 60-Hz line (mains) frequency artifacts. The latter should be applied carefully in order to avoid distortions that can occur when significant signal components are affected by the notch filter. The superior performance of digital filters over analog filters — especially regarding their perfectly linear phase characteristics — as well as some typical features of filters are discussed in detail in the EEG chapter of this book. Digital filtering is usually applied continuously on-line immediately after digitization by the ADC. By setting the filter coefficients appropriately, the bandwidth can be easily be adapted to the EP modality and EEG quality. Within certain limits, filters may also be applied after averaging, for instance, in order to remove residual high frequency noise.

5.2.6 Data Display

For routine applications, EP evaluation is still based exclusively on visual inspection. In the past, the average EP traces were written on paper strips with limited adjustability regarding the scaling of the

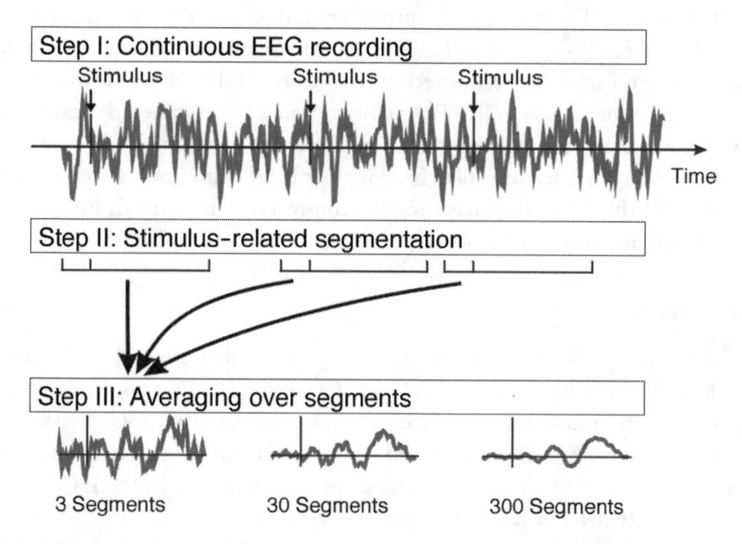

FIGURE 5.11 Principle of stimulus-related averaging. Triggered by the stimulus sequence epochs of fixed duration are extracted from the ongoing EEG. All these epochs are averaged (omitting artifacts) to obtain the low amplitude EP embedded in the high amplitude background EEG.

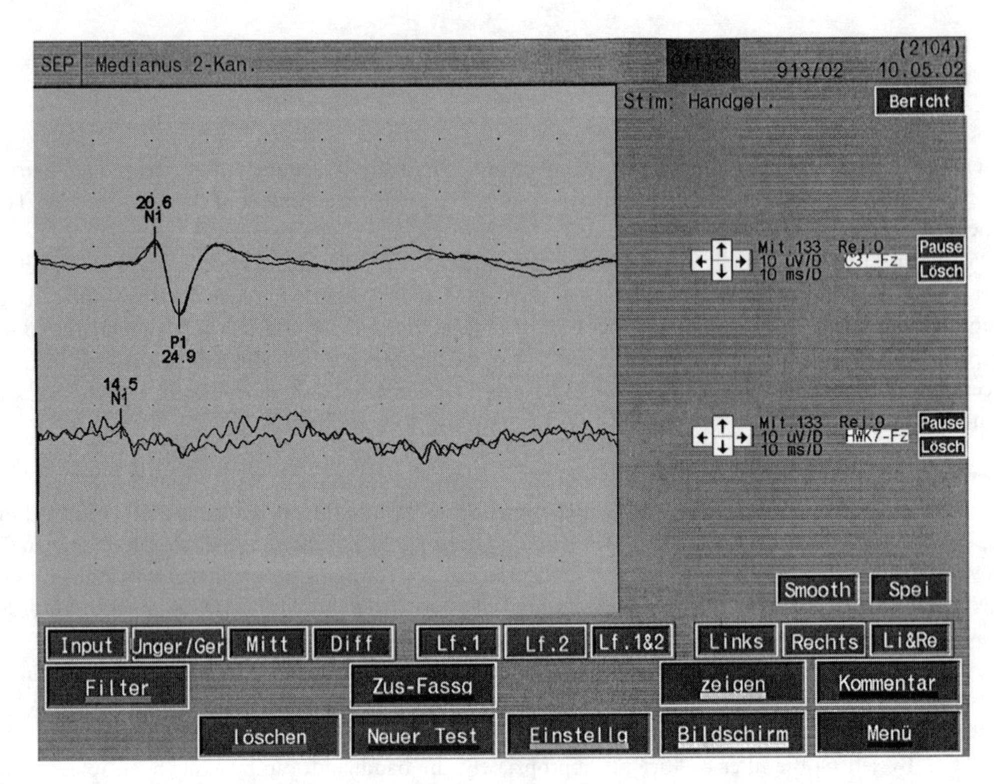

FIGURE 5.12 Screen shot taken from a recording EP device.

waveform. With the advent of digital, graphical computer screens and high resolution printers, the average waveform can be displayed with much higher quality in terms of graphic resolution. A practical example is given in Figure 5.12. The incoming raw data may also be displayed with high graphical quality, and may even be separately digitally filtered for display purposes only.

Latency and amplitude measurements are greatly assisted by cursors continuously indicating the amplitude and latency values where they are positioned. Using double cursors, peak-to peak-latencies and amplitudes are also easily measured. The evaluation is further supported by automatic peak detectors. These tools work well with VEPs, and can also be used with SEPs, depending on the signal quality, but are less reliable with BAEPs. The main problem with peak detection is to distinguish real peaks from noise components. This is a serious problem, especially with BAEPs, where a certain EP component is sometimes missing (e.g., due to fusion with an adjacent component), or where the component amplitudes are close to the noise floor. During EP evaluation it is often helpful to have another EP at hand (for instance, a previous recording of the same patient) that should be displayed simultaneously. For this purpose, most current EP systems can open additional graphic windows and display a separate EP in each window.

5.2.7 Data Storage

According to official regulations, the EP data or figures must be safely stored for 10 years or longer. The data volume per EP is in the range of a few kilobytes. Therefore, a huge number of EP datasets may be stored on current long-term mass storage devices like optical disks or CDs. Compared to optical disks, CDs are less reliable because they are not housed in their own cartridges. The long-term use of pure magnetic media such as floppy disks and magnetic tapes is discouraged in the IFCN recommendations for digital EEG recorders (Nuwer et al., 1998), because the risk of losing data cannot be controlled unless the environmental conditions of the storage room (e.g., temperature, dust, magnetic fields) are well controlled. Alternatively, only the printed EP figures may be stored. Care should be taken if a thermo-transfer printer is used for this purpose, because the resulting documents lack long-term stability.

5.2.8 Post-Processing

In routine applications, quantitative analyses techniques for EPs have not gained great importance. As mentioned before, some simple quantitative post-processing is applied in the context of long-term monitoring, for which continuous EP recordings are made over hours or days. Automatic peak detectors are helpful for documenting slowly varying latencies or amplitudes in terms of trend curves. In order to gain further insight into the underlying physiological processes, *source analysis* techniques (Fuchs et al., 1999; Scherg et al., 1999) are useful in order to identify the cerebral origin of certain EP components. However, this technique requires many more than two EP channels and, consequently, is mainly applied in research rather than in routine clinical applications.

5.2.9 Event-Related Potentials

Event-related potentials (ERPs) are obtained from a generalization of the EP method. ERPs reflect the specific brain electrical activity associated with cognitive tasks. The term ERP, rather than EP, is used because the relevant brain events are elicited in response to internal mental events, not just in response to external sensory stimuli (Picton et al., 2000). A simple example is the so-called *auditory oddball paradigm*, in which the subject is presented a long sequence of auditory tones of a particular frequency (e.g., 1000 Hz), which contains rarely occurring tones of a slightly deviant frequency (e.g., 1100 Hz), positioned at random within the sequence. The subject must press a button when he or she detects the deviant stimuli. If the brain potentials are selectively averaged for the frequent and rare stimuli, different waveforms result for the two stimulus classes, with a specific and reproducible difference at about 300 msec after stimulus onset. This so-called *P300* component reflects stimulus *processing* rather than mere perception; it reflects the subject's detection of stimulus deviance in comparison to a norm, and not just the physical discrepancy in frequency between the frequent and rare tones. Thus the basic idea with ERPs is to vary the brain's response by varying the subject's cognitive processing. The difference between the corresponding average potentials is assumed to represent a brain response specific to a particular mental process.

A huge variety of ERP experiments have been designed and performed in the past 20 years (for a review, see Münte et al., 2000). Some topics that have been addressed with this technique are visual and auditory perception and attention, music perception and processing, memory, language, and emotion. Because of their millisecond resolution, ERPs are particularly suitable for revealing and contrasting the time-course of different mental processes. By means of source analysis techniques (see above), the approximate spatial location of the neural generators involved in these processes can also be identified. ERPs are usually acquired as multichannel recordings (with current recorders, typically 32 or more channels), with the electrodes distributed widely over the scalp. In amplification and recording, the lower cut-off frequency has to be reduced to about 0.01 Hz (corresponding to a time constant of a few seconds), because many ERP components are characterized by spectral components in this frequency range. In certain cases, a bandpass down to DC is used, because slow shifts in brain potentials (e.g., related to cognitive stategies that extend over substantial periods) are of specific interest. Presumably, because of the more cognitive processes involved, ERPs are less reliable (i.e., less consistently evoked) than EPs, and thus more subject to noise problems. For a review of recording and publication standards for ERPs, see Picton et al. (2000).

5.3 Detecting of Malfunctions

EPs are the method of choice to test the integrity of sensory pathways and, in the case of SEPs and VEPs, to test the integrity of cortical sensory processing. As a general principle, axonal lesions as well as demyelinization can be detected and distinguished using EPs. An axonal loss leads to an amplitude reduction of certain peaks whereas demyelinization primarily causes latency shifts, and sometimes extended peak widths and amplitude reductions. In addition, damage to inhibitory or excitatory afferent fibers acting on the sensory nerve may indirectly affect the EP, leading to a slightly degraded morphology. Regarding the differentiation of normal and pathological EPs, the question of the appropriate normal reference EP arises. In case of longer observation periods (i.e., long-term monitoring), the EP history of the patient may serve as a reference in certain situations. Another solution may be to use the EP on the side opposite to the suspect EP, evoked by opposite-side stimulation. Sometimes, however, predetermined normal values are needed for a valid evaluation. Although a large number of articles have published possible normative values, the most appropriate way of establishing normative values is to do so in the local laboratory, because the precise values may depend on a wide variety of factors specific to the laboratory. These factors include the type of electrode, the lower and upper cut-off frequencies, and the kind of artefact rejection employed.

The remaining paragraphs describe some typical diagnostic applications of the EP method. For further reading see, for instance, Cracco and Bodis-Wollner (1986).

5.3.1 SEP

Here we sketch some malfunctions that can be observed with SEPs derived from stimulation of the median or tibial nerve. In the case of peripheral axonal lesions, the early components observed at cervical electrode sites are depressed or even completely missing. Depending on the severity of the lesion, later cortical peaks may also be depressed or missing. Cervical grey matter lesions usually lead to an amplitude reduction of the early component (N13) of the median nerve SEP, whereas the corresponding cortical peaks are still normal. A spinal cord injury syndrome can be differentially diagnosed by means of tibial SEP. In the case of a complete section of the spinal cord, the early cervical as well as the cortical peaks are completely missing, whereas an incomplete section causes an amplitude reduction and/or latency shift of these components. Pathological brainstem processes (for instance, vascular lesions) leave the early component (N13 in the tibial SEP) intact, but may lead to a delayed peak latency and/or an amplitude reduction. Lesions of higher neural structures usually cause similar effects. If the somatosensory cortex is affected, the corresponding component (N19 in the median and P37 in the tibial SEP) is depressed or even missing. Median or tibial nerve SEPs can also serve as an indicators in brain-death diagnosis. A missing main cortical component (N19 in the median and P37 in the tibial SEP) on both sides, both observed with contralateral stimulation, provides evidence for brain death, given further support from additional clinical signs.

5.3.2 BAEP

Objective hearing tests rely primarily on BAEPs, because various pathogenetic mechanisms can be identified from different specific variations of some or all of the BAEP peaks. Depending on the specific peaks affected, the BAEP can especially distinguish between a malfunction of the cochlea or the primary acoustic nerve, both affecting the early components, and a brainstem lesion, leading to latency shifts or amplitude reductions of later components. Impaired hearing associated with *acusticus neurinoma* is usually characterized by delayed peaks and/or reduced amplitudes of later components. Therefore, BAEPs are valuable indicators for specific function monitoring during surgical therapy of this tumor.

5.3.3 VEP

Various reasons for impaired vision can be discriminated by means of the VEP. Beyond variations of the VEP components (amplitude reduction or latency shift of the N75, P100, or N145), it is also important for diagnosing whether one or both eyes are involved. On the other hand, the VEP may be normal in the case of cortical blindness, and may thus help to identify this pathomechanism. VEPs are also a valuable indicator for multiple sclerosis (MS) diagnosis, because the optic nerve already suffers from demyelinization in the early stage of the disease. Consequently, a delayed latency of the P100 is consistent with MS. VEPs are also sensitive with respect to a maculo-papillar degeneration; the P100 latency is then specifically shifted to around 135 msec.

References

Altenmüller, E., Diener, H.C., and Dichgans, J., Visuell evozierte Potentiale (VEP), in *Evozierte Potentiale*, 2nd ed., Stöhr, M., Dichgans, J., Diener, H.C., and Buettner, U.W., Eds., Springer, Berlin, 1989.

Celesia, G.G. and Brigell, M.G., Recommendation standards for pattern electroretinograms and visual evoked potentials, in Recommendations for the Practice of Clinical Neurophysiology: Guidelines of the International Federation of Clinical Neurophysiology, Deuschl, G. and Eisen, A., Eds., Suppl. 52 to *Electroencephalogr. Clin. Neurophysiol.*, Elsevier, Amsterdam, 1999.

Cracco, R.Q. and Bodis-Wollner, I., Eds., *Evoked Potentials*, Alan R. Liss, New York, 1986.

Deuschl, G. and Eisen, A., Eds., Recommendations for the Practice of Clinical Neurophysiology: Guidelines of the International Federation of Clinical Neurophysiology. Supplement 52 to *Electroencephalogr. Clin. Neurophysiol.*, Elsevier, Amsterdam, 1999.

Epstein, C.M. and Boor, D.R., Principles of signal analysis and averaging. *Neurol. Clin.*, 6(4), 649–656, 1988.

Fuchs, M., Wagner, M., Kohler, T., and Wischmann, H.A., Linear and nonlinear current density reconstructions, *J. Clin. Neurophysiol.*, 16(3), 267–295, 1999.

Jasper, H. H., The ten-twenty system of the International Federation, *Electroencephalogr. Clin. Neurophysiol.*, 10, 371–375, 1958.

Kandel, E.R., Schwartz, J. H., and Jessell, T. M., *Principles of Neural Science*, 4th ed., McGraw-Hill, New York, 2000.

Münte, T., Urbach, T.P., Düzel, E., and Kutas, M., Event-related brain potentials in the study of human cognition and neuropsychology, in *Handbook of Neuropsychology*, Vol. 1, Boller, F. and Grafman, J., Eds., Elsevier, Amsterdam, 2000, pp. 139–236.

Nuwer, M.R., Comi, G., Emerson, R., Fuglsang-Frederiksen, A., Guerit, J.M., Hinrichs, H., Ikeda, A., Luccas, F.J.C., and Rappelsberger, P., IFCN standards for digital recording of clinical EEG, *Electroencephalogr. Clin. Neurophysiol.*, 106, 259–261, 1998.

Picton, T.W., Bentin, S., Berg, P., Donchin, E., Hillyard, S.A., Johnson, R., Jr., Miller, G.A., Ritter, W., Ruchkin, D.S., Rugg, M.D., and Taylor, M.J., Guidelines for using event-related potentials to study cognition: recording standards and publication criteria, *Psychophysiology*, 37, 127–152, 2000.

Scherg, M., Bast, T., and Berg, P., Multiple source analysis of interictal spikes: goals, requirements, and clinical value, *J. Clin. Neurophysiol.*, 16(3), 214–224, 1999.

Additional Recommendations and Standards

A comprehensive set of further recommendations is available via internet from the *International Federation of Clinical Neurophysiology (IFCN)*-home page at *http://www.ifcn.info/.*

International Electrotechnical Commission, Geneva, Switzerland, IEC 601 standard "Medical electrical equipment", Part 2-26: Particular requirements for the safety of electroencephalographs (IEC 601-2-26), 1994.

International Electrotechnical Commission, Geneva, Switzerland, IEC 601 standard "Medical electrical equipment," Part 2-40: Particular requirements for the safety of electromyographs and evoked response equipment (IEC 60601-2-40), 1998.

Noachtar, S., Binnie, C., Ebersole, J., Maugière, F., Sakamoto, A., and Westmoreland, B., A glossary of terms most commonly used by clinical electroencephalographers and proposal for the report form for the EEG findings, in Recommendations for the Practice of Clinical Neurophysiology: Guidelines of the International Federation of Clinical Neurophysiology, Deuschl, G. and Eisen, A., Eds., Suppl. 52 to *Electroencephalogr. Clin. Neurophysiol.*, Elsevier, Amsterdam, 1999.

6

Electroencephalography

Hermann Hinrichs
University of Magdeburg

CONTENTS

6.1 Basic Operational Mechanisms

The electrical potentials generated by the brain's neural activity can be observed at the scalp using appropriate amplification techniques. The measured signal is called the electroencephalogram (EEG). It reflects *global brain function*, rather than brain function related to the performance of specific cognitive tasks. Within the framework of everyday neurological examination, therefore, the EEG serves to provide initial information about global brain condition. For clinical examination purposes, the EEG is recorded over a period of approximately 15 to 20 min, with the patient sitting relaxed in a comfortable chair, keeping his or her eyes closed as illustrated in Figures 6.1 and 6.2.

The activity thus measured is called the *background EEG*, to distinguish it from activity measured while the patient is engaged in processing of specific external or internal stimuli. Advanced applications of EEG recording such as sleep staging, brain function monitoring in the intensive care unit, and so forth can lead to recording periods of several hours or even days. Additionally, with certain special patient groups, the brain's electrical signal may even be recorded from the surface of the cortex or from inside the brain, but discussion of such specialized recordings is beyond the scope of this chapter.

In order to serve as an index of the function of a spatially distributed neural network, the EEG must be recorded from multiple measurement positions distributed over the scalp, resulting in a number of different measured signals. For routine applications, the measurement positions are arranged according to an international standard called the 10-20 system (Jasper, 1958; see Figure 6.3). This standardized system facilitates the comparison and interpretation of EEG from different recording sessions and/or patients. The 10-20 system comprises 19 scalp electrodes and 2 ear electrodes. Accordingly, modern EEG devices record at least 21 different EEG signals, referred to as *channels*. For advanced applications, systems with 32 channels or even more (up to 512) are on the market. The American Electroencephalographic

0-8493-1140-3/04/$0.00+$1.50

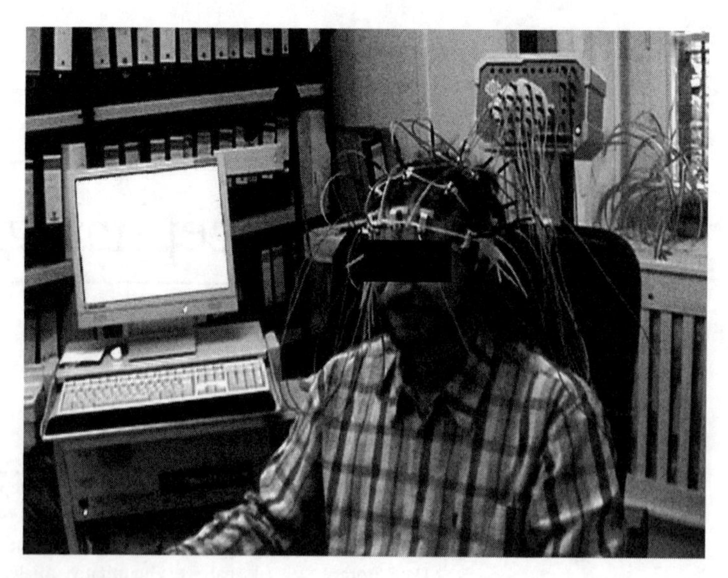

FIGURE 6.1 Recording an EEG.

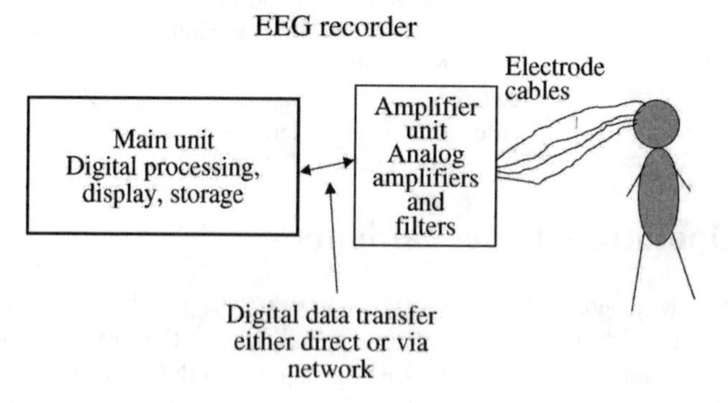

FIGURE 6.2 Basic components of an EEG device.

Society (1994) has published guidelines for the nomenclature of electrode locations that goes beyond the 10-20 system of Jasper.

Figure 6.4 shows some typical normal background EEG waveforms. The fluctuations in the waveforms typically cover an amplitude range of 50 μV, peak to peak. In certain cases, however, voltage fluctations may exceed 200 μV. While the EEG contains random noise, it also contains systematic frequency components, with the main component in most cases being a frequency of about 10 Hz (the so-called *Alpha rhythm*). For clinical applications, EEG frequency components ranging from 0.5 to 30 Hz are typically of most interest. To achieve proper signal representation and interpretation, therefore, a recording system bandwidth of 0.5 to about 70 Hz is required. The recording of the tiny scalp voltages requires both a low-noise large-gain amplifier and a stable, low-resistance electrical contact between the amplifier and the scalp tissue. The latter can be attained using appropriate electrodes either glued or mechanically fixed on the skin. With modern components and electronics, the necessary amplifier specifications can be reached even with restrictive safety limits protecting the patient from potential risks arising from failure of the electronics or the system operator.

The voltages observed at the electrodes are actually a combination of the EEG and potentials induced by the ambient environment. Among these external potentials are the 50- or 60-Hz line (mains) frequency and electrostatic charging of the patient's body. In addition, static electrode potentials also contribute to the total voltage picked up at the amplifier input. The amplitude of these external potentials usually exceeds the EEG by several magnitudes. Therefore, *differential amplifiers* are employed that magnify only the differences between EEG signals picked up at pairs of electrodes, and not the absolute amplitudes (see Figure 6.5).

10-20 electrode positioning system

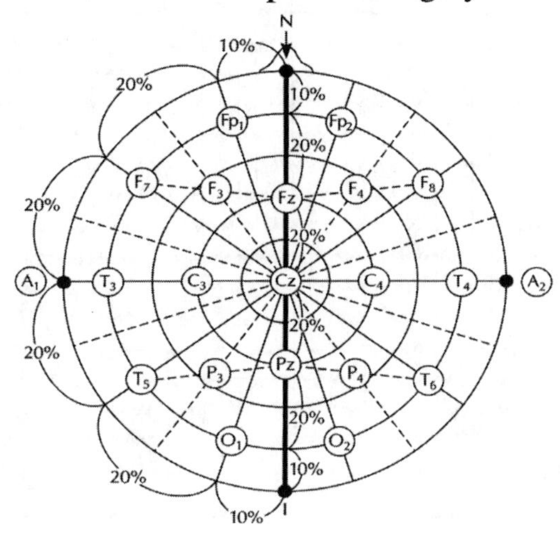

FIGURE 6.3 Schematic diagram of the international 10-20 system (Jasper, 1958) for electrode placement and labeling. The term "10-20" refers to the relative distances between adjacent electrodes as indicated in the figure.

The external potentials therefore tend to cancel each other out because they are almost identical at all electrode sites. There are no electrically neutral points on the surface of the head, or anywhere else on the body, so there is no physiologically canonical way of combining the various electrodes into pairs. Instead, the EEG has been examined using a number of different *electrode montages*, meaning that the EEG can be recorded with different types of electrode pairings. Each type of pairing yields different measured EEG signals, and thus a different view of EEG topography.

Although the set of montages used within a particular clinical EEG laboratory is typically standardized, there are still no standard montages with international acceptance across laboratories. Traditionally there are two groups of montages that are called *bipolar* and *unipolar* With bipolar montages, arbitrary pairs of electrodes are formed for the difference amplification process. With unipolar montages, all electrodes in a particular hemisphere are paired with one common electrode (which is usually located at the mastoid or at the ear lap) per hemisphere. The *referential* scheme is a variant of the unipolar montage in which all electrodes, regardless of hemisphere, share one common reference electrode. During recording, the reference electrode is often placed on the mastoid or earlobe. Given the use of modern digital EEG devices, however, the recorded voltage differences may be recalculated after the recording with respect to a virtual reference electrode, derived by averaging across all electrodes (a so-called *common average reference*). EEG recordings based on a referential montage (often called *reference recordings*) are preferable for this reason, because any other montage can be derived from the signals by mere recalculation.

Regarding the electrical contact between the skin and the amplifier input, the impedance should be (1) negligible with respect to the amplifier input resistance, and (2) almost constant over the relevant frequency range, especially toward low frequencies that approach direct current (DC). To meet these requirements, electrically conducting electrodes (usually made of metal) are fixed on the skin by various techniques. An electrolyte typically consisting of paste or gel provides a low resistance between the electrode surface and the skin. As an inevitable side-effect, this electrochemical system acts like an electrical battery generating a constant voltage of its own, the size of which depends on the electrode material. The difference in this constant voltage between different electrode types can be in the range of volts. Therefore, only identical electrodes must be used for EEG recording in order to prevent the differential amplifiers from being overloaded when fed with voltages that vary widely between pairs of electrodes.

Further external signal components are often superimposed on the EEG, corrupting the measured signal. There are both biological and technical sources of these so-called *artifacts*. Some examples are

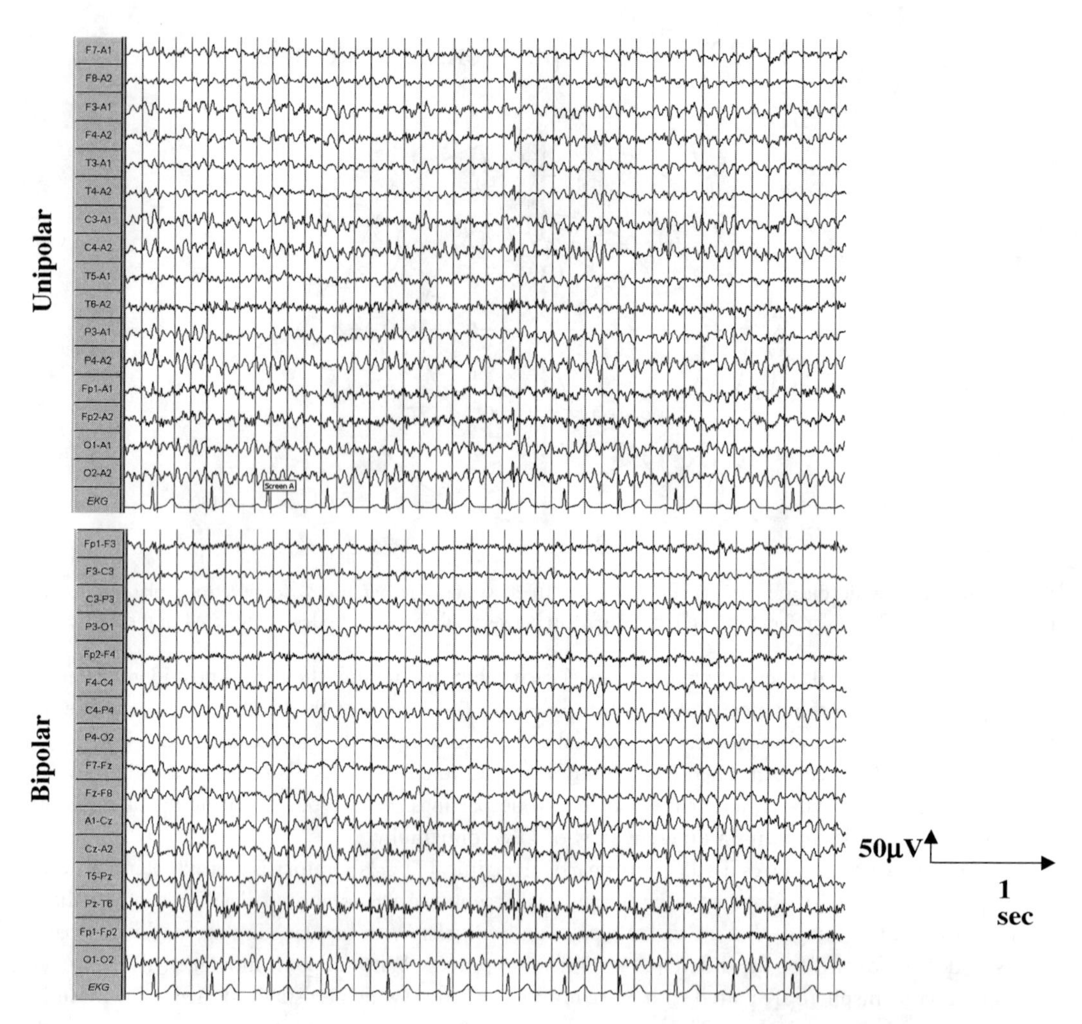

FIGURE 6.4 Example of a normal human multichannel EEG. (Upper) Display according to a *unipolar* recording, i.e., all signals refer to the electrical potential at either the left or right ear electrode (A1 and A2, respectively). (Lower) Same EEG-epoch after re-referencing according to a *bipolar* montage (according to the electrode labels seen at the left margin).

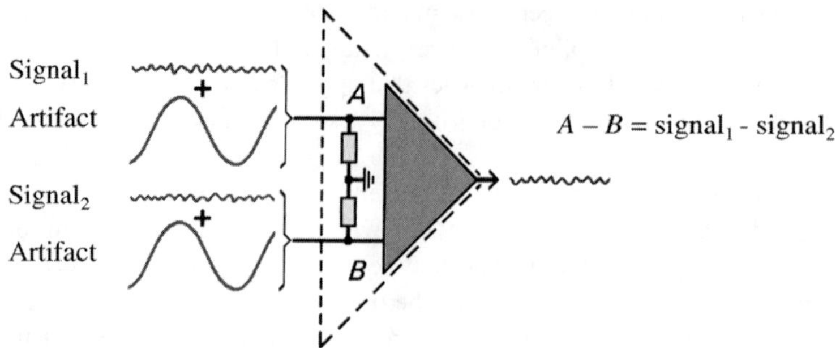

FIGURE 6.5 Principle of differential amplifier as used in EEG recorders to remove superimposed common high voltage activity form pairs of EEG signals.

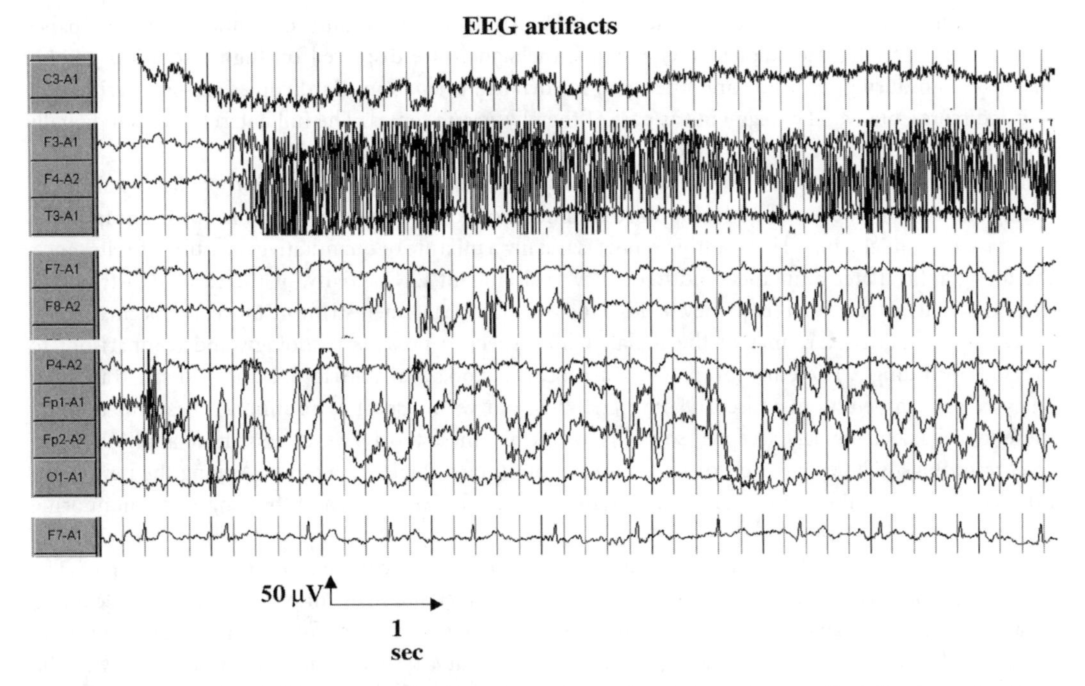

FIGURE 6.6 Examples of different types of artifacts (shown only selected channels per artifact): line (mains) artifact, i.e., 50 Hz activity; electromyogram (EMG) acitivity generated by scalp muscles if the subject isn't sufficiently relaxed; movement of electrodes on the skin; eye movements: the moving eye — as an electrical dipole — generates slowly varying electrical potentials which are picked up by the EEG electrodes; electrocardiographic (ECG) activity embedded in the ongoing EEG.

shown in Figure 6.6. Among the biological artifacts are residual electrocardiogram (ECG), electromyogram (EMG) generated by muscles in the vicinity of the electrodes, electro-oculogram (EOG) resulting from eye movement, and slowly fluctuating electrode voltages induced by transpiration, which influences the electrochemical conditions of the electrodes. Technical artifacts have a variety of causes, including inductive nonsymmetric coupling of the 50/60 Hz line (mains) frequency, which can occur when electrode impedances are too large, movement of the electrodes causing fluctuating electrode voltages, distortions of the ambient electrostatic field due to movement of the patient or the technician, unstable electrical contact between electrode and amplifier input, and bad electrode material due, for instance, to insufficient cleaning of the electrodes. Despite using differential amplifiers, these artifacts often significantly exceed the amplitude of the ongoing EEG, and can sometimes completely hide it. The 50/60-Hz artifacts and the EMG can be particularly problematic in this respect. EEG recording systems are usually designed to record moderately distorted EEG without clipping, although the signal display may still exhibit clipping, depending on the graphical scaling used to display the recorded voltages.

If artifacts cannot be avoided despite taking measures such as electrode replacement, the interpretability of the EEG can sometimes be improved if low- or high-frequency components of the recorded waveform are filtered out, thereby reducing the impact of the artifact. However, unusual low- or high-frequency EEG activity may be indicative of pathology, and so it may be advantageous instead to extend the frequency band compared to the routine setting. Whichever the case, the bandwidth of EEG recorders can be interactively adjusted by modifying both the lower cut-off frequency f_l (traditionally specified in terms of the corresponding *time constant*, defined as $1/2f_l$) and the upper cut-off frequency. Also, if line (mains) frequency artifacts cannot be removed by improving the electrode impedance, an appropriate notch filter helps to selectively suppress this component. From a technical point of view, adjustment of these filter specifications may be done by switching the corresponding amplifier settings or by modifying parameters of the internal digital post-processing algorithms. With modern EEG systems, digital solutions are usually preferred.

Traditionally, EEG signals were written continuously in real-time onto continuous z-folded paper strips. Since the advent of digital EEG systems, the signals are displayed on high-resolution graphic displays, both during recording and afterward for detailed evaluation. Hard copies are only written for selected representative EEG segments as part of the physician's report. The full dataset is stored digitally on modern mass storage devices, which serve as stable long-term EEG archives.

For routine applications the EEG evaluation is still based on a visual inspection of the signal traces, taking into account the spatial and temporal distribution of both the spectral structure and the amplitudes of the multichannel signal. The resulting report is usually a mixture of quantitative measures (for instance, the topographical area amplitude and frequency of dominant EEG activity, or the relative distribution of EEG activity over several frequency bands) and qualitative statements (for instance, the occurrence of specific signal patterns, ratings of the signals with respect to possible pathology, and comparisons to previous recordings). There are now many post-processing tools available (for instance, for spectral power analysis, pattern detection, and correlation analysis), but with respect to routine applications none of these tools has been widely accepted so far. Nevertheless, these tools have extended the applicability of EEG recordings well beyond their original application in neurological diagnosis. Among the new applications for EEG are the analysis of the action of cerebrally active drugs, and the long-term monitoring of cerebral function (see below).

Regarding the technical structure of modern EEG systems, different concepts are on the market. The system may consist of either (1) a front-end signal-preamplifier and main amplifier sending the acquired data via a dedicated cable to a dedicated computer providing the further functionality needed for data storage and evaluation (stand-alone system); or (2) the same system as just described, but with the dedicated computer connected to a central dataserver via a regular network, and with the server also being used as a *reader station* (i.e., for data display, or to allow further computers to access the data for evaluation); or (3) a front-end system sending the data via network connection directly to a server displaying and storing the data and/or distributing them to other systems linked via the same network. Moreover, EEG devices are increasingly being integrated into larger IT networks combining various biomedical techniques and at the same time organizing patient data management. Finally, there is a growing tendency to extend the functionality of EEG systems to include other neurophysiological methods like evoked potentials (EP), electromyography (EMG), or neurography.

6.1.1 Photic Stimulation

One of the main applications of EEG is the diagnosis of epilepsy. Specific spike-like EEG signals, often accompanied by a subsequent slow wave forming a so-called *spike wave complex*, indicate a risk of epileptic seizure. Therefore, these patterns carry a high level of diagnostic information. However, in many patients the spikes occur only rarely requiring an unacceptably long recording period to pick up at least a few spikes. It is known that some of these patients are sensitive with respect to repeated flashlight exposure. Under these circumstances a seizure may be provoked thereby improving the chances of picking up a large number of epileptic EEG patterns. Therefore, EEG recorders are usually equipped with a flashlight generator, with a flash frequency tunable over a range of approximately 0.1 to 30 Hz. This generator may be triggered either by the EEG recorder or by an internal clock. The flash onset is recorded and displayed simultaneously with the EEG so as to be able to correlate it with EEG variations during evaluation. Besides provoking epileptic EEG activity, the photic stimulation, if presented at an appropriate frequency, sometimes provokes synchronized EEG activity at the same frequency. This phenomenon is known as *photic driving*.

6.2 Signal Processing

In this section the main elements of modern digital EEG recorders will be described in more detail. Older analog devices that recorded the signals directly on endless paper strips will not be discussed. An excellent overview of the traditional analog techniques was provided by Cooper et al. (1981). As shown in Figure 6.7, EEG recording may be subdivided into the following logical stages:

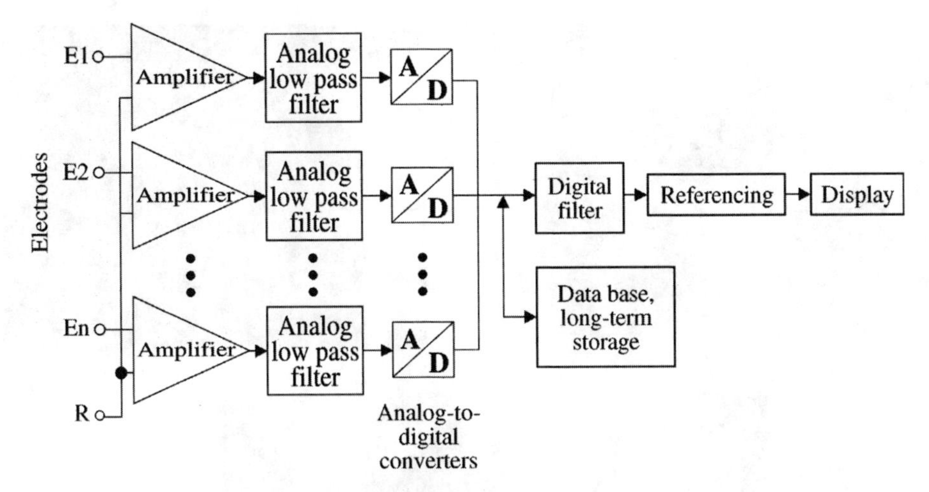

FIGURE 6.7 Technical block diagram of an EEG recorder. Rather than spending separate analog-to-digital converters (ADC) for each channel, some manufacturers provide just one ADC scanning all channels periodically by means of an analog multiplexer located between the ADC and the low pass filters. During recording the incoming actual EEG is displayed on the screen. For later evaluation, arbitrary multiple sets of EEG signals can be fetched from the archive and displayed in separate windows.

- Electrodes
- Analog preamplifier; safety considerations
- Analog-to-digital conversion
- Digital signal processing
- Signal display on screen and on paper
- Long-term data storage and retrieval

The remainder of this section is arranged according to this list of topics.

6.2.1 Electrical Coupling of Tissue/Skin and Electronics

Measuring the EEG requires the setting up of a closed loop passing current from its neuronal source through the various intervening layers of tissue to the electronic amplifier and back again through the head tissue to the neuronal source. Within this circuit, the coupling between skin surface and amplifier input plays a critical role; in contrast to the brain tissue, the skin itself usually exhibits a high resistance and therefore electrodes must be used in combination with a wet electrolyte in order to bridge this junction.

Standard electrodes consist of a metal plate covering an area of a few square millimeters. The electrolyte (saline solution) is either contained in liquid form in a pad wrapping the electrode or it is bound in a gel or paste filling the gap between electrode and skin. Various methods of fixing the electrodes on the head surface are available: a grid of rubber strips, special caps with the electrodes being integrated into the cap textile, gluing using a collodium-acetone solution, paste (i.e., the paste providing the electrolyte also serves as a fixation aide).

Among the metals used for electrodes are platinum, silver, gold, tin, and refined steel. Although all these materials are good conductors, they become *polarized* for biochemical reasons if a constant or only slowly varying voltage is present. This means that an inverse voltage is generated that subtracts from the real signal resulting in a decrease of the observed voltage. These electrodes are less suitable for the transmission of low frequency EEG components (i.e., they act like high-pass filters). For this reason, silver electrodes coated with a thin silver chloride layer (Ag/AgCl electrodes) are the current standard for routine applications. The chloride layer fully prevents polarization. A special variant is made by sintering a mixed powder of Ag/AgCl onto the electrode rather than applying it as a discrete metal coating. This

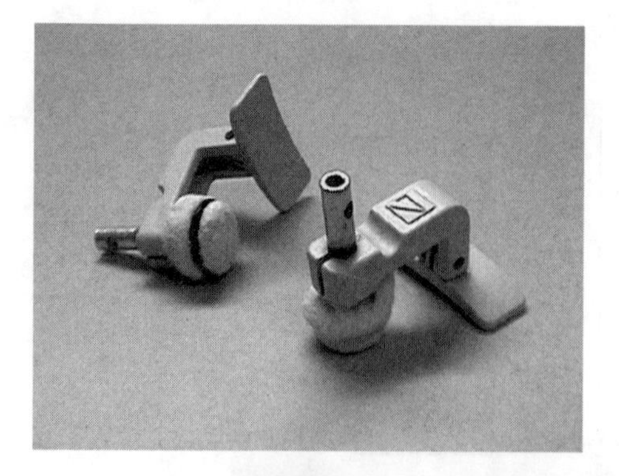

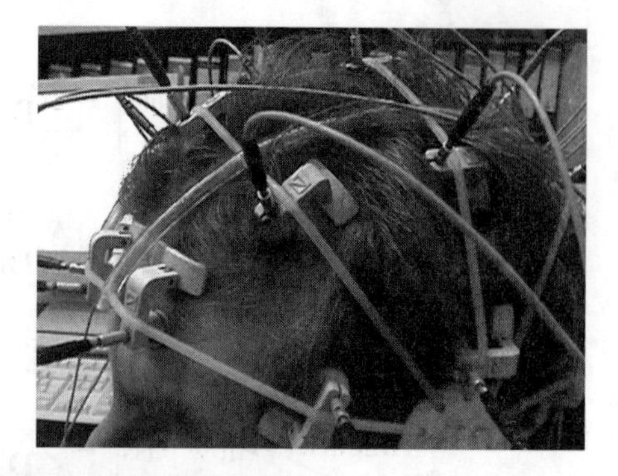

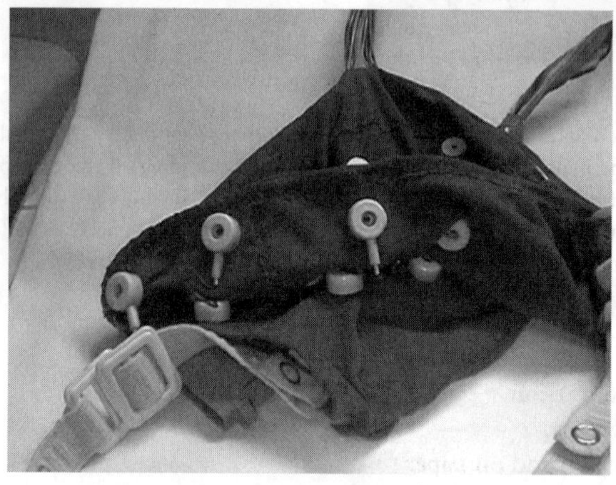

FIGURE 6.8 EEG recording electrodes. The electrodes shown in the upper row have to be applied individually using a dedicated flexible rubber frame (upper right). In contrast, electrocaps are available (lower) where all the electrodes are automatically placed at their right position once the cap is applied.

electrode requires less maintenance because, with the conventional Ag/AgCl electrode, the AgCl coating is easily damaged during routine use. If so, polarization occurs and the electrode needs to be re-coated with a new AgCl layer. Some electrode types are shown in Figure 6.8.

Special electrodes are available for particular critical applications: for example, for EEG recordings during operations, or in the intensive care unit, if patients are unconscious, it is important to apply the electrodes quickly and stably. For these purposes needles of refined steel are available that are pricked into the skin. In this context, the drawback of polarization is offset by ease of handling and stability of contact. For recording EEG in patients with certain types of epilepsy, *sphenoidal* electrodes consisting of either a steel, platinum, or Ag/AgCl wire are available. These are inserted through the muscle as close as possible to the anterior part of the brain's temporal lobe, permitting the recording of epileptogenic activity with greater sensitivity. Additional invasive electrode locations are often used for epilepsy diagnosis, such as the *nasopharyngeal* and *foramen* ovale electrode locations. In the context of presurgical epilepsy diagnosis, the recording of electrical activity at the cortex or even in deeper brain regions is sometimes required for precise localization of the epileptic focus. In these cases, recordings are made from electrodes arranged on a grid or strip, as well as multiple electrodes assembled on a single piece of wire, usually using platinum as the electrode material. Recently, graphite scalp electrodes have been introduced that have special advantages for EEG recordings made during magnetic resonance tomography (MRI).

As previously mentioned, another electrochemical effect, in addition to polarization, results from the fact that the unit composed of the electrolyte and electrode is — physically speaking — an electrochemical element like a battery, generating a DC voltage. This DC voltage is uniquely defined by the kind of electrode metal, and is several orders of magnitude larger than the EEG voltage. Given identical electrode types for all recording sites, this DC voltage cancels out as long as differential amplifiers are used. Cancellation of this voltage is a prerequisite for being able to amplify the EEG by a factor of approximately 10,000 without blocking the amplifiers. However, if different electrode metals are used simultaneously (leading to different electrode potentials), the difference between the electrode potentials will not be negligible and may provoke amplifier overload, or drive the amplifier into amplitude ranges in which linearity is not guaranteed. Mixing of electrode types should therefore be avoided. Alternatively, if different electrode types cannot be avoided, the total gain may be reduced, at the cost of a reduction in signal-to-noise ratio.

For a good quality recording, the impedance of the electrode-skin junction should be kept below 5 kΩ. However, this limit is sometimes too strict for applications in which patients cannot tolerate a long preparation phase. As a rule of thumb, keeping the impedance below 20 kΩ still results in acceptable recording quality. The importance of keeping impedances as low as possible derives from the following facts:

1. The amplitude of the EEG as measured at the amplifier's input depends on the ratio of the electrode impedance and the amplifier input impedance. Osselton (1965) has shown that the relative drop of the measured EEG amplitude is (R1 + R2)/(Rin + R1 + R2), where R1 and R2 are the impedance of the two electrodes whose voltage difference is being amplified, and *Rin* is the amplifier's input impedance. However, with modern EEG recorders the input impedance is usually much better than 10 MΩ resulting in a signal loss below 1% even for electrode impedances up to 50 kΩ.
2. By the general rules of physics, a resistor R generates a thermal noise voltage *Vn* which is specified by the equation

$$Vn_{eff} = \sqrt{4kTBR}$$

over the spectral bandwidth *B*, where *k* is the Boltzman constant and *T* the absolute temperature. With large resistances, this additional noise contributes significantly to the total measurement noise, thus degrading the signal-to-noise ratio.
3. Due to electromagnetic and electrostatic coupling, the line (mains) frequency (50 or 60 Hz) can be coupled into the measurement setup. When the electrode impedances are large, the resulting currents generate a 50/60 Hz AC voltage at these impedances, thus causing an artifact superimposed on the EEG signal. Due to the fact that the differential amplifiers (see above) record the *difference* between two voltages picked up at two electrodes, this effect is most pronounced if the impedances of the two electrodes used for the measurement differ greatly; it does not depend so much on the absolute values of the electrode impedances.

The ability to measure electrode impedances is usually included as a special function in modern EEG recorders. For this purpose, a constant alternating current (AC; usually 10 Hz) is fed from the recording electronics to the electrodes. According to Ohm's law, the voltage observed under these conditions directly reflects the resistance. Depending on the various recorder types and suppliers, graphical or alphanumerical methods are used to display the actual resistance values for all electrodes at a glance. For practical reasons, it is advantageous to have this display at the preamplifier located close to the patient's head, rather than only at the main recording unit.

6.2.2 Amplifier

Standard low noise operational amplifiers with high input impedance (>10 MΩ) are used to amplify the voltage differences between pairs of electrodes. The amplifier is split into two modules, with the first stage providing a modest gain of about 10. Before entering the second stage the signals pass a coupling capacitor that removes potential residual high voltage DC potentials that might occur if electrode potentials are not equal over the electrodes involved (which in practice usually cannot be avoided). The overall gain in most EEG systems is on the order of 10,000 to 20,000, yielding an EEG amplitude of about 1 volt at the amplifier's output. Due to the DC-blocking capacitor between the two modules, the amplifier has a high pass characteristic with a low frequency cutoff that is defined by the capacitor. Traditionally, the time constant of this circuit is specified, rather than the lower cut-off frequency. Usual values are 0.03, 0.1, 0.3 (standard), 1, and 3 sec, corresponding to 5, 1.6, 0.5, 0.16, and 0.05 Hz. Short-time constants facilitate the interpretation of EEG signals when there are large superimposed low frequency components, due either to artifacts or pathological activity. However, if pathological activity at low frequencies needs to be evaluated with high sensitivity, for instance, for brain death diagnosis, larger time constants are required. EEG recorders therefore allow switching between different settings. On the amplifier side, this is accomplished by hardware switches that select between various capacitor values. An alternative (in many available systems, additional) approach is to change the effective time constants by modifying the coefficients of the digital filters during signal post-processing (see below).

Besides providing adequate signal transmission, the amplifiers must be designed to match the safety demands specified by the *IEC 601* standard as formulated by the International Electrotechnical Commission, Geneva, Switzerland (1994). The main goal is to rule out the possibility that the current flowing from the amplifier input through the tissue exceeds 100 μV, even in the case of a failure of the electronics. Such protection can be achieved using appropriate resistors between the electrode cable and amplifier's input pins. In addition, modern EEG amplifiers usually provide full electrical insulation (using optical transmitters) of the front-end amplifier from subsequent electronics in order to prevent high voltages entering into the front end. Such decoupling is known as *floating input*, because there is no stable relation between the absolute signal amplitude within the preamplifier and the ground potential of the subsequent stages.

For special applications *DC recording* units are available that transmit the input difference signals without any frequency limitations, that is, without any DC-suppressing coupling capacitor. In order to avoid excessively large amplitudes that would exceed the amplifier's dynamic range, it is necessary to provide an individual DC voltage for each channel that is subtracted from the difference signal, thus compensating for the residual DC component attributable to fluctuating electrode potentials. From time to time these recorders need to be reset interactively in order to adapt the voltage of this DC compensation signal. Alternatively, a slow voltage follower may track the fluctuating DC, adapting the compensation signal automatically. However, in a strict sense, this is no longer a pure DC recorder.

Modern EEG systems are designed as referential recorders, meaning that all electrodes are measured with respect to one common reference electrode placed somewhere on the head. Accordingly, this electrode is internally connected to the inverting input pins of all the difference amplifier channels. One important characteristic of these difference amplifiers is their *common mode rejection* (CMR) characteristics, which are defined by the ratio g1/g2, where g1 is the gain applying to the difference voltage at the two input pins, and g2 is the gain applying to the common voltage at both input pins. A large CMR is a prerequisite for efficient suppression of noise components present at both input pins. Modern EEG amplifiers achieve a CMR of 80 dB or even better, thereby reducing common noise components by at least 1:10.000.

The intrinsic noise level of modern EEG amplifiers is about 0.5 μV_{eff} at a bandwidth of 100 Hz before amplification Adding the noise originating at the electrodes, a total noise floor up to 0.7 μV_{eff}, corresponding to an approximate peak-to-peak level of 2 to 3 μV (Gaussian amplitude distribution), is realistic.

6.2.3 System Calibration

Although modern operational amplifier electronics are very stable with respect to their specifications, it is still good practice to calibrate the total system each time an EEG is recorded. For this purpose a highly stable reference signal is provided that can be internally connected to all amplifier inputs on demand. Using a 1-Hz square wave signal (which is offered by most systems), the main features of the amplifier and all post-processing steps including filters can be checked at a glance.

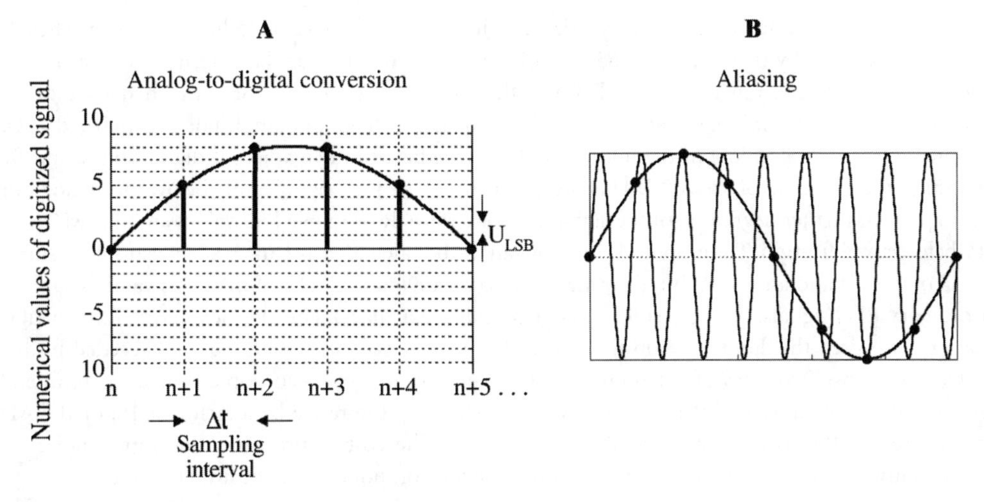

FIGURE 6.9 (A) Principle of analog-to-digital conversion. The continuous analog signal is converted into a sequence of numbers (indicated on the y-axis) representing the signal amplitudes at discrete points in time with a limited number of different amplitude values. The resulting temporal and amplitude resolution are labeled as Δt and U_{LSB} in the figure. The sampling rate thus is $1/\Delta t$. (B) Aliasing: A high frequency component (dotted line) mimics a low frequency component (straight line) if sampled with too low a rate.

6.2.4 Analog-to-Digital Converter (ADC)

Conversion from analog-to-digital signal representation (see Figure 6.9A) requires constraints to be placed on (1) the spectral bandwidth, (2) the amplitude resolution, and (3) the amplitude range. The sampling rate and the number of bits/sample (sometimes called the *resolution*) then needs to be adapted appropriately. According to the *Shannon Nyquist theorem*, the minimum sampling rate *fs* for adequate digital representation of analog signals is 2*fn, where fn is the highest frequency occurring in the signal. If this rule is violated (i.e., fs< 2*fn), a component at frequency f > fn will result in a spurious frequency component of a lower frequency after digitization, with the frequency of the spurious component being given by fn-(f-fn). This effect is known as *aliasing* (see Figure 6.9B). To prevent such distortion, analog low-pass filters (*anti-aliasing filters*) with an appropriate cut-off frequency are used to suppress high frequencies before digitization. Due to the limited steepness of the roll-off characteristic of the filter, the sampling rate should be slightly higher than twice the cut-off frequency fc. Typical values for fc and fs are 100 and 256 Hz, respectively. This bandwidth is larger than would be necessary for the EEG alone. However, high frequency artifacts such as electromyographic (EMG) activity sometimes can only be distinguished from EEG with the use of this larger bandwidth. Some EEG systems extend the analog bandwidth and the sampling rate even further and go down to the lower rate only after digital filtering and subsequent down sampling (i.e., sampling rate reduction, also known as *decimation*) as illustrated in Figure 6.10. Once the signals have been digitized with a sampling rate of fs, all further digital processing occurs within the limited frequency range of 0 to fn Hz.

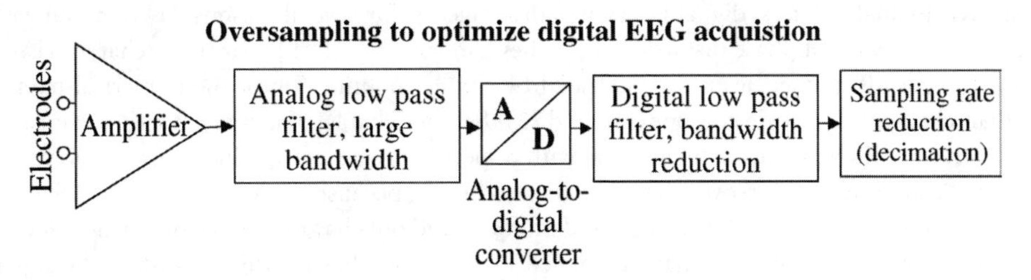

FIGURE 6.10 After passing an analog filter of large bandwidth, the signals are digitally sampled with a correspondingly high rate. A subsequent digital filter substantially reduces the bandwidth. Finally, the digital data rate is reduced accordingly. Usual reduction ratios (the *decimation factor*) are 1:4 or 1:16.

Current commercial EEG recorders provide a resolution *r* of either 12 or 16 bit per sample. The ADC input range covered by these 4,096 or 65,536 different code words must be determined by a trade-off between the amplitude range to be coded and the *least significant bit* (LSB), which determines the additional *quantization noise* generated by the ADC. The LSB is the input amplitude step (labeled as U_{LSB} in Figure 6.9B) corresponding to the numerical difference between two adjacent digital codes, and thus determines the precision of the ADC. This precision should be kept significantly below the analog noise level to prevent further degrading of the signal-to-noise ratio. Reasonable LSB values are thus well below 1 μV before amplification. The amplitude range R can the be calculated as $LSB*2^{r-1}$. For example, assuming an LSB of 0.5 μV and an *r* of 12 bit, the range is R = 0.5*4096 μV or ±1.024 mV. This value is sufficient for ordinary EEG signals, but may still clip large amplitude artifacts. For instance, severe EMG artifacts occasionally exceed this limit. Also, in the case of DC recordings this bound may be exceeded in unfavorable situations. Two ways of extending the ADC amplitude have been implemented in commercial systems: either the larger 16-bit resolution is used, extending the range by a factor of 16, or the ADC input range is arbitrarily shifted toward larger values, at the cost of precision/digitization noise. The second solution is only acceptable if low amplitude signal components are of little interest.

6.2.5 Digital Signal Processing

Once the EEG has been digitized, all the basic functions of the EEG recorder can be realized by using numerical algorithms and data transfer operations executed either by the main processor or by dedicated signal processors. The main functions are: (1) digital filtering and (2) calculation of virtual EEG signals corresponding to various electrode montages. Filtering is sometimes necessary to facilitate visual EEG evaluation in cases where abnormal pathological or artifactual signal components at certain frequency bands overlay (and thereby hide) the background activity under consideration.

6.2.5.1 Digital Filtering

With respect to EEG recording, filtering aims at the suppression of selected frequency ranges, either toward the upper frequencies (*low-pass* filtering) or the lower frequencies (*high-pass* filtering). In addition, a dedicated filter is usually provided for the selective suppression of one fixed frequency component (*notch filter*) with the goal of rejecting line frequency artifacts (50 or 60 Hz). Ideally, a filter transmits frequency components within its *passband* with a gain of 1 (i.e., perfect transmission) and frequencies within its *stopband* with a gain of 0 (i.e., perfect suppression). However, for various reasons, real-world filters do not achieve this perfect performance. Instead, the characteristics of real-world filter algorithms can be described as follows (see Figure 6.11). Within the passband the gain stays in a range $1 \pm \varepsilon$, where ε is known as the *passband ripple*, whereas throughout the stopband the gain is below $\delta << 1$, where δ is known as the *stopband ripple*. The frequency range between the passband and the stopband is named *transition band*, within which the gain monotonically decreases from 1 to 0. The steepness of this decreasing characteristic is specified by the *roll-off* value, usually given in terms of the logarithmic attenuation (decibel [dB]) per octave. The frequencies defining the edges of the passband and stopband are also called *cut-off frequencies*.

Compared to analog filters, digital filters are advantageous for several reasons: (1) they can easily be designed to work without phase distortions (i.e., they can have a perfect linear phase characteristic); (2) changing the cut-off frequencies is accomplished by simple modification of the numerical parameters rather than changing hardware components; and (3) the filter characteristics are strictly identical for all channels, whereas different analog filters differ with respect to their exact specifications, due to variability in electronic components. Moreover, digital filters are cheaper because the only investment needed is the design, which is easily accomplished using standard tools, and only has to be done once when developing the EEG recorder. Digital filtering may be applied in real-time, that is, while recording the signals, as well as later during data analysis and evaluation.

The general algorithm of a linear phase digital filter calculates the filtered signal samples as a weighted average of a limited number of subsequent samples of the input signal. The type of filter is defined by

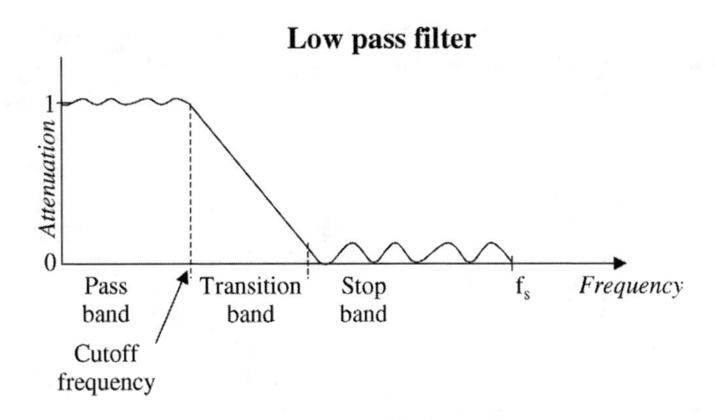

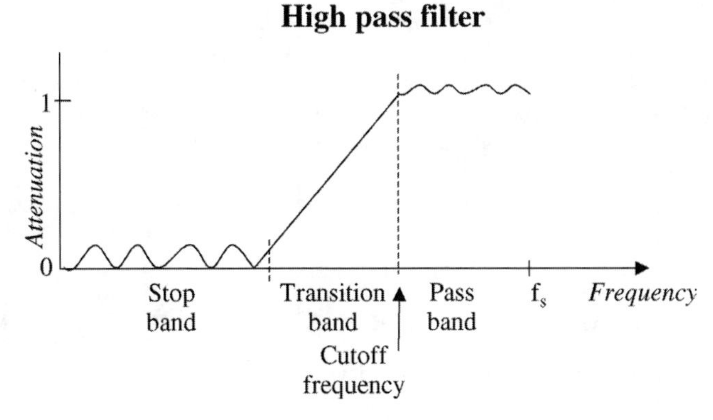

FIGURE 6.11 Schematic frequency responses of digital low pass (upper figure) and high pass (lower figure) filters. The Nyquist frequency is indicated by *fs*. The frequency characteristic repeats periodically toward higher frequencies because the corresponding signals cannot be distinguished from low frequency components due to aliasing (see above).

the sequence of weighting factors. For instance, if all the factors are all more or less similar, the output signal will come close to a moving average of the input signal. This filter thus resembles a low-pass filter. Alternatively, if the successive weighting factors have alternating signs, the filter will behave like a difference operator (which suppresses slowly varying signal components) and thus act like a high-pass filter.

The formal definition is as follows:

$$y_i = \sum_{j=0}^{p-1} a_j * x_{i-j}$$

where $a_j = a_{p-j}$, the filter output being designated by y_i, the filter coefficients by a_j (i.e., the weighting factors mentioned before), the filter order by p, and input data by x_i. The subscript i indicates the time step (i.e., the recording time between samples is $i^*\Delta t$, with Δt specifying the sampling interval 1/fs). From a numerical point of view, the various filter types differ only in the filter coefficients a_j and the filter order p. The latter mainly determines the computational effort needed to apply the filter. Large filter orders are necessary to realize filters with very small passband and stopband ripples, a narrow transition band and other rigid features. Therefore, the filter characteristic needs to be carefully defined in order to keep the computational demands within reasonable limits. In addition, with very narrow transition bands (resulting in steep roll-off slopes, which is optimal in terms of frequency characteristic; see previously), the filter output tends to overshoot (i.e., distortions) in case of steep signal gradients if the order p is too low. With respect to the EEG, this aspect is especially important for notch filter design.

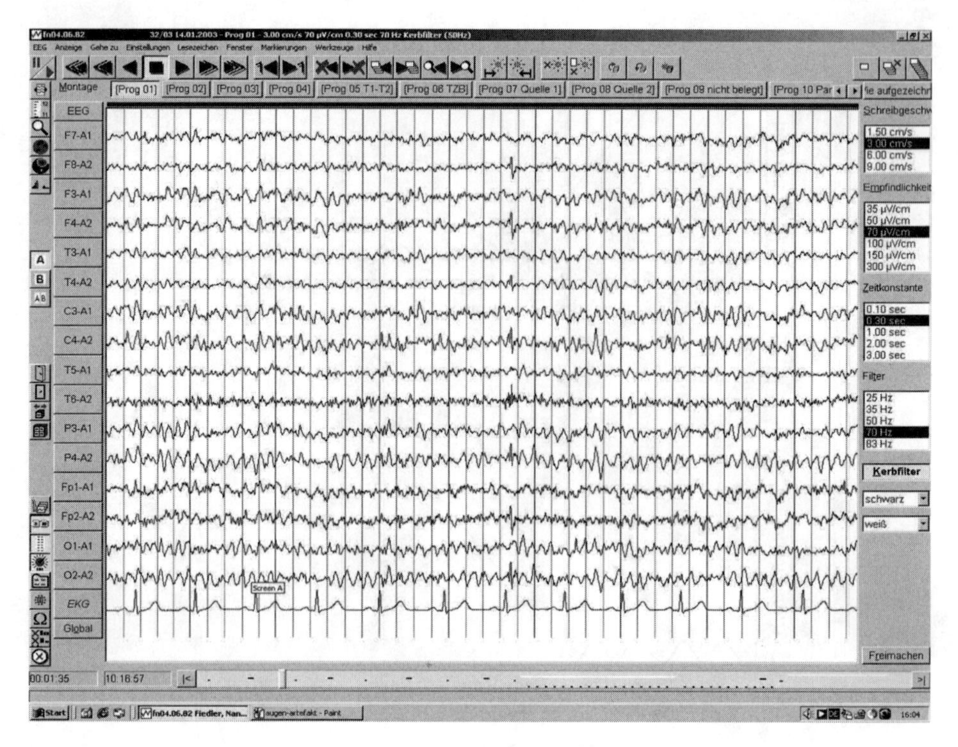

FIGURE 6.12 Screen shot taken from a recording EEG device.

Although digital filters in principle have completely flexible adjustment of cutoff frequencies, commercial EEG recorders usually provide a few preset cut-off frequencies for the passband. Typical examples are 15, 30, and 70 Hz for the upper cut-off, and 0.053, 0.16, 0.53, and 1.6 Hz for the lower cut-off (the latter corresponding to time constants of 3, 1, 0.3, and 0.1 sec, respectively).

6.2.5.2 Re-Referencing EEG Signals according to Various Electrode Montages

As previously mentioned, with older analog EEG recording devices, the electrode montage used during the recordings determined the electrode montage to be used for display and evaluation of the signals. By contrast, with modern digital EEG recorders, the signals are stored in a form that permits subsequent reprocessing. Given that the signals have been recorded with a referential electrode montage to begin with, it is then possible to recalculate the signals to simulate any other possible electrode montage.

To illustrate how to calculate an arbitrary EEG difference signal from the raw data, let us consider how the signals resulting from a bipolar electrode montage can be computed from the signals obtained from the original referential recording. If we assume that $E1_i - R_i$ and $E2_i - R_i$ (where i denotes the sequence of time points 1, 2, etc.) are the digital representations of two referentially recorded EEG channels picked up at electrodes $E1$ and $E2$, with R denoting the reference electrode, the difference signal $E1_i - E2_i$ is easily computed as

$$E1_i - E2_i = (E1_i - R_i) - (E2_i - R_i)$$

More complicated montages comprising channels from more than just two electrodes can be derived as well by such simple numerics. Alternatively, virtual references may be generated by combining a group of electrodes. The popular *common average reference* is a special example in which the average over all recorded EEG channels is taken as the reference, thus representing a spatial average EEG. The detailed definition of this type of reference varies among EEG laboratories.

6.2.6 Data Display

For routine diagnostic applications, EEG evaluation is still based exclusively on visual inspection. In the past, the EEG traces were continuously written on continuous z-folded paper strips, with a more or less fixed temporal and amplitude scaling of 3 cm/sec and 70 μV/cm, respectively, 10 sec of traces recorded per page. Different scalings were available for special applications. With modern systems, the EEG is analyzed using high resolution computer screens to display the signals. Usually the graphical resolution is better than 1024 by 768 pixels, thus allowing for a quality that is almost — although still not fully — comparable to the traditional paper recording. The advantages of this technique over paper recordings are obvious: signals can be displayed repeatedly at different scalings, color coding permits different signals to be distinguished, especially if the signals cross each other when there are large amplitudes, the different channels can be arbitrarily arranged on the screen, and measurement of amplitude and period duration is supported by providing interactive cursors, and so forth. In Figure 6.12 a snapshot of an EEG recorder screen is displayed.

Regarding real-time display, the operator can mark several event types (for instance, patient movement, eye movement, artifact, etc.) by pressing certain buttons or clicking the mouse. The number and meaning of different event codes can usually be defined by the user. Of course, all this marker information is stored with the raw data so as to be available during later evaluation. During EEG evaluation it is often helpful to have another EEG at hand (for instance, a previous recording of the same patient) that can be displayed simultaneously. For this purpose most current EEG systems can open additional graphic windows and display a separate EEG in each window. This feature may also be used to compare different sections of the same EEG during evaluation. In addition to the screen display, hard copies may be generated from selected parts of the EEG in order to serve as traditional printed documents in an EEG evaluation report. Conventional inkjet or laser printers clearly provide sufficient resolution to print the EEG traces with high quality.

6.2.7 Amplitude Mapping

The traditional way of displaying the observed EEG is to draw the amplitude of the n channels over time as n separate traces. This method allows for an excellent temporal analysis but is less suitable for topographical evaluations. Therefore, a complementary method has been developed showing the amplitudes of all channels at one instant in time, or averaged across a short time interval, for the topographical region covered by the electrode set (assuming a reference montage). Figure 6.13 shows an example of such a *topographic map*. Amplitude values between electrodes are estimated from the measured values by interpolation techniques, for example, by two-dimensional spline algorithms (see Perrin et al., 1987). The amplitude values are color or grayscale coded. Alternatively, equipotential lines may be used to

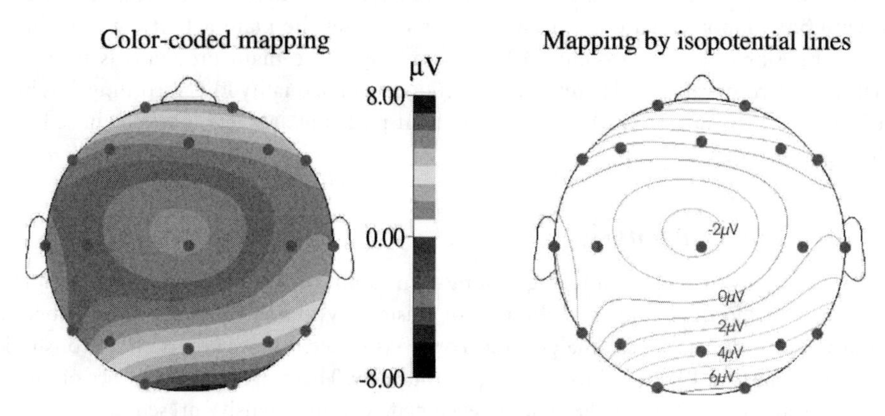

FIGURE 6.13 Display of spatial amplitude distributions applying mapping techniques. Amplitudes between electrodes (marked by dots in the figure) are estimated by means of spatial interpolation algorithms.

display the spatial amplitude distribution. A sequence of maps derived for different time points provides a concise overview of the spatiotemporal evolution of the EEG.

A crucial issue with amplitude mapping is the selection of the reference electrode. Maps derived using different reference signals (for instance, the central electrode Cz vs. a common average reference) may look completely different. Also, artifacts may lead to substantially corrupted maps, with the consequent risk of a severe misinterpretation if only the map is used for evaluation, rather than using it in conjunction with the raw underlying signals.

6.2.8 Data Storage

According to official regulations, clinical EEG data must be safely stored over 10 years or longer. The data volume per EEG session is typically about 10 MB (assuming 21 channels, a 256 Hz sampling rate, 2 bytes per sample, and a 15-min recording time). Despite the constantly growing capacity of magnetic disk storage devices, this medium is still not large enough to hold all EEG records acquired over several years. In addition, magnetic disks may "crash" and thus are not acceptable with respect to data safety. Therefore, current EEG devices are equipped with long-term storage devices. The IFCN recommendations for digital EEG recorders (Nuwer et al., 1998) encourage users to use optical disks to archive data, rather than magnetic tape media. The latter are less stable due to suboptimal mechanical and magnetic characteristics; in particular, there is a risk of erasing data due to ambient magnetic fields in the vicinity of strong electric currents. Recently, recordable CDs have become popular as storage devices. The stability of this medium may be sufficient for a 10-year period, but care must be taken to properly handle and store the CDs because they are not as well mechanically shielded as regular optical disks, which are permanently housed in individual cassettes.

As a general recommendation, the raw data should be stored on disk without any further processing. The patient information as well as the all relevant technical parameters, plus event marks, should be kept within the same file. This guarantees that a particular patient's EEG file can be retrieved even if the patient database crashes.

6.2.9 Visual Analysis

In routine clinical EEG applications, the focus of the visual analysis is on (1) the spectral structure of the EEG, (2) the topographical distribution of the various frequency components, (3) potential hemispheric asymmetries, (4) focused abnormal activity, and (5) spikes or a complex of spikes with a subsequent slow wave, especially in the context of EEG recorded from epileptic patients. The spectral evaluation concentrates on estimating the main amplitude and frequency in four basic frequency bands: *Delta* (0.5–4 Hz), *Theta* (4–8 Hz), *Alpha* (8–13 Hz), and *Beta* (13–30 Hz). These bands are accepted with only minor variations worldwide. In most cases the main activity of the adult EEG is observed in the Alpha band at around 10 Hz. Often one of the main problems is to discriminate artifactual activity from real EEG. Therefore, in addition to a high quality EEG recording, it is important to get sufficient information from the technician about potential artifacts that may have been introduced during recording.

6.2.10 Quantitative Analysis

Advanced applications such as monitoring of long-term brain function, sleep staging, evaluating the effects of drugs on the EEG, and so forth are not feasible by means of visual analysis because this method does not involve statistical analysis. Moreover, visual techniques are too time consuming and prone to error if hours of EEG need to be analyzed routinely. Therefore, a large variety of quantitative computer-based analysis techniques have been developed. A comprehensive presentation of all relevant methods exceeds the scope of this paper. Here, though, some methods are sketched that have gained some practical importance.

6.2.10.1 Spectral Analysis

This technique aims at estimating the spectral distribution of the signal power. Depending on the application, the result is just one power spectrum per channel, or a sequence of short-term spectra per channel. For further processing, the spectral data (some 100 numbers per spectrum) are usually concentrated in band-power values representing the average power and the median frequency in a small set of frequency bands. Various approaches to estimating the spectra have been proposed. Among these are (1) calculating and averaging the short-term spectra of consecutive signal segments using the fast Fourier transform (FFT); (2) parametric spectral analysis by fitting stepwise constant or time-varying linear stochastic models to the data; and (3) wavelet-based time-varying spectral analysis. A typical EEG power spectrum derived with method (1) is shown in Figure 6.14.

Spectral analysis is not restricted to the separate analysis of individual signals, but may be used to analyze the *joint* spectral power in pairs of signals, resulting in *cross spectra.* A special normalized variant of this technique results in *coherence spectra* which reflect the spectrally resolved correlation between pairs of signals. Coherence spectra have been used by a variety of authors to analyze functional connectivity between different brain regions.

6.2.10.2 Pattern Recognition

One of the paramount applications of the EEG is supporting the diagnosis of epilepsy. EEG spikes, and/ or spikes combined with a subsequent slow wave, are highly specific in indicating a risk of epileptic seizures. In many epileptic patients these patterns occur only very rarely or in an unusual morphology, even under photic stimulation. Hours or even days of continuous EEG recordings are sometimes required to pick up a sufficient number of spikes for a valid evaluation. Visual inspection is hardly feasible for these long-term EEG traces. In order to recognize these patterns, automatic procedures have been developed that detect steep slopes, sudden amplitude increases, unusual local spectral structure, and so forth. Once these patterns have been identified, a second important step is to discriminate true patterns from artifacts that frequently mimic these patterns.

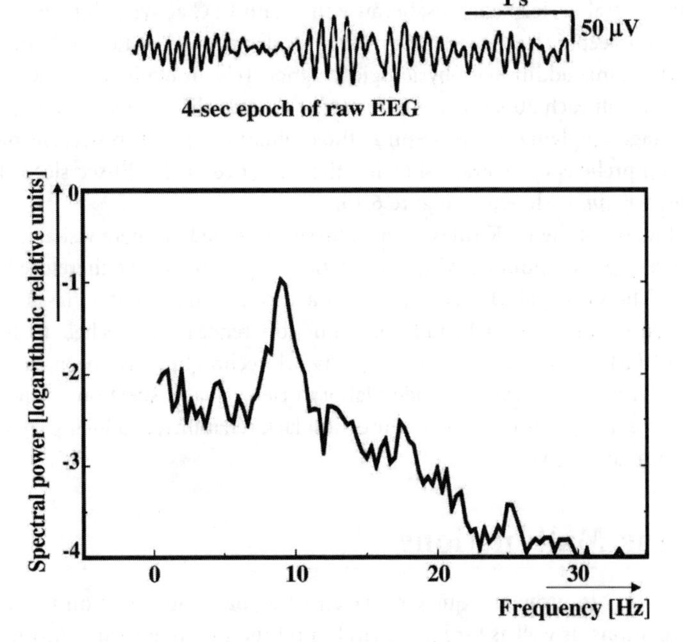

FIGURE 6.14 Example of an EEG power spectrum (representing one channel) estimated by averaging over 20 short-term spectra calculated from subsequent 4-sec epochs (one example shown in the upper trace). Note the peak near 10 Hz representing the dominating 10 Hz background activity seen in most nonpathological EEG recordings.

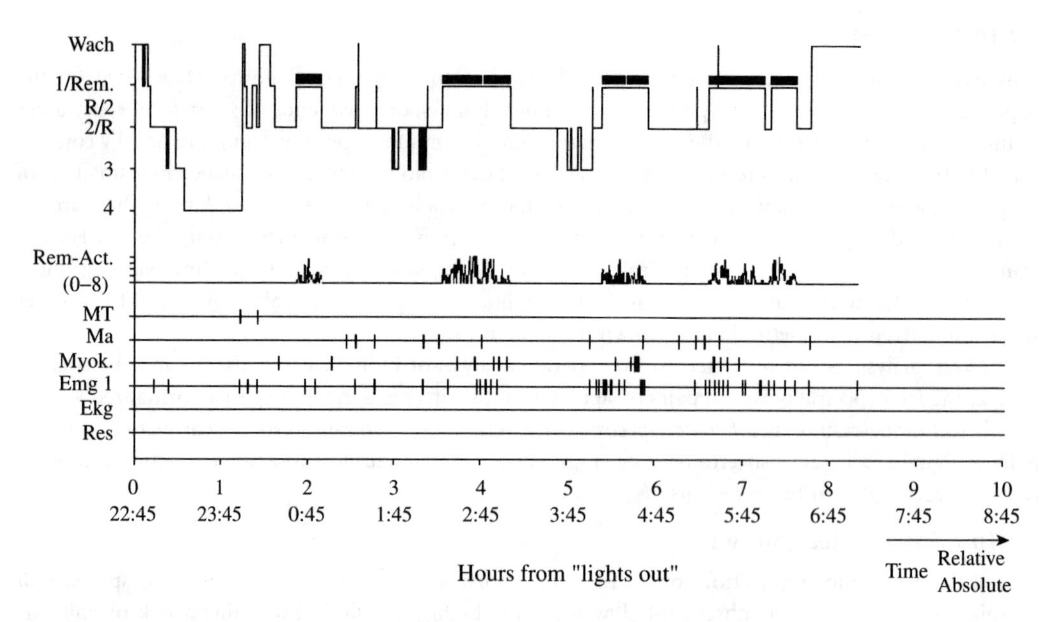

FIGURE 6.15 Example of a hypnogram (upper trace) resulting from an evaluation of a whole night recording according to the Rechtschaffen and Kales rules. Besides several channels of EEG, additional signals are included, among them the electrooculogram (EOG) and an electromyogram (EMG). Each step represents a 30-sec epoch classified into one of five different sleep stages (plus wakeness). Note the almost periodic repetition of low and deep sleep stages. In the lower part of the figure some additional results are shown like phases of rapid eye movements (REM, defining a sleep stage of its own), EMG activity, etc.

6.2.10.3 Sleep Staging

EEG recordings are central in sleep analysis, because the main EEG activity shifts more and more toward lower frequencies with deeper sleep stages. According to rules defined by Rechtschaffen and Kales (1968) (R&K), the EEG plus some additional physiological signals (electrooculogram [EOG], EMG) are rated in 30-sec steps. As a result each 30-sec period is assigned to four different sleep stages, plus the *rapid eye movement* (*REM*) stage. Applying this procedure, the evaluation of an 8-h sleep recording can be compressed into one comprehensive diagram showing the sequence of the 30-sec sleep stages. An example of this so called *hypnogram* is shown in Figure 6.15.

Since the introduction of the R&K rules, sleep analysis has relied on mere visual inspection, with each such analysis requiring several hours of visual inspection. Algorithms have therefore been developed for automatic analysis. The principal idea is to perform a spectral analysis and classify the low frequency activity using a discriminant function. In addition, some coherence measures help to discriminate normal sleep activity from REM activity. Recently, neural network techniques have been successfully applied in classifying sleep activity. Nevertheless, in many laboratories visual inspection of the signals is still the gold standard, because many automatic procedures still lack reliability, producing conclusions that differ from those of the human expert.

6.3 Detecting Malfunctions

The capacity of the EEG to provide a quick overview of global brain function is exploited for routine neurological examinations, as well as for long-term brain function monitoring during operations and in the intensive care unit. Here some typical applications are briefly discussed. A more comprehensive description is found in Niedermeyer and Lopes da Silva (1998).

6.3.1 Detecting Focused Malfunction

In a routine neurological examination, the EEG is often used either to exclude or to prove topographically focused central functional disturbances. For this purpose, the physician looks for topographically abnormal frequency distributions (especially frequencies below 8 Hz) occurring at a limited number of electrode sites, thus reflecting a limited brain area. The EEG is not only sensitive to such disturbances, but can also provide an estimate of severity of malfunction. However, conclusions as to the reason for the malfunction (which might be a tumor, an edema, a brain contusion, etc.) cannot be based on the EEG alone. A classical application for the EEG is estimation of the severity of head injuries. Also, following head injury the course of central nervous system function can be noninvasively monitored over hours, days, or weeks in the intensive care unit. Encephalitis is one of the rare diseases for which the EEG alone can provide strong evidence for its differential diagnosis, based on specific patterns of focused abnormalities over the temporal lobe that are almost unique to this disease.

6.3.2 Epilepsy

Two prominent issues in the context of epilepsy diagnoses are (1) to classify the type of epilepsy, and (2) to identify the epileptic focus driving the pathological activity. Both issues are important for selecting an appropriate therapeutic approach. The EEG is capable of addressing both questions. In general, most epileptic patients exhibit specific EEG patterns in a restricted brain area, which can be observed in a subset of skull electrodes located near these areas. These patterns usually comprise one or several subsequent spikes (duration < 100 msec), which are sometimes followed by a slow wave (duration = a few hundred milliseconds). Several variants of this so-called *spike wave complex* are specific to particular variants of epilepsy, permitting the use of EEG for differential diagnosis.

In addition, the topographical distribution of the abnormal activity can help to localize the epileptic focus. *Source analysis* techniques may further support this localization. Given a high signal-to-noise ratio, they are able to relate the surface voltage distribution to the underlying intracerebral neural sources. One of the main problems here is to observe a sufficient number of interictal spikes within a routine EEG recording session of only 15 to 20 min. Therefore, long-term EEG recording techniques are available that use ambulatory devices to pick up these EEG sequences. However, in severe cases in which only surgical therapy can help, depth recordings may be required to identify the epileptic focus with sufficient precision.

6.3.3 Coma Staging

In comatose patients, both adequate therapy and prognosis depend on the coma depth and its development. The EEG is a sensitive measure for evaluating these. Again, certain morphological and topographical EEG patterns provide specific evidence of various coma stages.

6.3.4 Brain Death Diagnosis

The spontaneous EEG is one of the most sensitive measures available for brain death diagnosis. According to official German recommendations, the EEG can prove brain death if (1) there is clinical evidence for this pathological status, (2) no brain-related electrical activity can be recorded even at an increased amplifier gain (or larger scale factor for the screen display), and (3) the low cut-off frequency is extended to 0.16 Hz and the recording time is extended to 30 min. However, artifacts obscuring the underlying brain electrical activity often preclude a valid EEG interpretation. Also, certain drug states (for instance, due to barbiturate abuse) as well as a low body temperature may simulate a brain-death EEG, and these factors must be taken into consideration before EEG recording.

6.3.5 Intraoperative Brain Function Monitoring

Intraoperative EEG monitoring mainly focuses on two fields of application: control of anesthesia and general brain function monitoring during operations in the brain. Pichlmayr and Lips (1983) and others have shown that the depth of anesthesia is significantly reflected in specific EEG patterns, which can be automatically detected and classified in real-time by appropriate computer algorithms. As direct measures of brain function, in contrast to epiphenomena such as blood pressure and heart rate, these indices allow for a more sensitive and immediate control of the depth of anesthesia, thereby saving drugs and reducing side effects. In addition, the risk of unintended wake-ups is minimized.

During surgery on brain vessels (for instance, arteria carotis endarterectomy), a temporary clamping of the vessel is sometimes required. In such situations, the EEG allows one to check whether the missing oxygen supply is tolerated by the brain. Potentially impaired brain function can be detected immediately from pathological EEG signs like decreased amplitudes and/or slowing in the relevant topographical area. Monitoring of the EEG can be done visually. However, for longer-term monitoring, support from automatic computer-based procedures is advantageous. Special devices have been developed for these applications. In principle, all these algorithms analyze the time-varying spectral distribution of the EEG individually for each channel. The critical parameters extracted from this spectral analysis are plotted in terms of a trend curve, thus providing significant data reduction and noise removal. However, a human interpreter still has to make the final decision regarding the presence of pathological changes in brain activity.

References

American Electroencephalographic Society, Guideline thirteen: guidelines for standard electrode position nomenclature, *J. Clin. Neurophysiol.*, 11, 111–113, 1994.

Cooper, R., Osselton, J.W., and Shaw, J.C., *EEG Technology*, 3rd ed., Butterworth-Heinemann, Oxford, 1981.

International Electrotechnical Commission, Geneva, Switzerland, IEC 601 standard "Medical electrical equipment," Part 2-26: Particular requirements for the safety of electroencephalographs (IEC 601-2-26), 1994.Jasper, H.H., The ten-twenty system of the International Federation, *Electroencephalogr. Clin. Neurophysiol.*, 10, 371–375, 1958.

Niedermeyer, E. and Lopes da Silva, F., *Electroencephalography: Basic Principles, Clinical Applications, and Related Fields*, 4th ed., Williams & Wilkins, Baltimore, 1998.

Nuwer, M.R., Comi, G., Emerson, R., Fuglsang-Frederiksen, A., Guerit, J.M., Hinrichs, H., Ikeda, A., Luccas, F.J.C., and Rappelsberger, P., IFCN standards for digital recording of clinical EEG, *Electroencephalogr. Clin. Neurophysiol.*, 106, 259–261, 1998.

Osselton, J.W., The influence of bipolar and unipolar connection on the net gain and discrimination of EEG amplifiers, *Am. J. EEG Technol.*, 5, 53, 1965.

Perrin, F., Pernier, J., Bertrand, O., Giard, M.H., and Echallier, J. F., Mapping of scalp potentials by surface spline interpolation, *Electroencephalogr. Clin. Neurophysiol.*, 66, 75–81, 1987.

Pichlmayr, I. and Lips, U., EEG monitoring in anesthesiology and intensive care, *Neuropsychobiology*, 10(4), 239–248, 1983.

Rechtschaffen, A. and Kales, A., A manual of standardized terminology, techniques and scoring system for sleep stages of human subjects, Natl. Inst. Neurol. Dis. Blind (NIH Publ. 204), Bethesda, MD, 1968.

Additional Recommendations, Standards, and Further Reading

American Electroencephalographic Society, Guidelines for writing EEG reports, *J. Clin. Neurophysiol.*, 1, 219–222, 1984.

Chatrian, G.E., Bergamasco, B., Bricolo, A., Frost, J., and Prior, P., IFCN recommended standards for electrophysiologic monitoring in comatose and other unresponsive states, *Electroencephalogr. Clin. Neurophysiol.*, 99, 103–126, 1966.

Ebner, A., Sciarretta, C.M., Epstein, C.M., and Nuwer, M., EEG instrumentation, in *Recommendations for the Practice of Clinical Neurophysiology: Guidelines of the International Federation of Clinical Neurophysiology*, Deuschl, G. and Eisen, A., Eds., Suppl. 52 to *Electroencephalogr. Clin. Neurophysiol.*, Elsevier, Amsterdam, 1999.

Noachtar, S., Binnie, C., Ebersole, J., Maugière, F., Sakamoto, A., and Westmoreland, B., A glossary of terms most commonly used by clinical electroencephalographers and proposal for the report form for the EEG findings, in *Recommendations for the Practice of Clinical Neurophysiology: Guidelines of the International Federation of Clinical Neurophysiology*, Deuschl, G. and Eisen, A., Eds., Suppl. 52 to *Electroencephalogr. Clin. Neurophysiol.*, Elsevier, Amsterdam, 1999.

Nunez, P.L., Electrical Fields of the Brain, Oxford University Press, New York, 1981.

Nuwer, M.R., Quantitative EEG. I. Techniques and problems of frequency analysis and topographic mapping, *J. Clin. Neurophysiol.*, 5, 1–43, 1988.

Nuwer, M.R., The development of EEG brain mapping, *J. Clin. Neurophysiol.*, 7, 459–471, 1990.

A comprehensive set of further recommendations is available via the Internet from the *International Federation of Clinical Neurophysiology (IFCN)*-home page at *http://www.ifcn.info/*.

7

Hearing and Audiologic Assessment

CONTENTS

Herbert Jay Gould
The University of Memphis

Daniel S. Beasley
The University of Memphis

The traditional role of audiologic assessment has been twofold: to determine the effects of hearing loss on a person's verbal communication ability and to establish the site of difficulty within the auditory system. Assessment of communication skills leads to the implementation of strategies for improving quality of life through use of assistive listening devices, hearing aids or alternative communication modes such as sign language. Determination of the site of the lesion within the auditory system assists in decisions regarding medical treatment plans for the alleviation of hearing problems. Historically, the primary tools for both of these tasks have been the pure tone audiogram and speech recognition testing.

Today, these two measures, although still important in the assessment process, have been joined by increasingly sophisticated measures designed to better pinpoint the site of lesion within the auditory system. Previously, a diagnosis of a "sensorineural" hearing loss indicated that the lesion could be located anywhere within the cochlea (sensory) through the VIIIth cranial nerve (neural). With today's advanced technology and related diagnostic techniques, audiologists can now determine damage at the cellular level within the cochlea per se, separating inner hair cell damage from outer hair cell damage.

0-8493-1140-3/04/$0.00+$1.50

In this chapter an overview of the auditory system, basic acoustics and audiologic assessment will be presented. Sources will be provided to allow the readers to expand their knowledge beyond this introductory commentary to specific areas of interest.

7.1 Structure of the Auditory System

The auditory system can be broken down into four major subsystems. These subsystems include: (1) an outer ear that collects and funnels the sound, (2) a middle ear that matches the airborne sound impedance to that of the fluid-filled cochlea, (3) an inner ear that converts the energy to neural impulses and (4) the central auditory nervous subsystems that perform complex perceptual judgments on the incoming information. Each of these subsystems contains a number of complex components that can affect an individual's hearing ability.

7.1.1 The Outer Ear

The outer ear consists of the pinna (auricle) and external auditory meatus (ear canal) as shown in Figure 7.1. The complex shape of the outer ear provides two functions. First, the pinna collects the sound signal and then amplifies the sound through resonance in the ear canal. The canal is approximately 25 mm in length and functions as a tube closed on one end (the eardrum). This provides a resonance peaking at approximately 3500 Hz. This resonance, when combined with the resonance effects of the head, torso and pinna, creates an approximate 15-dB sound pressure level (SPL) boost in the signal level striking the tympanic membrane for frequencies in the 2000- to 6000-Hz region.

The second major role of the outer ear system is to provide a protective function to the middle ear system by placing the tympanic membrane (eardrum) deep inside the skull. Cerumen (earwax) helps in this protective function and moves debris to the outside. The small guard hairs within the ear canal point laterally and help prevent the entrance of miniscule inert and biologic matter.

7.1.2 The Middle Ear

The middle ear provides a transformer function. Sound is principally transmitted through the air, while the nerve endings in the inner ear are contained in a fluid bath. The difference in density between the

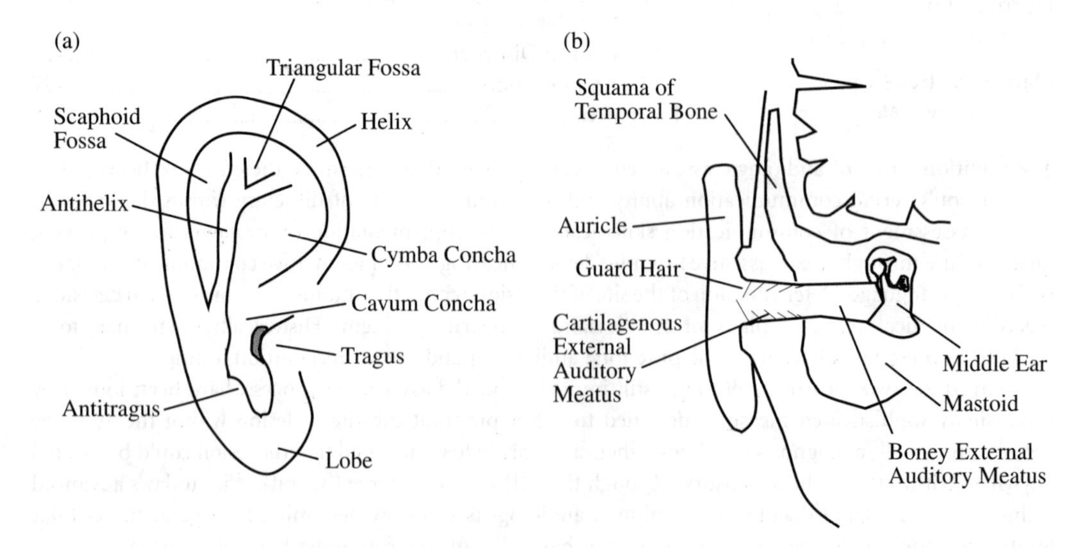

FIGURE 7.1 (a) Lateral view of the auricle; (b) coronal cut through the external and middle ear, looking in an anterior to posterior direction.

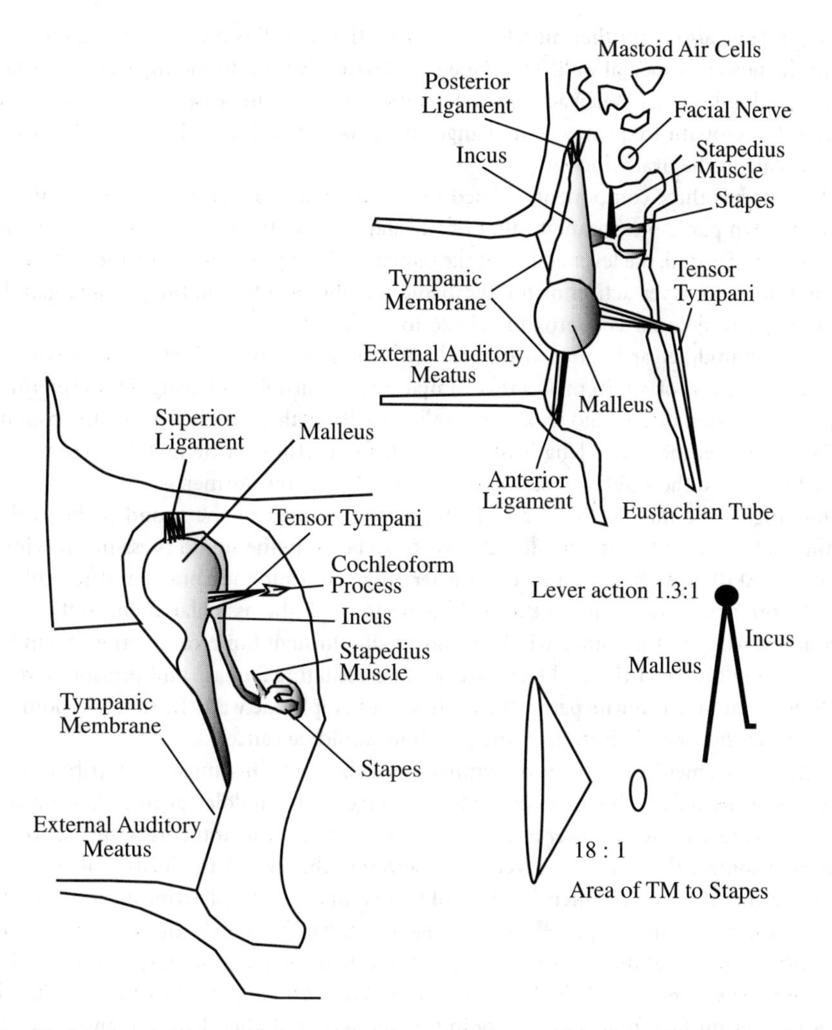

FIGURE 7.2 (Top) Coronal cut through the middle ear space, looking in an anterior-to-posterior direction. (Lower Left) Transverse cut through the middle ear space looking from superior to inferior. Note the axis that is formed from the anterior to posterior ligaments through the malleus and incus. (Lower Right) The middle ear mechanism provides a boost in signal pressure through the area difference of the tympanic membrane and stapes footplate as well as the lever formed by the malleus and incus through the axis of rotation.

air and fluid creates an impedance mismatch. To transmit the sound effectively to the nerve endings, the air/fluid impedance mismatch must be overcome.

The main structures of the middle ear are designed to perform this transformer function (Figure 7.2). The entry point to the middle ear is the tympanic membrane, which seals off the middle ear from the external auditory meatus. Within the middle ear is the ossicular chain comprised of a group of three tiny bones: the malleus, the incus and the stapes. The ossicular chain is suspended within the middle ear space. The chain connects the tympanic membrane to the oval window, which is the entry point to the inner ear, or cochlea. The malleus is attached to the tympanic membrane laterally, and ligaments suspend it anteriorly and superiorly. The tensor tympani muscle projects from the cochleariform process on the medial wall of the tympanic cavity and connects to the medial aspect of the malleus. Contraction of this muscle can modify ossicular chain motion; however, this modification appears to be of greater importance in animals than in humans.

The posterior aspect of the head of the malleus is attached to the body of the incus. The incus, through its long and lenticular processes, provides a bridge to the stapes. The stapes inserts into the oval window of the inner ear. Here also is another muscle attachment, the stapedius muscle, linking the head/neck of the stapes to the posterior medial wall. The stapedius muscle also acts to modify ossicular chain motion in the presence of loud sounds. When activated, the stapedius muscle increases the stiffness of the ossicular chain, raising the resonant frequency, and changes the axis of rotation and reduces the velocity of the stapedius footplate in the oval window.

The middle ear has three components related to its function as a transformer mechanism. The area difference of the tympanic membrane to that of the stapedial footplate provides a pressure increase of approximately 18:1. Second, the lever action of the ossicular chain provides a 1.3:1 mechanical advantage. Finally, there is a minor lever action of the tympanic membrane. Overall, the pressure gain because of the function of the middle ear is approximately 26 to 30 dB SPL.

This gain of the middle ear is often compared with the loss associated with transmission at an air/water boundary. The loss of 30 dB makes this comparison intuitively satisfying. However, the cochlea is not an expanse of water, but a fluid in a hard-walled cavity with two relief ports, the round and oval windows. Furthermore, the entire length of the cochlea is partitioned by internal structures. Durrant and Lovrinic[1] provide a thorough discussion of the middle ear transformer.

When thinking of the middle ear, it also is important to think of the sound paths to the cochlea. Although the middle ear provides a modest 20- to 30-dB boost to the sound pressure entering the inner ear, losses up to 60 dB are often seen in cases where the tympanic membrane and ossicular chain are disrupted. The three paths of sound to the cochlea are through the ossicular chain to the oval window, airborne sound directly to the round window, and finally through bone conduction. Sound enters the inner ear on different sides of the cochlear partition, necessitating a phase and pressure level difference between the ossicular and airborne paths. If the phase and amplitude were the same on both sides of the partition, the traveling wave deflection of the partition would be canceled.

The muscle arrangement of the tensor tympani and the stapedius muscle contribute to an action known as the acoustic reflex. This reflex provides a change in the middle ear impedance characteristics when the muscles are activated.[2] Wever and Lawrence listed four general theories for the acoustic reflex: (1) the intensity-control theory, (2) the frequency-selection theory, (3) the fixation theory, and (4) the labyrinthine pressure theory. The intensity-control theory, in a simplified form, suggested that the reflex is related to a protective function preventing damage to the ear from high sound levels. The frequency-selection theory suggests that the eardrum/middle ear mechanism frequency response is regulated by the tonus of the middle ear muscles. This theory, in its original form, appears incorrect in that the muscle system does not permit fine frequency tuning in the middle ear. Rather, Dorman and co-workers[3] have suggested that the broad upward frequency shift might play a role in speech perception in noise. They suggest that the reflex shifts the middle ear resonant frequency to slightly higher frequencies, an important element for understanding speech, while suppressing low frequencies, which are more characteristic of noise. However, this role is still being debated.[4] The fixation theory suggests that the middle ear muscles provide part of the supportive mechanism for the middle ear and contribute to the strength and rigidity of the ossicular chain. The final theory of labyrinthine pressure regulation has been rejected.

It is necessary for the resting middle ear pressure to be equal to that of the surrounding atmosphere for it to work optimally. If there is a pressure imbalance, the tympanic membrane will be moved from its normal rest position, resulting in a change in hearing. A passage known as the eustachian tube traveling from the middle ear cavity into the nasopharyngeal cavity regulates middle ear pressure. The eustachian tube exits the anterior wall of the middle ear space and opens at the posterior lateral aspect of the nasopharyngeal area adjacent to the adenoid. The eustachian tube is normally closed, opening only when the muscles raising the soft palate, at the rear of the oral cavity, are activated, such as during swallowing or yawning. The typical "stuffy ear" feeling when flying is due to the tube not being able to adjust rapidly enough to the large changes in atmospheric pressure. During childhood, as the bones of the face grow, the eustachian tube angle changes significantly, up until about 9 years of age. This change in angle results in an associated change in the vector of the muscles opening it. This, coupled with a reduction of the size of the adenoids with age, are primary factors accounting for the relatively low incidence of middle ear problems in adults, relative to that seen in early childhood.

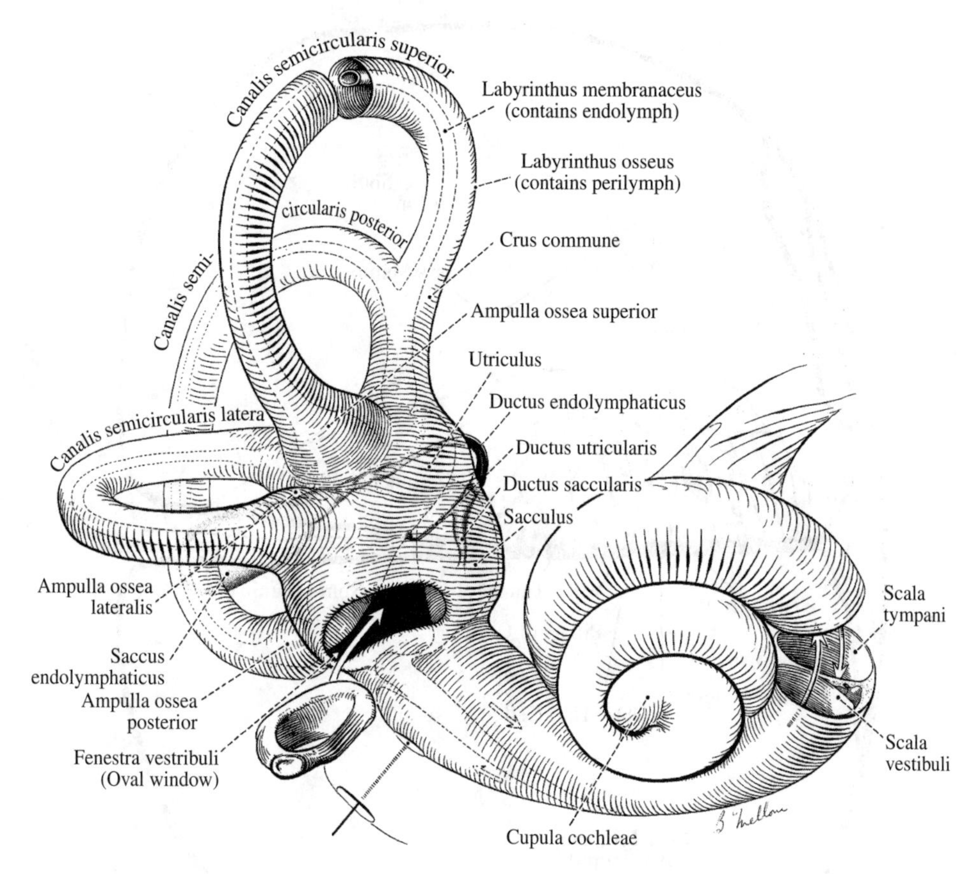

FIGURE 7.3 The stapes footplate enters the inner ear in the vestibule at the juncture of the cochlea and semicircular canals. (Drawing by Biaglio John Melloni, as shown in *Some Pathological Conditions of the Eye, Ear and Throat*, courtesy of Abbott Laboratories, North Chicago, IL.)

The view that middle ear pressure regulation is solely the realm of the eustachian tube is a simplification of a complex process that is still not fully understood. Since the *hydrops ex vacuo* theory was proposed by Politzer in the late 1800s, a significant body of work has accumulated on middle ear gas exchange.[5–14]

7.1.3 The Inner Ear

The inner ear combines the end organ for hearing and the end organ for balance. They share a common vestibular space and fluid arrangement (Figure 7.3). Due to the focus on the auditory system in this chapter, a description of the vestibular system will be omitted. However, it should be noted that hearing and balance problems are often related. The reader is referred to Shepard and Telian[15] as well as Jacobson et al.[16] for additional information on balance disorders and assessment.

As depicted in Figure 7.3, the cochlea starts at the vestibule of the inner ear and travels as a spiral tube within the temporal bone at the base of the skull. It is divided into three fluid-filled chambers: scala vestibuli, scala media and scala tympani (Figure 7.4). The scala vestibuli and scala tympani are joined at the apex of the spiral through an opening called the helicotrema. The scala media is formed between the other two scala by two membranous structures, Reissner's membrane and the basilar membrane. The organ of Corti lies on top of the basilar membrane and is shielded superiorly by the tectorial membrane.

The basilar membrane is critical to the function of the cochlea. The membrane varies in width and stiffness along its length, thereby providing the initial impetus to sort sounds tonotopically (by frequency). High frequencies establish deflections at the stiff base of the basilar membrane, while lower frequencies move progressively apically (toward the apex) as the stiffness lessens. This forms the basis for the traveling

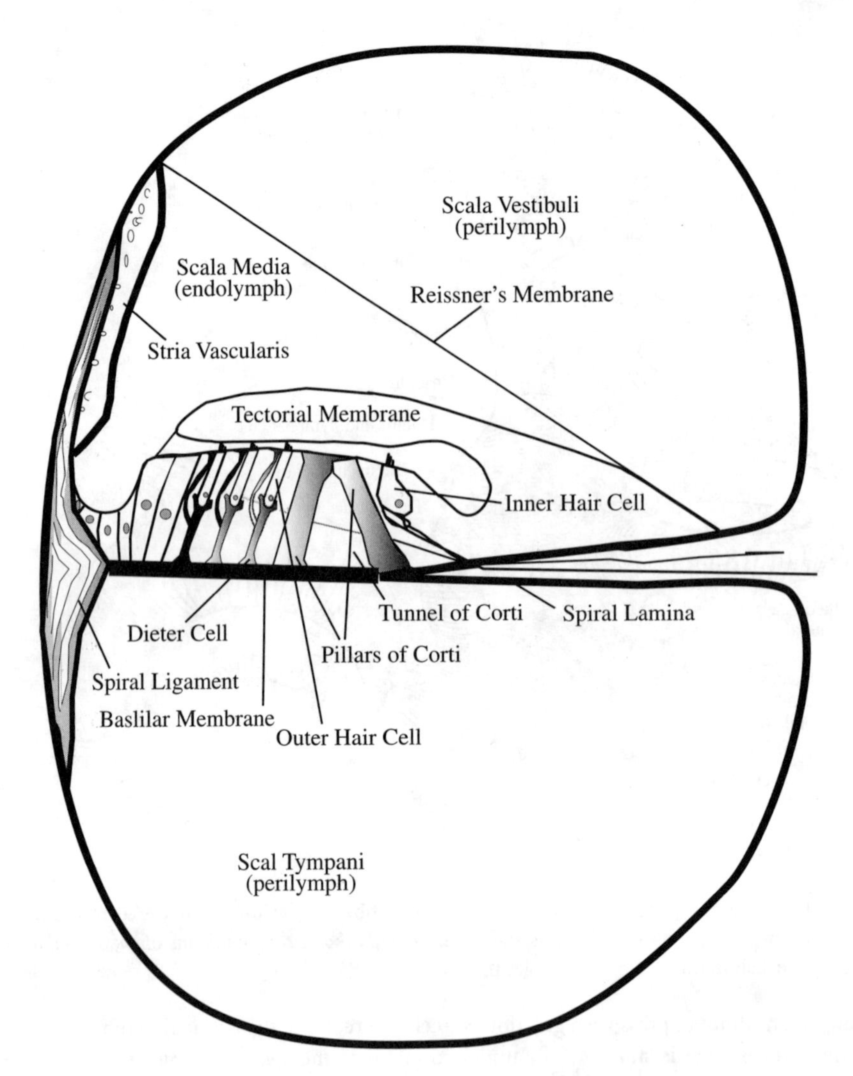

FIGURE 7.4 The cochlea is a three-chambered structure with the end organ of hearing, organ of Corti, located in the medial chamber. The high concentration of potassium which is required for the cells to function is produced by the stria vascularis on the lateral wall.

wave theory of hearing which is attributed to Georg von Békésy in his text *Experiments in Hearing*.[17] This theory states that signal frequency is encoded at the location of maximum deflection in the traveling wave, and loudness as the amplitude of that deflection. This theory was originally conceived with a passive inner ear system. However, it is now known, movement of the basilar membrane is modified by the outer hair cells in the organ of Corti.[18]

The Organ of Corti contains the sensory cells for hearing, cells that provide an amplification/tuning function and supporting cells (see Figure 7.4). The sensory cells are the inner hair cells while the outer hair cells provide amplification and tuning of incoming acoustic signals. These two cell types are located on either side of the pillars of Corti. Inner hair cells are located medial to the pillars while the outer hair cells are located lateral to the pillars. The inner hair cells form a single row of closely spaced cells. Supporting cells surround the inner hair cells. In contrast, the outer hair cells form three rows of cells with each row separated by a space. Each outer hair cell is supported by a Dieters cell. The Organ of Corti is bounded laterally by cells of Henson, Claudius and Boettcher.

Outer hair cells are long test tube-shaped structures with cilia (hairs) located at the top. For each cell, the lateral-most cilia tips are attached to the tectorial membrane. The point of motion for the tectorial membrane

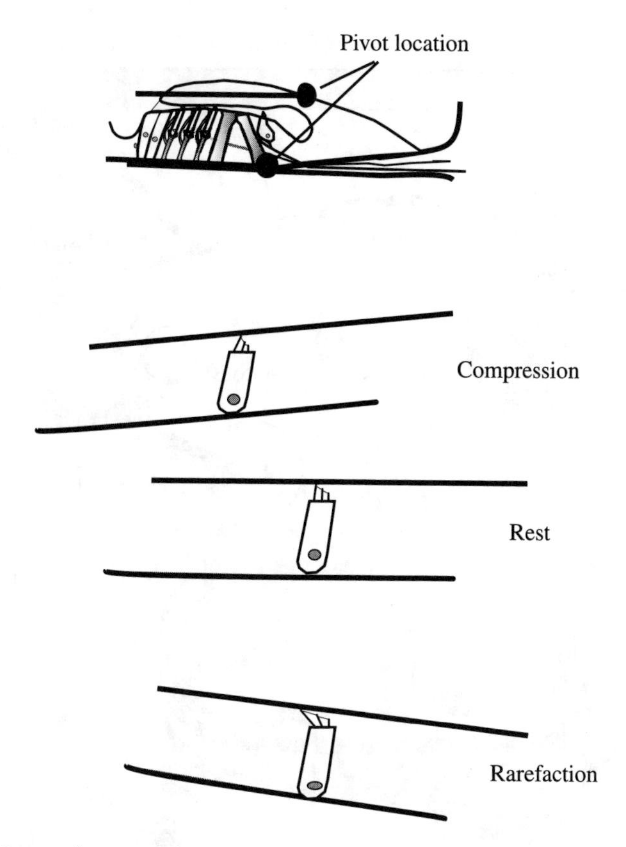

FIGURE 7.5 The basilar membrane and the tectorial membrane have different points of pivot. This difference creates a shearing action on the outer hair cells opening a mechanical gate and allowing potassium to enter the cell. The gate is open for one half the cycle during a rarefaction of sound pressure and is closed during the compression phase of the cycle.

is medially displaced from that for the basilar membrane on which the hair cell rides (Figure 7.5). The difference in motion between the basilar membrane and the tectorial membrane spreads the cilia bundle and opens a mechanical gate within the cilia. This gate regulates the flow of potassium into the cell. When the gate is opened, and potassium enters, the cell will shorten. When the gate is closed, the cell expands as the potassium is pumped out of the cell. The outer hair cells have been referred to as the cochlear amplifier and are essential for hearing low intensity sounds. Damage to the outer hair cells is a major factor in many cochlear hearing problems. The active role of the outer hair cells also results in a much steeper and narrower deflection of the basilar membrane at lower intensity levels, thereby providing greater frequency resolution within the cochlea.

The inner hair cells have a gourd-like shape with a narrower apex than base. The inner hair cells are the actual sensory receptors that will initiate activity within the central nervous system in the presence of auditory stimuli. Operation of both inner and outer hair cells is dependent upon a strong concentration of potassium that is generated on the lateral aspect of the scala media in the stria vascularis. The potassium appears to be circulated from the stria vascularis through the hair cells and back to the stria by way of the supporting cells in the organ of corti. The transport mechanism is the connexin 26 protein that forms a gap junction between adjacent cells. Approximately 30% of congenital nonsyndromic deafness is now thought to be related to a failure of connexin within the inner ear, which leads to diminished potassium levels within the scala media.[19,20]

7.1.4 Central Auditory Nervous System

The central auditory nervous system is comprised of both afferent (incoming) and efferent (outgoing) neuronal structures. It is probably the most complex subcortical sensory processing system in humans. The system is bilaterally represented and has multiple nuclei within the brain stem.

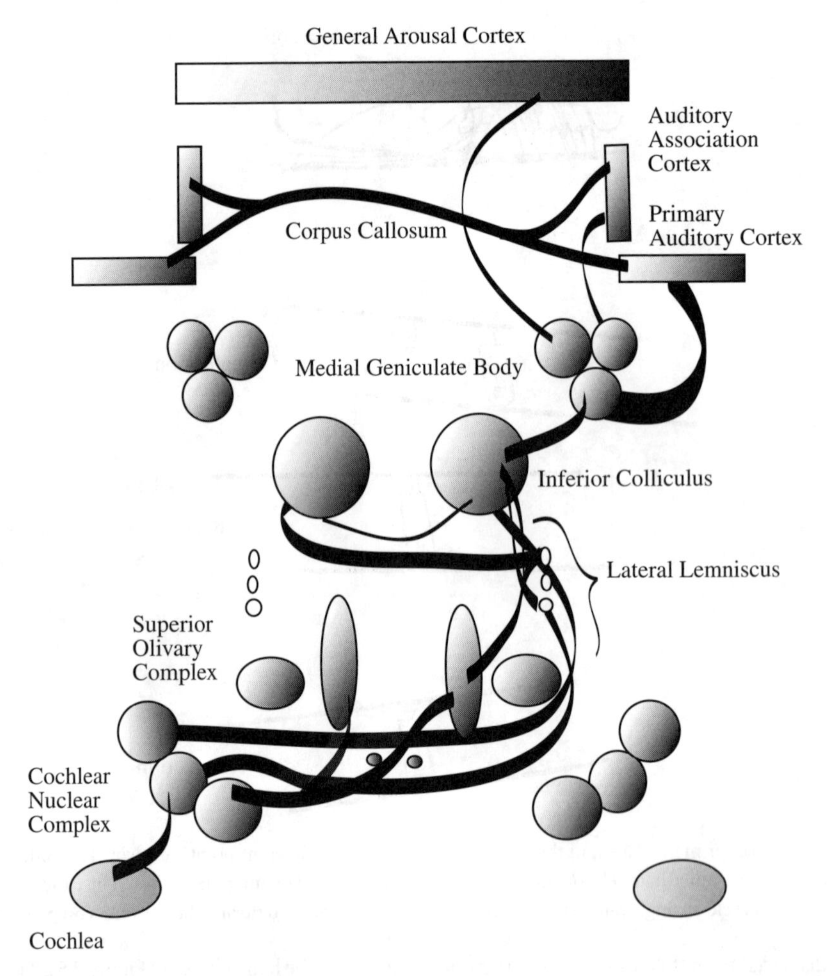

FIGURE 7.6 The ascending auditory pathway is primarily crossed. For clarity the figure only traces the right pathway from the cochlea to the cortex for low frequency information.

The afferent system begins at the base of the inner hair cells (Figure 7.6), as the auditory portion of the VIIIth cranial nerve, and passes through a boney opening, known as the internal auditory meatus, into the cranial vault. The internal auditory meatus also serves as a passage for the vestibular (balance) portion of the VIIIth nerve, the facial nerve and a blood vessel supplying the inner ear. Schwannomas (benign growths) are common within the internal auditory meatus, typically arising from the vestibular portion of the VIIIth cranial nerve.

The neural arrangement is different for the inner and outer hair cells. Each inner hair cell communicates with approximately ten afferent (ascending) neurons. Each neuron, however, only communicates with a single inner air cell. This provides a significant redundancy of neural response for activation of each sensory cell. The neurons exhibit a tuning curve that is similar to that seen for the hair cell. In contrast, outer hair cells primarily receive efferent (descending) input with each neuron connecting to multiple cells over approximately one quarter turn to the cochlea.

The VIIIth cranial nerve enters the posterior lateral aspect of the brain stem and connects to the cochlear nuclear complex (CNC). In the CNC, basic timing and pitch extraction are initiated. There are several intricate neuronal feedback loops within the nuclei as well as connections from the efferent system. These connections appear to help in sound localization and noise suppression.

Auditory information leaves the CNC by three distinct pathways. The anterior most pathway (anterior acoustic stria) enters another nuclear body, the superior olivary complex (SOC), bilaterally. The SOC has a major role in auditory localization. Output from the SOC is primarily to the ipsilateral (same side) lateral lemniscus. The lateral lemnisci have several nuclei and there is a shunting of some neurons across the midline at the Bundle of Probst. The intermediate and dorsal acoustic stria bypass the SOC and enter the lateral lemniscus, which is a major ascending pathway, primarily on the side contralateral (opposite) to the ear receiving the signal. There is also a small ipsilateral projection. The lemnisci enter into the inferior colliculus on the posterior aspect of the brain stem.

The inferior colliculus is a major way station in the pathway. Most neurons synapse at this point and some of the neurons cross the midline through a pathway called the anterior commissure. Several studies have suggested that processing of amplitude and frequency modulation may occur at this level.[21–26] Neurons leave the inferior colliculus through a pathway, the brachium of the inferior colliculus, and enter the medial geniculate body of the thalamus.

The medial geniculate body can be broken down into three major areas: ventral, dorsal and medial. Fibers leaving the medial geniculate body carry information to the cortical areas of the brain. The ventral medial geniculate projects to the primary auditory cortex though the internal capsule and contains about 90% of the fibers leaving the structure. The dorsal medial geniculate body projects to the auditory association cortex through the internal capsule. The medial portion of the geniculate receives input from both ventral and dorsal medial geniculate structures as well as other nuclei of the thalamus associated with other sensory systems. The cortical projections from the medial portion of the geniculate are widely distributed and are thought to be associated with alerting and arousal.

The primary auditory cortex is situated on the posterior superior surface of the temporal lobe on the transverse gyrus of Heschl. The superior temporal gyrus and Wernike's area also are associated with auditory processing. The auditory areas in the right and left temporal lobes of the brain are connected by a bundle of neurons that passes through the corpus callosum. This connection permits the bilateral transfer of information at the cortical level.

The complex arrangement of the auditory pathways allows information to be processed bilaterally in an efficient manner. The parallel processing of information that is initiated at the lower brain stem level is integrated at higher levels such as at the inferior colliculus and in the cortex. The redundancy inherent in information transfer through this maze of interactive subsystems insures accuracy in perception and communication skills even in light of neurologic insults and injury.

7.2 Sound and the Decibel

Hearing is the conscious interpretation of vibration as sound. Sound requires three key elements: (1) a source of vibratory energy, (2) a medium in which to transmit the vibration and (3) a receiver. Sounds can be quantified based on their physical frequency, complexity, and sound pressure level (SPL).

The frequency of sound is measured in Hertz (Hz) which is the number of 360 phase shifts per second. The frequency response characteristic of the ear is significantly impacted by the anatomic and physiologic characteristics of the outer and middle ear systems.[27] The range of frequencies processed by different species varies greatly. Elephants, for example, respond down into the human subsonic frequency range,[28] whereas bats can respond in the human ultrasonic range.[29,30] The normal frequency range for humans is 20 to 20,000 Hz.

The complexity of sound is based on the number of frequencies present and the physical combinations of those frequencies. At the simplest level, when a single frequency is present it is referred to as a pure tone. As additional frequencies are added, the sound becomes more complex. Complex sounds that have a regular repetition of the combined frequencies take on a tonal quality. At the other extreme, frequencies in a sound that have a truly random pattern are perceived as noise. The frequency structure of a sound also is related to the duration of the sound and its rise and fall time characteristics. Short duration electrical signals used to generate sounds will have a band of frequencies associated with them. This is referred to as the frequency bandwidth (BW) and is represented as

$$BW = 1/\text{Duration}$$

The bandwidth is modified by the characteristics of the transducer used to convert the electrical energy to sound. Similarly, sound frequency is affected by the durational rise and fall characteristics of the signal. Sounds that come on abruptly will have broader frequency ranges than those that have slower onset times or ones that are gated (shaped) to reduce the amount of frequency spread. For example, the Blackman window is a common gating function used to reduce frequency spread in short duration tones generated for auditory brain stem response (ABR) measurement.[28,31,32]

Most mammalian auditory systems are able to receive and process a broad range of energy that is measured in terms of pressure. In normally hearing humans, a pressure of 20 μPa causes the eardrum to move approximately 1/1,000,000,000th of an inch, resulting in the perception of sound. As pressure increases, the sound is perceived as becoming increasingly louder, up to a pressure level that is 10^{14} times greater than the softest sound pressure perceived. In order to deal with such a broad range of numbers, SPLs are expressed as a logarithmic ratio with a specific reference value.

Most sound level measurements in the environment as well as hearing aid specifications are reported in terms of SPL, referenced to 20 μPa, and measured as decibels (dB). dB SPL is represented by the formula:

$$dB \ \text{SPL} = 20\log\frac{\text{Pressure measured}}{\text{Pressure reference}}$$

This formula illustrates that 0 dB SPL is not the absence of sound. Sound can, and often does, fall into the negative dB range.

Figure 7.7 shows the minimum audible pressure map for the human ear. Such maps for other species will vary depending on the structure of their outer and middle ear systems. As can be seen, different SPLs are required at each frequency to be just audible. To account for the ears differing sensitivity by frequency, a number of different dB scales have been created. These scales are based on dB SPL but have a weighting factor for each frequency (ANSI-S1.4–1983).[33]

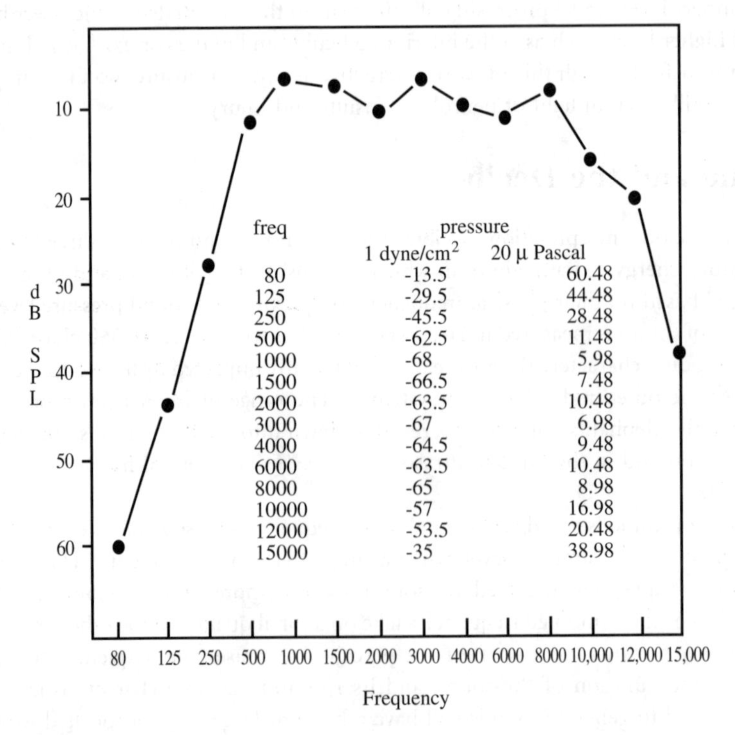

FIGURE 7.7 The minimum audible pressure (MAP) curve originally determined by Dadson and King in 1952.[1] The original data expressed in dynes/cm square have been converted by the author to the now commonly used reference of 20 μPa.

The three most common scales used are dBA, dBB and dBC. The dBA scale has its primary use in the area of noise damage-risk assessment. The dBA scale is based on a single sound level measurement that is taken across the frequency spectrum. This scale applies correction factors to the SPL value at each frequency that makes up the sound to account for the responsiveness of the human ear. The dBA scale uses a weighting factor that is based on the inverse of a 40-phon curve, where a phon is defined as the perceived equal loudness level across frequencies. The 40-phon curve equates loudness at all audible frequencies to that of a 40-dB SPL, 1000-Hz tone.

The dBB scale is seldom used. It reflects human hearing in a manner similar to the dBA scale except that the weighting factor is based on a smoothed inverse of the 70-phon curve. The loudness function represented by the 70-phon curve is flatter than that seen for the 40-phon curve. This reflects the underlying tuning curve for hair cells, which tends to flatten with increased sound pressure.

The dBC scale is used when a very low, inaudible frequency is present that may distort the overall sound pressure measure being taken of sounds in the audible range. There is virtually no weighting of the response throughout the audible portion of the frequency spectrum. The reader is referred to Durrant and Lovrinic,[1] Lipscomb,[34] Yost[35] and ANSI S1.4[33] for expanded discussion of these measurement scales.

Audiograms are graphic representations of the basic hearing ability of humans, reflecting the threshold at which a frequency becomes just audible. Sound level for human hearing measurements on the audiogram also have had correction factors applied. The audiogram specifies hearing in terms of dB HL. The 0 dB HL level at each frequency corresponds to a different SPL value (ANSI 3.6-1996).[36] These differences are due to the audibility differences between the frequencies as well as the physical characteristics of the transducer coupling with the ear. Specifically, each earphone and cushion arrangement used to measure hearing will alter these correction factors based on the relative amount of air space enclosed between the diaphragm and the tympanic membrane (eardrum). Because of the physical variability associated with the devices and even the testing environment, very precise calibration measurements must be made and maintained.

Decibels used to express values relative to an individual's hearing threshold are measured in terms of sensation level (SL). Thus, if a person had a hearing threshold of 40 dB HL and you presented a sound to them at 70 dB HL, that tone would be at 30 dB SL. That is, the sensation level of presentation was 30 dB greater than threshold for the signal. The SL measure is often referred to when performing audiometry using speech materials.

7.3 Assessing the Auditory System

Audiometric assessment of the auditory system is not pathology specific. Its main goals are to locate the site of a disruption in the system and to determine the severity of that disruption. The traditional categories of hearing loss have been conductive, sensorineural, mixed and functional. The sensorineural component can now be subcategorized into cochlear and retrocochlear, and in many instances even finer delineation is provided within these subcategories.

The severity of a disruption in the auditory system can be viewed in several ways, including degree of loss for specific tonal frequency, loss in speech intelligibility or, more generically, the amount of disruption to everyday activities as a result of communicative difficulty. Predictions can be made from one view of the loss to another, and variations between the prediction and the measured value may point to possible sites of auditory lesions.

7.3.1 Transducers

Acoustic signal generation for hearing assessment requires the use of transducers to generate the auditory signals. Loudspeakers are used to generate signals in a sound field. When using loudspeakers in a room, care must be taken in maintaining the orientation of the subject relative to the speaker as well as fixing the subject location. Variations in location and orientation may significantly alter the signal level at the ear. Use of pure tones when testing with loudspeakers is inadvisable due to the creation of standing waves in the testing environment.

Specific ear measurements are performed either with supra-aural headphones or with insert earphones. TDH-39 and TDH-49 supra-aural headphones mounted in MX41AR cushions traditionally have been the most common transducers used for measuring hearing. Recently, the use of earphones inserted into the ear canal, such as the ER3-A, have gained in popularity. Such earphones are particularly useful for evoked potential audiometric measurement because of their reduced shielding needs. The ER3-A earphone has several advantages in that it is lightweight, provides a greater inter-aural attenuation and generates a smaller electrical artifact than the TDH headphone.

When using headphones it is imperative that the diaphragm of the earphone be placed directly over the external auditory meatus. Without proper placement, the signal can be attenuated due to blockage by the tissue of the ear and face. It also is necessary to insure that the external auditory meatus does not collapse under headphone pressure. A collapse of the meatus will result in elevated thresholds with significant variability, particularly in the low frequency region. On visual inspection, ear canals that have a narrow oval appearance tend to collapse. It has been estimated that collapse of the ear canal will occur in 3 to 4% of the population while undergoing hearing testing using supra-aural headphones.[37–39]

The headphone band should be snug holding the headphone cushions securely in place in order to maximize attenuation between ears. With properly fit TDH-type headphones, a nominal 40-dB value is accepted as the amount of interaural attenuation. The cables from the headphone should be directed down the back of the subject to prevent extraneous noise generated by their rubbing on clothing.

Insert earphones are advantageous in auditory assessment of young children. The bulky TDH headphones and cushions are uncomfortable for many young children and will often provide a poor fit. Normal attenuation between ears (interaural attenuation) appears to be improved as the foam ear tip seals the ear canal.[40] Again, the cables should be directed behind the subject to prevent extraneous noise.

Insert earphones have several advantages when used to generate stimuli during electrophysiologic tests such as the ABR. First, there is a lower electrical noise associated with the inserts than with the headphones. This means that complex and heavy metal shielding is not required. Second, the insert transducer is separated from the head by a length of tube, creating a time delay between the electrical impulse to the earphone and the arrival of the sound at the ear. This helps separate any remaining electrical artifacts from the desired response.

When performing electrophysiologic tests, care should be taken to have the transducer body located away from electrodes and the electrode cables to prevent pickup of the electrical signals that are generated. The insert transducer tube should not be altered; it provides a resonance that is calculated as part of the earphone's response characteristic.

7.3.2 Pure-Tone Audiometry

The mainstay of audiometric measurement has been the pure-tone audiogram. Pure-tone audiometry provides a method for separating conductive losses, located in the outer and middle ear, from sensorineural losses associated with problems in the cochlea and central nervous system. Pure-tone audiometry is performed using both air conducted signals that pass through the outer and middle ears as well as bone conducted signals that are generated by an oscillator pressed against the mastoid or forehead. Bone conducted signals pass through the skull and bypass the outer and middle ear structures providing the signal directly to the cochlea. Typically, a problem in the outer or middle ear is suspected when the air conduction results are poorer than the bone conduction results. If lowered bone conduction scores are seen with the reduced air scores, a mixed loss is present indicating both an outer/middle ear problem and a simultaneous inner ear disorder.

7.3.2.1 Method

Test instructions for pure-tone audiometry should be brief, simple and to the point in order to minimize error-producing confusion on the part of the test subject. Typical instructions are: "You will hear a series of sounds, some will be very soft. Raise your hand whenever you hear the sound." The use of "tones" or "whistles" are often substituted for the more generic word "sound."

The pure-tone audiogram is obtained at octave intervals from 250 through 8000 Hz. Signals are initially presented at 30 dB HL for 2 sec at the frequency being tested. Longer signals increase the probability of a false positive response. Signals shorter than 1 sec will not allow the proper rise and fall times of the signal. If signals have very short durations (less than 500 msec), there will be inadequate sensory integration leading to higher threshold levels. The signal is lowered by 10 dB HL until no response is given, followed by raising the signal in 5 dB HL steps until a response is given. The signal is then lowered by 10 dB HL and the steps repeated. Once the subject responds two out of three times, at the same level, on the ascending signal increments, threshold is obtained and the process repeated at a new frequency. Standard audiometric test frequencies are 250 to 8000 Hz at octave intervals. Typically, the better hearing ear, by subject report, is measured first, commencing at 1000 Hz. After all frequencies have been measured, the test is repeated at 1000 Hz. The subject should have a threshold within 5 dB of the previous score for the measure to be considered reliable.

If the subject has a hearing loss greater than 30 dB and does not respond on the initial signal presentation, the signal level should be raised in 20-dB steps until a response is obtained. At that point the process of bracketing the threshold begins as described above.

7.3.3 The Audiogram

The audiogram is used for recording the individual's auditory thresholds. It is constructed such that the distance of 20 dB on the *y*-axis is equivalent to one octave on the *x*-axis. Right ear air-conducted thresholds are represented by a red circle while left ear air-conducted thresholds are represented by a blue X. Scores between 0 and 25 dB HL are considered to be within the normal range. Figure 7.8 provides an example of an audiogram.

There are often a number of different symbols on the audiogram; boxes, brackets [ ] and arrows < > represent different tests such as bone conduction testing and the use of masking. Each audiogram should have a legend listing the symbols and their interpretation.

7.3.3.1 Masking

Masking is the use of a noise to prevent hearing of a specified signal. It is typically employed to prevent the nontest ear from responding to a signal presented to the test ear. As mentioned earlier, interaural

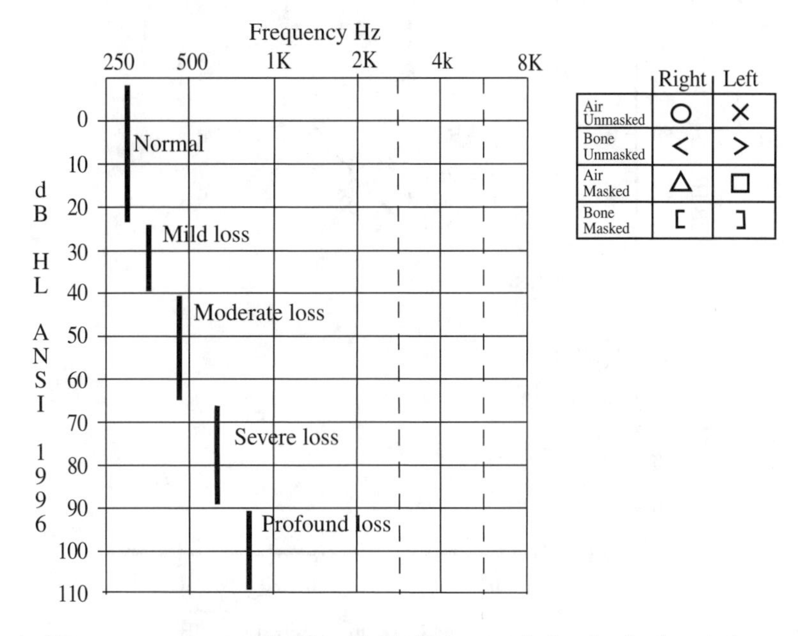

FIGURE 7.8 Audiograms are constructed with each 20-dB increase in hearing level equivalent to a one-octave increase in frequency. The common descriptive terms for hearing loss based on the pure tone average are shown with range bars to the left of the descriptor.

attenuation for air-conducted signals is approximately 40 dB. Therefore, a signal that is presented to one ear at 50 dB will cross the head and be received by the opposing ear at a level of 10 dB.

The crossing of signals from one ear to another can create significant problems if there are hearing differences greater than 40 dB between the ears for air-conducted signals. A "shadow" audiogram will often be seen where the poorer ear will yield thresholds that are 40 to 50 dB worse than the hearing ear if masking is not appropriately applied. For bone conduction measurements, whereby a vibrator is placed on the skull, usually over the mastoid process, interaural attenuation is 0 dB. Therefore, masking during bone conduction testing becomes critical in any test situation where there is a 10-dB or greater difference in hearing between the ears for air conduction.

The ideal masker would be a signal that is exactly the same as the test signal. However, such a signal would lead to confusion as to what to respond to by most subjects. Therefore, noise signals are employed for masking purposes. Most audiometers have different noise types to choose from when selecting a masker. The goal in choosing the most appropriate noise masker is to concentrate the maximum energy into the area of the test signal. In a flat spectrum signal the level per cycle (LPC) can be calculated from the overall signal level (OL) and the signal bandwidth (BW):

$$\text{LPC} = \text{OL} - 10 \text{ Log}_{10} \text{ BW}$$

For pure tones, narrow band maskers are most efficient, whereas speech signals require wider band maskers.

A secondary problem occurs when masking. The masker has the same interaural attenuation as the original signal and can cross back to the test ear. When this happens, overmasking has occurred. To avoid overmasking an ear, formulas have been established for calculating appropriate masking levels.[41]

Figure 7.9 graphically illustrates the masking concept. The *y*-axis represents the threshold in the test ear and the *x*-axis represents the masking applied to the nontest ear. If masking noise is inadequate, every 10-dB increase in the masker will result in a similar change in the threshold in the test ear. Once adequate masking is achieved, the test ear threshold will stabilize or plateau until the masker signal crosses to the test ear. This should be through a range of 30 to 40 dB of masker increase, i.e., the amount of interaural attenuation. Once the masker crosses to the test ear, the threshold will again rise in a linear fashion with increases in masker presentation level.

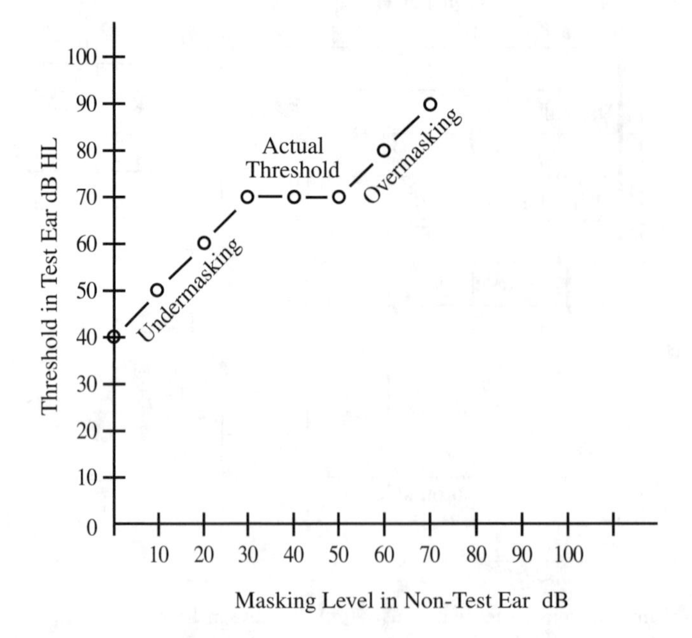

FIGURE 7.9 Under masking occurs when the masker is too weak to prevent crossover of the test stimulus to the nontest ear. Over masking occurs when the masker is too loud and crosses to the test ear.

7.4 Degree of Loss

Degree of hearing loss is often categorized as normal, mild, moderate, severe and profound (Figure 7.8). This description is based on the pure tone average (PTA), which is the average loss at 500, 1000 and 2000 Hz. These frequencies were chosen based on their contribution to the understanding of speech. "Normal" hearing is an average less than or equal to 20 dB HL; individuals with this degree of loss should not experience a great deal of difficulty in normal listening situations. Individuals with a mild loss have a pure tone average between 20 and 40 dB HL. These individuals typically will have only mild difficulty in most listening situations. They should be able to carry on a conversation in quiet at 3 ft. However, as distance or competing noise increases, their difficulty will become more apparent.

Moderate hearing loss is a pure tone average ranging from 40 to 70 dB HL. Individuals with a moderate loss will experience difficulty in conversation at 3 ft in quiet and will rely on visual cues to help in communication.

Severe loss is a pure tone average of 70 to 90 dB HL. Because conversational speech is generally in the 60- to 70-dB SPL range, a listener with a severe loss will miss most, if not all, of conversational level speech even in quiet. Individuals with moderate and severe hearing losses typically benefit from the use of assistive listening devices and hearing aids.

Profound hearing loss is a pure tone average of 90 dB HL or greater. Individuals with a profound loss may experience benefit from hearing aids but will often still have difficulty in oral communication situations. Frequency transposition aids and multichannel cochlear implants often provide significant levels of help.[42,43]

It should be noted that, though generalizations about daily function can be made based on the pure tone average, there is a great deal of individual variability. Some individuals with moderate hearing loss will experience significantly more difficulty than others with severe to profound hearing losses.

7.5 Speech Reception Threshold

The speech reception threshold (SRT) is the signal level at which a person can correctly identify spondaic word stimuli 50% of the time. Spondaic words are two syllables in length and have equal stress on both syllables (e.g., baseball). The PTA and SRT should correlate well and be within 8 dB HL of each other for the audiogram to be considered reliable. Gaps larger than this may be seen in steeply sloping losses where there is a precipitous loss across the speech range and into the upper frequencies. In such cases, a two-frequency average at 500 and 1000 Hz will be a better reflection of the SRT.

A discrepancy between the PTA and SRT also is seen in cases of functional hearing loss. Functional loss occurs when an individual hears better than audiometric test results indicate. Individuals with functional loss may or may not be aware of this problem. Because the individual may not be aware of the functional nature of the loss, as in cases of hysterical deafness, the term pseudo-hypoacousis is now used rather than the more pejorative designation "malingering." As hearing measurements, technology and procedures have evolved, the SRT, although still routinely used by many audiologists, is taking on a less vital role in hearing measurement. It is often used for determining the presentation level for a speech word recognition test, though this is just as easily and accurately set using the PTA. The SRT is probably most useful in testing young children for whom the audiogram is thought to be questionable or is impossible to obtain.

7.5.1 Method

Instructions should be kept simple. The subject should be instructed to repeat the word that they hear and, if they are not sure of the word, they should be instructed to guess. A typical instruction would be: "Please read the list of words on the sheet in front of you. You will be hearing these words through the earphones. Some of the words will be very quiet. I want you to repeat the word that you hear. If you are unsure of a word make a guess."

The subject should be familiarized with the word list prior to the beginning of the procedure by either letting them read the list or presenting it at 40 to 60 dB SL re PTA. The familiarization list order should be random, relative to the final test format. There have been several different methodologies for performing the SRT measure. Those advocated by the ASHA[44] as well as one recommended by Martin and Dowdy[45] are two methods that appear to provide good reliability. The difference is that Martin and Dowdy use a 5-dB step rather than the 2-dB step used in the ASHA method. The procedure starts by presenting one spondee at 30 dB HL and lowering the presentation level in 10-dB steps until the first spondee is missed. Each successive spondee is presented at 5-dB increments until one is correctly identified. The level is then lowered by 10 dB, and the process is repeated until three correct responses have been obtained at a given level.

7.6 Speech Recognition Testing

Speech and language recognition is a complex cognitive task requiring a relatively intact central auditory nervous system to function normally. There is a significant body of literature surrounding both the task and methods for testing the various processes that are used in recognizing speech. Research in this area can be traced back to Campbell in 1910 using nonsense syllables to assess telephone circuit performance.[46] However, it was research performed during World War II on speech recognition in normal individuals in order to improve battlefield communication that signaled the modern era of speech perception research. An early outgrowth of this research was the development of the articulation index (AI).[47,48]

The articulation index is a mathematical model for estimating the intelligibility of speech based on the acoustical characteristics of the stimulus and the transmission medium. The method has been standardized as ANSI 3.5.[49] This standard has been helpful in the study of communications systems, thereby eliminating the need for large groups of listeners to provide perceptual judgments of changes.

If the audiometric threshold is considered a special case of a filter in the transmission line, the AI can be used to predict speech recognition scores based on the stimulus material and audiometric configuration.[50–53] Deviations between the predicted value and the actual recognition score obtained for a subject provide clinical insight into cochlear function and central processing of auditory information. Unfortunately, the acoustical characteristics of each stimulus set must be precisely known for prediction to approach any degree of accuracy.

A second outgrowth of the World War II research was the establishment of the field of audiology. An initial focus of the field was in assessment and rehabilitation of returning veterans with hearing loss. Part of this assessment process required estimating the effects of a loss on speech communication. To assess speech recognition, the word lists and procedures originally used during the war for assessing communication systems were employed. As problems with these materials were uncovered, they were replaced with the recorded CID W-22 word lists. The CID W-22 word recognition test remains in common clinical practice to this time. Another list, the Northwestern University Auditory Test number Six (NU-6), is also commonly used as a substitute for the CID W-22.

Unfortunately, there are problems in using both of these lists for assessment of communication ability. They are administered in quiet, while we live in a noisy world. They are single words, while we listen to connected discourse. They are presented in optimal conditions, while we often function in less than ideal conditions. Because of these and other problems, numerous other measures have been created for assessing speech communication function.

Today, assessment of speech encompasses a wide range of materials. These materials are designed to assess everything from simple perception to more complex language processing strategies. Stimuli include nonsense syllables, words and sentences. The material can be presented monaurally (to one ear), or dichotically as competing messages. In assessing central auditory function, degraded speech stimuli are often used because they task the system sufficiently to identify problems in auditory processing. Popular methods of degrading speech include the use of filtering, time compression, distortion or competing signals. The reader is referred to Mendel and Danhauer[46] (1997) for a more thorough overview of speech perception and assessment.

7.7 Otoacoustic Emissions

An otoacoustic emission is an acoustic signal that has been generated by active processes in the inner ear and that is recorded from the ear canal. The emission has been linked to the expansion and contraction of outer hair cells participating in the active processes within the cochlea. Gold conjectured that an active cochlear process would produce a low-level tone emitted into the ear canal.[54] Unfortunately, amplifier sensitivity and noise levels did not permit him to successfully record an emission. The otoacoustic emission, however, was successfully recorded by Kemp 30 years later.[55] Since then there have been numerous articles on the topic. The four types of emissions are spontaneous, transient evoked, distortion product and stimulus frequency. This classification scheme is based on the stimulus type used to elicit the response. All otoacoustic emissions are believed to result from the movement of outer hair cells and require an intact outer and middle ear to be successfully recorded. For an excellent review of this topic see Robinette and Glattke[56] and Hall.[57]

7.8 Spontaneous Otoacoustic Emissions (SOAE)

Spontaneous otoacoustic emissions (SOAE) require no external stimulus. At present, SOAE can be recorded in approximately 70% of ears in normal hearing individuals.[58] This number has steadily risen over the past few years due to improvements in recording technology. Microphone sensitivity and noise floor levels are critical in the recording because the low levels of the response are easily missed or masked by outside noise. The presence of SOAEs appears to vary with racial group and gender, but age does not appear to be a factor through young adulthood.[59–62] However, there may be a decreased presence of SOAEs in individuals over 60 even with normal hearing.[63]

SOAEs have narrow bandwidths and relatively stable amplitudes and frequencies.[64] It is common for SOAEs to be present at multiple frequencies within an ear, and these frequencies are not necessarily the same in both ears of a single subject. They are only seen in relatively normal cochlea and are not recorded if there is a hearing loss greater than 30 dB HL. It has been conjectured that there may be natural imperfections in the organ of corti that might cause a perturbation and reverse the traveling wave.[65] SOAEs do not appear to be associated with tinnitus although there are a few anecdotal reports to the contrary.[66,67]

All otoacoustic emissions (OAE) must be transmitted from the cochlea back through the middle ear system before being recorded. Therefore, it is important to know the effects of the middle ear system on the OAE response. Middle ear pressure changes can cause a shift in SOAE frequency of up to 50 Hz. Although these shifts are typically upward in frequency, some downward shifts have been noted. There is typically a reduction in amplitude of the response as the pressure is moved from ambient. These shifts are consistent with changes in middle ear function. Stiffening of the tympanic membrane causes an upward shift in the resonance of the middle ear system. In addition, the change in stiffness makes it more difficult for the tympanic membrane to move and results in lower amplitude deflections and reduced input to and from the cochlea.

7.9 Transient-Evoked Otoacoustic Emissions

In contrast to SOAEs, which occur in a passive state, transient-evoked otoacoustic emissions (TEOAE) are elicited by brief duration stimuli. The emission was reported by Kemp (1978), who introduced the first commercially available unit for recording the response.[55] Many of the published studies have used this equipment and its default parameters for recording the TEOAE.

TEOAEs are present in all ears with thresholds better than 30 dB HL. TEOAEs provide an efficient screening tool because the emission disappears if a mild hearing loss is present. However, it is not possible to predict audiometric threshold levels from the TEOAE amplitude.

The small amplitude of the TEOAE necessitates a signal processing paradigm to extract the response from stimulus artifact and background noise as shown in Figure 7.10. Because the TEOAE is a deterministic signal in a relatively random background noise, a signal averaging strategy can be employed to

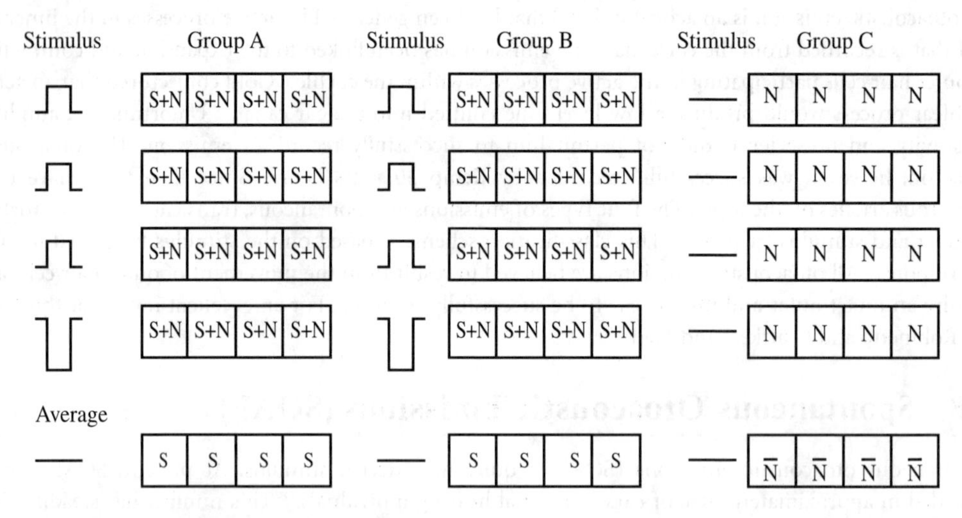

FIGURE 7.10 The paradigm for analyzing the responses during the TEOAE evaluation. Averaging within Groups A and B provides for cancellation of stimulus artifact. Correlation of Groups A and B demonstrates the responses reliability. Comparison of the FFT from Groups A and B to Group C provides a measure of OAE strength compared to background noise.

elicit the response. Using an averaging paradigm, stimuli are presented and the data averaged until the background noise is significantly attenuated. This is similar to the strategy used for evoked potential measurements discussed elsewhere in this book. Unlike evoked potentials, both the stimulus and the response are acoustic, thereby requiring a different strategy to eliminate the stimulus artifact.

Fortunately the largest part of the stimulus artifact occurs before the response is emitted from the cochlea back into the ear canal. This means that the response collection system can simply turn off during this time frame or, alternatively, discard the data in this time frame post hoc. Nonetheless, during the time frame of interest, there will still be a small, lower level stimulus artifact that may remain and obscure the data. This problem is managed as shown in the stimulus column in Figure 7.10. The stimuli are presented in chains of four, and the chain is repeated until an acceptable signal to noise ratio is reached. More specifically, the stimulus chain presents three stimuli of one polarity and a fourth stimulus 180° out of phase and equal in intensity to the sum of the previous three. This results in the stimulus artifact summing to zero.

Fortunately, the TEOAE is a nonlinear response from the cochlea. Therefore, when the polarity of the signal is reversed, the TEOAE response does not equal the sum of the previous three responses. This means that, although part of the response is canceled, a measurable portion remains in the average.

The TEOAE system also permits evaluation of the response repeatability by collecting stimuli into two separate analysis groups, labeled Group A and Group B in Figure 7.10. Stimulus chains and responses are alternately assigned to each group during the collection process. Once an average is obtained, the groups can be correlated for a statistical measure of similarity. If the responses are similar, the averages can be combined, thereby increasing the signal-to-noise ratio.

If a repeatable response is observed, it is important to know the frequency content and to determine if the frequency content is consistent with the stimulus and different from the background noise. To obtain the estimate of background noise, the data collection system maintains a third buffer, Group C (see Figure 7.10), which is collected during times of no stimulus presentation. To evaluate the frequency content, the system performs FFTs on the combined TEOAE response data, the noise data and finally the stimulus. The FFT should show larger amplitudes at stimulus frequencies for the TEOAE data than for the background noise data if a response is present.

The TEOAE in infants is approximately 10 dB larger than that seen in adults. Kok and coworkers reported a 78% prevalence of TEOAEs in newborns less than 36 h of age; however, this increased to 99% by 108 h of age.[68] Current reports of 90% success rate now often documented in clinical data may reflect that the subject was screened more than once during the first 36-h period. In adults, there appears to be little variation in response amplitude with age. However, it has been found that the right ear has a slightly larger response than the left, and that female responses are larger than males.

The TEOAE response is affected by stimuli that are presented in the contralateral ear.[69–71] The reduction in response amplitude that is seen is due to input to the cochlea from the efferent auditory neurological subsystem, most likely the crossed olivocochlear bundle. A similar effect is seen with the VIIIth nerve response during electrocochleography, where the N1 response (first negativity) is reduced in the presence of bilateral stimulation.

7.10 Distortion Product Otoacoustic Emissions

Distortion Product Otoacoustic Emission (DPOAE) measurements were introduced by Kemp in 1979. The emission is the result of an intermodulation between two frequencies presented to the ear. The stimulus frequencies, called primaries, are typically labeled f1 (lower frequency) and f2 (higher frequency). If the two primary frequencies are presented to the ear such that the f2/f1 ratio is 1.2:1.22, distortion byproducts are created in the inner ear. The cochlea produces a number of distortion byproducts simultaneously at areas that can be mathematically determined.[72] However, the largest of these is at the frequency 2f1-f2 and is known as the cubic-difference tone, as depicted in Figure 7.11.

The primary frequencies (f1 and f2) have associated presentation levels of L1 and L2. L1 and L2 presentation levels are either equal in SPL or with L2 presented at a level lower than L1. The optimum L1/L2 level is dependent upon frequency and on the L1 absolute level.[73] It is relatively common in clinical situations to place L2 approximately 5 dB below L1.

The DPOAE response, similar to that seen for TEOAE, is small, ranging between 5 to 15 dB SPL and, like the TEOAE, requires a processing strategy to extract it from the background noise. Unlike the TEOAE, the stimulating frequencies are distant to the DPOAE frequency response. Therefore, the stimulus artifact will not interfere with the response and there is no need to remove it from the recording.

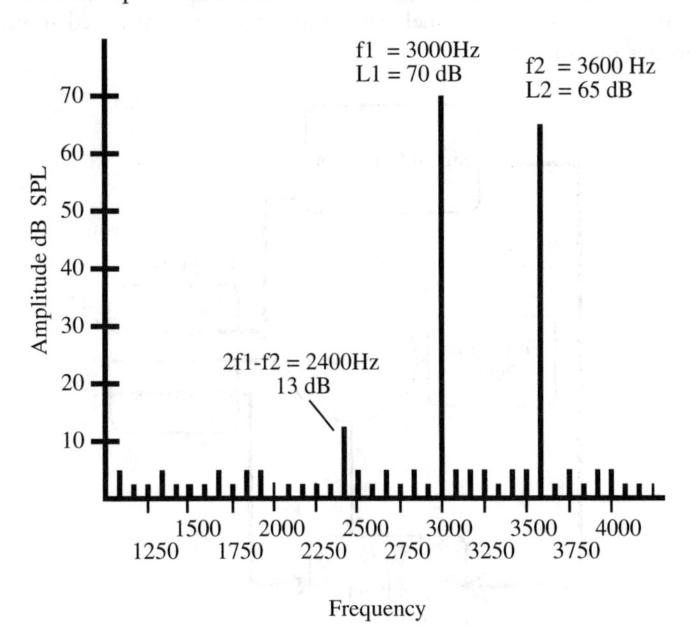

FIGURE 7.11 The distortion product otoacoustic emission is generated by the interaction of two primary tones labeled f1 and f2. The interaction of the tones creates the emission which is recorded at 2f1-f2.

7.11 Stimulus Frequency Otoacoustic Emissions

Stimulus frequency otoacoustic emissions (SFOAE) are elicited by a frequency glide presented to the test ear. When the response is present, an out-of-phase signal will be returned into the ear canal. The recording of this response is technically difficult, and therefore SFOAEs are not currently used in clinical settings. Shera and Guinan argue that the TEOAE and SFOAE should be joined conceptually because they occur at the stimulation frequency, whereas the DPOAE occurs at a frequency that is not present in the evoking stimuli.[74] They further argue that the underlying mechanism is different for the responses, with the former dependent on a linear coherent reflection of the signal while the latter depends on a nonlinear distortion. They suggest that, because the underlying mechanism is different, there should be differences in the manner in which they react to different cochlear pathologies.

7.12 Immittance Audiometry

Acoustic immittance audiometry, within limits, assesses middle ear pressure, impedance/admittance and function of the acoustic reflex. This battery of measures provides useful clinical information on middle ear status and can provide information regarding central auditory nervous system function up to the level of the superior olivary complex.

The history of acoustic immittance measures dates to Lucae in 1867.[75] He, along with later researchers, used mechanical acoustic impedance bridges until the development of the electromechanical bridge in the early 1960s. This development led to increased research into middle ear function and to eventual incorporation of these measures to clinical practices. Because early electromechanical bridges used either impedance or its reciprocal, admittance, some confusion in terminology developed. Now all measures are referred to as immittance, and terminology and procedures have been standardized (ANSI S3.39-1987).[76]

The basic system for acoustic immittance is diagrammed in Figure 7.12. The system generates a probe tone into a sealed ear canal. A portion of this tone's sound pressure will pass through the tympanic membrane and middle ear to the cochlea. The remaining pressure will be retained within the external ear canal. The microphone in the probe picks up the amount of retained pressure and passes it to the analysis circuit of the bridge. The immittance is indirectly measured by the sound pressure of the probe tone in the ear canal. The more pressure transmitted through the tympanic membrane, the greater the immittance.

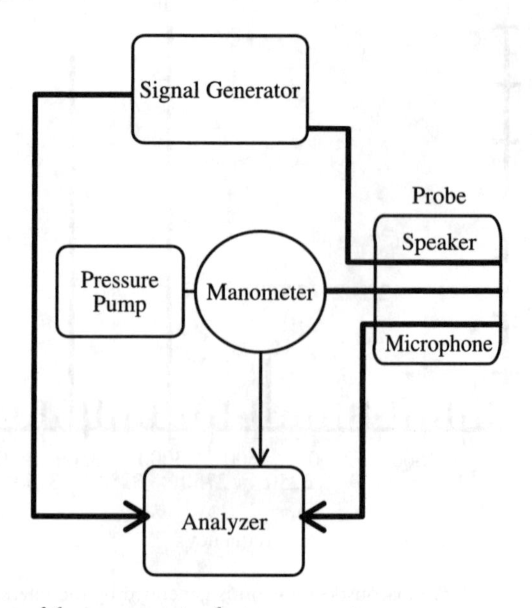

FIGURE 7.12 Block diagram of the components of a tympanometer.

The immittance measure is confounded by the size of the external ear canal and the depth of insertion of the probe tube. Different volumes will result in different pressures. To remove this confounding variable, pressure is applied within the sealed external auditory meatus. This pressure increase tightens the tympanic membrane, thereby preventing passage of sound pressure into the middle ear system. Subtracting the pressurized measure from the unpressurized measure provides the static immittance value for the middle ear system. Typically, a pressure of +200 mmH_2O, relative to ambient, is sufficient to isolate the ear canal from the middle ear.

Unfortunately, static immittance exhibits a large variation in the normal population. Both the sensitivity and the specificity of the measure are low, but as part of the diagnostic battery, they provide important information.

The tympanogram demonstrates acoustic immittance over a range of external auditory meatus pressure values. Measurements are typically acquired over a range of ±200 mmH_2O relative to ambient. Lower pressures, down to –400 mmH_2O, may be used in the case of some middle ear disorders. The resulting shape of the tympanogram is dependent on the middle ear status and the frequency of the probe tone. Tones in frequency ranges of 600 Hz and above result in multipeaked configurations that are often hard to interpret. Use of a 220-Hz probe tone results in a single peaked function that was classified by Jerger.[77] In this system, shapes are classified as A, B or C depending on the location of the immittance peak on the tympanogram (Figure 7.13). The classification system was originally developed during a period before immittance measures were expressed routinely in mmhos, and many impedance bridges provided data in arbitrary units. Therefore, the classification system is qualitative and is dependent on the experience and quality of the examiner's judgment. That being said, the system is in widespread clinical use.

All type A tympanograms have a peak compliance occurring within the normal pressure range, which is considered to be ambient to –100 mmH_2O. The lower limit can vary depending on the clinical setting and is often extended down to –150 mmH_2O. On occasion slight positive pressures may be seen, though this is atypical.

There are two subclassifications of type A tympanograms that are based on the compliance level at the tympanogram pressure peak. The first subtype is a deep configuration (A_d), the pattern of which suggests an excess amount of energy flow into the middle ear system at the pressure peak. Type A_d is typically associated with very flaccid tympanic membranes or with breaks in the ossicular chain. The second subtype is a shallow configuration (A_s), which reflects a lack of energy flow into the middle ear system. Type A_s tympanograms are associated with heavily scarred tympanic membranes or with ossicular fixation, particularly at the point of stapes footplate entrance to the oval window of the inner ear.

The type C tympanogram has a pressure peak less than –100 mmH_2O relative to ambient. To be classified as a type C, a peak must be seen, although it may be somewhat rounded. The peak may be in the normal admittance range or it may be reduced. Type C tympanograms indicate a problem with pressure regulation in the middle ear and are typically related to a failure of the eustachian tube. Children are particularly susceptible to eustachian tube problems due to the angle of the tube and the position of the adenoid adjacent to the opening into the nasopharynx.

It should be noted that the pressure peak on the tympanogram is only an approximation of the true middle ear pressure. As the ear canal pressure changes, the position of the tympanic membrane changes, either increasing or decreasing the volume of the middle ear space. Because pressure and volume are constant according to Boyle's law, the changes in volume will introduce a related pressure change.

Type B tympanograms are flat, exhibiting no peak and little if any change in compliance across the pressure range. These tympanograms will have very low static immittance values. Low immittance values, with small to normal canal size values, indicate that there is little energy flow into the middle ear space. This condition is seen when the middle ear space has fluid in it. In contrast, a type B tympanogram with a low static immittance value and a high canal size value suggests a perforation of the tympanic membrane. In effect the perforation opens up the volume of the middle ear space and mastoid air cell area. As the pressure freely enters the middle ear space, there is no displacement of the tympanic membrane as canal pressure is changed.

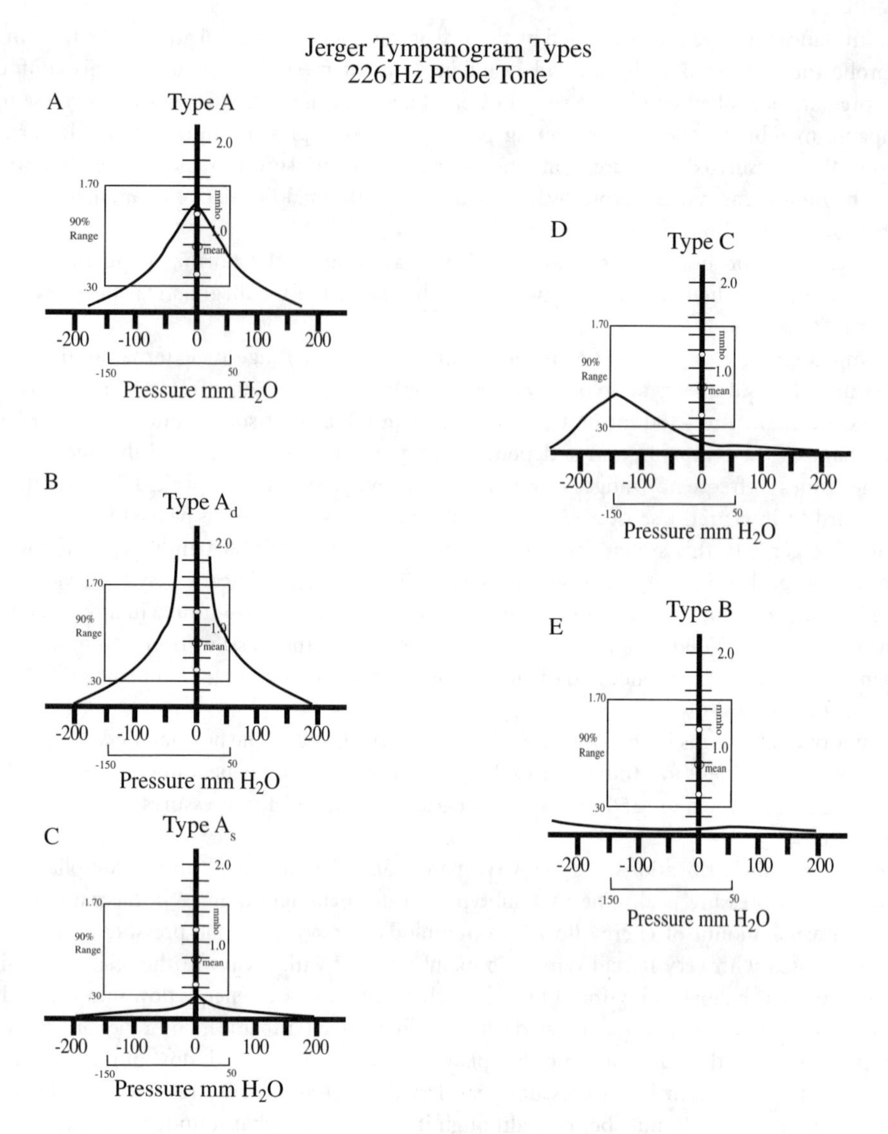

FIGURE 7.13 Tympanogram configurations. A through C represent type A tympanograms indicating normal pressures in the middle ear space. D represents a type C tympanogram normally associated with eustachian tube failure and beginning otitis media. E represents a flat tympanogram representative of tympanic membrane perforation or middle ear fluid.

7.13 Acoustic Reflex

The acoustic reflex also can be measured using immittance audiometry. The reflex is a contraction of the stapedius and tensor tympani muscles caused by a sound louder than approximately 80 dB SPL. Contraction of the muscles alters the immittance of the middle ear system. The reflex is bilateral, simultaneously affecting both ears equally.

The stimulus level required to elicit the acoustic reflex is relatively constant at approximately 80 to 90 dB SPL for individuals with cochlear hearing losses below 55 dB HL. This means that as hearing loss increases, there is a decrease in the sensation level (SL) required to elicit the response. After approximately 55 dB HL, there is a relatively linear increase in SPL required to elicit the response. The decreased SL phenomenon is related to loudness recruitment. Loudness recruitment is an abnormally fast growth in loudness for increasing SPLs and is reflective of abnormal cochlear function.

The immittance change is time locked to the stimulus onset and should be sustained for tones less than 2000 Hz for at least 30 sec. At 500 and 1000 Hz, a decrease in the reflex value by 50%, over a 10-sec period, at 5 dB SL re acoustic reflex threshold is suggestive of VIIIth nerve lesion.

7.14 Common Pathologic Conditions of the Auditory System

It would be impossible to cover all of the diseases, ototoxic effects and traumas that could alter hearing function in a chapter such as this. Also, as stated earlier, audiology is site specific rather than pathology specific. Thus, various pathologies may reflect large variations in auditory function depending on how the pathology is impinging upon the auditory system. In this section several common disease states seen in each of the auditory subsystems will be presented along with typical audiometric configurations associated with them.

In a conductive hearing loss, threshold by bone conduction is better than threshold by air conduction for a given signal. Conductive losses are associated with the external and middle ear systems that transport the sound to the cochlea.

The external ear is relatively resilient to conductive problems and typically requires a complete blockage of the external auditory meatus before significant changes in threshold are seen. If the meatus is blocked, losses up to 60 dB with flat configurations are typical.

Pathology of the tympanic membrane (TM) results in a complex array of findings. Small perforations of the TM can result in little or no loss. Losses associated with larger perforations will vary with their extent and location. Tympanometric measures for perforations demonstrate flat tympanogram and large (greater than 2 cc) ear canal volume with extremely low static compliance.

Scarring of the TM, known as tympanosclerosis, is seen via otoscopy as an area of white calcification. This rarely causes significant change in thresholds unless a majority of the TM is affected. In these cases, shallow tympanograms (type A_s) with reduced compliance may be observed. A similar finding is observed in otosclerosis, a disease discussed later in this section.

Monomeric tympanic membranes lack the fibrous middle layer of the TM. Mild to maximum conductive losses may be seen in these cases, and tympanometry yields a deep tympanogram (type A_d) with large static compliance. Similar tympanometric findings are seen for ossicular discontinuity.

Middle ear pathology again covers a broad range of structural malformations and pathologic agents. These can have little to no effect on the audiogram or may result in a maximum conductive loss. The most common problem in childhood is otitis media, with or without effusion.

Otitis media often starts as a pressure imbalance between the middle ear space and the outside atmosphere due to a failure of the Eustachian tube to open properly. As air is absorbed in the middle ear space, a pressure gradient develops across the tympanic membrane which results in a "stiffness tilt" to the audiogram. Figure 7.14a demonstrates an audiogram with a larger conductive loss in the lower frequencies than in the higher frequencies. As the disease process continues, fluid enters the middle ear space, adding mass to the system. This typically results in a drop in the high frequency region as shown in Figure 7.14b. The fluid will eventually thicken and the configuration of the hearing loss will flatten as shown in Figure 7.14c. This process can result in a maximum conductive loss of approximately 60 dB HL.

Tympanometry in otitis media will first present as a type C tympanogram with relatively good static compliance. As pressure drops in the middle ear space and fluid accumulates, the pressure peak will become more negative and present reduced static compliance values. The end result is a type B flat tympanogram with normal canal volume and a low static compliance value. As the condition is treated, the process reverses itself to a type C tympanogram and progresses to the normal type A.

In adulthood, otosclerosis is a well-known pathologic process. Otosclerosis is the slow change in the normal bone of the stapes footplate and surrounding cochlea to a softer spongy bone. Fixation of the stapes footplate in the oval window of the cochlea results from this bone remodeling. The pathologic

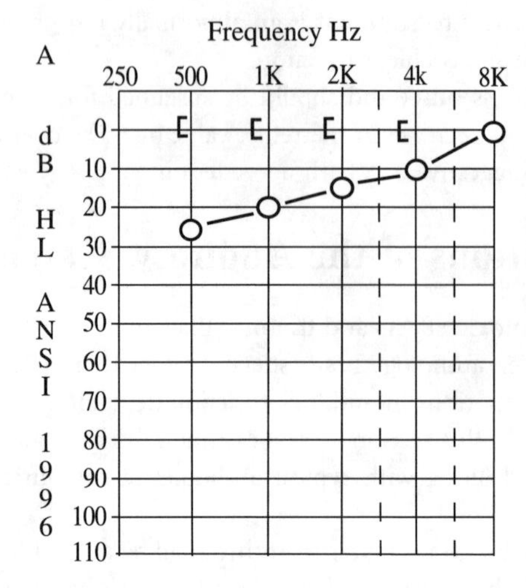

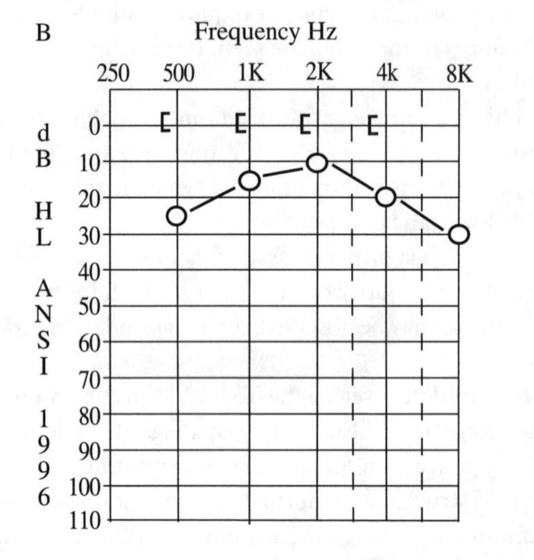

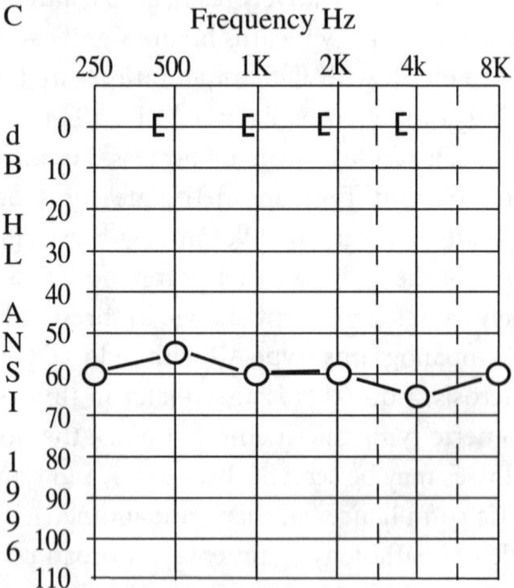

FIGURE 7.14 Air and bone conduction audiometric thresholds for the right ear demonstrating (A) a typical stiffness tilt audiogram often seen in early otitis media. (B) As fluid accumulates in the middle ear space a mass tilt is superimposed on the stiffness tilt seen in (A). (C) Flat, maximum conductive loss seen in otitis media once middle ear fluid has thickened.

process with eventual fixation of the stapes causes a conductive loss that is progressive over time. There also will be a small drop in bone conduction threshold at 2 kHz. This drop, known as Carhart's notch, as well as the conductive loss can be rectified with replacement of the stapes with a prosthetic strut. The tympanogram associated with otosclerosis is typically type A_s, with an absent stapedial reflex. Occasionally a small reflex is seen, but traveling in the opposite direction than expected. This is thought to occur from action of the tensor tympani muscle. Other ossicular fixations and, as noted previously, tympanosclerosis will present with similar findings.

Ossicular discontinuity is a break in the ossicular chain, usually occurring at the incudo-stapedial joint. This can result from head trauma or from bone necrosis in long-standing cases of otitis media. If any linkage remains between the parts of the ossicular chain, such as bands of fibrous scar tissue, hearing loss can range from mild to maximum conductive loss. The tympanogram is type A_d and the acoustic reflex is absent. As in otosclerosis, a small reverse reflex from the tensor tympani can occasionally be observed.

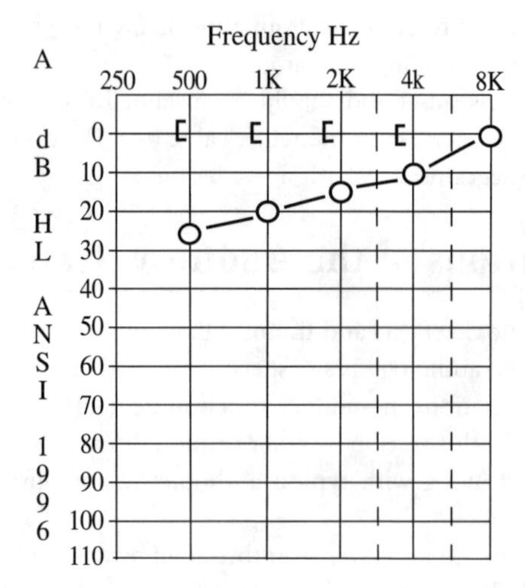

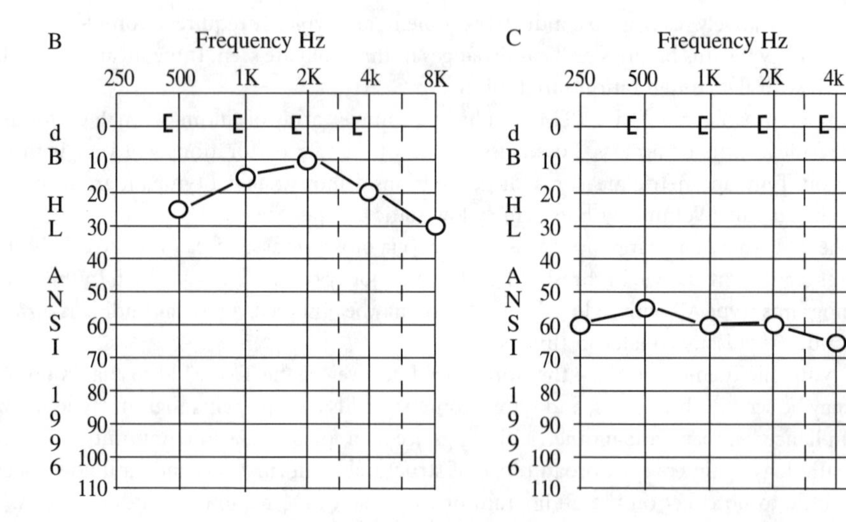

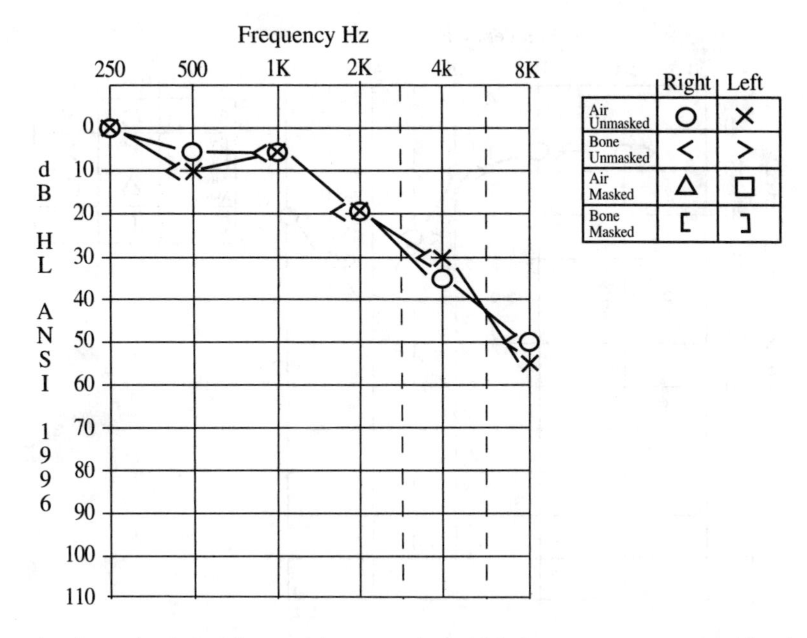

FIGURE 7.15 An air conduction audiogram, demonstrating a high frequency sensory-neural hearing loss. As the unmasked bone score interweaves with the air conduction scores, no masking is necessary.

7.15 Sensory-Neural Loss

Sensory-neural loss is defined as a loss in which there is no gap between the air-conducted and bone-conducted threshold responses to a given signal (Figure 7.15). Such losses typically reflect cochlear and, to a lesser extent, neural pathologies. Several sites have been identified within the cochlea as potential points of disruption to the auditory signal. Given today's technology and the improvements in audiometric testing procedures and materials, the term sensory-neural should now be divided into the categories of cochlear loss and neural loss.

A principal site of auditory disorder in the cochlea is the amplification system of the outer hair cells. Outer hair cells appear to be more susceptible to damage than inner hair cells and are particularly susceptible to insult from the environment. Noise and ototoxicity are two common environmental factors leading to hearing loss in adults.

7.15.1 Noise-Induced Loss

Noise is a major factor in modern life and is a significant contributor to outer hair cell damage. Noise-induced hearing loss has a characteristic notch in the 4000- to 6000-Hz region for both air- and bone-conducted scores (Figure 7.16). This notch progresses with exposure and, in older individuals, will combine with presbycusis (loss associated with aging) to render significant high frequency impairments.

The Occupational Safety and Health Administration (OSHA) has set limits for noise exposure for American workers.[78] Their damage-risk criteria suggest that repeated exposure to 90 dBA over an 8-h period could eventually lead to hearing loss. The risk criteria establishes a relationship between duration and level of exposure, with each 5-dBA increase in SPL cutting the exposure time in half. Exposure to 95 dBA should therefore be limited to no more than 4 h in a 24-h period and 100 dBA to no more than 2 h. Similarly, 85 dBA would only be permitted for 16 h.

Noise in modern-day life is not limited to the workplace. Many recreational activities now include use of power tools and engines that produce high levels of potentially damaging noise.[79–84] Properly fit hearing protection in the form of ear muffs and ear plugs are effective in preventing noise-induced losses and should always be worn in situations in which noise is present.

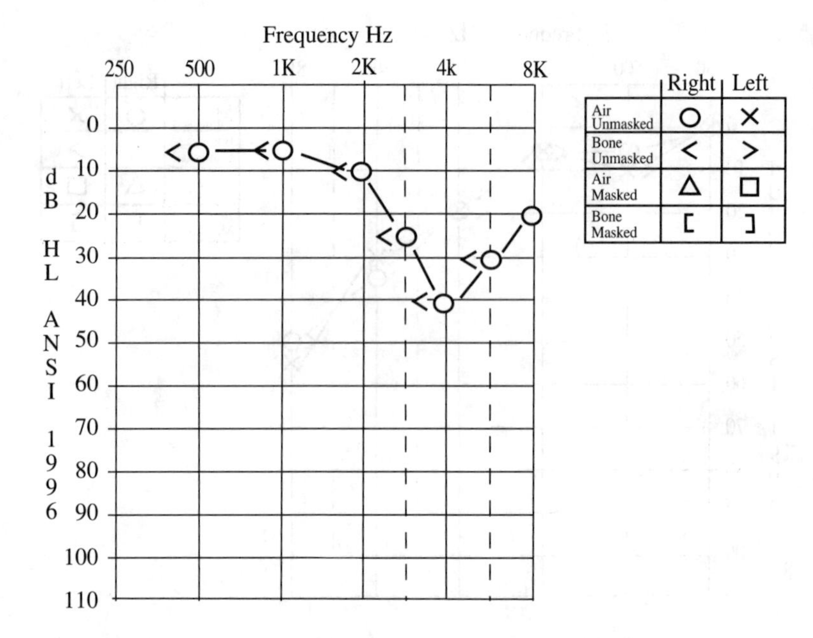

FIGURE 7.16 The audiogram demonstrates right ear thresholds seen in a noise-induced hearing loss. The notch in the 4000-Hz region, with improved thresholds at higher frequencies is characteristic of noise damage to the cochlea.

Presbycusis is hearing loss due to aging and is one of the most common forms of loss. Prevalence estimates suggest that approximately 25% of the population age 65 to 70 years old experiences hearing loss. This increases to approximately 40% for those over age 75. Such losses lead to decreases in the quality of life for older individuals, and this social problem will increase as the average life span increases. There are multiple physiologic etiologies for presbycusis, including outer hair cell loss, inner hair cell loss, metabolic changes associated with degeneration of the stria vascularis, and loss of neural elements.[85,86] Remediation of the loss and fitting of appropriate amplification remains a challenge.[87]

A relatively new disorder is auditory neuropathy or auditory dys-synchrony. This disorder reported by Starr and colleagues is a disruption of the inner hair cells, inner hair cell/neural junction or a conduction problem of the VIIIth nerve.[88] Advent of otoacoustic emission testing led to the discovery and diagnosis of the disorder, which is characterized by an absent ABR, absent acoustic reflexes and strong outer hair cell function with OAEs. For individuals exhibiting auditory dys-synchrony, hearing aid use is not recommended in most instances. There have been some reports of improved function with cochlear implants. A cochlear implant is an electronic device that receives acoustic input, encodes it and then transmits the coded signal to an array of electrodes that have been surgically threaded into the cochlea.[89]

Meniere's disease is a constellation of symptoms and includes fluctuating sensory neural hearing loss, vertigo and tinnitus, and a feeling of fullness in the ear.[90] These symptoms appear to be from failure to regulate fluid appropriately in the scala media. The term endolymphatic hydrops is often used in place of Meniere's disease. Hearing loss is typically unilateral (>80%) and more severe in the low frequency region. As the disease progresses, the hearing loss configuration tends to flatten and become more severe. One common measure for Meniere's disease is electrocochleography (EcochG).[91,92] With EcochG, the ratio of the summating potential to the action potential is evaluated and, as a rule of thumb, values larger than 0.4 are considered abnormal. This figure is dependent on a number of factors including the presence of symptoms at the time of test and the depth of electrode insertion. A second measure used in assessing Meniere's is the glycerol test.[93,94] Pure tone and speech discrimination scores are obtained and the patient is then given a diuretic, typically glycerol. Hearing is then measured 2 hours after taking the diuretic. If either a 12-dB improvement in the pure tone average or a 16% improvement in speech recognition scores is observed, the results are positive for the disease.

Modern antibiotics, chemotherapeutics, analgesics and environmental treatments can be toxic to the inner ear. Mycin antibiotics, for example, are known as toxic to hair cell structures in both the cochlea and vestibular systems. They can produce profound hearing loss and balance problems.

Cis-platinum is a widely used chemotherapy agent for certain cancers. Hearing loss related to *cis*-platinum ototoxicity is bilateral, typically symmetrical, progressive and irreversible. Degree of loss is dependent on dosage, route of administration, age, previous exposure to cranial irradiation, and any previous cochlear damage.[95,96]

Salicylates (aspirin) are also ototoxic.[97] However, the effects are reversible. High dose levels of aspirin, as used for arthritis pain relief, can result in tinnitus and sensory neural loss. Stopping the use of aspirin normally reverses the hearing loss and relieves the tinnitus.

7.16 Central Disorders

The most common problems with audition in the CNS are generically known as acoustic nerve tumors. This term is only somewhat accurate in that many of the growths are vestibular schwanomas. Nevertheless the effects on audition are the same: the growth disrupts normal transmission in nerve conduction from the cochlea. Often there is little or no loss of hearing for pure tones in the affected ear in the early stages. Speech recognition is often affected and, if lower than expected scores are observed relative to the pure tone average, a problem is suspect. A hallmark of VIIIth nerve involvement is abnormal auditory adaptation or fatigue. Tone decay procedures and Bekesy audiometry were initially used as part of the test battery for the detection of VIIIth nerve lesions. These measures were replaced by acoustic reflex decay testing and, more recently, by ABR tests. ABR in turn has largely been supplanted by the use of magnetic resonance imaging (MRI). However, a new variant of the ABR test may significantly improve diagnostic efficiency of this measure.[98]

Problems central to the auditory nerve that impinge upon the auditory system can also result in auditory dysfunction. These include, but are not limited to, multiple sclerosis, ischemic attack, vascular disorder and neoplasms. In general, these entities have very subtle effects on audition due to the highly redundant and broadly distributed nature of the auditory nervous system. Therefore pathology in one part of the system may be compensated for by the remaining unaffected areas. Similarly, most auditory signals themselves have a built-in redundancy. Thus, a general rule in behavioral assessment of the central auditory nervous system suggests both the neurologic system and the acoustic signal must have a reduction in their redundant characteristics before a problem is uncovered. This requires that behavioral auditory measures for central disorders involve complex manipulations of the auditory signal in order to stress the auditory pathways employed in the processing of those signals.

7.17 Amplification

Although there are numerous pathologic processes resulting in hearing loss, a vast majority of individuals with moderate to profound loss have cochlear losses that are not correctable by medical or surgical means. For these individuals amplification and assistive listening devices typically provide significant improvement in their ability to hear and understand speech.

Hearing aids come in a number of styles and circuit designs. The style and design most appropriate for any individual is dependent on numerous factors such as hearing thresholds, dynamic range, speech comprehension, life style, cognitive ability and dexterity. The fitting of a hearing aid must be part of a total rehabilitative package that will permit the person to make maximum use of any residual hearing. Some individuals adapt well to amplification while others have significant difficulty.[99–102]

There are several basic hearing aid styles in use today. The body aid style is not frequently used except for young children and where large amounts of power are required, e.g., bone conduction. The body aid is smaller than a package of cigarettes and the earphone is connected electrically with a cord. This positions the microphone and speaker, known as a receiver in hearing aid parlance, at a distance from one another. This separation reduces the problem of feedback, which produces a loud squeal. The behind-the-ear

(BTE) aid is a small aid that is placed behind the auricle. The microphone is typically mounted at the top of the aid and the receiver situated inside the aid and coupled acoustically to the ear by a tube. The in-the-ear (ITE) style of hearing aid fits into the ear canal with the electronics situated in the area of the concha. These small aids are popular but require manual dexterity for placement and operation of their small controls. The final style is a completely-in-canal (CIC) aid. These aids are fit down into the ear canal and take advantage of the resonant characteristics of the auricle. CIC aids require dexterity for insertion and a canal morphology that is large enough to permit placement of the electronics into the area.

The circuits in hearing aids come in both analog and digital form and offer varied filtering and signal compression characteristics. The digital designs offer significantly more flexibility in fitting than their analog counterparts; however, there is a significant cost differential. Signal filters in the digital designs are narrower and provide greater control in the final signal configuration.

Signal compression helps prevent distortion, discomfort and damage to the cochlea through overamplification. If a linear circuit is used, peak clipping of the signal will occur at the maximum signal output. This peak clipping creates distortion in the output signal and lowers speech intelligibility. Loud sounds that occur in our modern environment also can create a problem by overamplifying a signal, thereby creating discomfort and possible additional noise damage to the cochlea. Signal compression establishes a nonlinear amplification, such that amplification for louder sounds is reduced until at high signal levels, little if any amplification is present.

Microphone arrays providing directionality have provided a significant improvement in hearing aid design. This design on BTE and ITE aids typically permits amplification of signals located to the front of the listener while suppressing sounds of less significance from the sides and back of the listener. Thus, background noise, a major problem for the hearing aid user, is significantly reduced. For further information on hearing aid design and fitting, the reader is referred to Valente[103] and Sandlin.[104]

Cochlear implants are a relative newcomer to the area of auditory rehabilitation. The implant is an array of electrodes that is threaded into the cochlea. The electrodes send electrical signals to the tonotopically organized VIIIth nerve spread along the length of the cochlea. There is a signal processor connected to the electrode array that codes the electrical signals based on the acoustic input. This code activates combinations of electrodes to represent the incoming sounds. Implants have been successful in providing hearing function to the profoundly hearing impaired. Ethical considerations have been raised within the deaf community concerning the use of implants with some believing that deafness is not a handicap/disability and that the implant should not be used.[105–107]

The cochlear implant requires that the auditory portion of the VIIIth nerve is intact and the cochlea will permit entry of the electrode array. However, some pathologies, such as meningitis, can result in calcification of the cochlea, thereby preventing insertion of the electrode. Surgical intervention for other pathologies, such as neurofibromatosis, can result in sectioning of the VIIIth nerve thereby severing the connection from the cochlea to the brain. For these cases a new device, the brain stem implant, is currently being developed.[108–111] This device places the electrode array on the posterior lateral surface of the brainstem over the cochlear nuclear complex. Initial trials with this device have shown successes similar to those seen with early single channel cochlear implants.

References

1. Durrant, J.D. and Lovrinic, J.H., *Bases of Hearing Science*, 3rd ed., Williams & Wilkins, Baltimore, 1995, p. cm.
2. Wever, E.G. and Lawrence, M., *Physiological Acoustics*, Princeton University Press, Princeton, NJ, 1954.
3. Dorman, M.F., Lindholm, J.M., Hannley, M.T., et al., Vowel intelligibility in the absence of the acoustic reflex: performance-intensity characteristics, *J. Acoust. Soc. Am.*, 81, 562–564, 1987.
4. Phillips, D.P., Stuart, A., and Carpenter, M., Re-examination of the role of the human acoustic stapedius reflex, *J. Acoust. Soc. Am.*, 111, 2200–2207, 2002.
5. Ingelstedt, S., Mechanics of the human middle ear, *Acta Oto-Laryngol.*, Suppl. 228, 1–57, 1967.

6. Jones, M., Pressure changes in the middle ear after altering the composition of contained gas, *Acta Oto-Laryngol.*, 3, 1–11, 1961.
7. Magnuson, B., Physiology of the eustachian tube and middle ear pressure regulation, in *Physiology of the Ear*, Jahn, A. and Santos-Sacchi, J., Eds., San Diego, Singular-Thomson Learning, 2001, pp. 75–99.
8. Murphy, D., Negative pressure in the middle ear by ciliary propulsion of mucus through the eustachian tube, *Laryngoscope*, 89, 954–961, 1979.
9. Sade, J., Halevy, A., Hadas, E., and Saba, K., Clearance of middle ear effusions and middle ear pressures, *AORL*, 85(Suppl. 25), 58–62, 1976.
10. Sade, J. and Hadas, E., Prognostic evaluation of secretory otitis media as a function of mastoid pneumotisation. *Arch. Otorhinolaryngol.*, 225, 39–44, 1979.
11. Sade, J., The buffering effect of middle ear negative pressure by retraction of the pars tensa, *Am. J. Otol.*, 21, 20–23, 2000.
12. Flisberg, K., Ingelstedt, S., and Ortegren, U., On middle ear pressure, *Acta Oto-Laryngol.*, 182(Suppl.), 43–56, 1963.
13. Flisberg, K., Determination of the airway resistance of the eustchian tube, *Acta Oto-Laryngol.*, 224(Suppl.), 376–84, 1967.
14. Flisberg, K., The effects of vacuum on the tympanic cavity, *Otolaryng. Clin. N. Am.*, 3, 3–13, 1970.
15. Shepard, N.T. and Telian, S.A., *Practical Management of the Balance Disorder Patient*, Singular Publ. Group, San Diego, 1996, pp. xi, 221.
16. Jacobson, G.P., Newman, C.W., and Kartush, J.M., *Handbook of Balance Function Testing*, Mosby Year Book, St. Louis, 1993, pp. xii, 439.
17. Von Békésy, G., *Experiments in Hearing*, McGraw-Hill, New York, 1960, p. 745.
18. Robles, L. and Ruggero, MA., Mechanics of the mammalian cochlea, *Physiol. Rev.*, 81, 1305–1352, 2001.
19. Spiess, A.C., Lang, H., Schulte, B.A., et al., Effects of gap junction uncoupling in the gerbil cochlea, *Laryngoscope*, 112, 1635–1641, 2002.
20. Kikuchi, T., Adams, J.C., Miyabe, Y., et al., Potassium ion recycling pathway via gap junction systems in the mammalian cochlea and its interruption in hereditary nonsyndromic deafness, *Med. Electron Microsc.*, 33, 51–56, 2000.
21. Giraud, A.L., Lorenzi, C., Ashburner, J., et al., Representation of the temporal envelope of sounds in the human brain, *J. Neurophysiol.*, 84, 1588–1598.
22. Eggermont, J.J., Between sound and perception: reviewing the search for a neural code, *Hearing Res.*, 157, 1–42, 2001.
23. Kiren, T., Aoyagi, M., Furuse, H., et al., An experimental study on the generator of amplitude-modulation following response, *Acta Oto-Laryngol.*, 511(Suppl.), 28–33, 1994.
24. Kollmeier, B. and Koch, R., Speech enhancement based on physiological and psychoacoustical models of modulation perception and binaural interaction, *J. Acoust. Soc. Am.*, 95, 1593–1602, 1994.
25. Lorenzi, C., Micheyl, C., and Berthommier, F., Neuronal correlates of perceptual amplitude-modulation detection, *Hear Res.*, 90, 219–227, 1995.
26. Muller-Preuss, P., Flachskamm, C., and Bieser, A., Neural encoding of amplitude modulation within the auditory midbrain of squirrel monkeys, *Hear Res.*, 80, 197–208, 1994.
27. Webster, D.B., *Neuroscience of Communication*, Singular Publ. Group, San Diego, 1995, pp. x, 316.
28. Reuter, T., Nummela, S., and Hemila, S., Elephant hearing, *J. Acoust. Soc. Am.*, 104, 1122–1123, 1998.
29. Guppy, A. and Coles, R.B., Acoustical and neural aspects of hearing in the Australian gleaning bats, *Macroderma gigas* and *Nyctophilus gouldi*, *J. Comp. Physiol. A*, 162, 653–668, 1988.
30. Coles, R.B., Guppy, A., Anderson, M.E., et al., Frequency sensitivity and directional hearing in the gleaning bat, *Plecotus auritus* (Linnaeus 1758), *J. Comp. Physiol. A*, 165, 269–280, 1989.

31. Gorga, M.P. and Thornton, A.R., The choice of stimuli for ABR measurements, *Ear Hearing*, 10, 217–230, 1989.
32. Purdy, S.C. and Abbas, P.J., ABR thresholds to tonebursts gated with Blackman and linear windows in adults with high-frequency sensorineural hearing loss, *Ear Hearing*, 23, 358–368, 2002.
33. American National Standards Institute, ANSI S1.4-1983, American National Standard Specification for Sound Level Meters, American Institute of Physics for the Acoustical Society of America, 1983, pp. vii, 18.
34. Lipscomb, D.M., *Hearing Conservation in Industry, Schools, and the Military*, Singular Publ. Group, San Diego, 1994, pp. vii, 332.
35. Yost, W.A., *Fundamentals of Hearing: An Introduction*, 4th ed., Academic Press, San Diego, 2000, pp. xiii, 349.
36. American National Standards Institute, ANSI S3.6-1996, American National Standard Specification for Audiometers, Acoustical Society of America, 1996, pp. vi, 33.
37. Bess, J.C., Ear canal collapse. A review, *Arch. Otolaryngol.*, 93, 408–412, 1971.
38. Chaiklin, J.B. and McClellan, M.E., Audiometric management of collapsible ear canals, *Arch. Otolaryngol.*, 93, 397–407, 1971.
39. Marshall, L. and Gossman, M., Management of ear canal collapse, *Arch. Otolaryngol.*, 108, 357–361, 1982.
40. Sobhy, O.A. and Gould, H.J., Interaural attenuation using insert earphones: electrocochleographic approach, *J. Am. Acad. Audiol.*, 4, 76–79, 1993.
41. Martin, F.N. and Clark, J.G., *Introduction to Audiology*, 8th ed., Allyn and Bacon, Boston, 2002, p. cm.
42. Davis-Penn, W. and Ross, M., Pediatric experiences with frequency transposing, *Hearing Instrum.*, 44, 27–32, 1993.
43. Tyler, R.S. and Tye-Murray, N., Cochlear implant signal-processing strategies and patient perception of speech and environmental sounds, in *Practical Aspects of Audiology: Cochlear Implants*, Cooper H., Ed., Singular Publ. Group, San Diego, 1991.
44. ASHA, Guidelines for determining the threshold level for speech, *Asha*, 30, 85–89, 1988.
45. Martin, F.N. and Dowdy, L.K., A modified spondee threshold procedure, *J. Aud. Res.*, 26, 115–119, 1986.
46. Mendel, L.L. and Danhauer, J.L., *Audiologic Evaluation and Management and Speech Perception Assessment*, Singular Publ. Group, San Diego, 1997, p. xii.
47. French, N.R. and Steinberg, J.C., Factors governing the intelligibility of speech sounds, *J. Acoust. Soc. Am.*, 19, 90–119, 1947.
48. Fletcher, H. and Galt, R., The perception of speech and its relation to telephony, *J. Acoust. Soc. Am.*, 22, 89–151, 1950.
49. American National Standards Institute, ANSI S3.5-1997, Methods for calculation of the speech Intelligibility Index, Acoustical Society of America, 1997, pp. iii, 22.
50. Halpin, C., Thornton, A., and Hous, Z., The articulation index in clinical diagnosis and hearing aid fitting, *Curr. Opin. Otolaryngol. Head Neck Surg.*, 4, 325–334, 1996.
51. Studebaker, G.A., Gray, G.A., and Branch, W.E., Prediction and statistical evaluation of speech recognition test scores, *J. Am. Acad. Audiol.*, 10, 355–370, 1999.
52. Studebaker, G.A., McDaniel, D.M., and Gwaltney, C., Monosyllabic word recognition at higher-than-normal speech and noise levels, *J. Acoust. Soc. Am.*, 105, 2431–2444, 1999.
53. Studebaker, G.A., Gray, G.A., and Branch, W.E., Prediction and statistical evaluation of speech recognition test Scores, *J. Am. Acad. Audiol.*, 10, 355–370, 1999.
54. Gold, T., Hearing. II. The physical basis of action if the cochlea, *Proc. R. Soc. London Ser. B: Biol. Sci.*, 135, 492–498, 1948.
55. Kemp, D.T., Stimulated acoustic emissions from within the human auditory system, *J. Acoust. Soc. Am.*, 64, 1386–1391, 1978.

56. Robinette, M.S. and Glattke, T.J., *Otoacoustic Emissions: Clinical Applications*, Thieme, New York, 1997.
57. Hall, J.W., *Handbook of Otoacoustic Emissions*, Singular Publ. Group, San Diego, 2000, pp. xi, 635.
58. Penner, M.J., Glotzbach, L., and Huang, T., Spontaneous otoacoustic emissions: measurement and data, *Hearing Res.*, 68, 229–237, 1993.
59. Martin, G.K., Probst, R., and Lonsbury-Martin, B.L., Otoacoustic emissions in human ears: normative findings, *Ear Hearing*, 11, 106–120, 1990.
60. Bilger, R.C., Matthies, M.L., Hammel, D.R., et al., Genetic implications of gender differences in the prevalence of spontaneous otoacoustic emissions, *J. Speech Hearing Res.*, 33, 418–432, 1990.
61. Strickland, E.A., Burns, E.M., and Tubis, A., Incidence of spontaneous otoacoustic emissions in children and infants, *J. Acoust. Soc. Am.*, 78, 931–935, 1985.
62. Whitehead, M.L., Kamal, N., Lonsbury-Martin, B.L., et al., Spontaneous otoacoustic emissions in different racial groups, *Scand. Audiol.*, 22, 3–10, 1993.
63. Stover, L. and Norton, S.J., The effects of aging on otoacoustic emissions, *J. Acoust. Soc. Am.*, 94, 2670–2681, 1993.
64. van Dijk, P. and Wit, H.P., Amplitude and frequency fluctuations of spontaneous otoacoustic emissions, *J. Acoust. Soc. Am.*, 88, 1779–1793, 1990.
65. Kemp, D.T., Otoacoustic emissions, travelling waves and cochlear mechanisms, *Hearing Res.*, 22, 95–104, 1986.
66. Penner, M.J., An estimate of the prevalence of tinnitus caused by spontaneous otoacoustic emissions, *Arch. Otolaryngol. Head Neck Surg.*, 116, 418–423, 1990.
67. Penner, M.J. and Glotzbach, L., Covariation of tinnitus pitch and the associated emission: a case study, *Otolaryngol. Head Neck Surg.*, 110, 304–309, 1994.
68. Kok, M.R., van Zanten, G.A., Brocaar, M.P., et al., Click-evoked oto-acoustic emissions in 1036 ears of healthy newborns, *Audiology*, 32, 213–224, 1993.
69. Moulin, A., Collet, L., and Duclaux, R., Contralateral auditory stimulation alters acoustic distortion products in humans, *Hear Res.*, 65, 193–210, 1993.
70. Thornton, A.R.D. and Slaven, S., The effect of stimulus rate on the contralateral suppression of transient evoked otoacoustic emissions, *Scand Audiol.*, 24, 83–90, 1995.
71. Veuillet, E., Collet, L., and Morgon, A., Differential effects of ear-canal pressure and contralateral acoustic stimulation on evoked otoacoustic emissions in humans, *Hearing Res.*, 61, 47–55, 1992.
72. Gelfand, S.A., Hearing, in *An Introduction to Psychological and Physiological Acoustics*, 3rd ed., Marcel Dekker, New York, 1998, p. viii.
73. Whitehead, M.L., Stagner, B.B., McCoy, M.J., et al., Dependence of distortion-product otoacoustic emissions on primary levels in normal and impaired ears. II. Asymmetry in L1,L2 space, *J. Acoust. Soc. Am.*, 97, 2359–2377, 1995.
74. Shera, C.A. and Guinan, J.J., Jr., Evoked otoacoustic emissions arise by two fundamentally different mechanisms: a taxonomy for mammalian OAEs, *J. Acoust. Soc. Am.*, 105, 782–798, 1999.
75. Feldman, A.S. and Wilber, L.A., *Acoustic Impedance and Admittance: The Measurement of Middle Ear Function*, Williams & Wilkins, Baltimore, 1976, p. viii.
76. American National Standards Institute, ANSI S3.39-1987, American National Standard Specification for Instruments to Measure Aural Acoustic Impedance and Admittance (Aural Acoustic Immittance), American Institute of Physics for the Acoustical Society of America, New York, 1987, p. vi, 21.
77. Jerger, J., Clinical experience with impedance audiometry, *Arch. Otolaryngol.*, 92, 311–324, 1970.
78. OSHA, Occupational noise exposure: hearing conservation amendment, *Fed. Reg.*, 48, 9738–9785, 1983.
79. Bess, F.H. and Powell, R.L., Hearing hazard from model airplanes. A study on their potential damaging effects to the auditory mechanism, *Clin. Pediatr. (Philadelphia)*, 11, 621–624, 1972.
80. Shirreffs, J.H., Recreational noise: implications for potential hearing loss to participants, *J. Sch. Health*, 44, 548–550, 1974.

81. Molvaer, O.I. and Natrud, E., Ear damage due to diving, *Acta Otolaryngol., Suppl.*, 360, 187–189, 1979.
82. Chung, D.Y., Gannon, R.P., Willson, G.N., et al., Shooting, sensorineural hearing loss, and workers' compensation, *J. Occup. Med.*, 23, 481–484, 1981.
83. Plakke, B.L., Noise levels of electronic arcade games: a potential hearing hazard to children, *Ear Hearing*, 4, 202–203, 1983.
84. McClymont, L.G. and Simpson, D.C., Noise levels and exposure patterns to do-it-yourself power tools, *J. Laryngol. Otol.*, 103, 1140–1141, 1989.
85. Schuknecht, H.F. and Gacek, M.R., Cochlear pathology in presbycusis, *Ann. Otol. Rhinol. Laryngol.*, 102, 1–16, 1993.
86. Frisina, D.R. and Frisina, R.D., Speech recognition in noise and presbycusis: relations to possible neural mechanisms, *Hearing Res.*, 106, 95–104, 1997.
87. Cohn, E.S., Hearing loss with aging: presbycusis, *Clin. Geriatr. Med.*, 15, 145–161, viii, 1999.
88. Starr, A., Picton., T.W., Sininger, Y., et al., Auditory neuropathy, *Brain*, 119 (Pt 3), 741–753, 1996.
89. Cooper, H., *Practical Aspects of Audiology Cochlear Implants: A Practical Guide*, Singular Publ. Group, San Diego, 1991.
90. Mateijsen, D.J., Van Hengel, P.W., Van Huffelen, W.M., et al., Pure-tone and speech audiometry in patients with Meniere's disease, *Clin. Otolaryngol.*, 26, 379–387, 2001.
91. Ferraro, J.A. and Tibbils, R.P., SP/AP area ratio in the diagnosis of Meniere's disease, *Am. J. Audiol.*, 8, 21–28, 1999.
92. Storms, R.F., Ferraro, J.A., and Thedinger, B.S., Electrocochleographic effects of ear canal pressure change in subjects with Meniere's disease, *Am. J. Otol.*, 17, 874–882, 1996.
93. Thomsen, J. and Vesterhauge, S., A critical evaluation of the glycerol test in Meniere's disease, *J. Otolaryngol.*, 8, 145–150, 1979.
94. Mori, N., Asai, A., Suizu., Y., et al., Comparison between electrocochleography and glycerol test in the diagnosis of Meniere's disease, *Scand Audiol.*, 14, 209–213, 1985.
95. Berg, A.L., Spitzer, J.B., and Garvin, J.H., Jr., Ototoxic impact of cisplatin in pediatric oncology patients, *Laryngoscope*, 109, 1806–1814, 1999.
96. Nagy, J.L., Adelstein, D.J., Newman, C.W., et al., Cisplatin ototoxicity: the importance of baseline audiometry, *Am. J. Clin. Oncol.*, 22, 305–308, 1999.
97. Cazals, Y., Auditory sensori-neural alterations induced by salicylate, *Prog. Neurobiol.*, 62, 583–631, 2000.
98. Don, M., Masuda, A., Nelson, R., et al., Successful detection of small acoustic tumors using the stacked derived-band auditory brain stem response amplitude, *Am. J. Otol.*, 18, 608–621, discussion 82-5, 1997.
99. Mulrow, C.D., Tuley, M.R., and Aguilar, C., Correlates of successful hearing aid use in older adults, *Ear Hearing*, 13, 108–113, 1992.
100. Cox, R.M. and Alexander, G.C., Expectations about hearing aids and their relationship to fitting outcome, *J. Am. Acad. Audiol.*, 11, 368–382, quiz 407, 2000.
101. Alberti, P.W., Pichora-Fuller, M.K., Corbin, H., et al., Aural rehabilitation in a teaching hospital: evaluation and results, *Ann. Otol. Rhinol. Laryngol.*, 93, 589–594, 1984.
102. Malinoff, R.L. and Weinstein, B.E., Measurement of hearing aid benefit in the elderly, *Ear Hearing*, 10, 354–356, 1989.
103. Valente, M., *Strategies for Selecting and Verifying Hearing Aid Fittings*, 2nd ed., Thieme, New York, 2002.
104. Sandlin, R.E., *The Textbook of Hearing Aid Amplification*, 2nd ed., Singular Publ. Group, San Diego, 2000, p. xv.
105. Bryce, G., Cochlear implant and the deaf culture, *Am. J. Otol.*, 17, 496, 1996.
106. Lane, H. and Bahan, B., Ethics of cochlear implantation in young children: a review and reply from a Deaf-World perspective, *Otolaryngol. Head Neck Surg.*, 119, 297–313, 1998.

107. Lane, H. and Grodin, M., Ethical issues in cochlear implant surgery: an exploration into disease, disability, and the best interests of the child, *Kennedy Inst. Ethics J.*, 7, 231–251, 1997.
108. Nevison, B., Laszig, R., Sollmann, W.P., et al., Results from a European clinical investigation of the nucleus multichannel auditory brainstem implant, *Ear Hearing*, 23, 170–183, 2002.
109. Lenarz, M., Matthies, C., Lesinski-Schiedat, A., et al., Auditory Brainstem Implant. II. Subjective Assessment of Functional Outcome, *Otol. Neurotol.*, 23, 694–697, 2002.
110. Toh, E.H. and Luxford, W.M., Cochlear and brainstem implantation, *Otolaryngol. Clin. N. Am.*, 35, 325–342, 2002.
111. Lenarz, T., Moshrefi, M., Matthies, C., et al., Auditory brainstem implant. I. Auditory performance and its evolution over time, *Otol. Neurotol.*, 22, 823–833, 2001.

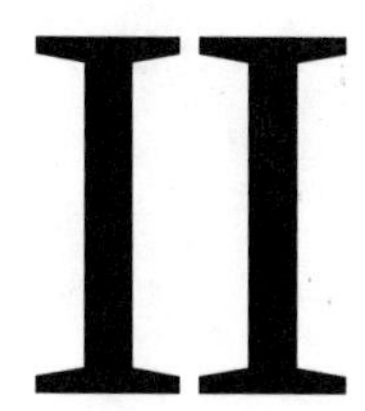

Imaging Techniques

Contributions of Technological Developments to Imaging

Imaging the interior workings of the human body has long been an elusive ambition of health-care providers. From the early drawings of Leonardo da Vinci, humans have aspired to visualize the body's machinery as accurately as possible. The development of x-ray imaging provided the first glimpse of a living human structure. This opened the door for visual diagnosis. The importance of such developments cannot be understated, given the degree to which humans rely on visual information.

Most imaging techniques aim to provide static images of hard and soft tissues. The use of contrast agents and multimodality imaging has greatly improved the resolution of the images obtained. However, recent technological and computational advances, along with the development of specific radiopharmaceuticals, have extended these capabilities to actual functional imaging. It is now possible to assess certain physiological processes and organ functions in real-time. The variety of imaging technologies available to clinicians is growing rapidly. The development of mesoscale imaging technologies has yielded devices that can be deployed inside the body via catheters to provide direct live images without contrast agents or ionizing radiation. Extraordinary advances in all areas of imaging technology have allowed clinicians to make accurate and efficient diagnoses, often in a noninvasive fashion.

This section includes the following chapters:

8. Magnetic Resonance Imaging
9. Ultrasonic Imaging
10. Emission Imaging: SPECT and PET
11. Endoscopy
12. Functional Brain Mapping Using Intracranial Source Imaging

II

Imaging Techniques

Contributions of Technological Developments to Imaging

8

Magnetic Resonance Imaging

Timothy P.L. Roberts
University of Toronto

Christopher K. Macgowan
University of Toronto

CONTENTS

8.1 Introduction

Magnetic resonance imaging (MRI) has evolved over the last three decades to become the method of choice for the vast proportion of noninvasive cross-sectional "scanning" in diagnostic radiology. Apart from simply "looking inside the body," the success and range of magnetic resonance imaging has built upon the variety of physiological and pathological insights available from different MRI approaches. That is to say, there is not "an MRI," but rather a broad variety of "MRI pulse sequences" that generate images whose appearance may reflect not merely tissue density (such as x-ray computed tomography [CT]), but also properties of the physicochemical microenvironment, such as fluid mobility, macromolecule (e.g., protein) content, metabolic products, blood flow and perfusion and so on. Mastery of this range of MRI techniques provides the radiologic "artist" with a broad "palette" of physiological sensitivities to exploit or deny as the image is created.

0-8493-1140-3/04/$0.00+$1.50

While many textbooks are devoted to magnetic resonance imaging, and even specific aspects thereof, the purpose of this chapter is to provide a swift overview of the MRI family of techniques, to discuss applications in the study of the brain and the heart and to introduce the varied roles of MRI in diagnostic radiology, in preclinical drug development and in basic science.

Founded on the science of nuclear magnetic resonance (NMR), the development of techniques for spatial encoding of NMR signals during the 1970s led to the birth and subsequent explosion of MRI. The MRI scanner thus consists of similar components to an NMR spectrometer, with the addition of systems for controlling the local magnetic field.

8.2 Hardware Components of an MRI Scanner

8.2.1 Magnet

The nuclear magnetic resonance experiment relies on placing the test sample (or in this case, patient) in a uniform and strong external magnetic field. In clinical practice the magnetic field strength may be as low as 0.2T or as high as 3T. Research systems for human imaging exist at field strengths as high as 8T, with 9.4T and higher systems in development. Smaller-bore experimental MRI systems exist with field strengths up to 20T. The static magnetic field strength of an MRI scanner is commonly referred to as B_0. Most systems employ superconducting technology, with liquid helium cooling.

8.2.2 Gradient Coils/Amplifier

The feature that distinguishes the MRI scanner from the NMR spectrometer is the ability to perform spatial encoding of detected signals for subsequent image formation. At the heart of this lies a requirement to control the "local magnetic field." Over and above the static (and uniform) magnetic field, B_0, an MRI scanner uses (three) magnetic field gradient coils to impose linear variations in magnetic field in any or all of the three Cartesian axes. Such magnetic field gradients are typically not in place throughout the image acquisition process but are "switched on" as required during the playing out of the MRI pulse sequence, a set of instructions controlling the timing of RF and gradient systems. Magnetic field gradient strengths on clinical MRI scanners are of the order of mT/m (some systems currently offer the capability of 60 mT/m) and may have 40 cm or more of spatial extent; magnetic field gradient coils are associated with powerful current amplifiers, leading to systems capable of slew rates up to 200 mT/m/msec. Interestingly, the characteristic acoustic noise of the MRI is a product of such rapid switching of magnetic field gradients.

8.2.3 RF Coils/Transmission and Reception System

With the sample placed in the static magnetic field, B_0, the MRI experiment continues by excitation and detection of the NMR response. Governed by the Larmor equation (Equation 8.1), excitation requires delivery of an oscillating magnetic field (at a frequency in the MHz range). Hence, a radiofrequency (RF) coil is used to transmit an RF wave into the sample (patient). Similarly, the same (or a second) coil is used to detect the weak NMR response, prior to preamplification and digitization.

$$\omega = \gamma \, B, \tag{8.1}$$

where ω is the Larmor or resonant frequency, γ is the gyromagnetic ratio ($\gamma/2\pi = 42.57$ MHz/T for the ^{1}H proton) and B is the *local* magnetic field. It is of critical importance that B relates to the local magnetic field, dominated by the static field B_0 but also sensitive to additional field influences (e.g., magnetic field gradients applied).

Thus, as with NMR, the origin of the signal used in MR imaging is the nuclear spin of the tissue constituent atoms. While NMR responses are detectable from a variety of non-zero spin nuclei (including biologically relevant nuclei such as ^{23}Na and ^{31}P), the vast majority of clinical MRI uses the ^{1}H proton as the source of signal. Not only does ^{1}H have the greatest sensitivity of all nuclei to the NMR experiment (with the exception of the nonrelevant tritium ion), but it must be remembered that the human body is composed of approximately 70% water (H_2O), each water molecule containing two ^{1}H protons in a liquid state optimal for NMR. Thus the ^{1}H signal source is present at concentrations of approximately 80 *M*. In fact, based on Boltzmann statistics relating the populations of nuclear spins in the two energy states associated with the application of the external field, it is clear that, even at 1.5 or 3T, the NMR experiment is extremely inefficient (with an excess population in the low-energy state of only a few spins per million). Thus the high available spin density of the ^{1}H in water molecules of the human body is fortuitous!

8.3 Image Encoding

While a detailed discussion of the process of image formation is beyond the scope of this text, an overview illustrating the main conceptual stages is worthwhile. Considering the ensemble of nuclear spins to be represented by a vector, M, initially aligned with the external magnetic field B_0, the first stage (RF excitation) involves rotating the vector M through an angle, α. This is achieved by applying a magnetic field oscillating at the Larmor frequency. The amplitude of the magnetic component of such an RF "pulse" is generally labeled B_1. The rotation or "flip" angle is predicted by the amplitude and duration of the RF pulse:

$$\alpha = \gamma B_1 t, \tag{8.2}$$

where α is the flip angle, γ the gyromagnetic ratio and t the pulse duration. After the B_1 field (RF pulse) is discontinued, the transverse component of the tilted vector M then undergoes circular motion (precesses) around the axis of the external field B_0. Since the magnetic vector M carries with it a tiny magnetic field, this also rotates. A conducting coil experiencing this changing magnetic field has an electrical current induced in it (Faraday's law of electromagnetic induction) and the NMR response has been detected. In practice, as discussed below, the amplitude of the detected oscillating signal decays over time (as the underlying spins contributing to the vector M lose phase coherence due to slightly different precession rates). Overall this damped oscillation — the NMR response — is known as the free induction decay (FID), "free" because it is no longer "forced" by the B_1 field, "induction" because of the mechanism of signal detection, and "decay" because of the signal's decreasing amplitude.

However, imaging requires that spatial information is encoded in the NMR response. How can that be achieved? In our three-dimensional spatial world, there are three mechanisms by which spatial information can be introduced into the process of magnetic resonance image formation: slice selection, frequency encoding, and phase encoding. We will deal briefly with these concepts (see Figure 8.1).

8.3.1 Slice Selection

If the RF field, B_1, is modulated in amplitude, it will cause excitation of spins resonant at a range of Larmor frequencies. If the amplitude modulation takes the form of a sinc function $(1/t)\sin(\pi t)$ envelope, then to a first approximation the frequency response profile takes the form of bandpass, with a narrow band of frequencies being uniformly excited and with spins whose resonant frequency lies outside the band being unaffected (and remaining aligned with the B_0 field, the nominal *z*-axis). But why would spins have different resonant frequencies? Simultaneously with the application of the sinc-modulated RF pulse, a linear magnetic field gradient is applied along one spatial axis, leading to a spatially varying local effective magnetic field and thus a spatially varying resonant frequency. If the gradient direction is the *z*-axis and the amplitude is G_z, the Larmor equation becomes modified to:

$$\omega(z) = \gamma (B_0 + G_z.z). \tag{8.3}$$

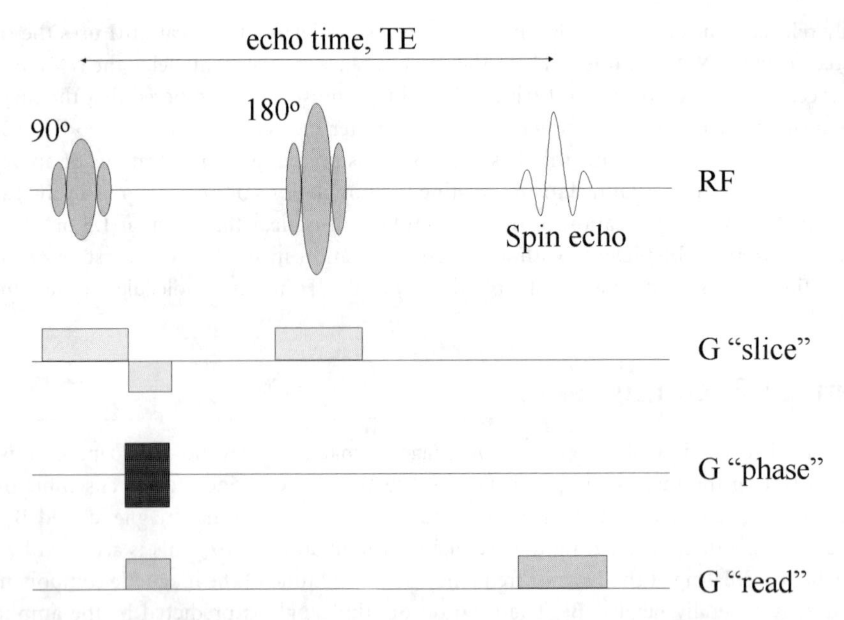

FIGURE 8.1 The timing diagram schematic for an MRI "spin-echo" pulse sequence. Essentially portraying the timing of instructions to the RF transmission system and each of the three spatial magnetic field gradient systems, this schematic illustrates the relative timing of 90 and 180 RF pulses (shown as sinc modulated) and subsequent spin echo formation at the echo time, TE. It also shows (as rectangles) the application of pulses of magnetic field gradient in the slice, phase-encode and readout spatial directions. Note the ladder representation of the phase encoding gradient pulse, implying that each time the shown RF excite/data readout module is repeated a different value of magnetic field gradient amplitude is used for phase encoding.

Thus a narrow band of frequencies excited has a direct interpretation as a narrow band of z-coordinates, or "slice." This interpretation is arrived at based on knowledge of the linear magnetic field gradient, G_z. Thus the gradient field application has transformed a mathematical property of "frequency selectivity" into the usable property of "spatial selectivity," and we have reduced the dimensionality of the image formation problem from 3 to 2.

8.3.2 Frequency Encoding

The NMR response can be restored as an echo (see below) time shifted with respect to the initial excitation. Response data (the induced current) must be collected during the echo formation, known as "readout." While the echo occurs at a constant time with respect to the initial excitation, the approach to the echo depends on the precessional frequency of the underlying spins. If the echo is acquired with the coincident application of a magnetic field gradient in one of the two remaining spatial directions, spin ensembles will be forced into formation of "lower frequency" and "higher frequency" echoes according to their spatial coordinate in this axis (e.g., x), which determines the effective local magnetic field they experience. Since these echoes are inherently summed in the echo acquisition process, some form of frequency analysis is required to resolve the frequency distribution of component echoes in the composite signal. Employing a one-dimensional Fourier transform of the echo, such a frequency abundance profile can be determined; with knowledge of the gradient field strength and orientation, this frequency abundance profile can be interpreted as revealing the one-dimensional spin distribution in space (since low frequencies are associated with low spatial coordinates in the direction of the applied magnetic field gradient because of the lower effective local magnetic field). This process is known as *frequency-encoding*.

8.3.3 Phase Encoding

A single, slice-selected, frequency-encoded NMR response can thus be interrogated to reveal a one-dimensional "projection" of a selected slice of the object under study. It does not, however, allow construction of a two-dimensional image. In fact there is insufficient information in a single echo to allow this. Consequently several echoes must be collected by repeated application of the RF excitation/data readout module. Note, in practice the sequence repeat time, TR, must be set to allow sufficient signal potential for subsequent cycles of the module. This ultimately limits most MRI acquisition rates. However, each collected echo is distinguished by its experience in terms of the remaining spatial axis. After spins have been excited by the RF pulse and during subsequent precession in the transverse plane, a magnetic field gradient is imposed for a short duration, aligned along this third spatial dimension (y). Spins undergo irrecoverable dephasing according to their spatial coordinate in this dimension and according to the magnitude of the gradient field, G_y. This is called *phase-encoding*. As the module is repeated, the magnitude of G_y is incremented (hence the ladder representation in the pulse sequence diagram). Consider a peripheral (high y-coordinate) distribution of spins — as G_y is increased, rapid dephasing occurs and spin-echo signal is strongly attenuated. Consider a more central (low y-coordinate) distribution: even increasing G_y only leads to slow dephasing, and subsequently spin echo amplitude persists, only weakly attenuated. Thus observing the rate of loss of spin-echo amplitude as a function of increasing G_y (phase encoding power), we can make an interpretation in terms of spin distribution in the y-direction.

8.3.4 k-space

A commonly employed representation is to portray the multiple (typically 128 or 256) spin echoes in a two-dimensional grid (where the *x*-axis scales with readout time) and the *y*-axis offset is proportional to the amount of phase encoding power. This "k-space" representation allows two-dimensional Fourier transformation (FT) to yield an interpretable image.* In general, the object of the MR pulse sequence is to fill "k-space" with data, for subsequent FT and interpretation. Thus, the pursuit of faster imaging approaches, for example, can be viewed conceptually as the pursuit of strategies to fill k-space faster. This has seen the evolution, beyond spin-echo imaging of gradient-recalled echo (GRE) imaging, fast spin-echo (FSE) imaging, spiral imaging and echo planar imaging (EPI). These are discussed at length in the suggested reading, but differ fundamentally as to how k-space is filled, either one "line" per excitation pulse (as discussed above, where image acquisition time depends strongly on TR since the RF excite/data readout module must be repeated many times at intervals TR), or multiple lines per excitation (FSE and, ultimately, EPI where the entirety of k-space may be filled with data from a single RF excitation, rendering TR largely irrelevant, image acquisition time being limited primarily by how fast the readout data can be digitized.

8.4 Endogenous Tissue Contrast

Magnetic resonance imaging has evolved into a powerful and, importantly, versatile tool in diagnostic radiology. This arises largely from the fact that the NMR signal detected is sensitive to a variety of factors of the local micro-environment of the ^1H protons. Often initially considered sources of signal loss and image "artifact," many of these sensitivities have been harnessed and may be exploited as sources of "image contrast" with appropriate construction of the MRI pulse sequence to allow weighted exposure

* In fact, the axes of k-space (k_x and k_y) are formed by considering integrated gradient field history in the pulse sequence timing. For a constant readout gradient G_x, $k_x(t)$ can be seen to equal $\gamma G_x.t$, such that the product of k_x and the x-coordinate will yield the phase angle of a spin population at coordinate x (note that for a constant gradient field amplitude, k_x is proportional to readout time, t). Similarly, the k_y coordinate is given by $\gamma G_y.t_p$, where t_p is the duration of the phase-encoding gradient pulse application.

or sensitivity to such factors. Although many exist, four categories of endogenous image contrast sources will be discussed, demonstrating the range of physiological inference that can be derived from sensitivity to such physical factors.

8.4.1 Relaxation Times

8.4.1.1 T_2*-Weighting

After excitation, the nuclear spins can be considered to rotate, or precess, in a transverse magnetization plane. As discussed above, this precession rate or frequency is dictated by the Larmor equation and is dependent on the local magnetic field. In the presence of a magnetic field gradient as in the "phase encoding" process, different precession rates lead to overall signal loss in the resultant observed signal, the degree of signal loss being related to the spatial distribution of nuclei in the direction of the applied gradient. However, it is not only application of external magnetic field gradients that lead to spatially varying local magnetic field and thus precessional dephasing and signal loss. Inhomogeneities in the magnetic field uniformity associated with magnet construction also contribute to dephasing of the precessing spins underlying the detected signal (free induction decay). The rate of loss of FID amplitude relates to the diversity of magnetic fields experienced by the excited nuclear spin population. Often approximated by an exponential decay, a single time constant (T_2*) can thus be used to characterize the rate of signal loss (and by inference field heterogeneity). T_2* is known as the "effective transverse relaxation rate," and typically takes values of the order of 10 to 100 msec in human tissues in clinical MRI scanners (1.5T), with uniform environments associated with longer T_2* values (more persistent FID). However, other sources of magnetic field heterogeneity dominate the effects of field construction. Different tissue types themselves become magnetized in the presence of an external field. The degree to which this magnetization occurs is governed by the tissue property of magnetic susceptibility, χ. Thus at interfaces between different tissue types (especially tissue/bone or tissue/air), local magnetic field homogeneity is disrupted by magnetic susceptibility differences. This can lead to signal voiding (often termed "magnetic susceptibility artifact") as well as signal mismapping on image formation (accumulated phase cannot be distinguished from deliberate "phase encoding").

$$S(FID) \propto -t/T_2^* \tag{8.4}$$

where S is the free induction decay signal amplitude, t is time and T_2* the effective transverse relaxation time constant. T_2*-sensitivity, although imposing sensitivity to the above "artifacts," can also be exploited by deliberately manipulating the local magnetic field homogeneity of tissue, for example by administration of a blood-borne magnetic contrast agent, which disturbs local field uniformity wherever it travels. This can be readily visualized on images acquired with T_2*-sensitivity and assessments of blood supply (perfusion) to a tissue can be made (see perfusion below). Furthermore, even without an exogenous contrast agent, transient changes in the balance of diamagnetic oxy-hemoglobin to paramagnetic deoxy-hemoglobin, arising as a consequence of neuronal activity can be detected (due to the field-disturbing effect of the deoxyhemoglobin). This contrast mechanism (conventionally referred to as BOLD, blood oxygenation level dependent) can be seen to simply be an extension of T_2*-weighted sensitivity in conjunction with a varying intravascular oxy/deoxy-hemoglobin balance (see fMRI below).

8.4.1.2 T_2-Weighting

However, to mitigate the effects of such spin dephasing and loss of signal in the free induction decay, a commonly employed MRI technique known as the "spin echo" was developed. After initial RF excitation and subsequent precession (with T_2* dephasing), a second RF pulse is applied to cause the nuclear spin magnetization to "flip" in the transverse plane. (See Figure 8.2.) The spatial location of nuclei is not changed, just the magnetization orientation. Thus spins continue to precess at different rates. However, where this previously led to *dephasing*, after the second (180°) RF pulse, the different precession rates now lead to *rephasing*. At a time after the 180° RF pulse equal to the time between initial RF excitation and the 180° RF pulse, spins will transiently realign, leading to recovery of signal, known as the *spin echo*.

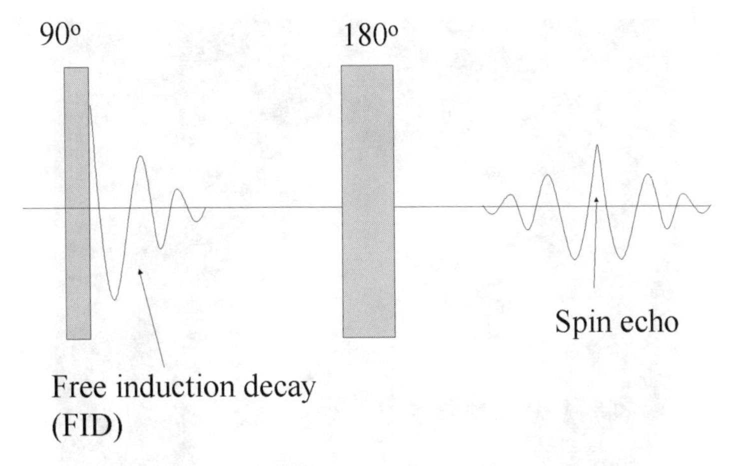

FIGURE 8.2 The free induction decay (FID) occurring after the initial 90° excitation exhibits rapid signal loss via T2*-dephasing. Application of a 180° refocusing RF pulse leads to formation of the spin-echo whose amplitude is restored. Note the amplitude at echo time TE is nonetheless attenuated, not by T_2^* mechanisms, but by T_2 decay. The degree of such attenuation depends on the tissue property of T_2 and can be a valuable contrast mechanism in (T_2-weighted) MRI.

The time between initial excitation and echo formation is known as the *echo time*, TE. However, the amplitude of the spin-echo does not retain the initial amplitude of the free induction decay. This is because the spin-echo mechanism refocuses or reverses the dephasing effects of *time-invariant* spatial magnetic field heterogeneity. But in addition to such heterogeneity, another mechanism exists by which local magnetic field variations, or fluctuations, occur due to the interaction of excited spins with each other. Consider the tiny magnetic field of an excited nuclear spin. As the water molecules diffuse, they may approach or depart from each other — transiently changing the effective local field each nuclear spin experiences in a random and irreversible fashion. Such irreversible transverse dephasing and subsequent signal loss in the spin echo is known as transverse or spin-spin relaxation, is a tissue-dependent property and is characterized by an exponential time constant, T_2, analogous to T_2^*.

$$S(\text{spin echo}) \propto \exp(-TE/T_2) \tag{8.5}$$

where S is the spin echo amplitude, TE the echo time, and T_2 the transverse relaxation time constant.

T_2-weighting (i.e., the sensitivity of the resultant MR image to T_2 effects) is thus controlled by choice of echo time, TE. Since species with long T_2 values (e.g., fluids such as cerebrospinal fluid, CSF) retain signal even at long TEs, while species with shorter T_2 values lose signal amplitude rapidly with increasing TE, choice of long TE values will introduce T_2-dependent contrast between tissues. This is generally referred to as *T_2-weighting*. The T_2-weighted image has become the mainstay of much clinical diagnostic radiology, in many cases revealing and delineating pathological tissues by hyperintensity associated with altered fluidity/water mobility. Of course, such contrast is gained at the expense of overall signal as in general signal is *lost* (just at different rates) with increasing TE. Commonly, MR images are described and evaluated in terms of a "contrast-to-noise ratio" (CNR) as opposed to the more typical signal-to-noise ratio (SNR).

8.4.1.3 T_1-Weighting

As discussed above, the process of phase encoding for image formation requires the repetition of the RF excite/data readout module to collect a set of typically 128 or 256 phase-encoded spin-echoes. Each module is separated by an interval, TR. During TR, nuclear spins, having been tipped out of their equilibrium magnetic alignment with the external field B_0, begin to recover or relax longitudinally. The longitudinal relaxation time is characterized as an exponential recovery process with time constant, T_1. T_1, like T_2, is a property of the tissue and reflects the ability of the excited spin system to "give back"

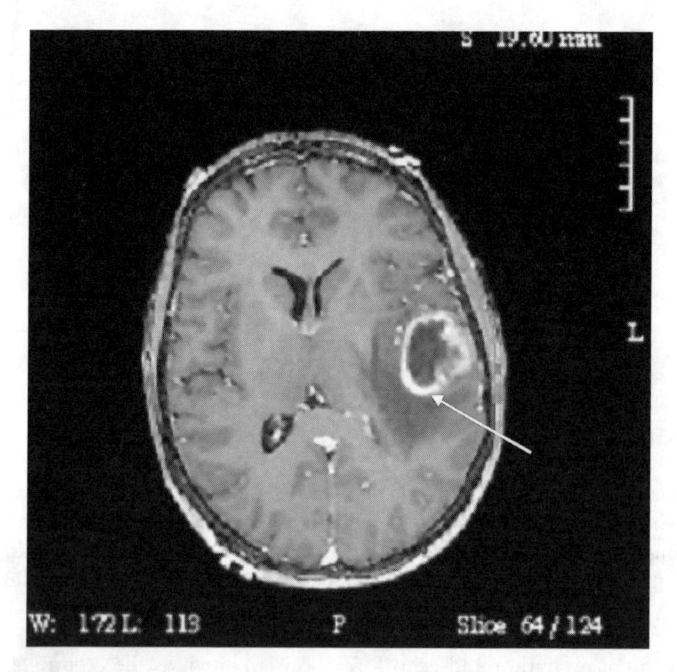

FIGURE 8.3 An axial T1-weighted image through a left hemispheric high-grade glioma after administration of Gd-based contrast medium shows characteristic "ring enhancement" of the lesion (associated with blood–brain barrier breakdown).

energy acquired during excitation. It is thus facilitated by magnetic interactions with microstructural and macromolecular entities in tissue (often referred to as the "lattice"). Thus free fluids are associated with long T_1 times and slow recovery. As a general rule of thumb, to approach asymptotic recovery, and allow full signal potential for subsequent RF excite/data readout modules of the pulse sequence, TR should be set to ~5^*T_1. To the extent that a given TR is less than 5^*T_1 for a given species, subsequent echoes will be attenuated by a factor that depends on T_1 and images are said to be T_1-weighted.

$$S(TR) \propto \{1 - \exp(-TR/T_1)\} \tag{8.6}$$

T_1-weighted imaging becomes especially valuable after administration of T_1-shortening Gd-based contrast agents. To the extent that these contrast agents undergo selective accumulation, there is regional T_1-shortening and consequent hyperintensity on T_1-weighted images (this is particularly useful for identifying areas of blood–brain barrier disruption, where intravascular contrast agent accumulates in the extravascular space of a lesion such as a brain tumor). (See Figure 8.3.)

A critical take home point from the above discussion of T_1- and T_2-weighting is that by deliberate manipulation of the pulse sequence parameters, specifically TR and TE, the user can control the sensitivity or weighting of the resultant image, in a manner not available to other cross-sectional imaging modalities such as computed tomography (CT). This represents both the power and the complexity of MRI as an imaging technique.

8.4.2 Flow

Bulk flow can also be visualized on MR images. Two phenomena exist that relate to the flow of blood water ^1H protons and their subsequent appearance: in-flow enhancement and flow-related dephasing (flow artifact). Both will be elaborated upon in the following discussion of MR angiography. However, they arise from different mechanisms. In-flow enhancement can be seen as a consequence of T_1-weighting (particularly of so-called gradient-recalled echo images). T_1-weighting is achieved as discussed above by using TR values that are considerable shorter than 5^*T_1 leading to signal suppression of longer T_1 entities.

This assumes that ^1H spins experience the repeated train of RF pulses. While this is indeed the case for stationary spins, in-flowing blood may not have experienced the full train of selective excitation pulses and may thus not be "T_1-weighted" but will rather deliver its full signal potential; thus vascular structures with in-flow appear hyperintense. If flow is too slow, the blood protons nevertheless experience a train of RF pulses and indeed exhibit signal suppression. Flow-related dephasing, on the other hand, describes the accumulation of phase relative to stationary spins arising from flow during the application of gradient field pulses. While a balanced pulse sequence design will lead to no net accumulation of phase in the slice select or readout directions (but only in the phase-encode direction), spins that relocate between gradient pulses in the pulse sequence module will acquire a net phase proportional to their velocity. This may be considered an artifact (since this accumulated phase will be misinterpreted by the image reconstruction and signals will be mismapped in the phase-encode direction), or exploited as a source of contrast, by observing the phase angle (retrievable from the complex acquired data), it is possible to deduce the flow velocity, or rather deliberately employ "flow encoding."

8.4.3 Diffusion

Exploiting (again) the spatially dependent accumulation of a "phase" angle by spins experiencing a magnetic field gradient pulse, the pulsed gradient spin-echo (PGSE) approach was developed for studying molecular diffusion in the time interval between application of matched magnetic field gradient pulses. A stationary spin would experience equal and opposite phase angles and so would be unimpeded by such a pulsed gradient pair. However, to the extent that there is relocation of spin position (by mechanisms such as, but not limited to, diffusion) during the interval separating the gradient pulses (typically ~40 msec), rephasing and dephasing will be imbalanced and there will be a net signal loss. The degree to which an imaging sequence is made sensitive to the processes of diffusion (more correctly, "apparent diffusion," since any form of displacement will contribute to signal loss) is defined by a quantity termed the *b-value*, which for rectangular gradient pulses of duration, δ, separation, Δ, and strength, G, is given by:

$$b = \gamma^2 \delta^2 G^2 (\Delta - \delta/3) \tag{8.7}$$

Additional signal loss on such diffusion-weighted images (DWIs) is approximated by a factor:

$$S \propto \exp(-bD), \tag{8.8}$$

where D is the apparent diffusion coefficient (ADC). Spatial maps of the ADC can be derived from two images acquired with different b-values (typically 0 and 1000 sec/mm^2).

The adoption of diffusion weighted imaging has seen a recent explosion due to the overcoming of hurdles limiting ultrafast image acquisition (to freeze effects of gross motion) as well as the appreciation of the sensitivity of DWI to acute pathophysiologic changes during acute ischemic stroke. In particular, the ADC has been observed to drop by as much as 50% in minutes to hours following an acute stroke, leading to a readily appreciated regional hyperintensity of the ischemic tissue on a diffusion-weighted image (see Figure 8.4). Furthermore, diffusion, or specifically "apparent diffusion," may exhibit directional preference. Such a phenomenon is termed *anisotropy* and can be assessed by comparing images acquired with diffusion sensitivity gradient pulses applied along different spatial axes. As such both the magnitude and preferred direction of anisotropic diffusion can be assessed. Recent developments in the field of diffusion tensor imaging (where the diffusion process is considered as a 3×3 matrix of diffusion coefficients) has allowed the following or tracking of anisotropic structures such as white matter fibers.

8.4.4 Magnetization Transfer

Another available contrast mechanism that shows considerable utility in the study of white matter development and disorders, and also in the study of cartilage exploits the phenomenon of magnetization

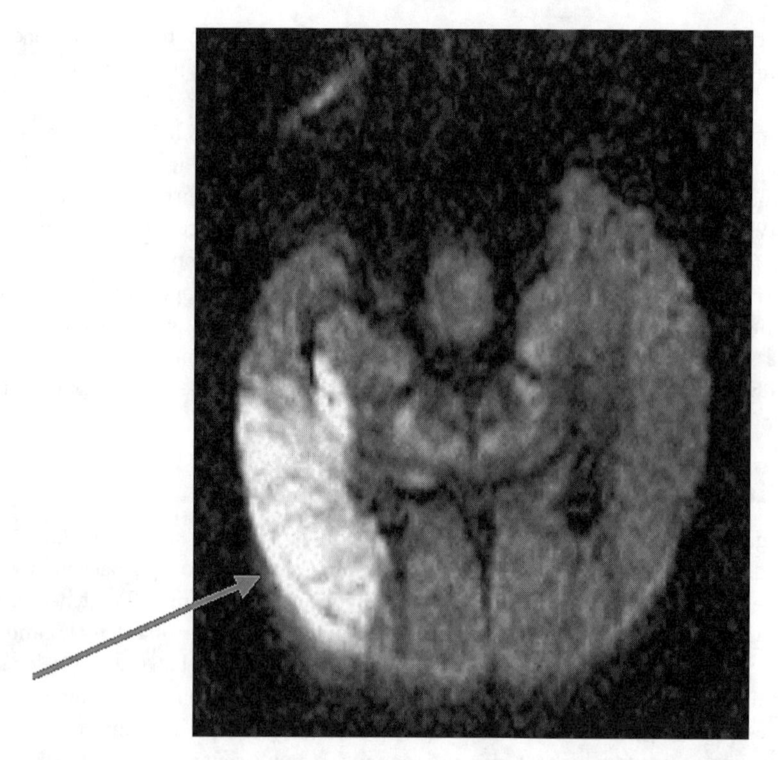

FIGURE 8.4 A diffusion weighted echo planar image (with diffusion sensitivity, b-value, of 1000s/mm^2) shows pronounced hyperintensity in the right posterior areas (arrow), associated with acute cerebral ischemia.

transfer to probe macromolecular or microstructural entities (e.g., myelin or collagen) that interact with free water protons. A simple model describes the protons of the macromolecular structure as "bound," while water molecule protons are "free." The bound state leads to sustained spin-spin interactions (see discussion of T_2 above) and a correspondingly broad spectral resonance. Consequently, the bound pool does not contribute directly to image intensity and only the free pool is interrogated. (The free water protons have a much longer T_2 and corresponding narrow spectral line.) As such, applying "off-resonance" irradiation (approximately 1 kHz from the nominal free water resonance) is expected to have no direct effect on the free water (narrow resonance) protons, and thus no direct effect on observed signal intensity, but would nevertheless magnetically saturate spins of the bound pool. This would not have particular significance without the phenomenon of chemical exchange in which protons from the free and bound pools may interact and indeed exchange with each other, provided the appropriate chemical environment is present (as in collagen or myelin). Such exchange leads to a decrease in the free water signal since some of the spins carry with them the saturation imposed upon them while they were in the bound state. The degree of such signal loss can be seen to reflect the density of such bound protons (and by extension, the concentration of macromolecular structures) and the opportunity for chemical exchange. While this signal loss can be substantial (~50%) in healthy white matter and/or cartilage, it decreases in demyelinating lesions and as an indicator of breakdown of the proteoglycan-collagen matrix in cartilage decay, e.g., in osteoarthritis.

8.5 Contrast Agents

Despite the above-discussed plethora of endogenous tissue contrast available to the MRI experiment, with associated "exquisite soft tissue contrast" in resulting images, there are occasions when exogenous contrast media (or tracers) are nonetheless beneficial.

8.5.1 Static Enhancement

The most widespread application of contrast-enhanced MRI is the delineation of pathological tissue by virtue of increased extravasation of a blood-borne contrast agent, or magnetic dye. The most common (and clinically approved) contrast media are based on small organic chelates of the gadolinium $(Gd)^{3+}$ ion with total molecular weights of 500 – 1000 Da (e.g., Magnevist™, Omniscan™ and Prohance™). As water approaches the Gd^{3+} ion, longitudinal relaxation of the water ^1H protons is facilitated. On T_1-weighted images this leads to elevated signal intensity and thus a regional probe of contrast agent distribution (see Figure 8.3).

8.5.2 Dynamic Enhancement: Perfusion and Permeability

The above "static" use of Gd-based contrast media does not fully exploit the opportunities of using an exogenous blood borne tracer. Drawing on the methodologies of nuclear medicine, it is possible to dynamically image or "track" the passage of contrast media after bolus injection. Typical injected volumes are of the order of 10 to 20 cm^3 (to achieve an overall dose of 0.1 mmol/kg BW with a 0.5 *M* stock solution). With power injectors delivering contrast media at a rate of up to 5 cm^3/sec, the bolus injection can be seen to be as short as 2 to 4 sec. To increase sensitivity to the low blood volume in the brain, imaging is typically performed with T_2*-weighting (to track the dynamic variations in field homogeneity disturbance associated with the paramagnetic Gd ion) (see Figure 8.5a). Signal intensity loss (Figure 8.5b) can then be related to change in effective transverse relaxation rate (ΔR_2*) where $R_2^* = 1/T_2^*$; this change is assumed proportional to instantaneous contrast agent concentration (Figure 8.5c,d). Interestingly, because the T_2* mechanism is a "field effect" the influence of the contrast agent extends beyond its immediate intravascular environment disturbing magnetic field homogeneity (and leading to signal loss) also in the neighboring parenchyma. This is the rationalization of the increased sensitivity of T_2*-based (or "negative enhancing") bolus tracking methods, compared to T_1-

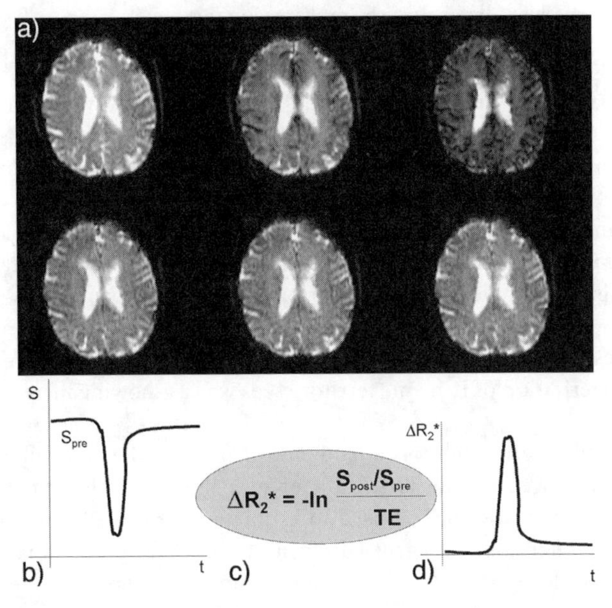

FIGURE 8.5 MR perfusion. (a) Six from a series of dynamic T_2*-weighted images acquired during passage of a bolus of Gd-based contrast agent (temporal resolution ~ 1 sec). In this example, the "negative enhancing" effect of the contrast agent can be seen as it passes through the brain and subsequently washes out (returning signal intensity toward pre-contrast levels). (b) Signal intensity time course can be converted via simple algebra (c) to a time course of ΔR_2* (the change is effective transverse relaxation rate). This quantity is assumed proportional to instantaneous tracer concentration and can be used in kinetic modeling.

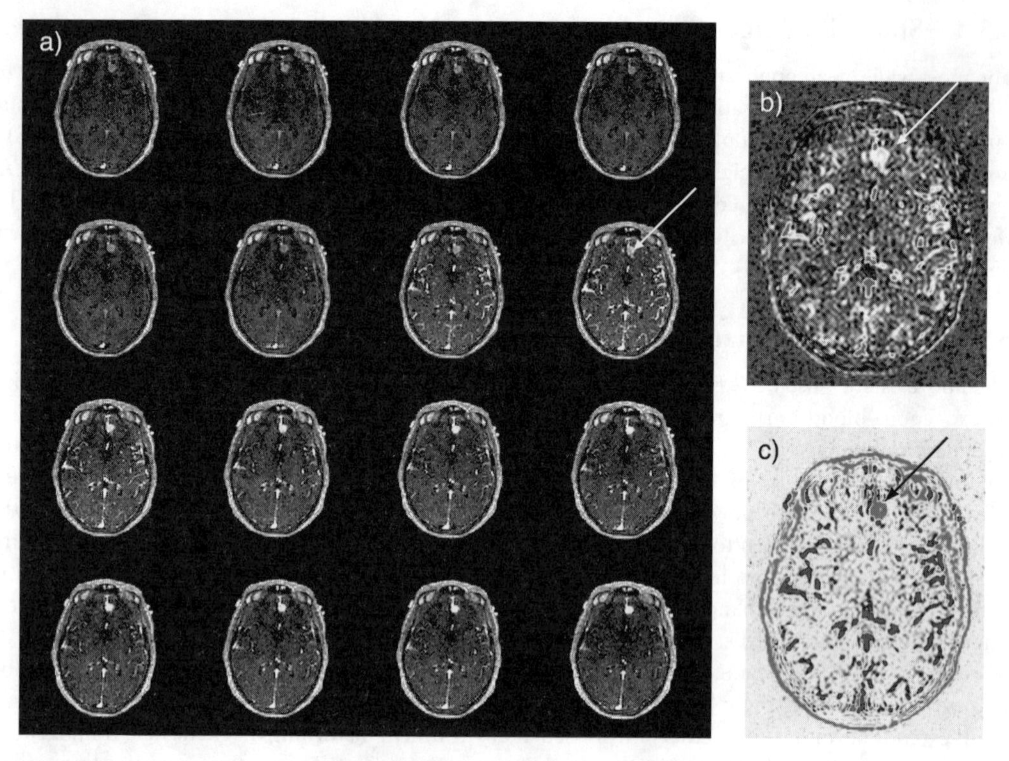

FIGURE 8.6 (See color insert following page 14-10.) MR permeability assessment. (a) 16 of a series of dynamic T_1-weighted images acquired during passage of Gd-based contrast agent in a patient with an intracranial tumor (arrow). Kinetic modeling of the progressive positive enhancement yields estimates of (b) fractional blood volume and (c) microvascular permeability, both of which are elevated in this tumor.

based ("positive enhancing") methods, which rely on close proximity of water ^{1}H protons to the contrast agent tracer. Dynamic T_1-weighted imaging, using the same contrast agent, may however also be used for perfusion assessment, as is typically the case in studies of e.g., myocardial perfusion. Dynamic imaging can be subsequently modeled using tracer kinetic techniques, to estimate parameters of perfusion including blood volume, blood flow and mean transit time. Quantitation accuracy is improved by inclusion in the model of an "arterial input function" which can be simultaneously measured in the imaging and reflects the timecourse of the contrast agent bolus in the feeding arterial structures (and thus accommodates any delay or dispersion that has occurred since the time of injection). Such assessments of perfusion, especially in the brain, have shown tremendous clinical promise in the characterization of ischemic territories, as well as showing increasing utility in the field of oncologic imaging.

Elevated microvascular permeability is a hallmark of many malignant tumors and a correlate of the phenomenon of *angiogenesis*, the formation of new blood vessels, critical for tumor growth. Dynamic contrast-enhanced MRI can be used to estimate microvascular permeability, since initial enhancement of tissue after contrast agent administration relates predominantly to contrast agent occupying the intravascular space (fractional blood volume), but *progressive* enhancement revealed on subsequent images occurs as a consequence of contrast agent extravasation beyond the compromised blood brain barrier and into the tumor interstitium. While multicompartment tracer kinetic modeling approaches are employed for the accurate estimation of microvascular permeability, an intuitive approach suggests that the *rate* (or slope) of such progressive enhancement relates to the rate of contrast agent leakage out of the intravascular space and thus the permeability of the vessel walls (Figure 8.6).

8.5.3 New Developments

A variety of novel contrast media are under development either with increased compartmental specificity (e.g., blood pool or intravascular agents) or with biochemical targeting (e.g., conjugated to antibodies specific for certain receptor expression) or even "smart" or switchable, in which the contrast medium is latent until biochemically "activated" — a reaction that leads typically to a conformational change and increased access of water to the relaxation enhancing moiety. While these developments are not yet a clinical reality, they appear poised to advance MRI into the emerging field of molecular imaging.

8.6 fMRI

Over the last decade, the field of human brain mapping has been revolutionized by the advent and development of the technique of functional magnetic resonance imaging (fMRI) (Figure 8.7). As discussed above in the description of T_2*, the blood oxygenation level dependent (BOLD) contrast mechanism is used to track changes in the balance of diamagnetic oxyhemoglobin to paramagnetic deoxyhemoglobin as a consequence of the phenomenon of neurovascular coupling and the electrical activity of neurons during stimulation or task performance. In fact, so intricate are the experimental paradigms currently being explored that it is possible to claim that where once we imaged the *brain*, we may now begin to image the *mind*.

The imaging methodology underlying BOLD fMRI is essentially identical to that of a dynamic contrast-enhanced perfusion study. Rapid (typically echo planar imaging, EPI) images are acquired (with T_2*-weighting) during alternating periods, or single events, of various stimuli, or control conditions. The central hypothesis is that regional neuronal activation leads to regional increase in oxy- to deoxyhemoglobin and thus regional increase in signal. The rapid imaging strategies allow this transient phenomenon

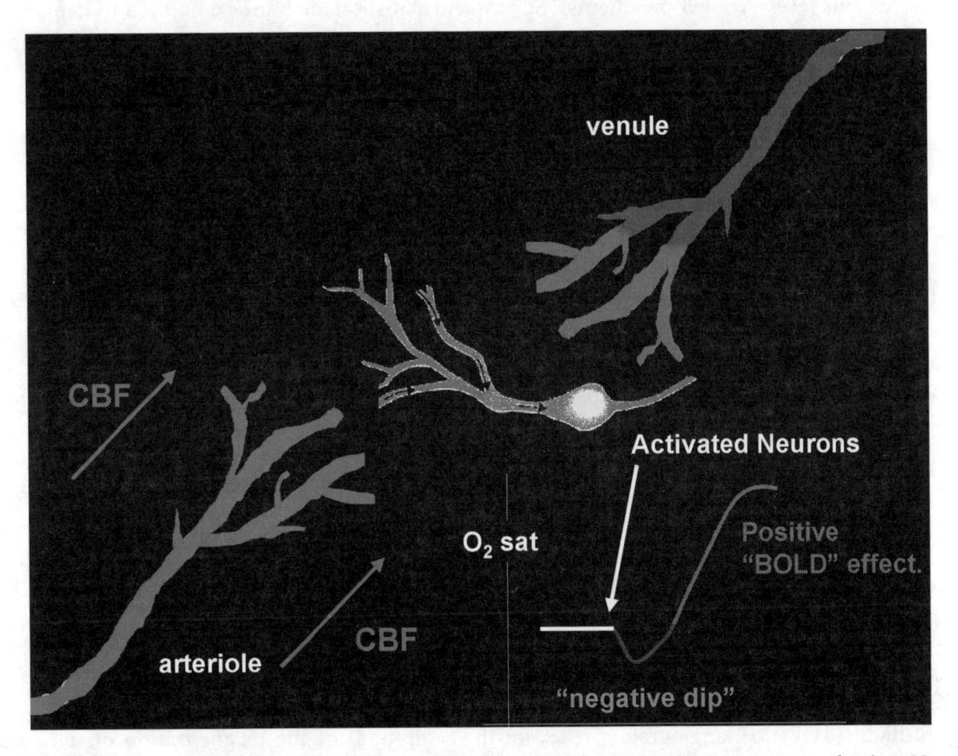

FIGURE 8.7 (See color insert following page 14-10.) Schematic of the fMRI BOLD contrast mechanism. Neuronal activation leads to an increase in regional CBF, without a concomitant increase in tissue oxygen consumption, leading to an increase in the oxygenation of the capillary bed and postcapillary venules. This increase in oxygenation can be visualized as an increase in signal on T_2*-weighted images, as paramagnetic deoxyhemoglobin is displaced.

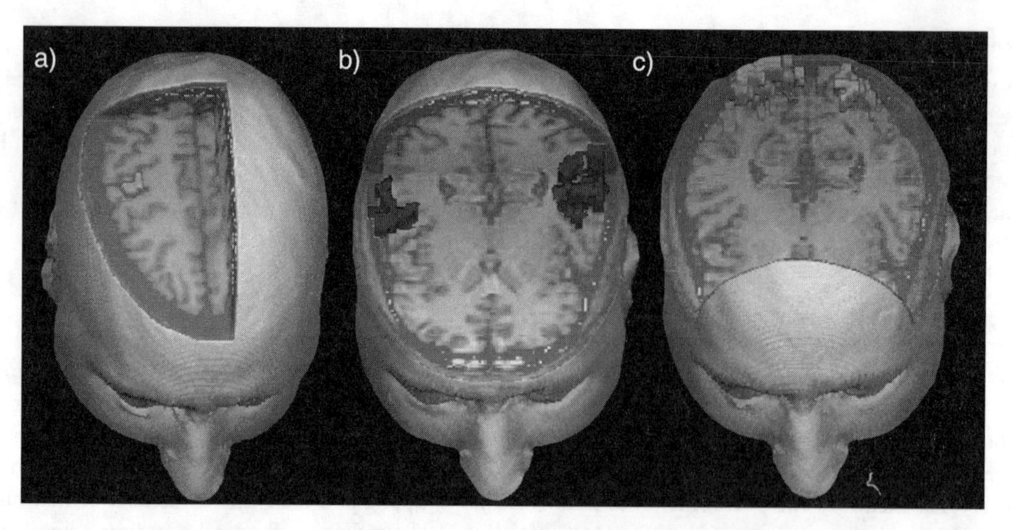

FIGURE 8.8 Human brain mapping. The BOLD fMRI experiment can be performed while stimulating various sensory (or cognitive systems) and corresponding pixels identified and highlighted on anatomic three-dimensional reconstructions. In this case, pixels of the (a) motor, (b) auditory, and (c) visual systems were identified in a single volunteer during repeated scanning with hand motor activity, auditory tone presentation, and checkerboard visual stimulation, respectively.

to be captured for subsequent analysis. Due to the small magnitude of the signal change, experimental paradigms conventionally require multiple repeated image acquisitions either during alternating "blocks" of stimulus and rest conditions (block design paradigms), or at specific times post-single stimulus (or cognitive) events (event-related paradigms). Subsequent statistical analysis is employed to define which of the observed signal intensity responses can be related to the parameters of the experimental model (e.g., stimulus time course). (See Figure 8.8.)

8.7 Magnetic Resonance Angiography and Flow Quantification

In the past, x-ray angiography and digital subtraction angiography were the standard diagnostic procedures for imaging vascular disease. The rapid advances over the past decade in three-dimensional magnetic resonance (MR) and computed tomography (CT) angiographic methods, however, allow physicians to obtain more detailed information about vascular anatomy and physiology. Multi-detector spiral CT can provide high resolution images of vessels quickly, but requires potentially high doses of radiation and contrast media. These may not be tolerated in a pediatric environment or in patients that need regular examination. As described in this section, MR angiography is a noninvasive alternative to CT angiography, and can also provide valuable physiological information ranging from the chemical composition of tissue to the oxygenation and flow of blood.

An ideal angiographic method is able to generate a strong signal, whatever that signal is, from within a vessel while also suppressing signal from tissue outside the vessel. Three methods for achieving this using MR are explained: time-of-flight angiography, contrast-enhanced angiography, and phase-contrast angiography. The benefits and drawbacks of each method are discussed. Flow quantification using phase-contrast imaging is also explained.

8.7.1 Time-of-Flight Angiography

Time-of-flight (TOF) MR angiography relies on the saturation[†] of the magnetization of static tissue within a repeatedly excited volume. Tissue outside the excited volume, including blood, remains highly

[†] Saturation refers to the demagnetization of tissue that results in suppression of the MR signal.

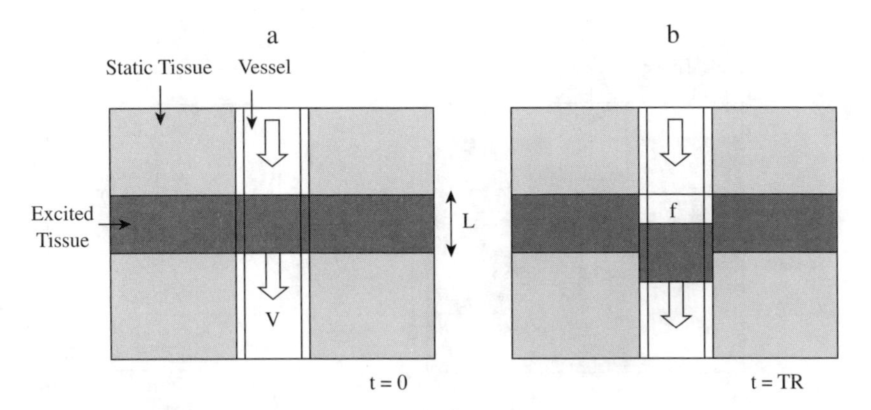

FIGURE 8.9 Explanation of two-dimensional TOF angiography. (a) A slice of thickness L positioned perpendicularly to a vessel of interest is repeatedly excited using an RF pulse with a flip angle of 90°. This leads to saturation of the signal within both the vessel and surrounding static tissue at time t = 0. (b) Blood flow at constant velocity v causes the movement of saturated blood out of the excited slice and fully magnetized blood into the slice. This inflow effect results in a bright signal within the vessel, relative to the surrounding tissue, depending on the fraction *f* of the slice thickness refilled at time t = TR when the signal is measured.

magnetized because it does not experience the same radio frequency (RF) excitations. Unsaturated blood that flows into the saturated volume will therefore appear brighter than the surrounding tissue. This so-called "inflow effect" is the basis of all TOF angiography (Figure 8.9).

Saturation of static tissue occurs when the time between successive RF pulses does not allow for complete T_1 decay of the magnetization. As a result, the magnetization will reach a reduced steady-state value after the application of numerous RF pulses. The steady-state magnetization, *M*, of static tissue imaged using a conventional‡ pulse sequence depends on the T_1-decay constant of the tissue and the TR of the pulse sequence according to the following expression:

$$M = M_0 \frac{(1-e^{-TR/T_1})\sin\alpha}{1-e^{-TR/T_1}\cos\alpha}, \tag{8.9}$$

where α is the flip angle of the RF pulse and M_0 is the maximum unsaturated magnetization of the tissue (Figure 8.10).

TOF MR angiography is designed to minimize *M* in static tissue while maximizing *M* in the moving blood. As shown in Equation 8.9, the saturation of static tissue can be increased by using a pulse sequence with a short TR or a flip angle near 90°, which makes static tissue appears darker in the acquired MR images. Assuming an RF pulse with $\alpha = 90°$ is used, Equation 8.9 simplifies to:

$$M = M_0(1-e^{-TR/T_1}). \tag{8.10}$$

The brightness of a vessel in an angiogram depends on the fraction of a voxel refilled with magnetized blood each TR, as depicted in Figure 8.9. Given constant plug flow in a cylindrical vessel oriented perpendicularly to the imaged slice, the fractional filling, *f*, of a voxel depends on the slice thickness, *L*, the velocity of blood, *v*, and the TR:

‡ For example, a spoiled gradient-echo pulse sequence.

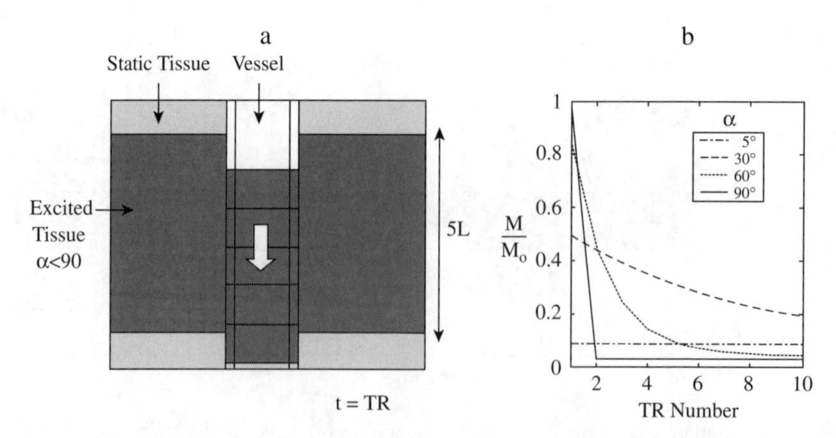

FIGURE 8.10 Explanation of three-dimensional TOF saturation effects. (a) Three-dimensional TOF angiography involves exciting thick slabs of tissue and spatially encoding all three dimensions of the resulting volume. A disadvantage of this approach is the progressive saturation of the blood as it propagates through the volume. Vessels in the resulting TOF angiogram will appear to be fading along the direction of flow. (b) Magnetization as a function of the number of applied RF pulses with T_1 = 1200 msec (i.e., typical of blood at 1.5 T) and TR = 40 msec, using different RF flip angles. Although the magnetization is initially large following a 90° RF pulse, the steady-state magnetization is much smaller than with the other flip angles shown. The flip angle that maximizes the steady-state signal is known as the Ernst angle, $\theta_E = \cos^{-1}(\exp(-TR/T_1))$.

$$f = \begin{cases} \mathrm{TR} \cdot \dfrac{v}{L} & v < L/\mathrm{TR} \\ 1 & v \geq L/\mathrm{TR} \end{cases} . \tag{8.11}$$

Vessel intensity will therefore increase relative to the surrounding tissue as TR increases or L decreases, and reach a maximum when the entire voxel is fully replenished between successive excitations. Since TR must remain short to ensure that static tissue remains well saturated, thin slices are typically imaged to increase f. This also improves the through-plane resolution of the vessel, but results in longer scans times.

A series of contiguous parallel slices imaged using this TOF approach can be stacked to form a three-dimensional angiogram. This three-dimensional spatial information is usually displayed as a two-dimensional projection of the data (see Figure 8.11). Alternatively, a three-dimensional surface of the vessels can be displayed (see Figure 8.12). In both visualization strategies, the anatomy can be rotated in real-time to assist in the interpretation of complex vascular anatomy.

Producing a spatially well-defined thin slice requires both a high-amplitude slice-selection gradient and a narrow-bandwidth RF pulse. Unfortunately, the simultaneous implementation of these two requirements leads to an increase in the duration of the excitation and adds to the minimum TR of the sequence. As shown in Equations 8.9 and 8.11, a longer TR results in a greater inflow of blood but also leads to an increase in background signal from static tissue (i.e., greater steady-state magnetization and less saturation).

Instead of collecting a series of parallel two-dimensional slices over a long period of time, three-dimensional MR data can be acquired. These data provide high spatial resolution by exciting a thicker slice and spatially encoding the through-plane dimension as well as the in-plane dimensions. This approach allows for a shorter TR but also results in the progressive saturation of the blood as it travels through the thick volume and experiences multiple excitations. As the saturation of the blood approaches that of the surrounding static tissue, image contrast between the vessel and the static tissue drops. Using smaller flip angle RF pulses reduces this saturation, but also reduces the saturation of the static tissue. Methods that combine a smaller flip angle with multiple overlapping thin three-dimensional volumes

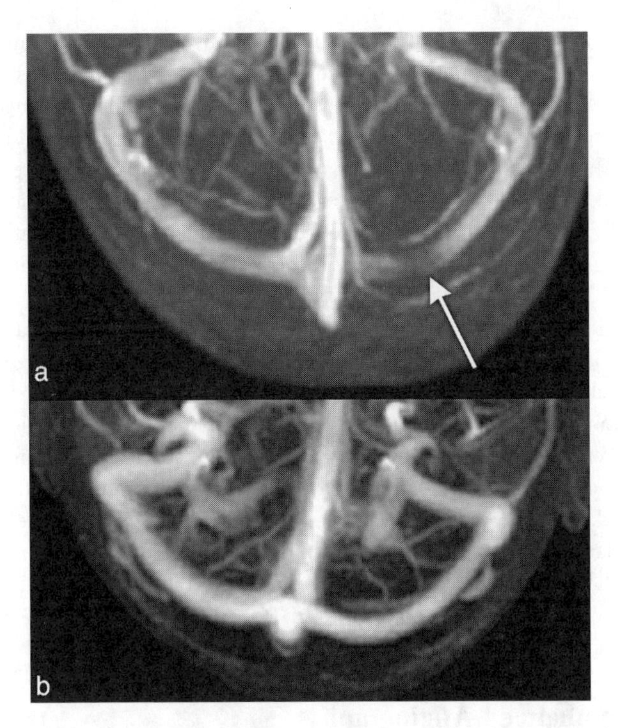

FIGURE 8.11 Comparison between (a) three-dimensional TOF and (b) three-dimensional contrast-enhanced angiography of the veins at the back of the head, displayed as (maximum-intensity) projections of the three-dimensional data. The improved resolution of (b) is apparent in the clearer depiction of the small cranial vessels and boundary of the large vein (cerebral sinus). A suspected left transverse thrombosis present in the TOF MR angiogram (white arrow) is not present in the contrast-enhanced image, indicating a blood-saturation artifact in (a). (Images courtesy of Dr. M. Shroff, Hospital for Sick Children and University of Toronto, Toronto, Canada.)

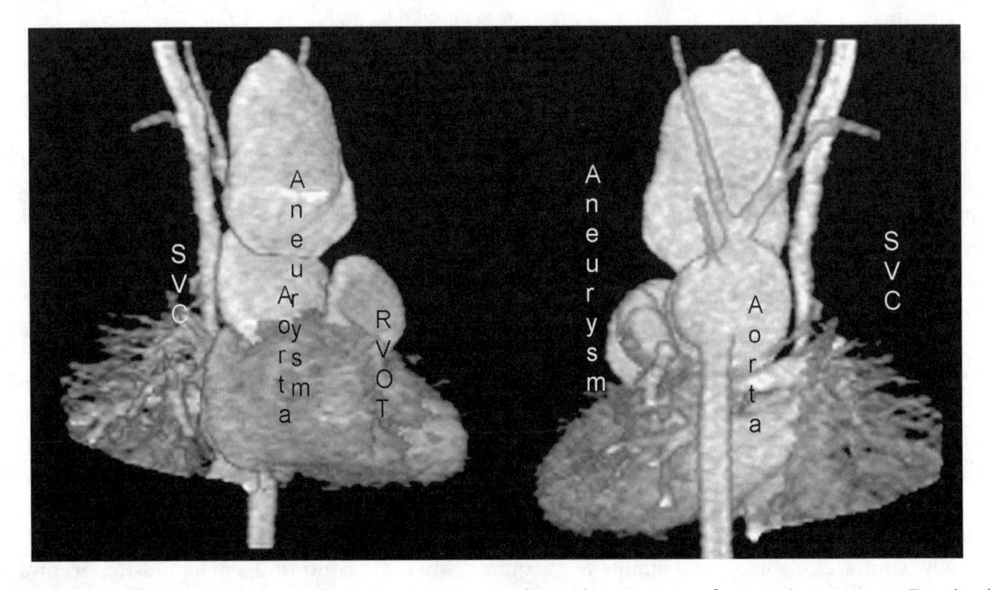

FIGURE 8.12 Two views of a surface-rendered contrast-enhanced angiogram of an aortic aneurysm. Despite the slow blood flow present in the aneurysm, the use of a contrast agent makes the aneurysm clearly visible. (Images courtesy Dr. Shi-Joon Yoo, Hospital for Sick Children and University of Toronto, Toronto, Canada.)

have been developed to avoid the blood saturation problem. Alternatively, ECG-gated selective inversion-recovery sequences have been implemented to image vessel in large three-dimensional volumes.

Another form of TOF angiography is known as arterial spin labeling. The method first tags blood using an inversion pulse applied to the upstream segment of a vessel. The tagged blood is then allowed to propagate through the vasculature before being imaged downstream. This process is repeated with the inversion pulse turned off, and the two images are subtracted to suppress static tissue. The resulting difference image ideally includes signal from the tagged blood only. Using different delays between blood tagging and image acquisition provides time-lapse information about the propagation of blood from the initial tagging site.

In general, TOF angiography provides a noninvasive measurement of vessel anatomy without the need for intravascular contrast agents. Despite its strengths, the dependency of TOF angiography on high flow rates limits its application in some vessel geometries. Vessels that curve into the plane of a two-dimensional acquisition, for example, will appear darker over that segment. This results from the fact that the longer blood remains within the imaging volume, the greater its saturation. Similarly, blood flow at the surface of a vessel is often slower than it is at the center. In this situation, flow at the edges of the vessel may appear darker due to increased saturation. This orientation-dependent artifact can mimic vessel narrowing similar to stenotic disease. Furthermore, small vessels and aneurysms can possess slow flow or no flow at all. The reduced inflow effect associated with these conditions limits the usefulness of TOF in such applications. Last, the long scan times of TOF angiography may preclude its use in vessels undergoing physiologic motion.

8.7.2 Contrast-Enhanced Angiography

Contrast-enhanced MR angiography involves the injection of an intravascular contrast agent to reduce the T_1 of blood. The resulting difference between the T_1 of the blood and of the surrounding tissue produces bright vessels in T_1-weighted images, with the degree of enhancement depending on the concentration of the agent and its relaxivity (change in relaxation rate per unit concentration of contrast agent, measured in sec^{-1} mM^{-1}).

Magnetic resonance contrast agents are normally injected intravenously, either manually or using a power injector. Rapid time-resolved imaging during contrast administration allows the passage of this injected bolus to be seen during its first pass through the vascular system. These images are often collected as projections of thick anatomical slices; however, newly developed methods using a variety of data acquisition and signal processing tricks are becoming available for time-resolved three-dimensional contrast-enhanced MR angiograms. (See Figure 8.12.)

Time-resolved angiography provides useful information about the flow patterns present in complex cardiovascular diseases such as congenital heart disease. Imaging during the first pass of the contrast agent is also important for generating angiograms of the arteries without venous enhancement. Alternatively, arteries and veins can be separated by their temporal rather than spatial characteristics through a pixel-by-pixel analysis of contrast enhancement curves.

Vessel brightness in an MR angiogram depends on the order in which k-space data are collected, and on the concentration of the contrast agent throughout the acquisition. For example, if data collection begins at the center of k-space (so-called "centric ordered" or "elliptic centric ordered" acquisitions) before the contrast agent has arrived, an abrupt increase in signal will occur when the contrast agent enters the imaging volume. An abrupt signal change in k-space produces ringing artifacts in the image, while the relatively brighter signal at the k-space periphery will lead to enhanced vessel edges in the angiogram. This intimate relationship between vessel appearance and acquisition timing makes the accurate estimation of contrast arrival time important to contrast-enhanced MR angiography.

Ideally, contrast-enhanced angiograms are acquired while the contrast agent is most concentrated within the vessels of interest. The transit time of the contrast agent from the injection site to the intended vessel has traditionally been estimated based on patient mass, heart rate and experience. Recently, improved estimation methods have been introduced. One such method involves the injection of a small test bolus of contrast agent. The transit time of the test bolus is measured using rapid imaging during injection. The measured transit time is then used as the delay between the full injection of contrast agent and the start of the angiographic acquisition. An extension of this method uses real-time MR imaging to detect the arrival of the full contrast bolus, which then automatically triggers the longer angiographic acquisition without the need for a test bolus.

The major advantage of contrast-enhanced angiography is its insensitivity to specific flow conditions. As a result, the method avoids many artifacts that affect other MR angiographic methods, including pulsatile flow artifacts, vessel-orientation saturation, slow-flow saturation, and patient motion. A disadvantage of the method is the need for a venous injection that is minimally invasive but requires patient preparation and relatively expensive contrast material.

8.7.3 Phase-Contrast Angiography

Both TOF angiography and contrast-enhanced angiography rely on changes in the magnitude of the MR signal to image vessels. Phase-contrast (PC) angiography instead uses differences in the phase of the signal between static and moving structures. The transverse magnetization of a structure moving through a magnetic-field gradient accumulates phase at a rate depending on the motion. This effect is the basis of phase-sensitive motion measurements and is a consequence of the Larmor frequency dependence on magnetic-field strength.

The precessional frequency, ω, of transverse magnetization moving through a magnetic-field gradient is given by:

$$\omega(t) = \gamma\, \vec{r}(t) \cdot \vec{G}(t) + \Delta\omega \,, \tag{8.12}$$

where γ is the gyromagnetic ratio and $\vec{r} = (r_x, r_y, r_z)$ is the position of the magnetization with respect to the motion-encoding magnetic-field gradient $\vec{G} = (G_x, G_y, G_z)$, both of which depend on time, t. $\Delta\omega$ represents all other sources of frequency variation, such as the difference in frequency between fat and water. Noting that frequency is simply the temporal derivative of phase ($\omega = d\theta / dt$) and expanding $\vec{r}(t)$ as a Taylor series produces the following expression for the phase of a moving structure gives:

$$\theta(t) = \gamma \int_0^t (\vec{r}_0 + \vec{v}_0 \tau + \frac{\vec{a}_0}{2} \tau^2 + \ldots) \cdot \vec{G}(\tau) d\tau + \Delta\theta \,, \tag{8.13}$$

where $\vec{r}_0$, $\vec{v}_0$ and $\vec{a}_0$ represent the position, velocity and acceleration at $t = 0$, respectively, and $\Delta\theta$ represents other constant sources of phase accumulation corresponding to $\Delta\omega$.

In PC angiography, blood flow is assumed to move at a constant velocity over the measurement period, making $\vec{a}_0$ and all higher-order terms of the Taylor series zero. As a result, Equation 8.13 simplifies to:

$$\theta(t) = \gamma (\vec{r}_0 \int_0^t \vec{G}(\tau)\, d\tau + \vec{v}_0 \int_0^t \vec{G}(\tau) \cdot \tau\, d\tau) + \Delta\theta \,. \tag{8.14}$$

If the goal of PC angiography is to highlight flowing blood based on its phase accumulation, then the first integral term in Equation 8.6 must be eliminated to prevent static tissue from dominating the phase calculation. This is accomplished by using a motion-encoding gradient with a net area of zero

$$\int_0^t \vec{G}(\tau)\, d\tau = 0 \,.$$

Finally, the phase errors amalgamated into the $\Delta\theta$ term are eliminated by performing two measurements, the first using a motion-encoding gradient of $\vec{G}(\tau)$ and the second using a gradient of $-\vec{G}(\tau)$. The phase difference between these two acquisitions (Figure 8.13), given by the following expression, produces a cancellation of $\Delta\theta$ and leaves:

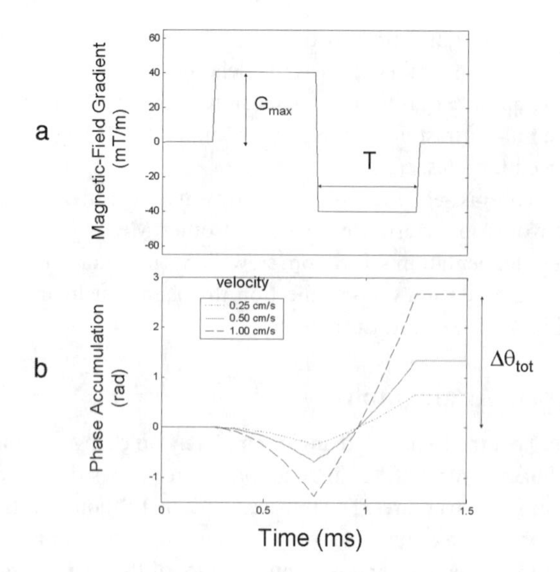

FIGURE 8.13 Phase accumulation due to flow through a magnetic-field gradient. (a) Bi-polar magnetic-field gradient applied to encode motion, with a total area of zero. (b) Phase accumulated by blood moving at constant velocity during the application of the gradient in (a). At the end of the application of the gradient, a net phase is accumulated which is proportional to the velocity: $\Delta\theta_{tot} = \gamma v T^2 G_{max}$. Above a critical velocity, known as the aliasing velocity ($v = \pi/\gamma G_{max} T^2$), a phase greater than π radians will be accrued by the flowing blood. This results in blood moving above this velocity appearing to move in the opposite direction. Such aliasing artifacts can be avoided using a weaker or shorter motion-encoding gradient.

$$\theta(t) = 2\gamma \cdot \vec{v}_0 \int_0^t \vec{G}(\tau) \cdot \tau \, d\tau \,. \tag{8.15}$$

The brightness of blood in PC angiograms depends only on the blood velocity, and does not require fully polarized blood entering the volume of interest. This allows large three-dimensional volumes to be imaged continuously. However, a limitation of PC angiography is its relatively long acquisition time compared with either TOF or contrast-enhanced angiography. The phase measurement described above provides motion sensitivity along only one dimension, which means that the creation of angiograms of complex vascular anatomy requires at least four complete sets of k-space data in order to detect flow in all three dimensions.

8.7.4 Phase-Contrast Flow Quantification

The same principles used to generate phase-contrast angiograms can be used to make quantitative measurements of blood flow. From time-resolved images of blood velocity, the velocity waveform, peak velocity or total volumetric blood flow can be calculated (see Figures 8.14, 8.15, and 8.16).

Phase-contrast imaging is normally performed using a single slice oriented perpendicularly to a vessel of interest. Time-resolved measurements are then made, typically with flow encoding applied parallel to the vessel only rather than in all three dimensions. In a uniform vessel, flow is directed primarily along the length of the vessel and may be encoded in this direction alone in order to reduce total scan time.

Volumetric flow measurements are useful for quantifying the total blood pumped by the heart each time it contracts, or the volume of blood provided to an organ. Volumetric flow measurements are obtained through post-processing of the time-resolved velocity measurements by calculating the average velocity over the vessel cross-section. This average velocity, multiplied by the area of the region of interest, represents the volume of blood crossing the imaged slice over that fraction of the cardiac cycle. Similar calculations performed over the entire cardiac cycle are summed to produce the total volume per cardiac cycle.

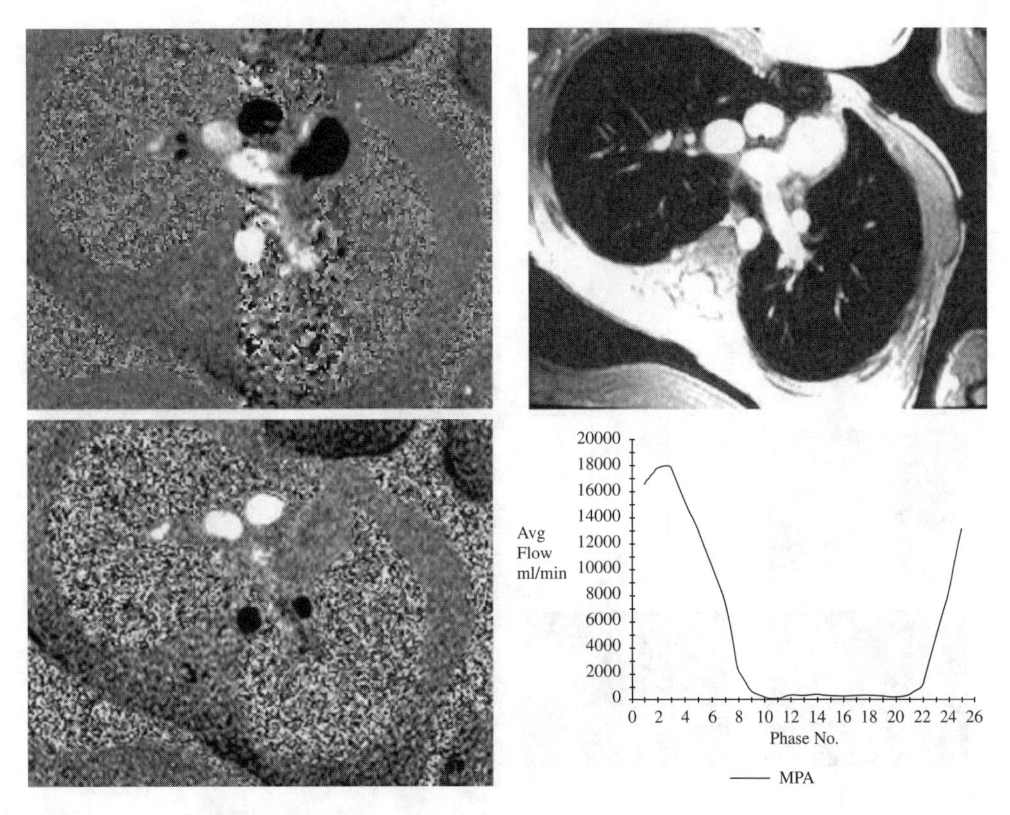

FIGURE 8.14 Phase-contrast images of flow through the main pulmonary artery (MPA). At the top right is an axial magnitude image of the chest, directly above the heart. At the left are two phase-contrast velocity images at the same location corresponding to different times in the cardiac cycle. The volume of blood passing through the MPA was measured in each velocity image to produce the graph at the bottom right. (Images courtesy Dr. Shi-Joon Yoo, Hospital for Sick Children and University of Toronto, Toronto, Canada.)

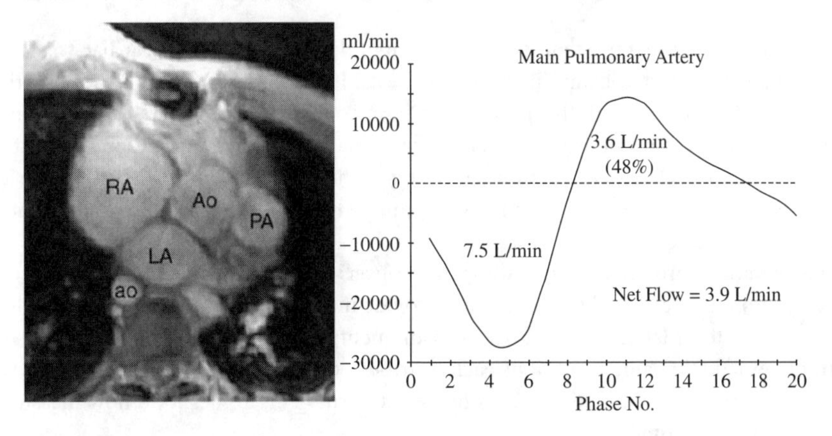

FIGURE 8.15 Pulmonary regurgitation in the pulmonary artery (PA) of a patient after surgery. Valves in the heart, when functioning properly, allow blood to flow in only one direction. As shown in the graph at the right, velocity measurements in the PA of this patient exhibit flow in both directions. In this graph, negative velocities represent flow in the proper physiologic direction toward the lungs, while positive velocities represent flow back into the heart. The total area under this curve represents the volume of blood pumped to the lungs each minute. The fraction of reversed flow (48%) provides a clinical estimation of valve dysfunction. MR is considered as the best method of evaluation of right ventricular function in conjunction with accurate simultaneous estimation of pulmonary flow. (Images courtesy Dr. Shi-Joon Yoo, Hospital for Sick Children and University of Toronto, Toronto, Canada.)

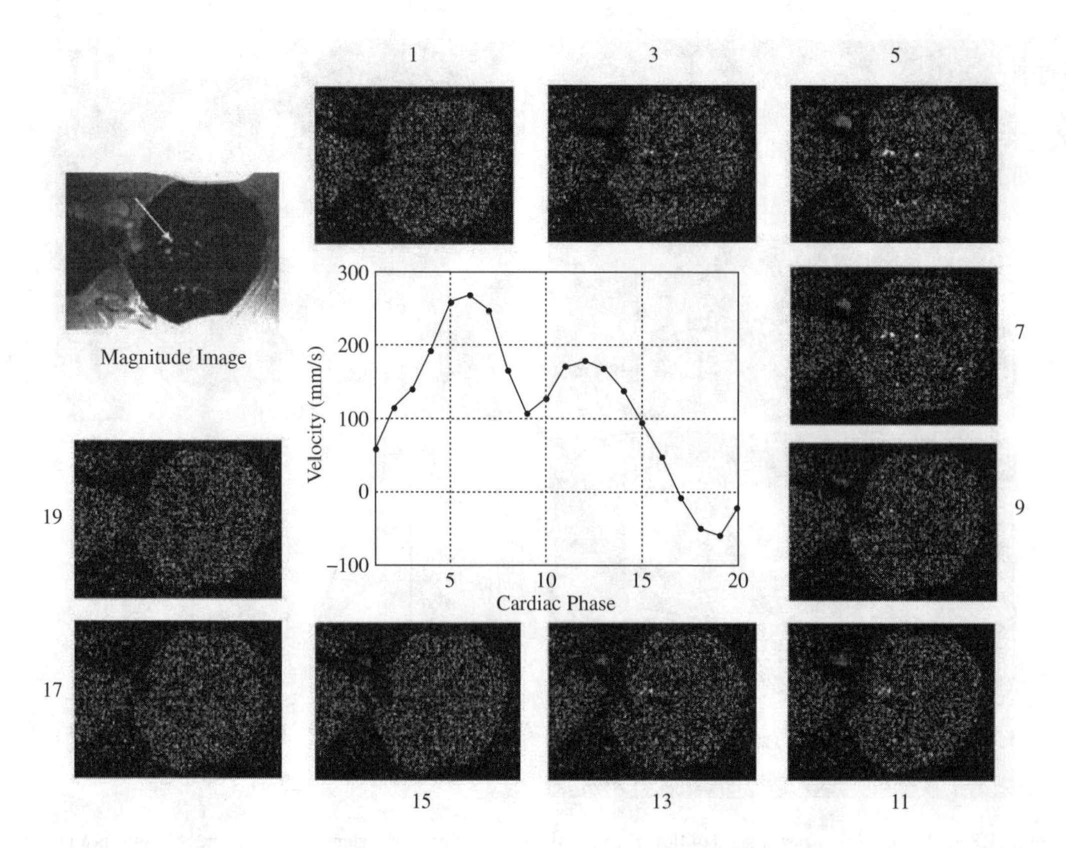

FIGURE 8.16 Phase-contrast measurements of blood velocity in a pulmonary vein. The upper left frame of this figure provides a magnitude image corresponding to an axial slice through the upper left lung of a healthy volunteer. The white arrow indicates a small pulmonary vein in which velocity was analyzed. The remaining images are phase-contrast velocity maps corresponding to the odd-numbered phases (labels) of the cardiac cycle, proceeding clockwise from the upper left. The central graph displays the velocity of the blood as measured from the phase-contrast data throughout the cardiac cycle.

In order to increase the effective temporal resolution of flow measurements, cardiac triggering is often used to combine data collected from different heartbeats. If the pattern of flow is not exactly the same following each cardiac contraction, this procedure can introduce errors to the flow measurement. These beat-to-beat changes may result from cardiac arrhythmia or changes in cardiac contraction due to respiration. Errors in the electrocardiogram triggering of the data acquisition also affect the accuracy of the data amalgamation. Triggering errors are compounded by respiration, which moves the heart and alters the received electrocardiogram signal.

A straightforward approach to eliminating this trigger error is to collect all the flow data in one heartbeat. Data from consecutive heartbeats then provide independent flow measurements that could be averaged together later. Magnetic resonance measurements of flow generally assume that the data is acquired under exactly the same conditions each heartbeat, or that beat-to-beat fluctuations will average to zero when the data are combined, which is not strictly true. This argues for a flow measurement that can be completed in real-time.

There are also immediate clinical benefits to fast MR measurements of blood flow. By reducing the total scan time of the study, patients may spend less time in the magnet. The risk of corrupted data due to patient motion is also reduced. Fast measurements reduce or eliminate the need for breath holding,** which can be difficult for cardiovascular or disoriented patients, or patients under general anesthesia.

** Breath holding refers to the practice of collecting MR data while the patient suspends respiration. The purpose of breath holding is to eliminate respiratory motion during data acquisition, which would otherwise corrupt the data.

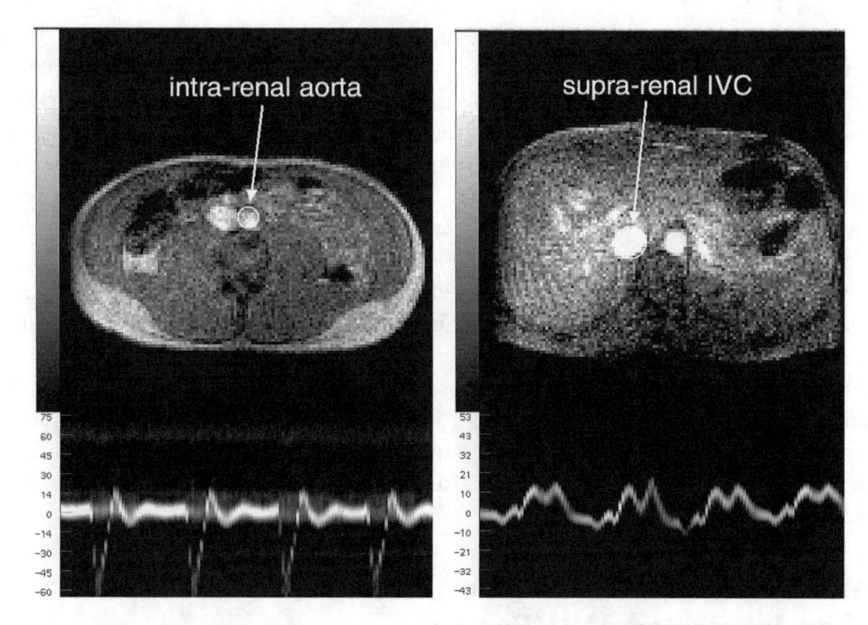

FIGURE 8.17 Real-time flow quantification using one-dimensional velocity encoding. The anatomical images at the top display the regions in which real-time flow measurements were performed (arrows to circled vessel). At the bottom are the corresponding measurements of the velocity spectra across four heartbeats, acquired at a temporal resolution of 42 msec.

Finally, measurements with high temporal resolution allow flow under changing physiological conditions to be investigated (e.g., during stress testing or pharmaceutical treatment).

There is a limit, however, to how quickly a flow-sensitive MR image can be acquired. This limit is due primarily to the speed with which the spatial distribution of the MR signals can be spatially encoded. One way to decrease scan time and increase temporal resolution is to discard some or all spatial information. By forcing the MR signal to emanate only from a volume of interest, the need for spatial encoding is reduced or eliminated. For this reason, methods have been developed using so-called volume-selective excitations to measure motion more quickly (see Figure 8.17).

8.8 MR Spectroscopy (MRS) and Spectroscopic Imaging (MRSI)

In addition to being dependent on physical factors that influence the local magnetic field, as described above, the NMR signal is also dependent on the local chemical environment of the ^1H protons. Indeed, the shielding effect of molecular electrons upon the ^1H nuclei and the subsequent characteristic "chemical shift" of the proton resonance according to its molecular environment (~CH_2 vs. ~CH_3, etc.) has been well known for many decades. In principle, molecules can thus be considered to have a "spectral" signature, with resonances at different frequencies (within a few parts per million [ppm], of the nominal 1H spectral peak), at intensities reflecting the abundance of protons in that environment (e.g., methyl, methylene, hydroxyl, etc.). Although a major component of structural organic chemistry, NMR spectroscopy has recently demonstrated convincing application in clinical use, especially in the area of brain tumors, Alzheimers disease and metabolic abnormalities of infant development. Beyond the brain, considerable utility is demonstrated in the study of prostate cancer and other branches of oncology. It seems likely that further applications will emerge.

In the field of intracranial brain tumors, in which MRS and its imaging analog, MRSI, have demonstrated most convincing utility, the technique focuses on relative quantitation of key metabolites and metabolic products. *N*-acetyl-aspartate (NAA), an amino acid and marker of neuronal integrity, is readily visualized in healthy brain at a chemical shift of 2.0 ppm (relative to the nominal proton resonance; the protons of water are, in fact, found to exhibit a resonance at 4.7 ppm). Creatine is visible at 3.0 ppm and free choline and choline-containing compounds are observed at 3.2 ppm. Other metabolites such as myoinositol, alanine and glutamate/glutamine are commonly reported as well, at clinical field strengths. In tumors, the link between pathology and metabolic function demonstrated by MRS is the general decrease in abundance of NAA, while the strength of the choline (Cho) resonance increases. While the quantitation may not necessarily allow assessment of tumor grade (aggression), it is proving sensitive for the prediction of future sites of tumor spread or recurrence (by identifying abnormalities in the spectral signature, prior to conventional imaging-based evidence of tumor).

Recent implementation of two- and three-dimensional MRSI allows (low-resolution) assessment of regional variations in NAA, Cr and Cho, including generation of MRS-derived "metabolite maps," indicating the regional abundance of each metabolite (and calculated by integrating intensity across the characteristic range of chemical shift frequencies associated with each metabolite) (Figure 8.18). Despite the potential utility of metabolic insights gained from MR spectroscopy, slow acquisition rates and low spatial resolution (~1 cm × 1 cm × 1 cm) have limited its application. Future promise of faster MRSI (by use of multiple echo and/or parallel imaging strategies) encourages the more routine adoption of higher resolution MRSI in clinical practice.

8.9 MR Evaluation of Cardiac Function: An Example of an Integrated MRI Exam

The evaluation of cardiac function and viability remains one of the most important diagnostic procedures in Western cultures due to the high mortality associated with heart disease. To diagnose cardiac problems, a variety of imaging modalities are enlisted, including MR imaging. This serves as an illustrative example of the combined use of several MRI-based approaches each with different sensitivities in the evaluation of a clinical situation. Many similar examples of the multiple capabilities of MRI can be found in characterization of the brain and other organ systems.

Magnetic resonance imaging is known for its excellent depiction of cardiovascular anatomy, but it is also sensitive to physiological information such as blood flow, the chemical composition of tissue, and the oxygen saturation of blood. This unique wealth of information from MR imaging, known as the "one-stop shop," makes it a growing method for evaluating many cardiac problems. Given the risky and expensive procedures needed to treat cardiac dysfunction, it is essential to have accurate diagnostic information. Two important aspects of an MR cardiac evaluation are described below: coronary angiography and myocardial function.

8.9.1 Myocardial Evaluation by MR

As with any mechanical pump, the performance of the heart depends intimately on its motion. Imaging of the contraction and relaxation of the heart provides a qualitative measurement of the mechanical health of the tissue. When injured, regions of the myocardium[††] may not contract as strongly as the surrounding healthy tissue. Furthermore, an efficient cardiac contraction requires that all four chambers of the heart contract in the appropriate sequence. Abnormalities in the electrical stimulation of the heart may result in an incorrect contraction pattern, which can also be diagnosed through MR imaging and subsequent analysis of myocardial wall thickness at each stage of the cardiac cycle, with subsequent determination of the degree of wall thickening associated with diastole (Figure 8.19).

A strength of MR imaging is its ability to measure the three-dimensional anatomy of the myocardium throughout the cardiac cycle. This is accomplished by acquiring a series of parallel slices that can be stacked together to form a three-dimensional volume at each point in the cardiac cycle. From these four-dimensional data, the change in volume of the heart can be measured during contraction. A small change

[††] Muscle of the heart.

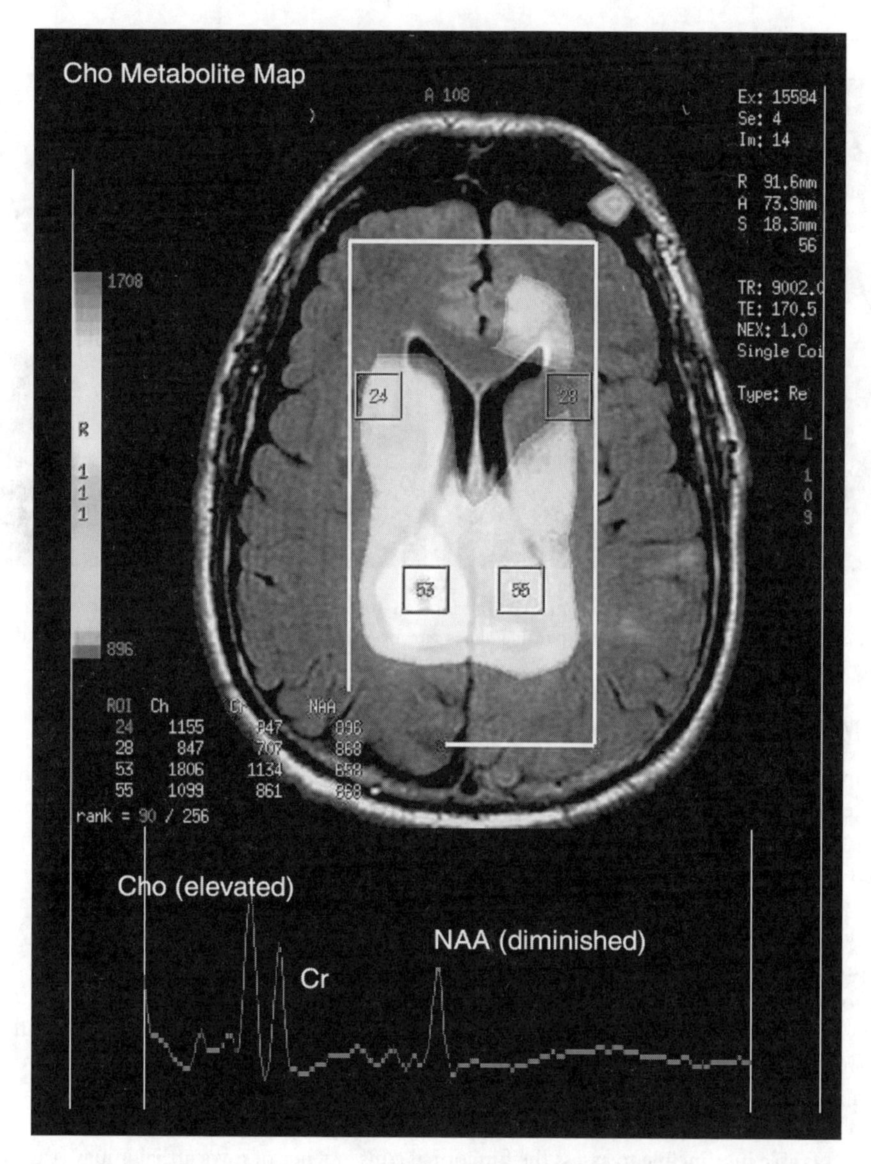

FIGURE 8.18 MR spectroscopy. Cho metabolite map from a patient with a right hemisphere glioma (hot spot on Cho color overlay). Below: representative voxel spectrum from tumor showing diminished NAA and elevated Cho.

in the volume of the cardiac chambers is associated with myocardial dysfunction that may be corrected surgically or with medication. The noninvasive nature of MR imaging allows it to be performed before and after such therapy in order to monitor its success.

When a mechanical dysfunction of the myocardium is detected, the next step is to determine if the muscle is dead or merely hibernating (or is "stunned") due to reduced blood flow, similar to having the muscles in a limb "fall asleep."

One method to measure myocardial damage with MR, known as "delayed enhancement," involves the injection of an intravascular contrast agent. This agent has been found to collect preferentially in damaged tissue several minutes after injection, making the damaged tissue appear brighter in the image. This effect is thought to result from damage to the capillaries in the affected muscle, causing them to leak contrast agent into the surrounding tissue. Conversely, rapid T_1-weighted imaging of the myocardium during the first pass of the contrast agent can provide information about myocardial blood flow, with regions receiving less blood appearing darker (less enhanced) in the MR images.

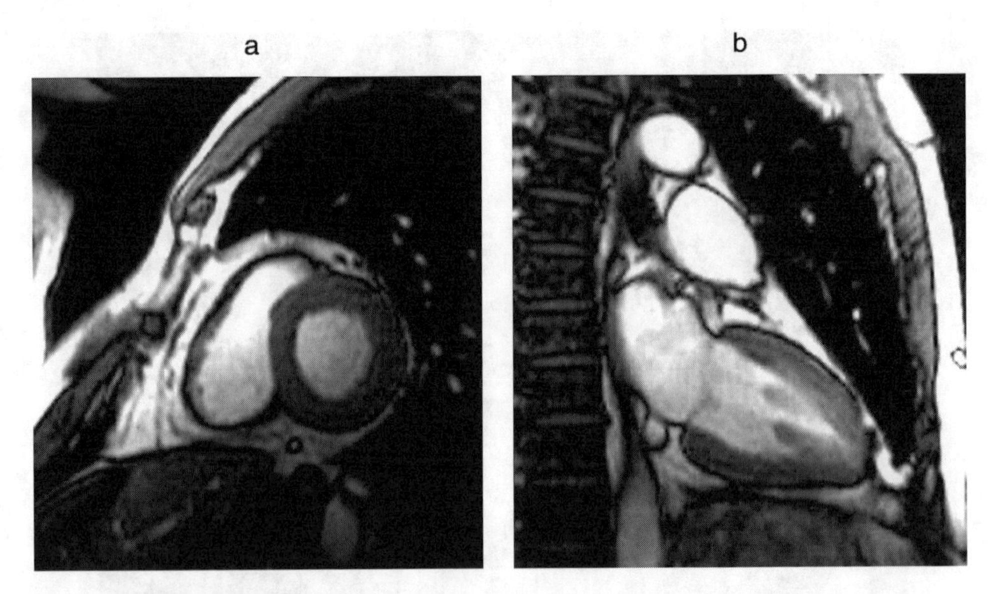

FIGURE 8.19 MR images of the heart from two standard anatomic views: (a) short-axis view and (b) long-axis view. Time-resolved images from multiple parallel slices can be combined to create four-dimensional data of the contracting heart.

8.9.2 MR Coronary Angiography

A common source of myocardial damage and dysfunction occurs when the blood supply to this muscle gets reduced or cut off completely. This can result from blockage of the vessel feeding the myocardium, known as the coronary vessels. Because the coronary arteries are small and moving, imaging of these vessels has represented one of the greatest recent challenges to cardiovascular MR.

Imaging of the coronaries requires the synchronization of the data acquisition to both the cardiac and respiratory cycles to ensure the vessels are in the same location throughout the acquisition. While the use of a pressure-sensitive belt strapped around the chest provides a reasonable measure of respiratory position for many clinical applications, this method is too inaccurate for high-resolution imaging of coronary vessel obstruction. Instead, MR methods (typically employing an additional "navigator" echo) that measure the displacement of the diaphragm or coronaries directly during the acquisition of high-resolution images have been developed and have resulted in the increasingly routine volumetric imaging of left and right coronary arteries.

Thus MRI is able in principle to assess the functional consequence of myocardial injury (through focal abnormalities in contractility), the nature of the injury (degree of ischemia, based on myocardial perfusion and/or late enhancement studies) and in principle the origin of the injury (an occlusion or stenosis of the relevant coronary artery). While MRI is by no means the only technique available for cardiac imaging, the integrated study it promises offers compelling argument for its adoption.

8.10 Conclusion

It is hoped that the above discussion has offered some insights into the versatility of the family of MRI techniques, their synergistic use in clinical diagnosis, prognosis and their potential role in characterizing response to interventional therapy in an increasingly physiologically specific manner. The field continues to evolve with exciting developments in hardware (e.g., higher field strength magnets, multiple RF coils, stronger and faster magnetic field gradient systems) and software (e.g., parallel imaging reconstruction algorithms, such as SENSE). These will no doubt contribute to developments in both increasing physiological specificity of MRI approaches and increasing utility of MRI in a real-time, or interactive manner.

Suggested Further Reading

Axel, L. and Dougherty, L., MR imaging of motion with spatial modulation of magnetization, *Radiology*, 171, 841–845, 1989.

Belliveau, J.W., Kennedy, D.N., McKinstry, R.C., et al., Functional mapping of the human visual cortex by magnetic resonance imaging, *Science*, 254(5032), 716–719, 1991.

Bryant, D.J., Payne, J.A., Firmin, D.N., and Longmore, D.B., Measurement of flow with NMR imaging using a gradient pulse and phase difference technique, *J. Comput. Assist. Tomogr.*, 8(4), 588–593, 1984.

Burstein, D., MR imaging of coronary artery flow in isolated and in vivo hearts, *J. Magn. Reson. Imaging*, 1, 337–346, 1991.

Duyn, J.H. and Moonen, C.T., Fast proton spectroscopic imaging of human brain using multiple spin-echoes, *Magn. Reson. Med.*, 30, 409–414, 1993.

Dydak, U., Weiger, M., Pruessmann, K.P., et al., Sensitivity-encoded spectroscopic imaging, *Magn. Reson. Med.*, 46, 713–722, 2001.

Einthoven, W., Fahr, G., and De Waart, A., On the direction and manifest size of the variations of the potential in the human heart and on the influence of the position of the heart on the form of the electrocardiogram, *Am. Heart J.*, 40, 163–193, 1950.

Farb, R.I., McGregor, C., Kim, J.K., Laliberte, M., Derbyshire, J.A., Willinsky, R.A., Cooper, P.W., Westman, D.G., Cheung, G., Schwartz, M.L., Stainsby, J.A., and Wright, G.A., Intracranial arteriovenous malformations: real-time auto-triggered elliptic centric-ordered three-dimensional gadolinium-enhanced MR angiography — initial assessment, *Radiology*, 220(1), 244–251, 2001.

Feinberg, D.A., Crooks, L., Hoenninger, J., III, Arakawa, M., and Watts, J., Pulsatile blood velocity in human arteries displayed by magnetic resonance imaging, *Radiology*, 153, 177–180, 1984.

Firmin, D.N., Nayler, G.L., Kilner, P.J., and Longmore, D.B., The application of phase shifts in NMR for flow measurement, *Magn. Reson. Med.*, 14, 230–241, 1990.

Haacke, E.M., Brown, R.W., Thompson, M.R., and Venkatesan, R., Eds., *Magnetic Resonance Imaging: Physical Principles and Sequence Design*, Wiley-Liss, New York, 1999.

Higgins, C.B., Hricak, H., and Helms, C.A., Eds., *Magnetic Resonance Imaging of the Body*, 3rd ed., Lippincott-Raven, Philadelphia, 1997.

Hu, B.S., Pauly, J.M., and Nishimura, D.G., Localized real-time velocity spectra determination, *Magn. Reson. Med.*, 30, 393–398, 1993.

Jack, C.R., Jr., Thompson, R.M., Butts, R.K., Sharbrough, F.W., Kelly, P.J., Hanson, D.P., Riederer, S.J., Ehman, R.L., Hangiandreou, N.J., and Cascino, G.D., Sensory motor cortex: correlation of presurgical mapping with functional MR imaging and invasive cortical mapping, *Radiology*, 190(1), 85–92, 1994.

Kim, J.K., Farb, R.I., and Wright, G.A., Test bolus examination in the carotid artery at dynamic gadolinium-enhanced MR angiography, *Radiology*, 206(1), 283–289, 1998.

Korin, H.W., Felmlee, J.P., Ehman, R.L., and Riederer, SJ., Adaptive technique for three-dimensional MR imaging of moving structures, *Radiology*, 177(1), 217–221, 1990.

Kucharczyk, J., Roberts, T., Moseley, M.E., and Watson, A., Contrast-enhanced perfusion-sensitive MR imaging in the diagnosis of cerebrovascular disorders, *J. Magn. Reson. Imaging*, 3(1), 241–245, 1993a.

Kucharczyk, J., Vexler, Z.S., Roberts, T.P., Asgari, H.S., Mintorovitch, J., Derugin, N., Watson, A.D., and Moseley, M.E., Echo-planar perfusion-sensitive MR imaging of acute cerebral ischemia, *Radiology*, 188(3), 711–717, 1993b.

Kwong, K.K., Belliveau, J.W., Chesler, D.A., et al., Dynamic magnetic resonance imaging of human brain activity during primary sensory stimulation, *Proc. Natl. Acad. Sci. U.S.A.*, 89, 5675–5679, 1992.

LeBihan, D., Ed., *Diffusion and Perfusion Magnetic Resonance: Applications to Functional MRI*, Raven, New York, 1995.

Li, D., Haacke, E.M., Mugler, J.P., III, Berr, S., Brookeman, J.R., and Hutton, M.C., Three-dimensional time-of-flight MR angiography using selective inversion recovery RAGE with fat saturation and ECG-triggering: application to renal arteries, *Magn. Reson. Med.*, 31(4), 414–422, 1994.

Lythgoe, M.F., Thomas, D.L., Calamante, F., Pell, G.S., Busza, A.L., King, M.D., Sotak, C.H., Williams, S.R., Ordidge, R.J., and Gadian, D.G., Acute changes in MRI diffusion, perfusion, T1 and T2 in a rat model of oligemia produced by partial occlusion of the middle cerebral artery, *Magn. Reson. Med.*, 44, 706–712, 2000.

Macgowan, C.K. and Wood, M.L., Motion measurements from individual MR signals using volume localization, *J. Magn. Reson. Imaging*, 9(5), 670–678, 1999.

Macgowan, C.K. and Wood, M.L., Fast measurements of the motion and velocity spectrum of blood using MR tagging, *Magn. Reson. Med.*, 45(3), 461–469, 2001.

Maki, J.H., Chenevert, T.L., and Prince, M.R., Three-dimensional contrast-enhanced MR angiography, *Magn. Reson. Imaging*, 8(6), 322–344, 1996.

Mazaheri, Y., Carroll, T., Du, J., Block, W.F., Fain, S.B., Hany, T.F., Aagaard, B.D., Strother, C.M., Mistretta, C.A., and Grist, T.M., Combined time-resolved and high-spatial-resolution three-dimensional MRA using an extended adaptive acquisition, *J. Magn. Reson. Imaging*, 15(3), 291–301, 2002.

Moonen, C.T.W. and Bandettini, P.A., Eds., *Functional MRI*, Springer-Verlag, Berlin, 1999.

Mori, S., Kaufman, W.E., Pearlson, G.D., et al., In vivo visualization of human neural pathways by magnetic resonance imaging, *Ann. Neurol.*, 47, 412–414, 2000.

Moseley, M.E., Kucharczyk, J., Mintorovitch, J., Cohen, Y., Kurhanewicz, J., Derugin, N., Asgari, H., and Norman, D., Diffusion-weighted MR imaging of acute stroke: correlation with T2-weighted and magnetic susceptibility-enhanced MR imaging in cats, *Am. J. Neuroradiol.*, 11, 423–429, 1990.

Nayler, B.L., Firmin, D.N., and Longmore, D.B., Blood flow imaging by CINE magnetic resonance, *J. Comput. Tomogr.*, 10, 715–722, 1986.

Nield, L.E., Qi, X., Yoo, S.J., Valsangiacomo, E.R., Hornberger, L.K., and Wright, G.A., MRI-based blood oxygen saturation measurements in infants and children with congenital heart disease, *Pediatr. Radiol.*, 32(7), 518–522, 2002.

Ogawa, S., Lee, T.M., Kay, A.R., et al., Brain magnetic resonance imaging with contrast dependent on blood oxygenation, *Proc. Natl. Acad. Sci. U.S.A.*, 87, 9868–9872, 1990.

Ogawa, S., Menon, R.S., Tank, D.W., et al., Functional brain mapping by blood oxygenation level-dependent contrast magnetic resonance imaging. A comparison of signal characteristics with a biophysical model, *Biophys. J.*, 64(3), 803–812, 1993.

Parker, D.L., Yuan, C., and Blatter, D.D., MR angiography by multiple thin slab three-dimensional acquisition, *Magn. Reson. Med.*, 17(2), 434–451, 1991.

Pohmann, R., von Kienlin, M., and Haase, A., Theoretical evaluation and comparison of fast chemical shift imaging methods, *J. Magn. Reson.*, 129, 145–160, 1997.

Pruessmann, K.P., Weiger, M., Scheidegger, M.B., and Boesiger, P., SENSE: sensitivity encoding for fast MRI, *Magn. Reson. Med.*, 42, 952–962, 1999.

Redpath, T.W. and Norris, N.G., A new method of NMR flow imaging, *Phys. Med. Biol.*, 29(7), 891–898, 1984.

Rosen, B.R., Belliveau, J.W., Vevea, J.M., and Brady, T.J., Perfusion imaging with NMR contrast agents, *Magn. Reson. Med.*, 14(2), 249–265, 1990.

Saeed, M., Wendland, M.F., Yu, K.K., Lauerma, K., Li, H.T., Derugin, N., Cavagna, F.M., and Higgins, C.B., Identification of myocardial reperfusion with echo planar magnetic resonance imaging. Discrimination between occlusive and reperfused infarctions, *Circulation*, 90(3), 1492–1501, 1994.

Sorensen, A.G., Buonanno, F.S., Gonzalez, R.G., Schwamm, L.H., Lev, M.H., Huang-Hellinger, F.R., Reese, T.G., Weisskoff, R.M., Davis, T.L., Suwanwela, N., Can, U., Moreira, J.A., Copen, W.A., Look, R.B., Finklestein, S.P., Rosen, B.R., and Koroshetz, W.J., Hyperacute stroke: evaluation with combined multisection diffusion-weighted and hemodynamically weighted echo-planar MR imaging, *Radiology*, 199(2), 391–401, 1996.

Stark, D.D. and Bradley, W.G., Eds., *Magnetic Resonance Imaging*, 2nd ed., C.V. Mosby, St. Louis, 1992.

Stejskal, E.O. and Tanner, J.E., Spin diffusion measurements: spin echoes in the presence of a time-dependent field gradient, *J. Chem. Phys.*, 42, 288–292, 1965.

Strecker, R., Scheffler, K., Klisch, J., Lehnhardt, S., Winterer, J., Laubenberger, J., Fischer, H., and Hennig, J., Fast functional MRA using time-resolved projection MR angiography with correlation analysis, *Magn. Reson. Med.*, 43(2), 303–309, 2000.

Stuber, M., Bornert, P., Spuentrup, E., Botnar, R.M., and Manning, W.J., Selective three-dimensional visualization of the coronary arterial lumen using arterial spin tagging, *Magn. Reson. Med.*, 47(2), 322–329, 2002.

Sussman, M.S., Stainsby, J.A., Robert, N., Merchant, N., and Wright, G.A., Variable-density adaptive imaging for high-resolution coronary artery MRI, *Magn. Reson. Med.*, 48(5), 753–764, 2002.

Turski, P.A., Korosec, F.R., Carroll, T.J., Willig, D.S., Grist, T.M., and Mistretta, C.A., Contrast-enhanced magnetic resonance angiography of the carotid bifurcation using the time-resolved imaging of contrast kinetics (TRICKS) technique, *Magn. Reson. Imaging*, 12(3), 175–181, 2001.

Van Bruggen, N. and Roberts, T.P.L., Eds., *Biomedical Imaging in Experimental Neuroscience*, CRC Press, Boca Raton, 2002.

Villringer, A., Rosen, B.R., Belliveau, J.W., Ackerman, J.L., Lauffer, R.B., Buxton, R.B., Chao, Y.S., Wedeen, V.J., and Brady, T.J., Dynamic imaging with lanthanide chelates in normal brain: contrast due to magnetic-susceptibility effects, *Magn. Reson. Med.*, 6, 164–174, 1988.

Warach, S., Chien, D., Li, W., Ronthal, M., and Edelman, R.R., Fast magnetic resonance diffusion-weighted imaging of acute human stroke, *Neurology*, 42(9), 1717–1723, 1992.

Wilke, N.M., Jerosch-Herold, M., Zenovich, A., and Stillman, A.E., Magnetic resonance first-pass myocardial perfusion imaging: clinical validation and future applications, *J. Magn. Reson. Imaging*, 10(5), 676–685, 1999.

9

Ultrasonic Imaging

CONTENTS

Elisa E. Konofagou
Harvard Medical School

9.1 Fundamentals of Ultrasound

In the past 30 years, ultrasound has become a very powerful imaging modality mainly due to its unique temporal resolution, low cost, nonionizing radiation, and portability. Lately, unique features such as harmonic imaging, three-dimensional visualization, transducer micro-machining, elasticity imaging, and the use of contrast agents have added to the higher quality and wider applications of diagnostic ultrasound images. In this chapter, a short overview of the fundamentals of diagnostic ultrasound and a brief summary of its many applications and methods are provided.

9.1.1 Ultrasound Echoes

Sounds with a frequency above 20 kHz are called ultrasonic, since they occur at frequencies inaudible to the human ear. When emitted at short bursts, propagating through media such as water with low reflection coefficient and reflected by obstacles along their propagation path, detection of the reflection, or *echo*, of the ultrasonic wave can help localize the obstacle. This principle has been used by sonar (SOund NAvigation and Ranging) and inherently used by marine mammals, such as dolphins and whales, that allows them to localize prey, obstacles, or predators. In fact, the frequencies used for "imaging" vary significantly dependent upon the application: from underwater sonar (up to 300 kHz), diagnostic ultrasound, therapeutic ultrasound, and industrial nondestructive testing (0.8–20 MHz) to acoustic microscopy (12 MHz to above 1 GHz).

9.1.2 The Wave Equation

As the ultrasonic wave propagates through the tissue, its energy and momentum are both transferred to the tissue. No net transfer of mass occurs at any particular point in the medium unless this is induced

0-8493-1140-3/04/$0.00+$1.50

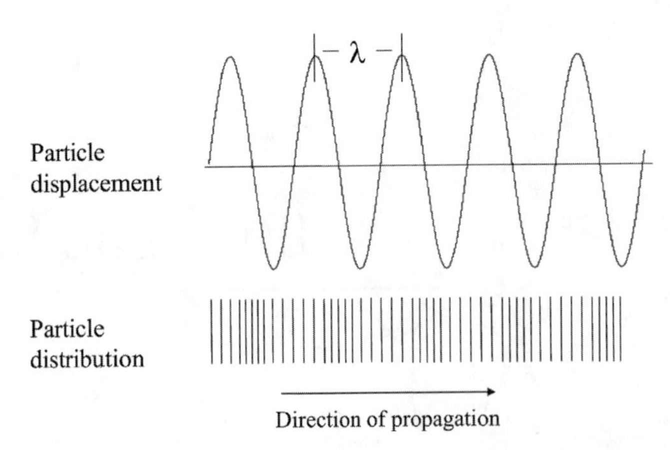

FIGURE 9.1 Particle displacement and particle distribution for a traveling longitudinal wave. The direction of propagation is from left to right. A shear wave can be created in the perpendicular direction, i.e., the particles would be moving in a direction orthogonal to the direction of propagation. (Adapted from Wells.[1])

by the momentum transfer. As the ultrasonic wave passes through the tissue, or medium, the peak local pressure in the medium increases. The oscillations of the particles result to harmonic pressure variations within the medium and to a pressure wave that propagates through the medium as neighboring particles move with respect to one another (Figure 9.1). The particles of the medium can move back and forth in a direction parallel (longitudinal wave) or perpendicular (transverse wave) to the traveling direction of the wave.

Let us consider the first case.

Assuming that a small volume of the medium that can be modeled as a nonviscous fluid (no shear waves can be generated) is shown on Figure 9.2, an applied force δF produces a displacement of $u+\delta u$ in the z-position on the right-hand side of the small volume. A gradient of force $\partial F/\partial z$ is thus generated across the element in question, and, assuming that the element is small enough so that the measured quantities within the medium are constant, it can be assumed as being linear, or

$$\delta F = \frac{\partial F}{\partial z}\delta z \tag{9.1}$$

and according to Hooke's law,

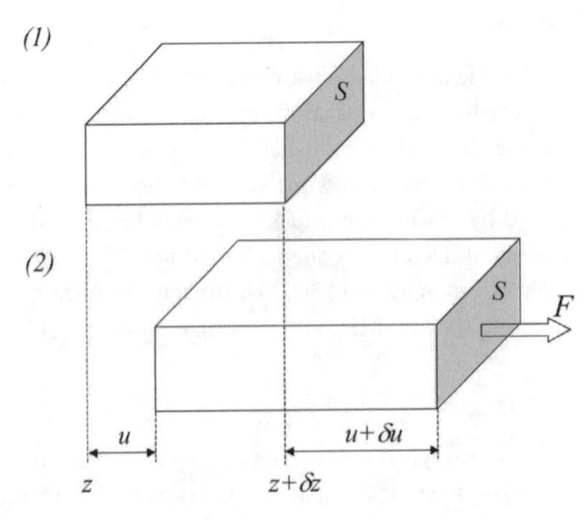

FIGURE 9.2 A small volume of the medium of impedance Z (1) at equilibrium and (2) undergoing oscillatory motion when an oscillatory force F is applied on its cross-sectional surface. (Adapted from Christensen.[7])

$$F = KS\frac{\partial u}{\partial z}, \tag{9.2}$$

where K is the adiabatic bulk modulus of the liquid and S is the area of the region on which the force is exerted. By taking the derivative of both sides of Equation 9.2 with respect to z and following Newton's second law, from Equation 9.1 we obtain the well-known "wave equation":

$$\frac{\partial^2 u}{\partial z^2} - \frac{1}{c^2}\frac{\partial^2 u}{\partial t^2} = 0 \tag{9.3}$$

where c is the speed of sound given by

$$c = \sqrt{\frac{K}{\rho}} = \sqrt{\frac{1}{\rho\kappa}},$$

where ρ is the density of the medium and κ is the compressibility of the medium. Equation 9.3 relates the second differential of the participle displacement with respect to distance to the acceleration of a simple harmonic oscillator. Note that the average speed of sound in most soft tissues is about 1540 m/s with a total range of ±6%. For the shear wave derivation of this equation please refer to Wells[1] or Kinsler and Frey[2] among others.

The solution of the wave equation is given by a function u, where

$$u = u(ct - z). \tag{9.4}$$

An appropriate choice of function for u in Equation (9.4) is:

$$u(t, z) = u_o \exp[jk(ct - z)], \tag{9.5}$$

where j is equal to $\sqrt{-1}$ and k is the wavenumber and equal to $2\pi/\lambda$ with λ denoting the wavelength.

9.1.3 Impedance, Power, and Reflection

The pressure wave $p(t, z)$ that results from the displacement generated and given by Equation (9.5) is given by

$$p(t,z) = p_0 \exp[jk(ct - z)], \tag{9.6}$$

where p_0 is the pressure wave amplitude and j is equal to $\sqrt{-1}$. The particle speed and the resulting pressure wave are related through the following relationship

$$u = \frac{p}{Z}, \tag{9.7}$$

where Z is the acoustic impedance defined as the ratio of the acoustic pressure wave at a point in the medium to the speed of the particle at the same point. The impedance is thus characteristic of the medium and given by

$$Z = \rho c. \tag{9.8}$$

The acoustic wave intensity is defined as the average flow of energy through a unit area in the medium perpendicular to the direction of propagation.[2] By following that definition, the intensity can be found equal to[3]

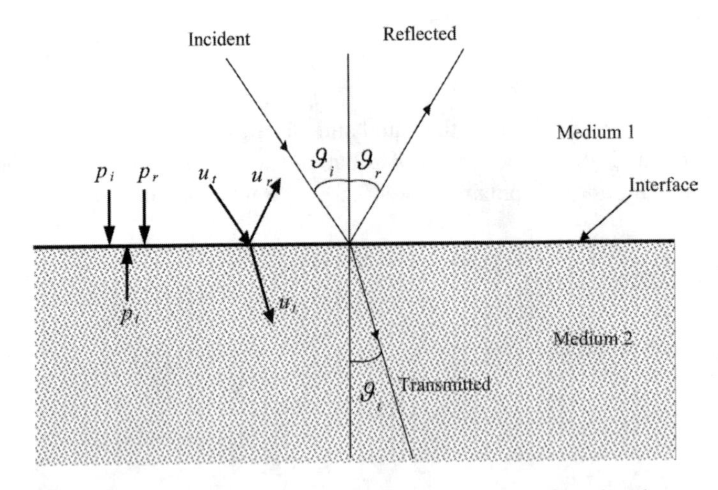

FIGURE 9.3 An incident wave at an impedance mismatch (interface). A reflected and a transmitted wave with certain velocities and pressure amplitudes are created ensuring continuity at the boundary.

$$I = \frac{p_0^2}{2Z} \tag{9.9}$$

and usually measured in units of mW/cm^2 in diagnostic ultrasound.

A first step into understanding the generation of ultrasound images is to follow the interaction of the propagating wave with the tissue. Thanks to the varying mean acoustic properties of tissues, a wave transmitted into the tissue will get partly reflected at areas where the properties of the tissue and, thus its impedance, are changing. These areas constitute a so-called "impedance mismatch" (Figure 9.3).

The reflection coefficient R of the pressure wave at an incidence angle of θ_i is given by

$$R = \frac{p_r}{p_i} = \frac{Z_2 \cos\vartheta_t - Z_1 \cos\vartheta_i}{Z_2 \cos\vartheta_t + Z_1 \cos\vartheta_i}, \tag{9.10}$$

where θ_t is the angle of the transmitted wave (Figure 9.3) also related to the incidence angle through Snell's law:

$$\lambda_1 \cos\vartheta_i = \lambda_2 \cos\vartheta_t, \tag{9.11}$$

where λ_1 and λ_2 are the wavelengths of the waves in medium 1 and 2, respectively, and related to the speeds in the two media through:

$$c = \lambda f \tag{9.12}$$

where f is the frequency of the propagating wave.

As Figure 9.3 also shows, the wave impingent upon the impedance mismatch also generates a transmitted wave, i.e., a wave that propagates through. The transmission coefficient is defined as

$$T = \frac{p_t}{p_i} = \frac{2Z_2 \cos\vartheta_i}{Z_2 \cos\vartheta_i + Z_1 \cos\vartheta_t}. \tag{9.13}$$

According to the parameters reported by Jensen[3] on impedance and speed of sound of air, water and certain tissues, the reflection coefficient at a fat-air interface is equal to –99.94% showing that virtually all of the energy incident on the interface is reflected back in tissues such as the lung. A more realistic example found in the human body is the muscle-bone interface, where the reflection coefficient is 49.25%, demonstrating the challenges encountered when using ultrasound for the investigation of bone structure. On the other hand, given the overall similar acoustic properties between different soft tissues, the reflection coefficient is too low when used to differentiate between different soft tissue structures ranging only between –0.1 and 0.1.

The values mentioned above determine both the interpretation of ultrasound images, or sonograms, as well as the design of transducers, as discussed in the sections below.

9.1.4 Tissue Scattering

In the previous section, the notions of reflection, transmission and propagation were discussed in the simplistic scenario of plane wave propagation and its impingement on plane boundaries. In tissues, however, such a situation is rarely encountered. In fact, tissues are constituted by cells and groups of cells that serve as complex boundaries to the propagating wave. As the wave propagates through all these complex structures, reflected and transmitted waves are generated at each one of these interfaces dependent on the local density, compressibility and absorption of the tissue. The groups of cells are called "scatterers", as they scatter acoustic energy. The backscattered field, or what is "scattered back" to the transducer, is used to generate the ultrasound image. In fact, the backscattered echoes are usually coherent and can be used as "signatures" of tissues that are, e.g., in motion or under compression, as it will be later shown.

An example of such an ultrasound image can be seen in Figure 9.4. The capsule (i.e., the outermost layer) of the prostate is shown to have a strong echo, mainly due to the high impedance mismatch between the surrounding medium, gel in this case, and the prostate capsule. However, the remaining area of the prostate is depicted as a grainy region surrounding the fluid-filled area of the urethra (dark, or low-scattering, area in the middle of the prostate). This grainy appearance is called "speckle", a term borrowed from the laser literature.[4] Speckle is produced by the constructive and destructive interference of the scattered signals from structures smaller than the wavelength, hence the appearance of bright and dark echoes, respectively. Thus, speckle does not necessarily relate to a particular structure in the tissue.

Given its statistical significance, the amplitude of speckle has been represented as having a Gaussian distribution with a certain mean and variance.[5] In fact, these same parameters have been used to indicate that the signal-to-noise ratio of an ultrasound image is fundamentally limited to only 1.91.[5] As a result, in the past, several authors have tried different speckle cancellation techniques[6] in an effort to increase the image quality of diagnostic ultrasound. However, speckle offers one important advantage that has rendered it vital in the current applications of ultrasound (Section 9.9). Despite it being described solely by statistics, speckle is not a random signal. As mentioned earlier, speckle is coherent, i.e., it preserves its characteristics when shifting from position. Consequently, motion estimation techniques that can determine anything from blood flow to elasticity are made possible in a field that is widely known as "speckle tracking". This is further discussed in later sections of this chapter.

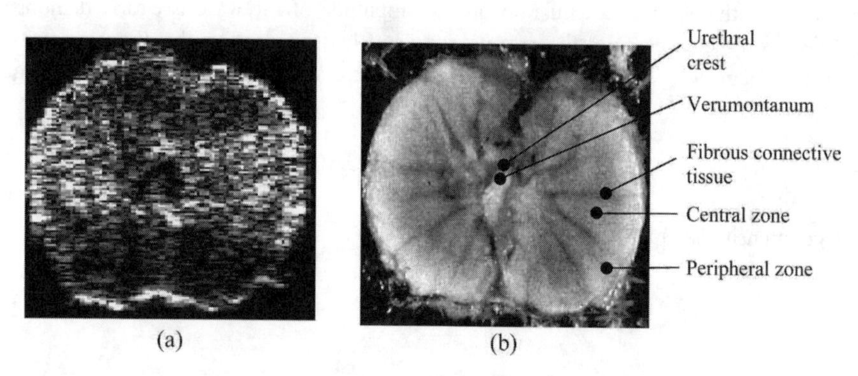

FIGURE 9.4 Sonogram of (left) an *in vitro* canine prostate and (right) its corresponding anatomy at the same plane as that scanned.

9.1.5 Attenuation

As the ultrasound wave propagates inside the tissue, it undergoes a loss of power dependent on the distance traveled in the tissue. Attenuation of the ultrasonic signal can be attributed to a variety of factors, such as divergence of the wavefront, reflection at planar interfaces, scattering from irregularities or point scatterers and absorption of the wave energy.[7] In this section, we will concentrate on the latter, being the strongest factor in soft (other than lung) tissues. In this case, the absorption of the wave's energy leads to heat increase. The actual cause of absorption is still relatively unknown but simple models have been developed to demonstrate the dependence of the resulting wave pressure amplitude decrease in conjunction with the viscosity in tissues.[8]

By not going into detail concerning the derivations of such a relationship, an explanation of the phenomenon is provided here. Let us consider a fluid with a certain viscosity that provides a certain resistance to a wave propagating through its different layers. In order to overcome the resistance, a certain force per unit area, or pressure, needs to be applied that is proportional to the shear viscosity of the fluid η as well as the spatial gradient of the velocity,[7] or

$$p \propto \eta \frac{\partial u}{\partial z} . \tag{9.14}$$

Equation 9.14 shows that a fluid with higher viscosity will require higher force to experience the same velocity gradient compared to a less viscous fluid. By considering Equations 9.2 and 9.14, an extra term can be added to the wave equation that includes both the viscosity and compressibility of the medium,[7] or

$$\frac{\partial^2 u}{\partial z^2} + \left(\frac{4\eta}{3} + \xi \right) k \frac{\partial^3 u}{\partial z^2 \partial t} - \frac{1}{c^2} \frac{\partial^2 u}{\partial t^2} = 0 , \tag{9.15}$$

where ξ denotes the dynamic coefficient of compressional viscosity. The solution to this equation is given by

$$u(t,z) = u_0 \exp(-\alpha z) \exp[jk(ct - z)] , \tag{9.16}$$

where α is the attenuation coefficient also given by (for $\alpha << k$)

$$\alpha = \frac{\left(\frac{4\eta}{3} + \xi \right) k^2}{2\rho c} . \tag{9.17}$$

From Equation 9.16 the effect of attenuation on the amplitude of the wave is clearly demonstrated. An exponential decay on the envelope of the pressure wave highly dependent on the distance results from the tissue attenuation (Figure 9.5). The intensity of the wave will decrease much faster, given that from Equation 9.9

$$I(t,z) = \frac{p_0^2}{Z} \exp(-2\alpha z) \exp[2jk(ct - z)] \tag{9.18}$$

or the average intensity is equal to

$$\langle I \rangle = I_0 \exp(-2\alpha z) . \tag{9.19}$$

Another important effect that tissue attenuation has on the propagating wave is a frequency shift. This is because a more complex form for the attenuation α is

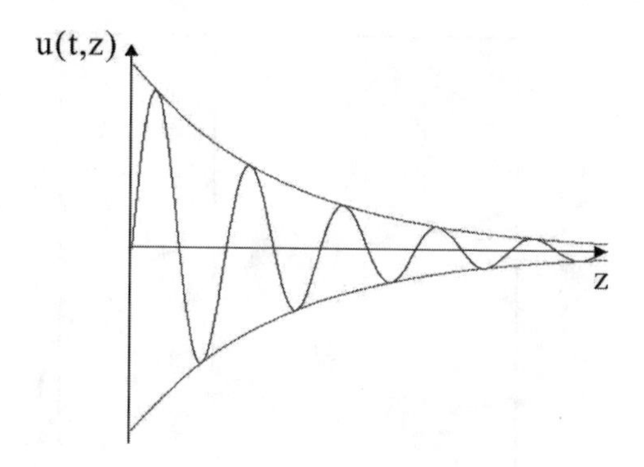

FIGURE 9.5 This is the attenuated wave of Figure 9.1. Note the envelope of the wave dependent on the attenuation of the medium.

$$\alpha = \beta_0 + \beta_1 f \tag{9.20}$$

where β_0 and β_1 are the frequency-independent and frequency-dependent attenuation coefficients.[3] In fact, the frequency-dependent term is the largest source of attenuation and increases linearly with frequency. As a result, the spectrum of the received signal changes as the pulse propagates through the tissue in such a way that a shift to smaller frequencies, or downshift, occurs. In addition, the downshift is dependent on the bandwidth of the pulse propagating in the tissue and the mean frequency of a spectrum (in this case Gaussian[3]) can be given by

$$\langle f \rangle = f_0 - \left(\beta_1 B^2 f_0^2\right) z, \tag{9.21}$$

where f_0 and B denote the center frequency and bandwidth of the transducer. Thus, according to Equation 9.21, the downshift due to attenuation depends on the frequency-dependent attenuation coefficient, the transducer center frequency, and its bandwidth. A graph showing the typical values of frequency-dependent attenuation coefficients (measured in dB/cm/MHz) is given in Figure 9.6.

9.2 Transducers

The pressure wave that was discussed in the previous section is generated using an ultrasound transducer, which is typically a piezoelectric material. "Piezoelectric" denotes the particular property of certain crystal polymers of transmitting a pressure ("piezo" means "to press" in Greek) wave generated when an electrical potential is applied across the material. Most importantly, since this piezoelectric effect is reversible, i.e., a piezoelectric crystal will convert an impinging pressure wave to an electric potential, the same transducer can also be used as a receiver. Such crystalline or semicrystalline polymers are the polyvinylidene fluoride (PVDF), quartz, quartz, barium titanate, and lead zirconium titanate (PZT).

A single-element ultrasound transducer is shown in Figure 9.7. Dependent upon its thickness (l) and propagation speed (c), the piezoelectric material has a resonance frequency given by

$$f_0 = \frac{c}{2l}. \tag{9.22}$$

The speed in the PZT material is around 4000 ms^{-1}, so for a 5-MHz transducer, the thickness should be 0.4 mm thick. The matching layer is usually coated onto the piezoelectric crystal in order to minimize the impedance mismatch between the crystal and the skin surface and, thus, maximize the transmission coefficient (Equation 9.13). In order to overcome the aforementioned impedance mismatch, the ideal impedance Z_m and thickness d_m of the matching layer are respectively given by

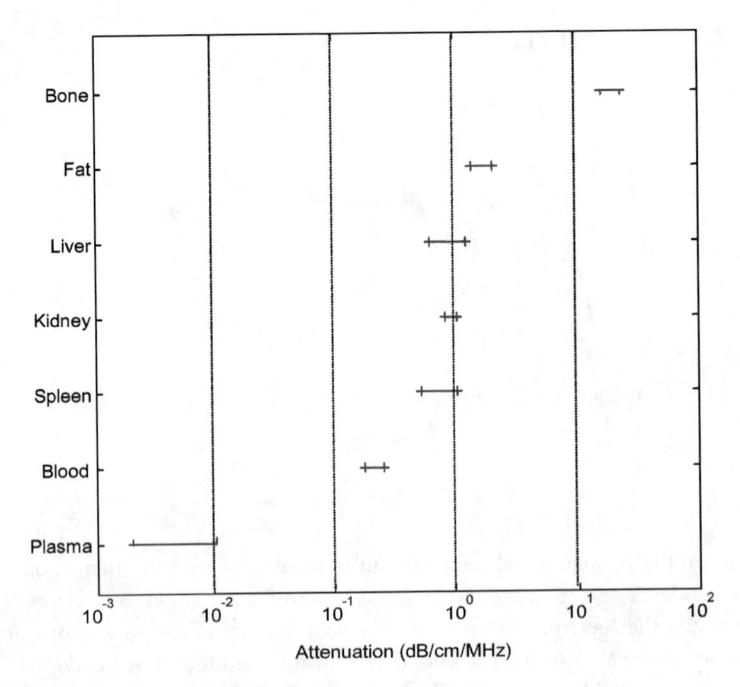

FIGURE 9.6 Attenuation values of certain fluids and soft tissues.[10]

$$Z_m = \sqrt{Z_T Z} \tag{9.23}$$

and

$$d_m = \frac{\lambda}{4} \tag{9.24}$$

with Z_T denoting the transducer impedance and Z the impedance of the medium.

The backing layers behind the piezoelectric crystal are used in order to increase the bandwidth and the energy output. If the backing layer contains air, then the air-crystal interface yields a maximum reflection coefficient given the high impedance mismatch. Another by-product of an air-backed crystal element is that the crystal remains relatively undamped, i.e., the signal transmitted will have a low bandwidth and a longer duration. On the other hand, as will be seen in Section 9.3.3, the axial resolution of the transducer depends on the signal duration, or pulse width, transmitted. As a result, there is a trade-off between transmitted power and resolution of an ultrasound system. Depending on

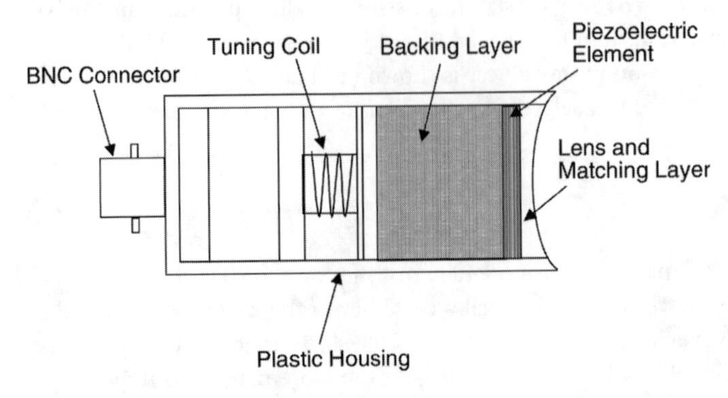

FIGURE 9.7 Typical construction of a single-element transducer.[3]

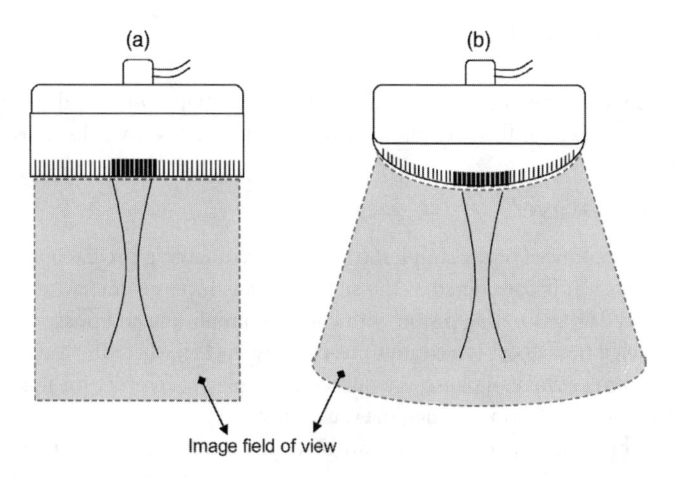

FIGURE 9.8 (a) Linear and (b) curved array transducer used for B-scan acquisition and according to the type of application.

the application, different backing layers are therefore used. Air-backed transducers are used in continuous-wave and ultrasound therapy applications. Heavily backed transducers are utilized in order to obtain high resolution, e.g., for high quality imaging at the expense of lower sensitivity and reduced penetration.

For imaging purposes, an assembly of elements such as that in Figure 9.8 is usually used and called an "array" of such elements. In an array, the elements are stacked next to each other at a distance equal to less than a wavelength for the minimum interference and reduced grating lobes (Section 9.3.2). The most common are shown in Figure 9.8. The linear array has the simplest geometry. It selects the region of interest by firing elements above that region (Figure 9.8a). The beam can then be moved on a line by firing groups of adjacent elements and then the rectangular image obtained is formed by combining the signals received by all the elements. A curved array is used when the transducer is smaller than the area scanned (Figure 9.8b). A phased array can be used to change the "phase," or delay, between the fired elements and thus achieve steering of the beam. The phased array is usually the choice for cardiovascular exams, when the window between the ribs allows for a very small transducer to image the whole heart. Focusing and steering can both be achieved by changing the pulsing delays between elements (Figure 9.9).

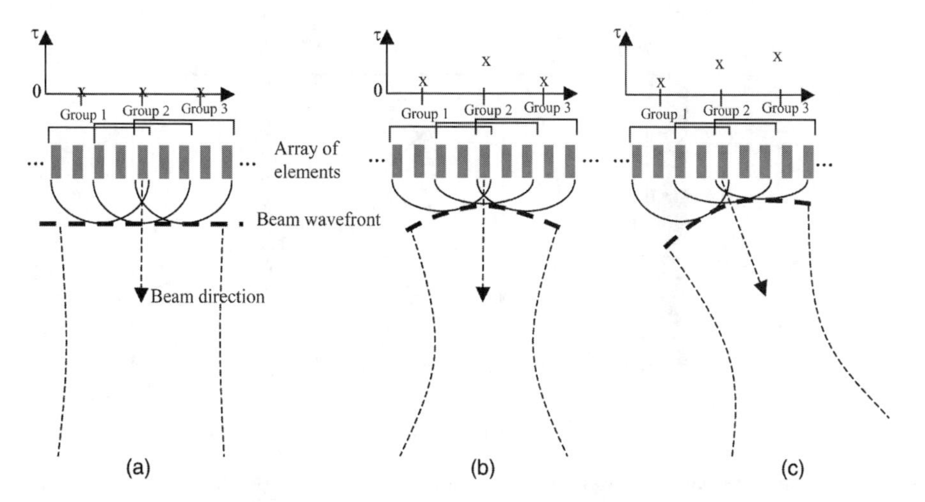

FIGURE 9.9 Electronic (a) beam forming, (b) focusing, and (c) focusing and beam steering as achieved in phased arrays. The time delay between the firings of different elements is denoted here by τ.

9.3 Ultrasound Fields

In the previous section, the different priorities of resolution and depth in pulsed-wave and continuous-wave practices were described. In this section, their distinct applications are discussed.

9.3.1 Continuous-Wave

Let us consider the field produced by the simplest transducer geometry: a circular aperture single-element transducer with a radius *r*. It is considered as the simplest transducer geometry, since the surface of the transducer can be viewed as a vibrating piston with constant amplitude and phase. The simplest kind of wave emitted from such a transducer is a continuous plane wave, i.e., where the wavefront, or the surface in which the motion is everywhere in phase, is assumed to be planar. In order for this to hold, the source of the wave has to be much smaller in size than the wavelength of the emitted wave. According to Huygen's principle, any wave can be considered as the sum of contributions from a particular distribution of sources, which have the suitable phase and amplitude to generate the wave in question. Therefore, the circular transducer can be assumed as being composed by several Huygen's sources all identical in size and at a uniform distribution.

In this case, a simple solution of the field distribution along the axis of symmetry of the source (Figure 9.10) can be found. The field, or beam, is found to have two distinct regions. The beam intensity along the central axis of the field $I(z)$ is given by

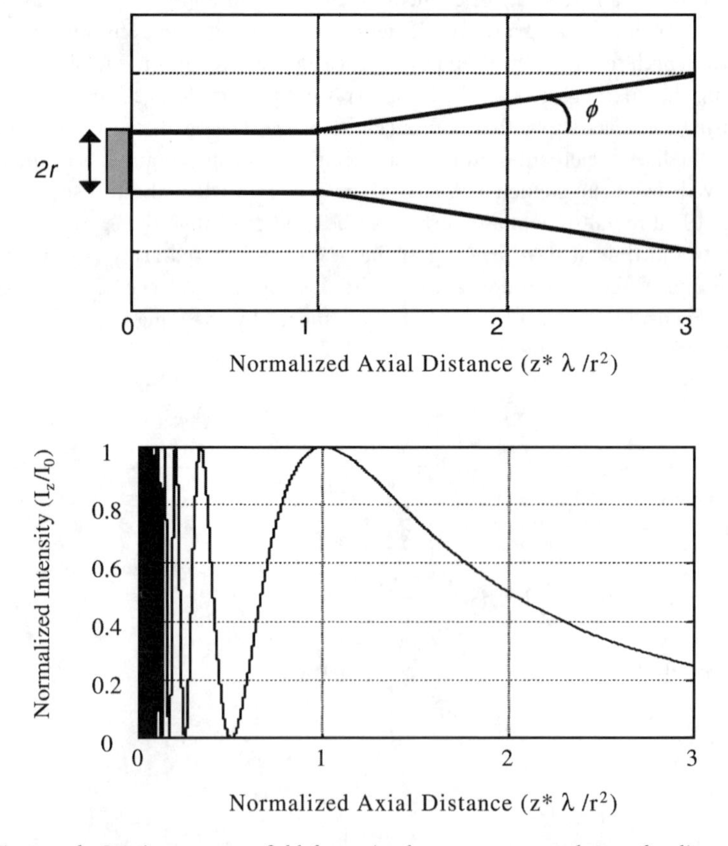

FIGURE 9.10 Top panel: Continuous-wave field for a circular aperture transducer of radius r and divergence angle ϕ. Bottom panel: Normalized intensity amplitude along the symmetry axis of the transducer shown on top at 5 MHz center frequency and 7 mm radius.

$$\frac{I(z)}{I_0} = \sin^2\left\{\frac{\pi}{\lambda}\left[\sqrt{r^2+z^2}-z\right]\right\}, \tag{9.25}$$

where I_0 is the maximum intensity. The maxima and minima of the field in Equation 9.25 are found at

$$z_m = \frac{4r^2-(2m+1)^2\lambda^2}{4(2m+1)\lambda}, \text{ m} = 0, 1, 2, \ldots \tag{9.26}$$

and

$$z_n = \frac{r^2-n^2\lambda^2}{2n\lambda}, \text{ n} = 1, 2, 3, \ldots, \tag{9.27}$$

respectively. The last axial maximum occurs at m = 0 when

$$z_0 = \frac{4r^2-\lambda^2}{4\lambda}$$

and, if $r^2 >> \lambda^2$,

$$z_0 = \frac{r^2}{\lambda}. \tag{9.28}$$

The region before z_0 is called the near field, or Fresnel zone, of the transducer and the region after z_0 is the far field, or Fraunhofer zone (Figure 9.10). Therefore, z_0 is called the transition point or transition distance beyond which the field becomes more uniform. The angle of divergence in the far field (Figure 9.10) is given by

$$\phi = \arcsin\left(0.61\frac{\lambda}{r}\right). \tag{9.29}$$

A slightly more complex but more applicable transducer geometry is that of a concave transducer (Figure 9.11). In that case, the variation in intensity is found by[9]

$$\frac{I(z)}{I_0} = kr^2 Jinc(kr\sin\phi) \tag{9.30}$$

where $Jinc(x) = J_1(x)/x$, $J_1(x)$ is the first-order Bessel function. The term $Jinc(kr\sin\varphi)$ is also known as the *directivity* factor. The beam profile is shown on Figure 9.12.

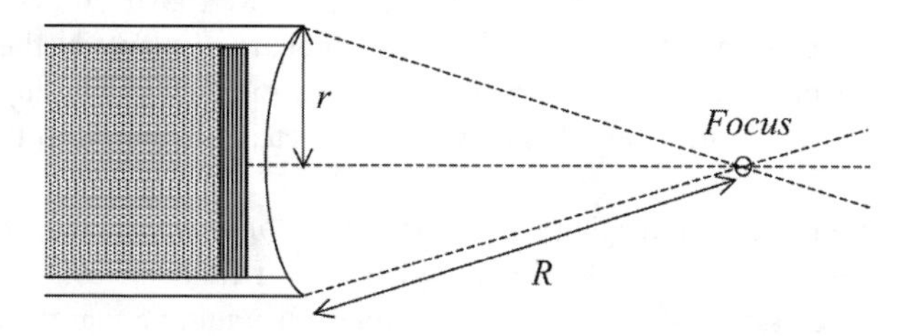

FIGURE 9.11 Field of view of a concave transducer with radius of curvature R and a radius of aperture r.

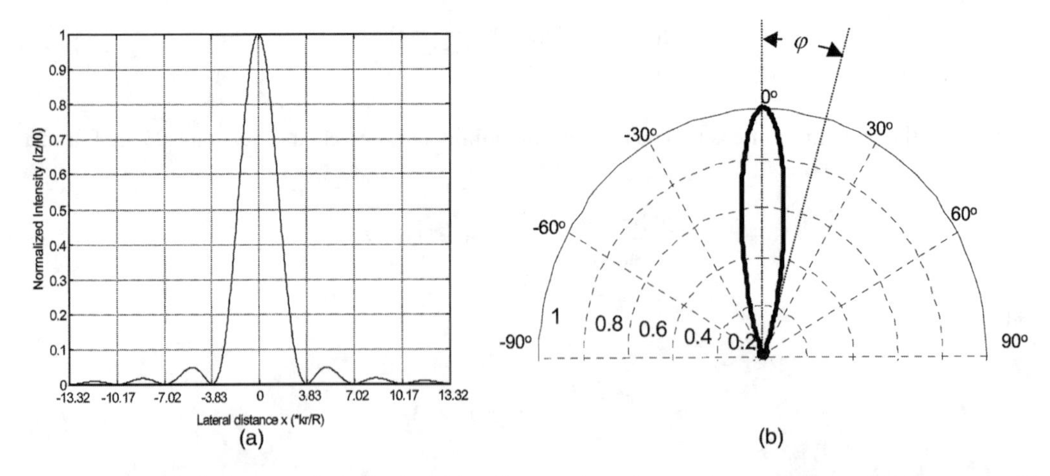

FIGURE 9.12 (a) The beam profile in the far field at distance z from the transducer of radius r. (b) The same profile in an angular plot.

9.3.2 Pulsed Pressure and Pulse Echo Fields

A pulsed pressure field can be generated either by spherical waves emitted by the aperture or by the intersection between spherical waves and the aperture. The latter observation is very important in treating the subsequent imaging in a systems approach.

As mentioned in Section 9.3, the reflected wave or signal is generated following the interaction of the transmitted wave with relatively small structures that cause a perturbation due to their density, compressibility, and absorption. The reflected wave can safely be assumed to be spherical in the case when the transmitted wave is backscattered and the scatterer-transducer distance is sufficiently large. In other words, when the same transducer is used for transmission and reception, the same impulse response can be used to describe the generation and reception of the scatterer field. By following a systems approach, the reflected waveform, $r(x,y,z)$, can be expressed as the convolution (denoted here by ⊗) of the wave field incident on the tissue structure, $p(x,y,z)$, and the impulse response, $f(x,y,z)$, that is associated with the acoustic properties of the tissue structure. That is,

$$r(x,y,z) = p(x,y,z) \otimes f(x,y,z), \tag{9.31}$$

where $p(x,y,z) = p_x(x) \otimes p_y(y) \otimes p_z(z)$ is also called the *point-spread function (psf)*, with $p_x(x)$ denoting the pulse-echo impulse response of the system along the axis of propagation, or axial direction, and is responsible for the radio frequency (RF) content of the signal, $p_y(y)$, the pulse-echo impulse response perpendicular to the axial direction but in the same plane, or lateral direction, and determines the *beam profile*, and $p_z(z)$ the pulse-echo impulse response perpendicular to the imaging plane, or elevational (azimuthal) direction[5] (Figure 9.13). A more complex relationship for the $r(x,y,z)$ can be obtained showing its time-dependence, or four-dimensional characteristics; the reader is encouraged to consult Section 2.5 in Jensen.[3]

The signal of Equation 9.31 is also called the "raw signal" or "RF signal" to denote the unprocessed ultrasonic tissue response received by the system. This is not the signal displayed by the ultrasonic scanners used in clinical environments and several processing and display methods can be applied on the received signal in order to obtain the physical and physiological parameters of interest to the clinicians. This is thoroughly discussed in Section 9.4.

As mentioned in Section 9.2, most imaging systems use arrays for faster and more controlled scanning. In this case, the fields are calculated based on the point-spread functions of the individual, usually identical, transducer elements. Following Huygen's principle and assuming that the wave propagation is linear, the individual impulse responses can be added according to

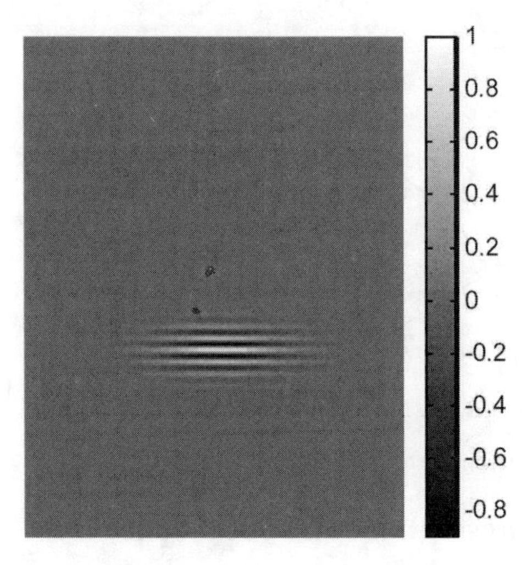

FIGURE 9.13 A two-dimensional version of the point-spread function $p(x,y,z)$.

$$p_a(x,y,z) = \sum_{j=0}^{N-1} p_j(x,y,z), \tag{9.32}$$

where N is the number of elements, $p_j(x,y,z)$ is the point-spread function for each element j and $p_a(x,y,z)$ is the point-spread function for the whole array at the tissue location of (x,y,z). If the elements are assumed to be very small, the field point far away from the array, the individual transducer elements can be assumed as having Dirac point-spread functions and for the example of a linear array of Figure 9.8a, the amplitude of the beam profile can be found equal to[3]

$$|P_a(f)| = \left| \frac{k}{d} \frac{\sin\left(N \dfrac{Dn\sin\vartheta}{c} f\right)}{\sin\left(\dfrac{Dn\sin\vartheta}{c} f\right)} \right| \tag{9.33}$$

where k is the wavenumber, d is the distance of the array to the field point, D is the distance between two neighboring elements in the array, and ϑ is the angle of divergence.

The main lobe of the beam profile of Equation 9.33 occurs naturally at $\vartheta = 0$ but other maxima of the response are found at

$$\varphi_g = \arcsin\left(\frac{n\lambda}{D}\right), \tag{9.34}$$

where n = 1, 2, …. For an array at 5 MHz with an element spacing equal to 0.15 mm, the angle φ_g for the next first maximum is equal to 11.8°. This means that the received signal will also be affected by scatterers that are off the image axis, in this case those positioned at 11.8° off the axis. These responses are naturally not desirable and are called *grating lobes* (Figure 9.14). Since the angle φ_g increases with a decreasing element spacing, one way to make sure they are out of the image plane (i.e., past 90°in Figure 9.14) is to ensure that the elements are separated by less than a wavelength (in the example mentioned above, it would mean that D < 0.3 mm). Typically, an element spacing equal to half a wavelength is chosen (like in the example above) so as to allow for steering of the beam. Steering, however, can move the grating lobes closer to the center of the beam, dependent on the steering angle.

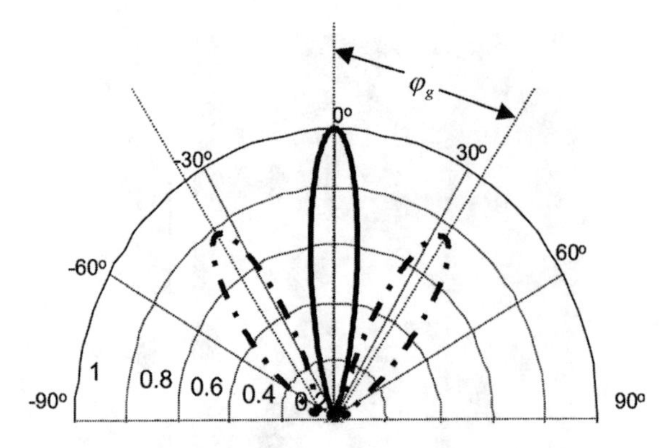

FIGURE 9.14 The beam profile from an N-element linear array.

9.3.3 Axial, Lateral Resolution, and Focal Spot Size

9.3.3.1 Axial Resolution

As explained earlier, different designs and trade-offs need to be considered depending on whether the application requires continuous-wave or pulsed-wave excitation. In the former case, a high efficiency is desired, while in the latter, high quality imaging should result. The transducer parameter that can best express the difference between the priorities in the two cases is the quality factor, or Q, defined as:

$$Q = \frac{f_0}{B}, \tag{9.35}$$

where f_0 is the center frequency of the transducer while B is the bandwidth of the spectrum of the pulse at the –3 dB level (Figure 9.15). Figure 9.15 shows the difference between two extreme cases of transducer designs. Since Q is inversely proportional to the bandwidth, high Q denotes long pulsewidth, or continuous-wave, while low Q denotes pulse-wave. Low Q, therefore, also denotes high axial resolution.

Axial, or longitudinal, resolution is defined as the minimum distance between two scatterers that can be discerned by the system (located along the axis of wave propagation). When the pulse is short, then the echoes successively reflected by the two scatterers can be better differentiated. When the pulse is too long, then the two echoes at reception blend together, making the differentiation between two scatterers impossible. Therefore, the axial resolution (AR) is directly proportional to the Q of the transducer and in fact is given by[7]

$$AR \approx \frac{Q\lambda}{4}. \tag{9.36}$$

9.3.3.2 Lateral Resolution and Focal Spot Size

Another important imaging parameter of an ultrasound transducer is the lateral resolution, defined as the minimum distance between two scatterers that can be discerned by the system and located perpendicular to the axis of wave propagation but in the imaging plane. Compared to the axial resolution, the lateral resolution is defined more by the lens than the pulse characteristics. The beamwidth of the transducer is often too wide to ensure good definition of lateral features in scanned objects. Therefore, a lens is often used as shown in Figure 9.11. The role of the lens is to direct waves entering at a certain angle ϕ to a particular distance in the focal plane x_0.[7] The lens in Figure 9.16 has a focal length given by

$$l_f = \frac{R}{1-n}, \tag{9.37}$$

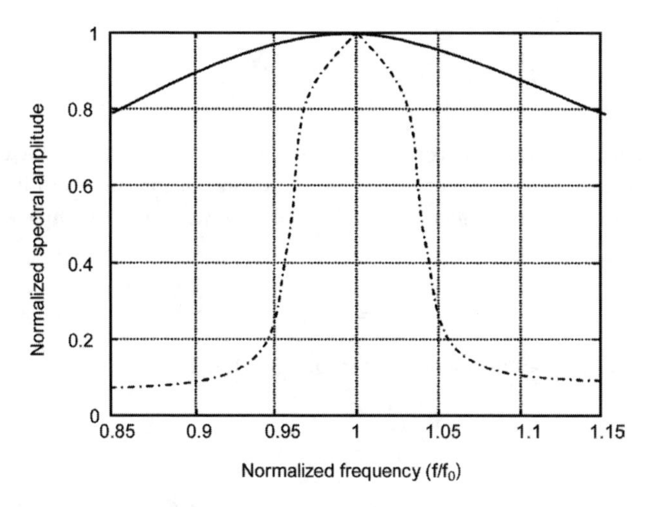

FIGURE 9.15 Two different frequency responses for Q = 2 (solid) and Q = 20 (dotted) transducers. (Adapted from Wells.[1])

where $n = (c/c_l)$ and c_l is the speed of sound in the lens and the "divergence angle" of the lens is given by

$$\sin\varphi = \frac{x_0}{l_f}. \tag{9.38}$$

Therefore, if a lens is placed in front of a circular disk transducer with a field given by Equation 9.30, from Equations 9.30 and 9.38 the directivity factor becomes equal to

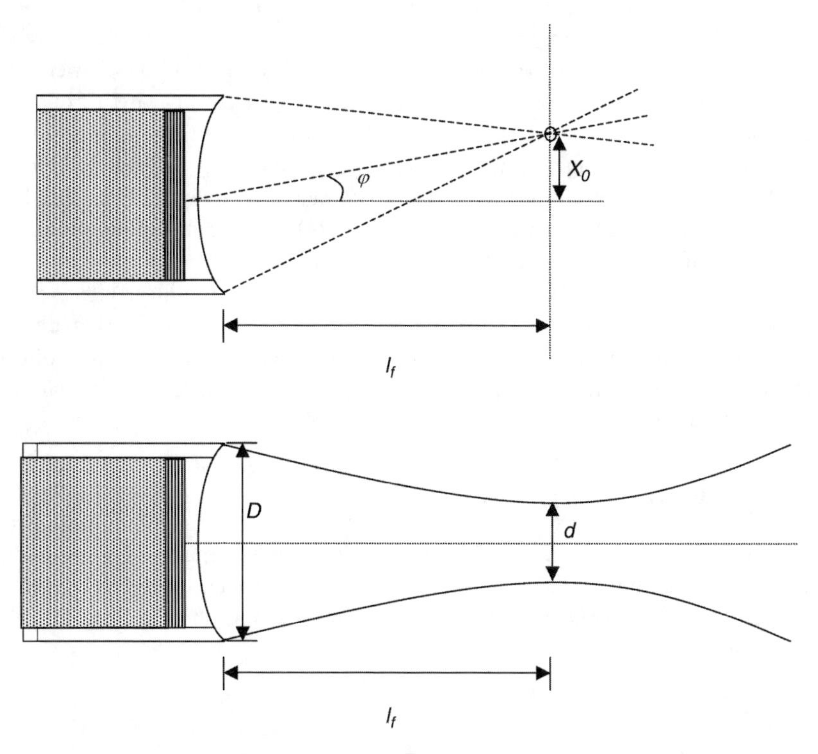

FIGURE 9.16 Top panel: The lens of the transducer has the property of focusing the waves at a distance x_0 from the focal point (to be compared with Figure 9.11). Bottom panel: The lens focuses the beam to a focal spot size equal to d.

$$H_l(x_0) = Jinc\left(kr\frac{x_0}{l_f}\right). \quad (9.39)$$

The field pattern of this focused transducer is exactly the same as the far field of the unfocused one with the same characteristics. The focused spot is the central portion of that field and its size is equal to the diameter of that portion, which is equal to the distance *d* between the two first zeros of the field in Equation 9.39 given by[7]

$$d = 2.44F\lambda, \quad (9.40)$$

where *F* is also known as the F-number of the transducer defined as

$$F = \frac{l_f}{D}. \quad (9.41)$$

The focal spot size (Equation 9.40) also determines the lateral resolution since two scatterers will be discernable in the lateral direction if they are separated by a distance at least equal to the focal spot size. Clearly, axial (Equation 9.36) and lateral (Equation 9.40) resolutions are determined by the wavelength, which sets their lower limits. For high quality imaging, short wavelengths need to be employed, thus denoting high transducer frequencies that are in turn limited by the resulting higher attenuation (Equation 9.20). This constitutes the well-known resolution vs. depth penetration trade-off that needs to be taken into account in the design of the optimal ultrasound system.

9.3.4 Nonlinear Effects

Until now, the tissue was assumed to respond linearly to the mechanical pressure applied by the propagating wave. This only applies to waves of very small amplitude. In fact, waves at higher amplitudes with pressures in the MPa range are routinely utilized in clinical scanners, clearly challenging the models presented until now. This means that, as the wave propagates through a nonlinear medium, it no longer has a constant speed but rather a speed dependent upon the local wave amplitudes. As a result, the propagating wave changes in shape as it propagates and the subsequent distortion introduces higher harmonics than the fundamental initially transmitted. These higher harmonics are more affected by attenuation (Equation 9.20) and the distortion increases with frequency, the nonlinearity of the medium, lower speed of sound, and lower attenuation coefficient. Compared to what was discussed in the previous subsections, the nonlinear effects will cause the wave to be absorbed faster, the point-spread function (Figure 9.13) to be more spatially variant, and the variability of the beam shape to be higher. There are, however, several advantages of utilizing this effect in certain applications, such as harmonic imaging and with contrast agents. These effects are further detailed in Section 9.5.

9.4 Ultrasonic Imaging

Ultrasonic imaging is usually known as *echography* or *sonography* depending on which side of the Atlantic Ocean one is scanning from. As mentioned earlier, the signal acquired by the scanner can be processed and displayed in several different fashions. In this section, the most typical and routinely used ones are discussed.

9.4.1 A-Mode

Figure 9.17 shows a block diagram of the different steps that are used in order to acquire, process, and display the received signal from the tissue.

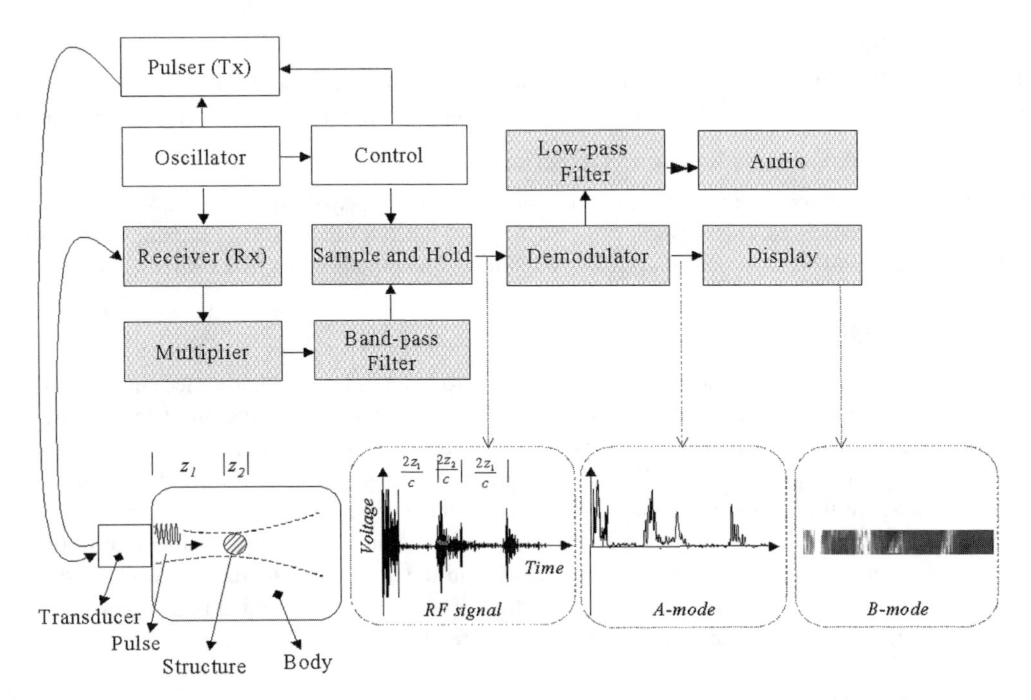

FIGURE 9.17 Block diagram of a pulsed-wave system and the resulting signal or image at three different steps.

9.4.1.1 Transducer Frequency

A pulse of a given duration, frequency, and bandwidth is first transmitted. As mentioned before, a trade-off between penetration (or low attenuation) and resolution exists. Therefore, the chosen frequency will depend on the application. Usually, for deeper organs such as the heart, the uterus, and the liver, the frequencies are restricted in the range of 3 to 5 MHz, while for more superficial structures, such as the thyroid, the breast, the testis, and applications on infants, a wider range of 4 to 10 MHz is applied. Finally, for ocular applications, a range of 7 to 15 MHz is determined by the low attenuation, low depth, and higher resolution required.

The pulse is usually a few cycles of that frequency long (usually 3 to 4 cycles) so as to ensure high resolution (Equation 9.36), and is generated by the transmitter through a voltage step sinusoidal function at a voltage amplitude (100 to 500 V) and a frequency equal to that of the resonance frequency of the transducer elements. For static structures, a single pulse or multiple pulses (usually used for averaging later) could be used at an arbitrary frequency. However, for moving structures, such as blood, liver, and the heart, a fundamental limit on the maximum pulse repetition frequency (PRF) is set by the maximum depth of the structure, or $PRF\ (kHz) = c/2D_{max}$. Typically, the PRF is in the range of 1 to 3 kHz.

9.4.1.2 RF Amplifier

The received signal needs to be initially amplified so as to guarantee a good signal-to-noise ratio. At the same time, the input of the amplifier should be devoid of the high voltage pulse in order to protect the circuits but also maintain its low noise and high gain. A typical dynamic range expected at the output is on the order of 70 to 80 dB.

9.4.1.3 Time-Gain Compensation (TGC)

As mentioned in Section 9.1.5, attenuation is unavoidable as the wave travels through the medium and it increases with depth. In order to avoid artificial darkening of deeper structures as a result, a voltage-controlled attenuator is usually employed, where a control voltage is utilized to manually adjust the system gain accordingly after reception of an initial scan. A logarithmic voltage ramp is usually applied that compensates for a mean attenuation level with depth.[6] The dynamic range becomes further reduced to 40 to 50 dB.

9.4.1.4 Compression Amplifier

The signals will ultimately be displayed as a grayscale on a cathode ray tube (CRT), where the dynamic range is typically only 20 to 30 dB. To this purpose, an amplifier with a logarithmic response is utilized.

9.4.1.5 Demodulation or Envelope Detection

Since the image is a grayscale picture, the amplitude of the signal is displayed. For this, the envelope of the RF signal needs to be calculated. This is usually achieved by using Hilbert transforms. The resulting signal is called a detected A-scan, A-line, or *A-mode scan* (A for Amplitude). An example of that is shown in Figure 9.17.

9.4.2 B-Mode

When the received A-scans are spatially combined after acquisition using either a mechanically moved transducer or the previously mentioned arrays and brightness-modulate the display in a two-dimensional format, the Brightness or B-mode is created, which has a true image format and is by far the most widely used diagnostic ultrasound mode. By default, sonogram or echogram refers to B-mode. Figure 9.18 a shows an image of the left ventricle imaged parasternally. One of the biggest advantages of ultrasound scanning is real-time scanning and this is achieved due to the shallow depth of scanning in most tissues and the high speed of sound. The frame rate is usually on the order of 30 to 100 Hz (while in the M-mode version it can be as fast the PRF itself; see below). The frame rate is limited by the number of A-mode scans acquired, N_A, and the maximum depth, i.e., frame ratemax $PRF_F = c/2D_{max}/N_A$.

9.4.3 M-Mode

Another fashion of displaying the A-scans is in function of time, especially in cases where tissue motion needs to be monitored and analyzed. In this case, only one A-scan from a particular tissue structure is displayed in brightness mode but followed in time depending on the PRF used, and is called Motion-, or M-mode scan. A depth-time display is then generated. A typical application of the M-mode display is used in the examination of heart-valve leaflets motion and Doppler displays (see later section). Figure 9.18b shows the M-mode version of the B-mode in order to follow the motion of the ventricle at the papillary muscle level.

9.4.4 C-Mode

The Constant-depth, or C-scan, is not used as widely as the aforementioned modes, mainly due to its distinct use of scanning. Instead of relying on the acquisition of reflected echoes from the medium, the

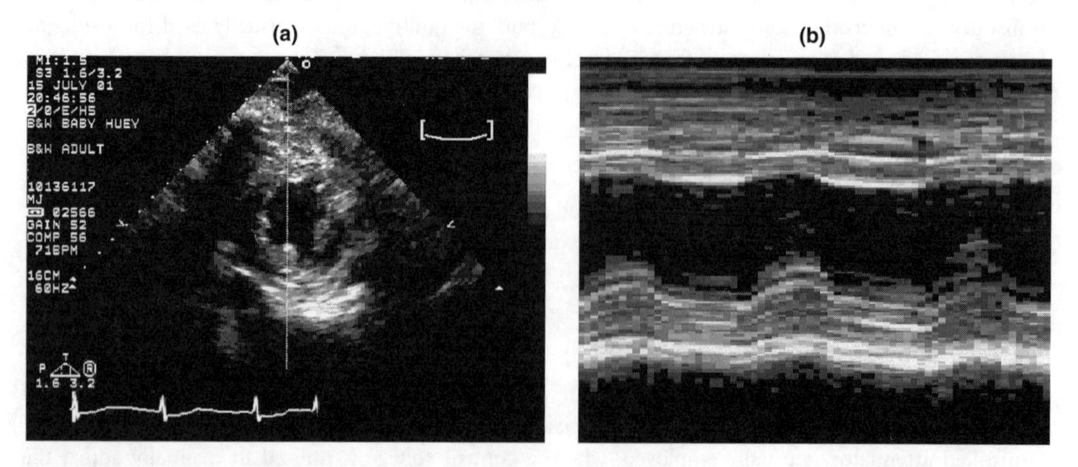

FIGURE 9.18 (a) B-scan of the left ventricle from an apical view; (b) M-mode image of the same view taken at the level of the papillary muscles shown in (left) over three cardiac cycles. (Images courtesy of Scott D. Solomon, Brigham and Women's Hospital, Boston, MA.)

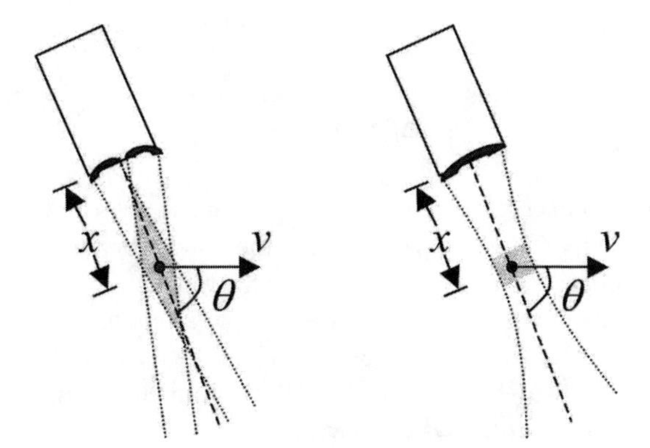

FIGURE 9.19 (Left) Continuous and (right) pulsed-wave systems.

pulse is transmitted from one side of the body by a transmitter to be received on the other side at the same depth by a separate transducer — borrowing from the x-ray CT scan principle. As a result, the scanning motion is perpendicular to the transmitted beam. The two main applications include attenuation measurement along the transmitted beam that depends on both the absorption by the tissue structures and reflection losses at the tissue interfaces, and measurement of the acoustical index of refraction defined as $n = c_w/c$, where c_w is the speed of sound in the water and c is the speed of sound in the tissue. The latter is achieved by measuring the time lapsing between pulse transmission and reception, or *time-of-flight*, in order to calculate the phase velocity of the tissue along the path that separates the two transducers. The C-scans have enjoyed applicability in tissues that are more superficial and relatively homogeneous so as to ensure travel of the echo through all the interfaces. Such an application is the human female breast.

9.4.5 Doppler

9.4.5.1 Doppler Equation

Let us consider the case of a scatterer, e.g., a red blood cell, as shown in Figure 9.19 at a distance x from the transducer and moving with constant velocity v and at an angle θ with respect to the transducer beam of frequency w = 2πf given by

$$u(t) = u_0 \cos(\omega t). \tag{9.42}$$

The received beam will be given by

$$u_r(t) = u_{r0} \cos\left\{\omega\left(t - \frac{2x}{c}\right)\right\}, \tag{9.43}$$

where *2x* is the round trip distance equal to $tv\cos\theta$ (Figure 9.19) and assuming $v << c$ we get

$$u_r(t) = u_{r0} \cos\left\{\omega\left(1 - \frac{2v\cos\theta}{c}\right)t\right\} \tag{9.44}$$

so that the frequency of the received signal is given by

$$f_r = f\left(1 - \frac{2v\cos\theta}{c}\right)$$

or

$$\Delta f = -\frac{2vf\cos\theta}{c} \tag{9.45}$$

that denotes the frequency shift caused in the received signal due to velocity v of the scatterer, which can have a positive or negative value (depending on whether the flow is forward or reverse, according to the conventions used) and at an angle θ to the central axis of the transducer beam. This shift is also known as the *Doppler shift* and Equation 9.45 is known as the *Doppler equation.* According to Equation 9.45, with a frequency f on the order of 2 to 10 MHz and $v\cos\theta$ in the range of 0 to 5 ms^{-1}, the Doppler shift varies usually in the range of 0 to 14 kHz, which is well within the human audio range and can be broadcasted through the speakers of the system (Figure 9.17).

There are several advantages and disadvantages in the formulation and use of the Doppler Equation. First, the formulation is very simple and easy to remember. However, the angle is very difficult to determine, thus making the accurate measurement of the velocity cumbersome. Second, the equation describes the motion of a single scatterer. In practice, a cloud of scatterers is moving with each scatterer at a different velocity, causing a different frequency shift. A spectrum is thus generated (Figure 9.20) that is typically changing during a cardiac cycle, especially when measuring pulsatile flow in key vessels inside the body. The multidimensionality of the Doppler spectrum allows the simultaneous observation of the distribution of blood velocities inside a vessel, their time variations, and their magnitudes. This constitutes a unique feature of ultrasound systems. The spectral characteristics also depend on the geometry of the vessel and the parameters of the beam. However, qualitative analysis of the Doppler spectra is capable of determining the type of flow inside a vessel, i.e., whether the flow is parabolic, turbulent, or other, by merely measuring the increase in the *bandwidth* of the Doppler spectrum, otherwise known as *spectral broadening*. The magnitude of the Doppler spectrum depends on the compliance of the vessel wall and the flow impedance.[3,6] However, stationary structures, e.g., within the vessel wall, usually constitute the main noise source in the velocity measurement, since they can generate disproportionally (often 10 to 100 times) larger echoes, or *clutter*, than the low backscatter echoes from blood. In addition, as discussed

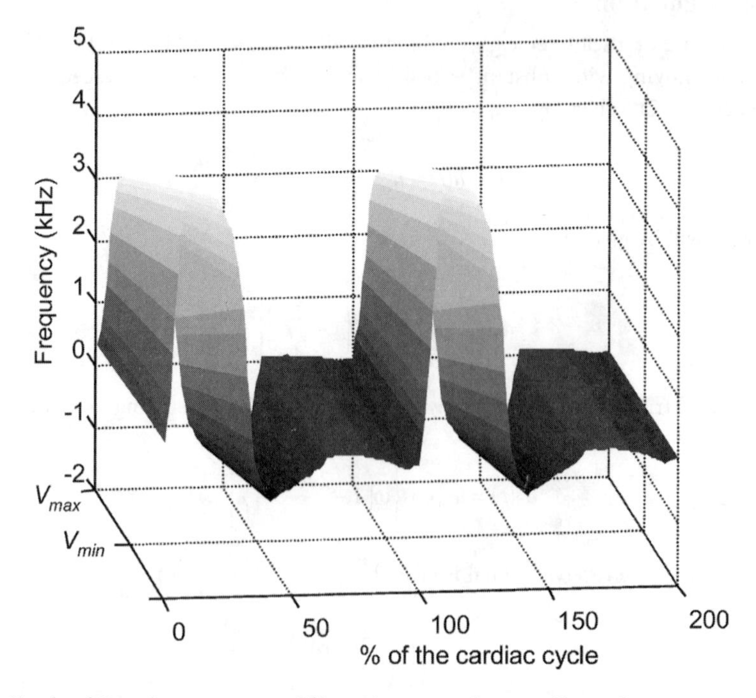

FIGURE 9.20 Simulated Doppler spectrum at different instances of two cardiac cycles.

earlier, attenuation also affects the received echo spectrum and often to a much larger extent than the Doppler effect.[3] On the other hand, the coherent interference of waves in a random medium, which was earlier defined as "speckle," also contains information on the motion of the scatterers in question. The expansive field of "speckle tracking" techniques is briefly discussed in Section 9.4.5.3. Finally, the Doppler equation does not take the beam finiteness into account and, as a result, when calculating the spectrum, frequency leakage occurs.[6] The well-known trade-off between spatial and frequency resolution also holds here. The aforementioned characteristics are only valid in the case of continuous-wave systems. As mentioned earlier, most imaging systems use pulsed-wave, or pulse-echo, methods to achieve higher resolution and those are discussed in the following section.

9.4.5.2 Continuous-Wave Velocity and Flow Detector

There are two types of Doppler systems, the continuous-wave and pulsed-wave (Figure 9.19). The continuous-wave system, as briefly discussed in the previous subsection, is the simpler of the two. A continuous pressure wave is transmitted by one transducer element while another receives the echoes scattered from the tissue during transmission. The frequency shifts, or differences in frequency, are measured using the A-scans and displayed and/or made audible. For those measurements, several methods have been developed over the years.[6] One technique of choice has been quadrature phase demodulation, in which the received echo (Equation 9.44) is multiplied by a quadrature signal with frequency equal to that of the transmitted wave (Equation 9.42) to yield

$$u_{rq}(t) = u_{r0}\cos\left\{\omega\left(1 - \frac{2v\cos\theta}{c}\right)t\right\}\cos(\omega t)$$

$$= \frac{u_{r0}}{2}\left[\cos\left\{\frac{2\omega v\cos\theta}{c}t\right\} + \cos\left(2\omega t - \frac{2\omega v\cos\theta}{c}t\right)\right] \tag{9.46}$$

A bandpass filter is used to remove the higher frequency component (second additive term in Equation 9.46) as well as the DC component introduced by stationary echoes.[3] After filtering, only the first additive term remains that contains the information on the frequency shift and the velocity (Equation 9.45). An example of such a display in a clinical environment is shown in Figure 9.21 and is also often called "sonogram."

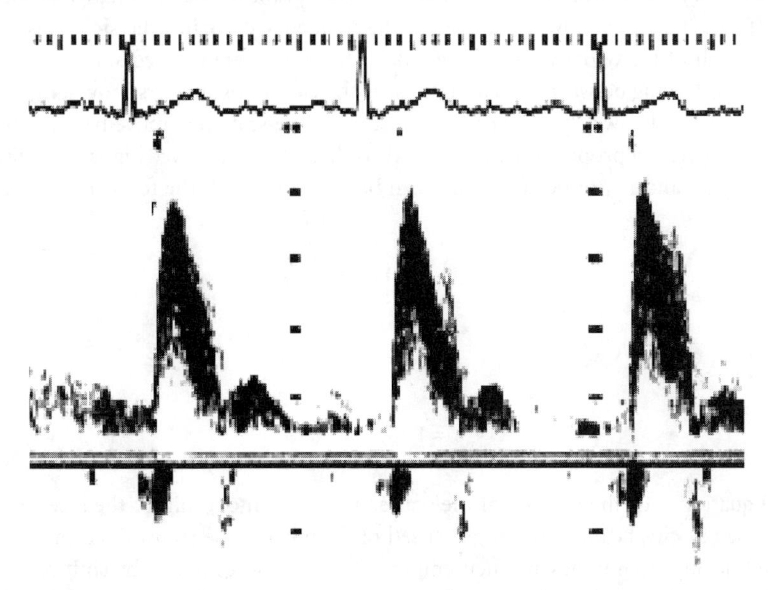

FIGURE 9.21 Continuous-wave (CW) Doppler sonogram with the corresponding EKG (top) of a normal aorta at the suprasternal notch over three cardiac cycles.

Since all Doppler frequencies fall in the audible human range, the Doppler spectrum can be listened to and judged by a clinician, and a very simple method that has been used in both old and current systems can provide a direct feedback regarding the blood flow characteristics. For example, a forward (reverse) flow occurs when the argument in the cosine term is positive (negative). It turns out[3] that the forward and reverse flows can be separated by shifting the phase of the Doppler signal by 90° and then adding its imaginary and real parts. The two flows are then heard over two individual speakers providing the flow direction (Figure 9.17). For more information on the subject as well as quantitative methods for flow measurements, the reader is encouraged to consult Jensen.[3]

9.4.5.3 Pulsed-Wave Velocity and Flow Detector

The previous subsection dealt with the application of the Doppler equation and the use of the Doppler spectrum for flow pattern detection and characterization. Despite its simplicity, a serious drawback of the continuous-wave approach is the lack of range, or depth, information due to the fact that transmit and receive elements are in close proximity. An inherent limitation of the technique is that there is non-uniqueness between a Doppler spectrum and a flow profile, rendering the method questionable for the reliable differentiation between normal and pathological cases. To overcome these limitations, pulsed-wave systems were developed that allow for the investigation of flow patterns in individual vessels or individual parts of a vessel (Figure 9.19). The pulsed-wave systems combine characteristics from pulse echo imaging and CW Doppler methods. A pressure wave of a certain frequency is emitted, similar to the CW system, but at short pulses and a certain PRF. RF echoes are then received by the same transducer following each pulse and then gated with an adjustable duration. This gate allows for the selection of the depth at which the velocity will later be measured.

An important limitation of the Doppler spectrum method is that, as briefly mentioned previously, the attenuation effect can be much more dramatic than the sought-after Doppler shift. For example, in the case where the vessel is at a depth of 5 cm from the transducer, the attenuation of the medium is at 0.5 dB/cm/MHz and the relative transducer bandwidth is at 80%, a downshift of the transducer center frequency equal to 16 kHz occurs. Assuming a velocity of 0.5 ms^{-1}, the Doppler shift will be on the order of 1 to 2 kHz, thus completely overshadowed by the downshift due to attenuation. In other words, in a pulsed-wave system, the classic Doppler effect is not utilized.

The Doppler effect is in fact interpreted in the time domain so as to avoid the undesirable and unavoidable frequency effects from other noise sources. Except for the scaling change of the signal in the time domain (following the bandwidth change in the frequency domain), the signal also experiences a time delay as a result of the velocity. In other words, if two pulses are emitted successively, according to the amount of time lapsing between the two pulses, as the cloud of scatterers moves, the received signal will also move accordingly, away or toward the transducer. The scatterers move between pulses that are emitted at a delay inversely proportional to the PRF, or T_{PRF}. If the received signals acquired at pulse 1 and 2 are given by u_{r_1} and u_{r_2}, respectively, they can be linked through the following equation:[3]

$$u_{r_2}(t) = u_{r_1}\left(t - \frac{T_{PRF}}{\alpha}\right), \tag{9.47}$$

where

$$\alpha = 1 - \frac{2v\cos\theta}{c}.$$

According to Equation 9.47, the velocity of the scatterers results into a shift of the received signal that is dependent on the velocity, beam-vessel angle, speed of sound, and the transmitted pulse delay. The so-called "speckle tracking" techniques are then employed in order to estimate the shift resulting from the scatterer motion that is equivalent to speckle displacement. No scatterer motion, or stagnant flow, will result to the two received waveforms being identical. Assumptions to obtain Equation 9.47 are that the displacement is relatively small, noise is negligible, and that transverse motion is not significant. The displacement can be safely assumed small in the case where $vT_{PRF} < b$, where b is the beamwidth.

An important limitation of a pulsed-wave Doppler system is that the frequency shift has to be at least smaller than half of the PRF. Otherwise, aliasing of the measured Doppler frequencies will occur. Since $PRF\ (kHz) = c/2D_{max}$ (from the pulse echo imaging section) and following Equation 9.45, the maximum velocity that can be measured without ambiguity at the maximum allowable gate depth, $D_{\max}$, is equal to

$$v_{\max} = \frac{c^2}{8f\cos\vartheta D_{\max}}. \tag{9.48}$$

This is otherwise known as the "range-velocity" trade-off. The inverse proportionality between velocity and center frequency and depth presents serious limitations to the pulsed Doppler systems for large depth applications. Several techniques have been developed in order to maximize performance and include an adjustable gate depth according to the PRF used and a sharp cut-off smoothing filter with an adjustable cut-off frequency, also dependent on the PRF. Finally, these shortcomings can also be avoided by combining the B-scan mode with the Doppler sonogram mode, otherwise known as *Duplex mode,* or the *Triplex mode* that is like the Duplex mode but with an additional color Doppler image superimposed on the B-scan (Figure 9.22). A user-defined line of site and range gate for the pulsed Doppler is overlapped onto a B-scan image, allowing for the identification of the vascular anatomy of interest (and possible artifacts in the Doppler estimate arising as a result) and for a more reliable and quantifiable Doppler estimate through angle θ and vessel diameter determination.

9.5 Current Developments

Despite the fact that diagnostic ultrasound is an older imaging modality compared to MRI and PET, it is very intriguing to see that it continues to expand as a field and to offer numerous applications. In the past decade, several leaps have been made with the advent of faster computer processors, contrast agents, the utilization of nonlinear wave propagation, signal processing techniques, and complex transducer architecture, to name a few. In this section, a short overview is presented of the key techniques that can routinely be used on ultrasound machines in the future, if not already.

9.5.1 Contrast Agents and Harmonic Imaging

During the wave interaction with tissues, besides the linear wave propagation discussed earlier, nonlinear effects also occur, especially at higher intensities (on the order of MPa) that are routinely used by

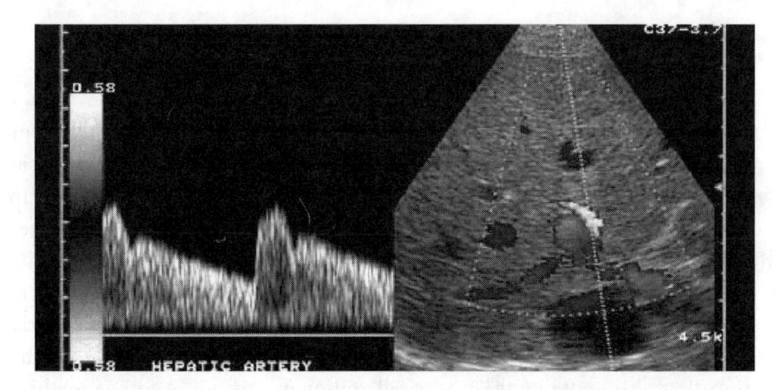

FIGURE 9.22 A triplex mode sonogram showing the PW Doppler sonogram (left) at the level of the hepatic artery in B-scan of the liver (right). Usually, the color (shown in this example on a grayscale) here indicates the direction of the flow, e.g., toward or away from the transducer. (Courtesy of CoreVision Pro, Toshiba Medical Systems, Irvine, CA.)

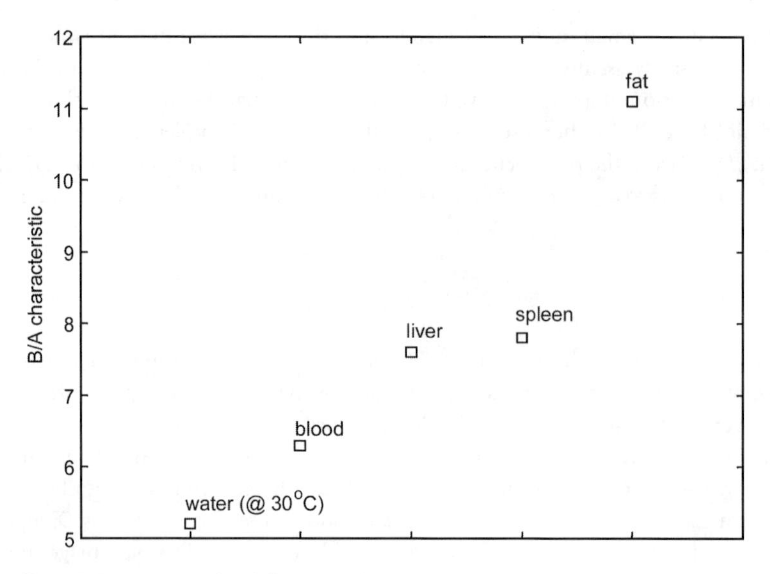

FIGURE 9.23 The B/A characteristic for different media.[3]

diagnostic scanners. This is because the pressure exerted by the beam can no longer be considered as negligible compared to the pressure of the medium. As a result, nonlinear waves can be generated that are dependent on the acoustic pressure, the medium characteristics and depth through which the beam travels. The medium characteristics can be given by the B/A parameter shown in Figure 9.23 for different media. Typically, the higher the B/A characteristic, the higher the nonlinearity term in the wave equation, and the higher the distortion in the resulting wave.

One of the main problems with the standard use of ultrasound arises from high attenuation in some tissues (Figure 9.6) and thus is most prominent in imaging of small vessels and velocity measurements, as described in the previous section. In order to overcome this limitation in the case of blood flow measurements, contrast agents are routinely employed. Contrast agents are typically microspheres of encapsulated gas or liquid coated by a shell, usually of albumin. Due to the high impedance mismatch created by the gas or liquid contained, the resulting backscatter by the contrast agents is a lot higher than that of the blood echoes.

An alternative method to generating higher backscatter due to the increased impedance mismatch is based on the harmonics generated by the bubble's interaction with the ultrasonic wave. This interaction results to a vibration of the latter at a resonance frequency f_r given by:[2]

$$f_r = \frac{1}{2\pi a}\sqrt{\frac{3\gamma P}{\rho}}, \tag{9.49}$$

where a is the radius of the contrast agent, γ is the adiabatic constant, P is the applied pressure, and ρ is the density of the bubble. The bubble vibration also generates harmonics above and below the fundamental frequency, with the second harmonic possibly exceeding the first harmonic. In other words, the contrast agent introduces nonlinear backscattering properties into the medium where it lies. Several processes of filtering out undesired echoes from stationary media surrounding the region, where flow characteristics are assessed, result in weakening of the overall signal at the fundamental frequency. Therefore, since residual harmonics will result from moving scatterers, motion characteristics can all be obtained from the higher harmonic echoes, after using a high-pass filter and filtering out the fundamental frequency spectrum that also contains the undesired stationary echoes. Another method for distilling the harmonic echo information is the more widely used phase or pulse inversion method. Figure 9.24 shows an example of how this method works. Instead of one, two pulses are sequentially transmitted with their phases reversed. Upon reception, the echoes resulting from the two pulses are summed up. A

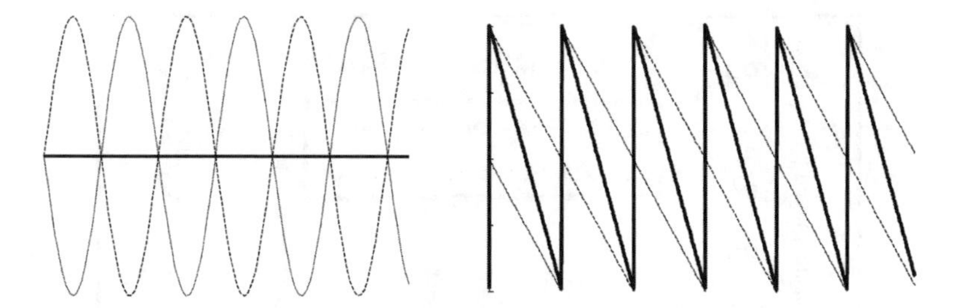

FIGURE 9.24 The pulse inversion method with (left) the transmitted pulses (initial in dashed and phase-inverted in dotted lines, respectively; summed waveform [bold solid] resulting in cancellation) and (right) the resulting potential sawtooths from the respective transmitted pulses of the left diagram. Note that the summed waveform (in bold solid) results in a sawtooth of twice the frequency.

sinusoid with a particular frequency f_0 will be cancelled at summation, while, for example, a sawtooth that contains a much higher amount of frequency content will have its fundamental at f_0 term removed with the extant components at $2f_0$, $4f_0$, etc. remaining.

Despite the fact that the idea of contrast agent use originated for applications in the case of blood flow, the same type of approach can be applied in the case of soft tissues as well. After being injected into the bloodstream, the contrast agents can also appear and remain on the tissues and offer the same advantages of motion detection and characterization as in the case of blood flow. An example of the contrast improvement provided by contrast agents in cardiac tissues is shown in Figure 9.25. However, it turns out that contrast agents are not always needed for imaging of tissues at higher harmonics, especially since backscatter from tissues can be up to two orders of magnitude higher than backscatter from blood. The nonlinear wave characteristic of the tissues themselves is thus sufficient in itself to allow imaging of tissues (Figure 9.23), despite the resulting higher attenuation at those frequencies. The avoidance of patient discomfort following contrast agent injection is one of the major advantages of this approach in tissues. Imaging using the harmonic approach (whether with or without contrast agents) is generally known as *harmonic imaging*. Compared to the standard approach, harmonic imaging in tissues offers the ability to distinguish between noise and fluid-filled structures, e.g., cysts and the gall bladder. In addition, harmonic imaging allows for better edge definition in structures and, therefore, is generally known to increase image clarity, mainly due to the much smaller influence of the transmitted pulse to the received spectrum. Harmonic imaging is now available in most clinical ultrasound systems. One of the main requirements for harmonic imaging is the large bandwidth of the transducer at the receiver so

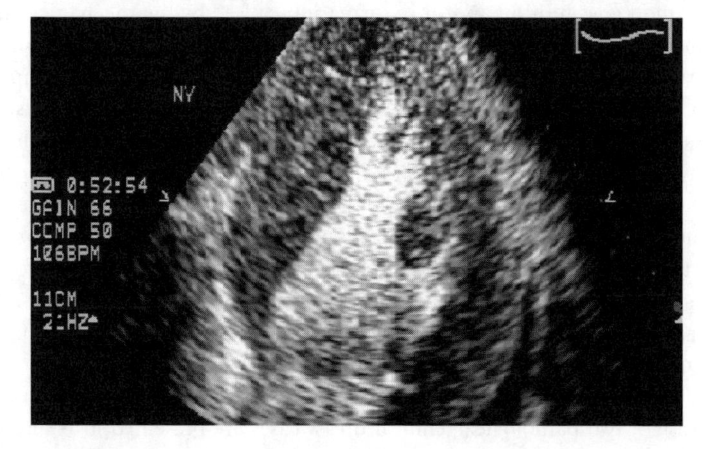

FIGURE 9.25 Long-axis echocardiogram of a left ventricle using harmonic imaging. Note the increase in resolution and image clarity as a result of the contrast agent introduction (to be compared to the echocardiograms without contrast of Figure 9.18). (Image courtesy of Scott D. Solomon, Brigham and Women's Hospital, Boston, MA.)

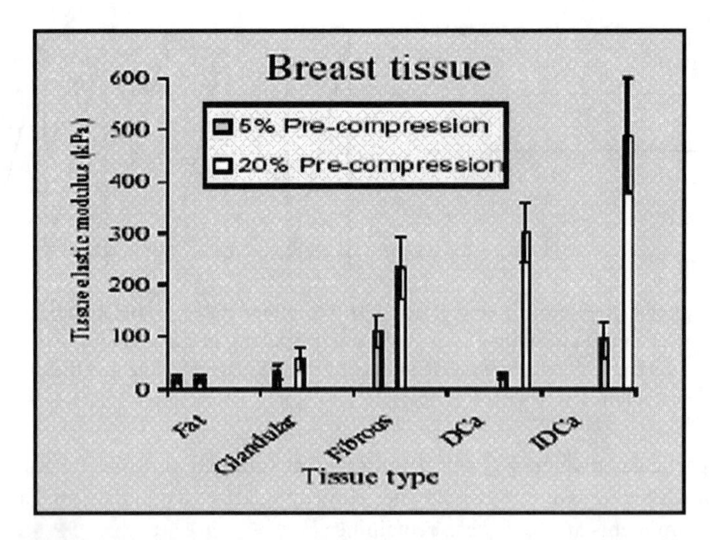

FIGURE 9.26 Elastic moduli (or stiffnesses) of normal and tumorous breast tissues. DCa, ductal carcinoma; IDCa, invasive ductal carcinoma. (Image courtesy of Tom Krouskop, Baylor College of Medicine, Houston, TX.)

as to allow reception of the higher frequency components. This is also in very good agreement with the higher resolution requirement for imaging.

9.5.2 Elasticity Imaging

Another field that, like harmonic imaging, has emerged out of ultrasonic imaging in the last decade is *elasticity imaging*. Its premise is built on two proven facts: (1) significant differences between mechanical properties of several tissue components exist and (2) that the information contained in the coherent scattering, or speckle, is sufficient to depict these differences following an external or internal mechanical stimulus. Figure 9.26 demonstrates the validity of the first fact by showing the range of elastic moduli for several different normal and pathological human breast tissues. Not only is the hardness of fat different than that of glandular tissue, but, most importantly, the hardness of normal glandular tissue is different than tumorous tissue (benign or malignant) by up to one order of magnitude. This is also the reason why palpation has been proven an infallible tool in the detection of cancer.

The second observation is based on the fact that coherent echoes can be tracked while or after the tissue in question undergoes motion and/or deformation caused by the mechanical stimulus, e.g., an external vibration or a quasi-static compression. Figure 9.27 shows the general concept behind the elasticity imaging techniques and, more specifically, the example of an applied compression to detect a harder lump in a method called *elastography*. Speckle tracking techniques are also employed here for the motion estimation. In fact, Doppler techniques, such as those used for blood velocity estimation, were initially applied in order to track motion during vibration (*sonoelasticity imaging* or *sonoelastography*). Parameters such as velocity and strain are estimated and imaged in conjunction with the mechanical property of the underlying tissue. The higher the velocity or strain estimated the softer the material and vice versa. In fact, these parameters can also be used for the recovery of the underlying tissue property but these methods have been proven cumbersome and unreliable in their numerous assumptions given the unknown stress distributions that often fail in the case of highly inhomogeneous tissues.

Examples of elastograms, or strain images, in the same *in vitro* prostate shown in Figure 9.4 (Figure 9.28) and in the case of two pathological, clinical breast cases are presented in Figure 9.29. In the case of the canine prostate, through comparison to Figure 9.4, complementary information based on the distinct mechanical responses and properties of the several anatomical structures of the prostate, such as the urethra and the peripheral zones, is provided. In the case of the breast, both benign and malignant

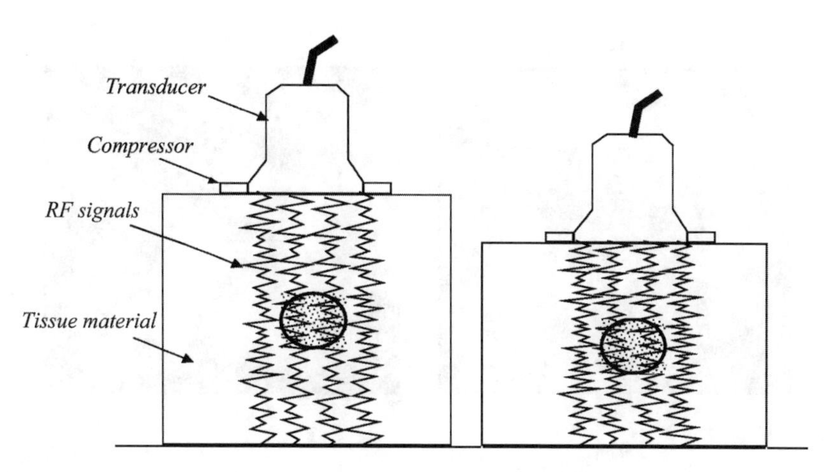

FIGURE 9.27 The principle of elastography. The tissue is insonified (left) before and (right) after a small uniform compression. In the harder tissues (e.g., the circular lesion depicted) the echoes will be less distorted than in the surrounding tissues.

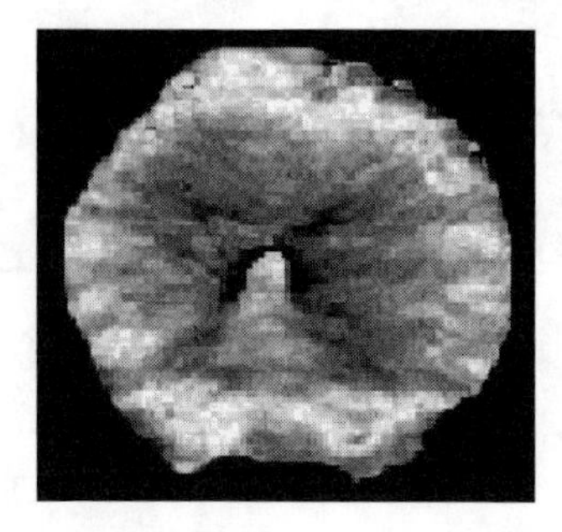

FIGURE 9.28 Prostate elastogram of the prostate in Figure 9.4. Black and white denote highest and lowest strains, respectively.[11]

tumors can be depicted in elastograms, whether visible on the sonogram or not. Through comparison between the sonographic and elastographic characteristics of the several tissue components, their malignancy type could be characterized.

Due to the vast impact that these techniques could have in imaging and characterization of tissues based on their mechanical attributes, a variety of very promising methods have recently developed, spanning from hand-held and real-time application of elastography to elastic modulus maps based on the wavelength of propagation through different tissues following an applied stimulus (*transient elastography*) and the use of the internal radiation force resulting from the pressure of the beam itself to locally displace (*remote palpation*) or vibrate (*ultrasound-stimulated vibroacoustography*), to name a few. This field has not been proven as applicable clinically as that of harmonic imaging due to its inherent, more complicated nature but all these techniques are on the brink of becoming readily applicable and very useful in conjunction with the standard, current use of ultrasonic imaging.

9.5.3 Three-Dimensional Imaging

Until now, only two-dimensional sonograms were presented and discussed. However, ultrasonic imaging has recently also expanded to three-dimensional imaging in clinical applications, especially cardiology and obstetrics. This is due to the advancement in transducer design, namely, the two-dimensional arrays, where beams are generated in all three planes (Figure 9.30c), but three-dimensional images can also be

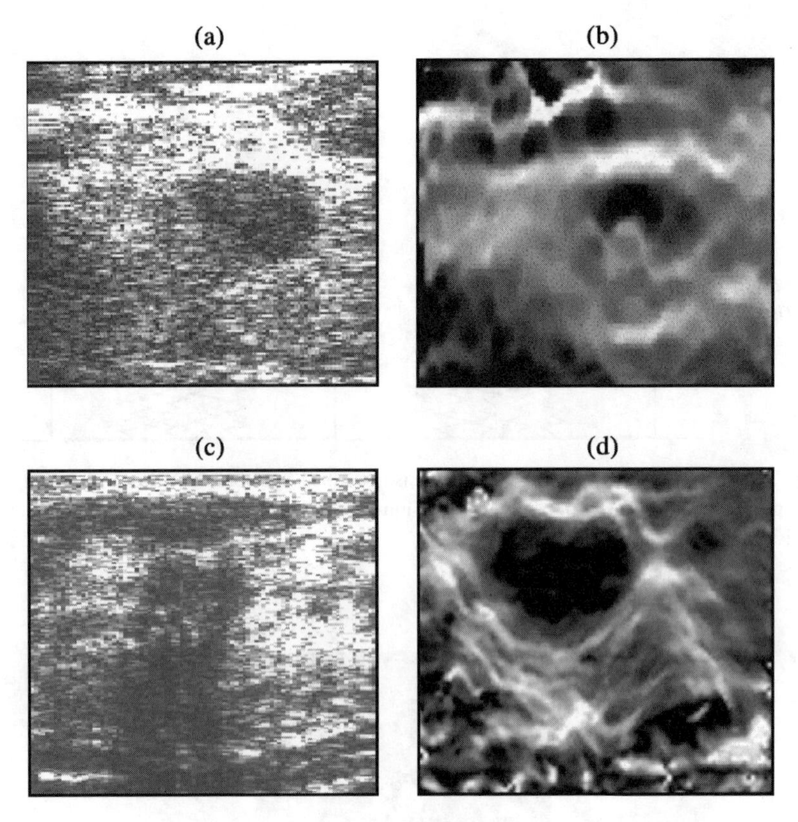

FIGURE 9.29 (a) Sonogram and (b) elastogram of an *in vivo* benign breast tumor (fibroadenoma); (c) sonogram and (d) elastogram of an *in vivo* malignant breast tumor (invasive ductal carcinoma). In these elastograms, black and white denote lowest and highest strains, respectively.

achieved with sweeping a linear or phased array out of plane (Figure 9.30a and b). An example of such a sonogram is shown in Figure 9.31.

9.5.4 Acoustic Microscope

As mentioned in Section 9.3.3.1, the resolution of ultrasonic imaging systems is ultimately limited by the wavelength used. Therefore, in principle, the smaller the wavelength or the higher the frequency (Equation 9.12), the better the resolution (Equations 9.36 and 9.40). The acoustic microscope uses much

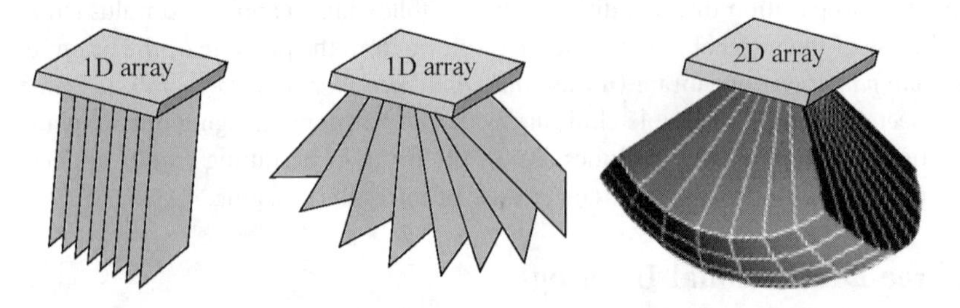

FIGURE 9.30 Three methods for three-dimensional ultrasonic imaging: (left) linear and (center) tilt mechanical scanning of standard (1D) array for the acquisition of a series of parallel two-dimensional images and three-dimensional image reconstruction; (right) two-dimensional ($N \times N$) array producing a pyramidal scan for the direct generation of three-dimensional images.

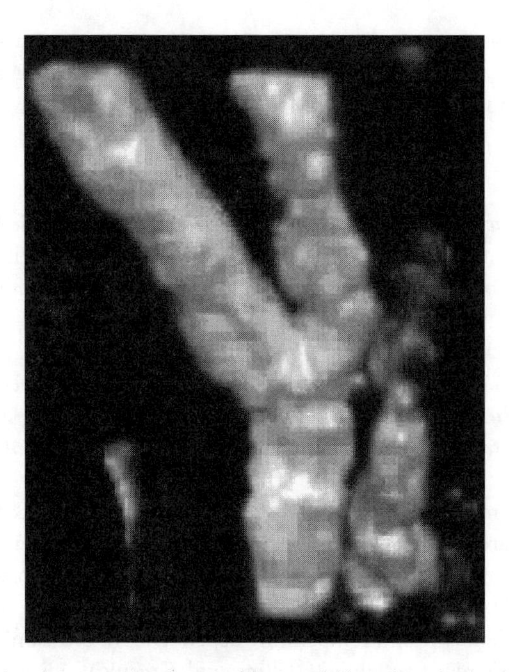

FIGURE 9.31 Three-dimensional sonogram of a carotid artery bifurcation obtained using Color Doppler Energy (EKG gated). The jugular next to the carotid is also evident in these images due to the nondirectionality of the CDE. (Image obtained using Acuson [Siemens] Sequoia and courtesy of John A. Hossack [University of Virginia, Charlottesville, VA, biomedical engineering], Sandy Napel [Stanford University, Stanford, CA, radiology], and R. Brooke Jeffrey [Stanford University, Stanford, CA, radiology].)

higher frequencies than those used in the medical imaging field in order to achieve resolution of the order of a micron — similar resolution to that of optical microscopes. The highest frequency currently used is on the order of 1.5 GHz with a corresponding wavelength equal to 1.0 μm.

The aforementioned trade-off between resolution and penetration applies here as well. Samples, thus, cannot be insonified at depths larger than a few microns. As a result, the acoustic microscope does not have the standard ultrasonic imaging applications. However, it provides the possibility of imaging tissues at the cellular level and allows observation of cell motion and interaction among other things. In addition, the acoustic microscope can provide completely different information on the tissues compared to the optical or electron microscopes, namely, it can show maps of attenuation as well as acoustic phase and

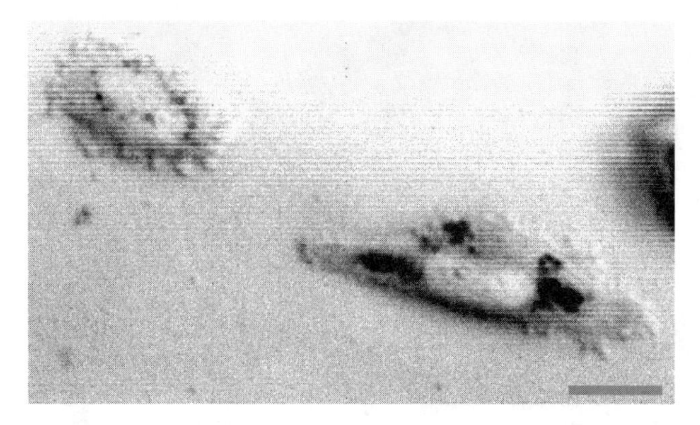

FIGURE 9.32 Acoustic microscope images obtained at 1 GHz of melanoma kidney cells. The bar is equal to 20 μm. (Image provided courtesy of C. Miyasaka and B. R. Tittmann, Department of Engineering Science and Mechanics, Pennsylvania State University, College Park, PA.)

impedance interfaces.[7] In other words, the acoustic microscope can depict tissue properties and characteristics that otherwise are unobtainable, even with other microscopes. An example of an acoustic microscope image is shown in Figure 9.32.

References

1. Wells, P.N.T., *Biomedical Ultrasonics*, Medical Physics Series, Academic Press, London, 1977.
2. Kinsler, L.E. and Frey, A.R., *Fundamentals of Acoustics*, 2nd ed., John Wiley & Sons, New York, 1962.
3. Jensen, J.A., *Estimation of Blood Velocities Using Ultrasound*, Cambridge University Press, Cambridge, U.K., 1996.
4. Burckhardt, C.B., Speckle in ultrasound B-mode scans, *IEEE Trans Son. Ultrason.*, SU-25, 1–6, 1978.
5. Wagner, R.F., Smith, S.W., Sandrik, J.M., and Lopez, H., Statistics of speckle in ultrasound B-scans, *IEEE Trans. Son. Ultrason.*, 30, 156–163, 1983.
6. Bamber, J.C. and Tristam, M., *Diagnostic Ultrasound*, Webb, S., Ed., IOP Publishing Ltd., London, 1988, 319–386.
7. Christensen, P.A., *Ultrasonic Bioinstrumentation*, 1st ed., John Wiley & Sons, New York, 1988.
8. Morse, P.M. and Ingard, K.U., *Theoretical Acoustics*, McGraw-Hill, New York, 1968.
9. Kino, G.S., *Acoustic Waves: Devices, Imaging and Analog Signal Processing*, Prentice-Hall, Upper Saddle River, NJ, 1987.
10. Haney, M.J. and O'Brien, W.D., Jr., Temperature dependence of ultrasonic propagation in biological materials, in *Tissue Characterization with Ultrasound*, Greenleaf, J.F., Ed., CRC Press, Boca Raton, FL, 1986, 15–55.
11. Ophir, J., Kallel, F., Varghese, T., Konofagou, E.E., Alam, S.K., Garra, B., Krouskop, T., and Righetti, R., Elastography, optical and acoustic imaging of acoustic media, *C.R. Acad. Sci. Paris*, Tome 2, Ser. IV, No. 8, 1193–1212, 2001.

10

Emission Imaging: SPECT and PET

Anthony J. McGoron
Florida International University

Juan Franquiz
Florida International University

CONTENTS

10.1 Introduction

Single photon emission computerized tomography (SPECT) and positron emission tomography (PET) are noninvasive medical imaging modalities that provide the three-dimensional distribution of a radiopharmaceutical in the human body. The radiopharmaceutical is a biological compound or drug that has been labeled with radioactive atoms. Other imaging studies using radiopharmaceuticals, such as dynamic and static studies, are based only on the projection of the three-dimensional distribution of radioactivity into two-dimensional planar images. In dynamic studies, a sequence of planar images displays the dynamic or kinetic behavior of the radiopharmaceutical; while in static studies, single planar images display the regional uptake of the radiopharmaceutical. All these imaging procedures are based on the external detection of gamma rays emitted from the patient and are commonly referred as emission imaging to be differentiated from those modalities based on the transmission of x-rays through the human body (e.g., radiographic imaging and x-ray computerized tomography). Since emission imaging is derived from the internal distribution of a radiopharmaceutical, the clinical information these images provide is related to those biochemical and physiologic processes in which the radiopharmaceutical is involved. The functional or metabolic information provided by emission imaging is the major characteristic that differentiates this modality from others that basically provide anatomical or structural

0-8493-1140-3/04/$0.00+$1.50

information. This advantage has been used for physicians for earlier diagnosis and management of diseases based on metabolic and physiological changes that can occur before structural or anatomical modifications may be noted. The wide range of clinical and research applications of emission imaging have been determined by progress in three important fields. One has been the radiopharmaceutical labeling of different drugs, substrates, monoclonal antibodies, ligands, neurotransmitters and blood cells with certain radioactive atoms that can be safely administered to humans. The second has been the technical advances in radiation detectors, electronics and associated instruments for the efficient detection of gamma rays and correction of physical effects degrading image quality and quantitative accuracy. The third factor has been the increasing power of affordable computers and the development of software algorithms for image processing and biokinetic modeling.

Detailed treatises of all aspects of emission imaging are available.[1] In this chapter, the current status of emission imaging is reviewed and a look into the future directions in the new millennium is described. Primary applications of emission imaging are in the areas of cardiology and oncology; thus, greater detail is dedicated to emission imaging applications to these two disciplines. However, since emission imaging has been applied to almost every organ group, the current status is reviewed for each system.

10.2 Radioisotopes

10.2.1 Atomic Structure and Radioactive Decay

10.2.1.1 Atomic Structure

Tightly bound protons and neutrons form the nucleus of an atom. Both types of particles within the nucleus receive the generic name of nucleons. According to the Bohr's atomic model, negatively charged electrons are located around the nucleus in orbits or shells of different binding energy levels. Protons have a positive electrical charge of the same magnitude as that of electrons and mass approximately 1840 times of that of the electron. Neutrons have the same mass as protons, but no electrical charge. Since nucleons include most of the atomic mass, the total number of nucleons in an atom is named the atomic mass number (A). The total number of protons, which is equal to the total number of orbital electrons, defines the unique position of the atom in the periodic table of elements and is named the atomic number (Z).

10.2.1.2 Isotopes

Those atoms having the same number of protons but a different total number of nucleons are named isotopes. The notation to represent isotopes is ${}_{Z}^{A}X$, where X is the chemical symbol of the element. Since there is a unique relationship between the atomic number and the symbol of the element, only the atomic mass number superscript is used to differentiate the isotopes of the same element.

10.2.1.3 Radioactive Decay

Nucleons are packed together in the atomic nucleus by the strong short-range nuclear forces among them. However, in certain combinations of protons and neutrons, electrostatic repulsion forces among protons predominate over nuclear forces and the nucleus becomes unstable. Unstable nuclei spontaneously transform to more stable combinations of neutrons and protons by releasing or absorbing energy in the form of subatomic particles or electromagnetic radiation of high frequency. This process has been given the name of radioactive transformation or radioactive decay. Upon a radioactive transformation, the resultant nucleus may be stable or it may still be unstable and subsequently transform again. The atomic nucleus prior to radioactive decay is named the parent, while the nucleus after transformation is named the daughter.

10.2.1.4 Radioisotopes

Those unstable isotopes of an element suffering radioactive decay are named radioisotopes. All nuclei with $Z > 82$ are radioactive, with the exception of ${}^{209}Bi$. Some others lighter natural nuclei ($Z < 82$) are also radioactive.

Table 10.1 Conversion of Units of Activity

1 Ci = 37 GBq
1 mCi = 37 MBq
1 μCi = 37 kBq
1 GBq = 27 mCi
1 MBq = 27 μCi
1 kBq = 2.7 x 10^{-2} μCi

10.2.2 Activity and Half-Life

10.2.2.1 Activity

The rate of radioactive decay, or disintegrations per unit of time of a radioactive sample, is named the activity of the sample. The classical unit of activity is the curie (Ci) defined as 3.7×10^{10} disintegrations per second (dps). The unit of activity of the System International (SI) is the Becquerel (Bq) defined as one disintegration per second. Activities in emission imaging are usually expressed in millicuries (mCi) and megabecquerels (MBq) or microcuries (μCi) and kilobecquerels (kBq). Table 10.1 shows the conversion between both units.

The activity of a sample at time t is proportional to the number of radioactive atoms in the sample ($N(t)$):

$$\frac{dN(t)}{dt} = -\lambda.N(t),$$

where λ is a proportionality constant named the decay constant, characteristic of each radioisotope. By solving the equation assuming N_0 radioactive atoms at $t = 0$:

$$N(t) = N_0 e^{-\lambda t},$$

which is the exponential law of radioactive decay.

Radioactive decay is a probabilistic phenomenon. From the exponential law, the probability that any specific atom does not decay at time t is given by $N(t)/N_0 = e^{-\lambda t}$, while the probability of decay is $1 - e^{-\lambda t}$. It is not possible to predict when a specific atom will decay, but from the half-life it is possible to predict when half of the atoms in a sample will decay.

10.2.2.2 Half-Life

The decay of a radioisotope is commonly expressed by its half-life. That is the time necessary for one half of the radioactive atoms of a sample to decay. The relationship between half-life ($T^1/_2$) and the decay constant can be easily demonstrated:

$$T_{1/2} = \frac{Ln2}{\lambda}$$

Table 10.2 shows the half-life of some radioisotopes commonly used in emission imaging.

10.2.3 The Energy of Nuclear Radiations

10.2.3.1 Electronvolt

The energy of particles or electromagnetic radiation involved in a radioactive decay process is expressed in a special unit named electronvolt (eV). It represents the energy acquired by an electron through an electric field of 1 V of potential difference. One electronvolt is equivalent to 1.6×10^{-19} Joules (J). Since this is a very small unit, the multiples kiloelectronvolt (keV = 10^3 eV) and megaelectronvolt (MeV = 10^6 eV) are commonly used.

Table 10.2 Principal Characteristics of Most Commonly Used Radioisotopes for Emission Imaging

Radioisotope	Half-life	Decay	Gamma energy used for imaging (keV)	Production
^{99m}Tc	6.02 h	IT	140	Generator
^{201}Tl	73 h	EC	70, 169	Cyclotron
^{111}In	68 h	EC	170	Cyclotron
^{131}I	8.04 d	β^-	362	Fission product
^{123}I	13.2 h	EC	158	Fission product
^{133}Xe	5.25 d	β^-	80	Fission product
^{67}Ga	78.3 h	EC	93, 185, 300	Cyclotron
^{81m}Kr	13 s	IT	190	Generator
^{18}F	110 m	β^+	511	Cyclotron
^{15}O	2.1 m	β^+	511	Cyclotron
^{13}N	10 m	β^+	511	Cyclotron
^{11}C	20.4 m	β^+	511	Cyclotron
^{82}Rb	1.3 m	β^+	511	Generator

IT: Isomeric transition; EC: Electron capture.

Particles carry energy in the form of kinetic energy of mass in motion, while the energy E_γ of electromagnetic radiation is expressed by:

$$E_\gamma = h.\nu\,,$$

where $h = 6.626 \times 10^{-34}$ J.s is the Planck's constant and ν is the frequency of the electromagnetic radiation expressed in s^{-1}.

10.2.3.2 Gamma Rays

Electromagnetic energy emitted by the atomic nucleus or annihilation processes is named gamma radiation. The energy of gamma rays can be from 50 keV to higher than 3 MeV, but for emission imaging, only gamma rays in the range from 60 to 511 keV are used. Frequency of gamma rays is usually higher than 3×10^{19} s^{-1} (Figure 10.1).

10.2.3.3 Characteristic X-Rays

Electromagnetic energy released from the transition of orbital electrons from an outer- to an inner-shell is named characteristic x-rays. Energy of characteristic x-rays is from 124 eV upward and usually overlaps the energy range of gamma rays. The frequency of characteristic x-rays is higher than 3×10^{17} s^{-1}.

10.2.4 Types of Radioactive Decay

The four major types of radioactive decay of interest in biomedical applications are alpha decay, beta decay, electron capture and isomeric transition.

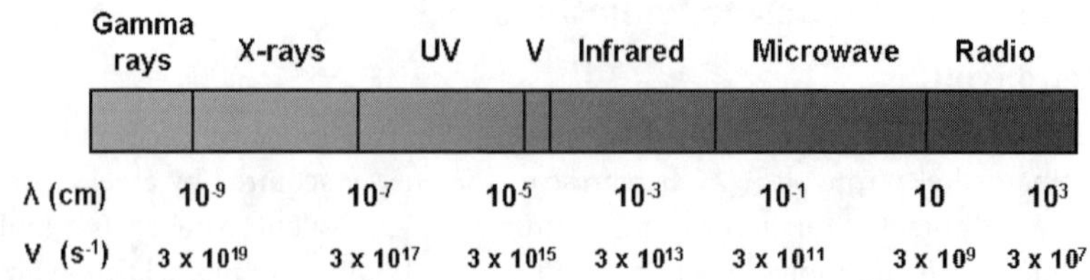

Gamma rays | X-rays | UV | V | Infrared | Microwave | Radio

λ (cm): 10^{-9} 10^{-7} 10^{-5} 10^{-3} 10^{-1} 10 10^{3}

ν (s^{-1}): 3×10^{19} 3×10^{17} 3×10^{15} 3×10^{13} 3×10^{11} 3×10^{9} 3×10^{7}

FIGURE 10.1 The electromagnetic radiation spectrum.

10.2.4.1 Alpha Decay

This is commonly limited to radioisotopes of high atomic number (Z > 82). The alpha particle consists of two protons and two neutrons and is equivalent to the nucleus of a Helium atom. Although the alpha particle is usually emitted with an approximate kinetic energy of 4 MeV, it is stopped by a few centimeters of air or by a few microns of tissue. Consequently, alpha emitters are not used for emission imaging but have been proposed and investigated for internal radiotherapy of cancer tumors. After an alpha decay, the atomic number of the daughter is two units less than that of the parent and the atomic mass is four units less than that of the parent:

$$ {}_{Z}^{A}X \rightarrow {}_{Z-2}^{A-4}Y + {}_{2}^{4}\alpha \ . $$

10.2.4.2 Beta Decay

This transformation consists in the nuclear emission of a particle of mass and magnitude of the charge equal to that of the electron and a neutral particle without mass. The particle may be negatively charged, in which case it is named negatron or beta minus (β^-). During β^- disintegration the atomic number of the daughter is increased by one unit:

$$ {}_{Z}^{A}X \rightarrow {}_{Z+1}^{A}Y + \beta^- + \overline{\upsilon} \ , $$

where $\overline{\upsilon}$ represents the neutral, without mass particle named antineutrino.

10.2.4.3 Positron Emission

In some radioisotopes (Table 10.2), the emitted particle may be positively charged. In this case the particle is named positron (β^+) and the atomic number of the daughter is reduced by one unit:

$$ {}_{Z}^{A}X \rightarrow {}_{Z-1}^{A}Y + \beta^+ + \upsilon \ , $$

the accompanying uncharged, without mass particle υ is named neutrino.

Both particles are stopped by a few millimeters of tissue and cannot be used directly for emission imaging. However, the positron has an important characteristic that makes it useful for emission imaging. After the positron loses most of its kinetic energy in some millimeters of tissue, the particle interacts with an electron at rest and the two particles undergo annihilation. In the annihilation process, the rest mass of each particle is converted into electromagnetic radiation in the form of two gamma rays of 511 keV, each emitted in opposite directions (Figure 10.2). The simultaneous detection of these two gamma rays is the foundation of PET imaging.

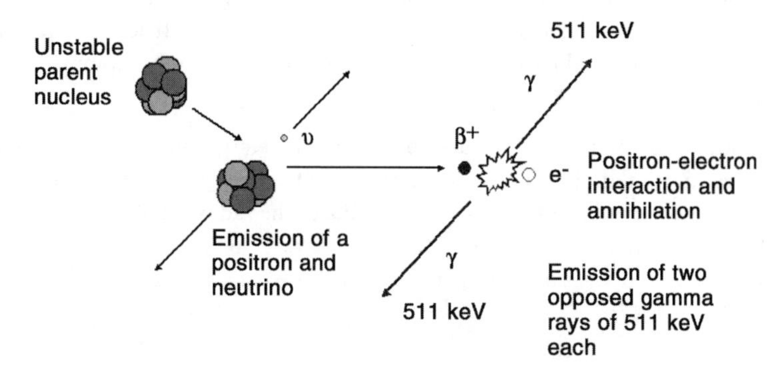

FIGURE 10.2 Annihilation of a positron and an electron, and emission of two gamma rays of 511 keV each in opposite directions.

Negatrons and positrons, the particles emitted during beta decay, are characterized by a maximum energy, but most particles are emitted with energies lower than the maximum. The difference in energy between the maximum and the specific energy of each particle is carried away by the neutrino or antineutrino particles. Consequently, beta decay yields a continuous energy spectrum of negatron or positron particles.

10.2.4.4 Electron Capture

This is a decay process in which an orbital electron is absorbed by an unstable nucleus. As a consequence of this process, the daughter nucleus reduces its atomic number in one unit, such as in the positron decay. The loss of an orbital electron produces a rearrangement of the orbital electrons to fill the vacancy. This rearrangement is usually accompanied by the emission of characteristic x-rays, with enough energy in some cases to travel out of the body and be used for emission imaging.

10.2.4.5 Isomeric Transition

This decay is produced when energetic excited nuclei transforms to a more stable state by emitting the excess of energy as gamma rays. Nuclear excited states usually occur after alpha, beta or electron capture decays. In isomeric transitions there is no change in the atomic or mass number. To differentiate the excited from the stable state, the letter m, meaning metastable, is added to the atomic mass of the parent:

$$^{99m}Tc \rightarrow {}^{99}Tc + \gamma(140\,keV)$$

An excited nucleus is named metastable when its half-life is higher than 10^{-6} sec. Gamma rays emitted in isomeric transitions have one or several specific energies, but not a continuous spectrum of gamma energies. In the above example, ^{99m}Tc has a half-life of 6 h and is produced by the beta decay of ^{99}Mo. The isomeric transition of ^{99m}Tc releases a gamma ray of 140 keV (Table 10.2).

10.2.5 Production of Radioisotopes

10.2.5.1 Natural Radioactivity

Natural radioactive nuclei are grouped into three radioactive decay series or chains. Each series starts with a long-lived parent and ends in a stable nucleus. The three radioactive series are the uranium series, which starts with ^{238}U ($T^1/_2 = 4.5 \times 10^9$ years) and ends with ^{206}Pb, the actinium series starting with ^{235}U ($T^1/_2 = 4.5 \times 10^9$ years) and ending with ^{207}Pb, and the thorium series starting with ^{232}Th ($T^1/_2 = 4.5 \times 10^9$ years) and ending with ^{209}Bi. There are 14 other lighter natural radioisotopes not members of these decay chains. Because natural radioisotopes decay by alpha or β^- emissions, have long half-lives or have no suitable chemical properties for labeling biological compounds, all radioisotopes used for emission imaging must be artificially produced.

10.2.5.2 Artificial Radioactivity

Artificial radioisotopes are created by nuclear reactions that modify the original composition of nucleons of a stable isotope named the target. Depending on the target and particles involved in the nuclear reaction, different types of artificial radioisotopes can be produced. The most common types of nuclear reactions are as follows:

- Neutron capture reaction (n,γ) is produced by bombarding target nuclei with neutrons in a nuclear reactor to produce a radioisotope with excess of neutrons decaying by β^- emission or electron capture (EC). The decay of this radioisotope produces the radionuclide of interest. Radiosotopes produced by this reaction are carrier-free because there are no radioisotopes of the target element. Examples of radioisotopes produced by this reaction are ^{131}I and ^{125}I:

$$^{130}Te + n \rightarrow {}^{131}Te + \beta^- \rightarrow {}^{131}I$$

$$^{124}Xe + n \rightarrow {}^{125}Xe + EC \rightarrow {}^{125}I$$

- Positive charged particle-neutron reactions are produced with medium-energy particle accelerators by bombarding targets with protons (p,n), alpha particles (α,n) or deuterons (d,n). These radioisotopes decay by positron and gamma emission (Table 10.2) and are separated from the target element by chemical reactions. The cyclotron is the most common type of accelerator used for radioisotope production using positively charged particles of low to medium energy (from 9 to 20 MeV). Small cyclotrons with related automated chemistry systems and ^{18}F-fluorodeoxy-D-glucose (^{18}FDG) synthesis units are commercially available for production of positron emitters of very short half-life (^{11}C, ^{13}N, ^{15}O) in medical institutions. Major producers of medical cyclotrons are General Electric Medical Systems (Milwaukee, WI), CTI Molecular Imaging Inc. (Knoxville, TN), EBCO Technologies Inc. (British Columbia, Canada) and IBA (Ion Beams Applications, Louvain, Belgium).
- Products of the fission of ^{235}U and ^{239}Pu in nuclear reactors, such as ^{99}Mo, ^{133}Xe and ^{131}I, can be separated from other fission products and used for emission imaging.

Because radioisotopes produced by positively charged particles and fission must be separated from other radioisotopes or the target itself by chemical means, the radionuclide purity must be controlled before its use in medical applications. Radionuclide purity is defined as the percentage of total activity in the form of the radionuclide of interest. Acceptable limits for radionuclide purity depend on the radioisotope.

10.2.6 Generators of Radioisotopes

Commercial generators based on the decay of a long half-life parent that yields a shorter half-life daughter are available for use in hospitals. The daughter is produced with a high radionuclide purity in a sterile and pyrogen-free solution ready for labeling and preparation of radiopharmaceuticals. When the half-life of the parent is longer than that of the daughter by a factor of 10 or more, there is a transient equilibrium in which the daughter decays with an apparent half-life equal to that of the parent. The parent-daughter activity relations are expressed by:

$$\frac{dN_1}{dt} = -\lambda_1 N_1(t)$$

$$\frac{dN_2}{dt} = \lambda_1 N_1(t) - \lambda_2 N_2(t)$$

where $N_1(t)$ and $N_2(t)$ are the number of radioactive atoms of the parent and the daughter, respectively. For initial conditions $N_1(t) = N_0$ and $N_2(t) = 0$, and for a decay constant of the daughter λ_2 more than ten times that of the parent λ_1 ($\lambda_2 \geq 10\lambda_1$), after a certain time t_m at which the daughter's activity reaches a maximum, the activity of the daughter can be approximated by:

$$\lambda_2 N_2(t) = \lambda_1 N_0 e^{-\lambda_1 t}$$

The most commonly used is the ^{99}Mo-^{99m}Tc generator, in which 86% of ^{99}Mo disintegrations decay to ^{99m}Tc. ^{99}Mo has a half-life of 67 hours, while ^{99m}Tc has a 6-h half-life. The parent ^{99}Mo is deposited on an alumina (Al_2O_3) column in the chemical form of ammonium molybdate. When the radioisotope decays to ^{99m}Tc, the decay product becomes $^{99m}TcO_4$ (pertechnetate) that is separated from the column by passing saline solution through it. The saline solution containing sodium-pertechnetate (Na-$^{99m}TcO_4$) is collected into a sterile, pyrogen-free, empty vial. This process is named elution of the column and the radioactive solution in the vial is named the eluate. The activity of ^{99m}Tc is removed by elution when it is needed for clinical imaging. After approximately 22 h, ^{99m}Tc is completely regenerated again by the decay of ^{99}Mo (Figure 10.3). Because about 50% of the maximum activity is reached after 8 h of eluating,

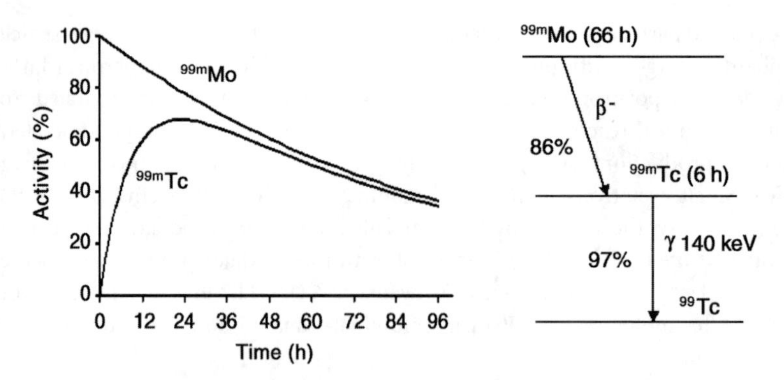

FIGURE 10.3 Activities of parent (^{99}Mo) and daughter (^{99m}Tc) as a function of time in a ^{99}Mo-^{99m}Tc generator. Right: A simplified radioactive decay scheme for ^{99}Mo.

the generator can be eluated every few hours if necessary. The availability of ^{99m}Tc 24 h/day, its physical properties, such as emission of exclusively gamma rays with a suitable energy (140 keV) for imaging, and the short half-life of 6 h have made this radioisotope the most convenient for gamma camera studies. In addition, its chemical properties allow labeling numerous compounds used for diagnostic studies of the thyroid gland, skeleton, kidneys, cardiac muscle, lungs and brain. For all theses properties, ^{99m}Tc is the most commonly used radioisotope for clinical studies with gamma camera.

Other commercially produced generators are the ^{82}Sr-^{82}Rb (Cardiogen-82, Bracco Diagnostics Inc.) and the ^{81}Rb-^{81m}Kr generators. The daughter ^{82}Rb is a positron emitter with a half-life of 1.2 min and has been used in myocardial perfusion studies using PET.[2] The parent ^{82}Sr has a half-life of 25 days. The ^{81}Rb-^{81m}Kr generator yields a radioisotope with a 13 sec half-life emitting gamma rays of 190 keV, while the parent ^{81}Rb has a half-life of only 4.7 h. It has been used for lung studies.[3] Other radioisotope generators have been investigated but not introduced into the clinical practice.

10.3 Radiopharmaceuticals

An estimated 10 to 12 million nuclear medicine diagnostic and therapeutic procedures are currently performed each year in the United States (Nuclear Medicine Society statistic). Unlike MRI and CT, nuclear medicine uniquely provides information about both the function and structure of organ systems within the body. While the introduction of ^{131}I for treating thyroid disease in 1946, followed a few years later by ^{131}I thyroid imaging, marks the beginning of nuclear medicine, it was the discovery of ^{99m}Tc in 1937 and the subsequent development of the first commercial ^{99m}Tc generator in 1964 that lead to the tremendous growth of nuclear medicine. For nuclear imaging, ^{99m}Tc has become the universal isotope because of its virtually ideal physical characteristics for scintigraphic applications (i.e., generator produced, 6-h half-life, 140 keV gamma radiation) and its versatile chemistry that can be manipulated to label a variety of ligands. The Mo/Tc generator can be shipped to laboratories for the production of single dose ^{99m}Tc radiopharmaceuticals on site making ^{99m}Tc by far the most utilized radioisotope in nuclear medicine. Other isotopes require cyclotron or reactor generation, which are more costly and less available for emergency or rapid administration.

Today, there are nearly 100 nuclear medicine imaging procedures available using various single photon emission isotopes and positron emission isotopes (Table 10.2). The characteristics required for an ideal radiopharmaceutical for nuclear medicine imaging are: (1) efficient accumulation and retention in the target organ, (2) rapid clearance from background (tissue and blood), (3) no accumulation in nontarget tissue, (4) no side effects, (5) low cost (^{99m}Tc), (6) easy preparation (kit formulation) and (7) discrimination between different types of the similar disease (high specificity).[4] Applications to specific organ systems, or for the diagnosis of various diseases, are described in the sections below, but it is by no means exhaustive. The availability of ^{18}F and, specifically, ^{18}F-fluorodeoxy-D-glucose (^{18}FDG) has allowed for the practical application of PET. The short half-life of most PET isotopes, with the exception of the 110-min half-life of ^{18}F, makes them impractical for routine use because they require a cyclotron on site at the hospital. Gamma emission imaging has been successfully applied to almost every organ of the body (brain, bone, heart, kidney, lung, neuroreceptors) as well as sites of inflammation, atherosclerosis, thrombosis and cancer. The molecular nature of nuclear medicine imaging leads to unique noninvasive pharmacokinetics modeling applications. Numerous examples of quantitation of neuroreceptor binding and distribution, blood flow and metabolism have been described in diverse clinical settings.[5-12] The future of nuclear medicine imaging radiopharmaceuticals lies primarily in the development of new ligands for ^{99m}Tc (for SPECT) and ^{18}F (for PET) to carry the radioisotope to the site of application without compromising the biological activity of the ligand molecule rather than in the development or discovery of new radioisotopes.

10.3.1 Cardiology

Nuclear cardiology imaging enables the examination of the heart at the tissue level. In addition to visualization of tissue perfusion, imaging with radionuclide tracers may reveal the functional consequences of an anatomic coronary artery stenosis and even differentiate viable myocardium from irreversible scar. For patients with suspected coronary disease, myocardial perfusion imaging has superior sensitivity and specificity compared to routine stress testing and provides information regarding the extent, severity and location of coronary artery disease (CAD).[13] Since the introduction of ^{201}Tl in the 1970s,[14] many agents have been examined clinically for the diagnosis of CAD. Many more agents have been tested in animals and humans and showed promise but failed to gain FDA approval. In addition to monitoring tissue perfusion, various agents have been investigated for measuring metabolism, viability, hypoxia/necrosis/infarct, atheroma and cardiac sympathetic nerves (Table 10.3). Single photon emission computed tomography (SPECT) is the mainstay of perfusion imaging while positron emission tomography (PET) continues to be the modality of choice for agents that track metabolism. This section will describe the state of cardiac radiopharmaceuticals and describe accepted criteria for the design of the ideal perfusion agent.

Table 10.3 Radiopharmaceuticals in Nuclear Cardiology

	SPECT (mechanisms)	PET (mechanisms)
Perfusion	^{201}Tl (potassium analogue)	^{38}K (potassium)
	^{99m}Tc-sestamibi (passive diffusion)	^{15}O water (difussion)
	^{99m}Tc-tetrofosmin (passive diffusion)	^{82}Rb (potassium analogue)
	^{99m}Tc-teboroxime (passive diffusion)	^{13}N ammonia (metabolic trapping)
	^{99m}Tc-furifosmin, Q12 (passive diffusion)	^{62}Cu PTSM (lipophilicity)
	^{99m}Tc-N-NOET (passive diffusion)	
	^{99m}Tc-albumin microspheres (blood flow)	
Viability	^{201}Tl (Na^+-K^+ ATP-ase)	^{18}F FDG (fluorodeoxy-D-glucose)
	^{99m}Tc-glucarate (cell damage)	^{13}N L-Glutamate (amino acid metabolism)
	^{99m}Tc-nitroimidazole (hypoxia)	^{18}F Misonidazole (hypoxia)
Metabolism	^{99m}Tc-fatty acid	^{11}C palmitate (fatty acid metabolism)
	^{123}I-BMIPP (fatty acid)	^{11}C acetate (oxidative metabolism)
	^{123}I-IPPA, (fatty acid)	^{11}C (^{13}N) amino acids (metabolism)
		^{18}F FDG (fluoro deoxy-D-glucose)
		^{15}O oxygen (oxygen consumption)
Sympathetic Innervation	^{123}I MIBG (norepinephrine analogue)	^{18}F metaraminol (adrenergic neuron density)
		^{11}C-HED, hydroxyephedrine (adrenergic neuron density)
Other	^{111}In platelets (thrombus)	^{11}C (^{13}N) amino acids (protein synthesis)
	^{111}In antimyosin (cell damage)	
	^{99m}Tc red blood cells (blood pool)	
	^{125}I and ^{123}I fibrinogen (thrombus)	

TABLE 10.4 Properties of ^{201}Tl and ^{99m}Tc

Advantages of ^{201}Tl	Disadvantages of ^{201}Tl	Advantages of ^{99m}Tc
Rapid myocardial extraction	Low energy emission (69–83 keV) attenuated by overlying tissue	The 140-keV gamma ray emission is ideally suited for imaging on a standard gamma camera
Minimal uptake by abdominal organs during exercise	Long physical half-life, unfavorable dosimetry and limited counting statistics	Less attenuated by soft tissue compared to the energy emissions of ^{201}Tl
Redistribution of ^{201}Tl permits differentiation of ischemia from scar	Cyclotron-generated, costly and difficult to maintain on hand for acute dosing in patients with chest pain	The shorter half-life (6 h) compared to ^{201}Tl (73 h) permits greater administered ^{99m}Tc activity and improved counting statistics
Not significantly affected by cardiac drugs	Slow redistribution results in long imaging sequences	Generator produced, more readily available for urgent use
Diagnostic and prognostic implications of ^{201}Tl lung uptake		

10.3.1.1 Single Photon Emission Agents

^{201}Tl, in the chemical form of thallous chloride, has been the principle tracer used in myocardial perfusion imaging for more than two decades. Its uptake closely follows that of potassium.[15] Since the early 1980s, numerous myocardial perfusion tracers have been developed that take advantage of the favorable physical imaging properties of ^{99m}Tc (listed in Table 10.4). The quality of images obtained with ^{99m}Tc-labeled radionuclides is superior to images obtained with ^{201}Tl because a dose 10 to 20 times higher of ^{99m}Tc can be administered, yielding images with higher count density. Additional information regarding left ventricular function (e.g., wall motion and ejection fraction) via ECG gating can be obtained simultaneously with myocardial perfusion imaging using ^{99m}Tc-labeled agents.[16] Figure 10.4 shows images from a typical nuclear myocardial perfusion protocol.

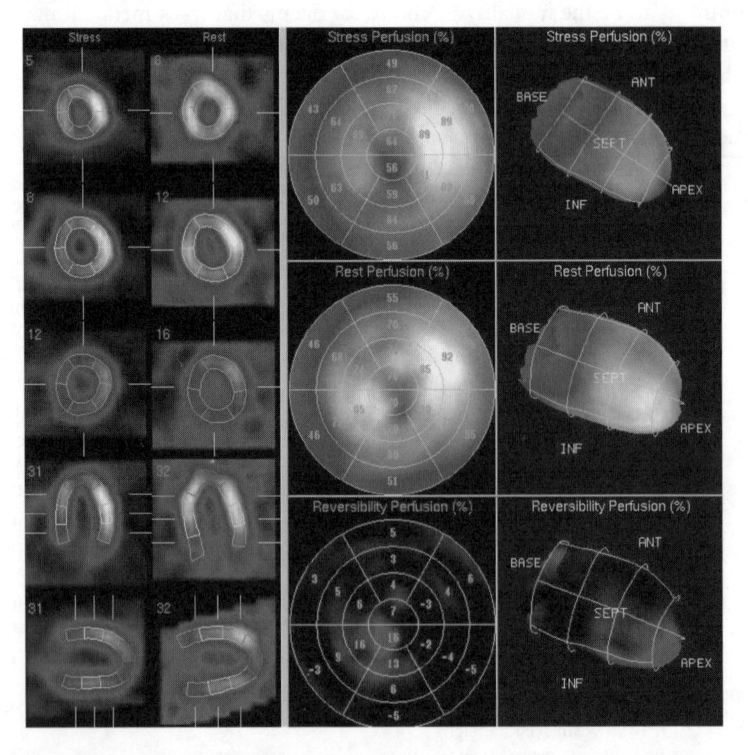

FIGURE 10.4 Myocardial perfusion SPECT with two radioisotopes (^{201}Tl for rest and ^{99m}Tc-sestamibi for stress) analyzed by using the Quantitative Perfusion SPECT (QPS) software. Images indicate probable infero-apical ischemia. (Courtesy of Dr. Jack Ziffer, Director of Cardiac Imaging, Baptist Hospital of Miami, Miami, FL.)

Table 10.5 Properties of an Ideal Myocardial Perfusion Tracer

1.	Uptake like a chemical microsphere (i.e., uptake closely related to myocardial blood flow over a wide range of normal, ischemic and augmented flows)
2.	Prompt uptake under temporary hemodynamic conditions, including peak exercise (i.e., high extraction fraction)
3.	Negligible interference with myocardial visualization from adjacent organs and tissues (i.e., Compton scatter)
4.	No significant attenuation of myocardial tracer activity by tissues between the heart and the activity detector
5.	Constant location and concentration of tracer in the myocardium during image acquisition
6.	Lack of interference with tracer uptake into the myocardium by pharmacological agents or impaired myocardial metabolism
7.	High photon flux detectable on standard imaging equipment
8.	Low tracer cost
9.	High tracer safety
10.	Rapid tracer availability for imaging patients with acute chest pain syndromes

^{99m}Tc is eluted from the ^{99m}Mo generator as pertechnetate (TcO_4^-) and injected in a different chemical form, achieved through commercially available kits, containing components to reduce pertechnetate to a lower oxidation state and form the desired technetium complex. Most cardiac ^{99m}Tc tracers are cationic (+1) complexes, though two neutral complexes have been introduced. The ^{99m}Tc agents were developed to mimic ^{201}Tl while taking advantage of the superior physical properties of ^{99m}Tc. While ^{201}Tl behaves as a potassium analogue and so is taken up via the Na^+-K^+-ATP-ase pump as well as by passive diffusion, most ^{99m}Tc agents do not appear to utilize Na^+-K^+-ATP-ase. For the case of the ^{99m}Tc myocardial perfusion agents, their uptake is by passive diffusion.[17] Other radioisotopes have been incorporated into tracers with cardiovascular SPECT applications but have had limited use either because of cost or instrumentation constraints, or both. For example, the chemistry of isotopes of iodine and indium is much less complex than that for technetium.[18] However, long physical half-life, emission energy, biological activity or cost has made them less desirable than technetium.

10.3.1.1.1 Experimental Models

When comparing the strengths and weaknesses of the various tracers, the properties of an ideal perfusion agent should be considered (Table 10.5). Various animal models have been used to compare and contrast the agents. Each model is designed to examine individual aspects of the tracer's characteristics.[19] Isolated cells and subcellular compartments (mitochondria, membranes) are useful for screening complexes with potentially favorable cell uptake and offer a measure of the apparent volume of tracer distribution independent of blood flow and plasma binding. Tracer extraction and retention during clinically relevant flows can easily be measured with the isolated perfused rat or rabbit heart. The influence of pharmacological agents on tracer uptake and retention can be examined with both isolated cell and organ models. The *in vivo* canine model allows for the examination of tracer kinetics in the presence of cardiac recirculation and allows the direct comparison of ischemic and nonischemic tissue in a single heart with endogenous blood plasma components. Each model is useful to characterize different properties of cellular tracers. Direct comparison between tracers has been hampered by methodological differences among experimental studies. For example, normalization of data plots of myocardial tracer activity vs. myocardial blood flow has varied substantially from study to study.[20,21] Flow rates and perfusate or suffusate in isolated heart and cell studies vary among labs. Additionally, methods for calculation of heart-to-organ tracer activity ratios have not been fully standardized.

10.3.1.1.2 ^{99m}Tc-sestamibi

^{99m}Tc hexakis-2-methoxyisobutyl isonitrile (^{99m}Tc-sestamibi) has been extensively studied clinically and in animal models. It is a monovalent cation consisting of a central Tc(I) core surrounded in an octahedral configuration by six identical methoxyisobutyl isonitrile ligands coordinated through the isonitrile carbon atoms. This structure is associated with sufficient lipophilicity to enable it to partition across biological membranes.[22] ^{99m}Tc-sestamibi is not actively transported across cell membranes but is strongly dependent on plasma and mitochondrial membrane potentials.[15] At 60 min after injection, approximately 1% of administered ^{99m}Tc-sestamibi is localized in the heart, 5.6% is localized in the liver, and 0.9% is localized in the lung.[23] High hepatic clearance requires rest images to be performed 60 min after administration and stress images performed 15 min after administration.

Lipophilicity is an essential property of first pass myocardial perfusion agents because it enhances the extraction efficiency by the heart and increases their blood clearance rate due to accumulation in the liver and skeletal muscle.[24] For ^{99m}Tc isonitrile compounds, it has been shown that increasing lipophilicity by adding alkyl groups can increase the myocyte uptake and accumulation of the agent.[25] However, increasing lipophilic properties too much results in greater nonspecific retention in the lung as well as increased accumulation in the liver,[26] which will interfere with the cardiac apex image. Chemical modifications of existing compounds have been made to modify the agents' metabolism. For instance, Barbarics et al. suggested that the substitution of an ethyl ether group into ^{99m}Tc-sestamibi may enhance substrate recognition by degradation enzymes and increase its potential for enhanced liver metabolism and thus hepatobiliary clearance.[22]

10.3.1.1.3 ^{99m}Tc-teboroxime

A second class of ^{99m}Tc myocardial imaging agents is the baronic acid adducts of technetium dioxime or BATO compounds. ^{99m}Tc-teboroxime has been approved for clinical use by the FDA but has not gained acceptance due to its rapid myocardial clearance. The kinetic properties of teboroxime translate into a requirement for rapid clinical imaging. As with ^{99m}Tc-sestamibi, ^{99m}Tc-teboroxime is highly lipophilic. Unlike ^{201}Tl and ^{99m}Tc-sestamibi, ^{99m}Tc-teboroxime has a neutral valence that permits it to diffuse rapidly back out of the myocardium after initial rapid uptake. ^{99m}Tc-teboroxime functions as a nearly pure myocardial blood flow tracer with little sensitivity to metabolic impairment compared with either ^{201}Tl or ^{99m}Tc-sestamibi.[27] A brief blood pool phase of approximately 0.5 to 1.5 min follows intravenous ^{99m}Tc-teboroxime injection. Myocardial uptake is apparent within 1 min after tracer injection. Although initially low, hepatic activity becomes prominent by 5 to 10 min after teboroxime injection and can interfere with visualization of the inferior wall of the left ventricle. Myocardial washout is rapid, with a half-time of approximately 6 to 12 min following intravenous injection.[28] Consequently, imaging should be started within 2 min following tracer injection and completed over approximately 10 min.

10.3.1.1.4 Radiochemical Basis of Imaging

The design of new ^{99m}Tc-containing tracers has been guided by observations of the relationships between basic biological and chemical properties and corresponding myocardial images. ^{99m}Tc-1,2-bis(dimethylphosphino)ethane $(DMPE)_2\ Cl_2$, the first ^{99m}Tc-containing myocardial imaging agent to be investigated in humans,[29] yielded excellent myocardial visualization in dogs, cats, rats and baboons, but virtually no detectable myocardial activity in pigs and highly variable activity in humans.[30] The Tc(III) complex, $(DMPE)_2\ Cl_2$, undergoes reduction *in vivo* to a neutral Tc(II) complex, allowing it to wash out of the heart rapidly and to be taken up into the liver.[31] Changes in oxidation state of ^{99m}Tc to the Tc(I) complexes, $(DMPE)_3$ and hexakis *t*-butylisonitrile (TBI) largely eliminated myocardial washout, but resulted in prolonged blood pool activity in the former and excessive tracer activity in the lungs for the latter.[32] A more successful approach to reducing excessive myocardial washout and hepatic uptake of tracer has involved the addition of ether functionalities. Addition of symmetric ether groups to the diphosphine backbone of $(DMPE)_2\ Cl_2$ led to the synthesis of ^{99m}Tc-tetrofosmin.[33] Replacement of the diphosphine backbone of $(DMPE)_2\ Cl_2$ with a Schiff base N_2O_2 ligand and moving the phosphorous atoms and ether functionalities to a separate pair of pendant ligands led to the mixed ligand complex, furifosmin (Q12) and related compounds.[34] In an attempt to design a compound that mimics the differential washout properties of ^{201}Tl, an ester pendant group was added to furifosmin.[35]

10.3.1.1.5 Second Generation ^{99m}Tc Myocardial Perfusion Agents

Similar to ^{99m}Tc-sestamibi, ^{99m}Tc-tetrofosmin and ^{99m}Tc-furifosmin (Q12) are cationic lipophilic complexes concentrated in the myocardial mitochondria.[36,37] Both have similar first pass extraction, minimal myocardial clearance and clear rapidly from the blood pool, which facilitates the use of rapid imaging protocols. Variations of the mixed ligand complexes have been introduced that show promise in animal studies.[19] *Bis*(*N*-ethoxy,*N*-ethyl-dithiocarbamato)nitrido Tc(V)^{99m} is a neutral lipophilic myocardial imaging agent referred to as TcN-NOET. TcN-NOET has been shown to have greater uptake into the myocardium, 3 to 5% of injected dose 60 min after tracer injection but blood clearance appears to be slower. The mechanism of TcN-NOET uptake is probably passive and it appears to remain trapped in the cell membrane.[38] Reversibility of perfusion defects with TcN-NOET has correlated well with ^{201}Tl redistribution.[39]

10.3.1.2 Positron Emission Tomography (PET)

Limitations inherent to the use of nonphysiologic single photon-emitting radiotracers have limited the quantitative power of SPECT. The use of positron emission radiolabeled tracers offers the potential for *in vivo* quantification of specific biological processes. With the introduction of PET, physiological tracers, which allow the synthesis of naturally occurring and biologically active compounds, have been developed (Table 10.3). Therefore, in addition to myocardial perfusion and function, the importance of energy metabolism in maintaining cardiac performance has been recognized.[16] PET imaging is uniquely quantitative, and allows for accurate attenuation correction of emission data, higher efficiency, more counts (better statistics) and better contrast resolution than single-photon systems. Substances of physiologic interest can be labeled so that perfusion and metabolically important biochemical pathways can be assessed.[40]

One PET tracer deserves special discussion. ^{18}FDG has become the most important radiopharmaceutical for the clinical application of cardiac PET. The mechanism of ^{18}FDG localization in cardiac (and cancer) cells is illustrated in Figure 10.5. Following the intracellular transport, ^{18}FDG is phosphorylated into ^{18}FDG-6-phosphate. Unlike glucose-6-phosphate, ^{18}FDG-6-phosphate does not react with glucose-6-phosphate isomerase. Because ^{18}FDG-6-phosphate does not enter glycolysis or participate in glycogen synthesis, the radioactivity in the tissue may represent the integral of glucose phosphorylation. Thus, imaging of tissue ^{18}FDG uptake permits the assessment of exogenous glucose utilization and has been considered the gold standard for tissue viability. PET remains a complex and costly procedure because of the need for a cyclotron or generator production of radioisotopes and radiochemical synthesis, the demands of the detection system and the complex biological behaviors of tracers. The technical difficulties of performing protocols with short half-lives and the high cost of maintaining PET instrumentation has limited the use of PET imaging to the largest institutions. Recently, multiple coincidence detection (MCD) imaging has allowed the detection of ^{18}FDG on a SPECT camera[41] and made the use of ^{18}FDG imaging more practical for many institutions.

10.3.1.3 Comparisons of Current SPECT Agents

Table 10.6 lists the properties of the current SPECT myocardial perfusion tracers. ^{99m}Tc myocardial imaging tracers are needed that permit convenient, brief imaging sessions and define accurately myocardial viability as well as perfusion. Second-generation ^{99m}Tc myocardial imaging agents, including tetrofosmin, furifosmin and ^{99m}TcN-NOET, were developed as an attempt to combine the favorable physical imaging properties of a ^{99m}Tc complex with improved target-to-nontarget tracer distribution

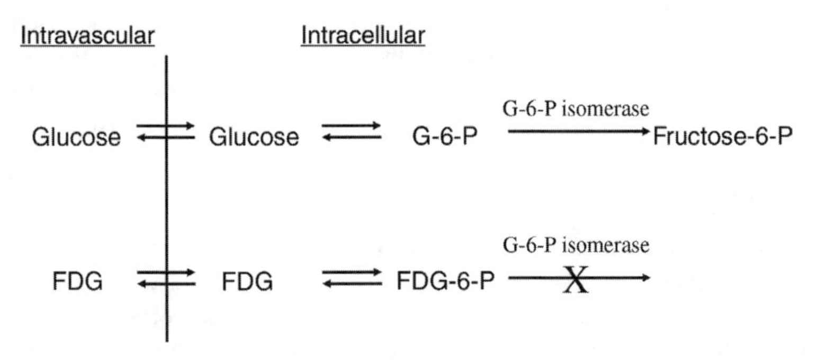

FIGURE 10.5 Mechanism of ^{18}FDG localization and uptake in cancer cells.

Table 10.6 Properties of ^{201}Tl and ^{99m}Tc Myocardial Perfusion Tracers

	^{201}Tl Element	Sestamibi Isonitrile	Teboroxime BATO	Tetrofosmin Diphosphine	Furifosmin Mixed Ligand	NOET Nitrido
Charge	Cation	Cation	Neutral	Cation	Cation	Neutral
Uptake	Active	Passive	Passive	Passive	Passive	Passive
Preparation	Cyclotron	Kit	Kit	Kit	Kit	Kit
Emax	0.69–0.73	0.39	0.72	0.24	0.26	0.54
Myocardial clearance	$T_{1/2}$ ~ 6 h	Minimal at 5 h	$T_{1/2}$ ~10 min	Minimal at 3 h	Minimal at 4 h	$T_{1/2}$ ~4 h
Injection to imaging time	1–15 min	15 min (stress) 60 min (rest)	1–2 min	~ 15 min	~ 15 min	30 min
Differential washout	Yes	Negligible	Yes	Negligible	Negligible	Yes
SPECT studies	Yes	Yes	Possible	Yes	Yes	Yes
Gated SPECT	No	Yes	No	Yes	Yes	No
% ID in heart (at 60 min rest)	1–2.7	1.0	Minimal, due to washout	1.2	1.2–2.3	3–5
Heart/liver (at 60 min rest)	2.6	0.3–0.6	Minimal, due to washout	1.4	1.0–1.6	0.6
Blood pool initial $T_{1/2}$	5 min	2.2 min	<2 min	<5 min	1.8 min	4.7 min
Effective dose equivalent	2.6 rem/ 2 mCi	1.1 rem/ 30 mCi	1.8 rem/ 30 mCi	0.8 rem/ 30 mCi	0.9 rem/ 30 mCi	0.7 rem/ 30 mCi
Clearance	Renal	Hepatic	Hepatic	Hepatic	Hepatic/ Renal	Hepatic/ Renal

to enable myocardial imaging early after tracer injection. These second-generation tracers may also provide valuable insights into the synthesis of future tracers, which, in addition to providing accurate assessment of myocardial perfusion, can accurately measure myocardial metabolism and viability. Gated SPECT with myocardial perfusion tracers may allow the evaluation of ventricular function in addition to perfusion, though gated SPECT evaluates function at the time of image acquisition and not at the time of injection. Potentially, a tracer could be developed that can track cardiac function at the time of injection, perfusion at the time of early uptake and tissue metabolism or viability by examining the fate of the tracer at later times.

^{201}Tl continues to be used widely for noninvasive detection of CAD and identification of viable myocardium. The physical imaging properties of ^{99m}Tc are clearly superior to those of ^{201}Tl, so that the challenge remains to develop a ^{99m}Tc myocardial tracer with biological properties that compare favorably to those of ^{201}Tl. Thus, ^{99m}Tc myocardial tracers are needed with: (1) improved tracer localization in the myocardium, (2) better tracer contrast between ischemic and normal myocardium, (3) improved detection of myocardial viability and (4) reduced interference from tracer activity in nontarget organs, particularly the liver and lungs. Progress has been made in developing ^{99m}Tc myocardial imaging agents that represent advances in these areas, but substantial further improvements in tracer development are needed.

10.3.2 Oncology

Nuclear medicine can be useful in the staging and therapy management of cancer. The earliest application of nuclear medicine imaging was in oncology using ^{32}P [42] and the first practical radioisotope for tumor imaging in humans was ^{67}Ga.[43] Nuclear medicine, particularly PET, is important in the diagnosis, treatment planning and the evaluation to treatment response in patients with cancer.[44,45] The radionuclide bone scan using ^{99m}Tc diphosphonate to diagnose the extent of metastases is the most frequently used

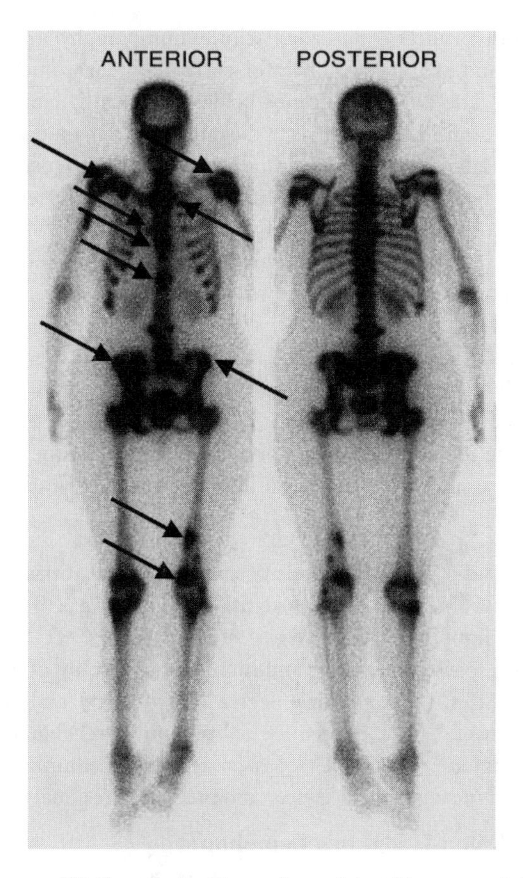

FIGURE 10.6 Planar bone scan of ^{99m}Tc-pyrophosphate of a patient with metastatic breast cancer. Note multiple lesions indicating metastatic tumors of the bone, only some of which are indicated by the arrows. (Courtesy of Dr. Jack Ziffer, Director of Cardiac Imaging, Baptist Hospital of Miami, Miami, FL.)

nuclear medicine procedure in cancer imaging (Figure 10.6). Tracer uptake is related to osteoblastic activity and local blood flow. It is highly sensitive and has the advantage of imaging the entire skeleton. The application includes evaluation of metastases, assessment of the response to therapy and guiding radiation therapy planning.[46] The whole-body bone scan is indicated to help stage cancer that is potentially metastatic, or in patients experiencing bone pain to help make decisions on treatment strategy and has a clinical role in detecting recurrent metastatic disease.[47] However, nuclear medicine lacks the anatomical detail of CT or MRI. Solid tumors are often first observed by CT, but treatment management is often compromised when relying on CT or MRI findings because the anatomical response often lags the metabolic response to cancer treatment. For instance, a reduction in tumor metabolic activity measured by ^{18}FDG PET may be an early indicator of tumor response to anticancer treatment and may be useful in evaluating the anticancer activity of new drugs. In addition, compared to other positron emitters, the half-life of 110 min of ^{18}FDG allows the time required to do whole body scan of patients searching for tumors and metastases. Experimental and clinical studies have demonstrated that ^{18}FDG uptake in cancer cells correlates with the tumor growth rate, tumor metastatic potential and the number of viable tumor cells. The Whole body scan is used to search for secondary tumors away from the primary tumor site. Such a procedure aids in the differentiation of metastatic from nonmetastatic, and therefore surgically resectable, tumors.[44]

10.3.2.1 Breast Cancer

While mammography is the standard method for diagnosing breast cancer, PET tracers such as ^{15}O, ^{62}Cu-PTSM, ^{11}C-L-methionine and ^{18}FDG have been used to detect, evaluate and assess treatment response of primary and metastatic breast cancer.[48] So-called scintimammography may be best used when x-ray mammography, ultrasound and MRI prove unhelpful, particularly for women with dense breasts or who have had previous surgery.[49] The differentiation of benign from malignant disease may possibly avoid needless and painful needle biopsies, and deliver a diagnosis quicker than waiting for biopsy results to return from the pathology lab. ^{201}Tl, ^{99m}Tc-sestamibi and ^{99m}Tc-tetrofosmin are useful in detecting primary tumor lesions of the breast, but ^{18}FDG PET imaging may have greater potential for differentiating malignant from benign legions and in monitoring metastatic disease.[49] ^{99m}Tc-sestamibi was used to monitor tumor angiogenesis, a prognostic indicator of breast cancer, and P-glycoprotein expression, associated with therapy response, in patients with breast cancer.[50-52] For breast cancer, the most powerful outcome is the degree to which axillary lymph nodes are involved.[53] Sentinel lymph nodes may be identified following interstitial injection of ^{99m}Tc-labeled colloids and then biopsied.[54] ^{18}FDG PET has been particularly useful in lung, breast and soft tissue sarcomas. ^{18}FDG PET with CT is useful to evaluate patients with lung nodules preoperatively. ^{18}FDG PET is also useful in determining the metastatic state of breast cancer since finding these tumors may not be possible using other imaging modalities.[55] ^{67}Ga-citrate has been found to be useful in the detection of primary breast lymphoma.[56]

10.3.2.2 Lung Cancer

Although radiography, CT and MRI are methods of choice, radiopharmaceuticals such as ^{67}Ga-citrate and ^{99m}Tc-labeled monoclonal antibodies, somatostatin analogues (e.g., ^{111}In octreotide and the recently approved ^{99m}Tc-depreotide), lipophilic cations (e.g., ^{99m}Tc-sestamibi, ^{99m}Tc-tetrofosmin) and PET tracers (e.g., ^{18}FDG) have been used to diagnose, stage and monitor the therapy of lung cancer.[57,58] Both ^{18}FDG PET and ^{99m}Tc-depreotide SPECT have a high degree of sensitivity and specificity in patients with suspected or known lung cancer.[59] ^{99m}Tc depreotide scintigraphy is reliable in detecting solitary pulmonary nodules of 1 cm in diameter.[58] ^{99m}Tc-MAA (macroaggregated albumin) used in conjunction with standard spirometry is useful in staging lung cancer and predicting residual function following surgery.[57]

10.3.2.3 Hodgkin's and Non-Hodgkin's Lymphoma

^{67}Ga has a high clinical value in the management of lymphoid patients, i.e., staging, diagnostic follow-up and as an indicator of prognosis. Diagnostic modalities such as CT and MRI appear to be inferior to ^{67}Ga scintigraphy in the evaluation of disease after treatment, for instance, in differentiating residual disease from scar.[60] Gallium scan predicted the survival of patients with diffuse large cell non-Hodgkin's lymphoma following chemotherapy. Scintigraphy with ^{67}Ga-citrate is important in the management of the disease by detecting residual disease or relapse after treatment, monitoring response during therapy and providing prognostic information, with sensitivity higher for Hodgkin's disease compared to non-Hodgkin's lymphoma.[61] ^{67}Ga scintigraphy has a sensitivity of 76 to 100% and specificity of 75 to 96% to determine if a residual mass detected by CT following therapy is residual cancer or made up only of fibrosis and necrosis.[62] So, while CT is the primary imaging modality for staging, if a tumor is ^{67}Ga avid before treatment, it can serve as its own control on serial examinations. Then, posttreatment, a negative ^{67}Ga image will indicate absence of disease.[62]

10.3.2.4 Brain Tumors

The uptake of tracers by brain tumors requires either a disruption of the blood-brain barrier or the presence of cells that are highly metabolic compared to surrounding tissue. Blood-brain barrier radiopharmaceuticals (e.g., Na-$^{99m}TcO_4$, ^{99m}Tc-DTPA, ^{201}Tl and ^{67}Ga-citrate) are excluded by normal brain cells, and so their uptake into the brain indicates a disrupted blood-brain barrier.[63] A disrupted blood-brain barrier is a characteristic of brain cancer, if not due to brain injury. If able to cross the blood-brain barrier, charged tracers such as ^{99m}Tc-sestamibi and ^{201}Tl are taken up by brain tumors with good specificity (91 to 100% for ^{201}Tl and ^{99m}Tc-sestamibi, respectively) but with slightly less sensitivity (about 71% for each).[64] ^{201}Tl SPECT was used to determine viability and ^{99m}Tc-DTPA human serum albumin was used to assess tumor vascularity during gamma knife radiosurgery in brain surgery.[65] Results showed that tumor viability occurs before tumor shrinkage, indicating earlier treatment success than might be detected by CT. Since tumors tend to have higher metabolic activity than surrounding tissue, the uptake of ^{18}FDG has provided prognostic information of primary brain tumors, though it may be more useful to evaluate the degree of malignancy and treatment effect.[66]

10.3.2.5 Head and Neck Cancer

^{201}Tl SPECT correctly identified positive nodes and was correctly negative when CT was falsely positive in a study of head and neck lesions, and also may be useful in the follow up of patients receiving radiation or chemotherapy.[67,68] It is useful in confirming the presence of local recurrence and metastases. Radio-guided sentinel lymph node biopsies following an interstitial injection of ^{99m}Tc-colloids may aid to stage cutaneous melanoma of the head and neck. ^{99m}Tc-sulfur colloid of 2.5 to 1,000 nm injected interstitially are engulfed by macrophages. Colloids less than 400 nm drain directly into the lymphatic system and will concentrate in the closest downstream lymph node. Metastatic cells of cutaneous melanomas, if present, should also be expected to collect in these nodes. Subsequently, nuclear scintigraphy identifies those nodes for needle biopsy. [69]

10.3.2.6 Special Conditions

Tumors are targeted due to their increased metabolic activity,[70] their high vascularity[71] and the leakiness of their capillary network.[51] The hypoxic fraction of tumors is likely to have a prognostic value since tumor hypoxia is associated with increased resistance to therapy.[72] Therefore, another potentially useful approach is to monitor the hypoxia state of the tumor using a hypoxic avid compound, such as the ^{99m}Tc-nitromidazoles or ^{18}F-misonidazole. Such compounds are trapped in hypoxic cells in their chemically reduced state, but are reoxidized in normally oxygenated cells and diffuse back out of the cell.[73] Measuring the tumor oxygenation with ^{15}O PET, either by inhalation of pure $^{15}O_2$ gas or after intravascular injection of ^{15}O-water, may also determine the resistance of a tumor to radio- or chemotherapy.[74,75] The presence of low oxygen areas within the boundary of a tumor may be an indication of the loss of vascularity of the tumor. Antiangiogenesis, the inhibition of the tumor to develop blood vessels, thus allowing the tumor to outgrow its blood supply, is a relatively new area of anticancer therapy. Therefore, angiogenesis or hypoxia imaging may further serve to evaluate the effectiveness of therapy, optimizing patient management,[76] though other, non-nuclear modalities have been investigated to assess tumor vascularity, including Doppler ultrasound, contrast enhanced MRI and CT.[71,77]

10.3.2.7 Mechanisms of Tracer Kinetics by Malignant Tissue

The uptake of agents such as ^{99m}Tc-sestamibi and ^{18}FDG is not specific to cancer cells, but also to a benign disease that may show abnormal metabolic activity. Therefore, the future of nuclear oncology is in cancer-specific imaging and therapy since the commonly used tracers (^{99m}Tc-methylenediphosphonate, ^{67}Ga-citrate and ^{18}FDG) are highly sensitive, but their specificity is low. Radiolabeled monoclonal antibodies may show high specificity and high sensitivity.[78] Tumor-specific agents are actively under development, and some have shown efficacy, for instance, ^{111}In-prostascint for prostate cancer.[79] Peptide-based ^{99m}Tc pharmaceuticals for cancer[80] have the potential for high specificity, a major limitation of most drugs. However, while there have been successes, the results have been largely disappointing due to low tumor accumulation and slow clearance from blood and nontarget tissue.[81] Localizing tumors through radio-labeled antibody binding to tumor-associated antigens is promising, but the problem of low specific activity remains. Nevertheless, with our expanding understanding of the targets expressed by cancer cells, much effort is expended toward understanding the chemistry of radiolabeling receptor-avid peptides.

The presence of the P-glycoprotein efflux system and multidrug resistance (MDR) protein family on the membranes of many cancer cells has been shown to act as the major factor in chemotherapy transport resistance.[82] The overexpression of the efflux systems leads to a decreased bioavailability of the chemotherapy drug leading to the failure of chemotherapy. ^{99m}Tc-sestamibi and ^{99m}Tc-tetrofosmin are substrates for the MDR proteins, due to their positive charge and lipophilicity, and thus may allow for clinical assessment of P-glycoprotein function in cancer patients and for the tailoring of chemotherapy regimens by predicting chemotherapy response.[52,83-85] The newer family of ^{99m}Tc-Q compounds shows even greater affinity for the MDR proteins.[86] The uptake of these compounds following chemotherapy treatment may indicate that the cells have developed drug resistant, and therefore unresponsive to common chemotherapy treatment. Thus, while ^{99m}Tc-sestamibi may be valuable in diagnosing untreated cancer on the one hand,[50] chemotherapy-induced toxicity may also allow for the increased accumulation of these tracers since the uptake of these lipophilic cationic agents is determined largely by the negative internal membrane potential, which is compromised by chemotherapy treatment.[87] Ultimately, these tracers may be valuable in the management of certain cancers, but this particular application is not in general practice.

10.3.3 Cerebral Imaging

SPECT and PET tracers have been employed for measuring blood-brain barrier permeability, cerebral perfusion and cerebral metabolism. The tight junctions between endothelial cells of the brain capillaries exclude many charged molecules[88] forming a protective barrier for the nervous system. Because compounds such as ^{99m}Tc-O_4^- (pertechnetate), ^{99m}Tc-DTPA, ^{99m}Tc-GHA, ^{201}Tl and ^{67}Ga distribute freely in the extracellular space but are normally excluded by the intact blood-brain barrier, their uptake into the brain indicates a disruption of this highly selective barrier.[63] The major PET radioisotope used in brain is ^{18}F. The glucose analogue ^{18}FDG has found wide use in measuring the metabolic activity of the brain.[7] ^{18}F-DOPA is an analogue of the drug L-DOPA used in the treatment of Parkinson's disease and has been used for imaging neurotransmission.[89] Other PET isotopes such as ^{11}C, ^{13}N and ^{15}O are also useful in the brain because they can be used to design a number of biologically active molecules, but due to their short half-lives they are not practical for general use. PET has also shown utility in diagnosing brain tumors,[63,90] epilepsy,[91] traumatic brain injury[92,93] and Alzheimer's.[94]

While magnetic resonance imaging (MRI) is usually the primary modality for epilepsy to detect structural causes associated with epilepsy, PET and SPECT may be used in patients where MRI is normal or conflicts with EEG or clinical findings.[66] The measurement of metabolism with PET is superior to blood flow in interictal studies, but because of the long uptake period of ^{18}FDG, PET is not suited for ictal imaging.[91] In fact, in SISCOM the anatomical MRI imaging is fused with the subtracted ictal and interictal SPECT blood flow image.[95] The SISCOM image may be further applied to the EEG to localize the epileptic focus. Pantano et al. quantitated cerebral blood flow in epilepsy patients with ^{133}Xe inhalation SPECT.[96] Matz and Pitts describe the evaluation of traumatic brain injury patients using clearance techniques, including ^{133}Xe.[97]

^{99m}Tc-ECD and ^{99m}Tc-HMPAO have been widely used for brain perfusion SPECT (Figure 10.7). Both are highly lipophilic neutral compounds that have the ability to cross the blood-brain barrier. ^{99m}Tc-HMPAO is widely available for routine use for cerebral blood flow imaging, but it is unstable *in vitro* unless stabilized with methylene blue, and must be used within 30 min of reconstituting the kit.[98] The tracer's uptake is very fast, followed by a transformation to a hydrophilic compound, which cannot return across the blood-brain barrier.[99] ^{99m}Tc-ECD was developed as an alternative to ^{99m}Tc-HMPAO and can be delivered from the

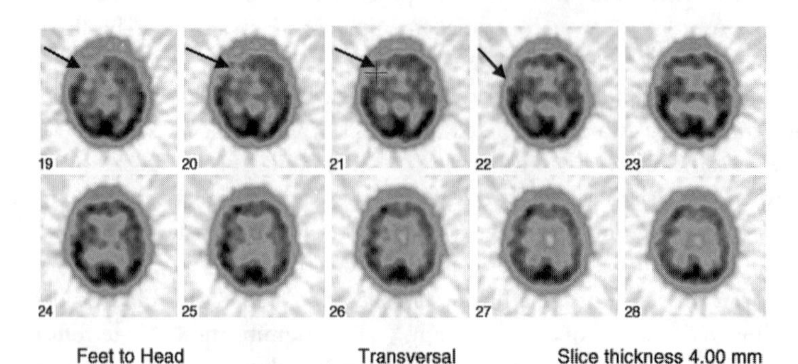

FIGURE 10.7 Transverse slices of a ^{99m}Tc-HMPAO brain SPECT scan showing diminished cerebral perfusion (arrow). (Courtesy of Dr. Jack Ziffer, Director of Cardiac Imaging, Baptist Hospital of Miami, Miami, FL.)

pharmacy as a dose due to its better *in vitro* stability.[100] ^{99m}Tc-ECD enters the brain by passive diffusion where it is hydrolyzed to a negatively charged complex, and thus stuck on the brain side of the blood-brain barrier.[101] Unlike PET, SPECT is inherently difficult to quantitate. As quantitative cerebral blood flow measurements are not practical with ^{15}O due to its short half-life, Murase et al. have reported a strategy for quantitative brain perfusion imaging with dynamic SPECT using ^{99m}Tc-HMPAO and ^{133}Xe.[102] The SPECT tracer useful in cardiac and oncology applications, the lipophilic cationic ^{99m}Tc-sestamibi, shows low uptake into the brain, possibly due to the presence of the multidrug resistance proteins on the luminal side membrane of the endothelial cells of the cerebral capillaries. Other neural applications of nuclear medicine include the neurotransmitter ^{123}I-MIBG used for neural blastomas[103] and dementia.[104]

10.3.4 Renal

Measures of renal function, such as glomerular filtration rate (GFR), effective renal plasma flow (ERPF) and renal tubular mean transit time (MTT) can be made noninvasively with nuclear medicine imaging.[105] Common radiopharmaceuticals for renal scintigraphy include ^{99m}Tc-diethylenetriamine pentaacetic acid (^{99m}Tc-DTPA) for GFR, and ^{123}I or ^{131}I ortho-iodohippuric acid (OIH) for ERPF. ^{99m}Tc-mercaptoacetyltriglycine (MAG3) is similar to OIH but with the more ideal radiotracer (^{99m}Tc), resulting in a lower radiation exposure and better quality images. Figure 10.8 shows a MAG3 renogram protocol. MAG3 is widely used for renal scintigraphy, quantitative measurement of ERPF, diuresis renography and evaluation of renal transplant but has higher protein binding and slower plasma clearance than OIH.[11] Following renal transplant, ^{99m}Tc-MAG3 provides prognostic, diagnostic and monitoring information.[106] An initial renal scintigraphic measure of ERPF following transplant predicts graft survival. Interestingly, the kinetics of ^{99m}Tc-ECD, the neutral lipophilic compound used for brain blood-flow imaging, and similar agents may be closer to OIH for renal imaging than are the kinetics of ^{99m}Tc-MAG3, but further investigation is necessary.[107] GFR may be measured with ^{99m}Tc-DTPA, but the uptake and clearance of MAG3 appear faster than DTPA and therefore may require lower doses. ^{99m}Tc-dimercaptosuccinic acid (DMSA) is used as a renal cortical imaging agent, primarily in infants and children, to assess renal track infection-induced chronic renal scarring, which can lead to hypertension, hyposthenuria, proteinuria and, in severe cases, chronic renal insufficiency.[108] The prolonged renal transit time resulting from renal artery stenosis may be measured with ^{99m}Tc-MAG3.[109] Efforts continue to develop new ^{99m}Tc-based compounds to evaluate renal function.[110] ^{99m}Tc labeled monocloncal antibodies have been studied for the diagnosis of tumors and, more recently, investigated for the diagnosis of liver and kidney functions.[111]

10.3.5 Pulmonary

In general, pulmonary scans are used to measure perfusion (e.g., ^{99m}Tc-macroaggregated albumin [MAA], ^{99m}Tc-DTPA or tracers specific for activated platelets), ventilation (using gases or aerosols) for the diagnosis of pulmonary embolism[112-114] or respiratory epithelial permeability (e.g., ^{99m}Tc-DTPA) to diagnose the efficiency of gas diffusion.[115] ^{99m}Tc-MAAs are micron-size biodegradable particles that, after being injected intravenously, lodge in the arteriocapillary beds during their first pass. Pharmaceuticals for pulmonary ventilation include ^{133}Xe gas, aerosols (e.g., ^{99m}Tc-Technegas, a carbon aerosol) or nebulized ^{99m}Tc-DTPA. These particles lodge in the alveoli and are cleared from the lung by diffusion into the capillaries. Smokers were found to have faster lung clearance of nebulized ^{99m}Tc-DTPA (of approximately 0.6 μm diameter), defined as the time for 50% clearance (t_{50}), as measured from dynamic planar lung images.[115] A combination perfusion/ventilation scan match or mismatch can be used to diagnose pulmonary embolism (Figure 10.9), but the timing of the two scans should be considered for an optimal ^{133}Xe ventilation image due to the different energy spectrum of the two isotopes.[116] ^{67}Ga imaging has been described for diagnosing pulmonary infections in HIV patients.[117] Nuclear medicine imaging is also employed to diagnose lung cancer using ^{99m}Tc-sestamibi, ^{99m}Tc-tetrofosmin or labeled ocreotide, which targets the somatostatin receptor.[112]

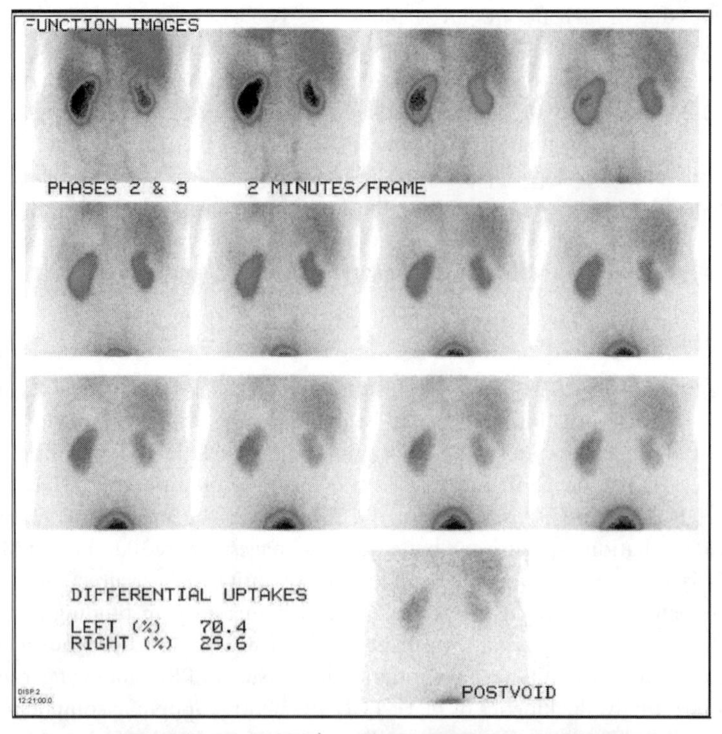

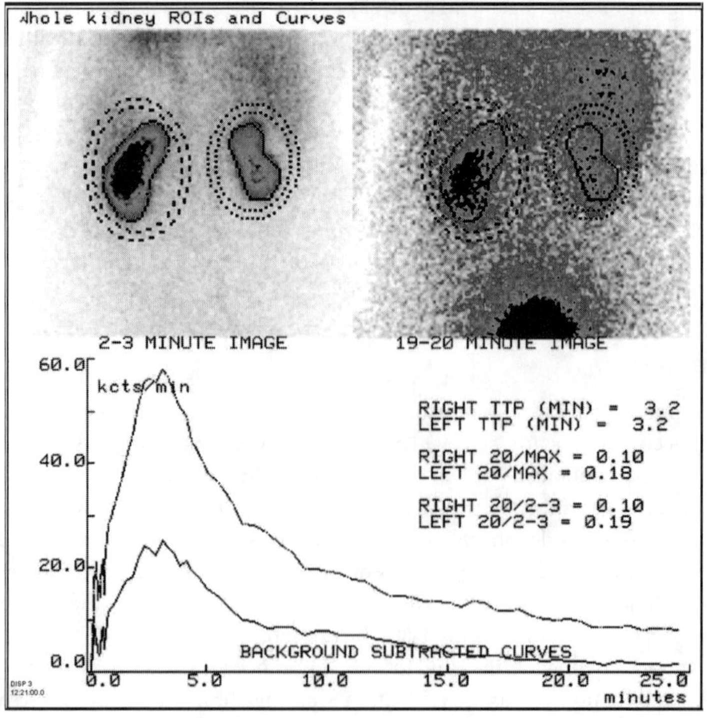

FIGURE 10.8 ^{99m}Tc-MAG3 kidney scan. Semi-quantitative analysis of perfusion and function from the dynamic planar images shows reduced function by the right kidney. (Courtesy of Dr. Jack Ziffer, Director of Cardiac Imaging, Baptist Hospital of Miami, Miami, FL.)

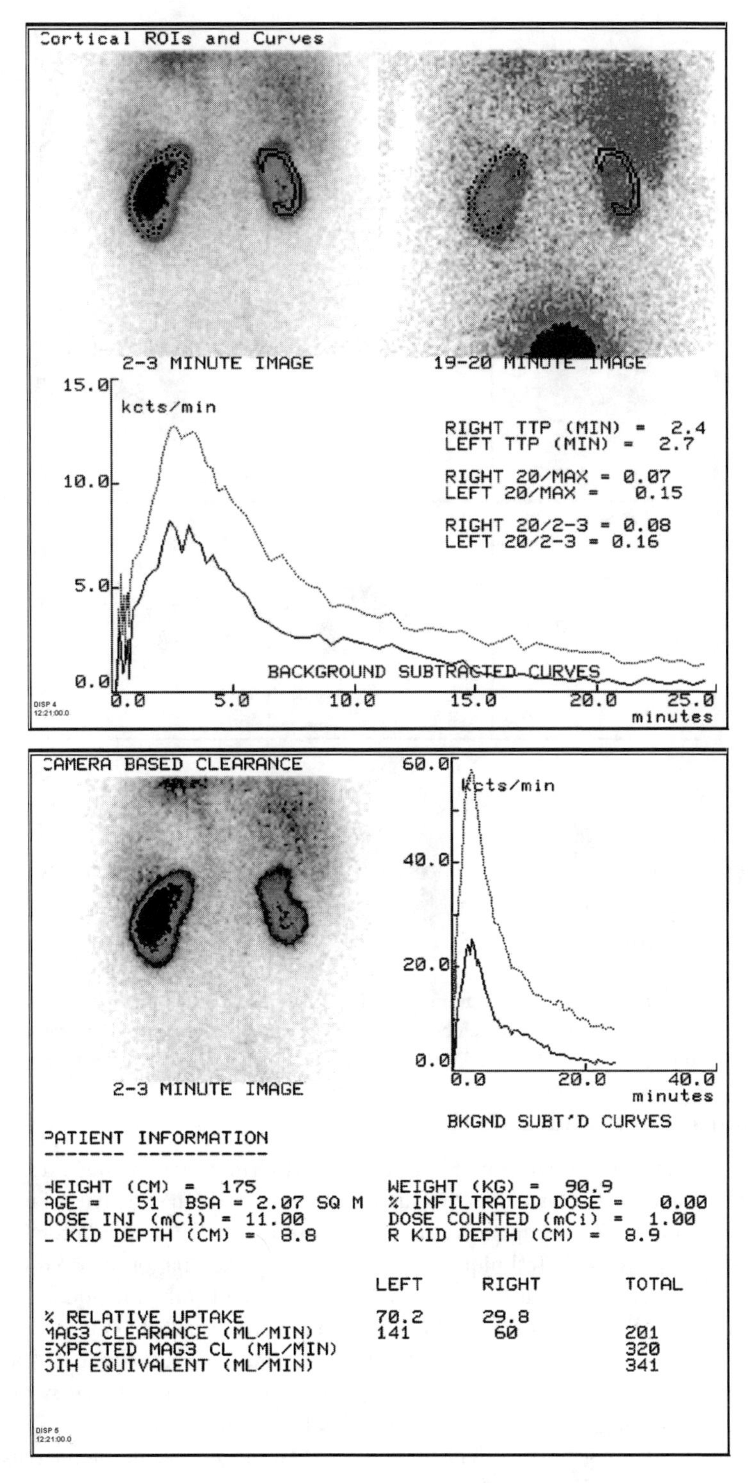

FIGURE 10.8 (CONTINUED) ^{99m}Tc-MAG3 kidney scan. Semi-quantitative analysis of perfusion and function from the dynamic planar images shows reduced function by the right kidney. (Courtesy of Dr. Jack Ziffer, Director of Cardiac Imaging, Baptist Hospital of Miami, Miami, FL.)

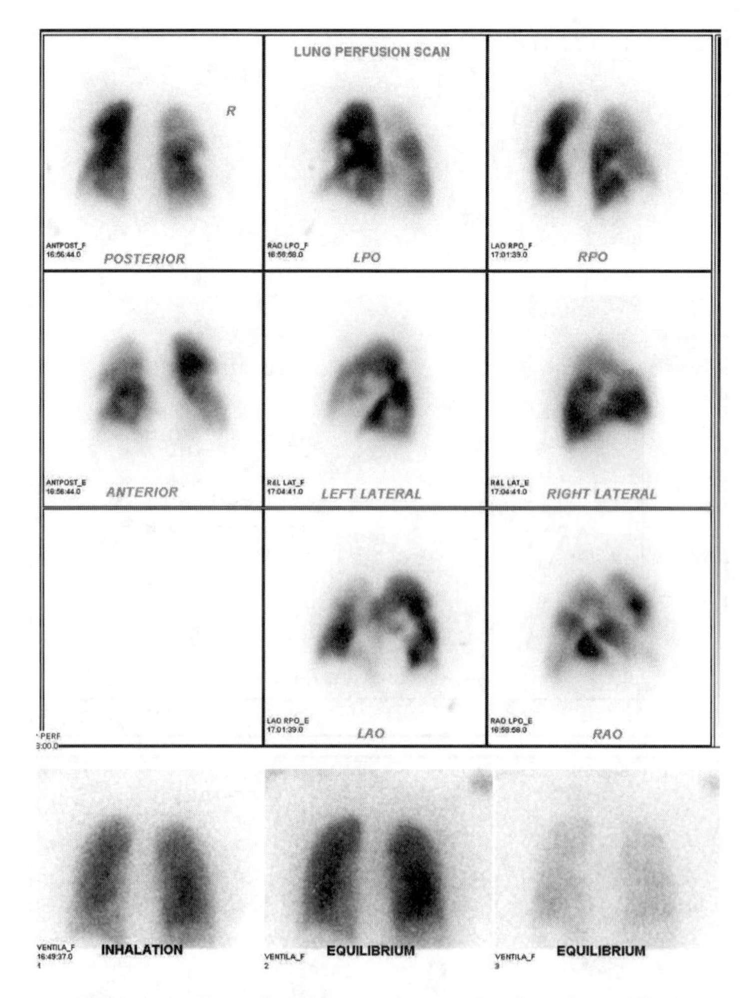

FIGURE 10.9 Lung perfusion (using ^{99m}Tc-albumin macroaggregates) and ventilation (^{133}Xe) scans showing reduced perfusion but normal ventilation. The mismatch between the perfusion and venitlation indicates the presence of a pulmonary emboli. (Courtesy of Dr. Jack Ziffer, Director of Cardiac Imaging, Baptist Hospital of Miami, Miami, FL.)

10.3.6 Inflammation and Infection

Early detection of infection and inflammation, and the determination of the extent, severity and localization of the disease may assist in directing their treatment. The high sensitivity of nuclear medicine imaging has led to a number of radiopharmaceuticals for this use[4,80,118,119] and is becoming useful in the management of AIDS patients.[120] Techniques for detection of inflammation is based on the injection of labeled autologous leukocytes that will be attracted to the site of inflammation, or the injection of radiolabeled compounds that accumulate in the inflammatory site, usually by nonspecific extravasation or binding of inflammatory components. ^{67}Ga-citrate, which binds to transferrin in leukocytes following injection, shows good sensitivity for the detection of chronic inflammation. It is easy to use because it does not require cell labeling, but it is not readily available, nonspecific and delivers a high absorbed radiation dose due to its long physical half-life (78 h).[11] Autologous white blood cells labeled with lipophilic ^{99m}Tc-HMPAO or ^{111}In-oxine for infection and inflammation imaging is also commercially available, but the process is labor-intensive and not suitable for rapid administration. Since all cell types will be labeled by these two compounds, the leukocytes must be separated from other cells, labeled and then reinfused. ^{111}In-oxine has the advantage that it irreversibly binds to cell membranes, while ^{99m}Tc-HMPAO is eluted about 7%/h.[118] Newer compounds employing 1-step ^{99m}Tc labeling methods, e.g.,

^{99m}Tc-labeled antigranulocyte antibodies, antibody fragments, nonspecific IgG, liposomes, chemotactic peptides, interleukins and chemokines, and antimicrobial peptides, have the advantage over autologous leukocyte techniques since they would not require *in vitro* cell isolation; the challenge is to label the peptide with the ^{99m}Tc isotope with high specific activity without modifying the biological activity of the peptide.[80,121]

10.3.7 Atherosclerosis, Thrombosis, and Vascular Imaging

A number of radiopharmaceuticals have been described for imaging thrombus and atherosclerosis.[80,122] Understanding plaque composition and morphology may lead to creative approaches for plaque imaging. While angiography remains the gold standard for the diagnosis of atherosclerosis, attempts have been made to image plaque morphology using ^{99m}Tc-, ^{125}I-, ^{123}I- or ^{111}In-labeled low-density lipoproteins (LDLs) that accumulate in the plaque. Another application is the use of autologous platelets labeled with ^{111}In-oxine, which accumulate at an athersclerosis or thrombotic site. However, similar to leukocyte labeling for infection imaging, it is a labor-intensive process unsuitable for rapid administration. A number of ^{99m}Tc-labeled peptide-based radiopharmaceuticals have been described for thrombus imaging, but clinical success remains elusive, particularly in the smaller coronary or even carotid arteries.[80] Various tracers have been developed to image the blood pool, including radiolabeled red blood cells, liposome blood cell surrogates and radiolabeled molecules bound to natural or artificial plasma proteins.[123]

10.3.8 Thyroid

The first application of nuclear medicine, for both imaging and therapy, was in the thyroid.[124] Iodine is an essential component of hormones produced by the thyroid and it has long been known to accumulate in the thyroid gland. Therefore, radiolabeled iodine, primarily ^{123}I and ^{131}I, is a highly specific radiotracer. Nuclear medicine, particularly ^{99m}Tc-sestamibi, has been used to diagnose hyperthyroidism, though most often accomplished by fine needle biopsy diagnosis, and the diagnosis of thyroid carcinoma, a more common endocrine application for nuclear medicine imaging.[63,125,126] The application of PET imaging with ^{18}FDG and ^{124}I or SPECT imaging with ^{131}I or ^{123}I has been described as a method to plan the dosimetry for ^{131}I therapy of thyroid cancer.[127] Nuclear imaging with ^{201}Tl or ^{99m}Tc-sestamibi is about 80% sensitive for residual and recurrent thyroid cancer of at least 1 cm, but with lower specificity than ^{131}I.[128] ^{201}Tl, ^{99m}Tc-sestamibi, ^{67}Ga and ^{18}FDG are useful for detecting differentiated thyroid cancer following therapy when the ^{131}I scintigram is negative, but are not considered ideal.[125,129] The somatostatin receptor analogue ^{111}I-octreotide, pentavalent ^{99m}Tc-DMSA, and ^{99m}Tc-sestamibi are useful for detecting medullary thyroid cancer, which makes up 5 to 10% of thyroid cancers.[125,129] Metaiodobenzylguanidine (^{131}I-MIBG or ^{123}I-MIBG, a norepinephrine analogue) was developed for adrenal medullae imaging, but is also taken up by many catecholamine-producing tumors.[130,131] High-resolution ultrasound may detect thyroid nodules, differentiated thyroid carcinomas and medullary thyroid carcinoma, but a potential advantage of nuclear medicine imaging, over other imaging methods, is that they allow for whole body imaging and may detect distant metastases.[125]

10.3.9 Methods of Quantitative Analysis of Tracer Kinetics

10.3.9.1 Renal Function

Molecular imaging is uniquely suited for tracer kinetics analysis, particularly by compartmental modeling.[5,132] The elimination of a drug by the kidney is described by the renal clearance, which is simply the volume of plasma that is totally cleared of the drug by the kidney per unit time. The gold standard for quantitative analysis of renal function is the plasma and urine sampling technique. If a substance (e.g., inulin, a 5200 mol wt polysaccharide) is freely filtered and is not reabsorbed or secreted by the renal tubules, then clearance (or GFR) is equal to the rate at which the substance is excreted in the urine × the volume of the urine divided by the plasma substance concentration. ^{99m}Tc-DTPA has suitable characteristics to measure GFR. Therefore, following the administration of a highly extracted tracer, serial blood samples are collected and tracer plasma clearance is calculated by the following equation:

$$Clearance = M_u(T)\int_0^{\infty} C_a(t)dt$$

where M_u is the amount of tracer that has entered the urine up to time T and Ca(t) is the arterial plasma time activity curve (PTAC), the plasma tracer concentration over time. If a substance is completely cleared from the plasma, and only by the kidneys, the clearance rate is equal to the ERBF. IOH and ^{99m}Tc-MAG3 have suitable characteristics to measure ERBF.

The multiple sample blood clearance technique provides only global information and is not considered practical for routine clinical use because it is technically complicated and invasive. Using external detection, regional, or individual kidney ERPF is measured by placing a region of interest (ROI) over the kidney and collecting serial images following tracer injection. ERBF using scintigraphic methods rely on either measuring the amount of a radioactive tracer arriving at the kidney on the first pass following a bolus injection, or on measuring the renal clearance of a tracer with high extraction fraction. The arterial tracer concentration, measured by a serial renogram of the arterial blood pool and corrected for actual plasma concentration, is integrated from 0 to 2.5 min. This is because the tracer is lost from the kidney into the ureter, violating the assumed characteristics of the tracer.[132] Therefore, the measure must be taken before tracer is lost. Renal scintigraphy for the measurement of ERPF, GFR and MTT requires dynamic (planar) imaging, serial imaging of the tracer in the kidneys over time. Though less accurate than collecting multiple plasma samples for plasma tracer activity, dynamic renal imaging is noninvasive, can generate data from individual kidneys, allows for the study of both structure and function, and does not require obtaining serial blood samples when a blood volume ROI (e.g., from the abdominal aorta) is included in the renogram image and used to generate the arterial concentration data.[133] A late plasma sample is, nonetheless, required to correlate the gamma camera counts to actual plasma tracer activity. Various completely camera-based methods have been introduced that do not require blood sampling, particularly important in pediatric imaging when multiple blood sampling is not practical, and requires only about 6 min of patient time. Automated analysis routines, such as the QuantEM® toolbox developed at Emory University, have been incorporated into commercial nuclear medicine systems (Figure 10.8).

GFR can be measured accurately using the Patlak graphical technique (also called the Patlak-Rutland technique).[88] Patlak et al. have described a model-independent approach for measuring the solute transfer flux.[137] With this method, the activity in the plasma and the activity in the tissue are integrated from 0 to T min. The following linear relationship is derived:

$$\frac{A_m(T)}{C_p(T)} = K_i \int_0^T \frac{C_p(t)dt}{C_p(T)}$$

where A_m is the tissue tracer amount and C_p is the plasma tracer concentration. The plot becomes a straight line, and the slope of the line is the tracer transfer flux K_i or, in this case, GFR.

The time for a tracer to pass from the blood to the urine following i.v. injection is called the mean transit time (MTT).[132] The MTT, the time for a bolus of tracer to pass through a volume, V, is related to the flow rate, Q, by MTT = V/Q. The MTT can be measured during dynamic imaging of the kidney using deconvolution analysis, which derives the renal time-activity curve that would be produced from an instantaneous arterial bolus injection.[138] MTT increases when GFR (tubular flow rate, Q) is reduced. Renal artery stenosis has the potential to reduce ERBF, reduce GFR and increase MTT. Other quantitative techniques for evaluating renal function have been reviewed.[11]

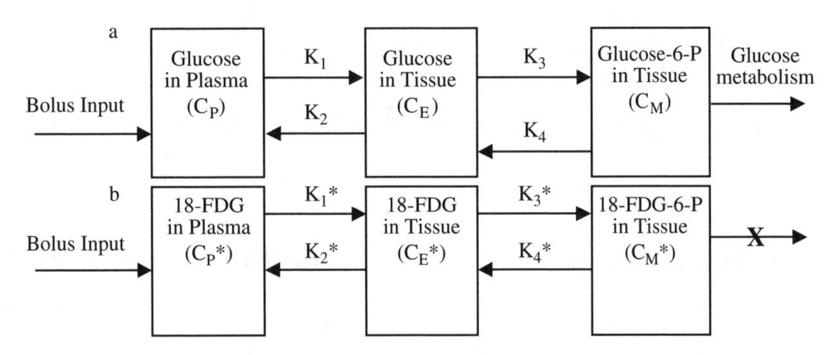

FIGURE 10.10 The three-compartment model for measurement of cerebral metabolic rate for endogenous glucose (a) and with ^{18}F-fluorodeoxy-D-glucose (^{18}FDG) (b). The superscript * denotes symbols that apply to ^{18}FDG, symbols without an asterisk apply to glucose. The parameters k_1* and k_2* refer to the capillary transport of ^{18}FDG between the physical compartments of the plasma and the tissue spaces. The parameters k_3* and k_4* refer to phosphorylation of ^{18}FDG and the dephosphorylation of ^{18}FDG-6-PO_4, respectively. The dephosphorylation of ^{18}FDG-6-PO_4 (k_4*) is often neglected.

10.3.9.2 Glucose Metabolism with ^{18}FDG

Sokoloff et al.[139] described the quantitative measure of cerebral metabolism rate of glucose (CMRglc) in rats using ^{14}C autoradiography, later adapted to PET by Phelps et al.[7] The properties of PET, i.e., the ability to directly measure and correct for photon attenuation, make it uniquely suited for quantitation of cellular tracer kinetics. Attenuation-corrected PET images can be calibrated by using a phantom of known dimensions and activity, to express the activity in each voxel in microcuries per milliliter, and is required to calculate absolute uptake rates of ^{18}FDG. The ^{18}FDG method for evaluating glucose metabolism is widely accepted in the clinical diagnosis of cardiac, cerebral and oncologic pathologies. The rate of ^{18}FDG phosphorylation, which is proportional to the glucose metabolic rate (CMRglc), may be estimated using the three-compartment model (1-plasma, 2-tissue ^{18}FDG and 3-tissue ^{18}FDG-6-PO_4, dephosphorylated ^{18}FDG in tissue [Figure 10.10]) containing four parameters (k1*–k4*). CMRglc is derived from the rate constants, and the plasma level of cold (nontracer) glucose, which is assumed to be in steady state. The mathematical description of the compartmental model is well defined and is described conceptually below.[7] The same abbreviations and symbols found in the literature are used here. The metabolic product of ^{18}FDG, ^{18}FDG-6-PO_4, is trapped in the cell and therefore its rate of accumulation in the cells is directly related to the cells glucose metabolic rate. The method requires dynamic imaging, multiple images of a ROI acquired over time (tissue time activity curve, TTAC), and also requires measuring plasma ^{18}FDG concentration over time (plasma time activity curve, PTAC). CMRglc is derived from the rate constants, and the plasma level of cold (nontracer) glucose, which is assumed to be in steady state.

The three-compartment mode for ^{18}FDG results in the following two differential equations:

$$\frac{dC_E{}^*}{dt} = k_1{}^*C_P{}^*(t) - (k_2{}^* + k_3{}^*)C_E{}^*(t) + k_4{}^*C_M{}^*(t)$$

$$\frac{dC_M{}^*}{dt} = k_3{}^*C_E{}^*(t) - k_4{}^*C_M{}^*(t)$$

From these two simultaneous linear differential equations, $C_E^*(t)$ and $C_M^*(t)$ can be solved in terms of $C_P^*(t)$, the ^{18}FDG in the plasma (PTAC) and $k1^*$–$k4^*$.[7] The ^{18}FDG image sequence from a region of interest (ROI), defined as the tissue time activity curve (TTAC, $C_i(t)$) is equivalent to $C_E(t)$ + $C_M^*(t)$. By measuring $C_i^*(t)$ with imaging and introducing the convolution operation of the PTAC, estimates of $k1^*$– $k4^*$ can be obtained:[7]

$$C_i^*(t) = \frac{k_1^*}{\alpha_2 - \alpha_1}[(k_3^* + k_4^* - \alpha_1)e^{-\alpha_1 t} + (\alpha_2 - k_3^* - k_4^*)e^{-\alpha_2 t}] \otimes C_p^*(t)$$

$$\alpha_1 = [k_2^* + k_3^* + k_4^* - \sqrt{(k_2^* + k_3^* + k_4^*)^2 - 4k_2^* k_4^*}]/2$$

$$\alpha_2 = [k_2^* + k_3^* + k_4^* + \sqrt{(k_2^* + k_3^* + k_4^*)^2 - 4k_2^* k_4^*}]/2$$

where $\otimes$ denotes the operation of convolution. The cerebral metabolic rate of glucose CMRglc can be calculated as

$$CMRglc = [k_1^* * k_3^* / (k_2^* + k_3^*)] * C_P / LC = K^* C_P / LC$$

where the lumped constant (LC) is a calibration term based on the difference in transport and phosphorylation kinetics between glucose and ^{18}FDG, considered to be constant for a specific region of the brain and CP is the plasma glucose concentration.

The rate constants are determined by iterative optimization using measured TTAC and PTAC. A simpler technique that does not depend on dynamic imaging is referred to as the autoradiographic imaging method because it requires only a single ^{18}FDG image, but does require knowledge of global average parameter values. This limitation is easily met for adult human brain glucose metabolism, but may not be strictly met for other applications, e.g., pediatrics or oncology. A disadvantage of this technique is that it requires an accurate measure of the clearance of ^{18}FDG from the plasma by arterial samples. This is clearly an undesirable procedure under any circumstances because it is dangerous and requires additional personnel and expertise, but is particularly unsuitable for pediatric cases. A number of groups have described methods using population average PTACs.[140-142] Nevertheless, quantitative analysis of glucose metabolism by ^{18}FDG imaging is not in general practice.

$$CMRglc = \frac{Cp[C_i^*(T) - \frac{k_1^*}{\alpha_2 - \alpha_1}[(k_4^* - \alpha_1)e^{-\alpha_1 t} + (\alpha_2 - k_4^*)e^{-\alpha_2 t}] \otimes C_p^*(t)}{(LC)\frac{k_2^* + k_4^*}{\alpha_2 - \alpha_1}[e^{-\alpha_1 t} - e^{-\alpha_2 t}] \otimes C_p^*(t)}$$

Patlak's graphical technique may also be applied to glucose metabolism.[137,143] Like the model described above, it requires serial plasma and tissue solute concentrations. However, the method is not specific to a particular compartmental model. Therefore, the method may be more suitable for measuring glucose metabolism in other tissues, i.e., malignant tissue. The ^{18}FDG methods developed originally for brain metabolism studies may also be applied to studying tumor metabolism due to the enhanced glucose metabolism of malignant cells.

10.3.9.3 Standardized Uptake Value (SUV)

Using attenuation-corrected PET images, quantitation of ^{18}FDG uptake in a lesion can be expressed by the standardized uptake value (SUV), which is defined for a voxel as the radiotracer concentration (μCi/ml) divided by the total injected dose and the patient weight[144]

$$SUV = C(t) / (Dose_{inj} * BW)$$

An SUV = 1 would be obtained everywhere if the entire ^{18}FDG distributes uniformly throughout the whole body. Normal SUV depends on the type of tissue. A direct relationship between tumor growth rate and SUV has been reported. Other important facts are that the SUV can differentiate benign from malignant lesions, and residual scar tissue from viable or recurrent cancer cells, and can be used to grade primary cancer lesions and for the follow-up of cancer response to therapy. The main clinical importance of quantitative PET imaging is that metabolic measures are more sensitive indicators of therapy injury to the tumor than changes in size determined by CT or MRI images.

The SUV is a semiquantitative method of evaluating tumor metabolic activity requiring only a single image, and is a compromise between the full kinetic analysis and the subjective visual evaluation. A change in the SUV following treatment is an indication of treatment success, as described for pancreatic carcinoma.[45] The simple SUV method is widely used in cancer diagnosis[45,145] and has also been evaluated in Alzheimer's disease.[146] An alternative method has been introduced that is a hybrid of the SUV method and the more accurate Patlak graphical approach and is described by the following equation:[147]

$$K_i = SUV * K_p(t) * V_0$$

where K_i is the fractional uptake rate (approximated by the Patlak slope), K_p is the plasma clearance rate at time T and V_0 is the initial distribution volume of ^{18}FDG defined by

$$V_0 = Dose_{inj} / (C_p(0) * BM)$$

$$K_p(T) = C_p(0) \Big/ \int_0^T C_p(t)dt$$

$C_p(0)$ is the initial plasma concentration of ^{18}FDG and is determined by extrapolating the relatively slow clearance phase of plasma ^{18}FDG data to zero on a semilogarithmic plot, assuming that in this period of time the intravascular and extravascular ^{18}FDG pool had reached steady state. The method was validated for patients with squamous cell carcinoma of the head and neck.

The three-compartment ^{18}FDG method developed originally for brain metabolism studies may also be applied to studying tumor metabolism. However, the compartmental model requires a homogenous tissue region with respect to blood flow, not satisfied for neoplasms, which are quite heterogeneous. The approach presented by Wu et al. is similar to that described above except that two regions of interest are required, i.e., tumor tissue and normal surrounding normal reference tissue, and six parameters compared to four.[12] The kinetics in the reference tissue is used to account for the normal cells in the cancer tissue region so that the kinetics in the cancer tissue region can be estimated.

10.3.9.4 Tracer Extraction Fraction

As described above in the section on cardiac perfusion applications, extraction fraction, the fraction of a tracer in the arterial supply that is removed in a single pass through the vascular bed, is a measure of the permeability of the capillaries in a tissue bed and is an important characteristic of a nuclear medicine tracer. More commonly, the permeability surface-area product (PS) is used to describe a tissue as it is not generally possible to determine either independently. In general, as the blood flow to a vascular bed increases, the uptake of the tracer increases. However, if the magnitude of the blood flow surpasses the rate at which tracer can be removed from the plasma, tracer extraction will not increase with blood flow, and therefore, extraction fraction falls. Substances with PS products that are very high relative to blood flow are referred to as perfusion limited or perfusion dependent and are useful as perfusion imaging agents. The relationship between *PS*, blood flow *Q* and E_{max}, the maximum instantaneous extraction fraction, is given by

$$PS = -Q * \ln(1 - E_{max})$$

This equation may be applied using experimental models to compare and contrast the characteristics of novel radiopharmaceuticals intended for analysis of tissue perfusion. The influence of pharmacological agents on tracer extraction and retention during clinically relevant flows can easily be measured with the isolated perfused organ or tumor models.[19,148] Compared to the isolated organ models, *in vivo* animal models allow for the examination of tracer kinetics in the presence of cardiac recirculation and allows the direct comparison of ischemic and nonischemic tissue or malignant and benign tissue in the same animal.

10.3.10 Future Directions of Radiopharmaceuticals for Emission Imaging

The molecular nature of nuclear medicine implies almost unlimited possibilities for new diagnostic and therapeutic discoveries, allowing for new and exciting opportunities for evaluating the efficacy of these treatment strategies, particularly as our understanding of peptide chemistry and cell surface protein chemistry improves.[70,123] As new gene and cell replacement therapies are developed, a methodology will be needed to track the bioretention and biodistribution of cell implants. Methods will be required for the *in vivo* monitoring of gene delivery and expression, and directly imaging of drug therapy, rather than simply imaging therapy response.[123,149] The availability of PET isotopes, such as ^{11}C, ^{13}N and $^{15}O_2$ as more hospitals install cyclotrons on site, will allow for the development of many new radiopharmaceuticals based on these biologically important molecules. However, in the short term, the advancement of the art of nuclear medicine and the introduction of new radiopharmaceuticals will largely be dependent on the discovery and development of new molecular ligands for ^{99m}Tc and ^{18}F.

10.4 Instrumentation for Emission Imaging

10.4.1 Gamma Camera

Anger designed the gamma camera in 1958[150] and although significant improvements have occurred in the last decades, the initial concept has remained basically unchanged. Emission images are created by the operation of four major components (Figure 10.11): (1) the multi-hole physical collimator, (2) the detection system, (3) the photon positioning circuitry and (4) the pulse height analyzer (PHA).

10.4.1.1 The Multi-Hole Collimator

A multi-hole collimator, made of a high atomic number substance, is attached to the external surface of the detector head (Figure 10.11). The collimator consists of an array of thousands of holes separated by walls (septa) made out of lead and tungsten. The shape of holes varies in different collimators, but the most common designs are circular and hexagonal shapes. Collimator septa prevent photons from

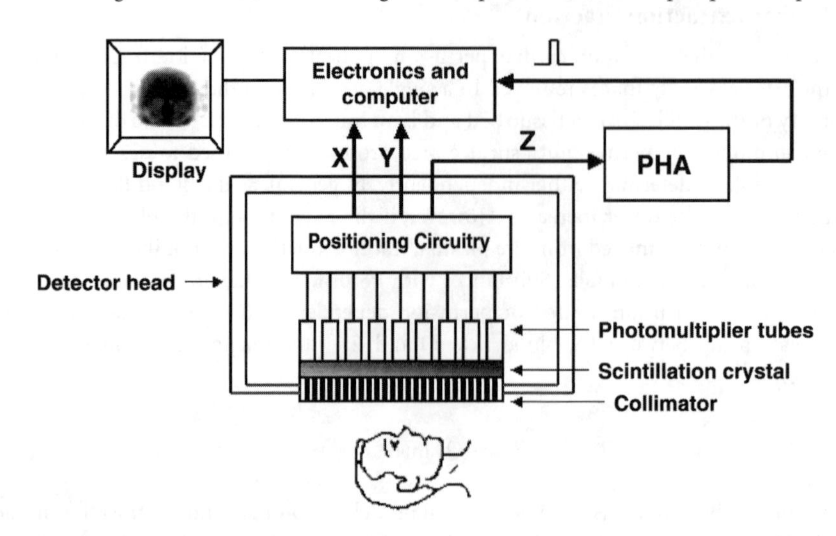

FIGURE 10.11 Simplified diagram of a gamma camera and its major components.

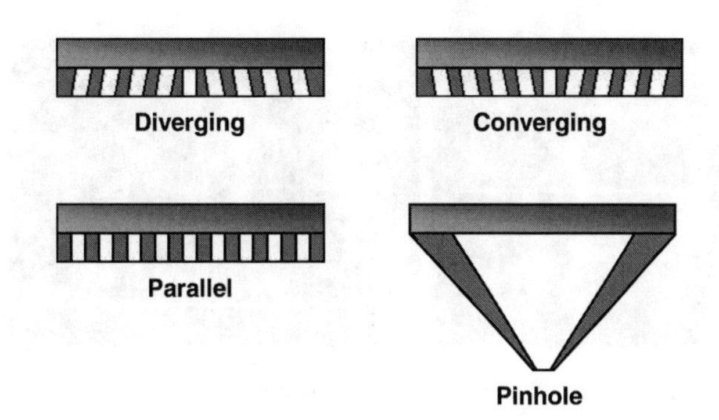

FIGURE 10.12 Types of collimators according to the direction of holes' angles and number of holes.

penetrating from one hole to another so that only those photons traveling parallel to the axes of the holes can reach the detector. Gamma rays traveling in a different angle are absorbed by septa and don't reach the detector surface. The collimator confines the direction of the incident gamma rays to an extremely small acceptance solid angle and makes a projection from the three-dimensional radioactive source onto the two-dimensional face of the detector system. The area of the patient's body that can be imaged by a single view receives the name field of view (FOV) of the gamma camera.

10.4.1.1.1 Collimator Types

The angle of the holes with respect to the detector surface can make the effective FOV equal, smaller or larger than the detector dimensions. According to the relationship between the effective FOV and the detector dimensions, collimators can be categorized in: diverging, converging, parallel and pinhole (Figure 10.12). The holes of the diverging collimator diverge from a common focal point located behind the detector. This collimator produces a minification of the object and consequently increases the effective FOV. This collimator is used when the organs to be imaged are larger than the detector dimensions. The converging collimator has its holes converging toward a common focal point in the direction of the patient. This collimator produces a magnification of the object and is used for imaging small organs or studying small infants. The parallel collimator has all its holes parallel to each other and perpendicular to the detector surface. This collimator projects an image of the same size as the object and is the most commonly used in clinical studies. Finally, the pinhole collimator consists of a cone with aperture in the tip. The image of the object is magnified and inverted with respect to the object. The magnitude of magnification increases as the object approaches the collimator. The pinhole collimator is used for high resolution imaging of small organs. The most common use of the pinhole collimator is for static imaging of the thyroid gland.

10.4.1.1.2 Geometric Efficiency and Spatial Resolution

The number of gamma rays passing through the collimator and reaching the detector depends on the number of holes, the acceptance solid angle and the septal thickness. The geometric efficiency and spatial resolution critically depend on these factors. The geometric efficiency is the percent of the gamma rays emitted by a point source that reaches the detector. Parallel hole collimators allow approximately 0.015% of the emitted gamma rays to reach the detector. Geometric efficiency can be improved by increasing the size of the collimator holes or by increasing the number of holes of smaller diameter but thinner septal thickness. Spatial resolution measures the ability of the gamma camera to identify the exact location at which a gamma ray has been emitted. This is commonly measured in terms of the full width at half-maximum (FWHM) of the line-spread function of the number of radiations or counts detected across the image of a line source (Figure 10.13). Although the spatial resolution also depends on the performance of other major components of the gamma camera, the FWHM is dominated by the collimator's geometric characteristics. The FWHM is a spatially variant function that rapidly broadens as the distance from source to collimator increases. Consequently, the best spatial resolution is nearest the collimator. At the typical organ depth of 10 cm, the FWHM is approximately 10 mm. The spatial resolution can be improved

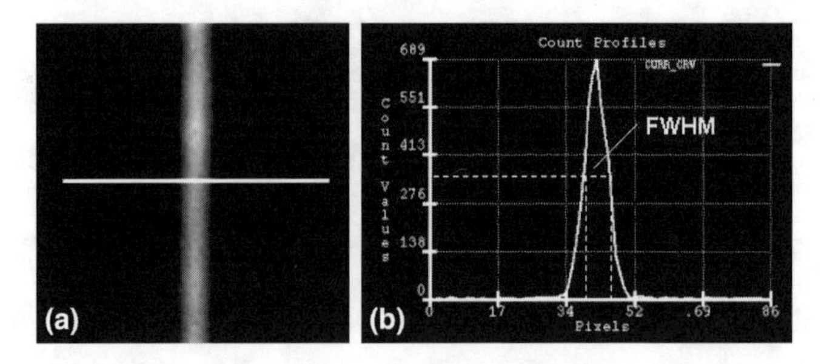

FIGURE 10.13 Determination of full width at half maximum (FWHM) from the counts profile through the image of a line source.

by reducing the size of collimator holes, but then the geometric efficiency is decreased. In theory, both geometric sensitivity and spatial resolution can be improved by increasing the number of holes of smaller diameter and thinner septal thickness. However, very thin septa leads to a high penetration of gamma rays between holes with the subsequent degradation of the spatial resolution. As a consequence of the penetration effect, a minimum septal thickness, determined by the energy of gamma rays, must be maintained. Any variation to collimator parameters to increase geometric sensitivity will degrade spatial resolution and vice versa. Commercially available collimators are designed to establish a trade-off between geometric sensitivity and spatial resolution. Table 10.7 shows some general characteristics of some types of collimators. Manufacturers provide specific characteristics of commercially available collimators. Collimators are constructed for septal penetration less than 5% of gamma rays with the energy at which the collimator has been designed. Low-energy collimators have septal thicknesses of only a few tenths of a millimeter. These septa can be damaged easily by any impact, but they provide the best geometric sensitivity and spatial resolution. Medium- and high-energy collimators require thicknesses of a few millimeters of lead. Larger septal thickness to prevent gamma ray penetration is one major factor limiting the useful energy range of gamma cameras to 360 keV (energy of gamma ray emissions of ^{131}I).

10.4.1.2 The Detector System

Detection is formed by a hermetically sealed scintillation crystal of NaI(Tl) and an array of photomultiplier tubes (PMTs). The scintillation crystal can be either circular with a diameter of 25 to 50 cm, or rectangular with dimensions of about 50 × 40 cm. Modern gamma cameras usually have rectangular crystals. The thickness of the crystal varies from 0.64 to 1.27 cm ($^1/_4$ to $^1/_2$ in.). The array of PMTs is attached to the internal surface of the scintillation crystal (Figure 10.11). The number of PMTs depends on the manufacturer, but in present-day gamma cameras it varies from 37 to 91, usually arranged in a hexagonal closed pack. The detection of a gamma ray starts with its interaction with the scintillation crystal. The gamma ray energy that is absorbed into the crystal is converted into scintillation light. The site at which scintillation light is emitted is identified by the positioning circuitry at the position at which a gamma ray impacted the crystal surface. The scintillation light strikes the photocathode of the

TABLE 10.7 Performance Characteristics of some Typical Parallel Hole Collimators used in Emission Imaging with Gamma Cameras

Collimator Type	Septa FWHM at 10 cm (mm) From the Collimator	Number of Holes	Maximum Energy (keV)	Geometric Sensitivity (%)
LEHR 7.4 mm	0.15	90,000	140	0.019
LEGP 8.8 mm	0.18	86,000	140	0.024
LEHS 13.4 mm	0.18	82,000	140	0.055
MEGP 12.3 mm	1.14	13,000	300	0.018
HEGP 12.5 mm	1.73	7,000	400	0.017

Note: LEHR: low energy high resolution; LEGP: low energy general purpose; LEHS: low energy high sensitivity; MEGP: medium energy general purpose; HEGP: high energy general purpose.

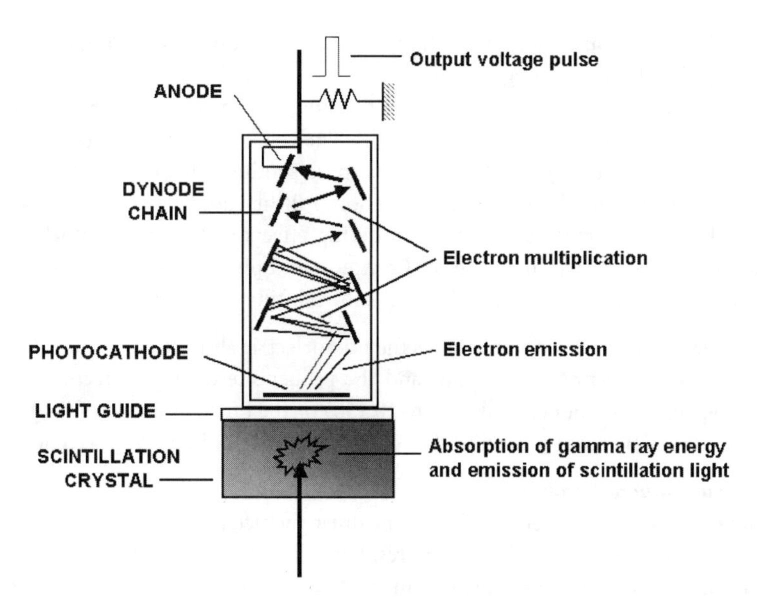

FIGURE 10.14 Operation of a photomultiplier tube coupled to a scintillation crystal.

PMTs nearest to the site of the gamma ray interaction (Figure 10.14). The amount of scintillation light received by each photocathode is inversely proportional to the distance from the PMT to the gamma ray interaction site. The photocathode of the PMT converts the scintillation light into electrons whose number is amplified by a sequence of dynodes to form an output voltage pulse proportional in height to the amount of scintillation light initially received by the photocathode (Figure 10.14). Some gamma camera models use a light guide between the crystal and the PMT array for minimizing loss of scintillation light in those areas not covered by PMTs and improving the light collection uniformity. In old analogue gamma camera models, the light guide was several centimeters thick to make more uniform the detection of those events not directly under a PMT. This effect improves the uniformity of the detector response but degrades the spatial resolution. Modern digital gamma cameras have thinner light guides, or don't have any light guide, and uniformity and other corrections are performed by microprocessors included into the detector head.

There are four possible events when a gamma ray goes through the collimator and reaches the scintillation crystal (Figure 10.15):

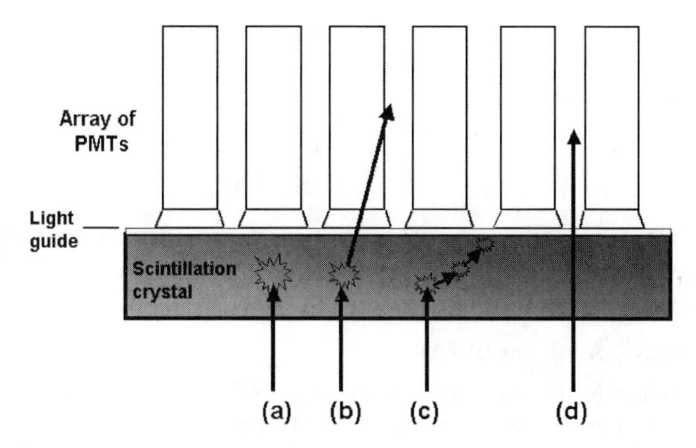

FIGURE 10.15 Probable events during the interaction of a gamma ray with a scintillation crystal: (a) photoelectric absorption, (b) Compton scattering, (c) multiple Compton and a final photoelectric absorption and (d) escape of the gamma ray.

1. Photoelectric absorption. The crystal in the site of interaction absorbs all the gamma ray energy. A fraction of the absorbed energy is converted into scintillation light.
2. Compton scattering. Only part of the gamma ray energy is absorbed in the site of interaction and a fraction of it converted into scintillation light. The rest of the gamma ray energy escapes from the crystal. One or more Compton scattering can be produced before the gamma ray escapes.
3. Compton scattering and photoelectric absorption. All the gamma ray energy is absorbed within the crystal by one or multiple Compton scattering effects and a final photoelectric absorption. Scintillation light is emitted in all sites of Compton and photoelectric interactions.
4. There is no interaction. The gamma ray crosses the scintillation crystal and no energy is absorbed.

The only desirable event for image formation is the photoelectric absorption (Figure 10.15a). This event identifies one radiation impacting the detector and the proper site of the interaction. Events involving Compton scattering either are not detected (Figure 10.15b) or the broad emission of light in multiple sites of interaction does not allow proper identification of the initial site of interaction (Figure 10.15c).

10.4.1.2.1 Gamma Camera Resolving Time

After each gamma ray is detected, there is a finite time during which a new gamma ray interaction cannot be detected as an independent event. This is the resolving time of the gamma camera, which is due to the scintillation and electronic processes involved in the detection of events. The major factor determining the resolving time in modern gamma cameras is the finite time required for the emission of the scintillation light (light decay time) by the scintillation crystal. The NaI(Tl) crystal has a decay time of 230 nsec, releasing the 98% of all scintillation light within 800 nsec. This decay time establishes a limit for the count rate that the gamma camera can resolve. Typical gamma camera resolving times are between 2 and 3 μsec. In present-day gamma cameras, a maximum of 50,000 counts per second (cps) can be recorded without significant loses.

10.4.1.3 Positioning Circuitry

The output signals of each PMT are processed by the positioning circuitry to determine a pair of signal coordinates X,Y corresponding to the gamma ray interaction site with the crystal, and a signal Z whose pulse height is proportional to the total gamma ray energy absorbed into the crystal (Figure 10.11). Former gamma cameras used analog positioning circuitry, but modern models use digital circuitry. In the image formation process, each PMT contributes to the generation of four position pulses or signals named X^+, X^-, Y^+, Y^-. In addition, the voltage output from each PMT is summed to obtain a pulse Z representing the total gamma ray energy absorbed within the crystal. The pulse Z is used to normalize the X and Y signal coordinates according to:

$$x = \frac{X^+ - X^-}{Z}$$

$$y = \frac{Y^+ - Y^-}{Z}$$

The Z normalization is needed to avoid spatial distortions due to statistical variations in pulse heights. If the position pulses are not normalized to the total energy pulse, the events will not be positioned at the same location, even though the interaction site is the same.

10.4.1.4 Pulse Height Analyzer (PHA)

Those gamma rays emitted by the source and absorbed within the crystal by photoelectric effect, produce scintillation light emission just in the site of interaction. This position can be exactly determined by the positioning circuitry and corresponds to the emission of a gamma ray in front of the detector and through the acceptance angle of the collimator's holes. However, some gamma rays can deviate from their original pathway by Compton scattering inside the body of the patient or in the collimator septa. These gamma rays

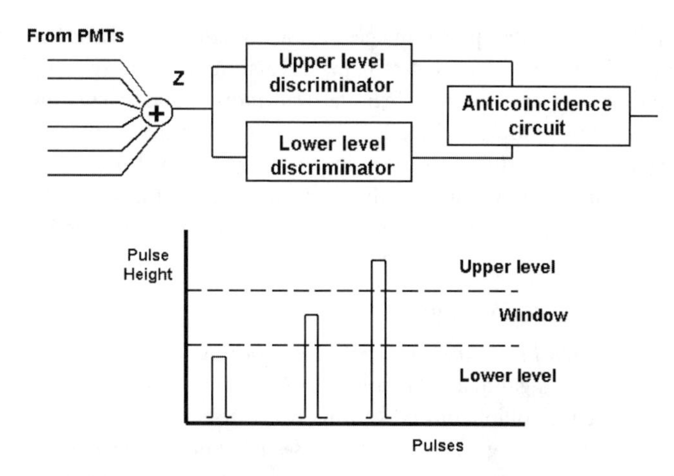

FIGURE 10.16 Operation of the pulse height analyzer. Only those pulses with height within the window should be accepted for counting.

reach the crystal with lower energy than that of the emission. Compton scattering can also be produced within the crystal (Figure 10.15b). All scattered events, if detected, give a mispositioning of the gamma ray emission and consequently degrade the spatial resolution of the gamma camera. Since scattered gamma rays have less energy than that of the original emission, they can be eliminated by using a PHA (Figure 10.16). The PHA eliminates those events whose Z pulse heights are out of a selected energy window. Current gamma cameras can have up to four single PHAs. They can be used singly for various radioisotopes in a multiradiotracer study or in conjunction with one another in the case of radioisotopes with various gamma emissions.

10.4.1.4.1 Energy Resolution

A finite energy window is needed because electronic statistical fluctuations in the detection system produce a gaussian distribution of those pulse heights corresponding to the gamma ray emission energy. The broader the distribution of pulse heights, the higher the probability to include scattered radiations in the energy window. To assess the spreading of the distribution, energy resolution is defined as the FWHM expressed as percentage of the average pulse height around the Gaussian peak. Energy resolution depends on the gamma ray energy, type, and quality of the crystal and associated electronics. For 140 keV and NaI(Tl) crystals, energy resolution varies from 10 to 15%.

10.4.1.5 Storage and Viewing Units

Finally, each gamma ray detected by the camera and accepted by the PHA is collected as a count in the digital storage unit of a computer system coupled to the gamma camera. Simultaneously, the event can create a dot on the viewing screen of a cathode ray tube used for monitoring the acquisition of images or positioning the patient. Other systems display on the computer screen the collection of counts in real-time. The collection and spatial distribution of thousands of counts create the emission image, which is stored digitally for further processing and viewing. Usually, images are collected or processed as a matrix of 64×64, 128×128, or 256×256 pixels. In dynamic studies that require a sequence of images at intervals of seconds or minutes, most common matrix formats are 64×64 or 128×128. Static images use 128×128 or 256×256 pixels. Rotational sequence of images for SPECT usually collects 64 images of 64×64 pixels. A typical SPECT study with 64 projections, 64×64 pixels each and 16 bits per pixel, should require 525 kb of storage space.

10.4.1.5.1 Gated Cardiac Studies

An additional type of study acquires data by dividing the cardiac cycle into 16 or 32 time bins, collecting images for each time bin. Since a time bin in a cardiac cycle is a very small time interval, the content of hundreds of cardiac cycles is added. The final result is a sequence of images corresponding to the variations of activity in the cardiac muscle or in the left ventricle cavity, depending on the radiopharmaceutical, during the cardiac cycle. Gated cardiac planar images are mostly used for studying left ventricular function by imaging the cavity with a radiotracer that remains circulating in blood (e.g., red blood cells labeled with ^{99m}Tc). This study allows assessing the regional wall motion and calculating the left ventricular ejection fraction. Planar images are usually taken in the 45° left anterior oblique (LAO), lateral and anterior positions. Gated cardiac SPECT is most commonly performed for the study of regional wall motion during perfusion imaging by using a radiopharmaceutical that is uptake by the cardiac muscle. During gated SPECT, each projection is divided into eight segments corresponding to eight time bins during the cardiac cycle.

10.4.1.6 Gamma Camera Performance

10.4.1.6.1 Intrinsic Detection Efficiency and Spatial Resolution

Major variables characterizing a gamma camera performance are the intrinsic detection efficiency and the spatial resolution. Since the collimator and gamma ray scattering in the source critically affect both variables, the basic performance of a gamma camera is assessed under scatter-free conditions and without collimator. Those variables determined without the influence of scattered radiations and without collimator are called intrinsic variables, while those determined under scattered radiations and with the collimator in place are called extrinsic variables. Intrinsic detection efficiency is defined as the number of counts per second per unit of activity detected from a point source at a distance of 1 m from the center of the crystal surface. Intrinsic spatial resolution is defined by the FWHM of a line spread function measured by imaging fine slits of a lead mask next to the detector when it is exposed to a distant source of gamma rays. Intrinsic detection efficiency mostly depends on:

1. The thickness of the crystal and the gamma ray energy. The detection efficiency of a $^1/_2$-in. thick NaI(Tl) crystal varies from 90% for 140 keV to about 13% for 511 keV photons. For 140 keV the loss in efficiency drops by 6% when the crystal thickness is reduced from $^1/_2$ to $^1/_4$ in. For higher energies the efficiency loss is more significant, e.g., for 364 keV the efficiency loss is 23% when the crystal thickness is reduced from $^1/_2$ to $^1/_4$ in. Increased detection efficiency can be achieved with thicker crystals. However, thicker crystals degrade spatial resolution due to a higher probability of multiple Compton scattering and a final photoelectric absorption (Figure 10.15c). An additional undesirable effect of thicker crystals is the diffusion of scintillation light over a longer path before reaching the PMTs. The best trade-off of sensitivity and resolution for imaging ^{99m}Tc or ^{201}Tl is a $^1/_4$-in. (0.6-cm) thick crystal. However, this thickness is inefficient for the higher gamma energies of ^{67}Ga, ^{111}In and ^{131}I (Table 10.2). Many manufacturers use $^3/_8$ in. (0.95 cm) thick NaI(Tl) crystals as a good compromise between efficiency and spatial resolution for the range of energies used with gamma cameras.
2. The energy window of the PHA. The wider the energy window, the higher the number of detected gamma rays. However, by widening the energy window, the number of detected scattered events is also increased resulting in degradation of the spatial resolution. Commonly energy windows used in clinical studies are ±10%, or ±15% around the gamma ray emission energy.

Intrinsic spatial resolution also depends on the quantum efficiency (Q.E.) of the PMT photocathode. The Q.E. is the percentage of incident scintillation photons converted to electrons in the photocathode. The number of electrons emitted by the photocathode per incident scintillation photons determines the statistical fluctuation of the PMT output signal. It has been determined that because of the noise uncertainty of current PMT used in gamma cameras, the lowest possible intrinsic FWHM is 4 mm.

10.4.1.6.2 Multidetector Gamma Cameras

Since there is an inverse relationship between detection efficiency and spatial resolution, any increase in intrinsic or extrinsic sensitivity degrades spatial resolution. Increasing the number of counts in an image by prolonging the collection time is not a practical solution because the possibility of patient involuntary motions can introduce image artifacts. In addition, the biokinetics of some radiopharmaceuticals don't allow long collection times. Increasing the amount of the radioisotope is not admissible above certain limits

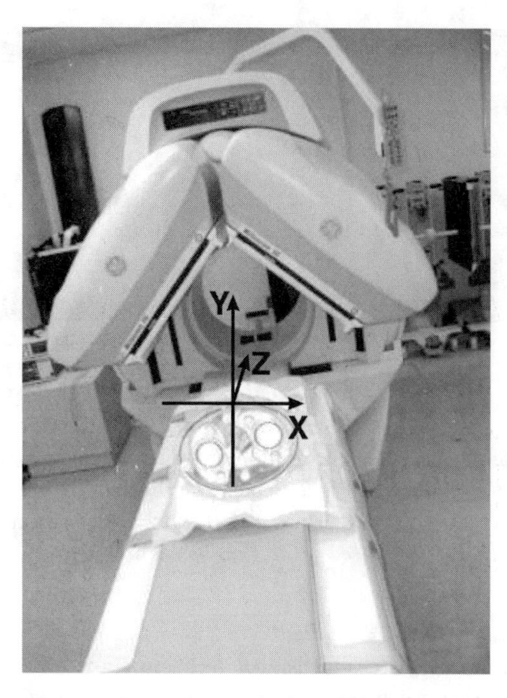

FIGURE 10.17 Dual-head rotating gamma camera with detectors at 90° angle. XY is the transaxial plane. Z is the axis of rotation.

because of dosimetry considerations and the resolving time of gamma cameras. The practical solution to increase both sensitivity and spatial resolution has been the development of multidetector gamma cameras. Two or three detectors can collect a higher number of counts in an acceptable time interval. The higher number of counts that can be collected with multidetectors also allows using high-resolution collimators even if they have a little lower geometric sensitivity. Trionix Research Laboratory and Picker International introduced three-detector systems for SPECT in the 1980s. Today the most commonly used systems are the dual-head variable angle gamma cameras. These systems facilitate the positioning of detectors at an angle of 180° or 90° (Figure 10.17). Detectors at an angle of 180° are used for whole body imaging acquiring simultaneously anterior and posterior views of the body and for SPECT of any organ by rotating the detectors 360° around the body of the patient. Detectors at 90° are used for cardiac SPECT by rotating the detectors 180°, from 45° right anterior oblique position (RAO) to 45° left posterior oblique (LPO) position.

10.4.2 Single Photon Emission Computerized Tomography

The first step in a SPECT study is the acquisition of a set of planar images or projections around the organ of interest by using a multi-detector rotating gamma camera. Detectors are mounted in a slip-rotating gantry (Figure 10.17), which is operated by microprocessor-controlled motors. Typical SPECT studies collect 60 or 64 projections at intervals of 6 or 5.6°. The gamma camera can orbit the patient in two different motion modes: step-and-shoot and continuous. In the step-and-shoot mode, no acquisition of counts is done during the time at which the detector is moving between two angles, while in continuous mode the gamma camera is acquiring data at all times. The mode most commonly used in clinical studies is the step-and-shoot. Projections are collected and stored with matrix format of 64×64 or 128×128.

10.4.2.1 The Filtered Backprojection Method (FBP)

This is the most commonly used method to obtain transaxial slices from projections around the body. The method is based on the application of two mathematical operators to the digital projection data. The first operator filters projections using a reconstruction low-pass frequency filter. The second operator,

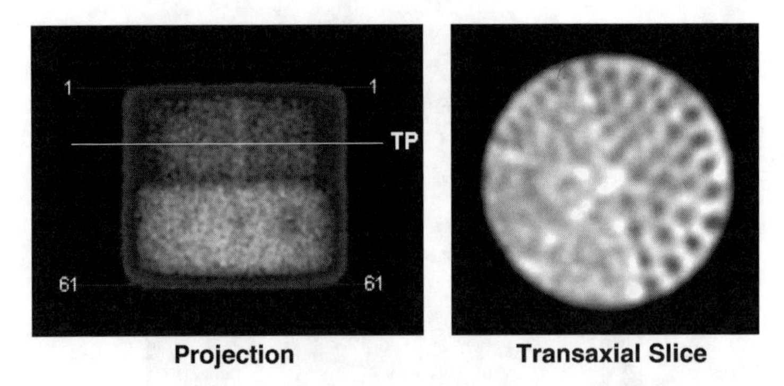

FIGURE 10.18 Projection of a Jaszczak phantom and reconstructed transaxial slice of the plane TP.

named backprojector operator, assigns each projection filtered pixel value, at the selected transaxial plane level (Figure 10.18), to all pixels along a perpendicular line through the reconstructed transaxial image plane. This is done for all pixels in the projection and over all projection angles. The reconstruction is achieved by the superposition of the filtered projection values for all angles. Coronal and sagittal slices are calculated from transaxial slices.

10.4.2.1.1 Degrading Effects in SPECT Studies

The FBP method yields accurate three-dimensional reconstructions of idealized projections free of degrading effects such as the depth-dependent geometric response of the detector, and attenuation and scattering of gamma rays within the patient. When the FBP method is applied to real projections, the reconstruction is significantly limited in terms of accurate quantitation and spatial resolution. The depth-dependent geometric response of the detector is the main cause of loss of spatial resolution. The major contributor of the depth-dependent geometric response effect is the collimator, which rapidly degrades the spatial resolution as the distance source-to-collimator increases. Proton attenuation is the most important source of inaccuracy in SPECT quantitations and the major cause of false positives in myocardial perfusion SPECT studies. Compton scattering is the dominant interaction in tissue for the energy range (50 to 360 keV) used in SPECT. Scattering of gamma rays accounts for approximately 45 and 65% of the total counts of ^{99m}Tc and ^{201}Tl myocardial SPECT studies, respectively. Although the PHA can eliminate scattered photons, the finite energy resolution and small count efficiency of gamma camera detectors require using window energy broad enough to include some scattered events. The presence of scattered photons degrades the reconstructed slices by lowering contrast.

10.4.2.1.2 Attenuation and Scatter Correction

Proper attenuation correction of SPECT studies has been an elusive goal for many years. However, recently, significant progresses have been achieved by using transmission attenuation maps and iterative reconstruction algorithms. These procedures include the transmission attenuation map into the reconstruction process. Attenuation maps are needed in those studies, such as myocardial perfusion SPECT, in which the organ to be imaged is surrounded by a nonuniform absorbing medium. In those SPECT studies in which the absorbing medium can be considered as homogenous and represented by a single attenuation coefficient value, the post-processing Chang's attenuation correction algorithm has demonstrated to be a good approach to the attenuation problem.[151] The Chang's method was designed to work with the FBP method and has been implemented in most commercial SPECT systems. The algorithm is based on dividing each reconstructed pixel by the average attenuation factor for that pixel. The Chang's average correction factor for any pixel (x,y) is given by:

$$c(x,y) = \frac{N}{\sum_{i=1}^{N} \exp(-\mu \cdot r_i)},$$

where N is the total number of projections, μ is the linear attenuation coefficient of the absorbing medium (e.g., soft tissue that can be approximated by water) and r_i is the distance between the pixel (x,y) and the boundary of the medium at the i-th projection. When the source is extensively distributed, the Chang's method can over- or subcorrect some parts of the image. In this case, projecting the corrected data to form a new set of projections performs a second correction. A set of error projections is obtained by substracting each corrected projection from its corresponding original projection. Error transaxial slices are reconstructed by the FBP method and added to the initially corrected slices to create the final attenuation corrected transaxial image.

There are two major types of scattering correction techniques: energy window-based techniques[152] and restoration-based corrections.[153] Energy window-based methods estimate the scatter component by using one or more energy windows abutted to the main energy window. These methods have been implemented by using different procedures, but basically the counts collected in energy windows corresponding to the energy of scattered photons are subtracted from those collected in the main energy window. Although these methods could increase noise, they have demonstrated acceptable clinical performance and are incorporated into many commercial SPECT systems. Restoration-based methods attempt to return scattered photons to their original emission sites. These methods require modeling the scattering process and include it into an iterative reconstruction algorithm. So far, the complexity of these methods and extensive computation required has made them impractical for clinical use.

10.4.2.2 Iterative Reconstruction

These methods are mostly based on the iterative creation of a set of transaxial slices by comparing the real projection data with those reprojected from the reconstructed slices. The initial transaxial slice is calculated by the FBP or from any other initial guess. From the difference between the acquired and calculated projections yields an error which is used to make corrections in the reconstructed slices. These are reprojected again and the same process continues until the difference between acquired and calculated projections is below some defined limit.[154] The most commonly used of these methods is the expectation maximization (EM) reconstruction that maximizes the probability of the reconstructed transaxial slices for the set of projection data.[155] The great advantage of iterative methods is that corrections to attenuation and depth-dependent detector response can be incorporated into the reconstruction process. Iterative methods were well known several years ago, but the required computer time to reach iterative convergence made them impractical for clinical studies. The availability of present-day, faster and more efficient computers has allowed introduction of iterative methods into the clinical practice. The EM method, and its faster variant, the ordered subset expectation maximization (OSEM) technique,[156] have been used for attenuation correction in cardiac SPECT with attenuation transmission maps acquired with point or line sources incorporated into the hardware of SPECT systems. Today, most vendors of SPECT have included into their systems collimated line sources for attenuation correction of cardiac SPECT using attenuation maps and iterative reconstruction methods.[157]

10.4.3 Quality Assurance of Gamma Cameras and SPECT

During the operation of gamma cameras and SPECT systems, several variables must be checked on a periodic basis. These variables are the extrinsic uniformity, spatial resolution and the test of the center of rotation.

10.4.3.1 Uniformity

This variable assesses that the detector yields a uniform image in response to a uniform flux of radiation. Extrinsic uniformity is assessed daily by using a ^{57}Co sheet source of 10 to 20 mCi yielding a count rate between 20 and 50 kcps. Ten million counts are collected to create the uniformity image. Visual inspection of the image can detect nonuniformities higher than 10%. However, a more detailed analysis is required for SPECT studies in which planar nonuniformities are amplified into reconstructed slices. Calculating the integral uniformity of the FOV and of the central FOV (CFOV) quantitatively assesses uniformity. The CFOV is the 75% of the central area of the FOV. Integral uniformity (IU) is defined as:

$$IU(\%) = \frac{Maximum\_pixel\_counts - Minimum\_pixel\_counts}{Maximum\_pixel\_counts + Minimum\_pixel\_counts} \times 100$$

Another variable is the differential uniformity defined by the same equation but only for a series of five consecutive pixels in the x and y directions. Acceptable limits for SPECT systems are:

Integral Uniformity UFOV < 5%
Integral Uniformity CFOV < 5%
Differential Uniformity UFOV < 4%
Differential Uniformity CFOV < 4%

10.4.3.2 Extrinsic Spatial Resolution

This test verifies that spatial resolution is satisfactory for clinical imaging and in good agreement with those benchmark images acquired at the time of the installation or after major reparation of the gamma camera. This test is performed weekly by using a ^{57}Co sheet source and a four-quadrant bar phantom with bar widths of 4.23, 3.18, 2.54 and 2.12 mm. This test is assessed by visual inspection of the bars image looking for distortions on the bars linearity or significant degradation in resolution compared to previous images (Figure 10.19).

10.4.3.3 Test of the Center of Rotation (COR)

This test checks the center of rotation (COR) offset and any tilt of the detector with respect to the axis of rotation. The COR is the intercept between the axis of rotation (Figure 10.17) and a normal from the center of the detector plane when the detector is parallel to the axis of rotation. If the normal doesn't intercept the axis of rotation, the COR offset is calculated as the distance between the normal from the center of the detector plane to the axis of rotation. The COR offset depends on the projection angle and the test calculates the mean and maximum COR offset of the SPECT system. The test is usually performed weekly, but some laboratories prefer a daily check. This is performed by using a point source with 1 to 3 mCi of ^{99m}Tc in a volume of less than 0.2 ml that is positioned at 1 or 2 cm from the axis of rotation. The mean difference between the positions of the point source in relation to the theoretical center of rotation for each projection is determined (mean COR offset). Acceptable limits for 64 × 64 projections

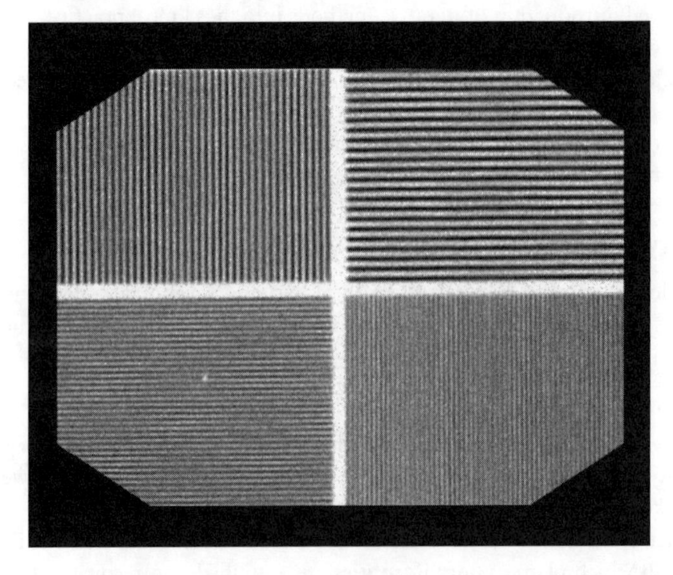

FIGURE 10.19 Image of a four-quadrant bar phantom for weekly quality control of extrinsic spatial resolution of gamma cameras.

are a mean offset of ± 0.2 pixels and a maximum error range of 0.5 pixels. COR offset out of this range can produce blurring and ring artifacts in reconstructed transaxial slices.

10.4.4 Positron Emission Tomography

10.4.4.1 Physical Basis of PET

Positron-emitting radioisotopes tend to be low atomic mass elements, many of them naturally found in the human body, such as carbon, oxygen and nitrogen. Radioisotopes of these elements and others of low atomic weight can label metabolically active compounds and be used for imaging a large number of physiologic and metabolic processes. In addition, the dual positron annihilation radiation of 511 keV (Figure 10.2) makes easier the localization of positron emission by external detectors. PET is based on the simultaneous detection of the two gamma rays emitted during positron annihilation (Figure 10.2). The two 511-keV gamma rays are detected by two opposite detectors and one event, or positron decay, is registered by a coincidence circuit (Figure 10.20) with a narrow acceptance time window (≈15 ns) for the two events. The method of coincidence detection doesn't require physical collimation, resulting in a greater sensitivity and resolution than those of SPECT. In addition, PET is a more quantitative technique allowing photon attenuation correction in a much easier way than SPECT. The total attenuation for the two 511-keV gamma rays is given by:

$$\text{Attenuation} = \exp[-\mu x] \cdot \exp[-\mu(d - x)]$$

$$\text{Attenuation} = \exp[-\mu d],$$

where d is the distance between boundaries in the line at which opposite gamma rays are emitted. Since total attenuation for coincidence events doesn't change anywhere in the line at which opposite gamma rays are detected, the attenuation correction is based on the total attenuation along the distance traveled by the two gamma rays and doesn't depend on the positron emission position. The major shortcoming of PET imaging has been the short half-life of positron emitters (Table 10.2), which has required the installation of a cyclotron in clinical institutions.

10.4.4.2 Development of PET Imaging

Brownell and Sweet at Massachusetts General Hospital obtained the first positron medical image in 1951.[158] They used two single NaI(Tl) detectors moved mechanically to detect brain tumors. The first positron tomographs were developed later using rectangular array of detectors or more advanced model

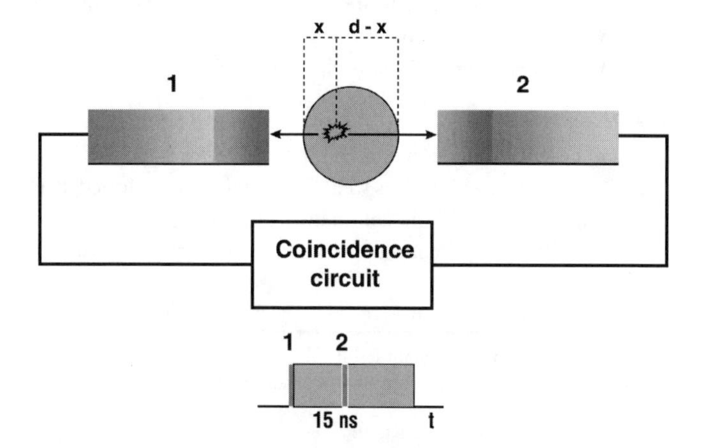

FIGURE 10.20 Coincidence detection of two gamma rays emitted in opposite directions during positron annihilation. An event or positron decay is registered when gamma rays are detected by detectors 1 and 2 within a time window in the coincidence circuit.

TABLE 10.8 Physical Properties and Application of Scintillation Crystals used for Emission and Transmission Imaging

	NaI(Tl)	BGO	LSO	GSO
Density (g/cm^3)	3.67	7.13	7.40	6.71
Effective Z	51	74	66	59
Light decay time (ns)	230	300	40	60
Relative light output	100	15	75	25
Energy resolution at 511 keV	9%	22%	26%	11%
Detection efficiency at 511 keV[a]	56%	82%	60%	74%
Hygroscopic application	Y	N	N	N
	SPECT	CT, PET	PET	PET

[a] Detection efficiency was calculated for thickness of 2.54 cm for NaI(Tl) and of 2.00 cm for BGO, LSO and GSO.

Note: NaI(Tl), thallium-doped sodium iodide; BGO, bismuth germanate; LSO, lutetium oxyorthosilicate; GSO, gadolinium oxyorthosilicate.

using hexagonal and circular array of detectors.[159] A significant improvement was the substitution of NaI(Tl) scintillation crystals by Bismuth Germanate (BGO) crystals[160] with better efficiency for the detection of 511 keV gamma rays (Table 10.8). The first cyclotron for medical use was installed at the Hammersmith Hospital, London, in 1955. A few years later, other cyclotrons were installed in institutions in the United States. All of these units were mostly dedicated to research.

10.4.4.2.1 ^{18}FDG

A significant impact in PET clinical applications was the development of ^{18}F-fluorodeoxy-D-glucose (^{18}FDG) at Brookhaven National Laboratory in 1976. This compound is a glucose analogue, metabolic imaging agent giving precise and regional information of energy metabolism in brain, heart, other organs and tumors (Table 10.9). In 1988 the Health Care Finance Administration approved the reimbursement for PET clinical studies of solitary pulmonary nodule and the staging of nonsmall cell lung cancer. Years later, the reimbursement for the diagnosis of other cancer locations, epilepsy and the study of myocardial viability was approved. Encouraged by the reimbursement of PET clinical studies with ^{18}FDG, centers for the production and regional distribution of the radiotracer have been created nationwide. Simultaneously with the development of regional centers for production of ^{18}FDG, PET instrumentation has been developed and expanded. Many institutions without PET facilities started using mobile PET units several days per week. Major vendors of SPECT systems adapted dual-head SPECT to perform PET by using coincidence circuitry. In recent years, dedicated PET scanners with a full ring of small detectors have been installed in many medical institutions. It is expected that the market for PET scanners surpass the SPECT market by 2003 with revenues of $800 million by 2007.

10.4.4.3 Dual-Head SPECT for PET

Dual-head SPECT with coincidence detection for PET has the advantages of lower cost ($500,000 to $700,000) and the capability to perform SPECT as well. Detectors are positioned at 180° from each other and rotate 360° around the patient. Multi-hole collimators are not used and photons can interact with the crystal at any angle. The position coordinates of gamma ray interactions in each detector are recorded

TABLE 10.9 Clinical Indications for ^{18}FDG-PET in Oncology

Differentiate benign from malignant lesions
Differentiate scar lesions from residual or recurrent malignancy
Monitor cancer therapy efficiency
Detect and identify distant metastasis
Improve cancer staging and consequently the therapeutic choices
Increases accuracy of radiation treatment planning by irradiating the most active tumoral cells with the highest radiation dose

when they occur within the coincidence time window (≈15 nsec). Other modifications to SPECT systems for PET imaging have been to expand the pulse height analyzer range to 511 keV, increase the lead thickness of the detector housing to prevent penetration of 511 keV photons, and implement high-counting rate capabilities. Major limitations are the lower sensitivity and high-count rate performance. The lower sensitivity of the gamma camera's $^3/_8$ in. thickness NaI(Tl) crystals for 511 keV (13%) requires an increase of the thickness of the crystal to $^5/_8$ or 1 in. at the expenses of reducing the resolution in SPECT studies with gamma emitters of lower energy. The absence of the collimator allows a very high flux of photons over the crystal that overwhelms the high count rate capability of gamma cameras. This results in lower quality noisy images. Prolonging the acquisition time to reduce image noise is not a practical solution in clinical studies. Other additional limitations are the higher scattering component and technical problems for correcting photon attenuation. A result of these limitations is that a significant number of lesions 2 cm or less in size cannot be detected. For these reasons, the Center for Medicare and Medical Services has declined reimbursement for most PET studies performed with dual-head SPECT. Consequently, the market for these systems has significantly declined in the United States.

10.4.4.4 Dedicated PET Scanner

The cost of these systems ranges from $1 million to $1.7 million. Sensitivity and high-count rate performance are much higher than those of dual-head SPECT, and corrections for scattering and attenuation allow quantitative studies with ^{18}FDG. Dedicated PET can also perform whole body scans with ^{18}FDG. The limit of lesion detection is between 5 and 7 mm. The scanner is formed by sequential rings of small detectors (~4 mm) that yield an axial field of view of approximately 15 to 20 cm (Figure 10.21). A coincidence event is created for any two detected single events in two opposite detectors within the coincidence time window. Each detector pair is referred to as a line of response (LOR). For each LOR the number of coincidence events is recorded. This information, which is equivalent to SPECT projections, is reconstructed into transaxial images. To avoid coincidences from detectors in different transaxial planes, small retractable septa are located to separate one axial plane of detectors from the others. This tomographic configuration receives the name of two-dimensional mode. Detectors are organized in blocks with 8×8 or 6×6 small crystals, according to the manufacturer. Four blocks form a bucket containing approximately 256 detectors (blocks of $8 \times 8 = 64$ detectors). One ring includes 16 buckets with 4096 detectors. Two rings of detectors in a typical dedicated PET may have, in total, 8192 small detectors (Figure 10.21). Recent advances in PET technology have been the development of lutetium oxyorthosilicate (LSO) and gadolinium oxyorthosilicate (GSO) scintillation crystals instead of BGO for detection of 511 keV gamma rays. LSO has a much lower light decay time and a much higher light output than BGO with a slightly lower detection efficiency at 511 keV (Table 10.8). Limitations of LSO are the intrinsic radioactivity of the material that produces a permanent background. Also, energy resolution is slightly worse than that of BGO. The other

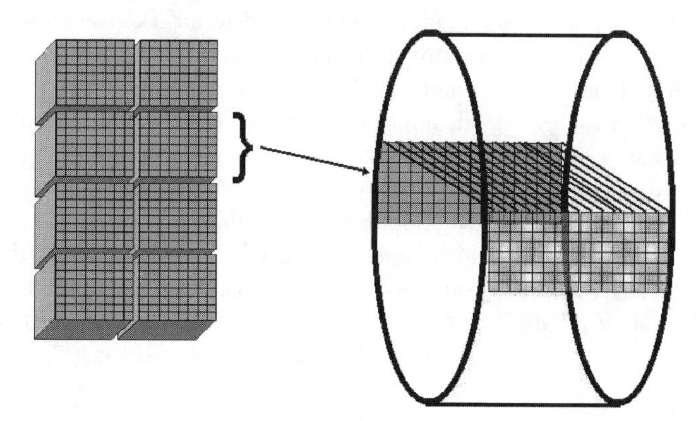

FIGURE 10.21 Axial field of view created by two rings of detectors. Eight detectors per ring width giving 16 axial image planes. Each block is formed by $8 \times 8 = 64$ detectors. Sixty-four blocks of detectors in the transaxial plane, form a whole ring around the patient.

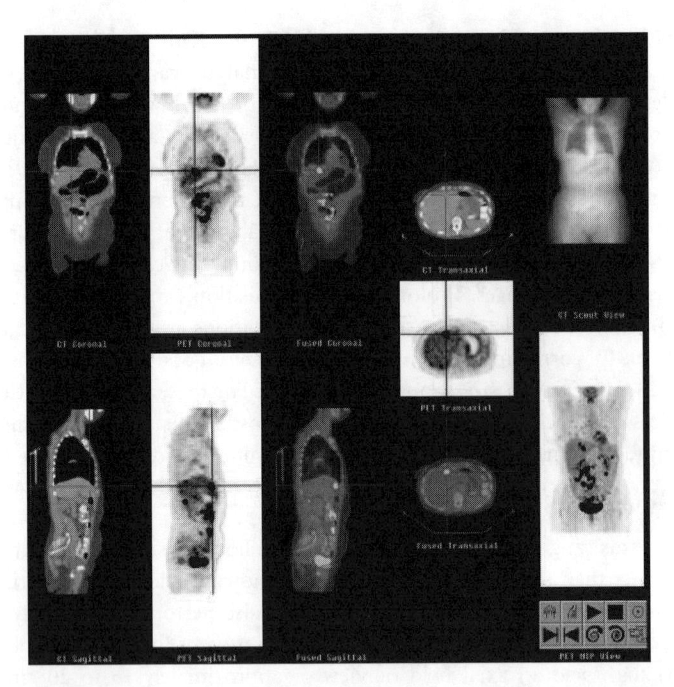

FIGURE 10.22 **(See color insert following page 14-10.)** PET whole body scan and CT anatomical reference. PET and fused PET/CT images indicate uptake of ^{18}FDG in liver and other abdominal areas. From left to right: CT, PET, and fused PET/CT coronal (top) and sagittal (bottom) views. The fourth column shows the transaxial images, from top to bottom: CT, PET, and fused PET/CT images.

scintillator, GSO, has a similar detection efficiency and light decay time, but smaller light output. One GSO advantage is better energy resolution that may reduce scattering artifacts.

Whole body PET images (Figure 10.22) are acquired in several axial steps or tomograph bed positions (the patient table moves in the axial axis) in order to scan most of the patient. The number of tomograph bed positions is determined by the size of the patient and the axial field of view of the scanner. Usually 5 beds are enough for most patients. The complete whole body scan may take 30 min. Faster detectors such as those constructed with LSO, and GSO may reduce the whole body scan time from 30 or 40 min to 20 min.

10.4.4.4.1 Spatial Resolution

Major factors limiting spatial resolution are (1) the range of positrons in tissue before annihilation, (2) the noncolinearity from 180° of annihilation photons and (3) the detector size. The positron range in tissue is due to the maximum emission energy of positrons. Previous to annihilation, positrons travel a finite distance between the emission and annihilation points. Higher positron emission energy yields a larger traveled distance and consequently, a higher degradation in spatial resolution. The noncolinearity from 180° of 511 keV is due to the fact that the momentum of the positron-electron pair just prior to annihilation may not be exactly equal to zero. This results in a slight deviation from 180° (±0.25°) and a slight deviation from 511 keV (±40 eV). The degradation in resolution due to noncolinearity of gamma rays increases with the diameter of the ring of detectors. For a ring diameter of 100 cm, the FWHM due to this effect is approximately 2.2 mm. Finally, larger detectors lead to coarser sampling and lower resolution. The FWHM can be estimated as equal to half of the detector width due to detector size. The combined effect of these three main factors can produce in a typical dedicated PET a FWHM of approximately 3 mm.

10.4.4.4.2 Degrading Effects

Two major degrading effects in dedicated PET are the scattered coincidence events and random coincidences. Scattered coincidences are produced when a 511-keV photon is separated from its trajectory by a Compton interaction within the patient and an event is registered as a false LOR. Random coincidence occurs at very high count rate at which two different positron annihilation events are detected within the same time window. The effect of these two artifacts is to reduce image contrast. Dedicated PET includes hardware and software components for correcting both degrading effects.

10.4.4.4.3 Attenuation Correction

Since attenuation only depends on the line at which opposite gamma rays are detected and not on the position of emission, attenuation correction factors can be easily estimated by measuring the attenuation of 511 keV around the human body. Use of one or two small rotating rods of ^{68}Ge performs this. The number of photons of 511 keV emitted by the annihilation of positrons from the ^{68}Ge source is registered without (blank scan) and with the patient in place (transmission scan). The ratio between the blank and transmission scans yields the attenuation correction factor for all the LOR around the body. Although this method has demonstrated good results in improving the quality of PET images, transmission images are affected by low number of counts that yields noisy attenuation correction factors. This error may be propagated to the attenuation-corrected PET images, affecting image quality and the accuracy of uptake quantitations.

10.4.4.4.4 Three-Dimensional PET

This technology doesn't use any septa between planes with rings of crystals. Under this configuration, any coincidence event is possible between two small crystals in different transaxial planes. The sensitivity can be increased by a factor of ten, but the contribution of scattered photons can be around 30%.

10.4.4.5 Improvement of PET Scanners

Major issues for improving the performance of PET scanners are (1) better resolution and quantitation of small lesions by correcting attenuation, scattering and partial volume effects, (2) monitoring and correcting involuntary patient motion, (3) compensating cardiac and respiratory motions by gating the register of activity, (4) increasing energy resolution by using scintillators with better energy resolution (e.g., GSO) and (5) reduction of PET scanner time by using scintillators with lower light decay time (e.g., LSO and GSO).

10.4.5 Computer Systems

Typical features of hardware associated to computer systems commonly used for SPECT and PET are at least 512 Mb of memory RAM, 20 Gb hard disk, display with 1024 × 1024 resolution for 256 gray levels and network connection with twisted-pair cabling and data transmission speeds of up to 100 Mb/sec. Software requirements include commercial software packages for reconstruction and processing, interfaces to radiology information systems (RISs) and other imaging modalities using the standard format DICOM. Most common and practical devices for permanent hardcopy of images are black and white laser printer with minimum resolution of 1200 dpi, thermal color printers and digital dry laser film printers.

10.4.6 Hybrid SPECT/CT and PET/CT Scanners

The recent trend in emission imaging has been to combine, in the same instrument image, emission and transmission capabilities. Major vendors have recently developed hybrid SPECT/CT and PET/CT scanners.

10.4.6.1 Hybrid SPECT/CT

The main motivation seems to be to solve the photon nonuniform attenuation problem in myocardial SPECT. The goal of nonuniform attenuation correction (AC) of myocardial SPECT has achieved considerable progress in the last decade. This progress has resulted from technical advances in transmission devices for acquiring patient-specific attenuation maps and the development of fast iterative reconstruction algorithms including attenuation correction. Initial attenuation transmission maps were acquired by using point or collimated line radioactive sources opposite to fan-beam collimated detectors in triple-head gamma cameras. Major disadvantages of these systems were image truncation in transmission images and the crosstalk effect between emission and transmission energies. Other procedures have used the scanning of line sources with parallel hole collimators for acquiring transmission maps previous to the emission scan. Although several initial clinical trials have demonstrated improved myocardial SPECT diagnostic accuracy with attenuation correction, some technical artifacts have led to questioning the clinical use of these methods. Technical factors affecting the quality of attenuation corrected images may depend on the configuration of the transmission system and reconstruction algorithms. However, some common technical problems of attenuation transmission maps with radioactive sources have been the noisy, low resolution and low quality transmission images, scattering of transmission sources, inaccuracy of attenuation coefficients, low activity, handling and preparation of the radioactive source and more technical complexity and time-consuming procedures for obtaining high quality studies. Recently, the commercial introduction of a hybrid SPECT/CT scanner has been a significant improvement in the acquisition of high quality patient-specific transmission maps.[161] The x-ray CT transmission scan yields a much higher photon flux and higher quality and resolution transmission images. SPECT and CT images are acquired sequentially by moving the patient table into the two imaging modalities. Transmission images are acquired and registered to the emission scan automatically, without the complexity of preparing or handling radioactive sources. There are no truncation or crosstalk effects and the map of attenuation coefficients for the photon emission energy is derived from the Hounsfield units (HUs) of the CT map.

So far, the only hybrid SPECT/CT scanner commercially available is the Hawkeye option, Millenium VG gamma camera, of GE Medical Systems. The hybrid scanner (Figure 10.23) is based on the integration of a low-cost, third-generation x-ray CT with a dual-head variable angle NaI(Tl) gamma camera. Both the SPECT and CT scanners are mounted on a slip-ring gantry with a 60-cm axial displacement between the centers of the two scanners. The same patient table is used for both imaging modalities and can travel an axial distance of 100 cm. The x-ray CT system includes a fan beam-

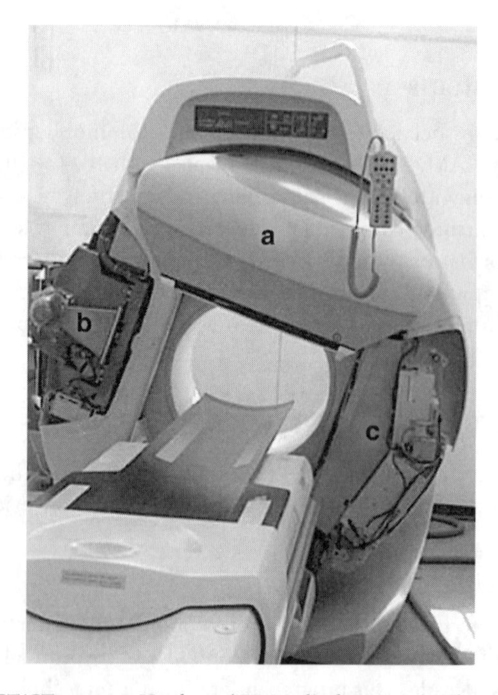

FIGURE 10.23 Hybrid SPECT/CT scanner Hawkeye (GE Medical Systems). The scanner combines a dual-head SPECT (a) with a low-cost, low-resolution x-ray CT, where (b) is the x-ray CT tube and (c) an array of 384 $CdWO_4$ x-ray detectors. Emission and transmission scans are performed sequentially. The images of both modalities are automatically registered.

collimated, low power, stationary anode x-ray tube and an array of 384 $CdWO_4$ detectors with dimensions of 1.8 × 28 mm arranged in an arc centered on the x-ray focal spot. The x-ray tube can operate in continuous mode up to a maximum of 140 kVp at 2.5 mA. The transmission scan acquires 40 transaxial slices of 1 cm thick each with spatial resolution of approximately 1 mm. A single slice is imaged in 13.8 sec. Total time of transmission scanning is 9.2 min. Transmission transaxial slices are reconstructed by the filtered backprojection method into frames of 128 × 128 or 256 × 256 pixels and used for the fusion of emission-transmission slices and for creating attenuation coefficient maps for attenuation correction. Attenuation coefficient maps are created by calculating, pixel by pixel, the linear attenuation coefficient of a material *x* at the photon emission energy E (μ(x,E)). This calculation is based on the HU of each pixel and the tabulated values of μ for air, water and bone at the emission energy according to the following.

For HU less than 0:

$$\mu(x,E) = \mu(water,E) + \frac{[\mu(water,E) - \mu(air,E)] \cdot HU}{1000}$$

For HU above 0:

$$\mu(x,E) = \mu(water,E) + \frac{[\mu(bone,E) - \mu(water,E)] \cdot HU \cdot \mu(water,kV_{eff})}{1000 \cdot [\mu(bone,kV_{eff}) - \mu(water,kV_{eff})]},$$

where kV_{eff} is the effective energy of the x-ray CT beam.

Transmission and emission scans are performed sequentially in any order. After completing the first scan, the patient table is moved automatically into the second scanner so that the axial field of view of both modalities exactly matches.

10.4.6.2 Hybrid PET/CT

In addition to better correct photon attenuation in PET studies, the need of an anatomical framework for interpreting the high uptake of ^{18}FDG has led to the development of hybrid PET/CT scanners. The high uptake of ^{18}FDG by the tumor produces very high-localized intensity PET images in which it is difficult to see other organs and structures. To evaluate the exact localization of the tumor, it is necessary that the anatomic framework be provided by the CT scan. The automatic motion of the patient table between them performs emission and transmission modalities sequentially. Emission and transmission images are registered automatically. PET/CT hybrid scanners have combined standard CT scanners with PET systems in such a way that CT can be used separately for clinical studies.[162] The first hybrid PET/CT introduced in the market was the Discovery LS (Figure 10.24) from GE Medical Systems. The instrument combines a GE Lightspeed CT scanner with the GE Advance PET scanner. The first Discovery LS was installed at the University Hospital, Zurich in March 2001. Other commercial PET/CT scanners already introduced into the market or that will be introduced soon are the Biograph PET/CT (Siemens), which is a combination of the ECAT EXACT HR+ PET and the SOMATON Emotion, and the Gemini PET/CT (Philips Medical Systems), which is a combination of the Allegro PET (former ADAC) and the CT MX8000 (former Marconi).

A current and very promising area of research and clinical application is the use of PET/CT images for radiation treatment planning. Modern radiotherapy treatments based on the concept of intensity modulated radiation therapy (IMRT) need to define precisely the location of the target volume, metabolic extension and heterogeneity of the tumoral tissue. By fusing the metabolic ^{18}FDG PET image with the CT structural information, the most metabolically active areas can be identified and improve the delivery of lethal radiation doses to these regions.

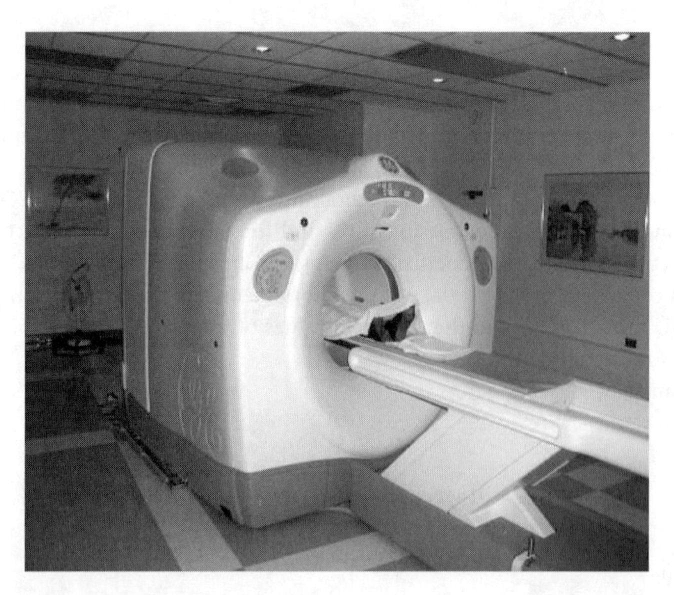

FIGURE 10.24 Hybrid PET/CT scanner Discovery LS (GE Medical Systems).

Acknowledgment

All clinical images were obtained by courtesy of Dr. Jack Ziffer, Director of Medical Imaging at Baptist Hospital of Miami, Miami, FL.

References

1. Henkin, R.E., M.A. Boles, G.L. Dillehay, J.R. Halama, S.M. Karesh, R.H. Wagner, and A.M. Zimmer, *Nuclear Medicine*, Vols. I and II, Mosby, St. Louis, 1996.
2. Stewart, R.E., M. Schwaiger, E. Molina, J. Popma, G.M. Gacioch, M. Kalus, S. Squicciarini, Z.R. al-Aouar, A. Schork, and D.E. Kuhl, Comparison of rubidium-82 positron emission tomography and thallium-201 SPECT imaging for detection of coronary artery disease, *Am. J. Cardiol.*, 67, 1303–1310, 1991.
3. Neumann, R.D., H.D. Sostman, and A. Gottschalk, Current status of ventilation-perfusion imaging, *Semin. Nucl. Med.*, 10, 198–217, 1980.
4. Boerman, O.C., H. Rennen, W.J. Oyen, and F.H. Corstens, Radiopharmaceuticals to image infection and inflammation, *Semin. Nucl. Med.*, 31, 286–295, 2001.
5. Ichise, M., J.H. Meyer, and Y. Yonekura, An introduction to PET and SPECT neuroreceptor quantification models, *J. Nucl. Med.*, 42, 755–763, 2001.
6. Slifstein M. and M. Laruelle, Models and methods for derivation of in vivo neuroreceptor parameters with PET and SPECT reversible radiotracers, *Nucl. Med. Biol.*, 28, 595–608, 2001.
7. Phelps, M.E., S.C. Huang, E.J. Hoffman, C. Selin, L. Sokoloff, and D.E. Kuhl, Tomographic measurement of local cerebral glucose metabolic rate in humans with (F-18)2-fluorodeoxy-D-glucose: validation of method, *Ann. Neurol.*, 6, 371–388, 1979.
8. Camici, P., E. Ferrannini, and L.H. Opie, Myocardial metabolism in ischemic heart disease: basic principles and application to imaging by positron emission tomography, *Prog. Cardiovasc. Dis.*, 32, 217–238, 1989.
9. Shulman, R.G., Functional imaging studies: linking mind and basic neuroscience, *Am. J. Psychiatry*, 158, 11–20, 2001.
10. Duncan, J.S., Imaging and epilepsy, *Brain*, 120, 339–377, 1997.

11. Itoh, K., 99mTc-MAG3: review of pharmacokinetics, clinical application to renal diseases and quantification of renal function, *Ann. Nucl. Med.*, 15, 179–190, 2001.
12. Wu, H.M., S.C. Huang, Y. Choi, C.K. Hoh, and R.A. Hawkins, A modeling method to improve quantitation of fluorodeoxyglucose uptake in heterogeneous tumor tissue, *J. Nucl. Med.*, 36, 297–306, 1995.
13. Mayo Clinic Cardiovascular Working Group on Stress Testing, Cardiovascular stress testing: a description of the various types of stress tests and indications for their use. *Mayo Clin. Proc.*, 71, 43–52, 1996.
14. Lebowitz, E., M.W. Greene, R. Fairchild, P.R. Bradley-Moore, H.L. Atkins, A.N. Ansari, P. Richards, and E. Belgrave, Thallium-201 for medical use. I, *J. Nucl. Med.*, 16, 151–155, 1975.
15. Piwnica-Worms, D., M.L. Chiu, and J. F. Kronauge, Divergent kinetics of 201Tl and 99mTc-SESTAMIBI in cultured chick ventricular myocytes during ATP depletion, *Circulation*, 85, 1531–1541, 1992.
16. Tamaki, N., E. Tadamura, T. Kudoh, N. Hattori, M. Inubushi, and J. Konishi, Recent advances in nuclear cardiology in the study of coronary artery disease, *Ann. Nucl. Med.*, 11, 55–66, 1997.
17. Meerdink, D.J. and J.A. Leppo, Experimental studies of the physiologic properties of technetium-99m agents: myocardial transport of perfusion imaging agents, *Am. J. Cardiol.*, 66, 9E–15E, 1990.
18. Thakur, M.L., Radiolabelled peptides: now and the future, *Nucl. Med. Commun.*, 16, 724–732, 1995.
19. McGoron, A.J., D. Biniakiewicz, R.W. Millard, A. Kumar, S.C. Kennedy, N.J. Roszell, M. Gabel, C. Huth, R.A. Walsh, and M.C. Gerson, Myocardial kinetics of 99m technetium-Q agents: studies in isolated cardiac myocyte, isolated perfused rat heart, and canine regional myocardial ischemia models, *Invest. Radiol.*, 34, 704–717, 1999.
20. Meleca, M.J., A.J. McGoron, M.C. Gerson, R.W. Millard, M. Gabel, D. Biniakiewicz, N.J. Roszell, and R.A. Walsh, Flow versus uptake comparisons of thallium-201 with technetium-99m perfusion tracers in a canine model of myocardial ischemia, *J. Nucl. Med.*, 38, 1847–1856, 1997.
21. Rosenbaum, A.F., A.J. McGoron, R.W. Millard, M. Gabel, D. Biniakiewicz, R.A. Walsh, and M.C. Gerson, Uptake of seven myocardial tracers during increased myocardial blood flow by dobutamine infusion, *Invest. Radiol.*, 34, 91–98, 1999.
22. Barbarics, E., J.F. Kronauge, C.E. Costello, G.A. Janoki, B.L. Holman, A. Davison, and A.G. Jones, In vivo metabolism of the technetium isonitrile complex [Tc(2-ethoxy-2-methyl-1-isocyanopropane)6]+, *Nucl. Med. Biol.*, 21, 583–591, 1994.
23. Wackers, F.J., D.S. Berman, J. Maddahi, D.D. Watson, G.A. Beller, H.W. Strauss, C.A. Boucher, M. Picard, B.L. Holman, R. Fridrich, et al., Technetium-99m hexakis 2-methoxyisobutyl isonitrile: human biodistribution, dosimetry, safety, and preliminary comparison to thallium-201 for myocardial perfusion imaging, *J. Nucl. Med.*, 30, 301–311, 1989.
24. Jones, A.G., M.J. Abrams, A. Davison, J.W. Brodack, A.K. Toothaker, S.J. Adelstein, and A.I. Kassis, Biological studies of a new class of technetium complexes: the hexakis(alkylisonitrile)technetium(I) cations, *Int. J. Nucl. Med. Biol.*, 11, 225–234, 1984.
25. Piwnica-Worms, D., J.F. Kronauge, B.L. Holman, A. Davison, and A.G. Jones, Comparative myocardial uptake characteristics of hexakis (alkylisonitrile) technetium(I) complexes. Effect of lipophilicity, *Invest. Radiol.*, 24, 25–29, 1989.
26. Kronauge, J.F., M.L. Chiu, J.S. Cone, A. Davison, B.L. Holman, A.G. Jones, and D. Piwnica-Worms, Comparison of neutral and cationic myocardial perfusion agents: characteristics of accumulation in cultured cells, *Int. J. Rad. Appl. Instrum. B*, 19, 141–148, 1992.
27. Maublant, J.C., N. Moins, P. Gachon, M. Renoux, Z. Zhang, and A. Veyre, Uptake of technetium-99m-teboroxime in cultured myocardial cells: comparison with thallium-201 and technetium-99m-sestamibi, *J. Nucl. Med.*, 34, 255–259, 1993.
28. Hendel, R.C., B. McSherry, M. Karimeddini, and J.A. Leppo, Diagnostic value of a new myocardial perfusion agent, teboroxime (SQ 30,217), utilizing a rapid planar imaging protocol: preliminary results, *J. Am. Coll. Cardiol.*, 16, 855–861, 1990.

29. Gerson, M.C., E.A. Deutsch, H. Nishiyama, K.F. Libson, R.J. Adolph, L.W. Grossman, V.J. Sodd, D.L. Fortman, J.L. Vanderheyden, C.C. Williams, et al., Myocardial perfusion imaging with 99mTc-DMPE in man, *Eur. J. Nucl. Med.*, 8, 371–374, 1983.
30. Deutsch, E., A.R. Ketring, K. Libson, J.L. Vanderheyden, and W.W. Hirth, The Noah's Ark experiment: species dependent biodistributions of cationic 99mTc complexes, *Int. J. Rad. Appl. Instrum. B*, 16, 191–232, 1989.
31. Vanderheyden, J.L., M.J. Heeg, and E. Deutsch, Comparison of the chemical and biological properties of trans-(Tc(DMPE)2)Cl2)+ and 1,2-bis(dimethylphosphino)ethane. Single-crystal structural analysis of trans(Re(DMPE)2Cl2)PF6, *Inorg. Chem.*, 24, 1666, 1985.
32. Gerson, M.C., E.A. Deutsch, K.F. Libson, R.J. Adolph, A.R. Ketring, J.L. Vanderheyden, C.C. Williams, and E.L. Saenger, Myocardial scintigraphy with 99mTc-tris-DMPE in man, *Eur. J. Nucl. Med.*, 9, 403–407, 1984.
33. Kelly, J.D., A.M. Forster, B. Higley, C.M. Archer, F.S. Booker, L.R. Canning, K.W. Chiu, B. Edwards, H.K. Gill, M. McPartlin, et al., Technetium-99m-tetrofosmin as a new radiopharmaceutical for myocardial perfusion imaging, *J. Nucl. Med.*, 34, 222–227, 1993.
34. Deutsch, E., J.L. Vanderheyden, P. Gerundini, K. Libson, W. Hirth, F. Colombo, L. Zecca, A. Savi, and F. Fazio, Development of nonreducible technetium-99m(III) cations as myocardial perfusion imaging agents: initial experience in humans [published erratum appears in *J. Nucl. Med.*, 29(3), 425, 1988], *J. Nucl. Med.*, 28, 1870–1880, 1987.
35. Rosenbaum, A.F., J. Lukes, D. Biniakiewicz, C. Fortman, A.J. McGoron, R.A. Walsh, and M.C. Gerson, Technetium-99m Q4 washout in human hearts [abstract], *J. Nucl. Med.*, 38, 165P, 1997.
36. Younes, A., J.A. Songadele, J. Maublant, E. Platts, R. Pickett, and A. Veyre, Mechanism of uptake of technetium-tetrofosmin. II. Uptake into isolated adult rat heart mitochondria [published erratum appears in *J. Nucl. Cardiol.*, 2(6), 560, 1995], *J. Nucl. Cardiol.*, 2, 327–333, 1995.
37. Roszell, N.J., A.J. McGoron, D.S. Biniakiewicz, et al., 99mTc-Q12 handling by isolated rat cardiac myocytes and mitochondria [abstract], *Circulation*, 92, I181, 1995.
38. Uccelli, L., M. Giganti, A. Duatti, C. Bolzati, R. Pasqualini, C. Cittanti, P. Colamussi, and A. Piffanelli, Subcellular distribution of technetium-99m-N-NOEt in rat myocardium, *J. Nucl. Med.*, 36, 2075–2079, 1995.
39. Fagret, D., P.Y. Marie, F. Brunotte, M. Giganti, D. Le Guludec, A. Bertrand, J.E. Wolf, A. Piffanelli, F. Chossat, D. Bekhechi, et al., Myocardial perfusion imaging with technetium-99m-Tc NOET: comparison with thallium-201 and coronary angiography, *J. Nucl. Med.*, 36, 936–943, 1995.
40. Gould, K.L., PET perfusion imaging and nuclear cardiology, *J. Nucl. Med.*, 32, 579–606, 1991.
41. Hasegawa, S., T. Uehara, H. Yamaguchi, K. Fujino, H. Kusuoka, M. Hori, and T. Nishimura, Validity of 18F-fluorodeoxyglucose imaging with a dual-head coincidence gamma camera for detection of myocardial viability [see comments], *J. Nucl. Med.*, 40, 1884–1892, 1999.
42. Lawrence, J.H., L.W. Tuttle, K.G. Scott, et al., Studies on neoplasms with the aid of radioactive phosphorus. I. The total phosphorus metabolism of normal and leukemic mice., *J. Clin. Invest.*, 19, 267–271, 1940.
43. Dudley H.C. and G.E. Maddox, Deposition of radiogallium (72Ga) in skeletal tissues, *J. Pharmacol. Exp. Ther.*, 96, 224–227, 1949.
44. Eary, J.F., Nuclear medicine in cancer diagnosis, *Lancet*, 354, 853-857, 1999.
45. Delbeke, D., D.M. Rose, W.C. Chapman, C.W. Pinson, J.K. Wright, R.D. Beauchamp, Y. Shyr, and S.D. Leach, Optimal interpretation of FDG PET in the diagnosis, staging and management of pancreatic carcinoma, *J. Nucl. Med.*, 40, 1784–1791, 1999.
46. Tryciecky, E.W., A. Gottschalk, and K. Ludema, Oncologic imaging: interactions of nuclear medicine with CT and MRI using the bone scan as a model, *Semin. Nucl. Med.*, 27, 142–151, 1997.
47. Bombardieri, E., F. Crippa, S.M. Baio, B.A. Peeters, M. Greco, and E.K. Pauwels, Nuclear medicine advances in breast cancer imaging, *Tumori*, 87, 277, 2001.
48. Wahl, R.L., Overview of the current status of PET in breast cancer imaging, *Q. J. Nucl. Med.*, 42, 1–7, 1998.

49. Buscombe, J.R., J.B. Cwikla, D.S. Thakrar, and A.J. Hilson, Scintigraphic imaging of breast cancer: a review, *Nucl. Med. Commun.*, 18, 698–709, 1997.
50. Yoon, J.H., H.S. Bom, H.C. Song, J.H. Lee, and Y.J. Jaegal, Double-phase Tc-99m sestamibi scintimammography to assess angiogenesis and P-glycoprotein expression in patients with untreated breast cancer, *Clin. Nucl. Med.*, 24, 314–318, 1999.
51. Scopinaro, F., O. Schillaci, M. Scarpini, P.L. Mingazzini, L. Di Macio, M. Banci, R. Danieli, M. Zerilli, M.R. Limiti, and A. Centi Colella, Technetium-99m sestamibi: an indicator of breast cancer invasiveness, *Eur. J. Nucl. Med.*, 21, 984–987, 1994.
52. Ciarmiello, A., S. Del Vecchio, P. Silvestro, M.I. Potena, M.V. Carriero, R. Thomas, G. Botti, G. D'Aiuto, and M. Salvatore, Tumor clearance of technetium 99m-sestamibi as a predictor of response to neoadjuvant chemotherapy for locally advanced breast cancer, *J. Clin. Oncol.*, 16, 1677–1683, 1998.
53. O'Doherty, M.J., PET in oncology I — lung, breast, soft tissue sarcoma, *Nucl. Med. Commun.*, 21, 224–229, 2000.
54. Tuttle, T.M., M. Colbert, R. Christensen, K.J. Ose, T. Jones, R. Wetherille, J. Friedman, K. Swenson, and K.M. McMasters, Subareolar injection of 99mTc facilitates sentinel lymph node identification, *Ann. Surg. Oncol.*, 9, 77–81, 2002.
55. Savelli, G., L. Maffioli, M. Maccauro, E. De Deckere, and E. Bombardieri, Bone scintigraphy and the added value of SPECT (single photon emission tomography) in detecting skeletal lesions, *Q. J. Nucl. Med.*, 45, 27–37, 2001.
56. Jing, J.M., E.E. Kim, L. Moulopoulos, and D.A. Podoloff, Primary breast lymphoma detected with SPECT using gallium-67-citrate, *J. Nucl. Med.*, 36, 236–237, 1995.
57. Chiti, A., F.A. Schreiner, F. Crippa, E.K. Pauwels, and E. Bombardieri, Nuclear medicine procedures in lung cancer, *Eur. J. Nucl. Med.*, 26, 533–555, 1999.
58. Menda, Y. and D. Kahn, Somatostatin receptor imaging of non-small cell lung cancer with 99mTc depreotide, *Semin. Nucl. Med.*, 32, 92–96, 2002.
59. Goldsmith, S.J. and L. Kostakoglu, Nuclear medicine imaging of lung cancer, *Radiol. Clin. North Am.*, 38, 511–524, 2000.
60. Draisma, A., L. Maffioli, M. Gasparini, G. Savelli, E. Pauwels, and E. Bombardieri, Gallium-67 as a tumor-seeking agent in lymphomas — a review, *Tumori*, 84, 434–441, 1998.
61. Rehm, P.K., Gallium-67 scintigraphy in the management: Hodgkin's disease and non-Hodgkin's lymphoma, *Cancer Biother. Radiopharm.*, 14, 251–262, 1999.
62. Front, D., R. Bar-Shalom, and O. Israel, The continuing clinical role of gallium 67 scintigraphy in the age of receptor imaging, *Semin. Nucl. Med.*, 27, 68–74, 1997.
63. Saha, G.B., W.J. MacIntyre, and R.T. Go, Radiopharmaceuticals for brain imaging, *Semin. Nucl. Med.*, 24, 324–349, 1994.
64. O'Tuama, L.A., S.T. Treves, J.N. Larar, A.B. Packard, A.J. Kwan, P.D. Barnes, R.M. Scott, P.M. Black, J.R. Madsen, L.C. Goumnerova, et al., Thallium-201 versus technetium-99m-MIBI SPECT in evaluation of childhood brain tumors: a within-subject comparison, *J. Nucl. Med.*, 34, 1045–1051, 1993.
65. Seo, Y., S. Fukuoka, J. Nakagawara, M. Takanashi, K. Suematsu, and J. Nakamura, Early effects of gamma knife radiosurgery on brain metastases: assessment by 201TlCl SPECT and 99mTc-DTPA-human serum albumin SPECT, *Neurol. Med. Chir. (Tokyo)*, 37, 25–30; discussion 30-1, 1997.
66. Barrington, S.F., Clinical uses of PET in neurology, *Nucl. Med. Commun.*, 21, 237–240, 2000.
67. Gregor, R.T., R. Valdes-Olmos, W. Koops, A.J. Balm, F.J. Hilgers, and C.A. Hoefnagel, Preliminary experience with thallous chloride T1 201-labeled single-photon emission computed tomography scanning in head and neck cancer, *Arch. Otolaryngol. Head Neck Surg.*, 122, 509–514, 1996.
68. Elgazzar, A.H., M. Fernandez-Ulloa, and E.B. Silberstein, 201Tl as a tumour-localizing agent: current status and future considerations, *Nucl. Med. Commun.*, 14, 96–103, 1993.

69. Mariani, G., M. Gipponi, L. Moresco, G. Villa, M. Bartolomei, G. Mazzarol, M.C. Bagnara, A. Romanini, F. Cafiero, G. Paganelli, and H.W. Strauss, Radioguided sentinel lymph node biopsy in malignant cutaneous melanoma, *J. Nucl. Med.*, 43, 811–827, 2002.
70. Phelps, M.E., PET: the merging of biology and imaging into molecular imaging, *J. Nucl. Med.*, 41, 661–681, 2000.
71. Delorme, S. and M.V. Knopp, Non-invasive vascular imaging: assessing tumour vascularity, *Eur. Radiol.*, 8, 517–527, 1998.
72. Chapman, J.D., E.L. Engelhardt, C.C. Stobbe, R.F. Schneider, and G.E. Hanks, Measuring hypoxia and predicting tumor radioresistance with nuclear medicine assays, *Radiother. Oncol.*, 46, 229–237, 1998.
73. Nunn, A., K. Linder, and H.W. Strauss, Nitroimidazoles and imaging hypoxia, *Eur. J. Nucl. Med.*, 22, 265–280, 1995.
74. Chapman, J.D., R.F. Schneider, J.L. Urbain, and G.E. Hanks, Single-photon emission computed tomography and positron-emission tomography assays for tissue oxygenation, *Semin. Radiat. Oncol.*, 11, 47–57, 2001.
75. Wiebe, L.I. and D. Stypinski, Pharmacokinetics of SPECT radiopharmaceuticals for imaging hypoxic tissues, *Q. J. Nucl. Med.*, 40, 270–284, 1996.
76. Libutti, S.K., P. Choyke, J.A. Carrasquillo, S. Bacharach, and R.D. Neumann, Monitoring responses to antiangiogenic agents using noninvasive imaging tests, *Cancer J. Sci. Am.*, 5, 252–256, 1999.
77. Miles, K.A., Tumour angiogenesis and its relation to contrast enhancement on computed tomography: a review, *Eur. J. Radiol.*, 30, 198–205, 1999.
78. Britton, K.E., Towards the goal of cancer-specific imaging and therapy, *Nucl. Med. Commun.*, 18, 992–1007, 1997.
79. Moul, J.W., C.J. Kane, and S.B. Malkowicz, The role of imaging studies and molecular markers for selecting candidates for radical prostatectomy, *Urol. Clin. North Am.*, 28, 459–472, 2001.
80. Okarvi, S.M., Recent developments in 99Tcm-labelled peptide-based radiopharmaceuticals: an overview, *Nucl. Med. Commun.*, 20, 1093–1112, 1999.
81. Hoffman, T.J., T.P. Quinn, and W.A. Volkert, Radiometallated receptor-avid peptide conjugates for specific in vivo targeting of cancer cells, *Nucl. Med. Biol.*, 28, 527–539, 2001.
82. Cordon-Cardo, C., J.P. O'Brien, D. Casals, L. Rittman-Grauer, J.L. Biedler, M.R. Melamed, and J.R. Bertino, Multidrug-resistance gene (P-glycoprotein) is expressed by endothelial cells at blood-brain barrier sites, *Proc. Natl. Acad. Sci. U.S.A.*, 86, 695–698, 1989.
83. Bart, J., H.J. Groen, N.H. Hendrikse, W.T. van der Graaf, W. Vaalburg, and E.G. de Vries, The blood-brain barrier and oncology: new insights into function and modulation, *Cancer Treat. Rev.*, 26, 449–462, 2000.
84. Del Vecchio, S., A. Ciarmiello, and M. Salvatore, Scintigraphic detection of multidrug resistance in cancer, *Cancer Biother. Radiopharm.*, 15, 327–337, 2000.
85. Ballinger, J.R., H.A. Hua, B.W. Berry, P. Firby, and I. Boxen, 99Tcm-sestamibi as an agent for imaging P-glycoprotein-mediated multi-drug resistance: *in vitro* and in vivo studies in a rat breast tumour cell line and its doxorubicin-resistant variant, *Nucl. Med. Commun.*, 16, 253–257, 1995.
86. Crankshaw, C.L., M. Marmion, G.D. Luker, V. Rao, J. Dahlheimer, B.D. Burleigh, E. Webb, K.F. Deutsch, and D. Piwnica-Worms, Novel technetium (III)-Q complexes for functional imaging of multidrug resistance (MDR1) P-glycoprotein, *J. Nucl. Med.*, 39, 77–86, 1998.
87. Piwnica-Worms, D., M.L. Chiu, and J. F. Kronauge, Detection of adriamycin-induced cardiotoxicity in cultured heart cells with technetium 99m-SESTAMIBI, *Cancer Chemother. Pharmacol.*, 32, 385–391, 1993.
88. Crone, C., Lack of selectivity to small ions in paracellular pathways in cerebral and muscle capillaries of the frog, *J. Physiol.*, 353, 317–337, 1984.
89. Thobois, S., S. Guillouet, and E. Broussolle, Contributions of PET and SPECT to the understanding of the pathophysiology of Parkinson's disease, *Neurophysiol. Clin.*, 31, 321–340, 2001.

90. Hawkins, R.A., M.E. Phelps, and S.C. Huang, Effects of temporal sampling, glucose metabolic rates, and disruptions of the blood-brain barrier on the FDG model with and without a vascular compartment: studies in human brain tumors with PET, *J. Cereb. Blood Flow Metab.*, 6, 170–183, 1986.
91. Spencer, S.S., The relative contributions of MRI, SPECT, and PET imaging in epilepsy, *Epilepsia*, 35, S72–89, 1994.
92. Abu-Judeh, H.H., M. Singh, J.C. Masdeu, and H.M. Abdel-Dayem, Discordance between FDG uptake and technetium-99m-HMPAO brain perfusion in acute traumatic brain injury, *J. Nucl. Med.*, 39, 1357–1359, 1998.
93. Bergsneider, M., D.A. Hovda, E. Shalmon, D.F. Kelly, P.M. Vespa, N.A. Martin, M.E. Phelps, D.L. McArthur, M.J. Caron, J.F. Kraus, and D.P. Becker, Cerebral hyperglycolysis following severe traumatic brain injury in humans: a positron emission tomography study, *J. Neurosurg.*, 86, 241–251, 1997.
94. Mazziotta, J.C., R.S. Frackowiak, and M.E. Phelps, The use of positron emission tomography in the clinical assessment of dementia, *Semin. Nucl. Med.*, 22, 233–246, 1992.
95. O'Brien, T.J., E.L. So, B.P. Mullan, M.F. Hauser, B.H. Brinkmann, C.R. Jack, Jr., G.D. Cascino, F.B. Meyer, and F.W. Sharbrough, Subtraction SPECT co-registered to MRI improves postictal SPECT localization of seizure foci, *Neurology*, 52, 137–146, 1999.
96. Pantano, P., C. Matteucci, V. di Piero, C. Pozzilli, M.T. Faedda, M.G. Grasso, C. Argentino, G. Cruccu, and A. Carolei, Quantitative assessment of cerebral blood flow in partial epilepsy using Xe-133 inhalation and SPECT, *Clin. Nucl. Med.*, 16, 898–903, 1991.
97. Matz, P.G. and L. Pitts, Monitoring in traumatic brain injury, *Clin. Neurosurg.*, 44, 267–294, 1997.
98. Sobal, G. and H. Sinzinger, Methylene blue-enhanced stability of (99mTc)HMPAO and simplified quality control — a comparative investigation, *Appl. Radiat. Isot.*, 54, 633–636, 2001.
99. Neirinckx, R.D., L.R. Canning, I.M. Piper, D.P. Nowotnik, R.D. Pickett, R.A. Holmes, W.A. Volkert, A.M. Forster, P.S. Weisner, J.A. Marriott, et al., Technetium-99m d,l-HM-PAO: a new radiopharmaceutical for SPECT imaging of regional cerebral blood perfusion, *J. Nucl. Med.*, 28, 191–202, 1987.
100. Koslowsky, I.L., S.E. Brake, and S.J. Bitner, Evaluation of the stability of (99m)Tc-ECD and stabilized (99m)Tc-HMPAO stored in syringes, *J. Nucl. Med. Technol.*, 29, 197–200, 2001.
101. Walovitch, R.C., T.C. Hill, S.T. Garrity, E.H. Cheesman, B.A. Burgess, D.H. O'Leary, A.D. Watson, M.V. Ganey, R.A. Morgan, and S.J. Williams, Characterization of technetium-99m-L,L-ECD for brain perfusion imaging I. Pharmacology of technetium-99m ECD in nonhuman primates, *J. Nucl. Med.*, 30, 1892–1901, 1989.
102. Murase, K., S. Tanada, H. Fujita, S. Sakaki, and K. Hamamoto, Kinetic behavior of technetium-99m-HMPAO in the human brain and quantification of cerebral blood flow using dynamic SPECT, *J. Nucl. Med.*, 33, 135–143, 1992.
103. Claudiani, F., P. Stimamiglio, L. Bertolazzi, M. Cabria, M. Conte, G.P. Villavecchia, A. Garaventa, E. Lanino, B. De Bernardi, and G. Scopinaro, Radioiodinated meta-iodobenzylguanidine in the diagnosis of childhood neuroblastoma, *Q. J. Nucl. Med.*, 39, 21–24, 1995.
104. Yoshita, M., J. Taki, and M. Yamada, A clinical role for [(123)I]MIBG myocardial scintigraphy in the distinction between dementia of the Alzheimer's-type and dementia with Lewy bodies, *J. Neurol. Neurosurg. Psychiatry*, 71, 583–588, 2001.
105. Peters, A.M., Scintigraphic imaging of renal function, *Exp. Nephrol.*, 6, 391–397, 1998.
106. Heaf, J.G. and J. Iversen, Uses and limitations of renal scintigraphy in renal transplantation monitoring, *Eur. J. Nucl. Med.*, 27, 871–879, 2000.
107. Moran, J.K., Technetium-99m-EC and other potential new agents in renal nuclear medicine, *Semin. Nucl. Med.*, 29, 91–101, 1999.
108. Rossleigh, M.A., Renal cortical scintigraphy and diuresis renography in infants and children, *J. Nucl. Med.*, 42, 91–95, 2001.

109. Russell, C.D., M. Japanwalla, S. Khan, J.W. Scott, and E.V. Dubovsky, Techniques for measuring renal transit time, *Eur. J. Nucl. Med.*, 22, 1372–1378, 1995.
110. Vanaja, R., S.V. Solav, S.H. Joshi, P. Kumar, and N. Ramamoorthy, Preparation of 99mTc-ethylene dicysteine (99mTc-EC) by transchelation using 99mTc-glucoheptonate (99mTc-GHA) and its evaluation for renal function studies, *Nucl. Med. Commun.*, 21, 977–982, 2000.
111. Xue, L.Y., A.A. Noujaim, T.R. Sykes, T.K. Woo, and X.B. Wang, Role of transchelation in the uptake of 99mTc-MAb in liver and kidney, *Q. J. Nucl. Med.*, 41, 10–17, 1997.
112. Salvatori, M., Advances in pulmonary nuclear medicine, *Rays*, 22, 51–72, 1997.
113. Rimkus, D.S., and W.L. Ashburn, Lung ventilation scanning with a new carbon particle radioaerosol (Technegas). Preliminary patient studies, *Clin. Nucl. Med.*, 15, 222–226, 1990.
114. Selby, J.B. and J.J. Gardner, Clinical experience with technetium-99m DTPA aerosol with perfusion scintigraphy in suspected pulmonary embolism, *Clin. Nucl. Med.*, 12, 1–5, 1987.
115. Morrison, D., K. Skwarski, A.M. Millar, W. Adams, and W. MacNee, A comparison of three methods of measuring 99mTc-DTPA lung clearance and their repeatability, *Eur. Respir. J.*, 11, 1141–1146, 1998.
116. Lu, H., J.B. Farison, and M.J. Dennis, Enhancement of Xe-133 ventilation lung scan image acquired after Tc-99m perfusion scan, *Biomed. Sci. Instrum.*, 33, 118–125, 1997.
117. Woolfenden, J.M., J.A. Carrasquillo, S.M. Larson, J.T. Simmons, H. Masur, P.D. Smith, J.H. Shelhamer, and F.P. Ognibene, Acquired immunodeficiency syndrome: Ga-67 citrate imaging, *Radiology*, 162, 383–387, 1987.
118. Becker, W. and J. Meller, The role of nuclear medicine in infection and inflammation, *Lancet Infect. Dis.*, 1, 326–333, 2001.
119. Chianelli, M., S.J. Mather, J. Martin-Comin, and A. Signore, Radiopharmaceuticals for the study of inflammatory processes: a review, *Nucl. Med. Commun.*, 18, 437–455, 1997.
120. O'Doherty, M.J. and T.O. Nunan, Nuclear medicine and AIDS, *Nucl. Med. Commun.*, 14, 830–848, 1993.
121. Boerman, O.C., E.T. Dams, W.J. Oyen, F.H. Corstens, and G. Storm, Radiopharmaceuticals for scintigraphic imaging of infection and inflammation, *Inflamm. Res.*, 50, 55–64, 2001.
122. Vallabhajosula, S. and V. Fuster, Atherosclerosis: imaging techniques and the evolving role of nuclear medicine, *J. Nucl. Med.*, 38, 1788–1796, 1997.
123. Bogdanov, A.A., Jr., M. Simonova, and R. Weissleder, Engineering membrane proteins for nuclear medicine: applications for gene therapy and cell tracking, *Q. J. Nucl. Med.*, 44, 224–235, 2000.
124. Hamilton, J.G. and M.H. Doley, Studies in iodine metabolism of the thyroid gland *in situ* by the use of radioiodine in normal subjects and in patients with various types of goiter, *Am. J. Physiol.*, 131, 135–143, 1940.
125. James, C., M. Starks, D.C. MacGillivray, and J. White, The use of imaging studies in the diagnosis and management of thyroid cancer and hyperparathyroidism, *Surg. Oncol. Clin. North Am.*, 8, 145–169, 1999.
126. Aguilar-Diosdado, M., A. Contreras, I. Gavilan, L. Escobar-Jimenez, J.A. Giron, J.C. Escribano, M. Beltran, A. Garcia-Curiel, and J.M. Vazquez, Thyroid nodules. Role of fine needle aspiration and intraoperative frozen section examination, *Acta Cytol.*, 41, 677–682, 1997.
127. McDougall, I.R., J. Davidson, and G.M. Segall, Positron emission tomography of the thyroid, with an emphasis on thyroid cancer, *Nucl. Med. Commun.*, 22, 485–492, 2001.
128. Maxon, H.R., Detection of residual and recurrent thyroid cancer by radionuclide imaging, *Thyroid*, 9, 443–446, 1999.
129. Sisson, J.C., Selection of the optimal scanning agent for thyroid cancer, *Thyroid*, 7, 295–302, 1997.
130. Wieland, D.M., L.E. Brown, M.C. Tobes, W.L. Rogers, D.D. Marsh, T.J. Mangner, D.P. Swanson, and W.H. Beierwaltes, Imaging the primate adrenal medulla with [^{123}I] and [^{131}I] meta-iodobenzylguanidine: concise communication, *J. Nucl. Med.*, 22, 358–364, 1981.

131. Von Moll, L., A.J. McEwan, B. Shapiro, J.C. Sisson, M.D. Gross, R. Lloyd, E. Beals, W.H. Beierwaltes, and N.W. Thompson, Iodine-131 MIBG scintigraphy of neuroendocrine tumors other than pheochromocytoma and neuroblastoma, *J. Nucl. Med.*, 28, 979–988, 1987.
132. Peters, M., Fundamentals of tracer kinetics for radiologists, *Br. J. Radiol.*, 71, 1116–1129, 1998.
133. Germano, G., B.C. Chen, S.C. Huang, S.S. Gambhir, E.J. Hoffman, and M.E. Phelps, Use of the abdominal aorta for arterial input function determination in hepatic and renal PET studies, *J. Nucl. Med.*, 33, 613–620, 1992.
134. Gates, G.F., Glomerular filtration rate: estimation from fractional renal accumulation of 99mTc-DTPA (stannous), *AJR Am. J. Roentgenol.*, 138, 565–570, 1982.
135. Itoh, K., K. Nonomura, T. Yamashita, K. Kanegae, M. Murakumo, T. Koyanagi, and M. Furudate, Quantification of renal function with a count-based gamma camera method using technetium-99m-MAG3 in children, *J. Nucl. Med.*, 37, 71–75, 1996.
136. Taylor, A., Jr., P.L. Corrigan, J. Galt, E.V. Garcia, R. Folks, M. Jones, A. Manatunga, and D. Eshima, Measuring technetium-99m-MAG3 clearance with an improved camera-based method, *J. Nucl. Med.*, 36, 1689–1695, 1995.
137. Patlak, C.S., R.G. Blasberg, and J.D. Fenstermacher, Graphical evaluation of blood-to-brain transfer constants from multiple-time uptake data, *J. Cereb. Blood Flow Metab.*, 3, 1–7, 1983.
138. Fleming, J.S. and P.M. Kemp, A comparison of deconvolution and the Patlak-Rutland plot in renography analysis, *J. Nucl. Med.*, 40, 1503–1507, 1999.
139. Sokoloff, L., M. Reivich, C. Kennedy, M.H. Des Rosiers, C.S. Patlak, K.D. Pettigrew, O. Sakurada, and M. Shinohara, The [14C]deoxyglucose method for the measurement of local cerebral glucose utilization: theory, procedure, and normal values in the conscious and anesthetized albino rat, *J. Neurochem.*, 28, 897–916, 1977.
140. Sandell, A., T. Ohlsson, K. Erlandsson, and S.E. Strand, An alternative method to normalize clinical FDG studies, *J. Nucl. Med.*, 39, 552–555, 1998.
141. Suhonen-Polvi, H., U. Ruotsalainen, A. Kinnala, J. Bergman, M. Haaparanta, M. Teras, M.a.a.P., O. Solin, and U. Wegelius, FDG-PET in early infancy: simplified quantification methods to measure cerebral glucose utilization, *J. Nucl. Med.*, 36, 1249–1254, 1995.
142. Shiozaki, T., N. Sadato, M. Senda, K. Ishii, T. Tsuchida, Y. Yonekura, H. Fukuda, and J. Konishi, Noninvasive estimation of FDG input function for quantification of cerebral metabolic rate of glucose: optimization and multicenter evaluation, *J. Nucl. Med.*, 41, 1612–1618, 2000.
143. Gjedde, A., High- and low-affinity transport of D-glucose from blood to brain, *J. Neurochem.*, 36, 1463–1471, 1981.
144. Oldendorf, W.H., Letter: expression of tissue isotope distribution, *J. Nucl. Med.*, 15, 725–726, 1974.
145. Calvo, R., J.M. Marti-Climent, J.A. Richter, I. Penuelas, A. Crespo-Jara, L.M. Villar, and M.J. Garcia-Velloso, Three-dimensional clinical PET in lung cancer: validation and practical strategies, *J. Nucl. Med.*, 41, 439–448, 2000.
146. Yamaji, S., K. Ishii, M. Sasaki, T. Mori, H. Kitagaki, S. Sakamoto, and E. Mori, Evaluation of standardized uptake value to assess cerebral glucose metabolism, *Clin. Nucl. Med.*, 25, 11–16, 2000.
147. Sadato, N., T. Tsuchida, S. Nakaumra, A. Waki, H. Uematsu, N. Takahashi, N. Hayashi, Y. Yonekura, and Y. Ishii, Non-invasive estimation of the net influx constant using the standardized uptake value for quantification of FDG uptake of tumours, *Eur. J. Nucl. Med.*, 25, 559–564, 1998.
148. Sevick, E.M. and R.K. Jain, Geometric resistance to blood flow in solid tumors perfused ex vivo: effects of tumor size and perfusion pressure, *Cancer Res.*, 49, 3506–3512, 1989.
149. Wunderbaldinger, P., A. Bogdanov, and R. Weissleder, New approaches for imaging in gene therapy, *Eur. J. Radiol.*, 34, 156–165, 2000.
150. Anger, H., Scintillation Camera, *Rev. Sci. Instrum.*, 29, 27, 1958.
151. Chang, L., A method for attenuation correction in radionuclide computed tomography, *IEEE Trans. Nucl. Sci.*, NS-25, 638–643, 1978.
152. Haynor, D.R., M.S. Kaplan, R.S. Miyaoka, and T.K. Lewellen, Multiwindow scatter correction techniques in single-photon imaging, *Med. Phys.*, 22, 2015–2024, 1995.

153. Moore, S.C., M.F. Kijewski, S.P. Muller, F. Rybicki, and R.E. Zimmerman, Evaluation of scatter compensation methods by their effects on parameter estimation from SPECT projections, *Med. Phys.*, 28, 278–287, 2001.
154. Gilland, D.R., R.J. Jaszczak, T.A. Riauka, and R.E. Coleman, Approximate three-dimensional iterative reconstruction for SPECT, *Med. Phys.*, 24, 1421–1429, 1997.
155. Tsui, B.M., G.T. Gullberg, E.R. Edgerton, J. G. Ballard, J. R. Perry, W.H. McCartney, and J. Berg, Correction of nonuniform attenuation in cardiac SPECT imaging, *J. Nucl. Med.*, 30, 497–507, 1989.
156. Meikle, S.R., B.F. Hutton, D.L. Bailey, P.K. Hooper, and M.J. Fulham, Accelerated EM reconstruction in total-body PET: Potential for improving tumor detectability, *Phys. Med. Biol.*, 39, 1689–1704, 1994.
157. Corbett, J.R. and E.P. Ficaro, Clinical review of attenuation-corrected cardiac SPECT, *J. Nucl. Cardiol.*, 6, 54–68, 1999.
158. Sweet, W.H., The use of nuclear disintegration in diagnosis and treatment of brain tumors, *N. Engl. J. Med.*, 245, 875–878, 1951.
159. Phelps, M.E., E.J. Hoffman, N.A. Mullani, and M.M. Ter-Pogossian, Application of annihilation coincidence detection to transaxial reconstruction tomography, *J. Nucl. Med.*, 16, 210–224, 1975.
160. Nester, O.H. and C.Y. Huang, Bismuth germanate: a high-z gamma-ray and charged particle detector, *IEEE Nucl. Sci.*, NS-22, 68, 1975.
161. Bocher, M., A. Balan, Y. Krausz, Y. Shrem, A. Lonn, M. Wilk, and R. Chisin, Gamma camera-mounted anatomical x-ray tomography: technology, system characteristics and first images, *Eur. J. Nucl. Med.*, 27, 619–627, 2000.
162. Kinahan, P.E., D.W. Townsend, T. Beyer, and D. Sashin, Attenuation correction for a combined three-dimensional PET/CT scanner, *Med. Phys.*, 25, 2046–2053, 1998.

11

Endoscopy

CONTENTS

Thomas D. Wang
Stanford University School of Medicine

George Triadafilopoulos
Stanford University School of Medicine

11.1 Introduction

Endoscopy is a powerful medical tool used for diagnosis and treatment of human diseases. Major developments in technology have paved the way for endoscopes to assume a key role in the practice of medicine.[1] Endoscopes have unparalleled ability to visualize lesions within internal organs with high resolution for minimally invasive medical purposes. These instruments can be inserted through natural body orifices (mouth, nose, anus, urethra) to access hollow organs, such as the oropharynx, esophagus, stomach, small intestine, colon, larynx, bronchial tree, and urinary bladder. This chapter will first present the fundamental concepts of endoscopy, including the optical, mechanical, and electronic designs required for proper function of an endoscope. Also, the basic theory of endoscopic image formation,

0-8493-1140-3/04/$0.00+$1.50

such as image detection, spatial intensity distribution, image resolution, signal to noise, and color image processing, will be elaborated. Finally, a brief description of new emerging endoscopic technology will be introduced with references to more detailed discussions. Numerous images are displayed to illustrate the features of each technology.

Technological innovation has significantly changed the practice of endoscopy in recent years. The first endoscopes consisted of crude, rigid tubes that provided only a limited view of easily accessible organs.[1] Recent developments have substantially upgraded the capabilities of endoscopes. First, fiber optic imaging bundles allowed for the development of flexible instruments that could be guided through tortuous organs to visualize deeply into the body. Next, miniaturized semiconductor detectors provided a substantial improvement in image resolution and a reduction of instrument size. Finally, ultrasound imaging has been combined with endoscopy to enable visualization beyond the tissue surface. However, medical endoscopy is still in the infant stage with many areas of active research and development. Conventional endoscopy is based on the detection of diffusely reflected white light from the tissue surface, using subtle changes in the color and shadows to reveal structural changes.[2] New advancements in optical imaging are going beyond white light, and take full advantage of light's properties. Several technologies that are being developed for clinical use include optical coherence tomography, high magnification endoscopy, chromoendoscopy, and fluorescence imaging. Also, wireless capsule and virtual endoscopy have demonstrated the potential to collect endoscopic images with minimal discomfort to the patient. Further technological improvements promise to improve the capability of endoscopes to visualize, diagnose, and treat human diseases, and are expected revolutionize the practice of medical endoscopy in the near future.

11.2 Basic Components of an Endoscope

In this section, an upper gastrointentinal endoscope, or esophagogastroduodenoscope, will be used to illustrate the basic components of an endoscope. An upper gastrointentinal endoscope is used to visualize the esophagus, stomach, and duodenum. A schematic diagram detailing the individual components of the endoscope is shown in Figure 11.1. The distal tip contains the optics required for illuminating and collecting endosocpic images, channels for delivery of instruments, and the mechanisms for providing air, water, and suction.[2] The bending section contains a set of hinges that allow the distal tip to deflect at large angles as high as 270°. The insertion tube comprises the distal part of the endoscope and is covered with a rugged plastic. The proximal end of the endoscope contains the entry into the instrument channel, the angulation control knobs for manipulating the distal end, a lock for maintaining distal tip deflection, air/water and suction valves, and remote switches for freezing, capturing, and storing images. An umbilical cord connects the endoscope to the video processor, and contains the light guide, electrical connectors, and conduits for air, water, and suction. The total length of the upper endoscope is about 1.5 meters, and can be longer for a colonoscope or enteroscope.

11.2.1 Distal End

The distal end of an endoscope contains the optics that form the endoscopic images. A cross section view of a forward-viewing endoscope is shown in Figure 11.2a, and displays the location of the objective lenses, illumination lenses, air/water conduit, and detector. The corresponding end-view is shown in Figure 11.2b, and two illumination lenses are located on either side of the objective to more uniformly illuminate the image. A large instrument channel is present for delivery of instruments, removal of tissue, and suction. The objective usually contains several optical elements, such as a diverging lens, intermediate lens(es), pupil, and an achromat. The air/water channel directs either water flowing across the outer surface of the objective to clear debris or air to insufflate and expand the organ being examined. The first endoscopes used a coherent optical fiber imaging bundle to transmit the image to the proximal end of the endoscope where it could be viewed directly by the endoscopist through an eyepiece. Because of recent advances in semiconductor technology, the imaging bundles have now

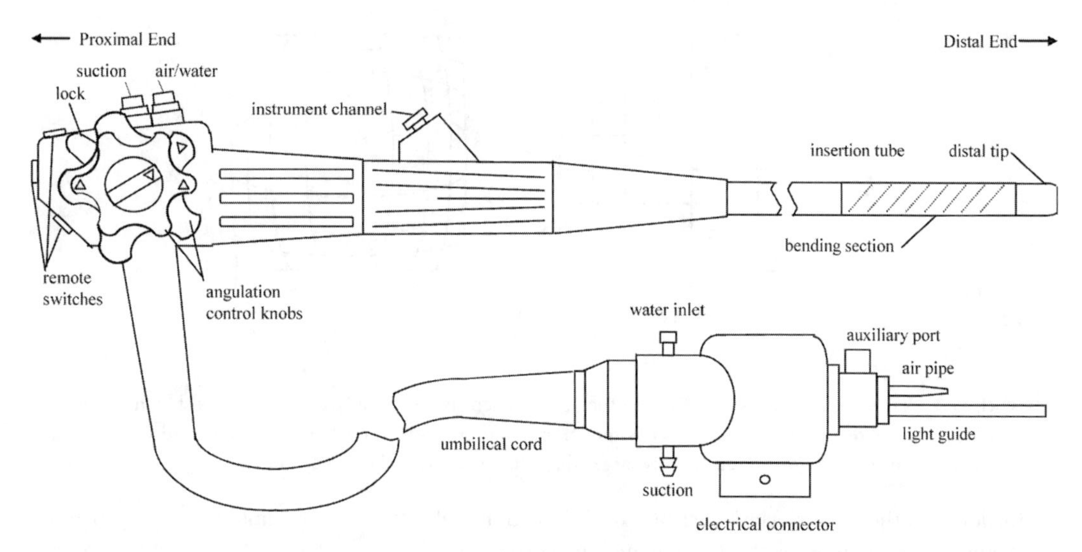

FIGURE 11.1 The basic components of a conventional endoscope is shown. The insertion tube is located on the distal end, and a short bending section connects to the distal tip. The proximal end contains the angulation control knobs, valves for suction, air, and water, and remote switches. The instrument channel is used to deliver accessories to the distal tip.

been replaced by miniaturized charge-coupled device (CCD) detectors located in the distal tip directly behind the objective lens to produce a video image.

11.2.2 The Objective Lens

The objective lens of the endoscope is designed to provide a large field of view with high image resolution. Since it is very difficult to achieve both of these requirements with a simple lens, endoscopes use multiple lenses to form the image. The design of these lens systems is complex, and is usually done with an optical ray tracing program. The optical train of lens elements required to produce the endoscopic image is shown in Figure 11.2a. The angle between a ray of light and the normal to the objective is defined as θ. A diverging lens (negative focal length) is needed to produce a large angle θ to maximize the field of view. A pupil is located behind the objective lens to block extraneous internal reflections. An intermediate lens helps focus the image onto the detector. An achromat corrects for chromatic aberrations so that all the colors in the visible spectrum will focus onto the same plane at the detector. The focal length of the objective is different in center of the image than in the periphery, and this design introduces barrel

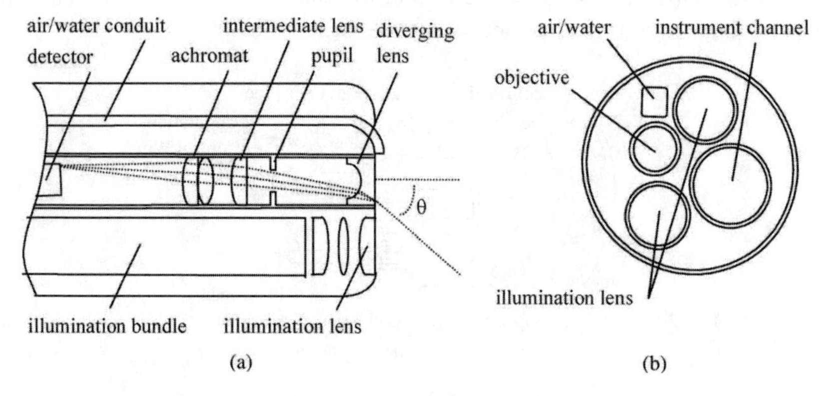

FIGURE 11.2 A detailed view of the distal tip. (a) A cross-section view shows the design of the optics, detector, and air/water conduits; (b) the end-view shows the relative location of these elements.

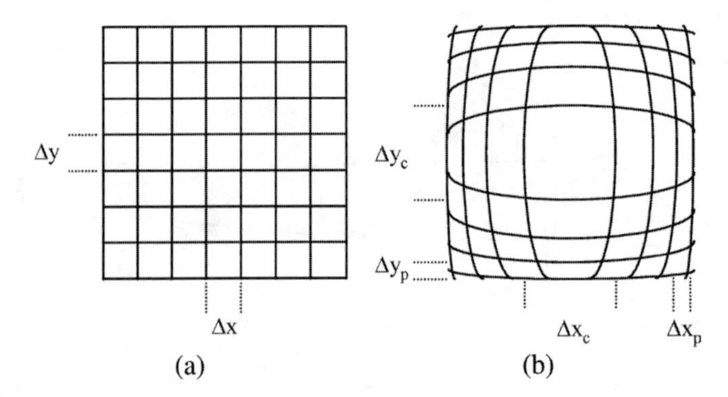

FIGURE 11.3 The effect of barrel distortion in the objective lens is illustrated. (a) An image is shown of a grid of boxes with no barrel distortion; (b) an image is shown with barrel distortion, where the height and width Δx_c and Δy_c in the center of the image are significantly larger than that in the periphery Δx_p and Δy_p.

distortion into the image.[3] The effect of barrel distortion is illustrated by an image of a grid of boxes with equal dimensions. In Figure 11.3a, there is no barrel distortion present and all of the boxes throughout the grid have the same width Δx and height Δy. For an objective lens with barrel distortion, the image magnification is higher in the center of the image than in the periphery. As shown in Figure 11.3b, the boxes in the center of the grid have significantly larger height and width dimensions, Δx_c and Δy_c, than those in the periphery, Δx_p and Δy_p. Because both fiber optic and video endoscopes are still in use, the term resel will be used to designate the smallest resolution element in image detection. A resel corresponds to either an optical fiber in an imaging bundle or a pixel (picture element) in a CCD array. The endoscopist can maximize the resolution of a region of interest by placing it in the center of the image where the density of image resels is the highest.

11.2.3 Insertion Tube

An exposed cross section of the insertion tube is shown in Figure 11.4.[2] The outside consists of a durable plastic covering capable of withstanding caustic bodily fluids, such as gastric acid and bile, and disinfectants for cleaning the instrument. Under the covering is a wire mesh that runs along the length of the tube to prevent twisting or stretching during use. Below the mesh are helically shaped steel bands that maintain the round shape and provide mechanical protection. The contents of the insertion tube include the light guide, imaging bundle, angulation control wires, air and water pipes, and instrument channel. The tube is designed with a stiffness that varies along the length of the endoscope in order to facilitate its insertion into the GI tract. The distal end can be manipulated to produce large bending angles that are needed for visualization of tissue located behind the endoscope (retroflexed view), and for fine movements to traverse tortuous internal organs, such as the intestines.

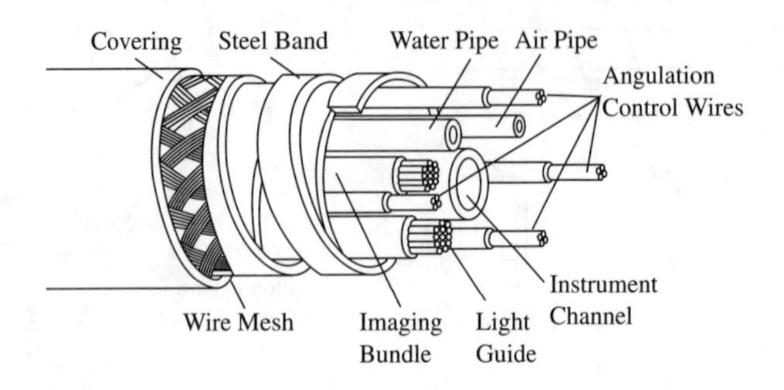

FIGURE 11.4 The contents of the insertion tube include the light guide, imaging bundle, angulation control wires, air and water pipes, and instrument channel, and are protected by a wire mesh and steel bands for mechanical protection.

11.2.4 Angulation Control

The angulation control of the distal end is performed by the left hand of the endoscopist, leaving the right hand free to hold and manipulate the insertion tube. These angulations are produced by a durable set of guide wires that deflect the distal end in four directions, termed up, down, left, and right, by convention. The angulation control knobs are connected to a sprocket that moves the guidewires connected to the distal tip. If desired, a brake can be applied to lock the position of the deflection. The second, third, and fourth fingers grip the proximal end of the instrument against the palm, leaving the left thumb to control the up/down knob and the left index finger to operate the air/water and suction valves. The right hand is used to torque and advance the insertion tube, insert accessories down the instrument channel, control the right/left knobs, and activate the remote switches.

11.2.5 Air, Water, and Suction Valves

A set of buttons and valves are located on the proximal end of the endoscope to deliver air and water or to suction intraluminal contents. When the small opening in the air/water valve is covered, air supplied by a pump within the video processor is emitted from the nozzle on the distal tip. Air is introduced into an organ, such as the colon or stomach, to expand the mucosal folds for better visualization. Air can also be removed from a distended organ for decompression. When the air/water valve is depressed, water is delivered from the pressurized water container located on the video processor and out the nozzle on the distal tip, and over the surface of the objective lens. Water is sprayed over the outer surface of the objective to remove debris that is obstructing the view. Intraluminal contents, such as fluid or stool, can be aspirated through the endoscope to a collection bottle via an external suction pump that provides negative pressure. The umbilical cord contains the connections for the light source, water container, suction pump, and electrical cord to safely return any leakage current. A vent on the connector allows the interior of an airtight and fluid-tight endoscope to be vented before the instrument is placed in an evacuated chamber for sterilization.

11.3 Endoscopic Imaging

11.3.1 Image Illumination

A variety of light sources such as metal halide, halogen, and xenon lamps can be used to provide image illumination. These light sources can provide an incident power $P_i(\lambda_i)$ at incident wavelengths λ_i over the visible and infrared band up to 300 W or more. Because of the intense heat generated by these light sources, filters are used to block the infrared portion, allowing only visible light to be delivered at the distal tip. In addition, large heat sinks and air circulation within the light source prevent excessive heating. The light guide consists of an incoherent fiber optic bundle that has a large numerical aperture (NA) lens at the proximal end to maximize the amount of illumination light collected. There is a diverging lens at the distal end that is designed to illuminate the field of view of the objective. The optical fibers in the light guide have high NA and high transmission efficiency. Also, they are made as large as possible without compromising their flexibility and durability in order to produce the highest possible packing fraction.

11.3.2 Image Detection

Image detection was first performed by the eye of the endosocpist viewing the proximal end of a fiberoptic imaging bundle through an eyepiece. Later, a camera was attached to the eyepiece to detect the image and display it on a video monitor. While this method is simple and effective, there have been several limitations.[4] First, if the endoscopist uses the eyepiece, no one else can view the image, and the images cannot be captured or stored. Second, a Moire pattern is produced by the superposition of the image from the fiber optic bundle and the detector array from the camera, resulting in the appearance of an

TABLE 11.1 Symbols Used in the Endoscopic Imaging Model

Symbol	Description
A_r	Area of tissue imaged per resel
c	Speed of light
d	Distance between endoscope and tissue
ε_t	Conversion efficiency of incident to return light
F_i	Incident illumination fluence
f_p	Packing fraction of detector
h	Planck's constant
θ	Angle from normal to endoscope
θ'	Angle from normal to tissue
θ_m	Maximum collection angle
λ_i	Wavelength of incident light
λ_r	Wavelength of returning light
η	Quantum efficiency of detector
N_r	Number of resolution elements
N_s	Number of signal photons
N_p	Number of photoelectrons
P_i	Incident illumination power
r	Radial distance between endoscope and tissue
r′	Radial distance between tissue and endoscope
r_L	Radius of objective lens
ρ_o	Distance between illumination and objective lenses
ρ'	Radial distance along tissue surface
r_i	Inner radius of resel
r_o	Outer radius of resel
T_o	Transmission efficiency of optical train
Δt	Exposure time of detector
z	Distance variable from endoscope to tissue

interference pattern artifact. Third, the fiber optic imaging bundle is inefficient in collecting light, requiring high power light sources. Finally, the number of optical fibers packed into the bundle, determining the image resolution, is limited by instrument size and stiffness. Also, the individual fibers may break over time, creating gaps in the image. In modern video endoscopes, a miniaturized CCD array located directly behind the objective lens detects the image, and eliminates many of these shortcomings.

11.3.3 Fiberoptic Endoscopy

Fiberoptic endoscopes use an imaging bundle for the transmission of images. An imaging bundle typically contains about 50,000 or more optical fibers, packed into a hexagonal array, as shown in Figure 11.5a. There is a practical upper limit to the number of fibers that can be used because of the associated increase in the diameter and stiffness of the insertion tube. The optical fibers are multimode and preserve the color and intensity of light. The spatial arrangement of the fibers at both the proximal and distal ends of the bundle is identical, resulting in a spatially coherent transmission of the image. For greater flexibility, only the two ends of the optical fibers are fused together (leached design). The overall diameter of the imaging bundle may vary between 0.5 to 3 mm, and may be over 2 m in length. Light is transmitted only through the core of the fiber, thus the area taken up by the cladding and dead space in between the fibers result in loss of light. This transmission factor is known as the packing fraction f_p. The inner and outer radii of the fiber are denoted by r_i and r_o, thus the fiber cores have an area of πr_i^2. Because of dead space in-between the fibers, the average area on the tissue is $2\sqrt{3}r_o^2$, by geometrical arguments. The packing fraction f_p for a fiber optic imaging bundle is given in Equation 11.1a. In the CCD array there is also a thin strip of dead space in-between the pixels, as shown in Figure 11.5b.[5] The distance from the center of the pixel to the edge of the active area is denoted r_i, and the distance to the middle of the dead zone is denoted r_o. The packing fraction for a CCD array is given by Equation 11.1b.

TABLE 11.2 Glossary of Terms

Term	Definition
Aberration	Imperfection in objective lens causing loss of focus
Achromat	Lens element that corrects focus for different wavelengths
5-ALA	5-Aminolevulinic acid, agent used for photodynamic diagnosis
Angulation control	Mechanism for steering distal tip of endoscope
ASIC	Application specific integrated circuit
Axial resolution	Ability to resolve detail with depth below tissue surface
Barrel distortion	Lens aberration that increases magnification in the center of the image
CCD	Charge coupled device semiconductor detector
CMOS	Complementary metal oxide semiconductor
Dark current	Charge generated in detector in the absence of light
Depth of field	Range of distance over which the image remains in focus
Distal	End of endoscope furthest from endoscopist
EGD	Esophagogastroduodenoscopy, esophagus, stomach, and duodenum
ERCP	Endoscopic retrograde cholangiopancreatography
EUS	Endoscopic ultrasound
Field of view	Diameter of region imaged by endoscope
Fluorescence	Spectroscopic light generated in visible spectrum
FNA	Fine needle aspiration for tissue histology
GI	Gastroenterology, study of stomach, liver, and intestinal disease
LED	Light emitting diode for image illumination
Moire	Wavy effect produced by the convergence of lines or patterns
Monochromatic	One color, or black and white
Mosaic	Repeated pattern of filters for producing color image
NA	Numerical aperture equal to sine of angle θ in free air
Objective	Group of lenses in endoscope that forms the image
OCT	Optical coherence tomography
Penetration depth	Distance light travels into tissue prior to attenuation
Pixel	Picture element
Photon	Individual package of light
Photoelectron	Charge produced by detected photon
Prism	Optical element for diverting image in side-viewing endoscope
Proximal	End of endoscope closest to endoscopist
Pupil	Aperture that blocks stray light
Read-out noise	Electronic noise involved in acquisition of charge from detector
Reflectance	Light diffusely scattered from tissue
Resel	Resolution element
RGB	Primary colors red, green, blue
Shift register	Memory for reading out a row of data in CCD array
SNR	Signal-to-noise ratio
Transverse resolution	Ability to resolve detail across tissue surface
US	Ultrasound
VHF	Very high frequency

$$f_p = \frac{\pi}{2\sqrt{3}}\left(\frac{r_i}{r_o}\right)^2 \tag{11.1a}$$

$$f_p = \left(\frac{r_i}{r_o}\right)^2 \tag{11.1b}$$

The maximum angle at which the imaging bundle will collect light is denoted by θ_m, and can be as high as 70°. The effective capture area of the lens is determined by the maximum light acceptance angle of the optical fiber, which can be up to 40° for glass fibers. The range of distances d over which the image remains in focus is called the depth of field, and typically ranges from 3 mm to as high as 100 mm. The

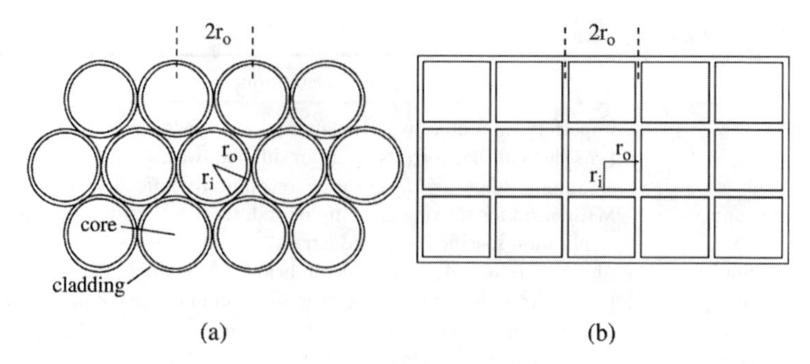

FIGURE 11.5 (a) The individual fibers of the imaging bundle are packed in a hexagonal array. The minimum distance between adjacent fibers determines the resolution of the bundle, and the ratio between the core area and the total bundle area defines the packing fraction. (b) There is thin strip of dead space in-between the pixels in the CCD array.

typical working distance of an endoscope is about 5 to 75 mm. The area of tissue imaged is circular in shape, and the diameter of this area is called the field of view.

11.3.4 Video Endoscopy

The CCD array is semiconductor detector made from silicon that is sensitive to light.[6,7] The surface of a CCD is divided into a two-dimensional array of pixels that may total over several hundred thousand in number. When a photon of light becomes incident on the surface of the silicon, electrons are generated and collected in potential wells. The amount of charge collected is proportional to the intensity of light detected. These charges accumulate over a period of exposure, and then are transferred out of the potential wells through a read-out process for storage and display. The schematic of the read-out process for a CCD array of size X by Y pixels is shown in Figure 11.6.[5] The total charge from each pixel in a row is transferred to the pixel located in the row directly below via a vertical shift register. Hence, the charges are coupled to one another as they move across the grid. The charge corresponding to the pixels in the last row is transferred by a horizontal shift register to the amplifier and converted into a voltage. This voltage signal is then transmitted electronically through the endoscope to the video processor. CCD detectors have several important features that make them well suited for image detection in endoscopy. In addition to low power requirements, high resolution, and good color reproduction, CCDs have a sensitivity and dynamic range greater than that of photographic film by a factor of 100 and 50 times, respectively. Further, CCDs are not susceptible to mechanical vibration and shock and are not damaged by bright illumination. New developments in semiconductor technology have enabled the miniaturization of the CCD arrays. These detectors can be fabricated small enough to detect the image directly behind the objective lens, providing better light transmission efficiency and increased image resolution. Thus, endoscopes can be designed with a smaller light guide and a larger field of view. Also, the number of pixels that could be packed onto a CCD was significantly higher than that of the fibers in an imaging bundle.[8–14]

11.4 Endoscopic Image Formation

The objective lens of the endoscope collects light returning from the tissue and forms an image. Because of the large angles involved in the delivery and collection of light, the intensity along a cross section of an image from a uniform plane of tissue is not uniform. Instead, the intensity peaks in the center of the image and decreases significantly in the periphery. In conventional endoscopy, the returning light is diffusely reflected from the tissue surface, and the signal is intense. However, in new endoscopic techniques such as fluorescence, the returning light, generated spectroscopically, is weak. These methods require quantitative analysis, and an understanding of the light distribution throughout the image is needed. A mathematical model for endoscopic image formation will be presented.[15]

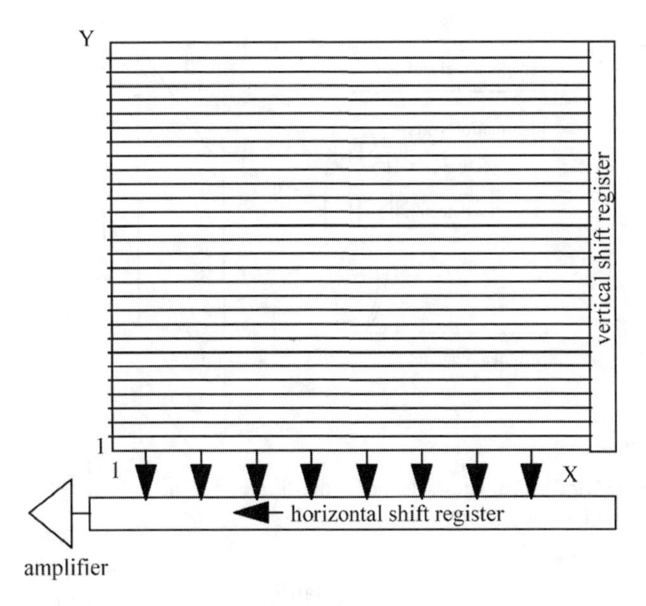

FIGURE 11.6 The read-out process for the CCD array. The total charge from each pixel in a row is transferred to the pixel located in the row directly below via a vertical shift register. The charge corresponding to the pixels in the last row is transferred by a horizontal shift register to the amplifier and converted into a voltage.

11.4.1 Spatial Distribution of Illumination Light

A set of spherical coordinates is defined at the distal end of the endoscope in Figure 11.7. The origin is located at the center of one of the illumination lenses, and has the distance variable r directed radially toward the tissue. The tissue is flat in shape, and oriented perpendicular to the endoscope at a distance d. The distance variable z defines the optic axis of the illumination lens, pointing perpendicularly through the tissue surface. The angle θ is defined between r and z. The variable ρ' represents the radial distance from the optic axis to an arbitrary region A_r in the plane of the tissue. The centers of the objective and illumination lenses are separated by a distance ρ_o. Light delivered from the illumination port has a maximum divergence angle of θ_m. The intensity of illumination light is assumed to be distributed in a Lambertian fashion, or uniformly over the surface of the illumination lens. The product of the incident power $P_i(\lambda_i)$ and the exposure time Δt determines the total energy incident onto the tissue. The incident fluence $F_i(\rho',d,\lambda_i)$, energy per unit area, valid for $0 \le \rho' \le d\tan\theta$, can be found to be as follows:

$$F_i(\rho',d,\lambda_i) = \frac{P_i(\lambda_i)\Delta t}{2\pi(1-\cos\theta_m)d^2\left(1+\left(\frac{\rho'}{d}\right)^2\right)^2} \tag{11.2}$$

Thus, the illumination energy on the tissue surface is not uniform, but it is maximum at the center of the image ($\rho' = 0$) and falls off toward the periphery ($\rho' = d\tan\theta$). The fluence produced by the other illumination port is similar.

11.4.2 Light Capture Efficiency

For either diffuse reflectance or fluorescence, the returning light is proportional to the incident light by a tissue factor ε_t. The total number of resels is designated N_r. For a fiber optic endoscope, N_r is the total number of fibers in the imaging bundle, and for a video endoscope, N_r is the product of the number of pixels X in each row and Y in each column of the CCD array. The average area A_r viewed per resel can be approximated by ratio of the total area imaged by the endoscope and the total number of resels N_r,

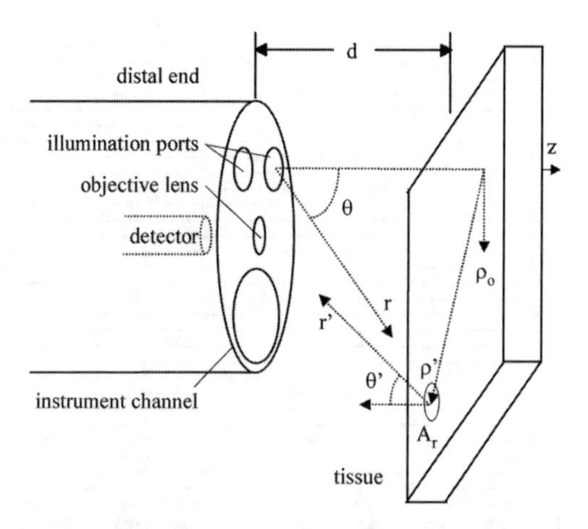

FIGURE 11.7 A set of spherical coordinates is defined at the distal end of the endoscope for the mathematical model of endoscopic image formation.

$$A_r = \frac{\pi\left(d\tan\theta_m\right)^2}{N_r} \tag{11.3}$$

As with the light from the illumination lens, the distribution of the light returning from the tissue region A_r is assumed to be Lambertian. At a distance r', the radiated energy can be taken to be uniformly distributed over the surface of a sphere whose area is given by $4\pi r'^2$. A fraction of the returning light, radiating isotropically toward the endoscope, is collected by the objective lens, which has a radius r_L and an area of $\pi r_L{}^2$. Thus, the fraction of the returning light that is collected is found from the ratio of the surface area of the lens with that of the sphere of radius r'.

11.4.3 Spatial Distribution of Returning Light

After the returning light is collected, it passes through the lenses in the objective with a transmission efficiency of T_o and incurs losses due to the packing fraction of the detector f_p. The approximate number of photons collected per resel can be determined from the collected light energy using the energy per photon of hc/λ_r as a conversion factor. The designation h is Planck's constant, c is the speed of light, and λ_r is the wavelength of the returning light. The total number of signal photons collected per resel, $N_s(\rho',d,\lambda_i,\lambda_r)$, valid for $0 \leq \rho' \leq d\tan\theta$, can be found to be as follows:

$$N_s(\rho',d,\lambda_i,\lambda_r) = \frac{K}{d^2\left(1+\left(\frac{\rho'-\rho_o}{d}\right)^2\right)^2\left(1+\left(\frac{\rho'}{d}\right)^2\right)^2}, \quad K = \frac{\lambda_r T_o f_p}{hc}\frac{r_L^2\varepsilon_t \tan^2\theta_m P_i(\lambda_i)\Delta t}{8(1-\cos\theta_m)N_r}. \tag{11.4}$$

As in the case of illumination, the spatial distribution of the returning light is not uniform, but is maximum at the center of the image ($\rho' = 0$) and falls off in the periphery ($\rho' = d\tan\theta$). The CCD detects the signal photons N_s, and they are converted into photoelectrons N_p with an efficiency η.

11.4.4 Experimental Validation of Model

The spatial distribution and distance dependence of an endoscopically collected image has been confirmed with fluorescence using a video colonoscope with following objective parameters of $\theta_m = 60°$, $r_L = 1.25$ mm, and $\rho_o = 6$ mm.[15] An argon laser with excitation wavelengths $\lambda_i = 351$ and 364 nm was used to excite autofluorescence over the spectral bandwidth from 400 to 700 nm from a flat specimen of resected

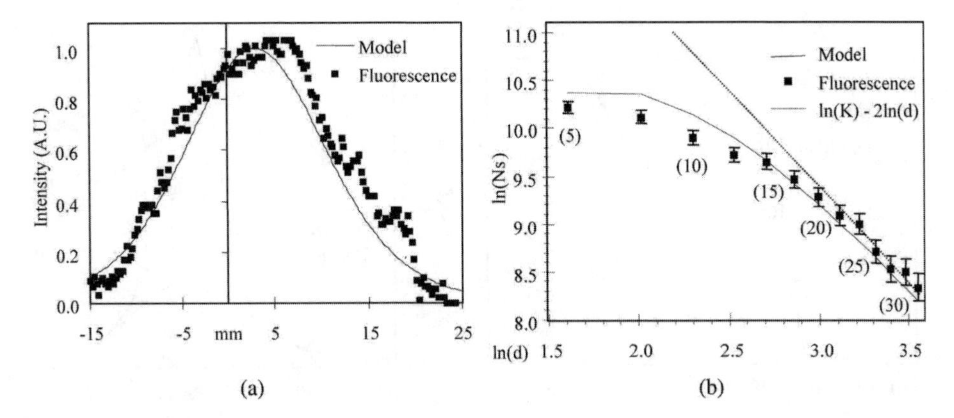

FIGURE 11.8 (a) A profile through the center of an endoscopically collected fluorescence image of colonic mucosa along at d = 20 mm is shown with the predicted model results. (b) The dependence of endoscopically collected fluorescence intensity over the range of distances between 5 and 35 mm is shown in a log-log plot.

colonic mucosa. In Figure 11.8a, the spatial distribution of fluorescence intensity collected is compared with that of the model, as predicted from Equation 11.4, for a distance of $d = 20$ mm, which is a typical operating distance. All values were ratioed by the peak intensity for normalization. As shown in Equation 11.4, the spatial profile of the detected image is not uniform but peaks near the center and falls off with ρ'. This nonuniform spatial distribution of collected light must be taken into account in quantitative methods for evaluating endoscopic images.

Furthermore, in Figure 11.8b the dependence of image intensity as a function of distance is shown on a log-log plot. The fluorescence intensity at $\rho' = 0$ is shown for distances d ranging between 5 and 35 mm in 2.5-mm increments from experimentally collected images is compared to the model results from Equation 11.4. The intensities at each distance d were divided by the value at $d = 20$ mm for normalization. The model predicts that the number of photons, N_s, will decrease with distance as $1/d^2$ for $d >> \rho_o$. In addition, the model shows that as d approaches 0, N_s reaches a maximum value. By taking the natural log of both sides of Equation 11.4, the results should approximate the line $\ln(N_s) = \ln(K) - 2\ln(d)$ for a $1/d^2$ dependence for large values of d. The experimental results shown in Figure 11.8b confirm the $1/d^2$ dependence for $d > 15$ mm. The corresponding distances in mm are shown in parentheses below the data points. For $d > 15$ mm, the measured values reach a maximum, as expected.

11.5 Endoscopic Image Resolution

The image resolution defines the level of detail that can be clearly seen on an endoscopic image. The transverse resolution is the smallest distance at which two objects located perpendicular to the optic axis (parallel to the surface of the tissue) can be distinguished while the axial resolution defines the smallest distance at which two objects located along the optic axis (into the tissue) can be distinguished. For conventional white light endoscopy, only the transverse resolution parameter is relevant because the light detected is reflected from the tissue surface and does not penetrate below. In other endoscopic methods where the light detected has penetrated with depth into the tissue, such as EUS and OCT, the axial resolution is also relevant. As discussed earlier, because of barrel distortion in the objective lens, the image resolution varies across the field of view. Thus, endoscopes are characterized by an average rather than an absolute transverse resolution. This average transverse resolution parameter can be approximated by geometric arguments to be the ratio of the total area imaged by the endoscope, $\pi(d\tan\theta_m)^2$ and the total number of resels N_r. This value is the same as A_t in Equation 11.3, which is valid over the depth of focus of the objective. In Figure 11.9a, a family of curves shows the average transverse resolution of endoscopic images as a function of distance d varying from 5 to 75 mm, the typical range of working distances. The total resels N_r vary from 50,000 to 200,000, and reflect typical values found in fiber optic

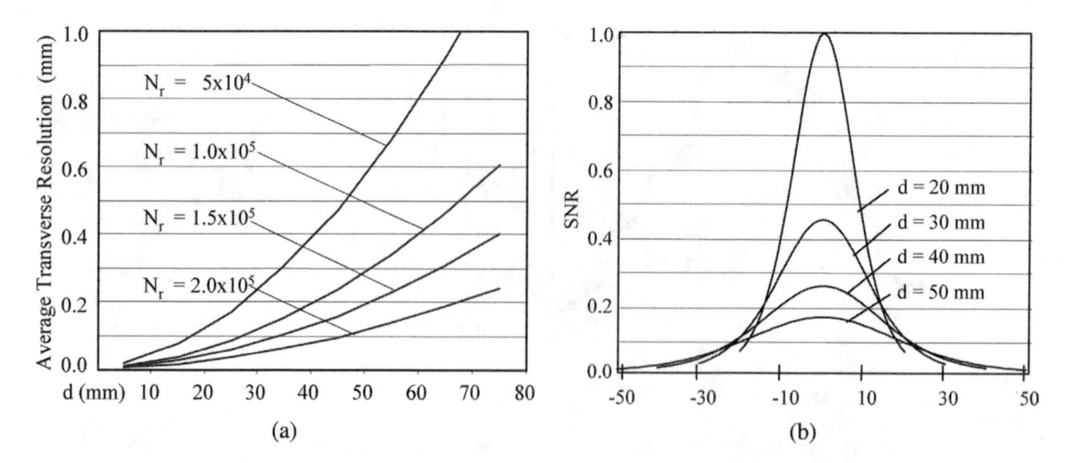

FIGURE 11.9 (a) A family of curves shows the average transverse resolution of endoscopic images as a function of distance d varying from 5 to 75 mm, the typical range of working distances, which improves as the distal end of the endoscope is moved in closer to the tissue surface. (b) A family of curves shows how the normalized SNR varies spatially for distances d ranging between 20 and 50 mm for a video endoscope.

and video endscopes. The total resels N_r is about 50,000 for fiber optic endoscopes and about 100,000 to 200,000 for video endoscopes. Because more pixels can be packed into a CCD array than optical fibers in an imaging bundle, the average resolution for video endoscopes is generally better. As shown in Figure 11.9a, the average transverse resolution for both fiber optic and video endoscopes is submillimeter over the depth of focus, and improves as the distal end of the endoscope is moved is closer to the tissue surface.

11.6 Endoscopic Image Signal-to-Noise Ratio

The signal-to-noise ratio (SNR) is another important imaging parameter in endoscopy. The SNR should be optimized in an endoscope so that smaller diameter light guides can be used to illuminate large fields of view. These designs result in thinner endoscopes that are more comfortable for patient use. The noise in an endoscopic image arises from dark current $D\Delta t$ and detector read-out noise N_{ro} in the detector, as shown in Figure 11.10. The conversion of signal photons to photoelectrons follows Poisson statistics, characterized by an average value $\overline{N}_p = \eta N_s$ and standard deviation $\sigma_p = \sqrt{\eta N_s}$. The expected output intensity $E(I)$ and variance σ_I^2 are given by the following:

$$E(I) = K\eta N_s \tag{11.5}$$

$$\sigma_I^2 = K^2[\eta N_s + D\Delta t] + N_{ro}^2 \tag{11.6}$$

The SNR is defined as the ratio of the expected intensity E(I), and the standard deviation of the signal σ_I is given by the following:

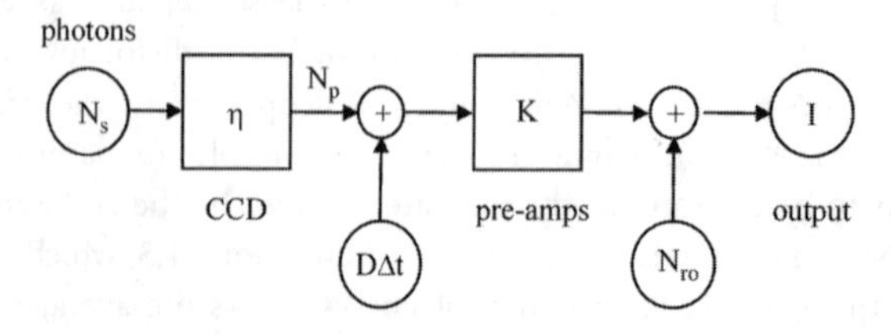

FIGURE 11.10 The noise in an endoscopic image arises from dark current $D\Delta t$ and detector read-out noise N_{ro} in the detector.

$$\mathrm{SNR} = \frac{E(I)}{\sigma_I} = \frac{\eta N_s}{\sqrt{\eta N_s + D\Delta t + \left(\frac{N_{ro}}{K}\right)^2}} \tag{11.7}$$

An intensified CCD detector may be used for fluorescence imaging, and the number of photoelectrons ηN_s is amplified by a large gain factor to suppress the instrument noise term

$$D\Delta t + \left(\frac{N_{ro}}{K}\right)^2$$

that can be ignored in the denominator of Equation 11.7. This condition is called shot-noise limited detection, and the SNR reduces to the following:

$$\mathrm{SNR} = \sqrt{\eta N_s} \tag{11.8}$$

A video endoscope can also be used for fluorescence imaging. In this situation, the instrument noise is usually much larger than the number of detected photoelectrons, and the photoelectron term ηN_s can be ignored in the denominator of Equation 11.7. This condition is called instrument-noise limited detection, and the SNR over the field of view can be approximated by the following,

$$\mathrm{SNR}(\rho, d) = \frac{K\eta}{d^2\left(1+\left(\frac{\rho-\rho_o}{d}\right)^2\right)^4 \sqrt{D\Delta t + \left(\frac{N_{ro}}{K}\right)^2}} \tag{11.9}$$

The family of curves in Figure 11.9b shows how the normalized SNR varies with ρ' for distances d ranging between 20 and 50 mm for a video endoscope.

11.7 Color Image Processing

11.7.1 RGB Color Wheel

CCD detectors are sensitive to light over the entire visible spectrum and generally produce monochromatic (black and white) images. Thus, image processing techniques, such as RGB sequential imaging or color filtering, are required to produce color images.[2] In the RGB sequential imaging method, a color wheel, shown in Figure 11.11a is placed in front of the light source in the video processor. The wheel contains a set of red, green, and blue filters, and rotates at approximately 30 Hz (video rate). The timing diagram shown in Figure 11.11b illustrates the read-out process. The times at which the start and end of the red filter is exposed to the light is designated t_{rs} and t_{re}, respectively. The CCD array will collect red light over this period of exposure. The intervening space between the red and green filters on the wheel is opaque and blocks any light from exposing the CCD detector during the time between t_{re} and t_{gs}. During this period, the data in the CCD array is read out and stored in the red page of image memory. This process is repeated in an identical fashion to produce the green and blue reflectance images. The time required to produces all three images takes about 1/30 sec. The red, green, and blue images located in memory are then superimposed to produce the color video image. The color images acquired with this method use the full resolution of the CCD array.

11.7.2 Color Filtering

Color images can also be produced with a colored filter placed over the CCD array rather than using a filter wheel. In this method, all of the color components are collected at the same period of exposure;

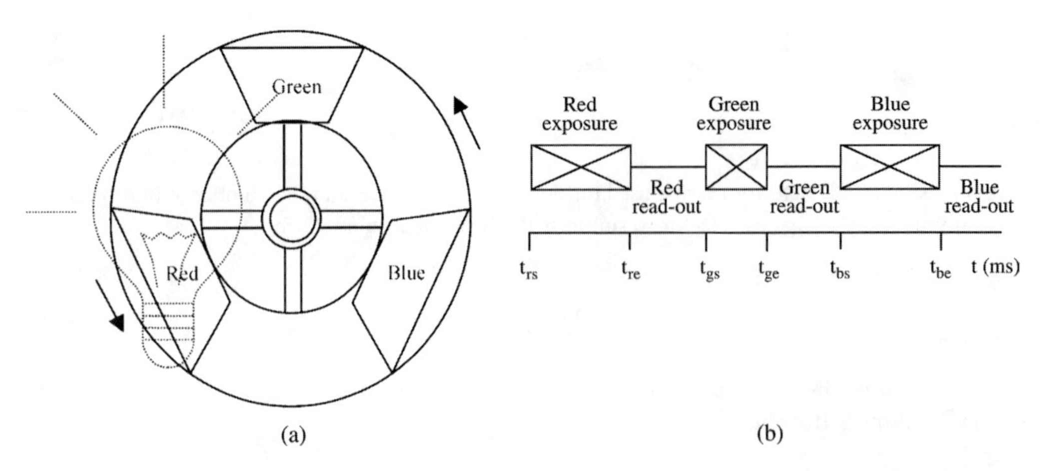

FIGURE 11.11 (a) In the RGB sequential imaging method, a color wheel is placed in front of the light source, located within the video processor. The wheel contains a set of red, green, and blue filters, and rotates at 30 cps. (b) The timing diagram of the red, green, and blue exposure and read-out periods is shown.

however, a loss of image resolution occurs as a trade-off. The two most common filters used are called RGB striped and mosaic. The array corresponding to an RGB striped filter, shown in Figure 11.12a, consists of three vertical filter columns, or stripes, that transmit red, green, and blue light in each column, respectively. The red filter allows reflected red light to pass and blocks green and blue. The green and blue filters work in a similar fashion. When an image is detected, the read-out process is performed as discussed before, but the columns of pixels corresponding to the red, green, and blue filters are separated into different pages of image memory. The images from the three pages in memory are then recombined for display purposes.

The array corresponding to a mosaic filter, shown in Figure 11.12b, has cyan (c), yellow (Y), and white (no filter) filters arranged in a 2 × 2 pixel pattern repeated over the array. These filters allow more of the light to pass than RGB striped filters, resulting in a higher SNR. The cyan filter allows blue and green light to pass, the yellow filter passes red and green light, and the white filter lets all of the light to pass.

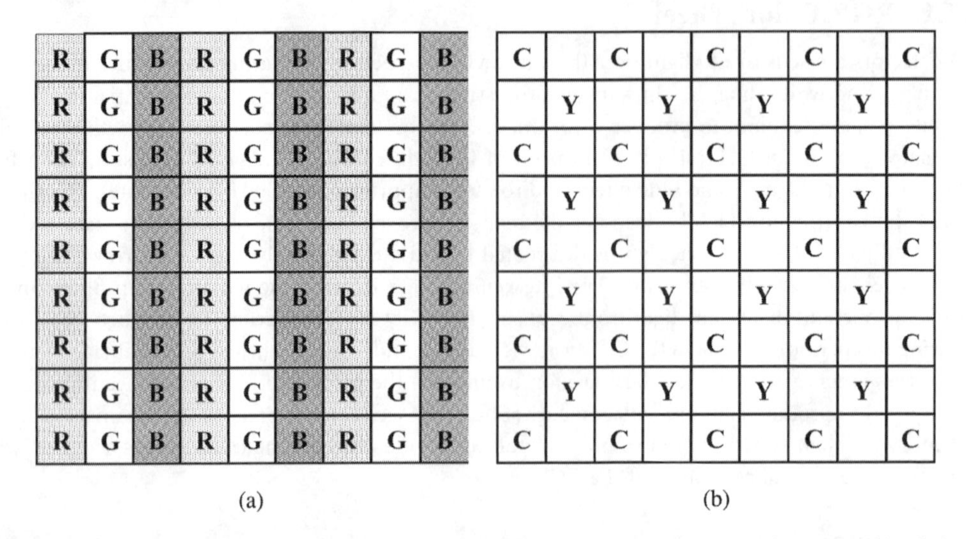

FIGURE 11.12 (a) A striped filter is shown with three vertical columns that transmit red, green, or blue light. (b) A mosaic filter is shown with cyan, yellow, and white (no filter) filters arranged in a 2 × 2 pixel pattern repeated over the CCD array.

By adding or subtracting the intensity of light detected from adjacent pixels, the individual red, green, and blue components can be obtained for each group of four pixels. For example, the intensity at pixel coordinates (x,y) on the array of the blue $I_B(x,y)$ is produced from the difference between the intensity of white $I_W(x,y)$ and yellow $I_Y(x,y)$. Similarly, the intensity of red $I_R(x,y)$ is obtained from that of white $I_W(x,y)$ and cyan $I_C(x,y)$. The intensities for the red, green, and blue components of the image at pixel location (x,y) are summarized in Equation 11.9.

$$I_B(x,y) = I_W(x,y) - I_Y(x,y) \tag{11.9}$$

$$I_R(x,y) = I_W(x,y) - I_C(x,y)$$

$$I_G(x,y) = I_W(x,y) - I_B(x,y) - I_R(x,y)$$

11.8 Endoscopic Retrograde Cholangiopancreatography

Tissue structures such as the pancreatic and biliary ducts are too small to directly insert an endoscope. Endoscopes can still be used to image these structures radiographically through fluoroscopy with a procedure called endoscopic retrograde cholangiopancreatography (ERCP). In ERCP, a cannula is inserted into the papilla, the site where the pancreatic and common bile ducts join, and contrast is injected. This contrast is viewed with delivery of x-rays onto a fluoroscopy monitor. Because the papilla, located within the Ampulla of Vater, is on the side wall of the duodenum, there is not enough space for a forward-viewing endoscope to maneuver and perform the cannulation. Instead, a side-viewing endoscope, or duodenoscope, is used. The optics for a side-viewing endoscope are designed for imaging tissue located along the parallel to the axis of the endoscope. In Figure 11.13a, a cross-section view shows an illumination bundle that is curved to deliver light to the side of the endoscope. Also, the objective collects returning light coming from the side using a prism to reflect the image to the detector. Furthermore, the side-viewing endoscope has a forceps raiser located in the instrument channel that elevates the catheter during cannulation, as shown in the side-view in Figure 11.13b. Only one illumination lens is located on the distal tip. Side-viewing duodenoscopes are about 120 cm in working length, and have a variety of instrument channel sizes, ranging from 2.8 to 4.0 mm. The larger diameter channels are useful for special instruments used in therapeutic biliary endoscopy, such as for endoscopic sphincterotomy, stone extraction, and stent placement. In Figure 11.15a, an image from a side-viewing duodeoscope is shown with a cannula inserted into the papilla. In Figure 11.15b, a radiograph shows the position of the duodenoscope with contrast filling the common bile duct (left) and the pancreatic duct (right).

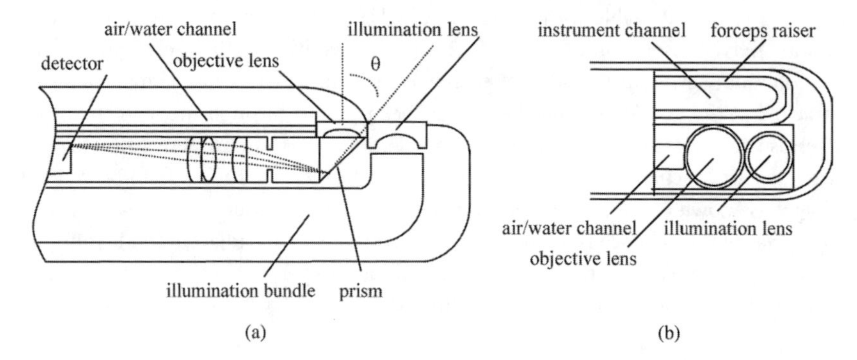

FIGURE 11.13 (a) A cross-section view of a side viewing endoscope shows the optics packaged to view images oriented parallel to the axis endoscope rather than perpendicular. (b) A side view shows one illumination lens and a forceps raiser to help guide cannulation.

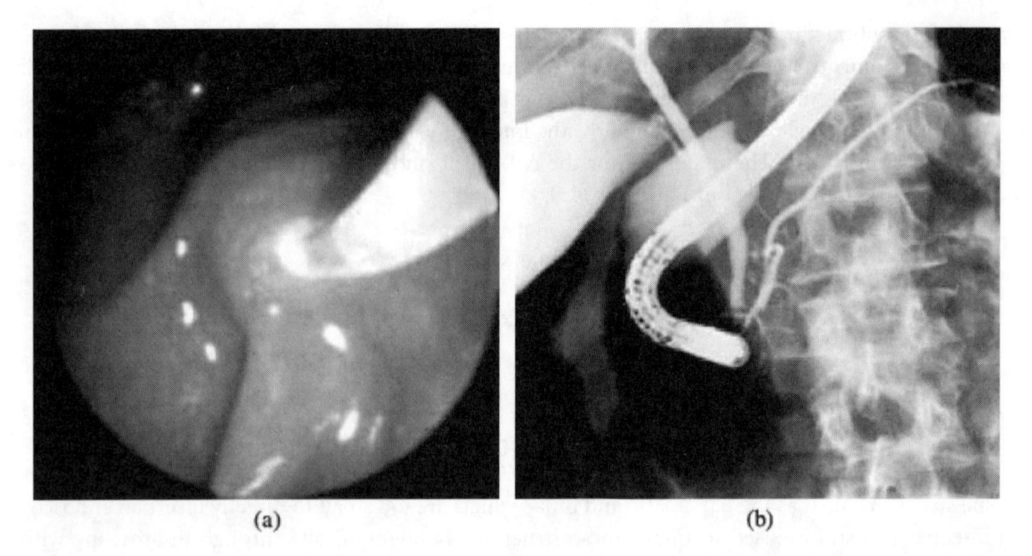

FIGURE 11.14 (a) A side-viewing duodenoscope is used to insert the cannula into the papilla. (b) A radiograph shows the position of the duodenoscope with contrast being injected into the papilla. The contrast is filling the common bile duct shown on the left and the pancreatic duct shown on the right.

11.9 Endoscopic Ultrasound

Endoscopic ultrasound (EUS) combines endoscopy with ultrasound (US), using a miniaturized US transducer attached to the distal tip. EUS collects ultrasound images with the transducer placed in close proximity to the structure being imaged, such as the esophagus, unlike transcorporeal ultrasound, where the sound travels through many layers of tissue.[16,17] The resolution obtained with EUS is significantly better because obstructing layers of bone and gas can be avoided and higher acoustic frequencies can be used. Since ultrasound imaging is described in another chapter, this section will discuss only technology specific to EUS. The clinical applications of these technological advances include determining the grade and stage of invading tumors and guiding fine needle aspiration (FNA) for tumor cytology. There are two modes of scanning, radial sector and linear array, and they are often used clinically in a complementary fashion.[18–23]

11.9.1 Radial Sector Scanning

Radial sector scanning provides ultrasound images in the plane oriented perpendicular to the axis of the endoscope. A radial sector echoendoscope uses a rotating acoustic mirror that can scan images in sectors of 360° or 180°. They are available with 7.5- and 12-MHz transducers that have a focal distance of 30 and 25 mm and an axial resolution of 200 and 120 μm, respectively, with a penetration depth of about 100 mm. The oblique-viewing echoendoscope, shown in Figure 11.15a, has a small radial sector echoprobe (e) attached at the distal tip. A needle (n) has been passed through the instrument channel, and an elevator (el) is used to maneuver the needle.[2] Radial scanning is usually performed first to determine the exact size, location, vacularity, and consistency of a lesion. An example of a 360° radial sector scan of the esophagus is shown in Figure 11.16a. The layers of the wall, mucosa (m), submucosa (sm), and muscularis propria (mp) can be seen clearly. The hyperechoic structure adjacent to the muscularis propria corresponds to the subserosa and the serosa. In addition, a hyperechoic tumor (t) can be seen in the submucosa. These findings are consistent with a lipoma.

11.9.2 Linear Array Scanning

Linear array scanning provides ultrasound images in the plane oriented parallel to the axis, and is useful for FNA. A linear array scanning echoendoscope uses an array of transducers that provides a wedge-shaped

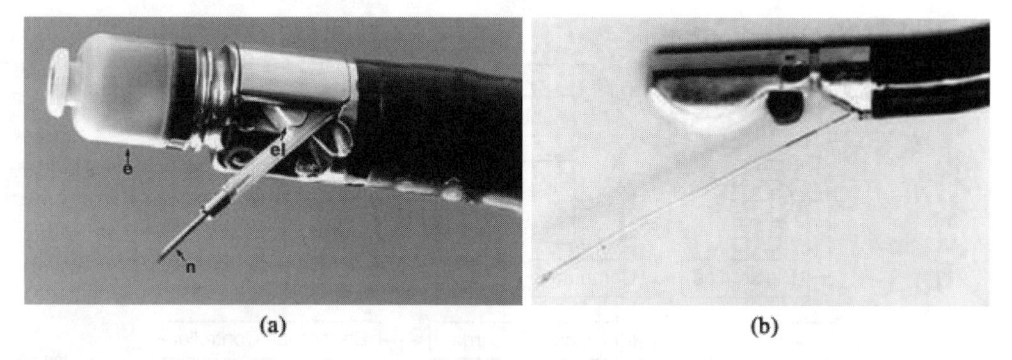

FIGURE 11.15 (a) An oblique-viewing endoscope has a small echoprobe (e) attached at the distal tip. A modified sclerosing needle (n) has been passed through the instrument channel where an elevator (el) is used to maneuver the needle. (b) An oblique-viewing endoscope has a curved linear array transducer located on the distal tip with a fine needle for aspiration protruding from the instrument channel.

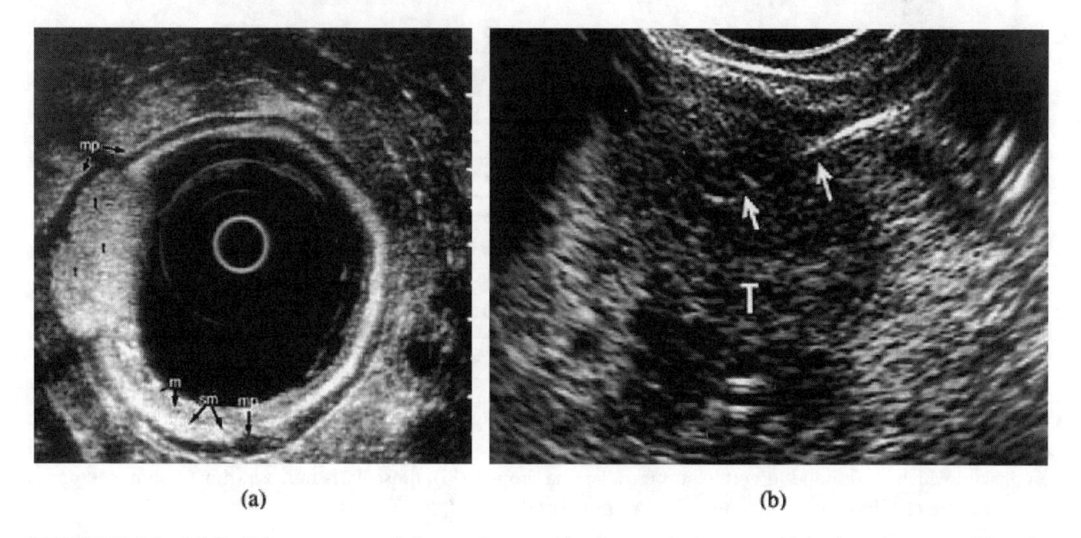

FIGURE 11.16 (a) Radial sector scan of the esophagus with a hyperechoic tumor (t) in the submucosa. The echo pattern of the tumor is more hyperechoic compared with that of the muscularis propria (mp). These findings are consistent with a lipoma. Note also the clear image of the mucosa (m), submucosa (sm), and muscularis propria. The hyperechoic structure adjacent to the muscularis propria corresponds to the subserosa and the serosa. (b) Linear array scan image of an EUS-guided FNA of a pancreatic tumor (T) with the arrows pointing to the needle.

image in sectors of 100 to 180°. They are available with 5- and 7.5-MHz transducers that have variable focal distances. The linear array can also provide color-flow mapping and Doppler imaging to locate blood flow in vessels for identifying landmarks and for assessing vascular invasion by tumors. In addition, this scanning mode provides continuous real-time visualization of a needle during EUS-guided FNA for cytology. The oblique-viewing echoendoscope, shown in Figure 11.15b, has a curved linear array transducer located on the distal tip with a fine needle for aspiration protruding from the instrument channel.[2] Figure 11.16b shows an endosonographic view of an EUS-guided FNA of a pancreatic tumor (T) with the arrows pointing to the needle.

11.10 Optical Coherence Tomography

Optical coherence tomography (OCT) performs cross-sectional imaging in a manner similar to that of EUS, except the phase property of light rather than the backscattering behavior of sound is used.[25–27] Moreover, OCT has up to 10 to 100 times better axial resolution than EUS at a penetration depth of up

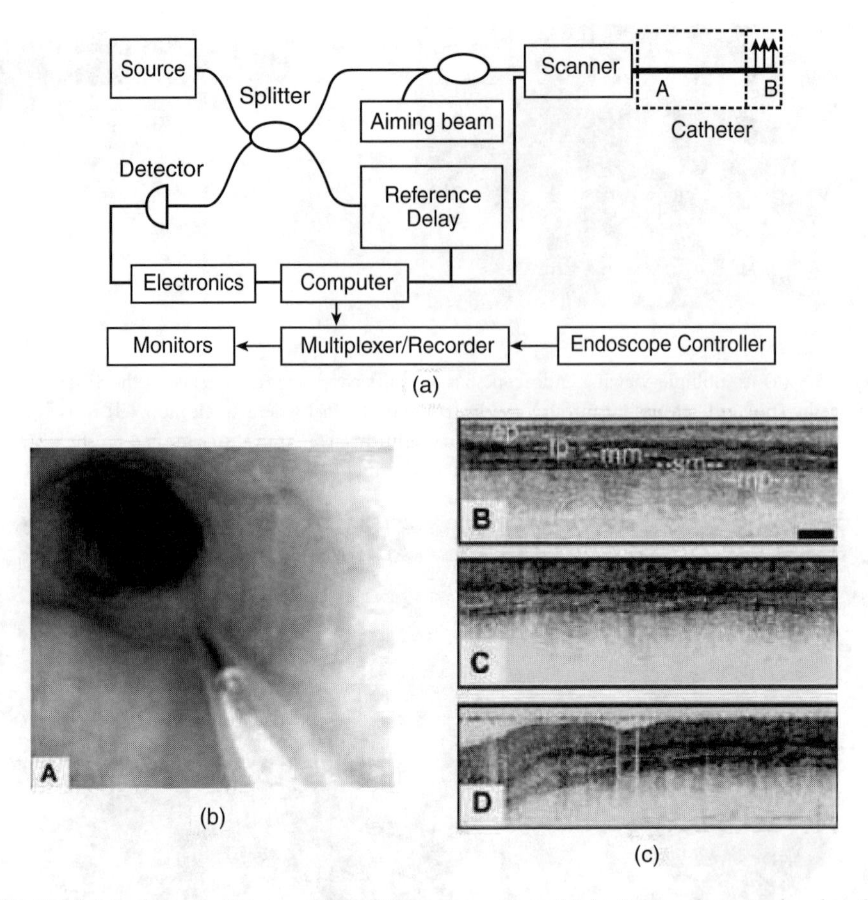

FIGURE 11.17 (a) A schematic diagram of an OCT imaging system. (b) An OCT catheter is placed in the lumen of the esophagus through the instrument channel of the endoscope. (c)–(e) OCT images show the layers of normal esophagus, which correspond to epithelium (ep), lamina propria (lp), muscularis mucosa (mm), submucosa (sm), and the inner, circular layer of the muscularis propria (mp).

to 1 mm. OCT is a technology that is being developed to assess tissue histopathology otherwise known as optical biopsy.[28,29] OCT has demonstrated the ability for distinguishing the layers of mucosa in the GI tract with potential to detect precancerous lesions such as dysplasia.[30–36] OCT uses an interferometer to compare the distance that light travels and becomes reflected from a layer of tissue in one optical path to that traveling along a reference path of nearly equal length. As shown in the schematic diagram in Figure 11.17a, light from a low-coherence laser diode source, 5 mW at $\lambda = 1300$ nm, is coupled into a single mode optical fiber, and divided by a beam splitter to the scanner and reference arms of a Michelson intereferometer.[33] The backscattered light from the tissue is recollected by the optical fiber in the catheter and then passed back through the splitter in the opposite direction. Similarly, light passing through the reference arm is reflected by a mirror and becomes coupled with that from the scanner. In the reference, a computer controls electronics that scan a mirror over a range of depths at which backscattering light will be measured, enabling an axial scan to be completed. Optical detection occurs if the difference in distance (phase) is within the coherence length of the source. By performing axial scans rapidly as the beam is swept across the tissue surface, a two-dimensional image is produced. The interferometer prevents multiply scattered light from being detected and significantly improves tissue resolution. In addition, contrast is provided by the difference in the reflectance of cellular and extracellular material present in each tissue layer.

In the OCT system described, the transverse and axial resolution at $\lambda = 1300$ nm is approximately 25 and 10 μm, respectively, and the light penetrates approximately 1 mm into the tissue.[33] The images are acquired in a manner similar to linear array scanning in EUS with image dimensions of 5.5 mm (512 pixels) in length and 2.5 mm (256 pixels) in depth with a frame rate of four images per second. An example of OCT image collection is shown in Figure 11.17b, where a 2-mm diameter OCT catheter is shown placed in the lumen of the esophagus through the instrument channel of the endoscope. In Figure 11.17c and 11.17d, an OCT image shows the layers of normal esophagus, which correspond to epithelium (*ep*), lamina propria (*lp*), muscularis mucosa (*mm*), submucosa (*sm*), and the inner, circular layer of the muscularis propria (*mp*). Furthermore, OCT imaging has demonstrated potential for other diagnostic purposes, such as the identification of premalignant tissue in the lung,[37] endometrium, and cervix,[38] measurement of blood flow via Doppler,[39] and the characterization of atherosclerotic plaque in coronary arteries.[40]

11.11 High Magnification Endoscopy

High magnification endoscopy is a new technology that visualizes the details of the mucosal surface to identify malignant from benign tissue.[41–44] While most raised mucosal lesions, such as polyps, can be identified easily with a conventional endoscope, there is increased evidence for the existence of flat lesions that have malignant potential.[45,46] These lesions cannot be seen easily on white light endoscopy. High magnification endoscopes have special intermediate lenses that can be inserted into the optical train of the objective to attain image magnifications as high as 170×, although most instruments operate at a magnification around 35×. In the high magnification mode, the depth of field is usually significantly reduced, and the endoscope must be placed very close to the mucosal surface. Also, the field of view decreases significantly, and the images are susceptible to motion artifacts. These endoscopes are often combined with high resolution CCD detectors to provide transverse resolution as low as 10 μm. In comparison, the naked human eye has a transverse resolution of approximately 125 μm. Conventional video endoscopes have CCDs with 100,000 to 200,000 total resels. The transverse resolution varies with distance as shown in Figure 11.9a. High magnification endoscopes can have total resels as high as 850,000. High magnification endoscopes are often used in combination with chromoendoscopy.

An example of high magnification endoscopy is illustrated with images taken of Barrett's esophagus, a premalignant condition for esophageal adenocarcinoma.[47] In Figure 11.18a, a standard endoscopic

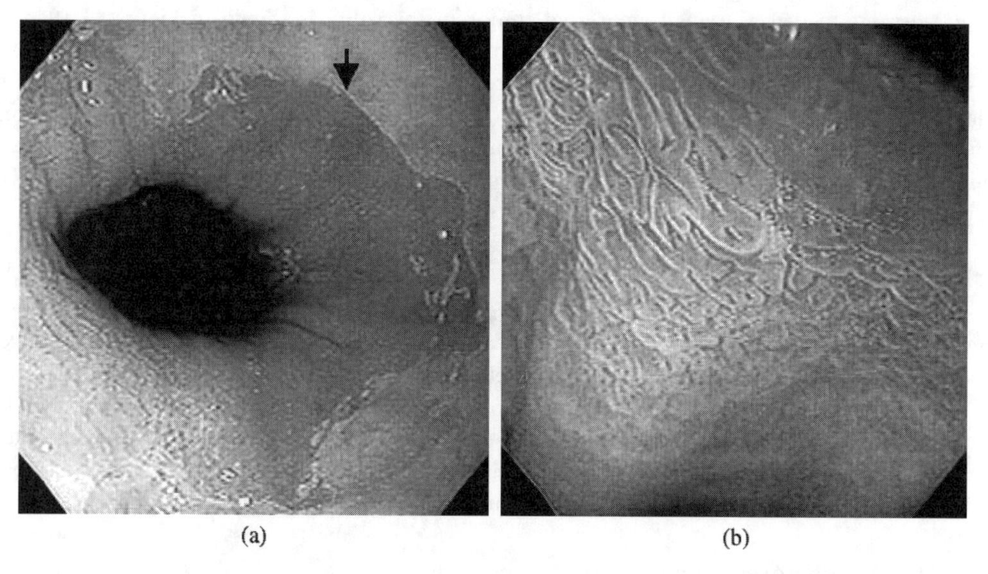

FIGURE 11.18 (See color insert following page 14-10.) (a) Normal endoscopic view of the distal esophagus after spraying with acetic acid, showing short extensions of columnar-appearing mucosa with squamous islands within Barrett's epithelium. (b) Enhanced magnification endoscopic view of the same field showing a fine villiform pit pattern.

image is shown of the gastroesophageal junction after being sprayed with acetic acid. Acetic acid reversibly denatures cytoplasmic proteins, and enhances the detail of small remnant islands of columnar epithelium.[48] The borders of the gastroesophageal junction are clearly visualized as well as the squamous islands within the Barrett's epithelium. The arrow indicates the region that is magnified at a power of 35× and shown in Figure 11.18b. The magnified view shows a fine villiform appearance that is classified into one of several characteristic pit patterns, (1) round pits with regular and orderly arranged circular dots, (2) reticular pits that are circular or oval and are regular in shape and arrangement, (3) villiform appearance with regular shape and arrangement, and (4) thick villous convoluted shape with a cerebriform appearance with regular shape and arrangement. These pit patterns have a high correlation with identification of Barrett's esophagus on histology.

11.12 Chromoendoscopy

Chromoendoscopy is an endoscopic technique that involves the application of tissue stains to highlight regions of interest in the mucosa, and is often used together with high magnification endoscopy.[49–51] The use of these methods is becoming more widespread for detection of flat lesions with malignant potential that are not apparent on conventional endoscopy. There are two common types of stains, contrast and vital stains. Contrast stains, such as indigo carmine and cresly violet, collect within the surface defects of the lesion and enhance the contrast in color.[52–54] These dyes are useful for identifying flat adenomas and carcinoma *in situ* in the colon and stomach. They are not absorbed by the mucosa, thus produce no systemic effects to the patient. Vital stains such as Lugol's iodine, methylene blue, and toluidine blue bind to the tissue and produce a chemical change. Lugol's solution contains iodine and potassium iodide and reacts with glycogen to produces a brown-black color.[55,56] This dye is used to enhance lesions such as squamous cell carcinoma and high-grade dysplasia of the esophagus, which are poor in glycogen. Methlyene blue is absorbed by the cytosol of the epithelium of the esophagus, and the small and large intestine.[57–61] This dye is particularly useful for staining the intestinal metaplasia associated with Barrett's esophagus, which turns a bright blue color and appears granular. Toluidine blue binds to the nucleus of cells, and highlights mucosa with increased DNA synthetic activity. This dye is also used for enhancing regions of Barrett's esophagus to screen for high-grade dysplasia. An example of chromoendoscopy with application of indigo carmine to detect a small, depressed tumor in the colon is shown in Figure 11.19.[54] On conventional endoscopy, these tumors have a faint reddish or whitish color, few vascular abnormalities, and a slight deformity in the mucosal surface. In Figure 11.19a, an 8-mm lesion is seen in the colon on a standard endoscopic view with a slightly depressed and reddish appearance and poorly defined borders. After indigo carmine is sprayed onto the lesion, the borders of the lesion are clearly defined, surface appears depressed, and the vasculature is enhanced, as seen in Figure 11.19b. The biopsy of this lesion confirmed adenocarcinoma.

11.13 Fluorescence Imaging

The endoscopic techniques discussed previously provide images of structural changes in the tissue. New endoscopic methods collecting fluorescence can determine the biochemical and molecular changes in the tissue. Fluorescence can originate from endogenous molecules, such as aromatic amino acids, NADH, FAD, and porphyrins, termed autofluorescence.[62] Also, fluorescence can be produced by exogenously administered drugs, such as hematoporphyrin derivative and 5-ALA, called photodynamic diagnosis. Both of these fluorescence methods are used to identify cancer at a early stage.

11.13.1 Autofluorescence

Autofluorescence images can be collected with either a fiber optic or video endoscope. Because no exogenous drugs are administered, these images can be acquired during routine endoscopy, and the

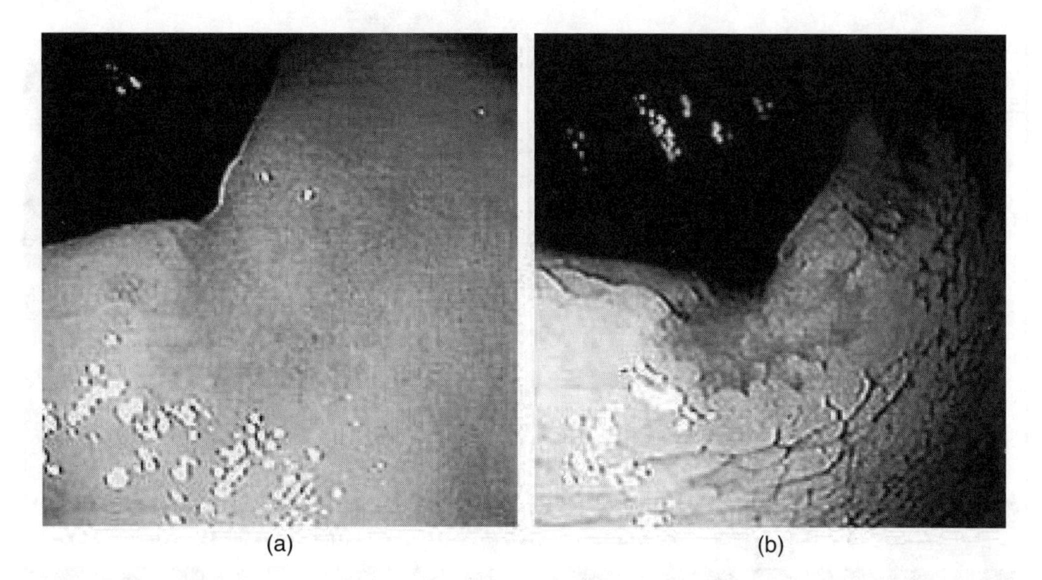

FIGURE 11.19 (a) A standard view on colonoscopy of an 8-mm flat colorectal cancer reveals a slightly depressed tiny, faint reddish lesion. (b) On chromoendoscopy, the depressed surface and surrounding slightly elevated mucosa is clearly revealed.

patients do not experience photosensitivity after the procedure. However, the fluorescence produced from endogenous molecules is much weaker than that from exogenous agents or from diffuse reflectance, by a factor of 1000 or more, and a laser is required for excitation (illumination). With a fiber optic endoscope, fluorescence can be separated into two or more spectral bands to ratio the images, which corrects for the spatial nonuniformity.[63–69] The optimal spectral regimes for collecting images are determined by fluorescence spectra collected from single point optical fiber probes.[70–73] Because the light passes through an optical train with many elements, the loss of fluorescence signal can be significant, and an intensified camera is needed for image detection.[74] A video endoscope can also be used to collect fluorescence. Because the CCD detector is located directly behind the objective, the fluorescence signal is much more intense.[75] Image processing algorithms are required to correct for spatial nonuniformity, and to identify regions of disease.[76]

An example of autofluorescence images of flat colonic adenomas is shown in Figure 11.20.[75] The schematic of a prototype video fluorescence imaging system is shown in Figure 11.20a. An argon laser delivers ultraviolet excitation light at 351 and 364 nm through an optical fiber placed in the instrument channel of a video colonoscope. A computer-controlled shutter is activated via a foot switch and delivered approximately 300 mW onto the mucosal surface for a period of 50 ms. The CCD detector collects fluorescence in the visible bandwidth, and detects both the white light and fluorescence images simultaneously. The standard endoscopic view in Figure 11.20b shows two flat adenomas identified by the arrows that are barely discernable on white light reflectance. These lesions appear as dark regions on fluorescence, as shown in Figure 11.20c. The fluorescence intensity at the site of the adenoma is approximately two times less than that of the surrounding normal mucosa. The fluorescence image was then processed using a moving average filter to predict regions of dysplasia to remove the spatial nonuniformity in the image. The unprocessed fluorescence image was divided by the moving average image, multiplied by 100 to form a percent ratio image. In Figure 11.20d, a color overlay shows the locations on the mucosa that have a high, medium, and low probability of containing dysplasia with the colors red, green, and blue, respectively. Note that the region of high probability (red) corresponds to the location of the two adenomas on the white light image. In addition to premalignant tissue in other areas of the GI tract,[76–82] autofluorescence imaging has also demonstrated the potential to detect lesions in the bladder,[83] head and neck,[84,85] larynx,[86,87] lung,[88–92] and nasopharynx.[93]

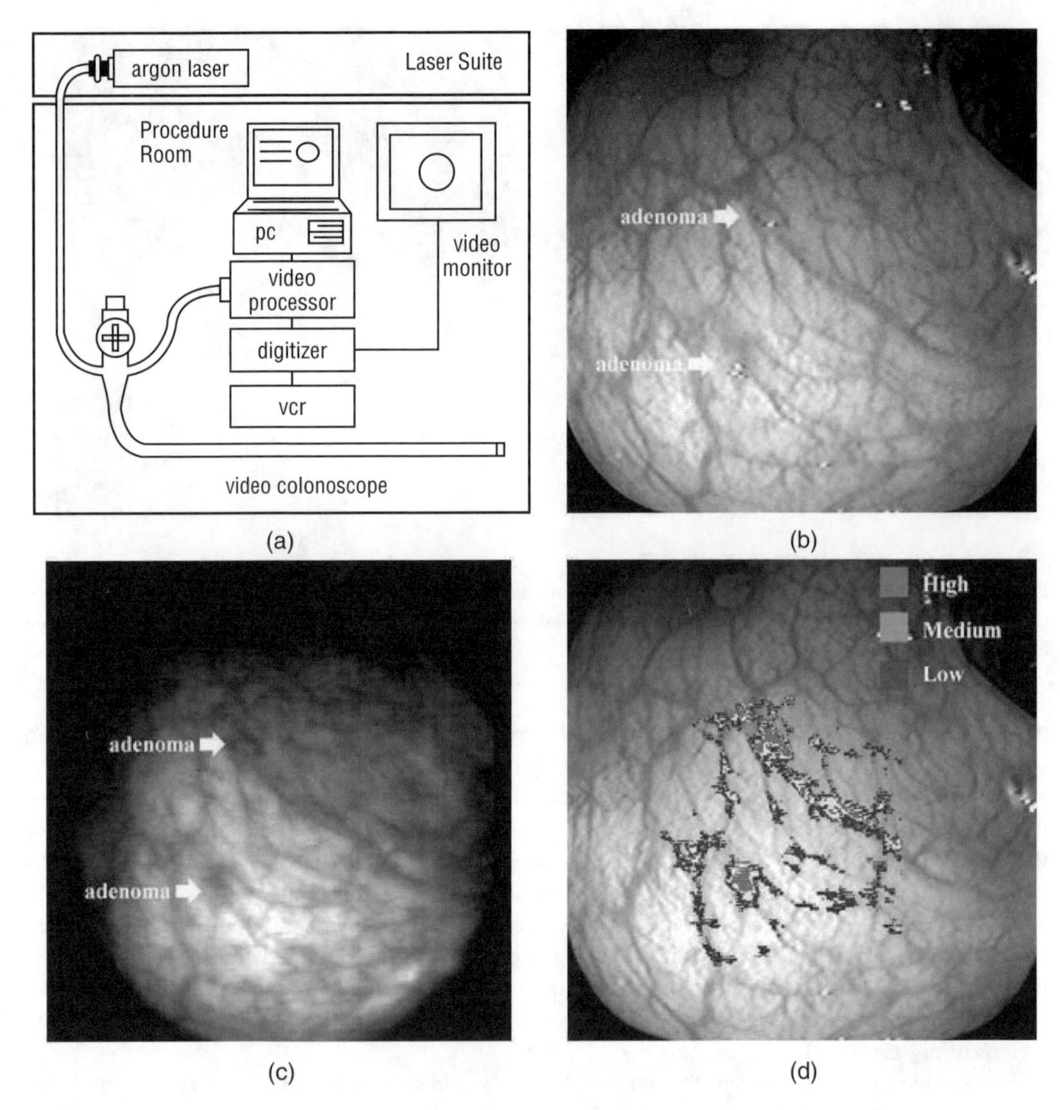

FIGURE 11.20 **(See color insert [Figure 11.20(d)] following page 14-10.)** (a) Schematic diagram of a video colonoscope for collecting autofluorescence images. (b) The standard endoscopic view shows two flat adenomas identified by the arrows that are barely discernable. (c) The lesions appear as dark regions on fluorescence, which is about 2 times less for the adenomas compared to that of the surrounding normal mucosa. (d) A color overlay shows the locations on the mucosa that have a high, medium, and low probability of containing dysplasia with the colors red, green, and blue, respectively. Note that the region of high probability (red) corresponds to the location of the two adenomas on the white light image.

11.13.2 Photodynamic Imaging

Photodynamic imaging collects fluorescence generated from externally administered agents, or prodrugs, which are internally converted and selectively taken up by cells that have higher metabolic activity.[94–98] A promising agent is 5-aminolevulinic acid (5-ALA), a porphyrin substrate in the heme biosynthetic pathway that induces the formation of protoporphyrin IX (PPIX), a compound with high fluorescence efficiency. 5-ALA has demonstrated potential to detect premalignant tissue in the bladder,[99–101] colon,[102] esophagus,[103–105] and oropharynx.[106] Excess exogenous application of 5-ALA leads to a three- to sixfold higher intracellular accumulation of PPIX in areas of high-grade dysplasia and malignant lesions compared with the surrounding mucosa. PPIX fluorescence is excited by blue light (peak of 405 nm), and the emission is

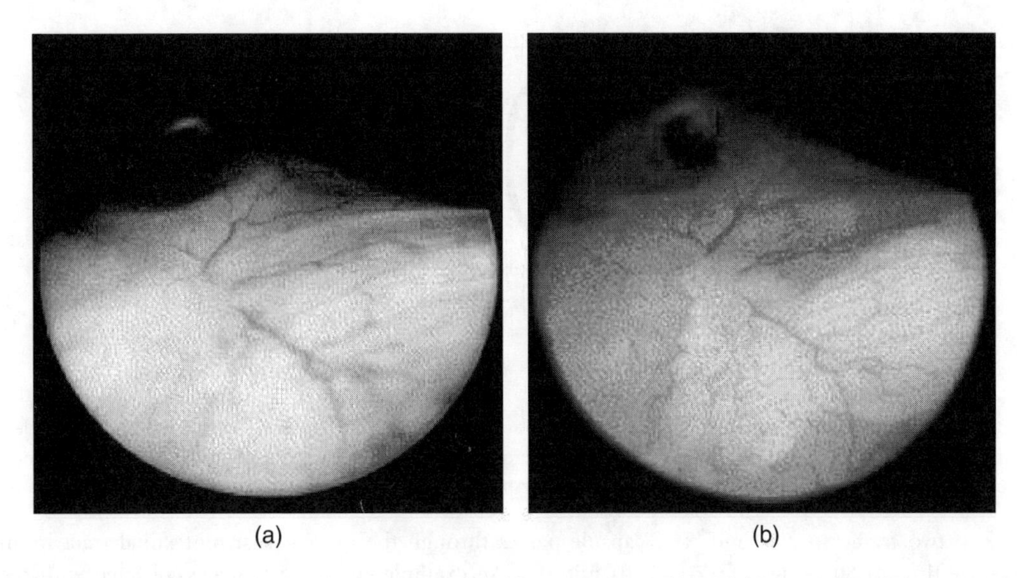

FIGURE 11.21 (a) A standard endoscopic view of bladder urothelium. (b) With blue excitation light activated, a region of red fluorescence is revealed. Subsequent biopsies confirmed that the regions of red fluorescence corresponded to transitional cell carcinoma on histology. (Figure is depicted here in black and white.)

red at wavelengths above 600 nm. ALA can be administered orally for systemic distribution, and the drug is cleared in about 48 h, and can produce mild skin photosensitivity and transient elevation of liver enzymes. ALA can also be administered intravesically for detection of transitional cell carcinoma (TCC) of the urinary bladder.[107] TCC is a flat urothelial lesion that has high malignant potential. These lesions are often missed on conventional endoscopy. An example of photodynamic imaging of fluorescence with 5-ALA is shown in Figure 11.21. Prior to the procedure, 5-ALA solution was instilled intravesically via a catheter for a dwell time of about 3 h. A short-arc xenon lamp produces 200 mW of blue excitation light in the spectral band between 375 and 440 nm. A 450 nm long pass filter is placed in the eyepiece of a cystoscope to collect the PPIX fluorescence. The images were detected with a color CCD with enhanced sensitivity above 600 nm. Figure 11.21a shows the standard endoscopic view of the bladder urothelium. Figure 11.21b shows the same view with blue excitation light activated, revealing a region of red fluorescence. Subsequent biopsies confirmed that the regions of red fluorescence corresponded to transitional cell carcinoma on histology.

11.14 Wireless Capsule

In addition to video endoscopes, the development of miniaturized detector technology has allowed for images to be collected with a wireless capsule.[108–111] All of the optics and electronics are contained within a small capsule that can be swallowed painlessly and passed throughout the gastrointestinal tract by peristalsis. There are no cables, wires, or optical fibers. This method of endoscopy is particularly suited for imaging regions of the GI tract that cannot be easily reached by conventional endoscopes, such as the small bowel. The illumination light is provided by battery powered white light-emitting diodes (LEDs). The images are collected by a low noise complementary metal oxide silicon (CMOS) detector that produce images with quality comparable to a CCD detector but with consumption of significantly less power. The images are transmitted from within the body via UHF band radio telemetry to aerials worn around the waist and stored on a portable solid state recorder. The integration of the detector, transmitter, and LEDs was performed by application specific integrated circuit (ASIC) design.

A schematic diagram of the capsule is shown in Figure 11.22a.[108] The capsule has dimensions of 11 × 30 mm. There is an optical dome that covers the four white LEDs, short focal length objective lens, and CMOS detector. Two silver oxide batteries provide all the required power for image illumination, detection, and transmission up to 6 h. The images are delivered via a transmitter and antenna at a

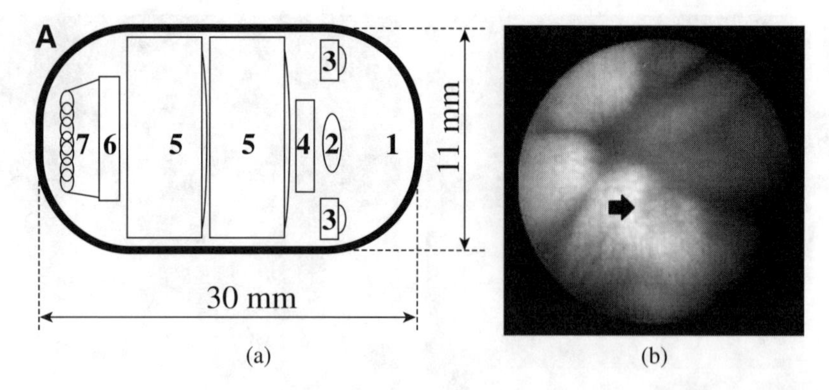

FIGURE 11.22 **(See color insert [Figure 11.22(b)] following page 14-10.)** (a) The schematic diagram of wireless capsule that has dimensions of 11 × 30 mm. There is an optical dome that covers the four white LEDs, short focal length objective lens, and CMOS detector. (b) An angiodysplastic lesion (arrow) has been found in the distal jejunum.

rate of two frames per second. The capsule passes through the human gastrointestinal tract in an average time of 80 (range of 17 to 280) minutes. An example endoscopic image collected with the wireless capsule is shown in Figure 11.22b, where an angiodysplastic lesion (arrow) has been found in the distal jejunum. The anatomic location of the capsule within the small bowel is determined by calculating the time of travel within the small bowel relative to the total small bowel transit time and the strength of the transmitted signal. The wireless capsule has potential for diagnostic use in occult gastrointestinal bleeding.

11.15 Virtual Endoscopy

All of the endoscopic methods discussed so far require an imaging instrument to be inserted into the patient. This process can cause significant patient discomfort and distress. Virtual endoscopy has the potential to provide high quality endoscopic images in cases where conventional endoscopy is incomplete or inadequate, such as in the presence of an obstructing lesion or patient noncompliance. Virtual endoscopy is a technology where images are acquired with a noninvasive imaging modality, such as computed tomography (CT), magnetic resonance imaging, or ultrasound, and are computer reconstructed to produce volumetric data.[112–118] This three-dimensional image is then projected with an endoluminal perspective to simulate an endoscopic image. Virtual endoscopy is most advanced with CT because of the development of the helical CT scanners that allow scans to be completed in only a few seconds. The fast image acquisition times minimize artifacts from patient respiration and motion. These scans are then post-processed to produce a set of complementary two- and three-dimensional images.[119]

The three-dimensional reconstructions can be performed with a mathematical process called surface or volume rendering. Surface rendering involves a preprocessing step that identifies iso-intense surfaces from an endoluminal perspective and reduces the data to a set of surface triangles. Data deep to the identified surfaces are discarded to reduce the data set and to increase the processing speed. Volume rendering generates images by assigning degrees of opacity to various structures within the image based on the attenuation coefficient of each voxel (volume element). The sense of depth and distance is achieved with perspective volume rendering where an object grows larger as the observer approaches. An example of images produced for virtual colonoscopy is shown in Figure 11.23.[120] In Figure 11.23a, an 8-mm-diameter polyp is identified on a two-dimensional axial CT scan of the colon. With volume rendering, the endoluminal three-dimensional view of the polyp is shown in Figure 11.23b. The virtual images of the polyp were confirmed on conventional colonoscopy performed the same day, shown in Figure 11.23c. Histologic evaluation of the biopsy revealed an adenomatous polyp.

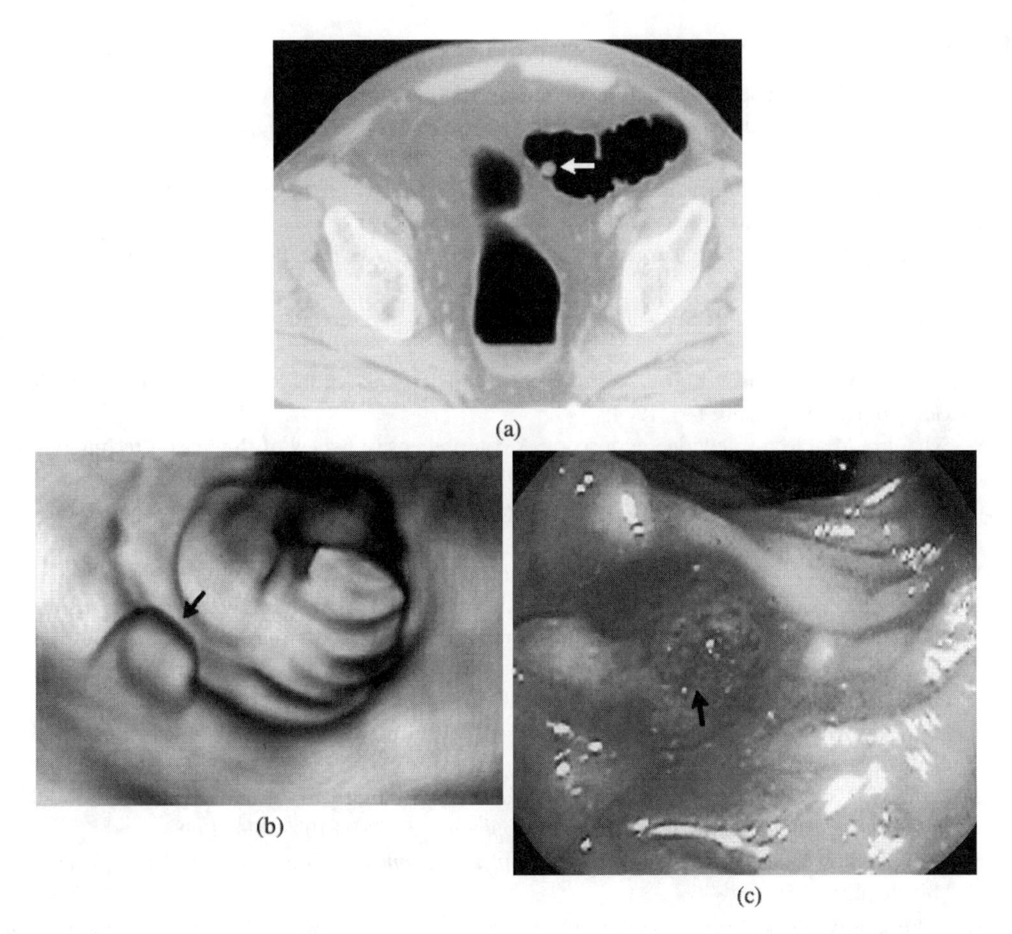

FIGURE 11.23 (See color insert [Figure 11.23(c)] following page 14-10.) (a) An 8-mm polyp was identified on an axial two-dimensional CT image of the colon and (b) on an endoluminal three-dimensional reconstruction. (c) The polyp was confirmed on conventional colonoscopy performed the same day. Histologic examination revealed an adenomatous polyp.

11.16 Summary and Conclusions

Endoscopy is a field that has undergone tremendous technological development in recent years, and new innovations promise to radically improve the capabilities of endoscopy in the near future. These technological improvements are very diverse and interdisciplinary. Advances in semiconductor technology have allowed detectors to become miniaturized, and have led to the development of video endoscopes and wireless capsules. These endoscopes can view larger areas with higher resolution. At the same time, the diameters of the insertion tubes are becoming smaller in size, which provides more patient comfort. The addition of ultrasound technology to endoscopy has allowed structural information to be collected beyond the tissue surface to depths of several millimeters and even into adjacent tissue structures. New methods are being developed to elicit even more diagnostic information from tissue. OCT provides morphologic information with subcellular resolution for real-time histopathology. Fluorescence spectroscopy, using endogenous fluorophores and photosensitizers, reveals biochemical and molecular information below the tissue surface. Magnification and chromoendoscopy provide high resolution details about the mucosal surface. The wireless capsule provides endoscopic images from previously uncharted territory such as the small bowel. Finally, virtual endoscopy provides endoluminal views without the endoscope. Thus, endoscopy is a highly technological field that promises exciting new developments in the near future.

References

1. Hopkins, H.H., The development of the modern endoscope, *Natnews*, 17(8), 18–22, 1980.
2. Sivak, M.V., *Gastroenterologic Endoscopy*, W.B. Saunders, Philadelphia, 2000.
3. Hecht, E., *Optics*, 2nd ed. Addison-Wesley, Reading, MA, 1987.
4. Reedy, R.P., Coherent fiber optics test techniques, *Opt. Eng.*, 19(4), 556–560, 1980.
5. Texas Instruments, Area Array Image Sensor Products, 1994.
6. Boyle, W. and Smith, G., Charge coupled semiconductor devices, *Bell Syst. Tech. J.* 49, 587–593, 1970.
7. Beyond, J.D.E. and Lamb, D.R., Charge-coupled devices and their applications, McGraw-Hill, New York, 1980.
8. Sivak, M.V. and Fleischer, D.E., Colonoscopy with a video endoscope, preliminary experience, *Gastrointest. Endosc.*, 30, 1–5, 1984.
9. Schapiro, M., Electronic video endoscopy. A comprehensive review of the newest technology and techniques, *Pract. Gastroenterol.*, 10, 8–18, 1986.
10. Demling, L. and Hazel, H.J., Video endoscopy: fundamentals and problems, *Endoscopy*, 5, 167–169, 1985.
11. Sivak, M.V., Video endoscopy, *Clin. Gastroenterol.*, 15, 205–234, 1986.
12. Knyrim, K., Seidlitz, H., Hagenmuller, F., and Classen, M., Videoendoscopes in comparison with fiberscopes: quantitative measurement of optical resolution, *Endoscopy*, 4, 156–159, 1987.
13. Knyrim, K., Seidlitz, H., Vakil, N., et al., Optical performance of electronic imaging systems for the colon, *Gastroenterology*, 96, 776–782, 1989.
14. Lux, G., Knyrim, K., Scheubel, R., and Classen, M., Electronic endoscopy — fibres or chips? *Z. Gastroenterol.*, 24(7), 337–343, 1986.
15. Wang, T.D., Janes, S., Wang, Y., Itzkan, I., Van Dam, J., and Feld, M.S., Mathematical model of fluorescence endoscopic image formation, *Appl. Opt.*, 37(34), 8103–8111, 1998.
16. Kremkau, F.W., *Diagnostic Ultrasound: Principles, Instruments and Exercises*, 3rd ed., WB Saunders, Philadelphia, 1989.
17. Goldstein, A., Physics of ultrasound, in *Diagnostic Ultrasound*, Rumack, C.M., Wilson, S.R., and Charboneau, J.W., Eds., Mosby-Year Book, St. Louis, 1991, pp. 2–18.
18. Menze, J., Domschke, W., Brambs, H.J., Frank, N., Hatfield, A., Natternman, C., et al., Miniprobe ultrasonography in the upper gastrointestinal tract: state of the art and prospects, *Endoscopy*, 28, 508–513, 1995.
19. Yanai, H., Tada, M., Karita, M., and Okita, K., Diagnostic utility of 20 megahertz linear endoscopic ultrasonography in early gastric cancer, *Gastrointest. Endosc.*, 44, 29–33, 1996.
20. Saitoh, Y., Obara, T., Einami, K., Nomura, M., Taruishi, M., Ayabe, T., et al., Efficacy of high-frequency ultrasound probes for the preoperative staging of invasion depth in flat and depressed colorectal tumors, *Gastrointest Endosc.*, 44, 34–39, 1996.
21. Chak, A., Canto, M., Stevens, P.D., Lightdale, C.J., Van de Mierop, F., Cooper, G., Pollack, B.J., and Sivak, M.V., Jr., Clinical applications of a new through the scope ultrasound probe: prospective comparison with an ultrasound endoscope, *Gastrointest. Endosc.*, 45, 291–295, 1997.
22. Adain, A.L., Han-Chuan, T., Casidy, M, Schiano, T.D., Liu, J., and Miller, L.S., High-resolution endoluminal sonography is a sensitive modality for the identification of Barrett's metaplasia, *Gastrointest. Endosc.*, 46, 147–151, 1997.
23. Chak, A., Isenberg, G., Mallery, S., Van Dam, J., Cooper, G.S., and Sivak, M.V., Jr., Prospective comparative evaluation of video US endoscope, *Gastrointest Endosc.*, 49(6), 695–699, 1999.
24. Huang, D., Swanson, E.A., Lin, C.P., Schuman, J.S., Stinson, W.G., Chang, W., Hee, M.R., Flotte, T., Gregory, K., Puliafito, C.A., and Fujimoto, J.G., Optical coherence tomography, *Science*, 254, 1178–1181, 1991.

25. Fujimoto, J.G., Bouma, B., Tearney, G.J., Boppart, S.A., Pitris, C., Southern, J.F., and Brezinski, M.E., New technology for high-speed and high-resolution optical coherence tomography, *Ann. NY Acad. Sci.*, 838, 95–107, 1998.
26. Bouma, B.E. and Tearney, GJ., Power-efficient nonreciprocal interferometer and linear-scanning fiber-optic catheter for optical coherence tomography, *Opt. Lett.*, 24, 531–533, 1999.
27. Izatt, J.A., Kulkarni, M.E., Wang, H.-W., Kobayash, K., and Sivak, M.V., Optical coherence tomography and microscopy in gastrointestinal tissues, *IEEE J. Select Topics Quant. Electr.*, 2, 1017–1028, 1996.
28. Tearney, G.J., Brezinski, M.E., Bouma, B.E., Boppart, S.A., Pitris, C., Southern, J.F., et al., In vivo endoscopic optical biopsy with optical coherence tomography, *Science*, 276, 2037–2039, 1997.
29. Brezinski, M.E., Tearney, G.J., Boppart, S.A., Swanson, E.A., Southern, J.F., and Fujimoto, J.G., Optical biopsy with optical coherence tomography. Feasibility for surgical diagnostics, *J. Surg. Res.*, 71, 32–40, 1997.
30. Tearney, G.J., Brezinski, M.E., Southern, J.F., Bouma, B.E., Boppart, S.A., and Fujimoto, J.G., Optical biopsy in human gastrointestinal tissue using optical coherence tomography, *Am. J. Gastroenterol.*, 92, 1800–1804, 1997.
31. Kobayashi, K., Izatt, J.A., Kulkarni, M.D., Willis, J., and Sivak, M.V., Jr., High-resolution cross-sectional imaging of the gastrointestinal tract using optical coherence tomography: preliminary results, *Gastrointest Endosc.*, 47, 515–523, 1998.
32. Rollins, A.M., Ung-Arunyawee, R., Chak, A., Wong, R.C.K., Kobayashi, K., Sivak, M.V., and Izatt, J.A., Real-time in vivo imaging of human gastrointestinal ultra-structure by use of endoscopic optical coherence-tomography with a novel efficient interferometer design, *Opt. Lett.*, 24, 1358–1360, 1999.
33. Bouma, B.E., Tearney, G.J., Compton, C.G., and Nishioka, N.S., High resolution imaging of the human esophagus and stomach in vivo using optical coherence tomography, *Gastrointest Endosc.*, 51, 467–474, 2000.
34. Poneros, J.M., Brand, S., Bouma, B.E., Tearney, G.J., Compton, C.C., and Nishioka, N.S., Diagnosis of specialized intestinal metaplasia by optical coherence tomography, *Gastroenterology*, 120(1), 7–12, 2001.
35. Poneros, J.M., Tearney, G.J., Shiskov, M., Kelsey, P.B., Lauwers, G.Y., Nishioka, N.S., and Bouma, B.E., Optical coherence tomography of the biliary tree during ERCP, *Gastrointest. Endosc.*, 55(1), 84–88, 2002.
36. Sivak, M.V., Jr., Kobayashi, K., Izatt, J.A., Rollins, A.M., Ung-Arunyawee, R., Chak, A., Wong, R.C.K., Isenberg, G.A., and Willis, J., High-resolution endoscopic imaging of the GI tract using optical coherence tomography, *Gastrointest. Endosc.*, 51, 474–479, 2000.
37. Pitris, C., Brezinski, M.E., Bouma, B.E., Tearney, G.J., Southern, J.F., and Fujimoto, J.G., High resolution imaging of the upper respiratory tract with optical coherence tomography, a feasibility study, *Am. J. Respir. Crit. Care Med.*, 157, 1640–1644, 1998.
38. Pitris, C., Goodman, A., Boppart, S.A., Libos, J.J., Fujimoto, J.G., and Brezinski, M.E., High-resolution imaging of gynecologic neoplasms using optical coherence tomography, *Obstet. Gynecol.*, 93, 135–139, 1999.
39. Chen, Z., Milner, T.E., Wang, X., Srinivas, S., and Nelson, J.S., Optical Doppler tomography, imaging in vivo blood flow dynamics following pharmacological intervention and photodynamic therapy, *Photochem. Photobiol.*, 67, 56–60, 1998.
40. Patwari, P., Weissman, N.J., Boppart, S.A., Jesser, C., Stamper, D., Fujimoto, J.G., et al., Assessment of coronary plaque with optical coherence tomography and high-frequency ultrasound, *Am. J. Cardiol.*, 85, 641–644, 2000.
41. Tada, M. and Kawai, K., Research with the endoscope, new techniques using magnification and chromoscopy, *Clin. Gastroenterol.*, 15, 417–437, 1986.

42. Stevens, P.D., Lightdale, C.J., Green, P.H., Siegel, L.M., Garcia-Carrasquillo, R.J., and Rotterdam, H., Combined magnification endoscopy with chromoendoscopy for the evaluation of Barrett's esophagus, *Gastrointest. Endosc.*, 40, 747–749, 1994.
43. Kudo, S., Tamura, S., Nakajima, T., Yamano, H., Kusaka, H., and Watanabe, H., Diagnosis of colorectal tumorous lesions by magnifying endoscopy, *Gastrointest. Endosc.*, 44, 8–14, 1996.
44. Siegel, L.M., Stevens, P.D., Lightdale, C.J., Green, P.H.R., Goodman, S., Garcia-Carrasquillo, R.J., et al., Combined magnification endoscopy with chromoendoscopy in the evaluation of patients with suspected malabsorption, *Gastrointest. Endosc.*, 46, 226–230, 1997.
45. Jaramillo, E., Watanabe, M., Slezak, P., and Rubio, C., Flat neoplastic lesions of the colon and rectum detected by high-resolution video endoscopy and chromoscopy, *Gastrointest. Endosc.*, 42(2), 114–122, 1995.
46. Jaramillo, E., Watanabe, M., Befrits, R., Ponce de León, E., Rubio, C., and Slezak, P., Small, flat colorectal neoplasias in long-standing ulcerative colitis detected by high-resolution video endoscopy, *Gastrointest. Endosc.*, 44, 15–22, 1996.
47. Guelrud, M., Herrera, I., Essenfeld, H., and Castro, J., Enhanced magnification endoscopy, a new technique to identify specialized intestinal metaplasia in Barrett's esophagus, *Gastrointest. Endosc.*, 53(6), 559–565, 2001.
48. Guelrud, M. and Herrera, I., Acetic acid improves identification of remnant islands of Barrett's epithelium after endoscopic therapy, *Gastrointest. Endosc.*, 47, 512–515, 1998.
49. Axelrad, A.M., Fleischer, D.E., Geller, A.J., Nguyen, C.C., Lewis, J.H., Al-Kawas, F.H., et al., High-resolution chromoendoscopy for the diagnosis of diminutive colon polyps: implications for colon cancer screening, *Gastroenterology*, 110, 1253–1258, 1996.
50. Siegel, L.M., Stevens, P.D., Lightdale, C.J., Green, P.H., Goodman, S., Garcia-Carrasquillo, R.J., and Rotterdam, H., Combined magnification endoscopy with chromoendoscopy in the evaluation of patients with suspected malabsorption, *Gastrointest. Endosc.*, 46(3), 226–230, 1997.
51. Saitoh, Y., Obara, T., Watari, J., Nomura, M., Taruishi, M., Orii, Y., Taniguchi, M., Ayabe, T., Ashida, T., and Kohgo, Y., Invasion depth diagnosis of depressed type early colorectal cancers by combined use of videoendoscopy and chromoendoscopy, *Gastrointest. Endosc.*, 48(4), 362–370, 1998.
52. Mitooka, H., Fujimori, T., Ohno, S., Morimoto, S., Nakashima, T., Ohmoto, A., Okano, H., Miyamoto, M., Oh, T., and Saeki, S., Chromoscopy of the colon using indigo carmine dye with electrolyte lavage solution, *Gastrointest. Endosc.*, 38(3), 373–374, 1992.
53. Mitooka, H., Fujimori, T., Maeda, S., and Nagasako, K., Minute flat depressed neoplastic lesions of the colon detected by contrast chromoscopy using an indigo carmine capsule, *Gastrointest. Endosc.*, 41(5), 453–459, 1995.
54. Kiesslich, R., von Bergh, M., Hahn, M., Hermann, G., and Jung, M., Chromoendoscopy with indigocarmine improves the detection of adenomatous and nonadenomatous lesions in the colon, *Endoscopy*, 33(12), 1001–1006, 2001.
55. Sugimachi, K., Kitamura, K., Baba, K., Ikebe, M., and Kuwano, H., Endoscopic diagnosis of early carcinoma of the esophagus using Lugol's solution, *Gastrointest. Endosc.*, 38(6), 657–661, 1992.
56. Yokoyama, A., Ohmori, T., Makuuchi, H., Maruyama, K., Okuyama, K., Takahashi, H., Yokoyama, T., Yoshino, K., Hayashida, M., and Ishii, H., Successful screening for early esophageal cancer in alcoholics using endoscopy and mucosa iodine staining, *Cancer*, 76(6), 928–934, 1995.
57. Canto, M.I., Setrakian, S., Petras, R.E., Blades, E., Chak, A., and Sivak, M.V., Jr., Methylene blue selectively stains intestinal metaplasia in Barrett's esophagus, *Gastrointest. Endosc.*, 44, 1–7, 1996.
58. Morales, T.G., Bhattacharyya, A., Camargo, E., Johnson, C., and Sampliner, R.E., Methylene blue staining for intestinal metaplasia of the gastric cardia with follow-up for dysplasia, *Gastrointest. Endosc.*, 48(1), 26–31, 1998.
59. Canto, M.I., Setrakian, S., Willis, J., Chak, A., Petras, R., Powe, N.R., and Sivak, M.V., Methylene blue-directed biopsies improve detection of intestinal metaplasia and dysplasia in Barrett's esophagus, *Gastrointest. Endosc.*, 51(5), 560–568, 2000.

60. Sharma, P., Topalovski, M., Mayo, M.S., and Weston, A.P., Methylene blue chromoendoscopy for detection of short-segment Barrett's esophagus, *Gastrointest. Endosc.*, 54(3), 289–293, 2001.
61. Kiesslich, R., Hahn, M., Herrmann, G., and Jung, M., Screening for specialized columnar epithelium with methylene blue: chromoendoscopy in patients with Barrett's esophagus and a normal control group, *Gastrointest. Endosc.*, 53(1), 47–52, 2001.
62. Campbell, I.D. and Dwek, R.A., *Biological Spectroscopy*, The Benjamin/Cummings Publishing Co., Menlo Park, 1984.
63. Profio, A.E., Doiron, D.R., and King, E.G., Laser fluorescence bronchoscope for localization of occult lung tumors, *Med. Phys.*, 6, 523–525, 1979.
64. Profio, A.E., Doiron, D.R., and Balchum, O.J., Fluorescence bronchoscopy for localization of carcinoma *in situ*, *Med. Phys.*, 10, 35–39, 1983.
65. Profio, A.E., Dorion, D.R., and and Sarnaik, J., Fluorometer for endoscopic diagnosis of tumors, *Med. Phys.*, 11, 516–520, 1984.
66. Andersson, P.S., Montan, S., and Svanberg, S., Multispectral system for medical fluorescence imaging, *IEEE J. Quant. Electron.*, QE-23, 1798–1805, 1987.
67. Baumgartner, R., Fisslinger, H., Jocham, D., Lenz, H., Ruprecht, L., Stepp, H., and Unsold, E., A fluorescence imaging device for endoscopic detection of early stage cancer — instrumental and experimental studies, *J. Photochem. Photobiol.*, 46, 759–764, 1987.
68. Brodbeck, K.J., Profio, A.E., Frewin T., and Balchum, O.J., A system for real time fluorescence imaging in color for tumor diagnosis, *Med. Phys.*, 14, 637–639, 1987.
69. Lam, S., MacAulay, C., Hung, J., LeRiche, J., Profio, A.E., and Palcic, B., Detection of dysplasia and carcinoma *in situ* with a lung imaging fluorescence endoscope device, *J. Thorac Cardiovasc. Surg.*, 105(6), 1035–1040, 1993.
70. Schomacker, K.T., Frisoli, J.K., Compton, C.C., Flotte, T.J., Richter, J.M., Nishioka, N.S., and Deutsch, T.F., Ultraviolet laser-induced fluorescence of colonic tissue: basic biology and diagnostic potential, *Lasers Surg. Med.*, 12, 63–78, 1992.
71. Cothren, R.M., Sivak, M.V., Van Dam, J., Petras, R.E., Fitzmaurice, M., Crawford, J.M., et al., Detection of dysplasia at colonoscopy using laser-induced fluorescence: a blinded study, *Gastrointest. Endosc.*, 44, 168–176, 1996.
72. Zonios, G.I., Cothren, R.M., Arendt, J.T., Wu, J., Van Dam, J., Crawford, J.M., Manoharan, R., and Feld, M.S., Morphological model of human colon tissue fluorescence, *IEEE Trans. Biomed. Eng.*, 43(2), 1–10, 1996.
73. Panjehpour, M., Overholt, B.F., Vo-Dinh, T., Haggitt, R.C., Edwards, D.H., and Buckley, F.P., Endoscopic fluorescence detection of high-grade dysplasia in Barrett's esophagus, *Gastroenterology*, 111, 93–101, 1996.
74. Wang, T.D., Van Dam, J., Crawford, J.M., Preisinger, E.A., Wang, Y., and Feld, M.S., Fluorescence endoscopic imaging of human colonic adenomas, *Gastroenterology*, 111, 1182–1191, 1996.
75. Wang, T.D., Crawford, J.M., Feld, M.S., Wang, Y., Itzkan, I., and Van Dam, J., In vivo identification of colonic dysplasia using fluorescence endoscopic imaging, *Gastrointest. Endosc.*, 49(4 Pt 1), 447–455, 1999.
76. Lim, J.S., *Two-Dimensional Signal and Image Processing*, Prentice Hall, Englewood Cliffs, NJ, 1990, pp. 533–536.
77. Chwirot, B.W., Kowalska, M., Sypniewska, N., Michniewicz, Z., and Gradziel, M., Spectrally resolved fluorescence imaging of human colonic adenomas, *J. Photochem. Photobiol. B*, 50(2–3), 174–183, 1999.
78. Izuishi, K., Tajiri, H., Fujii, T., Boku, N., Ohtsu, A., Ohnishi, T., Ryu, M., Kinoshita, T., and Yoshida, S., The histological basis of detection of adenoma and cancer in the colon by autofluorescence endoscopic imaging, *Endoscopy*, 31(7), 511–516, 1999.
79. Izuishi, K., Tajiri, H., Ryu, M., Furuse, J., Maru, Y., Inoue, K., Konishi, M., and Kinoshita, T., Detection of bile duct cancer by autofluorescence cholangioscopy: a pilot study, *Hepatogastroenterology*, 46(26), 804–807, 1999.

80. Mayinger, B., Horner, P., Jordan, M., Gerlach, C., Horbach, T., Hohenberger, W., and Hahn, E.G., Light-induced autofluorescence spectroscopy for tissue diagnosis of GI lesions, *Gastrointest. Endosc.*, 52(3), 395–400, 2000.
81. Abe, S., Izuishi, K., Tajiri, H., Kinoshita, T., and Matsuoka, T., Correlation of *in vitro* autofluorescence endoscopy images with histopathologic findings in stomach cancer, *Endoscopy*, 32(4), 281–286, 2000.
82. Kobayashi, M., Tajiri, H., Seike, E., Shitaya, M., Tounou, S., Mine, M., and Oba, K., Detection of early gastric cancer by a real-time autofluorescence imaging system, *Cancer Lett.*, 165(2), 155–159, 2001.
83. Koenig, F., McGovern, F.J., Enquist, H., Larne, R., Deutsch, T.F., and Schomacker, K.T., Autofluorescence guided biopsy for the early diagnosis of bladder carcinoma, *J. Urol.*, 159(6), 1871–1875, 1998.
84. Kulapaditharom, B. and Boonkitticharoen, V., Laser-induced fluorescence imaging in localization of head and neck cancers, *Ann. Otol. Rhinol. Laryngol.*, 107(3), 241–246, 1998.
85. Betz, C.S., Mehlmann, M., Rick, K., Stepp, H., Grevers, G., Baumgartner, R., and Leunig, A., Autofluorescence imaging and spectroscopy of normal and malignant mucosa in patients with head and neck cancer, *Lasers Surg. Med.*, 25(4), 323–334, 1999.
86. Zargi, M., Fajdiga, I., and Smid, L., Autofluorescence imaging in the diagnosis of laryngeal cancer, *Eur. Arch. Otorhinolaryngol.*, 257(1), 17–23, 2000.
87. Delank, W., Khanavkar, B., Nakhosteen, J.A., and Stoll, W., A pilot study of autofluorescent endoscopy for the in vivo detection of laryngeal cancer, *Laryngoscope*, 110(3 Pt 1), 368–373, 2000.
88. Kusunoki, Y., Imamura, F., Uda, H., Mano, M., and Horai, T., Early detection of lung cancer with laser-induced fluorescence endoscopy and spectrofluorometry, *Chest*, 118(6), 1776–1782, 2000.
89. Shibuya, K., Fujisawa, T., Hoshino, H., Baba, M., Saitoh, Y., Iizasa, T., Suzuki, M., Otsuji, M., Hiroshima, K., and Ohwada, H., Fluorescence bronchoscopy in the detection of preinvasive bronchial lesions in patients with sputum cytology suspicious or positive formalignancy, *Lung Cancer*, 32(1), 19–25, 2001.
90. Zellweger, M., Grosjean, P., Goujon, D., Monnier, P., van den Bergh, H., and Wagnieres, G., In vivo autofluorescence spectroscopy of human bronchial tissue to optimize the detection and imaging of early cancers, *J. Biomed. Opt.*, 6(1), 41–51, 2001.
91. Dhingra, J.K., Perrault, D.F., Jr., McMillan, K., Rebeiz, E.E., Kabani, S., Manoharan, R., Itzkan, I., Feld, M.S., and Shapshay, S.M., Early diagnosis of upper aerodigestive tract cancer by autofluorescence, *Arch. Otolaryngol. Head Neck Surg.*, 122(11), 1181–1186, 1996.
92. Kurie, J.M., Lee, J.S., Morice, R.C., Walsh, G.L., Khuri, F.R., Broxson, A., Ro, J.Y., Franklin, W.A., Yu, R., and Hong, W.K., Autofluorescence bronchoscopy in the detection of squamous metaplasia and dysplasia in current and former smokers, *J. Natl. Cancer Inst.*, 90(13), 991–995, 1998.
93. Qu, J.Y., Wing, P., Huang, Z., Kwong, D., Sham, J., Lee, S.L., Ho, W.K., and Wei, W.I., Preliminary study of in vivo autofluorescence of nasopharyngeal carcinoma and normal tissue, *Lasers Surg. Med.*, 26(5), 432–440, 2000.
94. Montan, S., Svanberg, K., and Svanberg, S., Multicolor imaging and contrast enhancement in cancer-tumor localization using laser-induced fluorescence in hematoporphyrin-derivative-bearing tissue, *Opt. Lett.*, 10, 56–58, 1985.
95. Lam, S., Palcic, B., McLean, D., Hung, J., Korbelik, M., and Profio, A.E., Detection of early lung cancer using low dose Photofrin II, *Chest*, 97, 333–337, 1990.
96. Kriegmair, M., Baumgartner, R., Knuchel, R., Stepp, H., Hofstadter, F., and Hofstetter, A., Detection of early bladder cancer by 5-aminolevulinic acid induced porphyrin fluorescence, *J. Urol.*, 155(1), 105–109, 1996.
97. Namihisa, A., Miwa, H., Watanabe, H., Kobayashi, O., Ogihara, T., and Sato, N., A new technique, light-induced fluorescence endoscopy in combination with pharmacoendoscopy, *Gastrointest. Endosc.*, 53(3), 343–348, 2001.

98. Bhunchet, E., Hatakawa, H., Sakai, Y., and Shibata, T., Fluorescein electronic endoscopy. A novel method for detection of early stage gastric cancer not evident to routine endoscopy, *Gastrointest. Endosc.*, 55(4), 562–571, 2002.
99. Koenig, F., McGovern, F.J., Larne, R., Enquist, H., Schomacker, K.T., and Deutsch, T.F., Diagnosis of bladder carcinoma using protoporphyrin IX fluorescence induced by 5-aminolaevulinic acid, *BJU Int.*, 83(1), 129–135, 1999.
100. Kriegmair, M., Zaak, D., Knuechel, R., Baumgartner, R., and Hofstetter, A., 5-Aminolevulinic acid-induced fluorescence endoscopy for the detection of lower urinary tract tumors, *Urol. Int.*, 63(1), 27–31, 1999.
101. Riedl, C.R., Daniltchenko, D., Koenig, F., Simak, R., Loening, S.A., and Pflueger, H., Fluorescence endoscopy with 5-aminolevulinic acid reduces early recurrence rate in superficial bladder cancer, *J. Urol.*, 165(4), 1121–1123, 2001.
102. Eker, C., Montan, S., Jaramillo, E., Koizumi, K., Rubio, C., Andersson-Engels, S., Svanberg, K., Svanberg, S., and Slezak, P., Clinical spectral characterisation of colonic mucosal lesions using autofluorescence and delta aminolevulinic acid sensitisation, *Gut*, 44(4), 511–518, 1999.
103. Messmann, H., Knuchel, R., Baumler, W., Holstege, A., and Scholmerich, J., Endoscopic fluorescence detection of dysplasia in patients with Barrett's esophagus, ulcerative colitis, or adenomatous polyps after 5-aminolevulinic acid-induced protoporphyrin IX sensitization, *Gastrointest. Endosc.*, 49(1), 97–101, 1999.
104. Mayinger, B., Reh, H., Hochberger, J., and Hahn, E.G., Endoscopic photodynamic diagnosis, oral aminolevulinic acid is a marker of GI cancer and dysplastic lesions, *Gastrointest. Endosc.*, 50(2), 242–246, 1999.
105. Endlicher, E., Knuechel, R., Hauser, T., Szeimies, R.M., Scholmerich, J., and Messmann, H., Endoscopic fluorescence detection of low and high grade dysplasia in Barrett's oesophagus using systemic or local 5-aminolaevulinic acid sensitisation, *Gut*, 48(3), 314–319, 2001.
106. Leunig, A., Betz, C.S., Mehlmann, M., Stepp, H., Arbogast, S., Grevers, G., and Baumgartner, R., Detection of squamous cell carcinoma of the oral cavity by imaging 5-aminolevulinic acid-induced protoporphyrin IX fluorescence, *Laryngoscope*, 110(1), 78–83, 2000.
107. Zaak, D., Kriegmair, M., Stepp, H., Stepp, H., Baumgartner, R., Oberneder, R., Schneede, P., Corvin, S., Frimberger, D., Knuchel, R., and Hofstetter, A., Endoscopic detection of transitional cell carcinoma with 5-aminolevulinic acid, results of 1012 fluorescence endoscopies, *Urology*, 57(4), 690–694, 2001.
108. Gong, F., Swain, P., and Mills, T., Wireless endoscopy, *Gastrointest. Endosc.*, 51(6), 725–729, 2000.
109. Iddan, G., Meron, G., Glukhovsky, A., and Swain, P., Wireless capsule endoscopy, *Nature*, 405, 417, 2000.
110. Appleyard, M., Glukhovsky, A., and Swain, P., Wireless-capsule diagnostic endoscopy for recurrent small-bowel bleeding, *N. Engl. J. Med.*, 344(3), 232–233, 2001.
111. Appleyard, M., Fireman, Z., Glukhovsky, A., Jacob, H., Shreiver, R., Kadirkamanathan, S., Lavy, A., Lewkowicz, S., Scapa, E., Shofti, R., Swain, P., and Zaretsky, A., A randomized trial comparing wireless capsule endoscopy with push enteroscopy for the detection of small-bowel lesions, *Gastroenterology*, 119(6), 1431–1438, 2000.
112. Hara, A.K., Johnson, C.D., Reed, J.E., et al., Reducing data size and radiation dose for CT colonography, *Am. J. Roentgenol.*, 168, 1181–1184, 1997.
113. Johnson, C.D. and Ahlquist, D.A., Computed tomography colonography (virtual colonoscopy): a new method for colorectal screening, *Gut*, 44, 301–305, 1999.
114. Vining, D.J., Virtual endoscopy, is it reality? *Radiology*, 200, 30–31, 1996.
115. Fenlon, H.M. and Ferrucci, J.T., Virtual colonoscopy: what will the issues be? *Am. J. Roentgenol.*, 169, 453–458, 1997.
116. Ahlquist, D.A., Hara, A.K., and Johnson, C.D., Computed tomographic colography and virtual colonoscopy, *Gastrointest. Endosc. Clin. N. Am.*, 7, 439–452, 1997.

117. Fenlon, H.M., Clarke, P.D., and Ferrucci, J.T., Virtual colonoscopy, imaging features with colonoscopic correlation, *Am. J. Roentgenol.*, 170, 1303–1309, 1998.
118. Dachman, A.H., Kuniyoshi, J.K., Boyle, C.M., et al., CT colonography with three-dimensional problem solving for detection of colonic polyps, *Am. J. Roentgenol.*, 171, 989–995, 1998.

12

Functional Brain Mapping Using Intracranial Source Imaging

George Zouridakis
University of Houston

Darshan Iyer
University of Houston

CONTENTS

12.1 Introduction

The treatment of certain complex neurological diseases, such as pharmacologically intractable epilepsy, brain tumors, and arteriovenous malformations, often includes surgical intervention. In all cases, accurate localization of the lesion to be resected is of paramount importance, and the margin between therapeutic treatment and debilitating side effects due to surgery is very narrow. Several additional factors contribute to the success of surgery, chief among which is the accurate identification of the cortical areas that are responsible for certain brain functions, such as sensation, movement, and speech. This latter procedure, known as functional brain mapping, is critical, because resection of such vital brain areas can have devastating results.

0-8493-1140-3/04/$0.00+$1.50

A number of noninvasive functional imaging modalities, including functional magnetic resonance imaging (fMRI) (Binder et al., 1997; Cuenod et al., 1995), positron emission tomography (PET) (O'Leary et al., 1996; Peterson et al., 1988), regional cerebral blood flow (rCBF) (Friberg, 1993), and single photon emission computed tomography (SPECT) (Gomez-Tortosa et al., 1994), can map brain functions with varying degrees of success. However, the most reliable approach to map the human brain still relies on direct electrical stimulation of the exposed cortex (Ojemann et al., 1989), a procedure that is highly invasive and unpleasant, and it is performed mostly intraoperatively on an awake patient.

Recently, however, completely noninvasive procedures have been successfully used for brain mapping (Breier et al., 2000; Ebersole and Wade, 1990; Gallen et al., 1994; Hamalainen et al., 1993; Papanicolaou et al., 1999; Zouridakis et al., 1998b). These procedures rely on the fact that performance of certain brain functions activates only a small population of cortical neurons whose activation gives rise to electromagnetic signals that can be recorded externally. The electrical aspects of brain activation are recorded in an electroencephalogram (EEG) by placing a set of electrodes on the scalp, while the corresponding magnetic aspects can be captured in a magnetoencephalogram (MEG) by placing an array of coils close to the head.

Electrical or magnetic source imaging (SI) refers to the localization of the intracranial sources that give rise to externally recorded electrical or magnetic signals, respectively. This procedure is a form of functional imaging and combines the neurophysiological EEG or MEG data with structural MRI scans. That is, while MRI alone provides information on the brain's anatomy, SI provides information about its function. Moreover, SI provides very high temporal and spatial resolution, which makes it far superior than any other functional imaging modality in that respect.

In this chapter we introduce the basic principles that make EEG- and MEG-based SI procedures possible, and the equipment used to accomplish it. Additionally, we provide a few concrete examples that demonstrate the usefulness of SI as a valuable clinical tool for functional brain mapping.

12.2 Neurophysiological Signals

12.2.1 Origin of Activity

When considering surface neurophysiological activity, two major aspects must be distinguished. The first one is the characterization of the sources underlying the observed signals. The human brain is composed of vast numbers of electrically active neurons and other supporting cells (e.g., glial cells) that are assembled in functional groups. In particular, the outer surface of the brain, the cerebral cortex, consists of a thin and highly compact intricate network of cells arranged in layers (Kandel et al., 1991). The average thickness of the cortex is 2.5 mm, and its density reaches an impressive 10^5 cells per millimeter which form approximately 10^{15} synapses. Conceptually, the building block of the cerebral cortex is a column, a structure of neurons arranged radially to the head surface, with a diameter of about 0.5 to 3 mm (Kelly, 1991). A specific type of neurons in a column, called pyramidal cells, have a linear structure with dendrites that are arranged parallel to each other. In the resting state, each of these neurons is negatively polarized relative to the surrounding electrolyte solution, because of the activity of the cell membrane. When a cell is in the active state, large quantities of positive and negative ions — namely, sodium (Na^+), potassium (K^+), and chloride (Cl^-) — cross the cell membrane, moving from the intracellular to the extracellular fluid, and vice versa. For all practical purposes, this ion movement is equivalent to a current flow, and it is responsible for all electrophysiological signals recorded externally. In particular, the electrical potentials and the magnetic fields recorded on the scalp as the EEG and MEG, respectively, result mainly from the temporal and spatial summation of postsynaptic activity generated along the apical dendrites of the pyramidal neurons. These fields represent the synchronous activation of a large number of neurons, estimated to be between 10^4 and 10^5 cells (Okada et al., 1992; Williamson and Kaufman, 1987).

The second aspect of surface neurophysiological activity is the influence of the tissues surrounding the active neurons, the so-called volume conductor effects. A detailed analysis of the relationship between the intracranial sources and the extracranially recorded signals is beyond the scope of this chapter, but excellent reviews can be found elsewhere (Hamalainen et al., 1993; Williamson and Kaufman, 1987). Briefly, neural activity can be represented mathematically as a current density in a closed volume of finite conductivity. Outside this volume, the conductivity and current density are zero. The intracellular currents give rise to an electric field outside the cells which, in turn, results in currents that flow passively through the rest of the conducting medium. Thus, the total current density can be divided into two components, primary (intracellular) and secondary (extracellular). The primary currents are more interesting in neurophysiology, because they are associated directly with cell activation. Under specific conditions (Lewine, 1990), that are fairly well approximated in many practical applications, it can be assumed that the electromagnetic fields recorded on the scalp as the familiar EEG and MEG are associated mainly with the primary (intracellular) currents, and thus they represent cell activation.

The relationship between the intracranial sources and the extracranially recorded biological signals can be computed as a function of the distance between the observation point and the source location. Both the magnetic field and the potential are inversely proportional to the square of this distance.

12.2.2 Localization of the Sources

Determining the extracranial potentials and magnetic fields that result from the intracranial current sources is known as the forward problem. Conversely, the inverse problem requires localization of the intracranial current sources that give rise to the externally recorded electrical potentials (EEG) and magnetic fields (MEG). Unfortunately, the inverse problem has no unique solution, as the corresponding mathematical equations can be satisfied by an infinite number of possible source configurations. To overcome this limitation, it is necessary to solve a "constrained inverse problem" and make assumptions for both the sources and the surrounding head tissues (Morse and Feshbach, 1963). These assumptions must be neurophysiologically based, otherwise the results computed and their interpretation may be completely erroneous (Jayakar et al, 1991; Nunez et al., 1991). A typical approach involves the so-called "quasi-static" approximation (Plonsey and Heppner, 1967) under which all potentials and currents at any given instant in time are determined by the properties of the sources at that time only. Moreover, the various brain tissues are assumed to be linear and completely characterized by their electrical conductivity, which is frequency independent. The medium can be inhomogeneous, if its conductivity is different for different compartments, and anisotropic, if the conductivity of the tissues is different along different directions in the three-dimensional space.

12.3 Mathematical Modeling

12.3.1 Source Models

Over the past several years, many different approaches have been developed to identify the sources that explain the fields recorded on the head surface. The most common approach has been to describe the activation of a well-localized (Nunez et al., 1991) small population of neurons at a particular point in time as a single equivalent current dipole. Indeed, when a neuron is activated, ion currents flow through it and this "electrical generator" can be modeled as a small current dipole, with a moment of about 10^{-13} A m. A schematic diagram of such an arrangement is shown in Figure 12.1.

However, to identify the sources that account for a complex field distribution over a time interval, a series of single dipoles is required (Supek and Aine, 1993). These dipoles can move in position and orientation over time, and when displayed on a single image, they appear as a moving dipole.[15,16] Another approach is to consider current distributions in the brain (Ioannides et al., 1990; Morse and Feshbach, 1963; Okada et al., 1992; Wang et al., 1992), and estimate several fixed dipoles at discrete points within a region of interest. Spatiotemporal source modeling (Baumgartner et al., 1991; Scherg, 1992; Scherg and von Cramon, 1985) is yet another approach that takes into consideration overlapping activity of multiple generators. In this case, dipoles are fixed in location and orientation, but they can vary over time in strength and polarity to explain the temporal evolution of the recorded fields.

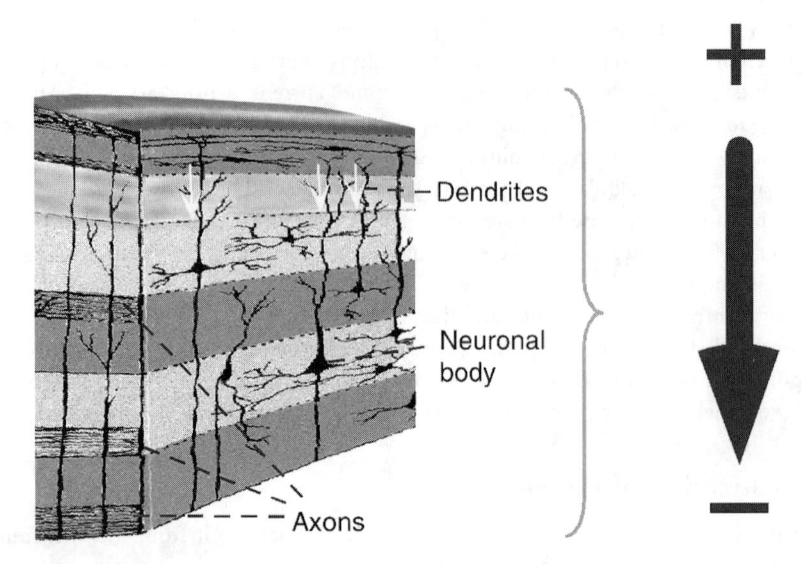

FIGURE 12.1 A well-localized small population of neurons, with pyramidal cells oriented radially to the head surface. The sum of currents (arrows on the cells) flowing in the apical dendrites can be modeled as a single equivalent current dipole.

In general, solutions for multiple-dipole sources are much less reliable than those for a single dipole (Cuffin, 1998), because in the former case the solutions provided are very sensitive to noise. Thus, most clinical applications still use single-dipole approaches.

12.3.2 Volume Conductor Models

Volume conductor models have evolved from extremely simple (Rush and Driscoll, 1978) to very realistic and computationally intensive ones (Fender, 1991). The first and simplest model was that of an infinite, homogeneous, isotropic medium. The next sophistication level considered a homogeneous but bounded medium (specifically, a sphere) as a head model (Wilson and Bayley, 1950). Later on, to account for the various tissue layers within the head, several concentric-sphere models were developed (Ruth and Driscoll, 1968; Schneider, 1972; Witner et al., 1972) that included three concentric spheres to account for the scalp, skull, and the brain. More recently, however, additional approaches, such as the eccentric-sphere model (Mejis and Peters, 1987) and the four-shell model, have been proposed. The latter uses a cerebrospinal fluid layer underneath the skull, and it is especially useful for hydrocephalic patients (Nishijo et al., 1996).

However, more realistic head models can be obtained if, instead of using arbitrary spheres, MRIs are employed to determine the curvature of a particular subject's head and fit the spheres of the multicompartment model (Lopes da Silva et al., 1991). More realistic models computed entirely from MRIs (Mejis and Peters, 1987) are implemented using numerical techniques, such as the boundary element method (BEM) (Mejis et al., 1989) and the finite element method (FEM). Finally, realistic head models that account also for the effects of anisotropy in the electrical conductivity have been developed (de Munck, 1988; Zhou and van Oosterom, 1991).

12.3.3 Source Estimation Procedure

Initially, inverse source localization procedures were implemented on spherical models (Rush and Driscoll, 1978; Smith et al., 1993) and they were later extended to work on realistic geometry. In the case of a single-current dipole, to identify the intracranial sources that explain the fields recorded on the head surface, the procedure takes the measured values from all sensors at a given instant in time and searches, using iterative minimization techniques, for an equivalent dipole within the head that could generate such fields (Henderson et al., 1975; Kavanagh et al., 1978; Schneider, 1972; Sidman et al., 1978). Techniques such as the brain electrical source analysis (BESA) (Jirsa et al., 2000) and CURRY (Neuroscan, El Paso, TX) are iterative with automatic picking of dipole sources and define one dipole for each point in time.

In more general cases, the localization procedure starts with some initial estimate of the distributed sources and then recursively enhances the strength of some of the elements, while decreasing the strength of the rest of the elements until they become zero. In the end, only a small number of elements will remain nonzero, yielding a localized solution. This method is implemented, for example, in the FOCUSS (Gorodnitsky et al., 1995) and LORETA (Pascual-Marqui et al., 1994) algorithms.

Another approach to source localization employs a spatiotemporal model, under the assumption that there are several dipolar sources that maintain their position and orientation fixed, while they vary only their amplitude as a function of time. Rather than fitting dipoles to measurements from one instant in time, dipoles are fitted by minimizing the residual least-square error over the entire time interval (Scherg and von Cramon, 1985). More advanced spatiotemporal approaches, such as the multiple signal classification algorithm (MUSIC) (Mosher et al., 1992), have also been developed, whereby the algorithm searches for a single dipole through the three-dimensional head volume. To localize the source, the user must search the head volume for local peaks. Extensions of this algorithm automate this search through a recursive approach (Mosher and Leahy, 1963).

12.4 Neurophysiological Recordings

12.4.1 Electroencephalography — EEG

The EEG is a record of the electrical aspects of neurophysiological activity. More specifically, a one-channel EEG represents the potential difference between two sites on the head, and requires two electrodes connected to the input of a differential amplifier — one active and one for reference. These electrodes are typically gold-plated or sintered Ag-AgCl, and they are attached to the scalp with a special glue (collodion) or electrolyte gel. Typically, the active electrode is placed close to the structures of interest, whereas the reference electrode is placed at a distant location (usually on the left or linked mastoids, behind the ears). This type of connection is called monopolar, or referential. When both the active and the reference electrodes are placed close to the structures of interest, the placement is called bipolar or differential. The advantage of this latter connection is that far-field activity common to both electrodes is cancelled and thus sharp localizations of events can be obtained. Alternatively, the reference electrode can be connected to a circuit that measures the average activity of all electrodes to obtain a recording with an average reference. The common electrical connection for the electrical circuitry of the recording equipment is called the ground, and all voltages are measured with reference to it. The patient is also connected to this point through a separate electrode typically placed on the patient's forehead. The potential differences in each channel are amplified by high-gain, differential amplifiers, and then it is either displayed on a monitor, saved on a hard disk, or simply plotted on paper, depending on the technology used.

For clinical recordings, electrodes are arrange on the head in a montage that follows the 10–20 international placement system and its extensions. Routine clinical equipment employs about 21 electrodes, whereas more recent systems specialized primarily for research may include hundreds of electrodes. In this case, arrays of electrodes are arranged on a cap for convenience, and these densely sampled recordings provide the so-called dense-array EEG, or dEEG. A system that uses 256 channels is described next.

12.4.1.1 EEG Recording Device

The latest dEEG systems incorporate several unique features: they offer high spatial sampling with up to 256 recording channels; they are portable, and often the complete set of 256 amplifiers is battery operated and is about the size of a book; they can use active electrodes for noise cancellation, in which case each electrode incorporates a micropreamplifier that preconditions the EEG signals before transmission to the main amplifiers through the electrode leads, and this eliminates the need for a shielded room; and finally, they provide very high sampling rates of up to 5 kHz per channel.

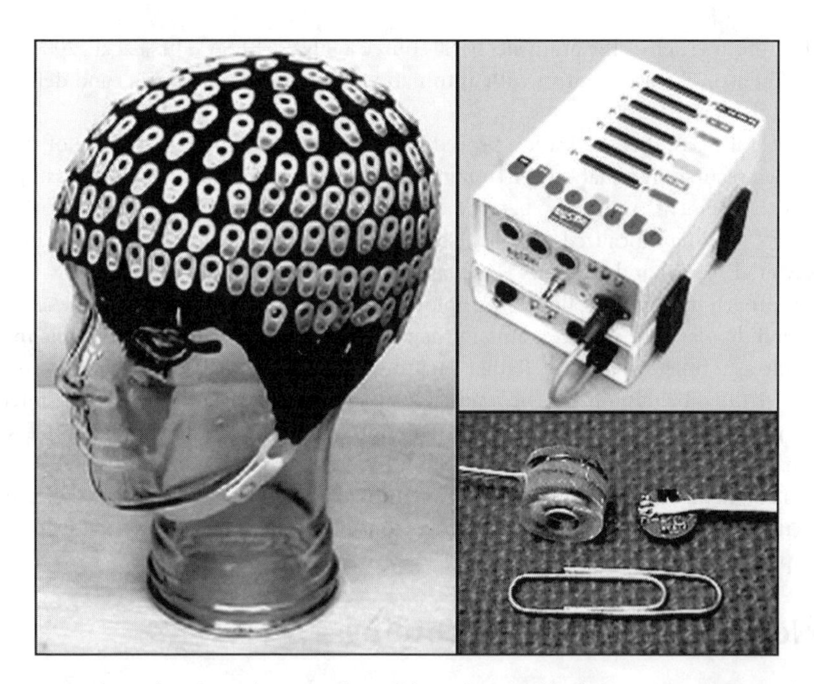

FIGURE 12.2 Active electrodes, electrode cap, and amplifiers of a portable dEEG system with 256 channels.

The active electrode is a sensor with a very low output impedance. By integrating the first amplifier stage with a regular electrode, extremely low-noise measurements are now possible without any skin preparation. The noise levels achieved can be as low as the thermal noise of the electrode impedance, which is the theoretically minimum level. Active electrodes eliminate all problems associated with high electrode impedances, cable shielding, capacitive coupling between the cables, and sources of interference, as well as any artifacts due to cable or connector movements. The amplifiers of a dEEG system (ActiveTwo, BioSemi, the Netherlands) available in our lab, along with an active electrode and a cap with the electrode holders, are shown in Figure 12.2.

12.4.2 Magnetoencephalography — MEG

The MEG measures the extracranial magnetic fields produced by intracranial electrical currents. Neuromagnetic signals are many orders of magnitude weaker than the ambient magnetic noise, which is due to the earth's field and to the presence of ferromagnetic objects and electrical instrumentation. Typical scalp-recorded magnetic fields have a peak amplitude of about 100 fT (Gomez-Tortosa et al, 1994; Lewine, 1990), whereas environmental electromagnetic noise in a hospital (power lines, elevators, MRI magnets, etc.) may be as high as 1 T (10^{15} fT) in extreme cases (Lewine, 1990). Therefore, to detect this kind of biological activity, it is necessary to use highly sensitive instrumentation and, at the same time, attempt to eliminate extraneous magnetic fields.

12.4.2.1 MEG Recording Device

MEG measurements were practically impossible before the introduction of superconductive instrumentation. The latest generation of biomagnetometers are composed of large arrays of pick-up coils, each of which is connected to a SQUID (superconducting quantum interference device) that acts as a very low noise, ultrahigh gain, current-to-voltage converter. The SQUIDs and induction coils are immersed in liquid helium to maintain a superconducting state. This type of device can detect even very small changes in magnetic flux, such as the one resulting from neurophysiological activity. Figure 12.3 shows a schematic diagram of a multisensor MEG system along with a detection coil and a SQUID of a single channel.

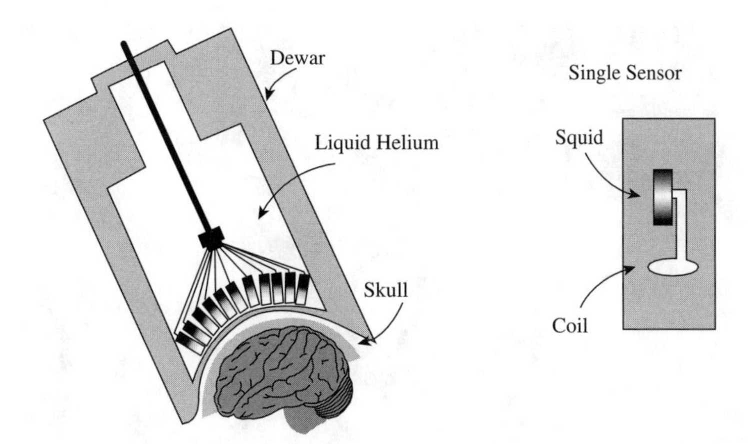

FIGURE 12.3 Schematic diagram of a multisensor MEG system (left) along with a detection coil and SQUID in a single channel (right).

To reduce the amount of extraneous magnetic noise, MEG systems are operated in specially designed magnetically shielded rooms (Gallen et al., 1994). Additional improvements in the quality of the MEG signals are obtained by selecting an appropriate type for the detection coils. Coils can be single-loop magnetometers that measure the magnetic field directly, and first-, second-, or third-order gradiometers that consist of two or more loops that measure spatial changes of magnetic field (Flynn, 1994). Various examples of coils for both planar and axial geometry are shown in Figure 12.4.

A gradiometer (Figure 12.4d) can selectively cancel out environmental magnetic noise, depending on its "baseline," i.e., the distance between the two coils; because the magnetic fields decrease very rapidly with distance from the source, fields generated by a neural source close to the gradiometer will be detected with different strengths in each loop, and therefore they will induce currents of different magnitude in the two loops, thus resulting in a nonzero net current in the gradiometer. On the other hand, fields generated far away from the gradiometer will be practically uniform in space and will result in zero net current.

Because of the sensitivity of MEG recordings to noise, patients implanted with electrically active medical devices such as cardiac pacemakers, neurostimulators, and infusion pumps cannot be studied with MEG, due to the electrical interference from the implanted devices. Also, equipment entering the room must be screened for large metallic components or electromagnetic activity that could introduce artifactual signals.

The cost and complexity of instrumentation led to the initial development of MEG systems containing only a few channels. Recently, however, whole-head systems with large arrays comprising 248 magnetometers have been developed (model 360WH, 4DNeuroimaging, San Diego, CA). An example of a 148-channel system is shown in Figure 12.5. The need for cryogenics, and for a shielded room and a rigid helmet-type sensor limit the scope of applications of the MEG-based mapping procedures.

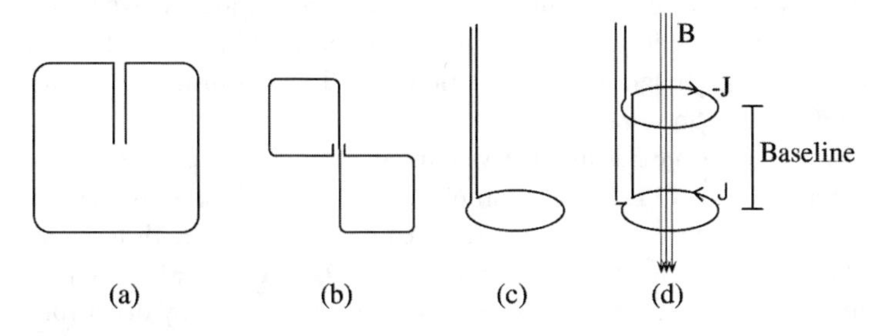

FIGURE 12.4 MEG detection coils include planar (a) magnetometers and (b) gradiometers, and axial (c) magnetometers and (d) gradiometers. In a gradiometer, a uniform field B creates currents J and –J of opposite polarity a produces a zero net signal.

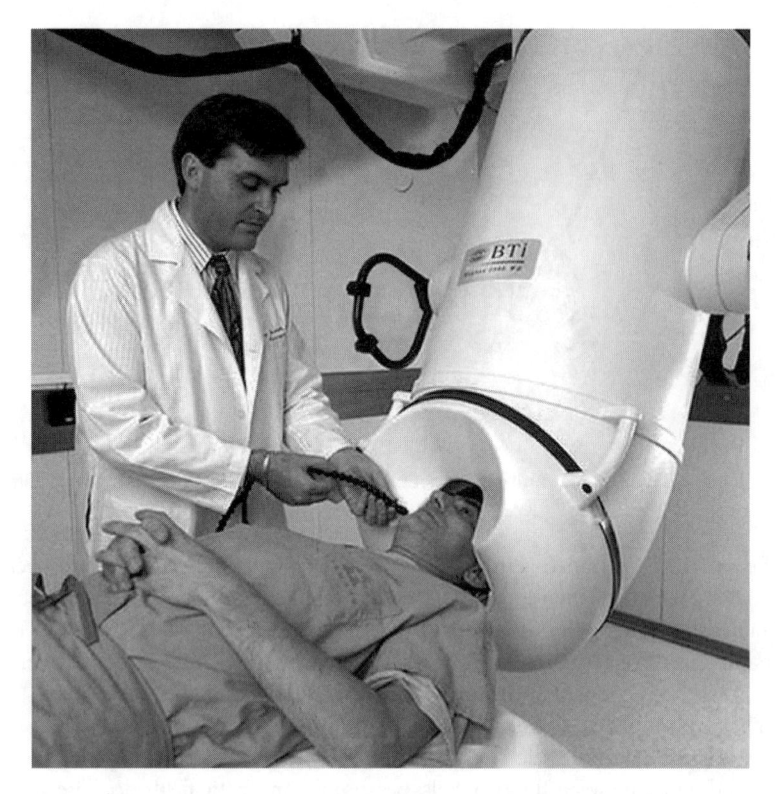

FIGURE 12.5 A whole-head MEG system with 148 recording channels operated in a magnetically shielded room.

12.5 Data Analysis

12.5.1 Surface Maps

Since both EEG and MEG activity have a common basis, their analyses can be carried out using similar methods. During the last 30 years, new techniques, such as color mapping of activity distribution over the scalp (Desmedt et al., 1987; Duffy et al., 1979), have shifted the focus from an analysis of waveforms, derived at selected scalp sites, to the spatial distribution over the entire scalp, at particular points in time. The recording sensors typically span a two-dimensional surface over the skull, and each sensor measures a time series. When these measurements are interpolated and color-coded to provide a spatially continuous representation of the measurements, a so-called topographic scalp map is obtained at each time point. Figure 12.6 shows the location of the sensors on the head and a three-dimensional map of the electrical fields corresponding to the peak of the N1 auditory component.

Topographic analysis is either done qualitatively, by interpreting focal maxima and minima in the map, or quantitatively by dipole localization methods (Brandt, 1992). Alternatively, a combined spatiotemporal approach, where topographic information over different instances in time, called a space-time series, is taken for source localization.

Recently, much effort has been made in the development of source imaging techniques based on high-resolution or dense-array EEG (dEEG). For example, techniques such as scalp Laplacian mapping and cortical imaging attempt to restore the high-frequency content of brain electrical activity that is smeared and distorted by the low-conductivity skull (Babiloni et al., 1996; He et al., 1995; Hjorth, 1975; Le et al., 1994). These techniques can enhance the spatial resolution of the EEG by deconvolving the low-pass spatial filtering effect of the head volume conduction (Freeman, 1980; He et al., 1996; Sidman et al., 1992). Since a surface cortical map lies closer to the actual sources, its potential distribution may provide more direct view of the neural sources (Fender, 1991; Jayakar et al., 1991).

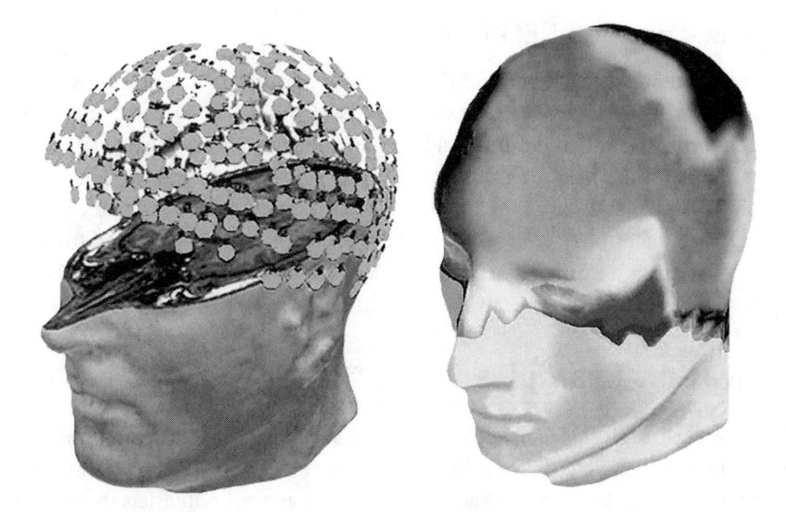

FIGURE 12.6 Example of three-dimensional topographic map. (Left) Arrangement of sensors on the head; (right) a three-dimensional map of the electrical fields obtained at the peak of the N1 auditory component.

12.5.2 Source Imaging Procedure

The SI procedure consists of several steps that culminate in the display of functional information obtained using MEG or EEG onto high-resolution anatomic images typically obtained by MRI. For this final step, it is necessary to translate EEG/MEG locations into MRI coordinates.

The precise location of the measurement points on the scalp is determined electronically with reference to a Cartesian coordinate system anchored on three landmarks (fiducial points) on each subject's head: two external ear canal points and the nasion. The line passing through the two pre-auricular points defines the y-axis of the system. The line perpendicular to the y-axis passing through the nasion defines the x-axis, and the line perpendicular to the x-y plane passing through the x-y origin defines the z-axis.

The EEG/MEG anatomic reference frame is established electronically: a set of three receivers triangulate the signal from a stylus-type transmitter placed successively at several reference points on the subject's head (typically the three fiducial points, the vertex, and the inion). Additionally, small vitamin E-containing capsules visible on MRI are placed on the fiducials. The locations of the common markers on the MR images and the EEG/MEG measurements serve for translating EEG/MEG locations into the MRI reference frame. Validation studies have shown that the accuracy of this approach can be as high as a few millimeters (Gallen et al., 1994). The same stylus transmitter can be used to define the curvature of the head by tracing its surface.

After the anatomic reference frame has been established, the fiducial points registered, and the patient's head digitized, the actual recordings are obtained. The latter consist of time-varying measurements at each detector position. The data undergo further analyses that allow the sources underlying the recorded activity to be localized.

The equivalent current dipole (ECD) model yields a description of the instantaneous current dipole in terms of its location, strength, and orientation, along with an estimate of its reliability (confidence volume). Even though there is some variation across labs regarding acceptance criteria for the dipole solutions, a high correlation between data and model and a small confidence volume are always desirable. It is, therefore, possible to select a set of "best-fitting dipoles" to describe the data.

Once the best fitting dipoles have been identified, they are co-registered onto the subject's MRI scan. The resulting images are then printed on MRI films with different symbols and colors, each corresponding to a distinct type of neurophysiological activity.

12.5.3 Mapping-Based on EEG or MEG

Both theory and experiment suggest that the MEG offers no significant advantage over the EEG (Cohen and Cuffin, 1991). MEG systems, however, are very expensive (total cost about $3 million); they require special cryogenic equipment, a magnetically shielded room, daily monitoring and maintenance, and they are available only in a handful of places around the world. Thus, the clinical usefulness of MEG can be very limited. On the contrary, in addition to the unique features mentioned earlier, the latest EEG systems incorporate several advantages: they are readily available in practically all clinical settings, and even the most sophisticated systems are much less expensive than MEG (total cost about $150,000). Therefore, successful brain mapping based on EEG can have a significant impact on patient care.

12.6 Application Examples

In general, the neurophysiological signals recorded on the surface of the head can be separated into two categories, spontaneous and elicited. For instance, epileptogenic discharges, such as interictal spikes, are events of the former type. The latter type of activity, known as evoked potentials in the case of EEG and evoked fields in the case of MEG, results from external stimulation of a specific sensory pathway, such as the auditory, the somatosensory, or the visual.

In the next sections we give examples from our studies during the past few years that illustrate the process of measuring surface activity and localizing the underlying sources.

12.6.1 Auditory Evoked Responses

The most prominent component of an evoked response obtained from transient auditory stimulation is the N1, which occurs at approximately 100 msec after stimulus onset. Due to the magnitude and consistency of the response, the sources underlying the N1 can be easily localized. Typically, neurophysiological signals are collected in "trials," each of which consists of a few hundred milliseconds of activity prior to and following the stimulus onset. Single-trial responses are contaminated by noise, and to improve the signal-to-noise ratio, many trials are collected and averaged (typically between 100 and 500), using the stimulus onset as a time reference. The averaging approach relies on the assumption that the neuronal responses to all stimuli are identical. Additionally, to eliminate artifacts from periodic events, such as arterial pulsations or the 60-Hz power line interference, the interstimulus interval is randomly varied within a predefined range.

A variety of stimuli can elicit this component. We used pure tones of 1-kHz frequency and 50 msec duration (10-msec rise/fall and 30-msec plateau) that were delivered binaurally at an intensity of 80 dB nHL, and a mean stimulus rate of 0.4/sec (Iyer et al., 2002). Figure 12.7 shows an example of the resulting evoked response. Each of the superimposed tracings represents the activity recorded on one of the 256 channels, while the highlighted area denotes the peak of the N1 component. The three-dimensional surface maps superimposed on the subject's MRI were reconstructed at the N1 peak, while the two dipoles indicate the cortical areas activated at that time.

The estimated sources underlying the N1 component were consistently found to be on the floor of the Sylvian fissure, i.e., in the area of the primary auditory cortex, as shown in Figure 12.8. The sources depicted correspond to activity during the highlighted interval around the N1 peak, as shown in Figure 12.7.

12.6.2 Somatosensory Evoked Responses

Localization of the central sulcus and the adjacent precentral and postcentral gyri is a fundamental objective in most mapping studies involving patients, when brain lesions are located in the parietal or frontal cortex. In a recent MEG study (Zouridakis et al., 1999), we used tactile stimulation to map the somatosensory cortex. Stimuli, i.e., bursts of compressed air, were delivered to a plastic diaphragm clipped to the patient's fingertip, lip, or toe (Benzel et al., 1993). Approximately 500 single trials were required,

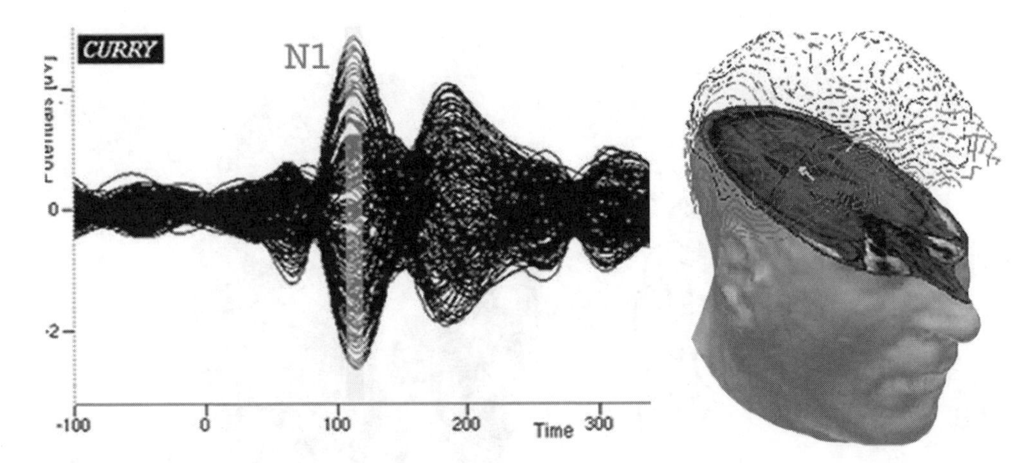

FIGURE 12.7 The N1 evoked potential resulting from auditory stimulation as recorded from 256 channels around the head (left), surface distribution of potentials at the N1 peak, and cortical areas activated during the highlighted portion of the N1 (right).

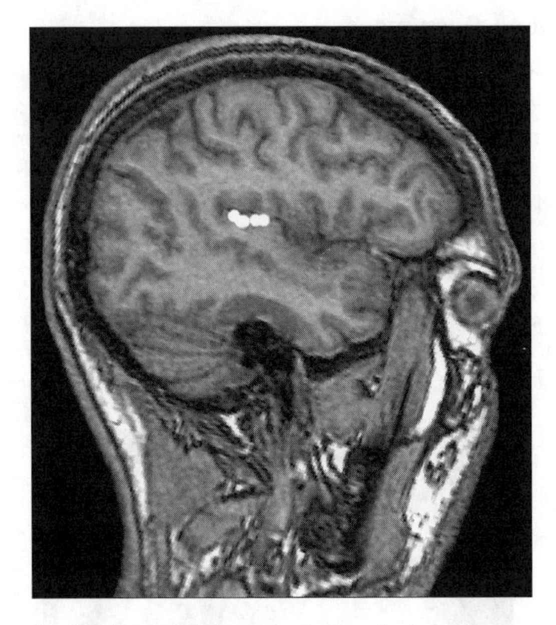

FIGURE 12.8 Localization of the auditory N1 component in the primary auditory area resulting from 1-kHz tone stimuli.

each composed of 100 msec of prestimulus and 100 msec of poststimulus activity. The interstimulus interval was approximately 500 msec. The average responses were digitally filtered with a bandpass filter between 2 and 40 Hz to eliminate high frequency noise, low frequency artifacts, and baseline drifts. At each time point between 30 and 75 msec following stimulus onset, dipole coordinates were obtained using a single-dipole model, and the ones with the best correlation between the measured and predicted fields were selected as the source location. Following this approach detailed mapping of the sensory homunculus can be achieved. In the case of EEG-based mapping, evoked responses are typically obtained using electrical stimulation. Figure 12.9 shows an example mapping, where left cortical areas are activated after stimulation of the subject's right toe, little finger, index finger, thumb, and lower lip. The topographic arrangement of the areas identified resembles the "homunculus" typically seen in textbooks.

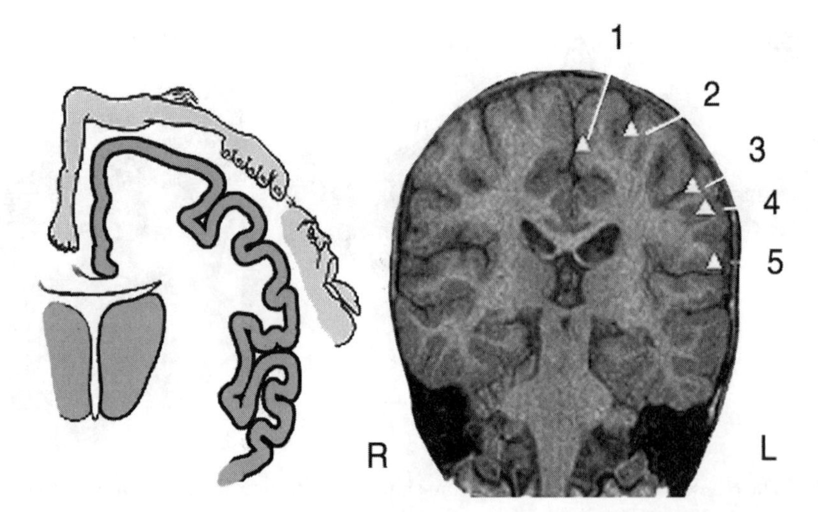

FIGURE 12.9 The cortical areas activated after stimulation of a patient's right toe (1), little finger (2), index finger (3), thumb (4), and lower lip (5) follow the well-known topography of a textbook "homunculus."

12.6.3 Visual Evoked Responses

In cases in which a lesion involves the occipital cortex, visual evoked responses can be used to assess preoperatively potential postoperative complications. Figure 12.10 shows an example of the cortical areas activated after stimulation of a patient's left hemifield of view with a checkerboard pattern (check size 1.4°, pattern reversal rate 1/sec). The maximum magnetic responses were obtained in the right hemisphere, at a latency of approximately 130 msec; this is indicated by a square in the figure.

12.6.4 Epileptogenic Spike Localization

Ictal events, such as spikes, are very important for localizing epileptogenic regions in the brain. During the past several years, MEG has been used in clinical settings as a noninvasive method for localizing the sources of ictal activity (Sutherling and Barth, 1989), and more recently, due to the availability of large-array sensors,

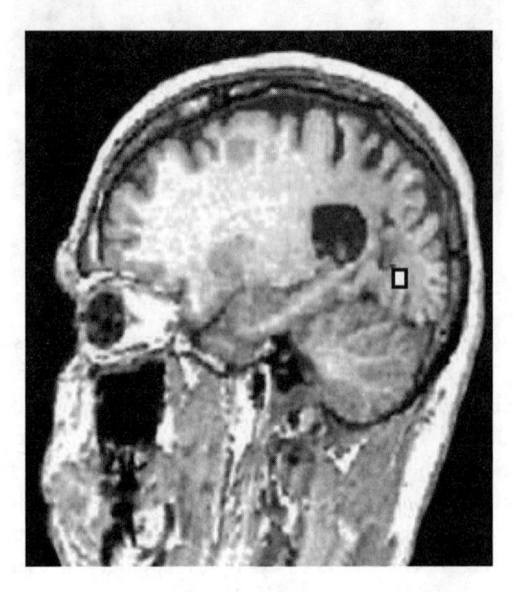

FIGURE 12.10 Cortical areas activated after stimulation of a patient's left hemifield of view with a checkerboard pattern stimulus.

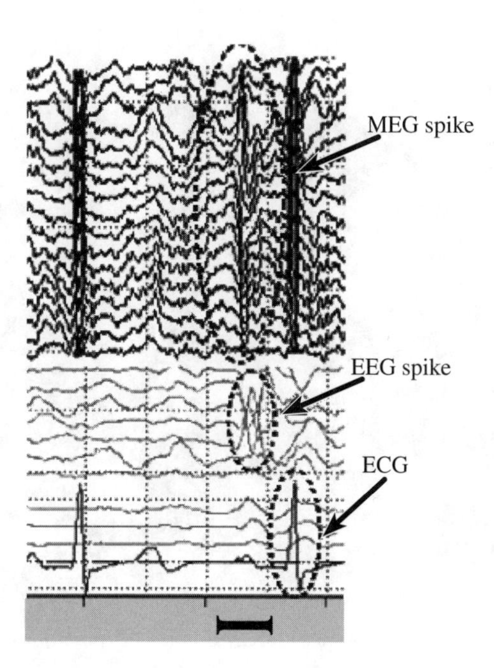

FIGURE 12.11 An epileptic interictal spike detected simultaneously on the MEG and EEG records, along with ECG artifacts.

the sources of interictal spikes (Aung et al., 1995; Papanicolaou et al., 1999). Several studies have suggested that noninvasive source imaging may reduce dependence on invasive electrophysiology for localization of epileptic foci (Papanicolaou et al., 1999; Smith et al., 1993; Zouridakis et al., 1999). Most MEG epilepsy studies report localizations of interictal activity only, because the large artifacts from muscle activity typically associated with seizures make localization of ictal sources extremely difficult. As an example, 2 sec of simultaneous MEG and EEG activity is shown in Figure 12.11 where, in addition to the artifacts resulting from the electrical activity of the heart, an interictal epileptic spike can be seen in both modalities.

Source localizations of several spikes obtained during this study are overlaid on MRI scans in Figure 12.12, where they are shown as triangles. In this case, a focal area of interictal epileptic activity over the lateral surface of the left posterior temporal lobe can be seen.

12.6.5 Language Mapping

Identifying brain regions involved in language functions is often an integral part of the evaluation that brain surgery patients. At present, this task is accomplished mostly through invasive techniques (Ojemann et al., 1989), but recently noninvasive techniques based on MEG have also been used. For example, using a task for continuous recognition of either printed or spoken single words, evoked responses were recorded for 1 sec after the onset of a word and the corresponding intracranial generators were modeled as single-current dipoles. The number of dipoles obtained in each hemisphere was used to quantify the extent of cerebral activation (Breier et al., 2000; Zouridakis et al., 1998a). The areas thus identified included the posterior part of the superior temporal gyrus, and the supramarginal and angular gyri. A characteristic MRI slice with the localized sources superimposed is shown in Figure 12.13, where the circles and triangles correspond to two repetitions of the same experimental task.

12.7 Concluding Remarks

The previous paragraphs give some examples of how SI is used for research and clinical purposes. Both MEG and EEG large-array systems have received Food and Drug Administration (FDA) approval for

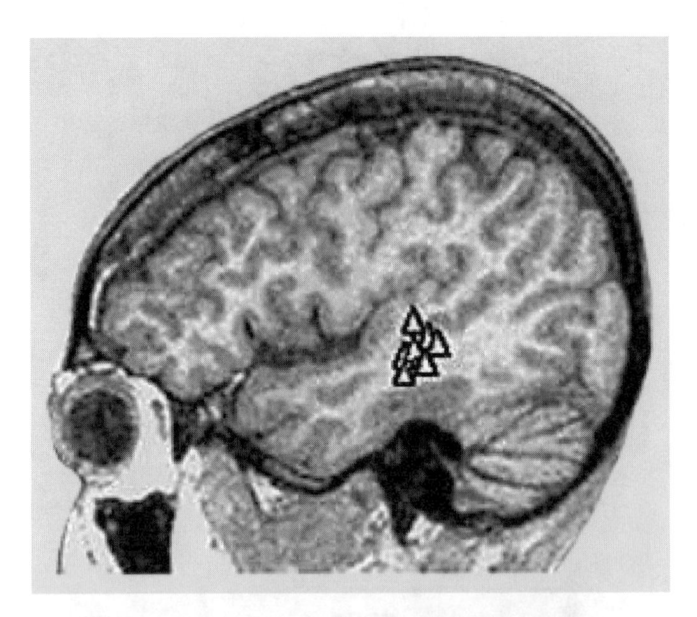

FIGURE 12.12 A cluster of epileptic interictal spikes localized in the left posterior temporal lobe.

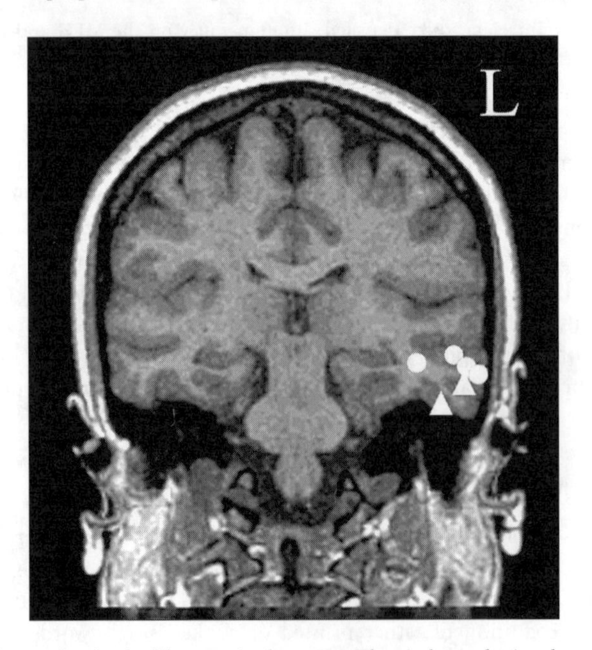

FIGURE 12.13 Cortical areas involved with receptive language. The circles and triangles correspond to two repetitions of the same experimental task.

clinical use, and they are gradually becoming available in many centers around the world. As new technological and computational advances come into existence, the clinical relevance of this technique becomes more apparent. In particular, in the case of epilepsy surgery, the usefulness of SI as a noninvasive tool to preoperatively delineate the extent of a lesion (to be resected) and of the eloquent cortex (to be preserved) has already been recognized (Breier et al., 2000; Gallen et al., 1994; Hamalainen et al., 1993; Papanicolaou et al., 1999; Zouridakis et al., 1998a, 1998b).

With the development of larger sensor arrays and of general source modeling algorithms, it is possible that future clinical applications of source imaging may be extended to include brain injury and stroke assessment, dementias, developmental disorders, as well as further characterization of higher cortical areas involved in attention, memory, and cognition. As a result, these procedures may lead to safer, faster, and more cost-effective clinical interventions.

References

Aung, M., Sobel, D.F., Gallen, C.C., et al., Potential contribution of bilateral magnetic source imaging to the evaluation of epilepsy surgery candidates, *Neurosurgery*, 37, 1113–1121, 1995.

Babiloni, F., Babiloni, C., Carducci, F., Fattorini, L., Onorati, P., and Urbano, A., Spline Laplacian estimate of EEG potentials over a realistic magnetic resonance-constructed scalp surface model, *Electroenceph. Clin. Neurophysiol.*, 98(4), 363–373, 1996.

Baumgartner, C., Sutherling, W., Di, S., and Barth, D.S., Spatiotemporal modeling of cerebral evoked magnetic fields to median nerve stimulation, *Electroenceph. Clin. Neurophysiol.*, 79, 27–35, 1991.

Benzel, E.C., Lewine, J.D., Bucholz, R.D., and Orrison, W.W., Jr., Magnetic source imaging: a review of the Magnes system of biomagnetic technologies incorporated, *Neurosurgery*, 33(2), 252–259, 1993.

Binder, J.R., Frost, J.A., Hammeke, T.A., Cox, R.W., Rao, S.M., and Prieto, T., Human brain areas identified by functional magnetic resonance imaging, *J. Neurosci.*, 17, 353–362, 1997.

Binder, J.R., Rao, S.M., Hammeke, T.A., Frost, J.A., Bandettini, P.A., Jesmanowicz, A., and Hyde, J.S., Lateralized human brain systems demonstrated by task subtraction functional magnetic resonance imaging, *Arch. Neurol.*, 52, 593–601, 1995.

Brandt, M.E., Topographic mapping of brain electromagnetic signals: a review of current technology, *Am. J. Physiol. Imaging*, 7(3–4), 160–174, 1992.

Breier, J.I., Simos, P.G., Zouridakis, G., and Papanicolaou, A.C., Lateralization of activity associated with language function using magnetoencephalography: a reliability study, *J. Clin. Neurophysiol.*, 17(5), 503–510, 2000.

Cohen, D. and Cuffin, B.N., EEG versus MEG localization accuracy: theory and experiment, *Brain Topogr.*, 4(2), 95–103, 1991.

Cuenod, C.A., Brookheimer, S.Y., Hertz-Pannier, L., Zeffiro, T.A., Theodore, W.H., and Le Bihan, D., Functional MRI during word generation using conventional equipment: a potential tool for language localization in the clinical environment, *Neurology*, 45, 1821–1827, 1995.

Cuffin, B.N., EEG dipole source localization, *IEEE Eng. Med. Biol. Mag.*, 17(5):118–122, 1998.

de Munck, J., The potential distribution in a layered anisotropic spherical volume conductor, *J. Appl. Phys.*, 64, 464–470, 1988.

Desmedt, J.E., Nguyen, T.H., and Bourguet, M., Bit-mapped color imaging of human evoked potentials with reference to the N20, P22, P27 and N30 somatosensory response, *Electroenceph. Clin. Neurophysiol.*, 68, 1–19, 1987.

Duffy, F.H., Burchfiel, J.L., and Lomroso, C.T., Brain electrical activity mapping (BEAM): a method for extending the clinical utility of EEG and evoked potential data, *Ann. Neurol.*, 5, 309–321, 1979.

Ebersole, J.S., EEG dipole modeling in complex partial epilepsy, *Brain Topogr.*, 4, 113–123, 1991.

Ebersole, J.S. and Wade, P.B., Spike voltage topography and equivalent dipole localization in complex partial epilepsy, *Brain Topogr.*, 3, 21–34, 1990.

Fender, D.H., Models of the human brain and the surrounding media: their influence on the reliability of source localization, *J. Clin. Neurophysiol.*, 8(4), 381–390, 1991.

Flynn, E.R., Factors which affect spatial resolving power in large array biomagnetic sensors, *Rev. Sci. Instrum.*, 65, 922–935, 1994.

Freeman, W., Use of spatial deconvolution to compensate for distortion of EEG by volume conductor, *IEEE Trans. Biomed. Eng.*, 27, 421–429, 1980.

Friberg, L., Brain mapping in thinking and language function, *Acta Neurochir. Suppl.*, 56, 34–39, 1993.

Gallen, C.C., Schwartz, B., Rieke, K., Pantev, C., Sobel, D., Hirschkoff, E., and Bloom, F.E., Intrasubject reliability and validity of somatosensory source localization using a large array biomagnetometer, *Electroencephal. Clin. Neurophysiol.*, 90, 145–156, 1994.

Gomez-Tortosa, E., Martin, E.M., Sychra, J.J., and Dujovny, M., Language-activated single-photon emission tomography imaging in the evaluation of language lateralization-evidence from a case of crossed aphasia: case report, *Neurosurgery*, 35, 515–519, 1994.

Gorodnitsky, I.F., George, J.S., and Rao, B.D., Neuromagnetic source imaging with FOCUSS: a recursive weighted minimum norm algorithm, *Electroencephalogr. Clin. Neurophysiol.*, 95(4), 231–251, 1995

Hamalainen, M., Hari, R., Ilmoniemi, R., Knuutila, J., and Lounasmaa, O., Magnetoencephalography — theory, instrumentation, and applications to noninvasive studies of the working human brain, *Rev. Mod. Phys.*, 65, 413–497, 1993.

Hari, R., Pelizzone, M., Makela, J.P., Hallstrom, J., Leinonen, L., and Lounasmaa, O.V., Neuromagnetic responses of the human auditory cortex to on- and off-sets of noise bursts, *Audiology*, 26, 31–43, 1987.

He, B., Chernyak, Y., and Cohen, R.J., An equivalent body surface charge model representative three-dimensional bioelectrical activity, *IEEE Trans. Biomed. Eng.*, 42(7), 637–646, 1995.

He, B., Wang, Y., Pak, S., and Ling, Y., Cortical source imaging from scalp electroencephalograms, *Med. Biol. Eng. Comput.*, 34(Suppl. 2), 257–258, 1996.

Henderson, C.J., Butler, S.R., and Glass, A., The localization of equivalent dipoles of EEG sources by the application of electrical field theory, *Electroenceph. Clin. Neurophysiol.*, 39, 117–130, 1975.

Hjorth, B., An on-line transformation of EEG scalp potentials into orthogonal source derivations, *Electroenceph. Clin. Neurophysiol.*, 39, 526–530, 1975.

Ioannides, A.A., Bolton, J.P.R., and Clarke, C.J.S., Continuous probabilistic solutions to the biomagnetic inverse problem, *Inverse Problems*, 6, 523–542, 1990.

Iyer, D., Boutros, N.N., and Zouridakis, G., Independent Component Analysis of Multichannel Auditory Evoked Potentials, 2nd Joint EMBS/BMES Conference, Houston, October 2002.

Jayakar, P., Duchowny, M., Resnick, T., and Alvarez, L.. Localization of seizure foci: pitfalls and caveats, *J. Clin. Neurophysiol.*, 8, 414–431, 1991.

Jirsa, V.K., Fink, P., Foo, P., and Kelso, J.A.S., Parametric stabilization of biological coordination: a theoretical model, *J. Biol. Phys.*, 6, 85–112, 2000.

Kandel, E.R., Schwartz, J.H., and Jessell, T.M., Eds., *Principles of Neural Science*, 3rd ed., Elsevier, New York, 1991.

Kavanagh, R.N., Darcey, T.M., Lehmann, D., and Fender, D.H., Evaluation of methods for three-dimensional localization of electrical sources in the human brain, *IEEE Trans. Biomed. Eng.*, 25, 421–429, 1978.

Kelly, J.P., The neural basis of perception and movement, in *Principles of Neural Science*, 3rd ed., Kandel, E.R., Schwartz, J. H., and Jessell, T.M., Eds., Elsevier Science, New York, 1991.

Le, J., Menon, V., and Gevins, A., Local estimate of surface Laplacian derivation on a realistically shaped scalp surface and its performance on noisy data, *Electroenceph. Clin. Neurophysiol.*, 90, 433–441, 1994.

Lewine, J.D., Neuromagnetic techniques for the noninvasive analysis of brain function, in *Noninvasive Techniques in Biology and Medicine*, Freeman, S.E., Fukushima, E., and Greene, E.R., Eds., San Francisco Press, San Francisco, 1990.

Lopes da Silva, F.H., Wieringa, H.J., and Peters, M.J., Source localization of EEG versus MEG: empirical comparison using visually evoked responses and theoretical considerations, *Brain Topogr.*, 4(2), 133–142, 1991.

Mejis, J.W.H. and Peters, M.J., The EED, EEG and MEG, using a model of eccentric spheres to model the head, *IEEE Trans. Biomed. Eng.*, BME-34, 913–920, 1987.

Mejis, J.W.H., Weier, O.W., Peters, M.J., and van Oosterom, A., On the numerical accuracy of the boundary element method, *IEEE Trans. Biomed. Eng.*, BME-36, 1038–1049, 1989.

Morse, P.M. and Feshbach, H., *Methods of Theoretical Physics I and II*, McGraw Hill, New York, 1963.

Mosher, J.C. and Leahy, R.M., Recursive MUSIC: a framework for EEG and MEG source localization, *IEEE Trans. Biomed.. Eng.*, 45(11), 1342–1354, 1998.

Mosher, J.C., Lewis, P.S., and Leahy, R., Multiple dipole modeling and localization from spatiotemporal MEG data, *IEEE Trans. Biomed. Eng.*, 39, 541–557, 1992.

Nishijo, H., Ikeda, H., Miyamoto, H., Endo, S., and Ono, T., Localization of an ictal onset zone using a realistic 4-shell head model of scalp, skull, liquor, and brain, *Soc. Neurosci. Abst.*, 22, 185, 1996.

Nunez, P. and Pilgreen, K., The spline Laplacian in clinical neurophysiology: a method to improve the EEG spatial resolution, *J. Clin. Neurophysiol.*, 38, 356–368, 1975.

Nunez, P.L., Pilgreen, K.L., Westdorp, A.F., Law, S.K., and Nelson, A.V., A visual study of surface potentials and Laplacians due to distributed neocortical sources: computer simulations and evoked potentials, *Brain Topogr.*, 4(2), 151–168, 1991.

Ojemann, G., Ojemann, J., Lettich, E., and Burger, M., Cortical language localization in left, dominant hemisphere: an electrical stimulation mapping investigation in 117 patients, *J. Neurosurg.*, 71, 316–326, 1989.

Okada, Y., Huang, J.C., and Xu, C., A hierarchical minimum norm estimation method for reconstructing current densities in the brain from remotely measured magnetic fields, in *Biomagnetism, Clinical Aspects*, Hoke, M., Ernd, S.N., Okada, Y.C., and Romani, G.L., Eds., Excerpta Medica, Amsterdam, 1992, pp. 729–734.

O'Leary, D.S., Andreason, N.C., Hurtig, R.R., Hichwa, R.D., Watkins, G.L., Ponto, L.L., Rogers, M., and Kirchner, P.T., A positron emission tomography study of binaurally and dichotically presented stimuli: effects of level of language and directed attention, *Brain Lang.*, 53, 20–39, 1996.

Papanicolaou, A.C., Simos, P.G., Breier, J.I., Zouridakis, G., Willmore, L.J., Wheless, J.W., Constantinou, J.E., Maggio, W.W., and Gormley, W.B., Magnetoencephalographic mapping of the language-specific cortex, *J. Neurosurg.*, 90(1), 85–93, 1999.

Pascual-Marqui, R.D., Michel, C.M., and Lehmann, D., Low resolution electromagnetic tomography: a new method for localizing electrical activity in the brain, *Int. J. Psychophysiol.*, 18(1), 49–65, 1994.

Peterson, S.E., Fox, P.T., Posner, M.I., Mintun, M., and Raichle, M.E., Positron emission tomographic studies of cortical anatomy of single-word processing, *Nature*, 1988, 331, 585–589, 1988.

Plonsey, R., The nature of sources of bioelectric and biomagnetic fields, *Biophys. J.*, 39, 309–312, 1982.

Plonsey, R. and Heppner, D., Considerations of quasistationarity in electrophysiological systems, *Bull. Math. Biophys.*, 29, 657–664, 1967.

Rush, S. and Driscoll, D., Current distribution in the brain from surface electrodes, *Anesth. Analg.*, 47, 717–721, 1978.

Scherg, M., Functional imaging and localization of electromagnetic brain activity, *Brain Topogr.*, 5, 103–112, 1992.

Scherg, M. and von Cramon, D., Two bilateral sources of the late AEP as identified by a spatio-temporal dipole model, *Electroenceph. Clin. Neurophysiol.*, 62, 32–44, 1985.

Schneider, M.R., A multistage process for computing virtual dipolar sources of EEG discharges from surface information, *IEEE Trans. Biomed. Eng.*, 19, 1–12, 1972.

Sidman, R., Vincent, D., Smith, D., and Lu, L., Experimental test of the cortical imaging technique-applications to the response to median nerve stimulation and the localization of epileptiform discharges, *IEEE Trans. Biomed. Eng.*, 27, 437–444, 1992.

Sidman, R.D., Giambalvo, V., Allison, T., and Bergey, P., A method for localization of sources of human cerebral potentials evoked by sensory stimuli, *Sensory Processes*, 2, 116–129, 1978.

Smith, D., Baker, G., Davies, G., Dewey, M., and Chadwick, D.W., Outcomes of add-on treatment with lamotrigine in partial epilepsy, *Epilepsia*, 34(2), 312–322, 1993.

Supek, S. and Aine, C.J., Simulation studies of multiple dipole neuromagnetic source localization: model order and limits of source resolution, *IEEE Trans. Biomed. Eng.*, 40, 529–540, 1993.

Sutherling, W.W. and Barth, D.S., Neocortical propagation in temporal lobe spike foci on magnetoencephalography and electroencephalography, *Ann. Neurol.*, 25(4), 373–381, 1989.

Wang, J., Williamson, S.J., and Kaufman, L., Magnetic source images determined by a lead-field analysis: the unique minimum-norm least squares estimation, *IEEE Trans. Biomed. Eng.*, 39, 665–675, 1992.

Williamson, S.J. and Kaufman, L., Analysis of neuromagnetic signals, in *Handbook of Electroencephalography and Clinical Neurophysiology*, Vol. 1, Gevins, A.S. and Remond, A., Eds., Elsevier, New York, 1987, pp. 405–448.

Wilson, F.N. and Bayley, R.H., The electric field of an eccentric dipole in an homogeneous spherical conducting medium, *Circulation*, 1, 84–92, 1950.

Witwer, J., Trezek, G., Jewett, D.L., and Yamashita, Y., The effect of media inhomogeneities upon intracranial electrical fields, *IEEE Trans. Biomed. Eng.*, BME-19, 352–362, 1972.

Yeh, G.C.K. and Martinek, K., The potential of an general dipole model in a homogeneous conducting prolate spheroid, *Ann. N.Y. Acad. Sci.*, 65, 1003–1006, 1957.

Zhou, H. and van Oosterom, A., Computation of the potential distribution in a four-layer anisotropic concentric spherical volume conductor, *IEEE Trans. Biomed. Eng.*, BME-38, 154–158, 1991.

Zouridakis, G., Simos, P.G., and Papanicolaou, A.C., Multiple bilaterally asymmetric cortical sources account for the auditory N1m component, *Brain Topogr.*, 10, 183–189, 1998a.

Zouridakis, G., Simos, P.G., Breier, J.I., and Papanicolaou, A.C., Functional hemispheric asymmetry assessment in a visual language task using MEG, *Brain Topogr.*, 11, 57–65, 1998b.

Zouridakis, G., Simos, P.G., Papanicolaou, A.C., and Breier, J.I., Magnetic source imaging: introduction and application examples, *J. Clin. Eng.*, 24, 51–61, 1999.

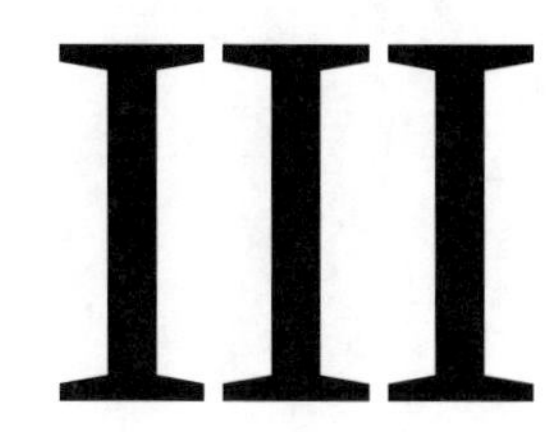

Biological Assays

Contributions of Technology to the Biological Revolution

Almost all disease states can be ultimately linked to some sort of dysfunction at the cellular or molecular level. The ability to identify abnormalities in the cellular content of diseased tissues has expanded clinical medicine. New technologies to manipulate these processes are emerging every day. At the frontline of this technology is the variety of assays used in clinical laboratories to examine the basis of human disease.

The development of these tools began almost immediately following the identification of cells as the basic building blocks of living beings. Microscopic assessment of tissues and cells, combined with various staining techniques, has greatly enhanced disease diagnosis. Many of these techniques have been fine-tuned to the point of almost total automation. As the biological revolution and information age continue to mature, the ability of clinicians to obtain accurate diagnoses will continue to increase.

This section includes the following chapters:

13

Molecular Biology Techniques and Applications

CONTENTS

Lidia Kos
Florida International University

Roman Joel Garcia
Florida International University

13.1 Introduction

The development and implementation of molecular biology techniques have had a major impact in both basic and applied biological research. Since its inception in the early 1950s, molecular biology has matured as a science. In the last 10 years many of the tedious, repetitive techniques have been automated; time-consuming multistep procedures have been converted into kits; high quality genomic and cDNA libraries are now commercially available, and improvements in the quality of reagents and enzymes have immensely benefited all nucleic acid manipulations.

All molecular biology techniques, from the most basic to those more sophisticated and novel, rely on the fundamental processes of molecular biology, DNA replication, transcription, and translation. DNA is a polymer of nucleotides organized as a double-stranded helix. The strands are antiparallel and the nitrogenous bases (adenine [A], cytosine [C], thymine [T], and guanine [G]) that constitute the nucleotides are held together by hydrogen bonding. DNA replication is semiconservative, meaning that each parent strand acts as a template for the synthesis of a new strand. Therefore, the resulting pair of DNA helices each contains one parent strand and one newly synthesized daughter strand. During replication, the enzyme DNA polymerase catalyzes the addition of nucleotides to the 3′end (free 3′ hydroxyl group) of each growing strand, thereby synthesizing these two strands in the 5′→3′ direction. The substrates for this polymerization are deoxyribonucleoside triphosphates, which are hydrolyzed as they are added to a given growing strand. The sequence of added nucleotides is dependent upon complementary base pairing with the template strands (As with Ts, and Gs with Cs).

0-8493-1140-3/04/$0.00+$1.50

The genetic information carried in DNA is expressed in two basic steps: DNA is first transcribed to RNA, and then RNA is translated into protein. In a given region of DNA, only one of the two strands can act as a template for transcription. Transcription from the DNA template strand occurs in a 5′→3′ direction and it is catalyzed by RNA polymerase (RNA polymerase II in eukaryotes) using riboses as substrates. RNA is generally single stranded, and it contains uracil pyrimidines instead of thymine bases. After transcription, the RNA molecule travels from the nucleus into the cytoplasm where translation occurs, thus its designation as "messenger RNA" (mRNA). During translation, amino acids are linked in an order specified by nucleotide triplets (codons) grouped within the mRNA. This is accomplished by an adapter transfer RNA (tRNA), which has an anticodon complementary to the mRNA codon, and which binds its corresponding amino acid. Specifically, a family of activating enzymes (aminoacyl-tRNA synthetases) attaches the amino acids to their appropriate tRNAs and subsequently form charged tRNAs. Translation is initiated when the charged tRNAs form a complex with the mRNA and ribosome. The ribosome moves along the mRNA one codon at a time, elongating the nascent polypeptide from the amino terminus toward the carboxyl terminus. After translation, proteins can undergo further modification by proteolysis, glycosylation, and phosphorylation.

This chapter provides an overview of the most commonly used and emerging molecular biology techniques, with a focus on the isolation and analysis of nucleic acids, especially as used in the examination of differences in gene expression. Changes in mRNA levels account for morphological and phenotypic manifestations and are good indicators of cellular responses to environmental signals. Establishing the expression patterns of multiple genes can elucidate the biochemical pathways and regulatory mechanisms that govern cell physiology. These types of studies also have the potential to identify the causes and consequences of diseases such as cancer, and aid in the development of drugs and their possible targets (Lockhart and Winzeler, 2000).

Although this chapter does not discuss the wide variety of protein assay techniques, such as western blots, two-dimensional gels, protein or peptide chromatographic separation and mass spectrometric detection, the use of specific protein-fusion reporter constructs and colorimetric readouts, or the characterization of actively translated polysomal mRNAs, these peptide-based protocols are the basis for several novel areas of research and they have recently garnered substantial attention (Pandey and Mann, 2000). A testament to this focus is reflected in the newly formed international alliance of industry, academic, and government members (HUPO: Human Proteome Organization) geared to drive a global effort aimed at determining the structure and function of all human proteins (Kaiser, 2002).

For readers who seek a wider range of exposure to molecular biology techniques or for those who require detailed laboratory protocols, such information can be found in the references cited within the sections of this chapter, or the literature within Sambrook and Russell (2001) and Ausubel et al. (2002).

13.2 Isolation of Nucleic Acids

13.2.1 DNA

The success of most molecular biology techniques depends on the quality of the starting nucleic acid preparation. In the case of DNA, the preparation should be free of contaminating RNA, proteins, lipids, and other cellular constituents that may disrupt the activity of the variety of enzymes used in these techniques. It should also be free of DNA nucleases, which can nick and degrade high-molecular-weight DNA. The isolation method also has to be gentle enough to forego levels of mechanical shear stress that can fragment large genomic DNA. The purification protocol generally starts with the use of a buffer containing one or several detergents (i.e., sodium dodecyl sulfate [SDS], Nonidet P-40, Triton X-100) in order to lyse the cells and disassociate the proteins from DNA. Incubation with proteinase K at high temperatures (56–65°) is used when further deproteinization is required. Following the proteinase K treatment, residual protein and contaminating lipids can be effectively removed by extraction with phenol and chloroform. Contaminating RNA can be degraded with DNase-free RNase, followed by a chloroform extraction. Pure DNA is then obtained by a simple precipitation with isopropanol or ethanol. Organic extractions can be avoided by employing a prolonged proteinase K incubation step followed by the addition of a saturated NaCl solution to precipitate proteins. Isolated DNA can be subsequently quantified in a spectrophotometer and evaluated for quality by agarose-gel electrophoresis.

One of the procedures that requires high quality pure DNA is the construction of a genomic DNA library. After isolation, genomic DNA is digested into small fragments with restriction endonucleases that cleave DNA at specific sites, defined by a sequence of bases (restriction site). A given fragment is ligated into a self-replicating vector that enables it to be maintained and propagated within bacterial cells such as *Escherichia coli* or yeast cells such as *Saccharomyces cerevisiae.* Such a library may be stored as a permanent source of representative sequences of a particular organism. They can then be used for screening to isolate a particular sequence of interest, or to determine the location and order of sequences in the genome from which the library was constructed (physical mapping).

13.2.2 RNA

There are various methods for isolating total cellular RNA, including some that allow for the simultaneous isolation of DNA. They are mostly based on solubilizing the cellular components, and inactivating intracellular RNases while maintaining biologically active RNA. Most isolation procedures combine the use of one or more reagents, such as organic solvents (phenol:chloroform), detergents (SDS, Nonidet P-40, sodium deoxycholate), or chaotropic salts such as guanidinium isothiocyanate (GITC). For pure RNA preparations, cesium chloride density gradients or precipitation of the RNA with LiCl are used to separate the contaminating cellular DNA. The most commonly used procedure was initially introduced by Chomczynski and Sacchi (1987). This method employs an extraction buffer containing GITC. The addition of N-lauroylsarcosine and B-mercaptoethanol in the mixture enhances the solubilization properties of GITC. The protocol involves an acidic phenol extraction that selectively retains cellular DNA in the organic phase and aids in the removal of proteins and lipids. The addition of chloroform further isolates lipids and establishes two distinct phases: an organic phase containing the DNA, proteins, and lipids, and an aqueous phase containing the RNA. In recent years, several commercial reagents based on this procedure, marketed as single-step RNA isolation solutions, have been made available. The intact RNA can then be used as a substrate for further manipulation in techniques such as Northern-blot analysis, RNase protection assay, and reverse transcription.

13.3 Analysis of Nucleic Acid

13.3.1 Hybridization-Based Techniques

Many of the applications aimed at the study of nucleic acids rely on the principles that govern molecular annealing (hybridization). Under appropriate conditions, two single-nucleic acid chains form a hybrid molecule to an extent that is largely dependent on the degree of their nucleotide complementarity. When coupled to suitable labeling and detection methods, this complementarity provides an important tool for identifying identical or related sequences of a reference nucleic acid sequence (probe). Among the various applications that take advantage of molecular annealing for nucleic acid analysis, the most frequently used techniques consist of hybridizing a labeled nucleic acid probe to a target nucleic acid immobilized on a solid support, typically a nitrocellulose or nylon membrane. Characteristic examples of these techniques are Southern blotting hybridization for the analysis of DNA, and Northern blotting, nuclease protection assays, and *in situ* hybridization for the analysis of RNA.

13.3.1.1 Southern Blot

In Southern blotting hybridization (Southern, 1975), DNA is digested with one or more restriction enzymes and the resulting fragments are separated according to size by gel electrophoresis. The fragments are then denatured into single-stranded molecules by treatment with alkali, neutralized, and transferred (blotted) to a hybridization membrane by capillarity using a high salt concentration buffer. After the

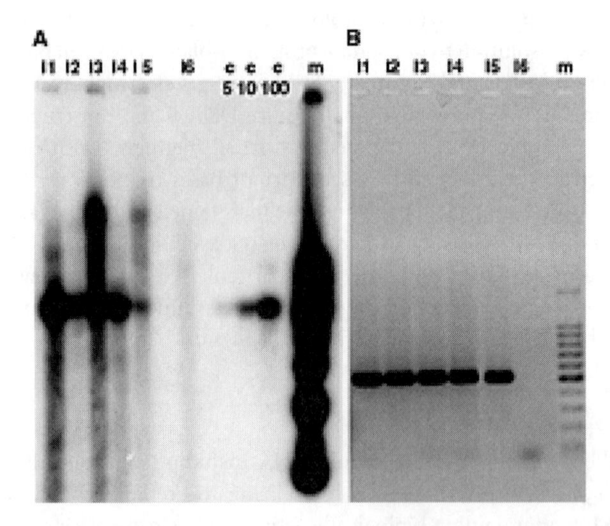

FIGURE 13.1 Identification of mouse lines (l1–6) carrying a specific transgene by Southern blot analysis (A) and PCR (B). (A) Genomic DNAs from six mice were digested with a restriction enzyme, gel-separated, blotted, and hybridized to an isotopically labeled probe corresponding to the transgene. (B) The same genomic DNAs were amplified with primers complementary to the transgene. Lines 1–5 are transgenic and line 6 is not. Southern blot analysis allows for the estimation of transgene copy numbers based on reference amounts of linearized plasmids containing the probe (c) corresponding to 5, 10, and 100 copies per genome. Lines 1–4 were estimated to have over 100 copies of the transgene and line 5 to have 10 copies. m, DNA size marker. (Images courtesy of A. Ittah, Florida International University, Miami.)

transfer, the DNA is UV cross-linked to the membrane thereby creating single-stranded target DNA molecules that are available for hybridization with a labeled single-stranded DNA probe. Probes can be labeled by incorporating radioactive or nonisotopic (fluorescent, biotinylated, digoxigenin) nucleotides into their nucleic acid structure. Following hybridization (generally overnight), nonspecific hybridization is removed by several washes, and the specific interactions that occur between the probe and target are detected through a range of procedures contingent upon the probe labeling method (autoradiography, phosphorimaging, fluorography, chemiluminescence, immunohistochemistry). Southern blotting has been used in a panoply of applications: to analyze gene organization, identify and clone specific sequences, study mutant and transgenic organisms (Figure 13.1A), characterize genotypes through restriction fragment length polymorphisms (RFLPs), allow genetic fingerprinting for both medical and forensic analyses, and diagnose genetic disorders and cancer.

13.3.1.2 Northern Blot

The procedure for Northern blot analysis, designed for RNA studies, was derived from Southern blot analysis (Alwine et al., 1977). RNA is separated according to size on an agarose gel under denaturing conditions (generally formaldehyde gels), transferred and irreversibly bound to a nitrocellulose or nylon membrane, and then hybridized with a labeled (generally radioactively with ^{32}P) nucleic acid probe. After washing the unbound and nonspecifically bound probes, target RNA molecules are revealed by autoradiography or phosphorimaging. Northern blot analysis detects the steady-state level of accumulation of a given RNA sequence in the sample being studied. Despite the development of increasingly sensitive techniques such as the RNase protection assay and reverse transcription PCR (RT-PCR), Northern analysis remains as one of the most commonly used procedures for gene expression studies. This technique has been widely employed to characterize cloned cDNAs, to study spatial (tissue/organ) and temporal specificity of gene expression (Figure 13.2A), and to analyze exogenous gene activity in transgenic organisms.

13.3.1.3 Nuclease Protection Assay

Nuclease protection assays are sensitive methods used to detect, quantify, and map (5′ and 3′ termini, exon-intron boundaries) specific RNAs in a complex mixture of total cellular RNA. These techniques

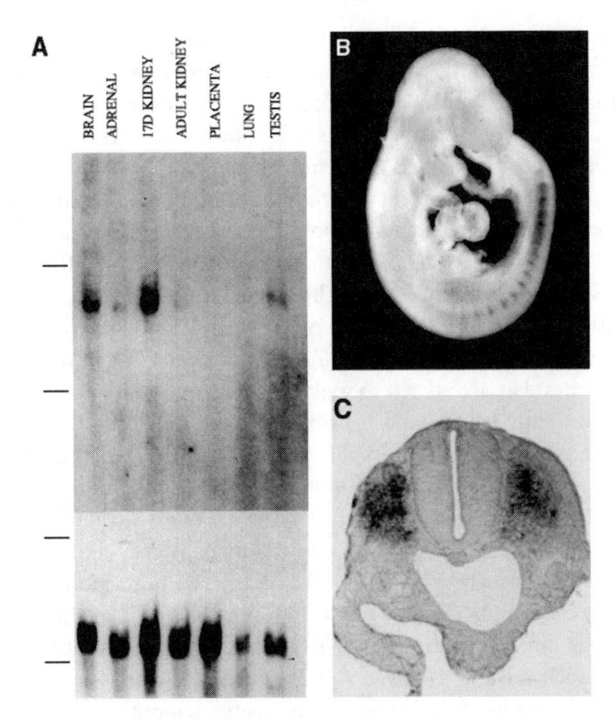

FIGURE 13.2 Analysis of gene expression by Northern blot (A) and *in situ* hybridization (B, C). (A) Total RNA was extracted from different mouse tissues as indicated, gel-separated, blotted, and hybridized with an isotopically labeled, specific transcription factor cDNA probe (top panel), and β-actin probe (bottom panel) for RNA normalization. The location of ribosomal bands is indicated on the left as horizontal lines for size estimation. This transcript is highly expressed in the 17-day kidney and brain. Low levels of expression are also detected in the adrenal, adult kidney, and testis. (B) A 9.5-embryonic day mouse embryo was hybridized with the same cDNA probe labeled with digoxigenin nucleotides. Detection was by immunohistochemistry using an anti-digoxigennin alkaline phosphatase tagged antibody. Transcripts are detected (purple color) in the developing somites. (C) Hybridization as in B directly to a frozen section allows for cellular localization of the transcript. (Figure is depicted here in black and white.)

include RNase protection and S1 mapping and are based upon solution hybridization (in contrast with the support-bound RNA targets in Northern blotting) and on the ability of RNA:RNA (RNase protection) and DNA:RNA (S1 mapping) hybrids to resist single-stranded specific nucleases. The assays depend upon the synthesis of a radioactively labeled probe that has partial complementarity to a portion of the target RNA. After hybridization, a mixture of nucleases is used to remove, by digestion, any remaining unhybridized probes and any single-stranded regions of hybridized probes. The nucleases are then inactivated and the remaining probe:target hybrids are precipitated. The products are separated on a denaturing polyacrylamide gel and are subsequently visualized by autoradiography.

These assays hold various advantages over Northern analysis. Solution hybridization tolerates high RNA input, and it is not affected by membrane transfer efficiency nor by the availability of support-bound RNAs. The signal-to-noise ratio is generally much better, since cross-hybridizing RNAs yield only short protected fragments. Finally, detecting hybridized probes on polyacrylamide gels is much more sensitive than doing so on agarose gels. However, one disadvantage of these assays is that the size of target RNAs cannot be determined.

13.3.1.4 *In Situ* Hybridization

In situ hybridization allows for the precise spatial characterization of a nucleic acid target, and, unlike hybridizations of solution-suspended nucleic acids to target sequences on membrane filters, the targets in this case are cross-linked and embedded in a complex matrix that decreases the access of the probe and the stability of the hybrids. The procedures employed are similar to those used in blotting techniques, but they incorporate extra permeabilization steps. Light or fluorescence microscopy is required for probe detection because the nucleic acid targets are bound to chromosomes, cells, or tissues. There are several techniques available for different applications (Choo, 1994; Wilkinson, 1995); probes can be double- or single-stranded DNA, cDNA, RNA, and oligonucleotides; the nucleotides can be labeled radioactively or conjugated with fluorochrome, biotin, or digoxigenin.

One of the most common applications of *in situ* hybridization is to localize genes on chromosomes for the cytogenetic analysis and detection of cancer-specific rearrangements. Introduction of fluorochrome labeled probes in the early 1980s (Bauman et al., 1980) overcame the problem of poor spatial resolution that was created by the use of isotopically labeled probes, and it made FISH (fluorescence *in situ* hybridization; Trask, 1991) a valuable tool for constructing physical maps. FISH is based on the same principle as Southern blot analysis. The target DNA is the nuclear DNA of interphase cells or the DNA of metaphase chromosomes that are affixed to a glass microscope slide. The test probe, generally large genomic clones, is fluorescently labeled and hybridized to the slide. The slide is washed of unbound-probe and processed for hybridized-probe visualization through fluorescence microscopy and powerful image processing software. FISH allows for the simultaneous analysis of multiple probes and it is therefore used to order and distance DNA markers. In particular, the use of extended chromatin fiber preparations has allowed the generation of precise long-range physical maps (Cai et al., 1995).

RNA analysis methodologies such as Northern blot and RNase protection assays require the homogenization of the tissue or cell sample, and as a result it is impossible to relate RNA expression to histology and cell morphology. The direct hybridization of RNA probes (generally labeled with digoxigenin and detected by immunohistochemistry) to tissue sections or whole embryos (Figures 13.2B and C) has become a powerful tool during the examination of the spatial/temporal expression patterns of genes at the cellular level and during embryonic development.

13.3.2 Polymerase Chain Reaction

Since its introduction in the early 1980s (Saiki et al., 1985; Mullis and Faloona, 1987), polymerase chain reaction (PCR) has revolutionized the field of molecular biology. This technique reproduces the basic mechanism of DNA replication and it enables large amounts of DNA to be produced from very small quantities of starting material (the template). PCR is also a simple, robust, extremely sensitive, and speedy technique. An enormous number of PCR variations and applications have been described, and an equally large number of books and journals have been devoted to this technique.

PCR is extensively used in molecular biology and genetic disease research (Figure 13.1B) in order to identify and clone novel genes; in clinical practice, to detect viral targets such as HIV; in evolutionary studies, to track sequences of degraded ancient DNAs; in crime labs, for forensic casework; and in microbial ecology analysis, for the identification and quantification of environmental and food pathogens.

13.3.2.1 Basic PCR

PCR is an *in vitro* DNA amplification method that involves the repetition of a cycle consisting of a number of defined stages. The reagents required for PCR include a thermostable DNA polymerase (*Taq* polymerase), each of the four deoxynucleoside triphosphates (dNTPs), a source of template DNA (such as genomic DNA or cDNA containing the target sequence), and two oligonucleotide primers designed to complement DNA sequences flanking the region of interest. The primers are usually 15 to 30 base pairs and although for certain applications they may be degenerate in their sequence, they are usually directly complementary to the flanking DNA sequences of a specific DNA stretch of interest.

The PCR procedure involves the repetition of a series consisting of three fundamental steps that define one PCR cycle: double-stranded DNA template denaturation at 94 to 96°C, the annealing of two oligonucleotide primers to the single-stranded template at 35 to 55°C (depending on the melting temperature of the primer:template hybrids), and the enzymatic extension of the primers at 72°C to produce copies that can serve as templates in subsequent cycles. As the cycles proceed, both the original template and the amplified targets serve as substrates for the denaturation, primer annealing, and primer extension processes. The three separate steps are usually repeated between 25 and 40 times. Since every cycle doubles the amount of target copies, an exponential amplification occurs. However, the process is self-limiting and amplification factors are generally between 10^5- and 10^9-fold. Excess primers and dNTPs help drive the reaction that commonly occurs in 10 m*M* Tris-HCl buffer (pH 8.3) containing 50 m*M* KCl (to provide proper ionic strength) and magnesium as an enzyme cofactor. Because of the inherent repetition involved in the procedure, PCR has been automated by the production and design of numerous automatic thermocyclers.

PCR has facilitated and increased the sensitivity of numerous techniques such as sequencing (Mitchell and Merrill, 1989; Bevan et al., 1992; Rapley, 1996), cloning, site-directed mutagenesis (Higuchi et al., 1988), detecting polymorphisms and mutations in restriction fragment-length polymorphisms (RFLPs) (Saiki et al., 1985), denaturing gradient gel electrophoresis (DGGE), temperature-gradient gel electrophoresis (TGGE) (Wartell et al., 1990), and single-strand conformational polymorphism (SSCP) (Dockhorn-Dworniczak et al., 1991). Recently, the cell-localization ability of *in situ* hybridization has been combined with the sensitivity of PCR in primed *in situ* hybridization (PRINS) (Hindkjaer et al., 1994). This procedure is based on the rapid annealing of an unlabeled DNA primer to its target sequence *in situ* (chromosome, tissue section). The primer serves as an initiator site for *in situ* chain elongation, which is dependent upon *Taq* polymerase and fluorescent, biotinylated, or digoxigenin labeled nucleotides. This technique labels the site of hybridization rather than the probe and the amplified signal remains localized to the site of synthesis.

13.3.2.2 Reverse Transcriptase-PCR

Reverse transcriptase-PCR (RT-PCR) is a method used to amplify cDNA copies of RNA. The basic technique initially involves converting RNA to a single-stranded cDNA template. An oligodeoxynucleotide primer (generally oligo [dT], which binds to the endogenous poly[A] tails of mRNAs) is hybridized to the mRNA and then extended by the enzyme, reverse transcriptase. The cDNA is then amplified by PCR using a second primer, preferentially gene-specific, and *Taq* polymerase. RT-PCR has a number of applications but it is especially useful for retrieving and cloning the 5′ and 3′ termini of mRNAs, generating cDNA libraries from small amounts of mRNA, and measuring gene expression levels.

A useful adaptation to RT-PCR is differential display (DD-RT-PCR). In DD-RT-PCR, cDNAs are made from two mRNA samples using short arbitrary primers in addition to the oligo (dT) primer with modified 3′ ends. The resulting pair of cDNA populations is compared on side-by-side tracks in a polyacrylamide gel where they are resolved as a complex pattern of bands. Each mRNA is represented as a single band and differential bands can be isolated and cloned (Liang and Pardee, 1992) (Figure 13.3). This technique identifies genes that are differentially expressed in the two mRNA populations.

RT-PCR and the procedure of subtractive hybridization are the bases of other methods developed to compare two mRNA populations and to identify differentially expressed genes. In one of these, representational difference analysis (RDA), mRNAs isolated from both populations are converted into double-stranded cDNA, digested with a restriction enzyme, and the resulting cut ends modified by attaching linkers. Amplification of the modified cDNA populations generates the "representations." After eliminating the linkers from one of the representations, the "driver," it is hybridized in excess against the other, the "tester." Subsequent amplification results in the removal of common hybridizing sequences and the exponential amplification of unique sequences in the tester (Hubank and Schatz, 1999).

13.3.2.3 Quantitative PCR

The PCR-based methods used to estimate the concentration of a particular DNA or RNA sequence provide a largely unlimited sensitivity for the detection of these nucleotides. However, they do not allow direct sequence-quantification, because PCR efficiency depends on the amount of template in the sample, and the amplification is exponential only at low concentrations of the template. Therefore, the amount of the amplification product is not a direct reflection of the original amount of the template; it is simply an end-point measurement. Additionally, subtle differences in the reaction conditions may cause significant sample-to-sample variation in the final yield of the PCR. To overcome these problems, an internal

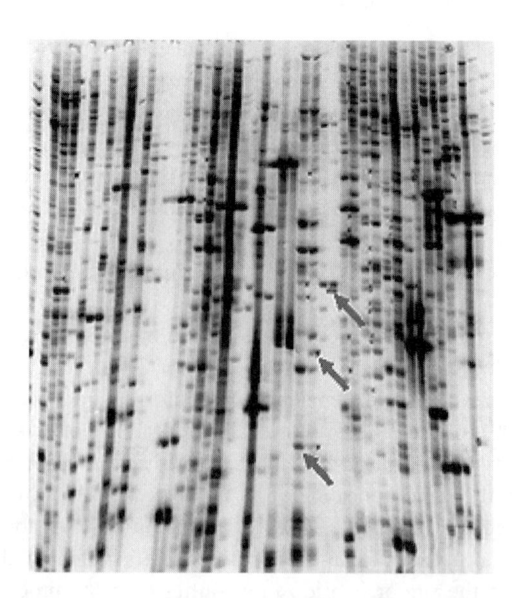

FIGURE 13.3 A portion of a differential display RT-PCR gel. cDNAs from two cell populations were generated, amplified with different sets of arbitrary primers, and ran side-by-side on the polyacrylamide gel. Examples of differentially expressed bands are indicated by the arrows. (Image courtesy of A. Ittah and S. Mandat, Florida International University, Miami.)

standard, which is as similar as possible to the target sequence and usually a housekeeping gene or its mRNA, is coamplified in the same reaction with the target sequence. For certain applications, it is sufficient to determine the relative amount of a target sequence compared to the standard. In order to determine the absolute amount of a target sequence, it is necessary to add a known amount of a standard to the sample before amplification.

Recently, an increasingly sophisticated method has been developed wherein the amplified DNA or RNA is quantified during the exponential phase of PCR, a time when none of the components of the reaction are limiting. This method, real-time PCR (Bustin, 2000), improves the precision of quantifying target sequences, and eliminates much of the variation associated with end-point measurements. Real-time PCR uses commercially available fluorescence-detecting thermocyclers to amplify specific sequences and measure their concentrations simultaneously. The earliest instruments used a fluorometer coupled to a thermocycler to measure the increase in fluorescence emitted by dyes (ethidium bromide or SYBR Green I) that intercalate into, or bind to the grooves of, double-stranded DNA during the exponential phase of the amplification. Because these dyes are universal, they do not guarantee an exclusive association with the amplified product. However, the development and use of fluorescently labeled oligonucleotide probes (Taqman, binary hybridization) in real-time PCR reactions has solved the specificity problem and has made this a powerful technique for the analysis of differential gene expression, and screening for mutations as well as single nucleotide polymorphisms.

13.3.3 High-Throughput Techniques

The genomes of 800 organisms have either been sequenced completely or are in the process of being sequenced (www.ncbi.nlm.nih.gov:80/entrez). There is also a large scale effort to collect DNA sequence information from all expressed genes. This is accomplished by methods predicated upon the random sequencing of partial cDNA clones generated from mRNAs; the predominant methodology in use is called expressed sequence tag (EST) analysis. EST sequences generally represent 200 to 800 base pairs of first-pass sequence information extending in from the mRNA 3′ ends. Sequences from the two large public EST projects, the EST project and the Cancer Genome Anatomy Project (www.ncbi.nlm.nih.gov/ncicgap/), are deposited into the databank dbEST (www.ncbi.nlm.nih.gov/dbEST/), a division of GenBank. Sequences stored in dbEST are subjected to an automated process called UniGene that compares ESTs and assembles overlapping sequences into clusters (www.ncbi.nlm.nih.gov/UniGene/).

Novel technologies have been developed in order to exploit this large and rapidly increasing amount of sequence information. Among the high-throughput, comprehensive genomic methods used to analyze mRNA expression levels, serial analysis of gene expression (SAGE) and array-based hybridization are currently the most common approaches. These techniques enable a characterization of the entire set of expressed genes — the "transcriptome" (Velculesco et al., 1997; 1999).

13.3.3.1 Serial Analysis of Gene Expression

In SAGE (Velculesco et al., 1995), cDNA synthesized from total cellular RNA is cut with specific restriction enzymes into short (10 to 14 base pairs) nucleotide sequence fragments. Each fragment, a tag, is able to uniquely recognize a transcript. These tags are then randomly concatenated, amplified through cloning, sequenced, and compared with genomic databases. The expression level of a given transcript is obtained by quantifying the number of times a particular tag is observed. SAGE analysis allows the obtainment of a gene expression profile for cells or tissues, as well as the identification of novel transcripts. The Cancer Genome Anatomy Project has created a database, SAGEmap, to provide quantitative gene expression data from various organisms (www.ncbi.nlm.nih.gov/SAGE/).

13.3.3.2 Array-Based Hybridization

Nucleic acid arrays are based on the same principles as conventional blotting techniques, labeled DNAs or RNAs (in solution) are hybridized to complementary sequences attached at specific locations on a select surface. The first arrays to be developed generally consisted of fragments of DNA with unknown sequences spotted on nylon membranes. The hybridized material was often radioactively labeled (Lennon and Lehrach, 1991; Southern et al., 1994; Zhao et al., 1995; Nguyen et al., 1995). The use of glass as a substrate, the development of technologies for synthesizing or spotting nucleic acids on glass slides at very high densities, and the employment of fluorescence for detection, have allowed the generation of much smaller arrays (microarrays) that harbor immense quantities of information (Fodor et al., 1993; Pease et al., 1994; Schena et al., 1995; Shalon et al., 1996). There are now two principle microarray types, those that consist of cDNAs and those comprised of oligonucleotides. The analysis of arrays with more than 250,000 oligonucleotides or over 10,000 different cDNAs is now commonplace in many biomedical applications.

Data obtained from arrays reveal changes in the expression pattern of a number of genes, thus allowing the identification of markers for disease characterization (Golub et al., 1999; Alizadeh et al., 2000), gene regulatory sequences (Wolfsberg et al., 1999), and drug targets (Marton et al., 1998). This technology is also being applied to genotyping and polymorphism detection (Roses, 2000), as well as to the quantification of DNA-protein interactions (Bulyk et al., 1999).

13.3.3.2.1 cDNA Microarrays

To generate cDNA microarrays, a collection of sequenced cDNAs (generally ESTs) are spotted by robotic deposition (contact printing) on a solid support (usually glass) in high-density arrays. This type of assay can be customized, so that arrays are generated for specific cell processes such as apoptosis and aging. One nanogram of a single cDNA fragment (located closer to the 3′ end of the gene) up to 1000 base pairs in length is spotted at intervals of 100 to 300 μm. The material used for hybridization is usually fluorescently labeled cDNA obtained from the two groups of cells/tissues to be compared. The two pools of cDNA are labeled with two different fluorophores (generally Cy3 and Cy5) and are then hybridized to the same array (Figure 13.4). After hybridization the array is scanned and digitally recorded. The recorded emission intensities are considered proportional to the original amount of mRNA on each spot. The two digitally recorded images are superimposed and the results are expressed as ratios of the intensity generated by each of the two fluorophores.

13.3.3.2.2 Oligonucleotide Arrays

This technique is based on microchip technology and it uses the principles of photolithography (Lipshutz et al., 1999) from the electronics industry (GeneChip). Approximately 10^7 copies of each selected oligo-

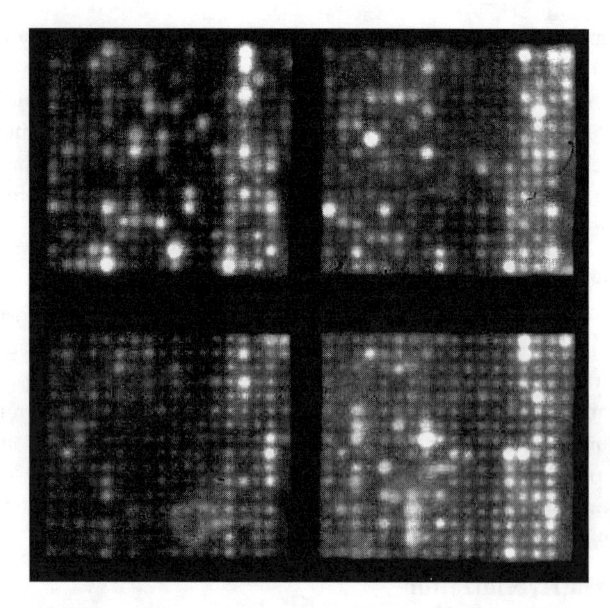

FIGURE 13.4 A portion of a mouse cDNA array hybridized with a red fluorescent–tagged experimental sample and a green fluorescent-tagged reference sample. (Figure is depicted here in black and white.)

nucleotide (short sequences of 20–25 base pairs of DNA) are directly synthesized, base by base, in hundreds of thousands of different 24×24 μm areas on a glass support. Each gene is represented by many sequences that span the entire length of its cDNA. Each oligonucleotide spot has a control for nonspecific binding, represented by a spot with a mismatch sequence that consists of a mutated central-nucleotide. The probe material is generally biotinylated complementary RNAs (cRNAs) synthesized from cDNAs that are derived from the cells/tissues under comparison. Both cRNAs are labeled with the same fluorophore (phycoerythrine-streptavidin) and hybridized onto different chips. The results are also digitally recorded and are expressed as units of fluorescent intensity.

13.3.3.2.3 Perspectives on Array-Based Hybridization

There are many variations and improvements on array-based techniques: the hybridization reaction may be driven by an electric field (Edman et al., 1997); the surface can be made of materials such as a gel, plastic, silicon, or gold, or be comprised of beads at the ends of fiber optic bundles (Walt, 2000). Protein, cDNA transfected cell clusters (Ziauddin and Sabatini, 2001), and tissue (www.nhgri.nhi.gov/DIR/CGB/TMA/) arrays are also being currently developed.

It is important to point out that these new approaches do not substitute conventional methods. Northern blot, nuclease protection assay, *in situ* hybridization, and RT-PCR should be used to complement these broader measurements and to follow up on genes undergoing functional analysis or being considered as drug targets, or as candidates for population genetics studies. Furthermore, although thousands of genes may be surveyed with these methods, the elaboration of a cell's/tissue's complete picture will be possible only when a comprehensive correlation between genomic and proteomic (the state of activation, level of activity, and sequence of protein–protein interactions) data are available (Celis et al., 2000).

13.4 Applications

13.4.1 Cardiovascular

Aberrant blood vessels of the cardiovascular system that populate the stroma in malignant tumors are a requisite for expansive tumor growth. A comparison between the transcriptional signatures of these circulatory vessels and the vasculature in homeostatic tissues should yield a valuable resource for clinical and basic studies. Kenneth Kinzler led a team (St. Croix et al., 2000) that generated such signatures using the mRNA populations of endothelial cells (ECs) from vessels and microvessels in one patient's neoplastic colorectal tissue (NEC) and normal colonic mucosa (MEC). A SAGE library was generated from both NEC and MEC populations comprising of 193,000 tags corresponding to more than 32,500 unique transcripts. A comparison between pairs of genes found in both MEC and NEC populations revealed that 79 expressed gene pairs had at least a tenfold expression difference. Of the 46 tag-pairs that were relatively overexpressed in NEC, some coded for angiogenic vessel markers and others for proteins involved in extracellular matrix construction; however, 14 tags had no functional description. Nine of these 14 tumor endothelial markers (TEMs) were investigated in neoplasms and subsequently found in primary cancers of the lung, pancreas, breast, and brain, with one, TEM7, found in the metastatic and primary cancers of each of these tissues. The nine TEMs were generally also found expressed in sites of normal neovasculature such as the corpus luteum and granulation tissue of healing wounds, suggesting that tumors recruit their vasculature through analogous molecular mechanisms.

Cardiovascular cells and tissues are also known to transduce mechanical forces into aberrant physiological responses such as hypertensive vascular disease and atherosclerotic plaque rupture. Describing the early molecular mediators of these responses may suggest new insight into several cardiovascular diseases. Thomas Wight and co-researchers (Lee et al., 2001) cultured human arterial smooth muscle cells (ASMCs), the primary source of arterial extracellular matrix, on a thin elastometric membrane resting on a plastic cylinder support. This membrane underwent cyclic tensile deformation as the platen assembly was moved sinusoidally, conferring a precise and uniform biaxial strain profile upon the ASMCs. Northern analysis was performed at 12-h intervals to quantify changes in the transcription levels of select proteoglycans whose hydrophilic properties allow cells to resist compression. The researchers found that biglycan and versican, known to serve as low density lipoprotein binding reservoirs, were up-regulated. The team stated these findings in light of the response-to-retention hypothesis that proposes that retention of atherogenic lipoproteins in the artery is a central process in atherogenesis, thus suggesting that atherogenesis arises as an adverse molecular mechanism that unfolds from an initial defense against prolonged mechanical stress.

13.4.2 Cerebral/Nervous

Medulloblastomas (MBs) are embryonal tumors of the central nervous system (CNS) and they are also the most common childhood brain malignancies, but their pathogenesis is not known, their classification relative to other embryonal CNS tumors is dubious, and patient response to therapy is difficult to predict. In order to address these problems, Golub and colleagues (Pomeroy et al., 2002) have developed a classification system based on microarray expression data from 99 patients.

The team began by generating an expression profile of several CNS embryonal tumors such as MBs, atypical teratoid/rhabdoid tumors (AT/RTs), and tumors from the primitive neuroectodermal (PNET). They then used signal-to-noise rankings, a "supervised learning method" of data analysis, to distinguish the tumor set. The data showed that medulloblastomas were clearly separable from malignant gliomas and PNETs. AT/RTs, which are associated with an extremely poor prognosis, were also easily distinguishable.

The researchers then focused on the molecular heterogeneity of MBs. In particular, they investigated desmoplastic MBs, a histological subtype of classical MBs found in a rare autosomal dominant disorder (Gorlin's syndrome) that results from a mutation in the sonic hedgehog (SHH) receptor; the SHH pathway is known to be mitogenic for cerebellar granular cells. The resulting desmoplastic gene signatures correctly classified 33 of 34 desmoplastic tumors and generated previously unrecognized evidence supporting the derivation of medulloblastomas from cerebellar granule cells through activation of the SHH pathway.

The researchers also investigated the heterogeneity of treatment responses in MB patients through an eight-gene model k-NN algorithm that uses gene expression to "learn" the distinction between successfully treated patients and those who eventually succumbed to their malignancy. Patients that were predicted to be survivors had a 5-year overall survival of 80% compared with 17% for patients predicted to have a poor outcome. A number of "molecular markers of outcome" were also generated from the microarray data, including genes characteristic of cerebellar differentiation and extracellular matrix proteins, that were associated with a favorable outcome, and genes related to cerebellar differentiation, which were under-expressed in poor-prognosis tumors. In summary, the authors state that these genomics-based outcome predictors will minimize unnecessary toxicity during therapy, and will allow earlier experimental treatment regimens for those patients portended not to respond to standard therapies.

Middleton et al. (2002) have also used cDNA microarrays, but to determine differential patterns of gene expression in the dorsal prefrontal cortex (PFC) of schizophrenia patients (SPs) and matched controls. In particular they looked at genes known to be nested within more than 71 metabolic pathways. The authors note that alterations in the metabolism of PFC schizophrenia patients are well documented and perhaps secondary changes to deleterious alterations in PFC synaptic structure and function.

The array results showed that SPs differentially expressed genes (all down-regulated) in only 5 of the 71 represented metabolic pathways. The researchers observe that these abnormal pathways involved decreases in energy shuttles and amino acid metabolism, fatty acid synthesis, neurotransmitter metabolism, and glycolysis.

In another set of experiments (meant to be controls for SP drug treatments), *in situ* hybridization (quantified by high-resolution scans of film images) conducted on haloperidol-treated monkeys revealed dramatic drug-associated increases in transcript levels of *malate dehydrogenase type 1* (*MAD1*), whose protein is found in the malate shuttle pathway and whose transcript levels were significantly reduced in SPs. These results revealed that diminished *MAD1* transcript levels in SPs are not attributable to drug treatment and suggested that *MAD1* may be a successful direct or indirect target for antipsychotic drug therapies. In general, the authors have shown that SPs have a highly specific pattern of metabolic alterations in the PFC affecting such pathways as the mitochondrial malate shuttle, and aspartate/alanine metabolism raising the possibility that normalizing these specific changes may exert a therapeutic effect.

13.4.3 Orthopedic

Osteoarthritis (OA) is the most common form of degenerative joint disease, diminishing the integrity and amount of articular cartilage over years. Understanding the sequence of molecular events that occur during chondrogenesis may reveal novel gene targets that will help normalize the increased intra-articular levels of collagenase, neutral proteases, degradative products of proteoglycans, and remodeling of subchondral bone seen in developed OA. Sekiya et al. (2002) have used microarrays to examine chondrogenesis in a simple *in vitro* system predicated upon adult bone marrow stroma stem cells (MSCs).

The investigators extracted mRNA from MSC micromass pellets on days 0, 1, 7, 14, and 21. These pellets were then cultured in the presence of known chondrocyte differentiation determinants such as bone morphogenetic protein 6. After determining the fold changes in gene expression over time, the researchers reported a chronology of molecular events: The mRNAs for macromolecules of the cartilage matrix (such as proteoglycans) were continuously increasing during all measured intervals; an angiogenic factor (*VEGF*) and a metalloproteinase (*MMP14*) had early roles in chondrogenesis; a transcription factor (*forkhead*) which is required for skeletal tissue development had intermediate stage roles; and collagens (*COL3A1* and *COL16A1*) had later roles in chondrocyte differentiation. Microarray analyses of this simple system may lay a temporal-based molecular foundation for novel arthritic therapies, and allow for studies of the gene profiles generated by potential drug candidates.

The extracellular matrix (ECM) degradation seen in both rheumatoid and osteoarthritis is enhanced by interleukin-1β (IL-1β), a secreted cytokine that is upstream of lytic enzymes such as the family of matrix metalloproteinases (MMPs). In an attempt to find the early response genes that mediate IL-1β–induced MMP secretion in resting cells, Vincenti and Brinckerhoff (2001) have stimulated a chondrocytic cell line (SW1353) with IL-1β for 2 h and then identified the expressed genes with microarray analysis. The results revealed a myriad of gene expression changes involving transcription factors, cytokines, growth factors and their receptors, adhesion molecules, proteases, and signaling intermediates.

Although the researchers confirmed changes in gene expression already known to be associated with IL-1β, their results also allowed them to identify new mechanisms for the decadence seen in the ECM of joint disease patients. For example, the down-regulation of *integrin* $\alpha 1$, a cell-adhesion molecule that chondrocytes use to bind to type II collagen, suggested that this might lead to a compromise in matrix adhesion. The microarray data also documented several other induced and repressed genes that have no known role in chondrocyte biology and that may serve as the basis for future joint disease treatments.

13.4.4 Muscular

Skeletal muscles serve as a minimally invasive tissue model for long-lived, high oxygen-consuming postmitotic cells, features shared with critical aging targets such as the heart and brain. Kayo et al. (2001) have used human high-density oligonucleotide arrays (7070 genes and ESTs) to investigate the effects of aging and caloric restriction (CR) (which extends the life span in rodents) on vastus lateralis transcripts in rhesus monkeys.

The researchers found that aged muscle cells up-regulated inflammatory/immune and oxidative stress response genes and down-regulated nuclear encoded proteins that function in mitochondrial energy metabolism. The authors suggest that reactive oxygen species (ROS) damage on the mitochondria, accrued over the life span, results in reduced mitochondrial function or biogenesis and the subsequent mitochondrial-related transcriptional signatures within the nucleus.

The major transcriptional class induced in middle-aged monkeys subjected to CR (30% food reduction for 9 years) was from genes encoding structural proteins such as collagens, known targets of growth factors (e.g., growth hormone). CR down-regulated certain genes involved in energy metabolism, which suggested that CR monkeys have reduced mitochondrial electron transport activity. However, this reduction is likely due to a hypometabolic state as opposed to ROS damage. By identifying 34 transcripts that were differentially expressed in aged and middle-aged monkeys, the researchers were able to determine how many of those were altered as a result of CR in the CR-middle-aged cohort. Interestingly, no age-related transcriptional markers were observed to change away from expression levels in aged monkeys. Nevertheless, the middle-aged primates did show physiological benefits from CR as defined by increased insulin sensitivity, reduced blood glucose, and reduced oxidative stress-induced cytokine expression by peripheral blood mononuclear cells. This seems to show that although CR does not retard the aging of transcriptional machinery, it may beneficially alter molecules involved in other cellular processes.

The extraocular muscles (EOMs) are responsible for voluntary and reflexive movements of the eyes and thus their function is critical for clear vision. The unique and dynamic range of eye movements is reflected in EOM biology, which is very different from other skeletal muscles. EOMs are spared from several types of muscular dystrophy; therefore, a transcriptional study of these cells may reveal gene products that confer this pathogenic resistance. Porter et al. (2001) have used high-density oligonucleotide arrays, consisting of 9977 genes (representing an estimated 25–35% of the mouse genome) to perform expression profiling on three putative muscle classes: limb, masticatory, and EOM. The cRNAs used as targets were derived from the mRNAs extracted from the masseter, EOM, and gastrocnemius/soleus cells of 8-week-old male mice.

The researchers found that although rodent masticatory and limb samples did not reveal statistically different allotypes, 400 genes had an EOM-specific expression pattern, genes that belonged to functional classes that reflected key aspects of muscle biology such as transcriptional regulation, sarcomeric organization, excitation-contraction coupling, intermediary metabolism, and immune response. One emerging theme of interest was that EOMs retain the expression of genes that are normally repressed during skeletal muscle development. *Pitx2*, which is expressed during embryonic days 8 to 12.5 in the mouse eye and which has an unknown role in myogenesis, appears to be such a gene. The authors point out that *Pitx2* mutations produce the ocular defects in Rieger's syndrome and that knockouts also exhibit EOM dysgenesis; they suggest that *Pitx2* or other differentially expressed transcription factors with an established developmental role may be involved in the resilience seen in adult EOMs.

13.4.5 Sensory

Volatile odorants are predominantly small organic molecules (<400 Da) that can be discriminated by different G protein-coupled odorant receptors (ORs), each of which is likely expressed uniquely in a given olfactory neuron (ON). Malnic et al. (1999) have identified dorsal nasal septum ORs for a set of aliphatic odorants (AOs) and have shown that the olfactory system uses a concentration-sensitive combinatorial receptor coding scheme to encode odor identities. The work conducted on these receptors may help generate novel treatments for hyposmia patients or the elderly, who have a decreased ability to detect odors.

The researchers first used Ca^{2+} imaging to detect an intracellular influx of Ca^{2+} into ONs (an ON response to odorants) after stimulation with four classes of AOs. Ninety eight of 647 ONs responded to these AOs. Positive ONs were then subjected to single-cell RT-PCR using degenerate primers matching conserved amino acid sequence motifs in mammalian ORs. These steps resulted in the amino acid sequences of 14 aliphatic ORs.

The odorant response profiles of the 14 ONs, corresponding to the 14 ORs, revealed that a single OR can recognize multiple AOs, that a given AO is recognized by multiple ORs, and that any two AOs are never recognized by the same combination of ORs. Additionally, AO concentration, carbon chain length, and functional group were "receptor code" determinants. The analysts note that differences in the sizes of odor codes might be relevant to specific anosmia. For example, if an odorant has only one OR in its receptor code, mutations in that OR would result in a particular anosmia. However, if an odorant is recognized by multiple ORs, mutations in one OR would generate a code change that would replace the original odor perception.

In another chemosensory study, Matsumani et al. (2000) identified a candidate bitter taste-receptor family (the TRBs) belonging to the G protein-coupled receptor (GPCR) superfamily. These receptors may eventually serve as targets for novel treatments aimed at individuals with ageusia, the inability to taste sweet, sour, bitter, or salty substances, or hypogeusia, where individuals show a reduced ability to sense these stimulants.

Based upon evidence that bitter and sweet receptors were coupled to a common intracellular G protein, and analogous evidence involving 1000 odor GPCRs, along with the premise that some taste receptor genes would be found at loci already associated with taste sensation, the researchers began a search for novel intramembrane GPCRs associated with taste. The team first used a mouse genome informatics database to locate the *SOA* locus, which codes for a protein involved in the detection of bitter tastes, and to correlate it to its syntenic region found on human chromosome 12p13. They then checked for cloned genes in the National Center for Biotechnology Information database that mapped close to this region in chromosome 12; the researchers used the Human Genome Sequence database to identify a focal set of genetic sequences that flanked the acquired cloned sequences. After searching this focus region with large sets of GPCR protein sequences garnered from a GPCR database, and finding no genes that appeared to code for GPCRs, they used a pheromone receptor (*V1R5*) to search the area. They were subsequently able to find a novel sequence encoding a distantly related protein with a seven-transmembrane domain structure characteristic of GPCRs (*hTRB2*). Using the *hTRB2* gene sequence to search the chromosome 12 database, the researchers found six more genes in the focal area that shared sequence motifs with *hTRB2*. They went on to find one more related gene on chromosome 5, and 4 more on chromosome 7.

The investigators subsequently used RT-PCR with degenerate primers matching conserved sequences in TRBs to isolate mRNAs within circumvallate and foliate taste papillae, which are located on the tongue and that contain taste buds that are clustered with taste receptor cells. *In situ* hybridization experiments further showed that TRB genes are probably selectively expressed in these gustatory cells.

13.4.5 Digestive

Colorectal cancer, nearly always a carcinoma, is the most common visceral cancer of the entire digestive system accounting for approximately 60,000 deaths in the United States every year, despite the fact that it produces symptoms relatively early and can be cured by resection. Metastatic liver lesions are usually responsible for the deaths of colorectal cancer patients. Using these metastatic liver lesions, researchers led by Bert Vogelstein (Saha et al., 2001) prepared a SAGE library of approximately 95,000 tags representing at least 17,324 transcripts. Of these, 144 were found to be previously inventoried, in high numbers, at metastasis libraries (relative to other SAGE libraries). Thirty-eight interesting transcripts were further investigated in varying metastatic tissues using real-time PCR. One gene, *PRL-3*, encoding a 22-kD tyrosine phosphatase (an enzyme that likely controls the activity of other proteins by removing a phosphate from them) was consistently overexpressed. This gene was not expressed in normal colorectal epithelium, intermediately expressed in advanced primary colorectal cancer tissue, and significantly expressed in metastatic lesions. *PRL-3* was found amplified in 3 of 12 metastases studied with an average of 29 copies per diploid genome, matching a characteristic trait of genes that play a causative role in metastasis.

The intestine is also a sight of a complex society of indigenous microbes whose particular population in an individual can affect their nutritional status, health and predisposition to certain diseases, and susceptibilities to food and other allergies. Jeffrey Gordon and co-workers (Hooper et al., 2001) used a gnotobiotic (pathogen free) mouse model inoculated with *Bacteroides thetaiotaomicron* to study how commensal bacteria affect our genes. Ileal mRNAs were isolated from mice that registered with $>10^7$ colony-forming units per milliliter of ileal contents. Biotinylated cRNA targets were generated from the mRNAs and applied to gene chips representing 25,000 mouse genes. High-throughput analysis showed that *B. thetaiotaomicron* colonization led to the increase of several noteworthy gene products such as transcripts for the *Na^+/glucose cotransporter* (*SGLT-1*), the *small proline-rich protein 2a* which appears to fortify the intestinal epithelial barrier (*sprr2a*), *angiogenin-3* which stimulates neovascularization, and *colipase*, a fatty acid binding protein (*L-FABP*). In general, the results revealed that *B. thetaiotaomicron* alters the expression of genes involved in nutrient absorption, mucosal barrier fortification, xenobiotic metabolism, angiogenesis, and postnatal intestinal maturation.

13.4.6 ENT

Squamous cell carcinomas of the head and neck (HNSCCs) arise from diverse anatomical locations, including the oral cavity, oropharynx, hypopharynx, larynx, and nasopharynx. However, they have in common an etiological association with tobacco or alcohol. The clinical course of these neoplasms is difficult to predict based on established prognostic clinicopathological criteria, and more than 30,100 cases and 7,800 deaths occur annually in the United States. Reed and colleagues (Villaret et al., 2000) have addressed these problems by searching for proteins that may serve as HNSCC markers and vaccine candidates.

The researchers began by generating a PCR-based subtracted library. Briefly, they hybridized "tester" cDNAs from HNSCCs to an excess of "driver" cDNAs from six histologically normal organs. The resulting unhybridized "target" nucleotides comprised of less abundant but differentially expressed genes in HNSCCs. These were separated and cloned into vectors to generate a library. A total of 985 cDNA fragments from individual library colonies were then PCR amplified and arrayed onto 2 × 2-in. glass slides (creating chips), which were used to examine the differential gene expression profiles of HNSCCs and normal tissues. The team then sequenced cDNAs that corresponded to low basal mRNA expression levels in the normal tissues and tenfold or greater levels in tumors. Thirteen genes were identified as having potentially useful expression profiles: nine of them were previously characterized keratinocyte genes, cell adhesion-related molecules, and metalloproteinases, while four were unknown. These genes will undergo full-length cloning for further analysis.

In a related study, Leethanakul et al. (2000) performed a differential expression analysis using human cancer-related cDNA microarrays on normal epithelium, five laser capture microdissected (LCM) HNSCCs, and one LCM hyperplasia lesion. A distinct expression pattern was found among normal, premalignant, and malignant HNSCC tissues. The team judged genes of biological significance to be those differentially expressed by at least twofold in at least three of the six cancer tissue sets. In general, these genes were involved with the control of cell growth and differentiation, matrix degradation, angiogenesis, apoptosis, and signaling; most were not previously implicated in HNSCC. For example, the hyperplastic tissue only overexpressed *cyclin D1* and DP_2, genes that might correlate with increased cell proliferation. In the HNSCCs, they noted a decrease in cytokeratins (which most likely reflects a loss of tumor cell differentiation) and an increase in genes involved in the *wnt* and *notch* signaling pathways, which have a putative role in maintaining an undifferentiated epithelium. These pathways were never before implicated in squamous cell carcinogenesis and their precise function in this context warrants further investigation. Based on their work, the researchers expect that the technologies they implemented will make it possible to define a pattern of gene expression in a tumor progression model of HNSCC, thereby potentially providing valuable markers to study premalignant lesions.

13.4.7 Pulmonary

Adenocarcinomas of the peripheral lung (AC) and the more centrally located squamous carcinomas (SCs) are the most common types of non-small cell lung cancer (NSCLC), a malignancy that accounts for nearly 80% of all lung cancers, the leading cause of cancer deaths worldwide. Nacht et al. (2001) have created a global picture of the genetic activities that distinguish AC and SC, and have described a screened set of highly differentially expressed genes that will likely provide new molecular targets for improved NSCLC diagnosis, prognosis, and therapy.

The researchers identified and quantified nine unique SAGE libraries comprising of 59,000 distinct transcript tags, from five different tissue libraries and cell lines derived from AC and SC samples as well as from normal epithelial cells (obtained from the small and large airways). Hierarchical clustering analysis based upon a selection of 3921 SAGE tags, which appeared at least 10 times in all nine libraries, generated a branching pattern that grouped normal and tumor tissues, and that distinguished the nine elements in these two sets. These groups were also described when only 115 statistically significant and highly differentially expressed tags were used.

An analysis of these SAGE tags showed that SCs overexpressed genes involved in cellular detoxification or antioxidation. The authors point out that their presence in these cancers most likely represents a cellular response by the bronchial epithelium to environmental carcinogenic insults. ACs were characterized by high-level expression of small airway-associated or immunologically related proteins. The researchers state that these genes may reflect the origin of tumors derived from known small-airway epithelial cells, a role in tumorigenesis, or B-cell and antigen-presenting cell infiltration into the tumors.

Pitti et al. (1998) have found a soluble decoy receptor, dubbed decoy receptor 3 (DcR3), that appears to be secreted by primary lung tumors to evade an immune-cytotoxic attack. The team began their investigations by searching for a set of related ESTs that showed homology to the tumor necrosis factor (TNF) receptor (TNFR) gene superfamily. TNFR is a transmembrane protein related to Fas, which triggers cell apoptosis when it encounters the Fas ligand (FasL), a protein expressed by immune-cytotoxic cells such as activated T-cells and natural killer cells.

Using PCR, with primers based on the consensus EST region in the discovered ESTs, the researchers screened human cDNA libraries and found a previously unknown full-length cDNA derived from human fetal lung tissue, encoding *DcR3*. The DcR3 amino acid sequence revealed that the protein lacked an apparent transmembrane sequence, suggesting that it was secreted; transfected cells confirmed that this was the case. To search for potential DcR3-ligand interactions, the team transfected cells with TNF-family transmembrane ligands. The results showed that DcR3 preferentially bound to cells transfected with FasL. The investigators went on to find that DcR3 blocked the activation-induced cell death of mature T lymphocytes and that DcR3 reduced the apoptosis of Jurkat T leukemia cells, an event induced by peripheral blood natural killer cells.

Because genomic amplifications frequently contribute to tumorigensesis, the team also analyzed *DcR3* gene-copy number by quantitative PCR in 35 primary lung and colon tumors (relative to DNA from normal peripheral blood leukocytes). Eight of 18 lung tumors showed a 2- to 18-fold *DcR3* gene amplification. *In situ* hybridization in primary tumor tissue sections revealed that 6 of 15 lung tumors expressed *DcR3* mRNA. Collectively, these results suggest that secreted DcR3 proteins allow lung neoplasms to escape immune-induced apoptosis.

13.4.8 Lymphatic

A challenge of malignant cancer treatment is to effectively administer specific therapies to genetically distinct tumor types while minimizing toxicity. Technological advancements in cancer classification have therefore been central to providing indemnity to cancer patients. Golub et al. (1999) have described systematic and generic approaches that discover and predict cancer classes based upon quantifying global gene expression. The researchers specifically define cancer class discovery as identifying unrecognized fundamental tumor subtypes, and class prediction as placing a tumor in defined classes, which could reflect "current states or future outcomes." The team used human acute leukemias, cancers that involve the neoplastic transformation of lymphoid (ALL) or myeloid (AML) pluripotent hematopoietic stem cells, as a test case.

To conduct their experiments, the researchers hybridized the mRNAs from 38 bone marrow samples (27 ALL and 11 AML) onto a 6817 human-gene high-density oligonucleotide microarray. Because there existed sufficient similarities and distinctions to classify AML and ALL as distinct acute leukemias based upon morphology, histochemistry, immunophenotyping, and cytogenetic analysis, the investigators were able to test if their analytical approaches would generate a molecular data set that matched these proven classification methods.

With the resulting microarray expression information, and algorithms that clustered their 38 initial leukemia samples, the investigators found that their class discovery approach automatically found the distinction between AML and ALL, as well as the distinction between B- and T-cell ALL. The authors note that in terms of basic biology and clinical treatment, these are the most fundamental distinctions known among acute leukemias. In order to "predict" cancer classes, the team used an algorithm based upon the "weighted votes" of a set of 50 informative genes (from thousands of genes) that best discriminated between AML and ALL. Using this methodology, they subclassified tumor samples as AML or ALL, and ALL samples as either T- or B-cell ALL. The investigators suggested that expression-based class predictors could be adapted to a clinical setting in order to aid an appropriate drug response-or-survival prognosis, while class discovery methods could be used to identify fundamental subtypes of any cancer and to search for mechanisms that cut across distinct cancer types.

Alizadeh et al. (2000) have looked at a different aggressive lymphatic malignancy, diffuse large B-cell lymphoma (DLBCL) which, if present in a patient, allows for only a 40% chance of prolonged survival after therapy. In order to generate a molecular profile of possible DLBCL subtypes, the researchers used clustering analysis on 1.8 million measurements of gene expression garnered from 128 "lymphochips," each carrying 18,000 cDNA clones corralled from libraries that had genes preferentially expressed in lymphoid cells and genes important to immunology or cancer biology. The researchers first found that the genes that distinguished germinal center B cells from other stages in B-cell ontogeny were also differentially expressed among DLBCLs, suggesting that B-cell differentiation genes may also be used to subdivide DLBCL. The team therefore clustered the DLBCL cases using only these transcript signatures. Two large branches were evident in the resulting dendrogram, categories that corresponded well with the overall survival of the patients concerned. The resulting groups were called GC B-like DLBCL (GBD) and activated B-like DLBCL (ABD). Their expression patterns suggested that ABD cells constitutively expressed genes in the signal transduction pathways of peripheral blood B cells undergoing activation and mitogenesis, and that GBD cells were characteristic of germinal center B cells. These categories reflected tumors arising from different stages in B-cell differentiation. GBD patients had a significantly better overall survival rate than those with ABD. A noteworthy gene in the GBD signature is *BCL-6*, a well-established germinal center marker that is overexpressed in these cells, while a notable feature of the ABD profile was the expression of *FLIP* and *BCL-2*, two genes whose products inhibit apoptosis.

13.4.9 Reproductive

Mutations in known sex-linked genes such as *Sry* (*sex-determining region gene Y*), whose protein helps organize the bipotential gonads into testes rather than ovaries, leads to a variety of intersex conditions, such as 46,XY dysgenesis. This disorder may result in dysgerminoma, a germ cell tumor that accounts for about 2% of all ovarian cancers, and gonadoblastoma, a sex cord–stromal tumor originating either from the sex cords of the undifferentiated embryonic gonad or from the stroma of the ovary.

However, not all 46,XY gonadal dysgenesis cases are described by mutations in known genes like *Sry*. Therefore, Perera et al. (2001) used representational difference analysis (RDA) in an attempt to find novel genes that trigger male sex determination. They started by studying mouse gonads at 13.5 days postcoitus (dpc), the time of early-stage testis differentiation. The subsequent sequencing of a set of differentially expressed genes, and a comparison of these sequences against DNA databanks using basic local alignment search tool (BLAST), identified one novel gene, later termed *tescalcin*, with a sequence homology to many members of the EF-hand family of Ca^{2+}-binding proteins, a subset of which are implicated in cell differentiation and cell cycle pathways.

Based upon the predicted tescalcin amino acid sequence, the investigators also discovered an *N*-myristoylation site and sequences suggestive of kinase phosphorylation sites. The enzyme *N*-myristoyltransferase covalently attaches the *N*-myristoyl lipid molecule to receptive proteins, which are then anchored, by *N*-myristoyl, to the cell membrane.

The team went on to use RT-PCR at tandem time intervals on male gonads and mesonephros, with specific primers for *tescalcin* and *Sry*, followed by Southern blot analysis. *Tescalcin* was first detected at a time synchronous with peak *Sry* expression.

Based on the findings generated by RDA, BLAST, amino acid sequence data, RT-PCR, and Southern blot analysis, the researchers appear to have found a novel protein that responds to Ca^{2+}, and a myristoyl switch, in order to subsequently modulate membrane-associated signaling processes that occur during the critical time of male sex determination. A subsequent functional and clinical analysis of this gene may lead to ties with intersex pathologies.

Although Mi et al. (2000) did not identify a novel gene, using the yeast signal sequence trap (YSST) they isolated a cDNA fragment from a human testis library encoding for a secreted protein they called syncytin, a retroviral peptide whose coding sequence is sequestered in the human genome. YSST is based upon the genetic selection of a *Saccharomyces cerevisiae* strain deleted for its invertase gene, which must be secreted if sucrose or raffinose is the sole carbon source. These strains are transformed with YSST vectors that carry invertase genes that lack their secretion signal peptides, and possible heterologous secreted genes that are fused upstream of this defective invertase and that provide the necessary signals to restore invertase secretion.

After isolating a full-length *syncytin* cDNA from the same human testis library, the team used protein homology searches to find that *syncytin* is an envelope gene transcribed in HERV-W[2] retroviruses. They also searched human DNA databases for *syncytin* cDNA and found multiple ESTs for it, supporting the case that a human *syncytin* gene is expressed in our genome. In yet another set of searches, the investigators found that chromosome number 7 contained a sequence with 100% homology to the *syncytin* cDNA.

Using a Northern blot of 23 human tissues, the researchers went on to find high *syncytin* expression only in the placenta. *In situ* hybridization revealed that *syncytin* mRNA is restricted to syncytiotrophoblasts, a fused cell type of fetal origin giving rise only to extraembryonic tissue. The results engendered by subsequent transfection experiments constantly showed that *syncytin* alone was capable of mediating cell fusion.

The researchers suggest that because of *syncytin's* ability to modulate the morphology of syncytiotrophoblasts, it may be involved during their invasion of the uterine wall and hence be a candidate gene involved in certain placental disorders. For example, the authors noted that uncontrolled syncytiotrophoblast invasion has been observed in choriocarcinoma and they went on to show that *syncytin* expression levels in BeWo cells (a choriocarcinoma-cell line), as revealed by Northern blot, were increased at least fivefold after induction by forskolin, a known choriocarcinoma "syncytiogen," thus suggesting a role for *syncytin* in the pathology of this neoplasm.

Acknowledgments

We thank Avner Ittah and Sean Mandat for the gels in Figures 13.1 and 13.3, and Erasmo Perera for helpful discussions.

References

Alizadeh, A.A., Eisen, M.B., Davis, R.E., Ma, C., Lossos, I.S., Rosenwald, A., Boldrick, J.C., Sabet, H., Tran, T., Yu, X., et al., Distinct types of diffuse large B-cell lymphoma identified by gene expression profiling, *Nature*, 403, 503–510, 2000.

Alwine, J.C., Kemp, D.J., and Stark, G.R., Method for detection of specific RNAs in agarose gels by transfer to diazobenzyloxymethyl-paper and hybridization with DNA probes, *Proc. Natl. Acad. Sci. U.S.A.*, 74, 5350–5354, 1977.

Ausubel, F.M., Struhl, K., Brent, R., Kingston, R.E., Moore, D.D., Seidman, J.G., and Smith, J.A., Eds., *Current Protocols in Molecular Biology*, Wiley Interscience, New York, 2002.

Bauman, J.G., Wiegant, J., Borst, P., and van Duijn, P., A new method for fluorescence microscopical localization of specific sequences by *in situ* hybridization of fluorochroome labelled RNA, *Exp. Cell Res.*, 128, 485–490, 1980.

Bevan, I.S., Rapley, R., and Walker, M.R., Sequencing of PCR-amplified DNA, *PCR Methods Appl.*, 1, 222–227, 1992.

Bulyk, M.L., Gentalen, E., Lockhart, D.J., and Church, G.M., Quantifying DNA-protein interactions by double-stranded DNA arrays, *Nature Biotechnol.*, 17, 573–577, 1999.

Bustin, S.A., Absolute quantification of mRNA using real-time reverse transcription polymerase chain reaction assays, *J. Mol. Endocrinol.*, 25, 169–193, 2000.

Cai, W., Aburatani, H., Stanton, V.P., Housman, D.E., Wang, Y.K., and Schwartz, D.C., Ordered restriction endonuclease maps of yeast artificial chromosomes created by optical mapping on surfaces, *Proc. Natl. Acad. Sci. U.S.A.*, 92, 5164–5168, 1995.

Celis, J.E., Kruhoffer, M., Gromova, I., Frederiksen, C., Ostergaard, M., Thykjaer, T., Gromov, P., Yu, J., Palsdottir, H., Magnusson, N., and Orntoft, T.F., Gene expression profiling: monitoring transcription and translation products using DNA microarrays and proteomics, *FEBS Lett.*, 480, 2–16, 2000.

Chomczynski, P. and Sacchi, N., Single step method of RNA extraction by acid guanidinium thiocyanate-phenol-chloroform extraction, *Anal. Biochem.*, 162, 156–159, 1987.

Choo, K., *Methods in Molecular Biology, Vol. 33: In Situ Hybridization Protocols*, Humana, Totowa, NJ, 1994.

Dockhorn-Dworniczak, B., Dworniczak, B., Brommelkamp, L., Bulles, J., Horst, J., and Bocker, W., Non-isotopic detection of single strand conformational polymorphism (PCR-SSCP): a rapid and sensitive technique in the diagnosis of phenylketoburia, *Nucleic Acids Res.*, 19, 2500–2502, 1991.

Edman, C.F., Raymond, D.E., Wu, D.J., Tu, E., Sosnowski, R.G., Butler, W.F., Nerenberg, M., and Heller, M.J., Electric field directed nucleic acid hybridization on microchips, *Nucleic Acids Res.*, 25, 4907–4914, 1997.

Fodor, S.P., Rava, R.P., Huang, X.C., Pease, A.C., Holmes, C.P., and Adams, C.L., Multiplexed biochemical assays with biological chips, *Nature*, 364, 555–556, 1993.

Golub, T.R., Slonim, D.K., Tamayo, P., Huard, C., Gaasenbeek, M., Mesirov, J.P., Coller, H., Loh, M.L., Downing, J.R., Caligiuri, M.A., et al., Molecular classification of cancer: class discovery and class prediction by gene expression monitoring, *Science*, 286, 531–537, 1999.

Higuchi, R., Krummel, B., and Saiki, R.K., A general method of in vitro preparation and specific mutagenesis of DNA fragments: study of protein and DNA interactions, *Nucleic Acids Res.*, 16, 7351–7367, 1988.

Hindkjaer, J., Koch, J., Mogensen, J., Kolvraa, S., and Bolund, L., Primed *in situ* (PRINS) labeling of DNA, *Methods Mol. Biol.*, 33, 95–107, 1994.

Hooper, L.V., Wong, M.H., Thelin, A., Hansson, L., Falk, P.G., and Gordon, J.I., Molecular analysis of commensal host-microbial relationships in the intestine, *Science*, 291, 881–884, 2001.

Hubank, M. and Schatz, D., cDNA representational difference analysis: a sensitive and flexible method for identification of differentially expressed genes, *Methods Enzymol.*, 303, 1999.

Kaiser, J., Public-private group maps out initiatives, *Science*, 296, 827, 2002.

Kayo, T., Allison, D.B., Weindruch, R., and Prolla, T.A., Influences of aging and caloric restriction on the transcriptional profile of skeletal muscle from rhesus monkeys, *Proc. Natl. Acad. Sci. U.S.A.*, 98, 5093–5098, 2001.

Lee, R.T., Yamamoto, C., Feng, Y., Potter-Perigo, S., Briggs, W.H., Landschulz, K.T., Turi, T.G., Thompson, J.F., Libby, P., and Wight, T.N., Mechanical strain induces specific changes in the synthesis and organization of proteoglycans by vascular smooth muscle cells, *J. Biol. Chem.*, 276, 13847–13851, 2001.

Leethanakul, C., Patel, V., Gillespie, J., Pallente, M., Ensley, J.F., Koontongkaew, S., Liotta, L.A., Emmert-Buck, M., and Gutkind, J.S., Distinct pattern of expression of differentiation and growth-related genes in squamous cell carcinomas of the head and neck revealed by the use of laser capture microdissection and cDNA arrays, *Oncogene*, 19, 3220–3224, 2000.

Lennon, G.C. and Lehrach, H., Hybridization analyses of arrayed cDNA libraries, *Trends Genet.*, 7, 314–317, 1991.

Liang, P. and Pardee, A.B., Differential display of eukaryotic messenger RNA by means of the polymerase chain reaction, *Science*, 257, 967–971, 1992.

Lipshutz, R.J., Fodor, S.P., Gingeras, T.R., and Lockhart, D.J., High density synthetic oligonucleotide arrays, *Nature Genet.*, 21, 25–32, 1999.

Lockhart, D.J. and Winzeler, E.A., Genomics, gene expression and DNA arrays, *Nature*, 405, 827–836, 2000.

Malnic, B., Hirono, J., Sato, T., and Buck, L.B., Combinatorial receptor codes for odors, *Cell*, 96, 713–723, 1999.

Marton, M.J., DeRisi, J.L., Bennett, H.A., Iyer, V.R., Meyer, M.R., Roberts, C.J., Stoughton, R., Burchard, J., Slade, D., Dai, H., Bassett, D.E., Jr., Hartwell, L.H., Brown, P.O., and Friend, S.H., Drug target validation and identification of secondary drug target effects using DNA microarrays, *Nature Med.*, 4, 1293–1301, 1998.

Matsunami, H., Montmayeur, J.P., and Buck, L.B., A family of candidate taste receptors in human and mouse, *Nature*, 404, 601–604, 2000.

Mi, S., Lee, X., Li, X., Veldman, G.M., Finnerty, H., Racie, L., LaVallie, E., Tang, X.Y., Edouard, P., Howes, S., Keith, J.C., and McCoy, J.M., Syncytin is a captive retroviral envelope protein involved in human placental morphogenesis, *Nature*, 403, 785–789, 2000.

Middleton, F.A., Mirnics, K., Pierri, J.N., Lewis, D.A., and Levitt, P., Gene expression profiling reveals alterations of specific metabolic pathways in Schizophrenia, *J. Neurosci.*, 22, 2718–2729, 2002.

Mitchell, L.G. and Merril, C.R., Affinity generation of single stranded DNA for dideoxy sequencing following the polymerase chain reaction, *Anal. Biochem.*, 178, 239–242, 1989.

Mullis, K.B. and Faloona, F.A., Specific synthesis of DNA *in vitro* via a polymerase chain reaction, *Methods Enzymol.*, 155, 335–350, 1987.

Nacht, M., Dracheva, T., Gao, Y., Fujii, T., Chen, Y., Player, A., Akmaev, V., Cook, B., Dufault, M., Zhang, M., Zhang, W., Guo, M., Curran, J., Han, S., Sidransky, D., Buetow, K., Madden, S.L., and Jen, J., Molecular characteristics of non-small cell lung cancer, *Proc. Natl. Acad. Sci. U.S.A.*, 98, 15203–15208, 2001.

Nguyen, C., Rocha, D., Granjeaud, S., Baldit, M., Bernard, K., Naquet, P., and Jordan, B.R., Differential gene expression in the murine thymus assayed by quantitative hybridization of arrayed cDNA clones, *Genomics*, 29, 207–216, 1995.

Pandey, A. and Mann, M., Proteomics to study genes and genomes, *Nature*, 405, 837–846, 2000.

Pease, A.C., Solas, D., Sullivan, E.J., Cronin, M.T., Holmes, C.P., and Fodor, S.P., Light-generated oligonucleotide arrays for rapid DNA sequence analysis, *Proc. Natl. Acad. Sci. U.S.A.*, 91, 5022–5026, 1994.

Perera, E.M., Martin, H., Seeherunvong, T., Kos, L., Hughes, I.A., Hawkins, J.R., and Berkovits, G.D., Tescalcin, a novel gene encoding a putative EF-Hand Ca^{2+}-binding protein, Col9a3, and Renin are expressed in the mouse testis during the early stages of gonadal differentiation, *Endocrinology*, 142, 455–463, 2001.

Pitti, R.M., Marsters, S.A., Lawrence, D.A., Roy, M., Kischkel, F.C., Dowd, P., Huang, A., Donahue, C.J., Sherwood, S.W., Baldwin, D.T., Godowski, P.J., Wood, W.I., Gurney, A.L., Hillan, K.J., Cohen, R.L., Goddard, A.D., Botstein, D., and Ashkenazi, A., Genomic amplification of a decoy receptor for Fas ligand in lung and colon cancer, *Nature*, 396, 699–703, 1998.

Pomeroy, S.L., Tamayo, P., Gaasenbeek, M., Sturia, L.M., Angelo, M., McLaughiln, M.E., Kim, J.Y., Goumnerova, L.C., Black, P.M., Lau, C., Allen, J.C., Zagzag, D., Olson, J.M., Curran, T., Wetmore, C., Biegel, J.A., Poggio, T., Mukherjee, S., Rifkin, R., Califano, A., Stolovitzky, G., Louis, D.N., Mesirov, J.P., Lander, E.S., and Golub, T.R., Prediction of central nervous system embryonal tumour outcome based on gene expression, *Nature*, 415, 436–442, 2002.

Porter, J.D., Khanna, S., Kaminski, H.J., Rao, J.S., Merriam, A.P., Richmonds, C.R., Leahy, P., Li, J., and Andrade, F.H., Extraocular muscle is defined by a fundamentally distinct gene expression profile, *Proc. Natl. Acad. Sci. U.S.A.*, 98, 12062–12067, 2001.

Rapley, R., Ed., *Methods in Molecular Biology, Vol. 65: PCR Sequencing Protocols*, Humana, Totowa, NJ, 1996.

Roses, A.D., Genetic susceptibility to cardiovascular diseases, *Am. Heart J.*, 140, S45–S47, 2000.

Saha, S., Bardelli, A., Buckhaults, P., Velculescu, V.E., Rago, C., St. Croix, B., Romans, K.E., Choti, M.A., Lengauer, C., Kinzler, K.W., and Vogelstein, B., A phosphatase associated with metastasis of colorectal cancer, *Science*, 294, 1343–1346, 2001.

Saiki, R.K., Scharf, S.J., Faloona, F., Mullis, K.B., Horn, G.T., Erlich, H.A., and Arnheim, N., Enzymatic amplification of β-globin genomic sequences and restriction site analysis for diagnosis of sickle cell anemia, *Science*, 230, 1350–1354, 1985.

Sambrook, J. and Russell, D.W., Eds., *Molecular Cloning. A Laboratory Manual*, Cold Spring Harbor Laboratory Press, Cold Spring Harbor, NY, 2001.

Schena, M., Shalon, D., Davis, R.W., and Brown, P.O., Quantitative monitoring of gene expression patterns with a complimentary DNA microarray, *Science*, 270, 467–470, 1995.

Sekiya, I., Vuoristo, J.T., Larson, B.L., and Prockop, D.J., In vitro cartilage formation by human adult stem cells from bone marrow stroma defines the sequence of cellular and molecular events during chondrogenesis, *Proc. Natl. Acad. Sci. U.S.A.*, 99, 4397–4402, 2002.

Shalon, D., Smith, S.J., and Brown, P.O., A DNA microarray system for analyzing complex DNA samples using two-color fluorescent probe hybridization, *Genome Res.*, 6, 639–645, 1996.

Southern, E.M., Detection of specific sequences among DNA fragments separated by gel electrophoresis, *J. Mol. Biol.*, 98, 503–517, 1975.

Southern, E.M., Case-Green, S.C., Elder, J.K., Johnson, M., Mir, K.U., Wang, L., and Williams, J.C., Arrays of complementary oligonucleotides for analyzing the hybridization behaviour of nucleic acids, *Nucleic Acids Res.*, 22, 1368–1373, 1994.

St. Croix, B., Rago, C., Velculescu, V., Traverso, G., Romans, K.E., Montgomery, E., Lal, A., Riggins, G.J., Lengauer, C., Vogelstein, B., and Kinzler, K.W., Genes expressed in human tumor endothelium, *Science*, 289, 1197–1202, 2000.

Trask, B.J., Fluorescence *in situ* hybridization: applications in cytogenetics and gene mapping, *Trends Genet.*, 7, 149–154, 1991.

Velculesco, V.E., Zhang, L., Vogelstein, B., and Kinzler, K.W., Serial analysis of gene expression, *Science*, 270, 484–487, 1995.

Velculesco, V.E., Zhang, L., Zhou, W., Vogelstein, J., Basrai, M.A., Basset, D.E., Hieter, P., Vogelstein, B., and Kinzler, K.W., Characterization of the yeast transcriptome, *Cell*, 88, 243–251, 1997.

Velculesco, V.E., Madden, S.L., Zhang, L., Lash, A.E, Yu, J., Rago, C., Lal, A., Wang, C.J., Beaudry, G.A., Ciriello, K.M., Cook, B.P., Dufault, M.R., Ferguson, A.T., Gao, Y., He, T.C., Hermeking, H., Hiraldo, S.K., Hwang, P.M., Lopez, M.A., Luderer, H.F., Mathews, B., Petroziello, J.M., Polyak, K., Zawel, L., Kinzler, K.W., et al., Analysis of human transcriptomes, *Nat. Genet.*, 23, 387–388, 1999.

Villaret, D.B., Wang, T., Dillon, D., Xu, J., Sivam, D., Cheever, M.A., and Reed, S.G., Identification of genes overexpressed in head and neck squamous cell carcinoma using a combination of complementary DNA subtraction and microarray analysis, *The Laryngoscope*, 110, 374–381, 2000.

Vincenti, M.P. and Brinckerhoff, C.E., Early response genes induced in chondrocytes stimulated with the inflammatory cytokine interleukin-1β, *Arthritis Res.*, 3, 381–388, 2001.

Walt, D.R., Bead-based fiber-optic arrays, *Science*, 287, 451, 2000.

Wartell, R.M., Hosseini, S.H., and Moran, C.P., Jr., Detecting base pair substitutions in DNA fragments by temperature gradient gel electrophoresis, *Nucleic Acids Res.*, 18, 2699–2705, 1990.

Wilkinson, D.G., Ed., *In Situ Hybridization. A Practical Approach*, IRL Press, Oxford, U.K., 1995.

Wolfsberg, T.G., Gabrielian, A.E., Campbell, M.J., Cho, R.J., Spouge, J.L., and Landsman, D., Candidate regulatory sequence elements for cell cycle-dependent transcription in *Saccharomyces cerevisiae*, *Genome Res.*, 9, 775–792, 1999.

Zhao, N., Hashida, H., Takahashi, N., Misumi, Y., and Sakaki, Y., High-density cDNA filter analysis: a novel approach for large-scale, quantitative analysis of gene expression, *Gene*, 156, 207–213, 1995.

Ziauddin, J. and Sabatini, D.M., Microarrays of cells expressing defined cDNAs, *Nature*, 411, 107–110, 2001.

14

Theoretical Considerations for the Efficient Design of DNA Arrays

Arnold Vainrub
University of Houston

Tong-Bin Li
University of Houston

Yuriy Fofanov
University of Houston

B. Montgomery Pettitt
University of Houston

CONTENTS

14.1 Introduction

The use of combinatorial or array-based detection (and synthesis) technologies has qualitatively changed many areas of bioscience in the last several years. These technologies include DNA, protein, and combinatorial chemistry arrays. Of these, DNA arrays, designed to determine gene content and expression levels in living cells, have shown the most potential. DNA arrays allow simultaneous, parallel measurement of thousands of interactions between target strands and genome-derived probes. Two areas of concern are the design and analysis of such experiments. Microarrays are rapidly producing enormous amounts of raw data. The bioinformatics solutions to problems associated with the analysis of data on this scale are a major current challenge. In addition, designing such experiments requires consideration of not only the genomic information required to answer a given problem but also consideration of the chemistry and physics of highly charged species near prepared surfaces.

On the medical side, DNA arrays may someday help us to better understand complex issues concerning human health and disease. Among other things, they should help us separate out the effects of ones genes vs. environment and life-style to help usher in the individualized molecular medicine of the future.

A current important practical application of DNA arrays is biosensors used to determine which organism a given DNA/RNA sample belongs. This use of microarrays is based on specific properties of viral and microbial genomes and the ability of arrays to provide information regarding the presence/absence of thousands of short subsequences in given genome simultaneously.

0-8493-1140-3/04/$0.00+$1.50

While DNA arrays will be an important tool for some time, it should be emphasized that DNA array technology is still at an early stage of development. It is cluttered with heterogeneous technologies and data formats as well as basic issues of signal to noise, fidelity, calibrations, and statistical significance that are still being sorted out. Until these issues are resolved and standardized, it will not be possible to define accurately the complete genetic regulatory network of even a well-studied prokaryotic cell system.

DNA arrays were introduced as a high throughput technology for performing hybridization assays based on formation of a double helix to a surface-immobilized single-strand DNA probe according to Watson-Crick pairing rules. In its current high-density format, in a single microarray experiment the hybridization is performed with up to hundreds of thousands of different probes, producing a tremendous volume of information on the assayed DNA sequence and their abundance in the tested target. Typically, a DNA microarray hybridization experiment contains 10^7 to 10^{10} DNA probe molecules of a sequence to be tested, immobilized in a ~50-μm-diameter spot on a prepared glass surface, and thus may include about 10^4 to 10^5 different probe spots per square centimeter. Usually, the probes are oligonucleotides of 8 to 80 bases long, tethered by one end through a linker molecule to the surface. DNA microbeads are similar to microarrays, but the probes are tethered to a micron size glass bead's surface (Brenner et al., 2000) similar to peptide technology.

The use of DNA microarrays in clinical practice is a rapidly growing area. In present work we will concentrate our attention on two tasks: electrostatic effects in solution DNA hybridization at surfaces and the ability of microarrays to serve as biosensors based on information of the presence or absence of certain subsequences.

14.2 Surface Design

14.2.1 Role of Interface Electrostatic Interactions

Electrostatic effects in solution DNA hybridization (formation of the double helix by two complimentary DNA single strands) are well known (Saenger, 1984, Bloomfield, 1999). They appear simply because the DNA is a negatively charged polymeric ion, and thus an electrostatic repulsion occurs that can be either between single strands (ssDNA) or double helices (dsDNA). Each phosphate group PO_2^- of the outer dsDNA backbone bears a single negative charge, and therefore typical dsDNA B-helix is often modeled by a 2-nm-diameter cylinder with a high negative surface charge of about six electron charges per nanometer of length. The repulsion diminishes when the added salt cations are present in solution and partly shield the electrostatic interactions. Thus, the dsDNA stability against a dehybridization into ssDNAs increases with the solution ionic strength; typically, the melting temperature of dsDNA increases from 10 to 20°C as the added salt concentration grows tenfold. For instance, in human blood plasma concentrations of approximately 150 m*M* for Na^+ and 2.5 m*M* for Ca^{2+} cations produce the electrostatic screening length about 1 nm and help make the chromosomal dsDNA stable.

In addition to the above-mentioned DNA-DNA repulsion, two new electrostatic interactions appear for a DNA microarray, namely, the DNA-surface interaction and repulsion between the assayed nucleic acid and the on-surface layer of DNA probes. The nucleic acid–surface interactions operate on surface-tethered DNA probes, the assayed nucleic acid (which is a biological RNA or prepared from it by a reverse transcription cDNA), and also dsDNA formed as their hybrid. Our theoretical analysis of this DNA-surface electrostatic interaction shows its possible important role in on-surface hybridization thermodynamics (Vainrub and Pettitt, 2000, 2003). Recent experiments (Heaton et al., 2001; Su et al., 2002) confirm the theory and demonstrate a complete control of hybridization and melting by applied electric potential to the oligonucleotide array on gold film surface. Indeed, the negative surface potential –300 mV induces the melting of prehybridized dsDNA whereas the positive potential promotes the hybridization of complimentary DNA targets (Heaton et al., 2001). The experiments can be simply understood (Vainrub and Pettitt, 2000, 2003) as a result of the electrostatic repulsion between both the negatively charged surface and ssDNA target tending to melt the dsDNA and remove the target from the surface; attraction to the positively charged surface stabilizes the dsDNA. It is important that the probe DNA is tethered to the surface (typically through the covalent bond and linker molecule) and thus dsDNA cannot be displaced or diffuse from the negatively charged surface and must be released by melting a mobile target ssDNA that can drift from the surface to decrease the electrostatic energy. Interestingly, the DNA-surface repulsion (attraction) occurs even for noncharged dielectric (metallic) surfaces due to the known electrostatic induction phenomena (Vainrub and Pettitt, 2000). Evidently, the DNA-surface electrostatics can be regulated by the surface charge and material (dielectric or metallic) as well as almost canceled by using long linker molecule and/or high ionic strength hybridization solution. In previous work (Vainrub and Pettitt, 2000, 2003) we considered in detail the DNA-surface electrostatics and its optimization in oligonucleotide microarrays.

Here we focus on another type of on-array electrostatic interaction, the repulsion between the assayed nucleic acid and array of surface tethered DNA probe that both bear the negative charge (Vainrub and Pettitt, 2002). First, we describe the origin of this interaction that is specific for on-array hybridization and does not occur in homogeneous solution hybridization assays. To obtain sufficient numbers of dsDNA hybrids for reliable detection, the oligonucleotide probe molecules are quite crowded on the array with the surface density typically from 10^{12} to 10^{14} probes per square centimeter corresponding to the mean distance between the neighbors on the surface from 10 to 1 nm, respectively. Therefore, a target cDNA closely approaches not only a hybridization partner, but also the surrounding probe oligonucleotides, which contribute into electrostatic repulsion of the target. Recently we considered this effect (Vainrub and Pettitt, 2002) and derived an equation for the on-array hybridization binding isotherm:

$$C_0 = \frac{\theta}{1-\theta}\exp\left(\frac{\Delta G_0}{RT}\right)\exp\left[\frac{V_S N_P(Z_P + \theta Z_T)}{RT}\right]. \tag{14.1}$$

Here θ ($0 < \theta < 1$) is the hybridization efficiency, i.e., the fraction of hybridized probes, C_0 is the assayed DNA concentration, $\Delta G_0 = \Delta H_0 - T\Delta S_0$ is the Gibbs free energy (ΔH_0 the enthalpy, ΔS_0 the entropy) of dsDNA formation in homogeneous solution, T is the temperature, and R is the universal gas constant. Z_P and Z_T denote the probe and target lengths (the number of nucleotides), and N_P is the probe surface density. V_S is the interaction strength, which is estimated (Vainrub and Pettitt, 2002) both theoretically and from the experiments as about 10^{-14} J m^2/mol for 25-mer long probe oligonucleotides in 1 *M* NaCl solution.

The array hybridization isotherm, Equation 14.1 as demonstrated in Figure 14.1, successfully explains the well-known experiments (Forman et al., 1998; Guo et al., 1994; Shchepinov et al., 1995), showing

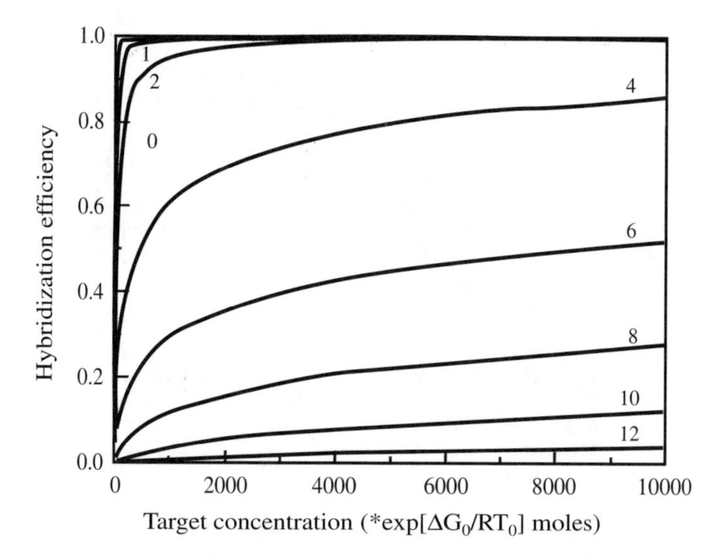

FIGURE 14.1 Hybridization binding isotherm at different surface density of 25-mer probe oligonucleotides. The curve number notes the surface density in 10^{12} probes/cm^2 units. The number 0 corresponds to the Langmuir isotherm.

the temperature decrease and strong broadening of the dsDNA melting on array compared to solution. Also, the theory quantitatively accounts for the recent 25-mer (Peterson et al., 2001) and 20-mer (Watterson et al., 2000) oligonucleotide array experimental data. Below we review how this theory can be used in microarray optimization. It should be noted that, in addition to the discussed electrostatic forces, the other interface interactions, e.g., hydration effects, van der Waals forces, and steric hindrance (packing), could contribute under specific array conditions. However, the interface electrostatic effects often dominate the interactions. In combination with understanding the probabilistic basis of the sequences for analysis (below), we now have the ability to bring some interesting concepts to bear on the design of biochips.

14.2.2 Sensitivity Enhancement

Considering the interaction-free energies involved in surface-bound DNA devices, several factors affecting binding and performance were apparent. We found that the concentration dependence of the electrostatic repulsion between the assayed target and probe array affects the sensitivity and dynamic range of DNA microarrays. Calculated from our theory, Figure 14.2 shows the number of hybrids θN_p as a function of the target concentration at different probe surface densities N_p assuming the same array parameters $Z = 25$, $V_s = 10^{-14}$ J m²/mol and room temperature $T = 25°C$ as in Figure 14.1. For microarray assays in the low target concentration regime, the strongest signals (curve 1 in Figure 14.2) correspond to a probe density of about 10^{12} cm^{-2}. As seen in the insert to Figure 14.2, the theoretical sensitivity peak is rather narrow suggesting that the probe density on the surface in microarrays should be thoroughly optimized for each surface preparation and solution condition. This result is in accord with experimental observations of a clear signal peak in a similar probe density range (Steel et al., 1998) and a weaker signal at higher probe densities (Peterson et al., 2001). This means the dynamic range near higher target concentrations can be expanded by an increase of the probe density at the expense of a substantial decrease in sensitivity. The width of the peak may have other factors that could be important under different conditions.

Explicit control of the electrostatic interactions by microscopic or macroscopic field generation is therefore of obvious importance for optimization of microarrays. Suppression of the Coulomb repulsion could, in favorable circumstances, increase the sensitivity. We predict this could be achieved using external fields, charged molecular surface preparations, and in three-dimensional arrays using probe immobilization in gels, which indeed show solution-like hybridization thermodynamics (Vasiliskov et al., 2001),

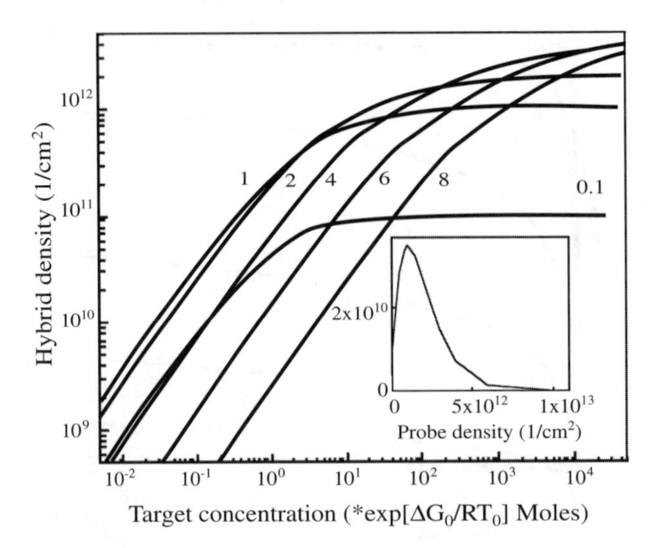

FIGURE 14.2 Number of hybridized probes as a function of the normalized target concentration at different surface density of 25-mer probe oligonucleotides. The curve number notes the surface density in 10^{12} probes/cm² units. Insert: Number of hybrids vs. probe surface density at the normalized target concentration 0.1.

but suffer from the slow hybridization and washing kinetics. For two-dimensional arrays use of multivalent counterions for enhancement of the Coulomb screening and repulsion reduction (Nguyen et al., 2000) may be important as well as the use of a positive electrostatic potential at the surface (Vainrub and Pettitt, 2000). In addition, replacement of DNA probes by noncharged peptide nucleic acids (PNA) (Nielsen, 2001) provides an interesting chemical way to lessen the unfavorable electrostatic interaction. Other complications arise to make a detailed analysis of such a hetero duplex beyond the scope of our present discussion.

14.2.3 Multiplexed SNPs Detection

In contrast to gene expression profiling, the Coulomb hybridization blockage plays a positive role in on-array single nucleotide polymorphism (SNP) genotyping and provides an interesting possibility for multiplexed SNPs detection. Given a reasonable estimate of the mean SNP frequency in a human chromosome DNA of about 1 per 1000 nucleotide sites (Cutler et al., 2001), the individual genomes may differ by several millions of SNPs. Therefore, highly multiplexed detection using microarrays is very important for high throughput large-scale SNP genotyping.

The principle of on-array multiplexed SNPs genotyping is demonstrated in Figure 14.3. For 20-mer perfectly matched duplexes with oligomer L 5′-CTGAA CGGTA GCATC TTGAC-3′ and oligomer H 5′-CTGAG CGGTA GCACC GCGAC-3′ the melting curves in solution at 5 nM oligonucleotide concentration with 1 *M* added NaCl salt are shown in Figure 14.3 (left side). The H duplex (T_m = 72.5°C, 70% of GC-bases) is more stable than the L duplex (T_m = 62.9°C, 50% of GC-bases) because of the higher GC-base content (SantaLucia et al., 1996). In addition to the matched L and H, Figure 14.3 shows also the melting curves for the L1 and H1 SNPs corresponding to the A for T single nucleotide replacement at the tenth position from the 5′-end. As a practical example, the conditions for an SNP detection are defined as at least 1% hybridization efficiency signal strength and 1.5 times discrimination ratio for the match/mismatch signals. The resulting detection temperature ranges of L and H SNPs are shown in Figure 14.3 by the bars. Since in solution L and H ranges do not overlap, the two SNPs cannot be detected

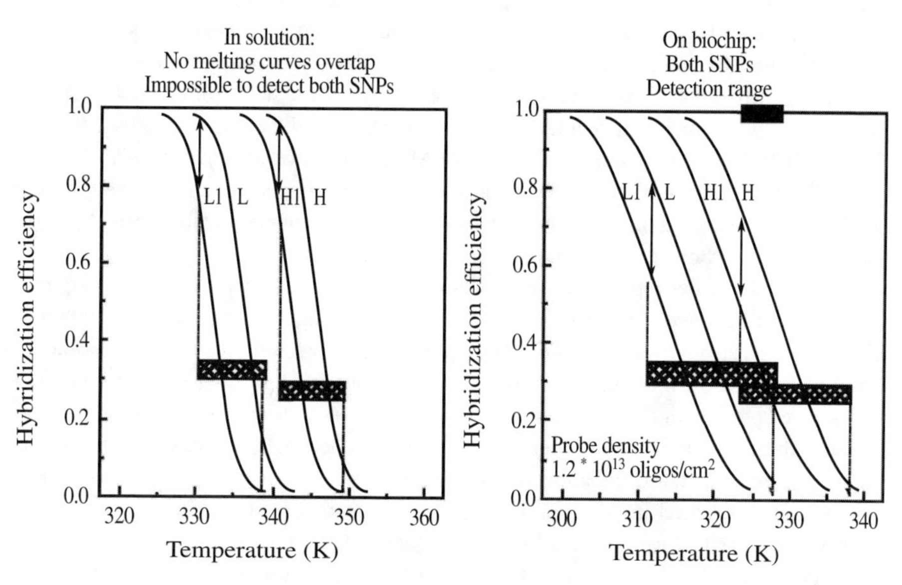

FIGURE 14.3 Principle of multiplexed SNPs detection on DNA biochip. The melting curves of matched 20-mers L and H and their single mismatches L1 and H1. The (L, L1) bar shows the temperature range where both detection and discrimination between L and L1 duplexes is possible (see text); the (H, H1) bar indicates the similar range for H and H1. In solution (left figure) the (L, L1) and (H, H1) ranges do not overlap, but on DNA biochip (right figure) the overlap occurs and allows detection of both (L, L1) and (H, H1) SNPs in a single fixed temperature experiment.

in a single temperature assay. However, on an array with a probe surface density $N_p = 1.2*10^{13}$ cm^{-2} the above-mentioned broadening of melting curve increases the detection ranges for L and H SNPs and makes them both detectable in the overlap temperature region as shown in Figure 14.3 (right side). This example illustrates the principle behind our suggested multiplexed detection of SNPs that differ by up to 10°C in the melting temperature. Further extensions of diversity of on-array genotyped SNPs can be achieved using higher probe surface density to make the melting transition even more broad.

14.3 DNA Biosensors

14.3.1 Presence of Short Subsequences in the Genomes

Statistical analysis of the appearance of short subsequences in different DNA sequences, from individual genes to full genomes is important for a variety of reasons. Applications include PCR primer (Fislage, 1998; Fislage et al., 1997) as well as microarray probe design (Southern, 2001). Several attempts (Deschavanne, et al., 1999; Karlin and Ladunga, 1994; Karlin and Mrazek, 1997; Nakashima et al., 1997; Nakashima et al., 1998; Nussinov, 1984; Sandberg et al., 2001) have been made to employ the frequency distribution of short subsequences (n-mers) to identify species with relatively short genome sizes (microbial). In such an approach, the shape of the frequency distribution for certain short subsequences, 2–4-mers (Deschavanne et al., 1999; Karlin and Ladunga, 1994; Karlin and Mrazek, 1997; Nakashima et al., 1997; Nakashima et al., 1998; Nussinov, 1984) and 8–9-mers (Deschavanne et al., 1999; Sandberg et al., 2001) has been used to decide what microbial genome one is dealing with, based on a given piece of genome or a whole genome.

Many sequencing projects are in progress and more full genomes have recently become available. The several hundred projects completed so far provide sufficient material to consider them from a statistical viewpoint. Yet, we are still far from having a complete or even reasonable statistical picture. There are simply too many species yet to be sequenced to obtain globally relevant statistical answers.

Recently (Fofanov et al., 2002a, 2002b) the comparative statistical analysis of the presence/absence of all possible short n-mers (7 to 20 nucleotides long) for more than 250 complete genomes was performed in this group. The set under consideration included 76 complete microbial genome sequences with sizes ranging from 0.58 to 7.04 Mb and 176 viral genomes (128 RNA containing viruses with genome sizes from 0.32 to 130.76 Kb and 48 DNA containing viruses with genome sizes from 2.0 to 671.19 kb) as well as complete genomes of five multicellular organisms: *Caenorhabditis elegans* (99.99 Mb), *Drosophila melanogaster* (119.98 Mb), *Oryza sativa* (Rice, 255.87 Mb), *Schizosaccharomyces pombe* (12.49 Mb), and *Homo sapiens* (human, 2.875 Gb) genomes. A complete list of genomes and all supplementary materials mentioned below can be found on the University of Houston Bioinformatics lab website http://www.bioinfo.uh.edu/publications/how_random_are_genomes.

Tables 14.1 and 14.2 show representative results for some of the analyzed genomes (microbial and viral), for $n = 8$ and 12 using our techniques. It is worth mentioning that as n increases, the total number of possible n-mers, 4^n, strongly exceeds the total sequence length M and most of the possible n-mers do not appear at all because the maximum number of n-mers contained in this sequence is $M - n + 1 \approx M$. Moreover, for a reasonably high ratio, $4^n/M$, most of the n-mers that appear tend to appear only once, in accordance with the fact that the number of present n-mers becomes very close to M (see Tables 14.1, 14.2, and supplementary data on the above-mentioned Web site). That is why it was decided to use the statistics for "presence/absence" in our method of analysis, instead of the usual "frequency of appearance," which is reasonable for short n-mers (total sequence length $M << 4^n$).

Let us consider the results obtained for different n-mers in the various genomes. Plotting the frequency of presence, f, of n-mers in genomes (the number of different n-mers present in a given genome over the total number of n-mers, 4^n) against the ratio $4^n/M$ gives a convenient view of the statistics. Figures 14.4 through 14.6 correspond to the microbial, RNA containing viruses and DNA containing viruses, respectively. The frequency of n-mers for different values of n is shown with different symbols. The analytical distribution that corresponds to the frequency of presence of n-mers in a purely random

TABLE 14.1 Frequency of Presence of 8-mers and Self-Similarity* for Several Viral Genomes

Accession	Genome	Total Sequence Length (bp)	Number of Present 8-mers	Frequency of Present 8-mers	Random Boundary	Self-Similarity
NC_001436	Human T-cell lymphotropic virus type 1	17,014	13,739	20.96%	22.86%	8.31%
NC_001707	Hepatitis B virus	6,430	5,963	9.10%	9.35%	2.64%
NC_001503	Mouse mammary tumor virus	17,610	14,307	21.83%	23.56%	7.35%
NC_001547	Sindbis virus	11,703	10,431	15.92%	16.35%	2.67%
NC_001434	Hepatitis E virus	7,176	6,517	9.94%	10.37%	4.12%
NC_003312	Swine hepatitis E virus	7,257	6,608	10.08%	10.48%	3.81%
NC_001489	Hepatitis A virus	7,478	6,543	9.98%	10.78%	7.42%
NC_001433	Hepatitis C virus	9,413	8,480	12.94%	13.38%	3.29%
NC_001653	Hepatitis D virus	1,682	1,608	2.45%	2.53%	3.17%
NC_001802	Human immunodeficiency virus type 1	9,181	7,725	11.79%	13.07%	9.83%
NC_003461	Human parainfluenza virus 1	15,600	12,242	18.68%	21.18%	11.82%
NC_001796	Human parainfluenza virus 3	15,462	11,506	17.56%	21.02%	16.46%
NC_003443	Human parainfluenza virus 2	15,646	12,702	19.38%	21.24%	8.74%

* See the definition in the text.

TABLE 14.2 Frequency of Presence of 12-mers and Self-Similarity for Several Microbial Genomes

Accession	Genome	Total Sequence Length (bp)	Number of Present 12-mers	Frequency of Present 12-mers	Random Boundary	Self-Similarity
NC_000964	*Bacillus subtilis*	8,429,628	5,346,103	31.87%	39.50%	19.32%
NC_002696	*Caulobacter crescentus*	8,033,894	3,399,234	20.26%	38.05%	46.75%
NC_000913	*Escherichia coli* K12	9,278,442	5,695,881	33.95%	42.48%	20.08%
NC_000916	*Methanobacterium thermoautotrophicum*	3,502,754	2,658,450	15.85%	18.84%	15.91%
NC_003197	*Salmonella typhimurium* LT2	9,714,864	5,821,910	34.70%	43.96%	21.06%
NC_002758	*Staphylococcus aureus* Mu50	5,756,080	3,398,622	20.26%	29.04%	30.25%
NC_003098	*Streptococcus pneumoniae* R6	4,077,230	2,992,091	17.83%	21.57%	17.34%
NC_002737	*Streptococcus pyogenes*	3,704,882	2,778,223	16.56%	19.81%	16.43%
NC_002578	*Thermoplasma acidophilum*	3,129,812	2,602,761	15.51%	17.02%	8.84%
NC_002689	*Thermoplasma volcanium*	3,169,608	2,590,718	15.44%	17.22%	10.30%
NC_000919	*Treponema pallidum*	2,275,888	1,978,453	11.79%	12.69%	7.04%
NC_000853	*Thermotoga maritima*	3,721,450	2,755,886	16.43%	19.89%	17.43%
NC_002162	*Ureaplasma urealyticum*	1,503,438	948,274	5.65%	8.57%	34.06%
NC_002505	*Vibrio cholerae* chromosome I, chromosome II	8,066,854	5,383,520	32.09%	38.17%	15.94%
NC_002488	*Xylella fastidiosa* 9a5c	5,358,610	3,996,398	23.82%	27.34%	12.88%

"genome" is also shown for comparison in all figures as a solid line. One can observe the extraordinary similarity between these plots. All of the different genomes form a well-defined pattern, when plotted against the ratio $4^n/M$ and not against the size of the genome or the length of the n-mer separately.

For much longer genomes of multicellular organisms, practically all n-mers for $n < 12$ are present. Therefore, we chose to calculate the number of distinct 13–20-mers present in each genome (see Figure 14.7 and Table 14.3). These results point to the conclusion that the presence of n-mers in all genomes

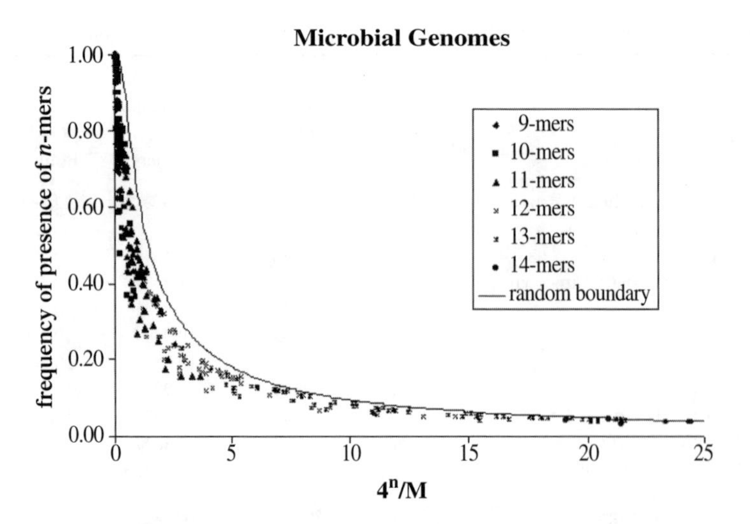

FIGURE 14.4 Frequency of presence of 9–14-mers in 76 microbial genomes.

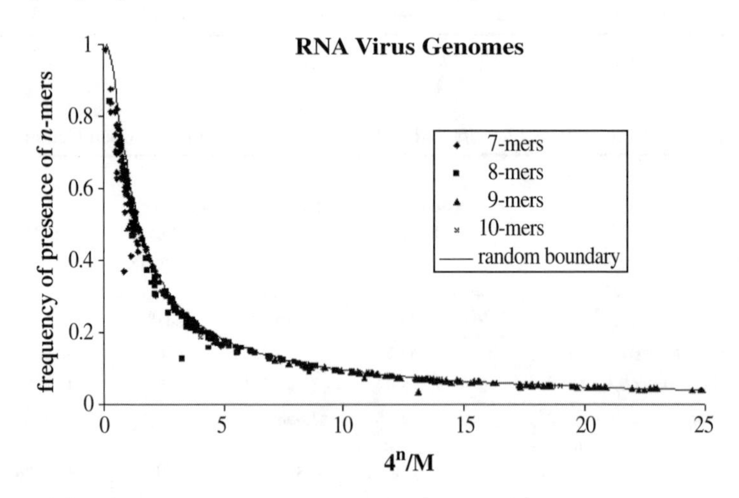

FIGURE 14.5 Frequency of presence of 7–10-mers in 129 RNA viral genomes.

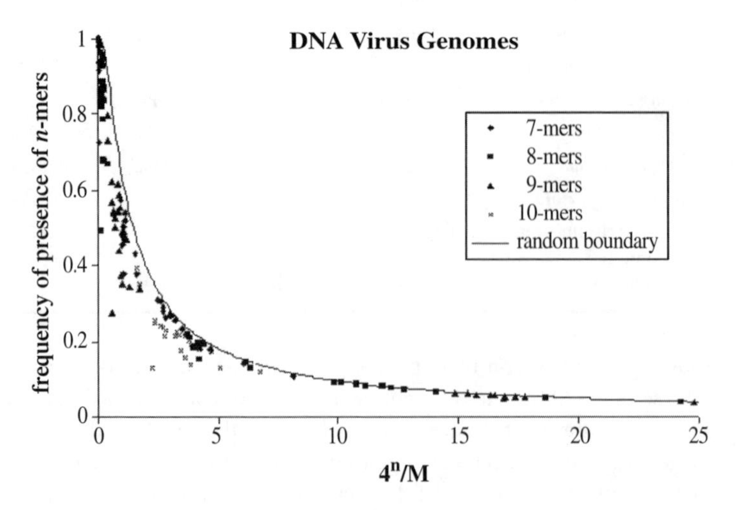

FIGURE 14.6 Frequency of presence of 7–10-mers in 48 DNA viral genomes.

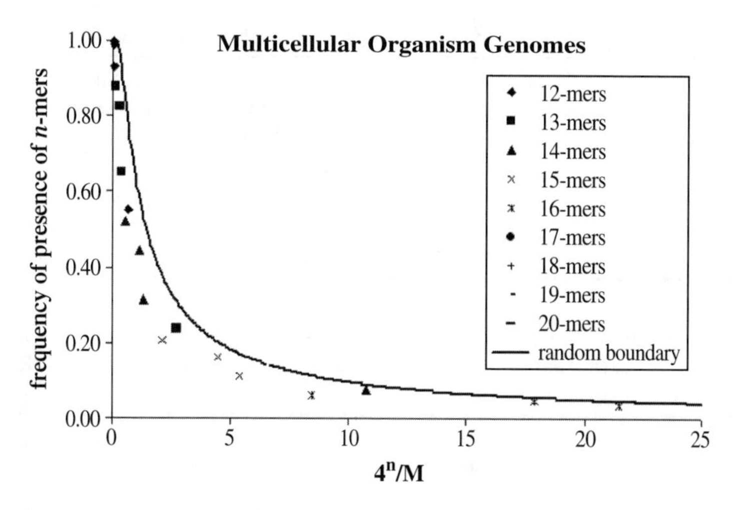

FIGURE 14.7 Frequency of presence of 7–10-mers in 48 DNA viral genomes.

TABLE 14.3 Frequency of Presence of *n*-mers and Self-Similarity for Several Genomes of Multicellular Organisms*

Genome	Total Sequence Length (bp)	Number of Present *n*-mers	Percent of Present *n*-mers	Random Boundary: (1–exp(–1/x))	Self-Similarity
Caenorhabditis elegans (14-mers)	199,980,344	83,915,577	31.26%	52.53%	40.5%
Drosophila melanogaster (14-mers)	239,963,692	119,253,045	44.43%	59.10%	24.8%
Oryza sativa (15-mers)	511,742,384	220,383,196	20.52%	37.91%	45.9%
Schizosaccharomyces pombe (12-mers)	24,980,160	9,256,101	55.17%	31.08%	28.8%
Homo sapiens (16-mers)	5,749,472,188	1,577,086,225	36.72%	73.78%	50.2%

* *n* is different for every genome.

considered (in the range of *n*, when the condition $M<<4^n$ holds, where *M* is the genome length) can be treated as a nearly random process.

This statistical property of genomes leads to the conclusion that a relatively small random subset of *n*-mers of particular size printed on the DNA microarray can be used for fast estimation of the genome size of unknown microorganisms. If future research shows similarity between presence/absence statistics in coding and noncoding regions in multicellular organisms, such DNA microarrays can be employed to estimate the size of the transcriptome (the expressed part genome) in different circumstances. However, it must be emphasized that the statistical quality of how random a random subset of *n*-mers is used may be critical to the success of such an approach.

14.3.2 Correlation of Presence of Short Subsequences between Genomes

Even if, as it is mentioned above, the presence of short *n*-mers in microbial/viral genomes can be treated as an almost random process, the correlations or simply the number of *n*-mers presented in different genomes simultaneously remains an open question. The interesting problem is to find out how independent/correlated the appearances of *n*-mers are in different genomes. One of the possible ways to approach this question is by using the well-known multiplication property for the joint probability of the intersection of events, according to which two events, *A* and *B*, can be treated as independent if $p(A \cap B) = p(A)p(B)$.

TABLE 14.4 The Frequency of Presence of 12-mers within the Three Microbial Genomes

Genome (G)	Genome Length	Total Sequence Length (bp)	Number of Different 12-mers Present in Genome: $N(12,G)$	$p = N(12,G)/4^n$
Salmonella typhi	4,809,037	9,618,074	5,813,330	34.65%
Mycobacterium tuberculosis H37Rv	4,411,529	8,823,058	4,361,508	26.00%
Bacillus subtilis	4,214,814	8,429,628	5,346,103	31.87%

TABLE 14.5 Actual and Predicted Simultaneous Presence of 12-mers within the Three Microbial Genomes: (1) *Salmonella typhi,* (2) *Mycobacterium tuberculosis* H37Rv, and (3) *Bacillus subtilis*

Case	Number 12-mers	$N(n, G_1, G_2)/4^n$	Calculated Probability Assuming Independence
Present in genomes (1) and (2)	1,943,814	11.6%	9.0%
Present in genomes (1) and (3)	2,335,710	13.9%	11.0%
Present in genomes (2) and (3)	1,334,288	8.0%	8.3%

Let us provide a simple example based on three different genomes: (1) *Salmonella typhi* (NC_003198), (2) *Mycobacterium tuberculosis* H37Rv (NC_000962), and (3) *Bacillus subtilis* (NC_000964). A complete set of n-mers would contain 4^n n-mers, which, for $n = 12$, is $4^{12} = 16{,}777{,}216$. Based on our analysis, Table 14.4 shows how many different 12-mers are contained in each of these three genomes. The number $N(n, G_1, G_2)$ of n-mers ($n = 12$) that appears in each pair of species genomes (G_1, G_2) is shown in Table 14.5. We can compare the probabilities of finding randomly picked 12-mers in each pair of genomes with probabilities calculated using the multiplication rule. As seen from Table 14.5, the actual and calculated (expected) probabilities do not differ greatly from each other, which allows us to treat the presence/absence of randomly picked 12-mers in these three genomes as statistically independent events.

Actual and expected pair-wise probabilities were calculated (Fofanov et al., 2002a, 2002b) in each of the above-mentioned groups of genomes (170,000+ pairs in total). We were especially interested in the range of n where $p^* = 5$ to 50% of the total possible number of n-mers occurred. This range is different for different genome sizes and can be determined from Figure 14.4. The analytic formula for the random boundary also can be used to estimate this range:

$$n^* = \frac{\log\left[M(1-p^*)/p^*\right]}{\log(4)} \quad . \tag{14.2}$$

Upper and lower bounds for sizes from 0.8 to 10 Mb, which are typical for microbial genomes, are shown in Table 14.6. In accordance with this, the value $n = 12$ seems to be the most reasonable one for all microbial genomes. For viral genomes, the value was found to be $n = 7$.

For all 2800+ pairs of microbial genomes and the value of $n = 12$, the average ratio of actual and expected probabilities was found to be 1.35 ± 0.61. For viral genomes and the corresponding value of $n = 7$, the average ratio of actual and expected probabilities was found to be 1.06 ± 0.10 for 1100+ genome

TABLE 14.6 The Optimal Length of n-mers (n^*) for Different Genome Sizes and Frequencies of Presence (p^*)

Total Sequence Length (bp)	n^* Determined for Frequency of Presence 50% ($p^* = 0.5$)	n^* Determined for Frequency of Presence 5% ($p^* = 0.05$)
0.8 Mb	9.80	11.93
2.0 Mb	10.47	12.59
10.0 Mb	11.63	13.75

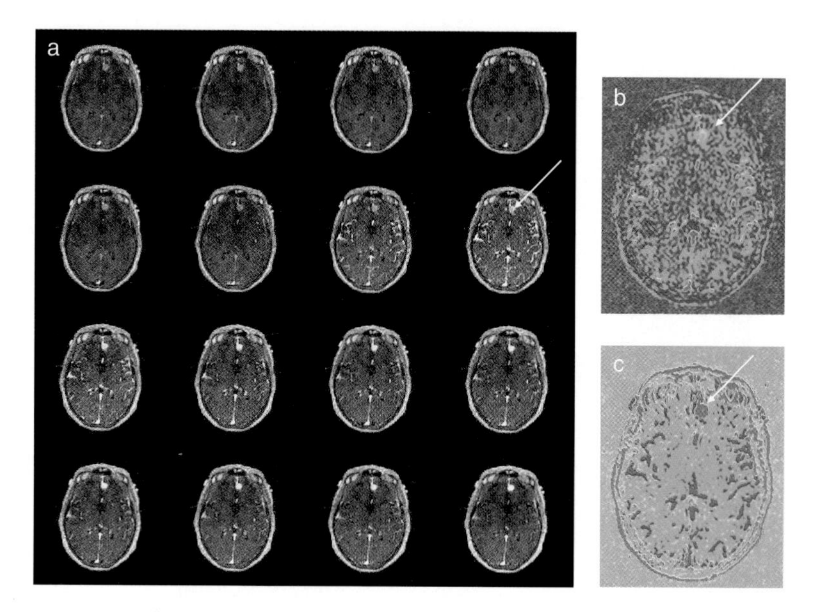

COLOR FIGURE 8.6 MR permeability assessment. (a) 16 of a series of dynamic T_1-weighted images acquired during passage of Gd-based contrast agent in a patient with an intracranial tumor (arrow). Kinetic modeling of the progressive positive enhancement yields estimates of (b) fractional blood volume and (c) microvascular permeability, both of which are elevated in this tumor.

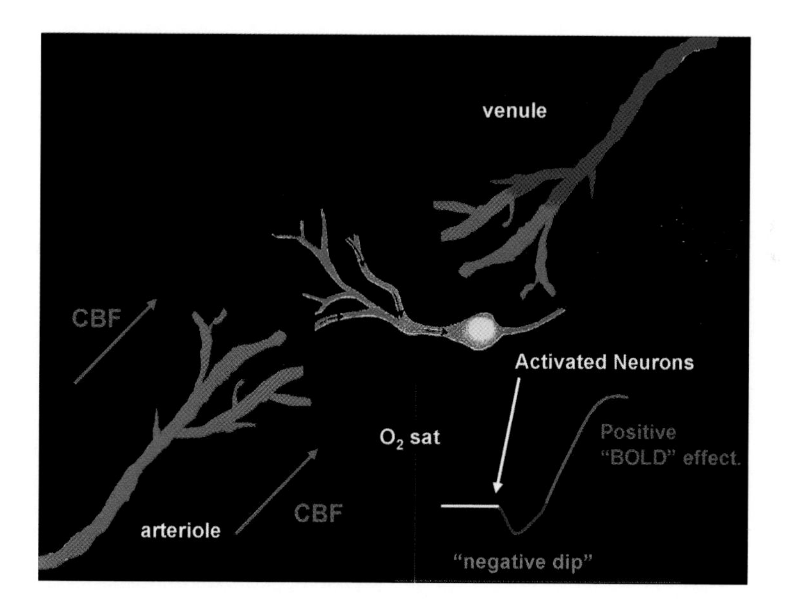

COLOR FIGURE 8.7 Schematic of the fMRI BOLD contrast mechanism. Neuronal activation leads to an increase in regional CBF, without a concomitant increase in tissue oxygen consumption, leading to an increase in the oxygenation of the capillary bed and postcapillary venules. This increase in oxygenation can be visualized as an increase in signal on T_2*-weighted images, as paramagnetic deoxyhemoglobin is displaced.

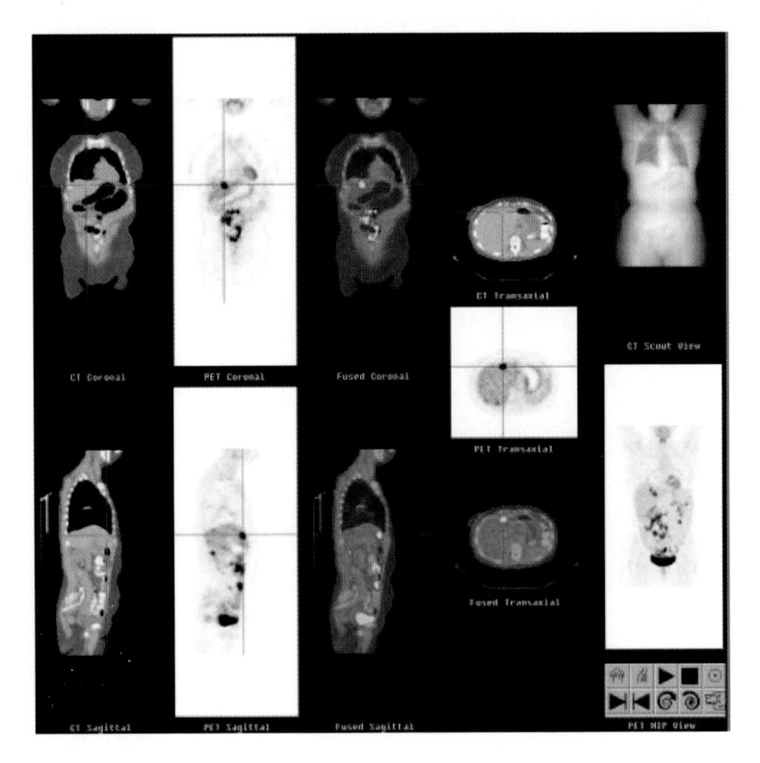

COLOR FIGURE 10.22 PET whole body scan and CT anatomical reference. PET and fused PET/CT images indicate uptake of ^{18}FDG in liver and other abdominal areas. From left to right: CT, PET, and fused PET/CT coronal (top) and sagittal (bottom) views. The fourth column shows the transaxial images, from top to bottom: CT, PET, and fused PET/CT images.

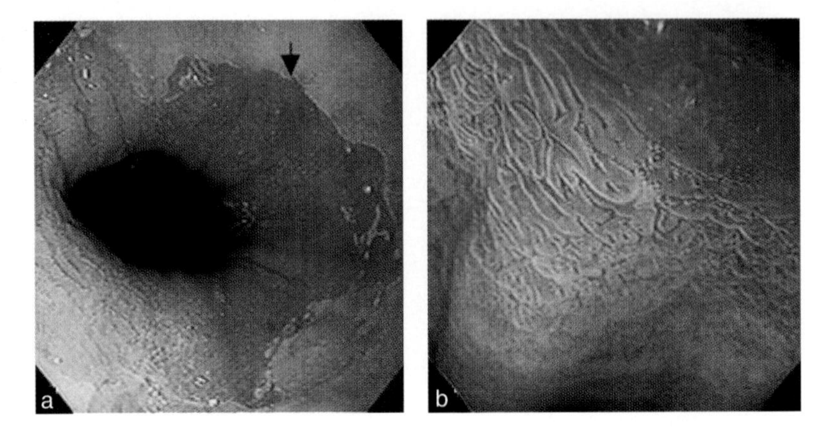

COLOR FIGURE 11.18 (a) Normal endoscopic view of the distal esophagus after spraying with acetic acid, showing short extensions of columnar-appearing mucosa with squamous islands within Barrett's epithelium. (b) Enhanced magnification endoscopic view of the same field showing a fine villiform pit pattern.

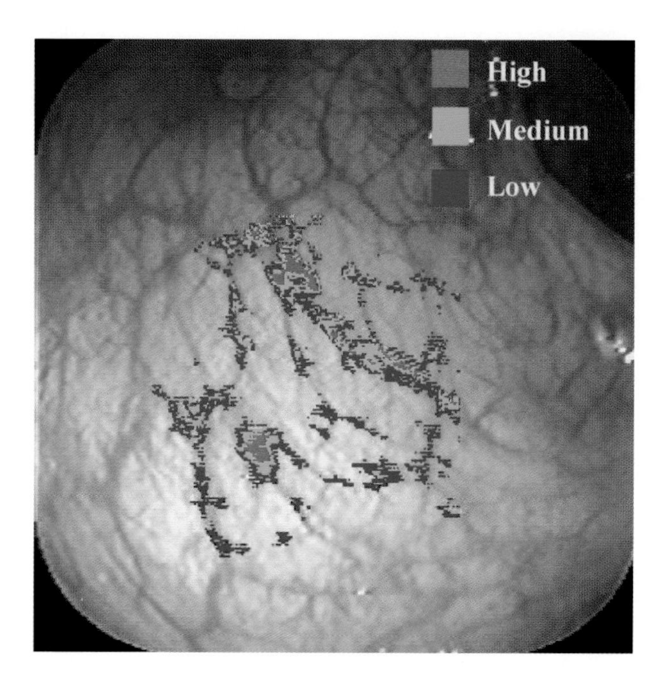

COLOR FIGURE 11.20(d) A color overlay shows the locations on the mucosa that have a high, medium, and low probability of containing dysplasia with the colors red, green, and blue, respectively. Note that the region of high probability (red) corresponds to the location of the two adenomas on the white light image.

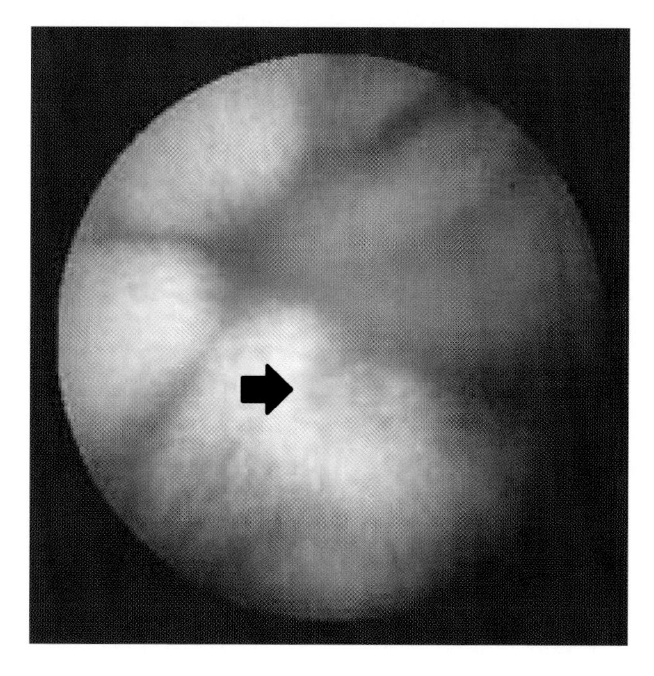

COLOR FIGURE 11.22(b) An angiodysplastic lesion (arrow) has been found in the distal jejunum.

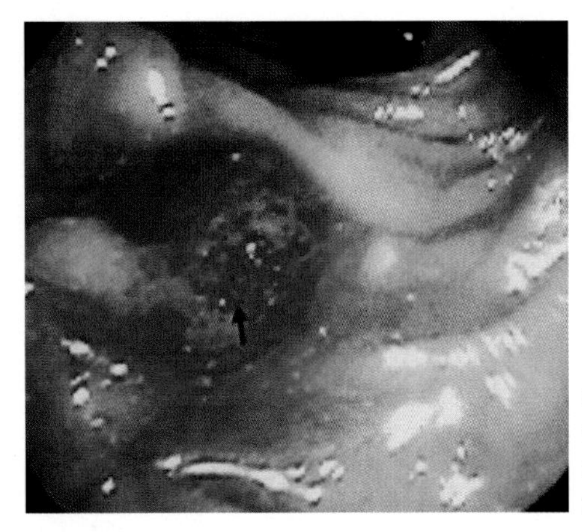

COLOR FIGURE 11.23(c) An 8-mm polyp was confirmed on conventional colonoscopy performed the same day [as (a) and (b)]. Histologic examination revealed an adenomatous polyp.

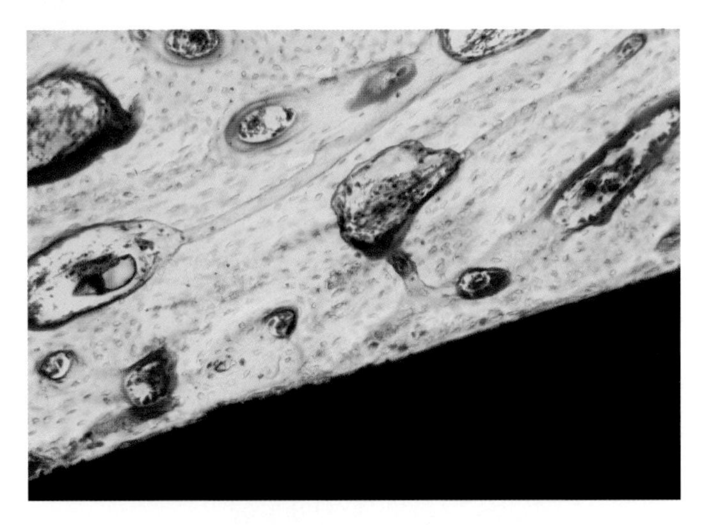

COLOR FIGURE 16.4 Section of the femoral head and adjoining stainless steel implant. Note the 'clean' interface between the tissue and the implant. Elliptical areas contain osteoclasts and osteoblasts, cells involved in the growth and remodeling of bone. (With thanks to Professor P. Revell.)

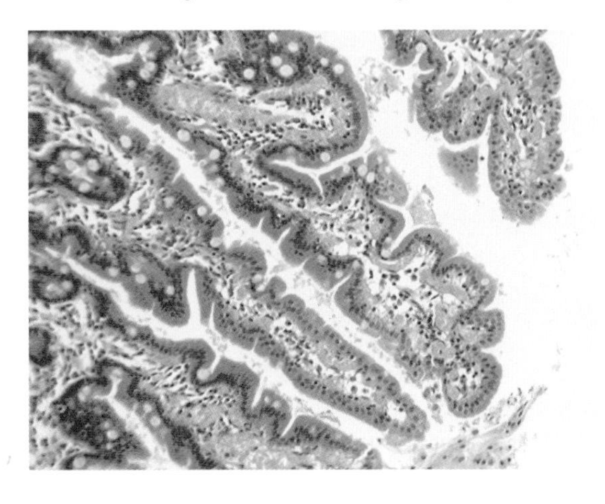

COLOR FIGURE 16.5 Section through the lining of the small intestine stained with hematoxylin and eosin.

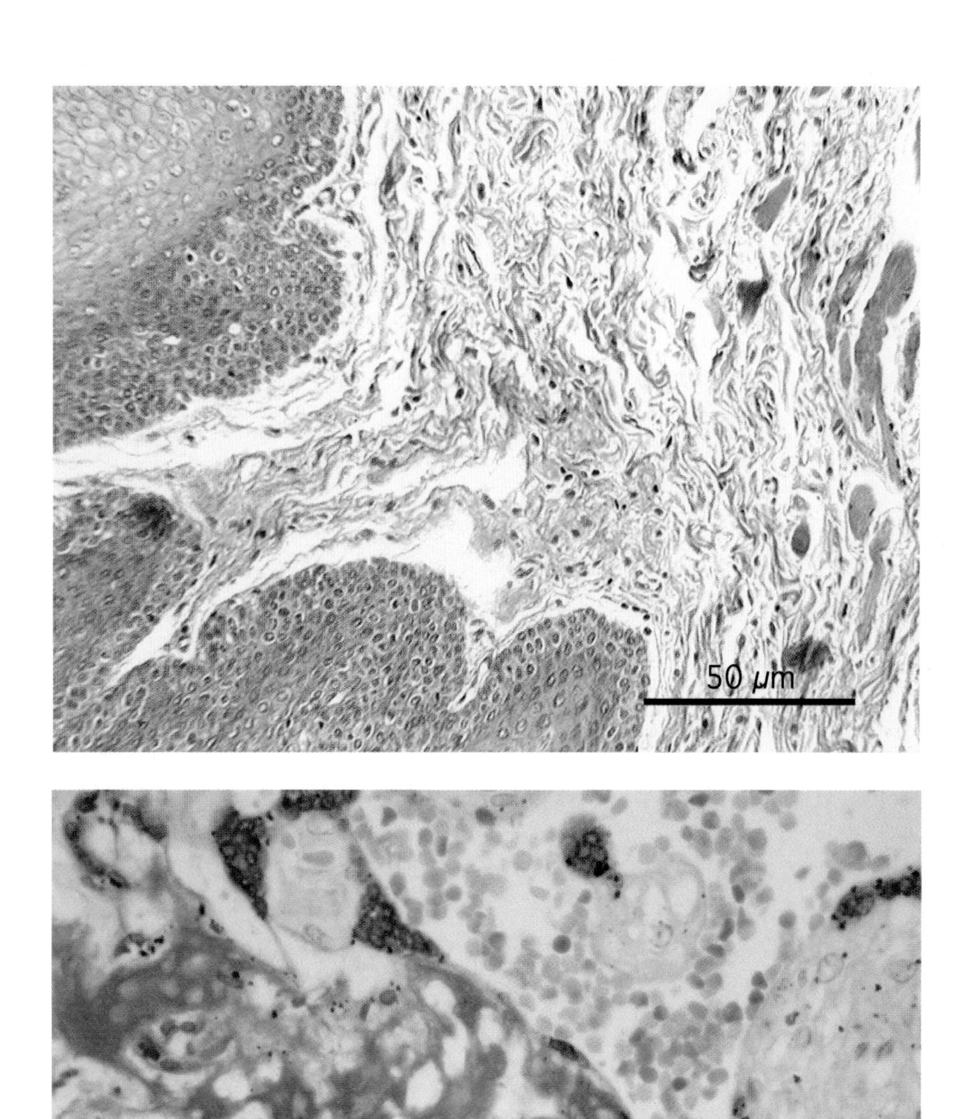

COLOR FIGURE 16.6 (Upper panel) Transverse section of the tongue treated with Masson's trichrome stain, showing muscle in red, connective tissue in blue/green, and cell nuclei in purple. (Lower panel) Section of placenta stained with MSB. With this stain, fibrin is red, other connective tissue is blue, and red blood cells are yellow.

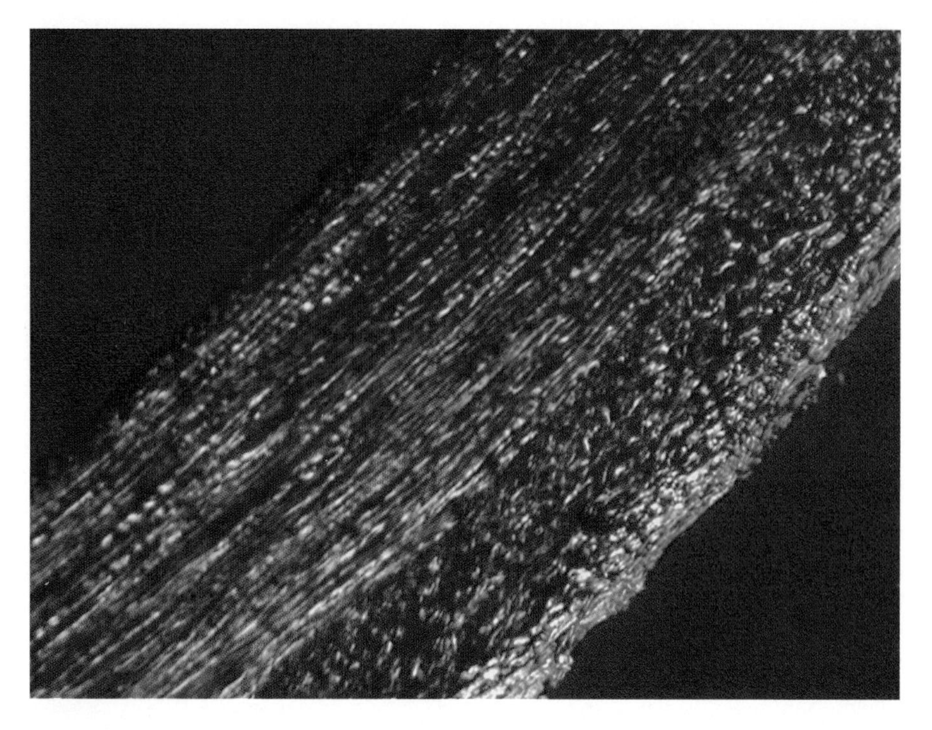

COLOR FIGURE 16.9 Transverse section of a porcine carotid artery viewed under polarized light. The birefringent collagen fibers appear bright against a dark background.

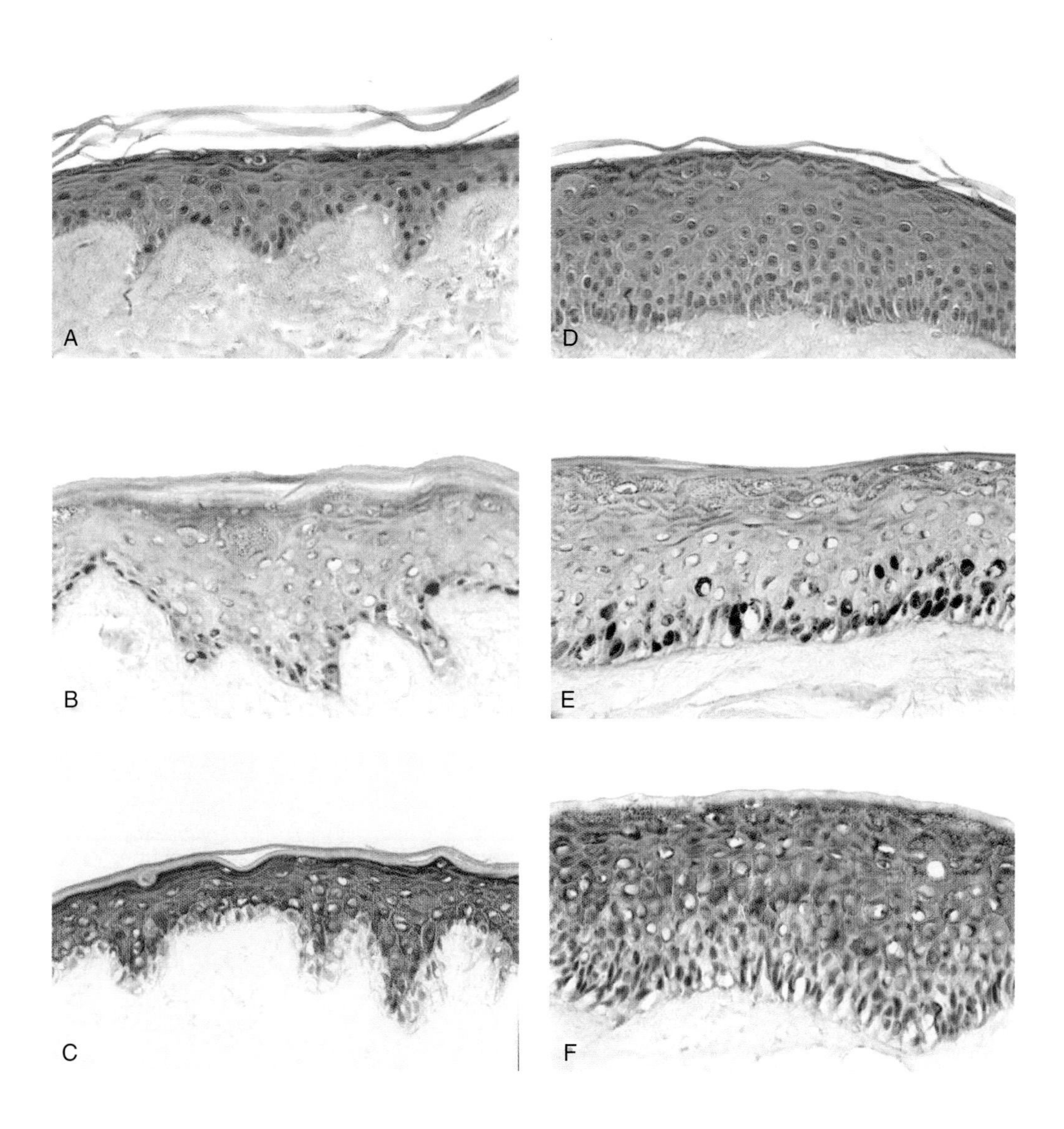

COLOR FIGURE 19.3 KGF induces hyperproliferation and delays differentiation in a skin equivalent model system. Sections of skin equivalents unmodified (A, B, C) and genetically modified to express KGF (D, E, F) were cultured for 7 days at the air/liquid interface. Cryosections were stained with hematoxylin and eosin (H&E; A, D), a nuclear proliferation antigen (Ki67; brown; B, E), and the differentiation marker keratin 10 (K10; brown; C, F). Ki67 and K10 sections were counterstained with hematoxylin (blue) (magnification 40×). Note the increased thickness and basal cell density of the KGF-modified tissues. Also note that in unmodified tissues proliferation is confined to the basal layer, while in KGF-modified tissues proliferating cells extend up to three to four suprabasal layers. The same suprabasal layers that contain proliferating cells are also negative for the differentiation marker K10, suggesting that KGF alters the spatial control of proliferation and differentiation in the genetically modified tissues.

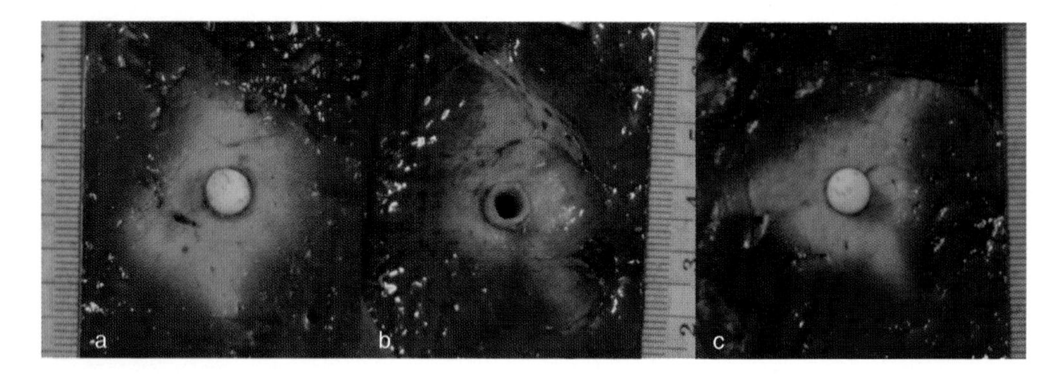

COLOR FIGURE 31.9 Examples of conformal thermal therapy with dual-frequency interstitial ultrasound heating applicator. Thermal lesions (shown transverse to the heating applicator) were created by varying the power, frequency, and rate of rotation during heating in excised liver. The ruler scales represent 1-mm increments and the location of the heating applicator is shown by the markers in each panel. Arbitrary thermal lesion geometries are possible with this applicator design.

pairs DNA-based viruses and 1.04 ± 0.05 for 8100+ genome pairs RNA-based viruses. This led us to the conclusion that for this range of n, the presences of n-mers in different genomes, to a good approximation, can be treated as independent events.

The highest deviations between expected and actual probabilities were found for closely related genomes. For 48 DNA-based viruses under consideration, using 7-mers, the highest ratio (185%) was found for *Duck hepatitis B virus* (NC_001344) vs. *Stork hepatitis B virus* (NC_003325) with 8.1% expected and 15.0% actual.

An example of closely related microbial genomes would be *S. aureus N*315 (NC_002745) vs. *S. aureus* Mu50 (NC_002758) with 4.0% expected and 19.7% actual or 491% higher than expected. Another extreme case was found for three microbial genomes: *Chlamydophila pneumoniae* CWL029 (NC_000922), *C. pneumoniae* AR39 (NC_002179), and *C. pneumoniae* J138 (NC_002491), which have the highest (eightfold) ratio of actual and expected probabilities for 12-mers (1.5% expected and 12.3% actual). For the group containing 24 human chromosomes, pair-wise ratios of actual and expected probabilities of 14-mers were found to be 1.91 ± 0.16, maximum ratio being found for $n = 20$ and Y-chromosomes (expectation 2.9% vs. actual 6.9%).

Assuming that results for 250+ genomes are statistically significant, we expect similar behavior from many different (as yet sequenced) genomes. Thus our analysis indicates that, in this case, one may use relatively small sets of randomly picked n-mers for differentiating between different viruses and organisms.

Let us further illustrate the idea by continuing our example for three microbial genomes. Let n^* be the size of n-mer, which fits the interval where from 5 to 50% of all possible n-mers show up for a desirable range of genome lengths. In accordance with Table 14.6, we may choose the value $n^* = 12$. Let us randomly pick L 12-mers (say, $L = 1000$). Given a genome G_1 with the frequency of presence of n-mers p_1, we expect that $K = p_1 L$ n-mers present in G_1 will appear also in our random set, forming a "fingerprint" of G_1 (in our example, we expect $50 < K < 500$). The probability, ε, that the fingerprint of G_1 will exactly coincide with the fingerprint of some other genome G_2 (with the frequency of presence of n-mers p_2) is (Fofanov et al., 2002a; 2002b):

$$\varepsilon = (1 - p_1 - p_2 + 2p_{12})^L. \tag{14.3}$$

Here p_{12} is the probability for the n-mer to be present in both genomes simultaneously.

Let us consider the numeric example mentioned in Tables 14.4 and 14.5 of two species that are far from each other, *Salmonella typhi* vs. *Mycobacterium tuberculosis* H37Rv; $p_1 = 0.3465$, $p_2 = 0.2600$, $p_{12} = 0.1160$; with $L = 1000$, a remarkable accuracy of $\varepsilon = 1.7*10^{-204}$ can theoretically be achieved.

Given a desirable probability of error, ε, one can determine the appropriate size, L, of a random set of n-mers that can be used for reliable identification of genomes as

$$L = \frac{\log \varepsilon}{\log(1 - p_1 - p_2 + 2p_{12})}. \tag{14.4}$$

For related organisms, the genomes may contain large common parts. This means that p_{12} may be close to p_1 and p_2. To give a numeric example of close relatives, let us consider *S. aureus N*315 vs. *S. aureus* Mu50. Now $p_1 = 0.198$, $p_2 = 0.203$, $p_{12} = 0.197$, and an accuracy of $\varepsilon = 10^{-10}$ can be achieved with $L = 4451$. We would like to stress that our analysis predicts a logarithmic dependence of the sampling or microarray size, L, on the error probability, ε. This feature is of principal importance for the estimation procedure under discussion.

Therefore, we can use practically any sufficiently random subset of n-mers of appropriate size for design a microarray to diagnose an organism to which a given DNA/RNA sample belongs. Different sizes of n-mers must be employed for recognition of different organisms based on their genome length. Values of n that correspond to given intervals of genome lengths can be easily calculated using above formulas. In fact, only 11 different n values, $7 \le n \le 17$, would be enough to cover a large variety of genome sizes from 1 kb to 9 Gb.

The important advantage of such an approach is that it can be used without *a priori* knowledge of the sequence itself. This implies there is no need to perform the expensive and time-consuming process of sequencing before array construction. It is enough to obtain the purified DNA, hybridize it on a sufficiently random microarray chip, and check which n-mers show up. Taking into account how accessible the DNA of thousands of microbes and viruses are, how easily each microarray can be produced, and the fact that we do not need to determine quantitative values of expression (we need only a yes/no answer), it should be possible to produce an essentially universal microbial/viral DNA chip.

14.4 Conclusions

In this article we have attempted to demonstrate how to use both physical and mathematical techniques to explore design criteria of relevance to modern genetic analysis. In particular, DNA arrays allow simultaneous, parallel detection and concentration measurement of thousands of target strands. In this article we have concentrated on two areas of concern in the design and analysis of such experiments: the information content of the polymer and the physical/chemical properties of the detection. Microarrays are now producing amounts of raw biological (and biophysical) data on a scale not seen before in the biological arena. The bioinformatics solutions to problems associated with the analysis of data on this scale will remain a challenge for some time. The physical design of efficient devices to conduct such experiments requires consideration of the chemistry and physics of often highly charged species near prepared surfaces as well as the sequence. This article was aimed at demonstrating the current state of theory in the hopes that many will find application of these principles.

ACKNOWLEDGMENTS

This work was partially supported by grants from NIH, Texas Coordinating Board, and the Robert A. Welch Foundation to BMP. TBL was a fellow at the Keck Center for Computational Biology. BMP and YF acknowledge the Texas Center for Learning and Computation for seed funding, and also NPACI for computing time and support at the San Diego Supercomputing Center. We also thank the Molecular Science Computing Facility (MSCF) in the William R. Wiley Environmental Molecular Sciences Laboratory, a national scientific user facility sponsored by the U.S. Department of Energy's Office of Biological and Environmental Research and located at the Pacific Northwest National Laboratory. Pacific Northwest is operated for the Department of Energy by Battelle. BMP and AV also thank Accelrys for providing visualization software through the Institute for Molecular Design.

References

Bloomfield, V.A., Crothers, D.M., and Tinoco, I., *Nucleic Acids: Structures, Properties and Functions*, University Science Books, Sausalito, CA, 1999.

Brenner, S., Johnson, M., Bridgham, J., Golda, G., Lloyd, D.H., Johnson, D., Luo, S., McCurdy, S., Foy, M., Ewan, M., Roth, R., George, D., Eletr, S., Albrecht, G., Vermaas, E., Williams, S.R., Moon, K., Burcham, T., Pallas, M., DuBridge, R.B., Kirchner, J., Fearon, K., Mao, J., and Corcoran, K., Gene expression analysis by massively parallel signature sequencing (MPSS) on microbead arrays, *Nat. Biotechnol.*, 18, 630–634, 2000.

Cutler, D.J., Zwick, M.E., Carrasquillo, M.M., Yohn, C.T., Tobin, K.P., Kashuk, C., Mathews, D.J., Shah, N.A., Eichler, E.E., Warrington, J.A., and Chakravarti, A., High-throughput variation detection and genotyping using microarrays, *Genome Res.*, 11, 1913–1925, 2001.

Deschavanne, P.J., Giron, A., Vilain, J., Fagot, G., and Fertil, B., Genomic signature: characterization and classification of species assessed by chaos game representation of sequences, *Mol. Biol. Evol.*, 16, 1391–1399, 1999.

Fislage, R., Differential display approach to quantitation of environmental stimuli on bacterial gene expression, *Electrophoresis*, 19, 613–616, 1998.

Fislage, R., Berceanu, M., Humboldt, Y., Wendt, M., and Oberender, H., Primer design for a prokaryotic differential display RT-PCR, *Nucleic Acids Res.*, 25, 1830–1835, 1997.

Fofanov, Y., Luo, Y., Katili, C., Wang, J., Powdrill, B.Y.T., Fofanov, V., Li, T.-B., Chumakov, S., and Pettitt, B.M., How independent are the appearances of n-mers in different genomes? Submitted, 2000a.

Fofanov, Y., Luo, Y., Katili, C., Wang, J., Powdrill, B.Y.T., Fofanov, V., Li, T.-B., Chumakov, S., and Pettitt, B.M., Short subsequences in genomes: how random are they? Submitted, 2002b.

Forman, E.J., Walton, I.D., Stern, D., Rava, R.P., and Trulson, M.O., Thermodynamics of duplex formation and mismatch discrimination of photolithographically synthesized oligonucleotide arrays, *ACS Symp. Ser.*, 682, 206–228, 1998.

Guo, Z., Guilfoyle, R.A., Thiel, A.J., Wang, R., and Smith, L.M., Direct fluorescence analysis of genetic polymorphisms by hybridization with oligonucleotide arrays on glass supports, *Nucleic Acids Res.*, 22, 5456–5465, 1994.

Heaton, R.J., Peterson, A.W., and Georgiadis, R.M., Electrostatic surface plasmon resonance: direct electric field-induced hybridization and denaturation in monolayer nucleic acid films and label-free discrimination of base mismatches, *Proc. Natl. Acad. Sci. U.S.A.*, 98, 3701–3704, 2001.

Karlin, S. and Ladunga, I., Comparisons of eukaryotic genomic sequences, *Proc. Natl. Acad. Sci. U.S.A.*, 91, 12832–12836, 1994.

Karlin, S. and Mrazek, J., Compositional differences within and between eukaryotic genomes, *Proc. Natl. Acad. Sci. U.S.A.*, 94, 10227–10232, 1997.

Nakashima, H., Nishikawa, K., and Ooi, T., Differences in dinucleotide frequencies of human, yeast, and Escherichia coli genes, *DNA Res.*, 4, 185–192, 1997.

Nakashima, H., Ota, M., Nishikawa, K., and Ooi, T., Genes from nine genomes are separated into their organisms in the dinucleotide composition space, *DNA Res.*, 5, 251–259, 1998.

Nguyen, T.T., Grosberg, A.Y., and Shklovskii, B.I., Screening of a charged particle by multivalent counterions in salty water: strong charge inversion, *J. Chem. Phys.*, 113, 1110–1125, 2000.

Nielsen, P.E., Peptide nucleic acid: a versatile tool in genetic diagnostics and molecular biology, *Curr. Opinion Biotech.*, 12, 16–20, 2001.

Nussinov, R., Doublet frequencies in evolutionary distinct groups, *Nucleic Acids Res.*, 12, 1749–1763, 1984.

Peterson, A.W., Heaton, R.J., and Georgiadis, R.M., The effect of surface probe density on DNA hybridization, *Nucleic Acids Res.*, 29, 5163–5168, 2001.

Saenger, W., *Principles of Nucleic Acid Structure*, Springer-Verlag, New York, 1984.

Sandberg, R., Winberg, G., Branden, C.I., Kaske, A., Ernberg, I., and Coster, J., Capturing whole-genome characteristics in short sequences using a naive Bayesian classifier, *Genome Res.*, 11, 1404–1409, 2001.

SantaLucia, J., Allawi, H.T., and Seneviratne, P.A., Improved nearest-neighbor parameters for predicting DNA duplex stability, *Biochemistry*, 35, 3555–3562, 1996.

Shchepinov, M.S., Case-Green, S.C., and Southern, E.M., Steric factors influencing hybridization of nucleic acids to oligonucleotide, *Nucleic Acids Res.*, 25, 1155–1161, 1995.

Southern, E.M., DNA microarrays — history and overview, *Methods Mol. Biol.*, 170, 1–15, 2001.

Steel, A.B., Herne, T.M., and Tarlov, M.J., Electrochemical quantitation of DNA immobilized on gold, *Anal. Chem.*, 70, 4670–4677, 1998.

Su, H.J., Surrey, S., McKenzie, S.E., Fortina, P., and Graves, D.J., Kinetics of heterogeneous hybridization on indium tin oxide surfaces with and without an applied potential, *Electrophoresis*, 23, 1551–1557, 2002.

Vainrub, A. and Pettitt, B.M., Surface electrostatic effects in oligonucleotide microarrays: control and optimization of binding thermodynamics, *Biopolymers*, 68, 265–270, 2003.

Vainrub, A. and Pettitt, B.M., Thermodynamics of association to a molecule immobilized in an electric double layer, *Chem. Phys. Lett.*, 323, 160–166, 2000.

Vainrub, A. and Pettitt, B.M., Coulomb blockage of hybridization in two-dimensional DNA arrays, *Phys. Rev.*, E66, art. no. 041905, 2002.

Vasiliskov, V.A., Prokopenko, D.V., and Mirzabekov, A.D., Parallel multiplex thermodynamic analysis of coaxial base stacking in DNA duplexes by oligonucleotide microchips, *Nucleic Acids Res.*, 29, 2303–2313, 2001.

Watterson, J.H., Piunno, P.A., Wust, C.C., and Krull, U.J., Effects of oligonucleotide immobilization density on selectivity of quantitative transduction of hybridization of immobilized DNA, *Langmuir*, 16, 4984–4992, 2000.

15

Biological Assays: Cellular Level

Clark T. Hung
Columbia University

Robert L. Mauck
Columbia University

CONTENTS

15.1 Introduction

The goal of this chapter is to provide general background information targeted to the researcher who is considering the incorporation of living cells into their research. With the challenges associated with understanding fundamental mechanisms of cell behavior at the complex *in vivo* level (most physiologic model), researchers have alternatively studied tissue explant cultures, cells cultured in three-dimensional cultures, and cells cultured in two-dimensional cultures (least physiologic model) (see Figure 15.1). Culturing cells *in vitro* facilitates manipulation of the cell and affords the ability to prescribe the environment of the cell with specificity (e.g., chemical and physical). We begin with an overview of tissue culture techniques relevant to the design and practice of growing cells in culture. Issues of cell source, culture medium, cell phenotypic characterization, two- and three-dimensional cultures, and cryopreservation are specifically addressed. The chapter then proceeds to describe a variety of powerful biological techniques including microscopy, flow cytometry, and molecular biology assays that are used to characterize and monitor cell function and intracellular activities of cells growing in culture.

15.2 Cell Culture

15.2.1 Cell Sources

Cells for experimental investigations can be obtained from a variety of sources including tissue-derived primary cell isolations, transformed cell lines, and clonal cell lines that are available from commercial

0-8493-1140-3/04/$0.00+$1.50

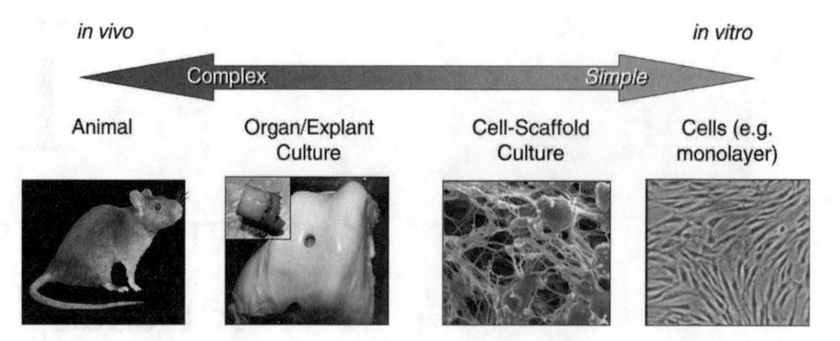

FIGURE 15.1 Schematic illustrating continuum of *in vivo* to *in vitro* models, which progress from the most physiologic condition to the least physiologic experimental condition.

cell banks (e.g., American Type Culture Collection and European Collection of Animal Cell Cultures). A cell line is derived from first passaged primary cultures. The choice of cell source is often dictated by the nature of the scientific question or application that is pursued. Established cell lines have been well studied and offer less experimental variability with the benefits of ease of procurement and maintenance. However, cell lines are considered to be further removed (with respect to primary cells) from the physiologic situation.

15.2.1.1 Primary Cells

Primary cells constitute a cell population that is directly isolated from the tissue source (e.g., fragment or whole living tissue or organ) and is a term used to refer to the original cell culture prior to passage or subculture. These "normal" cells typically have a finite life span, and exhibit contact inhibition, anchorage-dependence, and changes in characteristics with increased age in culture. These cells can also generally be passaged for several generations depending on the cell type (e.g., 50 for normal human fibroblasts). Transformed cells represent cells derived from tumors or that are genetically altered (using carcinogenic agents or viruses). Transformed cells commonly exhibit infinite life span (are immortal or continuous) and may express numerous altered characteristics.[1] The latter is not displayed by all immortalized cells.

15.2.1.2 Clonal Cell Lines

Clonal cell lines represent a population of cells that are derived from a single primary or transformed cell, resulting in a theoretically homogeneous phenotypic population. Over time, however, naturally occurring mutations can arise, causing inhomogeneity in the cell population, requiring recloning. Clonal selection permits a cell with specific characteristics to be isolated. In general, cloning of established cell lines is more successful than cloning of primary cells. While isolated primary cells behave most similarly to cells *in vivo*, since cell lines are maintained under artificial conditions *in vitro* (e.g., frozen or cultured), there exist several potential drawbacks associated with primary cells. Primary cultures rich in a particular cell type may be contaminated by extraneous cell types introduced during the isolation procedure, which gives rise to an inhomogeneous cell population. Progressive cell passaging may result in the propagation of the contaminant cells, permitting them to increase in proportion over time in culture. Although transformed cell lines are readily available, passaged routinely, and proliferate indefinitely, they may exhibit abnormal (e.g., nonphysiologic and loss of differentiated function) behavior as a result of their transformation.

Stem cells provide an alternate and continually expandable cell source. In particular, mesenchymal stem cells are pluripotent and have been isolated from bone marrow and a variety of other tissues, including perichondrium, periosteum, fat, and muscle.[2-7] Prompted by environmental cues (e.g., growth factors[8-10] and physical stimulation[11,12]), these highly proliferative cells can differentiate toward a number of different cell lineages. Alternatively, differentiated cells may be trans-differentiated to other cell types, as in the case of dermal fibroblasts exhibiting a chondrocyte-like phenotype in micromass culture in the presence of lactic acid.[13]

15.2.1.3 Cell Passaging

Cell passaging refers to the process of subculturing cells (plating, trypsinization, and replating of cells) and is a method by which the cell number can be expanded in culture. Upon culturing the cells on an intermediary surface (e.g., tissue culture ware) and then releasing the cells through disruption of cell-substrate attachments (using trypsin, mechanical cell scraping, or other agents such as versene or calcium-chelating molecules such as EGTA), the cells are deemed passaged (i.e., cell passage 1). Each subsequent subculture increases the cell passage number. Trypsinization requires rinsing of cell monolayer with a serum-free medium (serum proteins competitively inhibit enzyme activity) such as phosphate buffered saline or Hank's Balanced Salt Solution. Mild agitation may augment enzymatic activity. Cell lines are typically expanded (upon purchase) and then frozen down for storage (at low passage). Cells may then be thawed and expanded at low passage for future use as needed (see Section 15.2.4).

15.2.2 Techniques for Primary Cell Isolation

15.2.2.1 Enzymatic Cell Isolation Techniques

Enzymatic digestion techniques have been adopted for isolation of a variety of cell types, including Schwann cells,[14] smooth muscle bladder cells,[15] dermal fibroblasts,[16] endothelial cells,[17] and liver cells.[18] In general, the tissue of interest is removed aseptically (e.g., using betadine, prepodyne, ethanol wash of the external surface, and a biological hood) from the source and extraneous tissue dissected away. The tissue is typically minced so as to provide maximal surface area for subsequent enzymatic treatment. Enzymatic treatment, using an enzyme cocktail tailored to disrupt components of the particular tissue matrix with different levels of aggressiveness (trypsin, collagenase, hyaluronidase, protease, elastase, dispase), acts to dissociate the cells from their ECM. Agitation (e.g., orbital shaker, rocker plate, spinner flask) may also facilitate digestion of tissue. Different enzymes may be applied simultaneously or sequentially.

Enzymatic digestion protocols need to be optimized for cell yield and viability. Tissue debris is separated from cells using a series of filtering steps, with a filter pore size dependent on the cell type (e.g., for chondrocytes typically ~20-μm filter[19] and for osteoblast-like cells a ~45-μm filter[20]). Centrifugation of cells ($1000 \times g$) after filtering permits separation of the supernatant (enzyme solution) from the cells that have passed through the filter. The supernatant is aspirated and replaced with fresh serum-containing medium, and the cells resuspended via mild agitation to dislodge and disperse the cell pellet. Care must be taken to avoid overdigestion of tissue, which may result in decreased cell viability and altered function (e.g., from degradation of cell surface receptors). In some protocols a serial digestion is adopted, where sequential digestions are performed on the same harvested tissue, with differing cell populations released at varying time points. Extraction of osteoblast and osteoclast-like cells from neonatal rat calvaria (the skull cap) is an example of such a serial digestion.[21-23] After isolation of cells, contaminant cells or mixed populations can be separated using a variety of techniques, including selective permeabilization,[24] adherence/nonadherence to plating surfaces,[25] and cell sorting[14] (see Section 15.4, "Flow Cytometry"). If distinct cell populations are spatially distributed (e.g., stratified tissues such as articular cartilage), the tissue can be dissected in appropriate sections and digested.[26,27] Isolation techniques can also be designed to release units of cells and their associated matrix, such as chondrons that are found in articular cartilage.[28-30] Mechanical isolation of cells is an alternative mechanism, but may be more susceptible to cell damage and lower yields.

15.2.2.2 Cell Migration Isolation Techniques

Migration of cells out of tissue explants offers an alternative method for isolating primary cells. Minced tissue is plated onto tissue culture-treated dishes and, over time, cells will crawl from the tissue and migrate onto the dish. Partial enzymatic digestion of the tissue as well as addition of chemokinetic/chemotactic factors in the medium may further help to expedite outgrowth. The migration technique avoids cell damage associated with use of enzymes. However, if cells require subculture (such as for expansion), enzymatic exposure may be unavoidable. Cell isolation via migration has been used for a variety of cell types, including bone cells,[31-33] knee ligament fibroblasts[34-36] (see Figure 15.2), and skin

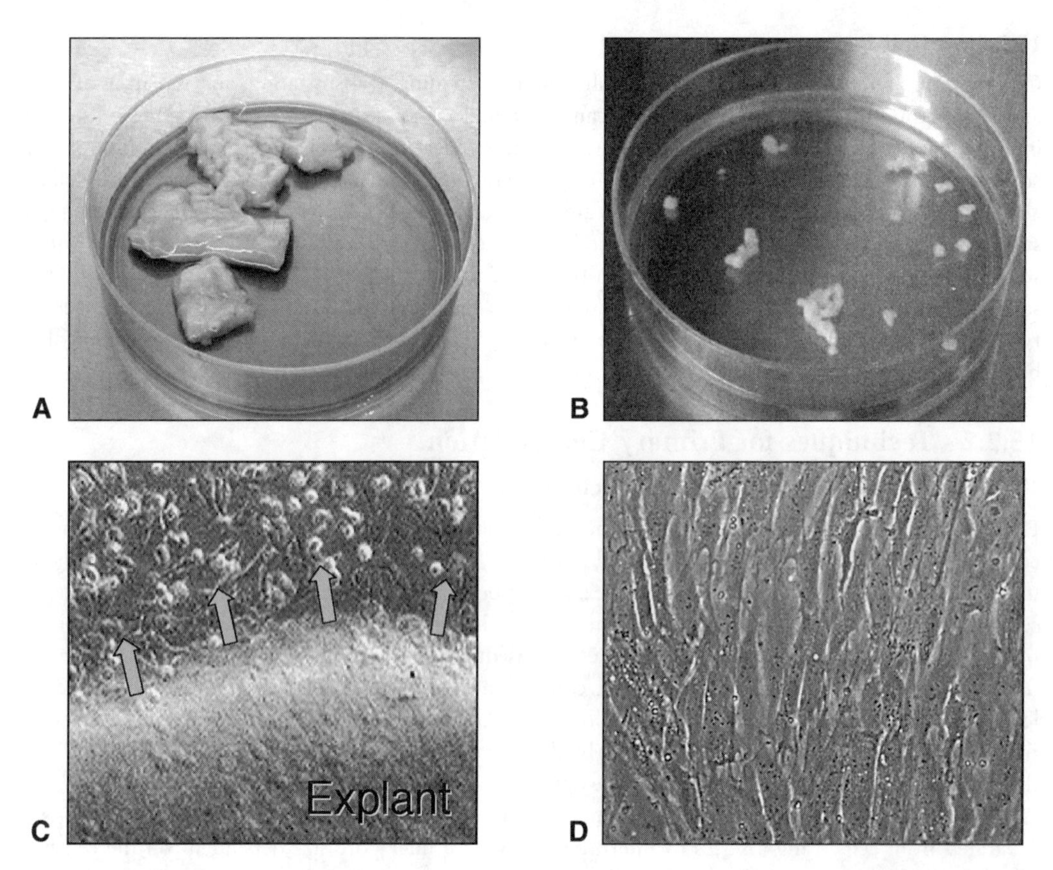

FIGURE 15.2 Isolation of medial collateral ligament (MCL) knee fibroblasts from (A) tissue explant; (B) minced ligament tissue on polystyrene culture dish; (C) MCL fibroblasts migrating out of tissue explant; (D) phase contrast image of confluent MCL fibroblast monolayer.

epidermal cells.[16] Whereas bone cells can be extracted from neonatal calvarial tissue using enzymatic digestion, bone cells from mature bone, which is not amenable to enzymatic digestion due to its mineralized content, are also isolated using explant outgrowth cultures.[31]

15.2.2.3 Phenotypic Characterization

Once cells are isolated, they should be characterized for their expression of markers consistent with the desired cell type. Purity of the cell population may be assessed using molecular, biochemical, and histological analyses. The phenotypic expression of cells is, however, influenced by culturing conditions, including medium constituents, nature of plating substrate, two- or three-dimensional cultures, and the physical environment. This characterization should also be performed periodically on passaged cells for the same reasons.

15.2.3 Culturing Techniques

15.2.3.1 Tissue Culture Media

Cells are cultured in an aqueous environment from which nutrients and wastes are exchanged via diffusion. A physiologic basal medium (e.g., for primary cells, Eagle's Medium, Dulbecco's modified Eagle's Medium, Alpha MEM, or Ham's F-12 is used, whereas cell lines are typically grown in RPMI 1640, Iscove's modified Dulbecco's Medium, or DMEM/F12) is used to provide an aqueous environment for cells in culture, with cell-specific additives that may include amino acids, glucose, vitamins, and serum. Serum, typically used at 10% volume/volume, contains a cocktail of growth factors needed for

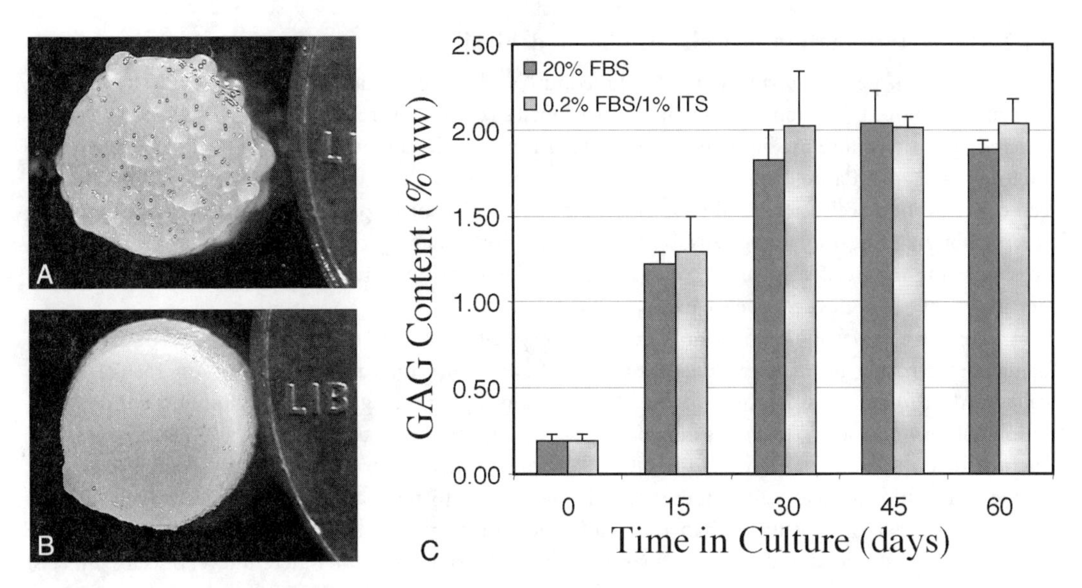

FIGURE 15.3 Chondrocyte-seeded agarose disks cultured in (A) DMEM supplemented with 20% FBS or (B) ITS (insulin, transferrin, and selenium) medium with 0.2% FBS after 45 days in culture; (C) although there were differences in the overall appearance of the disks over culture time, chondrocyte synthesis of glycosaminoglycans was comparable for each medium used (n = 3 constructs/group).

cell proliferation and maintenance, albumin (the major protein component of serum), transferrin (the major iron transport protein in vertebrates), anti-proteases, and attachment factors (e.g., fibronectin, laminin).[1] The use of serum has potential disadvantages, including batch-to-batch variations (e.g., variable absolute and relative amounts of constituents) as well as the potential for contamination by bacteria, fungi, mycoplasm, and viruses. For these reasons, serum-free medium is often desirable (commercialization or basic science studies where batch-to-batch differences are not acceptable).[37] These media are typically supplemented with factors such as growth regulators (e.g., insulin), transport proteins (e.g., transferrin), and trace elements (e.g., selenium)[38] (see Figure 15.3). Cultureware (not presterilized commercially) is sterilized using alcohol (70% ethanol) rinse, ultraviolet irradiation (~20 min), and ethylene oxide (caution should be used to ensure that the gas has completely dissipated before using); and growth media are typically sterilized via sterile filtering (typically ~0.2-μm pore size). Certain liquids used in tissue culture (e.g., water) can also be autoclaved (with slow venting).

Acid and base maintenance of the medium is regulated using organic buffers such as HEPES, TES, and BES. Sodium bicarbonate buffer-supplemented medium in conjunction with a carbon dioxide incubator is a common buffering system for tissue culture. Phenol red is a convenient indicator of medium pH, where a more orange appearance indicates an acidic environment and a violet appearance indicates an alkaline environment. Physiologic osmolality (typically ~300 mOsmol/kg) must also be maintained, with some studies using bovine serum albumin (major protein component of serum) in place of serum in studies where growth factors (in serum) are undesirable. Antibiotics such as penicillin/streptomycin/neomycin as well as antifungal agents (e.g., amphotericin, nystatin) can be added. Medium changes are typically performed daily or every other day depending on metabolic activities of the cultures. Tissue culture incubators add 5% carbon dioxide (95% air) and maintain a fully humidified environment at 37°C, thereby preventing medium evaporation and inadvertent changes to medium osmolality. Different oxygen tensions can also be used to create a hypoxic environment.[39,40] Medium supplementation with cell-specific agents may be added to promote cell expansion, and maintenance of cell phenotype-function, or to optimize cell function-synthetic activities.[16,25,41,42] Metabolites (e.g., glucose, proline), co-factors (e.g., ascorbate), and mineral salts (e.g., calcium/magnesium that are important for enzyme function and cell adhesion) are often added as well.[16]

15.2.3.2 Determination of Cell Number and Viability

Once cells are suspended, serum-containing medium is added to quench the enzymatic activity followed by centrifugation. Upon removal of the supernatant (enzyme-culture medium), the cells can be resuspended in tissue culture medium and counted. Counting of cells can be performed using the trypan blue exclusion assay with a light microscope and hemacytometer, yielding the percentage of viable cells and cell concentration (cells per milliliter). The molecular weight of trypan blue excludes it from crossing the membrane of healthy living cells, staining the interior of damaged or dead cells blue. Given the cell concentration for a cell suspension, cell plating (e.g., cells per unit area) or seeding densities (e.g., cells per unit volume) at desired levels can be achieved.

Assessment of cell viability in monolayer culture, explant tissues and tissue constructs can be performed using commercially available live/dead assays and fluorescence microscopy (see Section 15.3.2), where calcein-AM (excitation 495 nm/emission 520 nm) stains living cells green and propidium iodide (excitation 530 nm/emission 615 nm) stains dead cells red. This assay is useful for a variety of applications such as determination of nutrient limitations in three-dimensional culture or tissue impact loading studies.[43] For biochemical assays, there may also be a need to normalize cell activities by cell number rather than use absolute values. Changes or differences in the production of cell products, for example, may be due to variations in the cell number rather than differences in the inherent level of cell synthesis. Dyes that bind specifically to negatively charged DNA, such as Hoechst 33258 dye, require a cuvette or microplate fluorometer, or epifluorescence microscopy system equipped to quantify DNA. Using ultraviolet (365-nm wavelength) excitation, the bound Hoechst dye emits light at 465 nm. The fluorescence emission of Hoechst dye is 400-fold lower when bound to RNA than to DNA.[44] Cell number can be determined by using a conversion factor for DNA per cell (e.g., 7.7 pg of DNA per cell for chondrocytes[45]). Such techniques are applicable to cell monolayers and tissues.[44,45] PicoGreen (excitation 480 nm/emission 520 nm) is another readily available dye for DNA quantification.[46]

15.2.3.3 Two-Dimensional Cultures

Certain cells are anchorage dependent and will grow and function only when adhered to physical surfaces. Cell attachment on tissue culture plastic, glass, or porous filter membranes commonly used for cultivating anchorage-dependent cells relies in part on medium constituents (such as fibronectin or laminin found in serum) that adsorb to the substrate surface and promote cell-substrate binding via integrins[47] (see Figure 15.2d). Surface treatments such as gas-plasma discharge (e.g., tissue culture plastic) or acid wash can also make the surface more wettable. Surface coating with biopolymers (poly-D-lysine, poly-L-lysine) or purified matrix components (e.g., fibronectin, laminin, or collagens I and IV) are also used to enhance cell adhesion, spreading and proliferation on glass and plastic substrates. Biosubstrates such as the complex basement membrane extracellular matrix Matrigel can also be used.[1] Cell–cell interactions can be manipulated by cell seeding density (i.e., proximity of cells to one another). Preconfluent cultures are relatively sparse, while confluent cultures exhibit cell-to-cell abutment and limited cell division due to contact inhibition. Micropatterning techniques that permit selective spatial adsorption of cell substrates at the microscale have also been used to tailor design of cell shape, spatial organization of cells, and cell–cell interactions.[18,48,49,50-55]

15.2.3.4 Three-Dimensional Cultures

Behavior of cells in two- and three-dimensional culture may be different, with the latter representing in most instances a more physiologic environment.[56,57] Cells can be maintained in their physiologic three-dimensional environment (preserving *in situ* cell–matrix and cell–cell interactions) using explant cultures. In explant cultures, whole or fragments of tissue are cultured and sustained by the growth medium in which they are submerged. Calvarial cultures,[58] neuronal tissue slice cultures,[59] cartilage explants,[60] and flexor tendons[61] have been maintained in such a manner. However, the complexities of the native tissue (e.g., inhomogeneous properties and variable cell populations) may not be suitable for certain studies. In such cases, there are several potential options for studying cells using a three-dimensional culture system. Micromass cultures (adherent cells in high-density spot cultures) represent

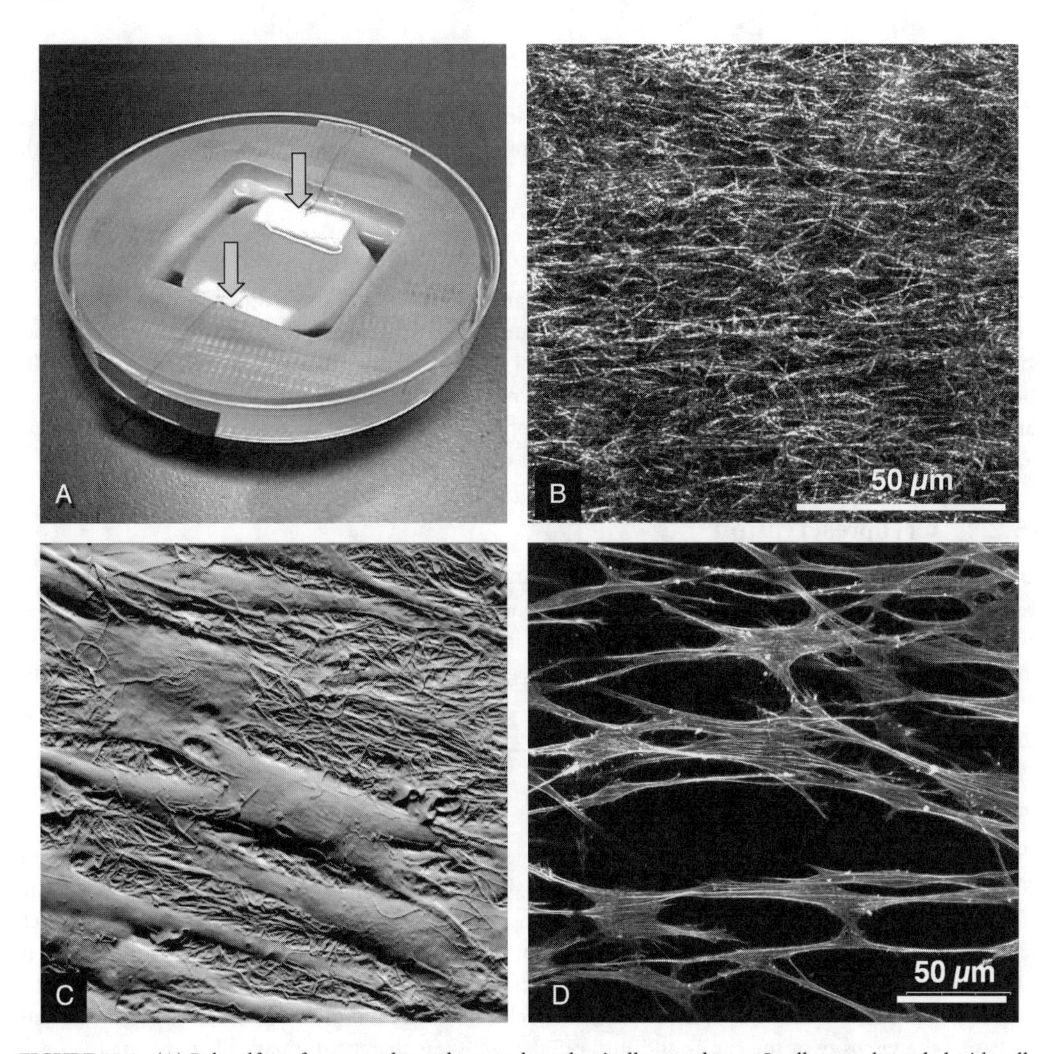

FIGURE 15.4 (A) Polysulfone frame used to culture and mechanically stretch type I collagen gels seeded with cells. Porous polyethylene anchors permit mechanical loading via tension applied to sutures (arrows) in order to study contractile response of dermal and cardiac fibroblasts to controlled loading. (B) Confocal reflectance microscopy of collagen gel formed by dermal fibroblast alignment (488 nm laser epi-illumination, PMT using blue reflection filter, 60× 1.4 NA oil immersion objective at 1024 × 1024 pixels). (C) Contact mode atomic force microscopy (Bioscope, Digital Instruments), deflection image with 100 × 100 μm scan size, of dermal fibroblasts in 3-D collagen gel matrix aligned as above. (D) Confocal microscopy image of rhodamine phalloidin labeling of actin cytoskeleton of dermal fibroblasts that were subjected to uniaxial tension (note parallel alignment with direction of loading). (Courtesy of Kevin D. Costa and Jeffrey Holmes, Columbia University, New York.)

transition from two-dimensional monolayer to three-dimensional culture systems.[62] Cells can be cultured as a cell suspension over a surface that discourages cell adhesion (e.g., tissue culture surface coated with agarose). Similarly, pellet cultures of centrifuged cells have been studied, permitting the study of three-dimensional cell–cell interactions.[25,29] Cells can also be suspended in biocompatible hydrogels (e.g., agarose) (see Figure 15.3) or sodium alginate,[63] fibrin,[64] and collagen[65-67] (see Figure 15.4), on commercially available microcarrier beads of various materials (e.g., collagen, dextran, polystyrene[68]), and on biodegradable scaffolds (e.g., PGA, PLLA) that have different properties and confer varying cell-matrix interactions. The latter will be reviewed in Chapter 19, and are designed to optimize diffusion of nutrients and cell function in a physiologic three-dimensional environment.[69] Cell expansion or tissue growth bioreactors can be used with cells alone or cells on carriers or seeded in scaffolds. Commercially available bioreactor systems for culturing cells include flow perfusion (e.g., hollow fiber)[70] or permeation systems,[71,72] rotating wall vessels (RWV),[73,74] spinner flasks, and mixing bioreactors.[75,76] These bioreactors are aimed at optimizing nutrient availability to cells and growing tissue constructs as well as providing a hydrodynamic environment conducive for cell/tissue growth (e.g., Gooch et al.[77]). Other bioreactors are aimed at the application of specific mechanical stimuli for study of cell physical regulation and long-term growth.[63,78]

15.2.3.5 Co-Cultures

Co-cultures of multiple cell types can also be maintained in two- and three-dimensional culture conditions, such as hepatocytes and 3T3 fibroblasts,[49] neurons and Schwann cells,[42] smooth muscle cells and chondrocytes,[79] smooth muscle cells and endothelial cells,[80] and endothelial cells and fibroblasts.[81] In these systems, culture conditions may need to be optimized for maintaining multiple phenotypes simultaneously. Co-culturing cells *in vitro* may reestablish physiologically relevant interactions or relationships between different types of cells that are necessary for optimal growth.

15.2.4 Cryopreservation

Cryopreservation is important for long-term preservation and storage of living cells and tissues.[82-84] When freezing cells, the number of passages from the original must be minimized (i.e., early passage material available for new working stock). Cryopreservation involves dramatic temperature drops (e.g., from a physiologic +37°C to the boiling point of liquid nitrogen –196°C) accompanied by significant cell water efflux mediated by differential intracellular and extracellular electrolyte concentration during the freezing process.[83] The application of cryoprotectant agents has been used to minimize cell injury and to control ice formation during cell freezing.

15.2.4.1 Crypoprotectants

The most common cryoprotective agents are the cell-permeating dimethylsulfoxide (DMSO) and glycerol (5 to 10% v/v reagent grade or better).[85] In general, cryoprotectants increase the osmolarity of the extracellular solution, thereby depressing the freezing point (to about –5°C) and encouraging greater dehydration of the cells prior to intracellular freezing (thereby reducing intracellular ice formation). It is thought that permeating cryoprotectants reduce cell injury due to solution effects by reducing potentially harmful concentrations of electrolytes in the cell, stabilizing cell proteins or cell membranes, and increasing the viscosity of the extra- and intracellular solutions thereby dramatically reducing the rates of ice nucleation and crystal growth.[83] In addition to these potential mechanisms above, DMSO and glycerol are thought to act by increasing the permeability of the membrane and thus the water flux across the cell membrane during the freezing and thawing process. The rate of water efflux is proportional to the magnitude of the driving force (i.e., the osmotic pressure difference across the membrane) and the permeability for the plasma membrane to water. Knowledge of the hydraulic permeability of the cell membrane is therefore useful in efforts to optimize protocols for cell freezing.[86-90] Glycerol may be sterilized by autoclaving for 15 min at 121°C and 15 psig. DMSO must be sterilized by filtration using a 0.2-μm nylon syringe filter. While glycerol is less toxic than DMSO for most cells, DMSO is more penetrating, and is usually preferred when using larger, more complex cells.

15.2.4.2 Freezing Process

Ice forms at different rates during the cooling process.[90] A uniform cooling rate of 1°C/min from ambient temperature is effective for cryopreserving a wide variety of cells and can be performed effectively using commercially available freezing containers (e.g., Nalgene "Mr. Frosty"[85]). Despite the control applied to the cooling of the cells, most of the water present will freeze at approximately –2 to –5°C. Cooling at rates too rapid is associated with intracellular ice formation, and membrane rupture due to osmotic fluxes. With too slow cooling, cell injury is thought to arise from exposure to highly concentrated intra- and extracellular solutions ("solution effects") or to mechanical interactions between cells and the extracellular ice.[91] Induction of gas bubble formation by intracellular ice, or osmotic effects due to the melting of intracellular ice during warming, may also give rise to cell injury. Generally, the larger the cell, the more critical slow cooling becomes. In practice, cell suspensions are mixed in equal parts with cryoprotectant solution followed by equilibration for ~15 min at room temperature. Cells can be aliquoted into cryovials (sealed airtight) using 0.5- to 1-ml volume for commonly used vial sizes (1 to 2 ml), frozen at –20°C for several hours, and then transferred to a –60 to –80°C freezer for 48 h (acceptable for temporary short-term storage). Last, for long-term storage, vials should be transferred to liquid nitrogen (<–130°C).[1]

15.2.4.3 Thawing Process

Cryoprotective chemicals can themselves be damaging to cells. For most cells, warming from the frozen state should occur as rapidly as possible until complete thawing is achieved. The contents of the vial should be transferred to fresh growth medium following thawing to minimize exposure to the cryoprotective agent. Furthermore, addition and removal of cryoprotectants before and after cryopreservation can cause damage to cells due to excessive osmotic forces. Accordingly, cryoprotectants are usually added and removed gradually, changing the concentration of the extracellular solution in a stepwise fashion. Thawing protocols using a gradual addition of medium to the frozen cells, dilution protocols or initial resuspension in medium containing impermeant solutes of similar tonicity as the crypoprotectant solution may facilitate diffusion of the cryoprotectant out of the cell during the thawing process.[1] Generally, the greater number of cells (typically 10^6 to 10^7 cells/ml) initially frozen down, the greater the recovery.[85] Ultimately, cell viability upon recovery will determine the efficacy of the cryopreservation protocol.

15.3 General Microscopy Principles

Various microscopy tools take advantage of interactions when light strikes an object, namely, that incident light waves can be absorbed, reflected, refracted, polarized, diffracted or cause resultant fluorescence. Several microscopy techniques that are commonly applied to the study of cells are presented in this section. Resolution of a microscope objective is defined as the smallest distance (R) that two distinct points on a specimen can be distinguished as such (Rayleigh criterion). Numerical aperture (NA) is a measure of the ability to gather light and resolve fine specimen detail at a fixed object distance. Resolution is given by the expression $R = 0.61\lambda/(NA_{obj})$, where $NA = n\sin\alpha$ where α is the aperture angle, n = refractive index ($n_{air} = 0.95$, $n_{oil} = 1.35 - 1.4$), and λ is the wavelength of light.[92] The limit of resolution is 100 to 250 nm, depending on the optics and wavelength of light applied.[93] For bright-field applications, brightness varies as $(NA)^2/(\text{magnification})^2$. The higher the NA of the total system, the better the resolution and the shallower the depth of field. Depth of field, related to the axial resolving power along the optical axis, is proportional to the inverse of $(NA)^2$ and is defined as the thickness of the optical section that can be brought into focus. Portions of the object out of this plane of focus (i.e., over and under the section) degrade the quality of the image. In practice, having a higher NA (horizontal resolving power) and magnification are accompanied by disadvantages of very shallow depth of field (more image degradation due to blurred background) and short working distance.

15.3.1 Light Microscopy

Brightfield microscopy, used with transmitted or reflected (epi-illuminated) light from a tungsten-halogen lamp source, is considered the most basic of the imaging modes, with illuminating rays entering the objective lens and "lighting up the background." The image results from illumination that falls on to the specimen emanating from within the aperture angle of the objective, while illumination from outside this angle provides a dark-ground image.[94] Since brightfield microscopy provides low intrinsic contrast, other techniques have been developed for contrast enhancement. Contrast is the degree to which the object of interest is separated from its background in terms of color and/or brightness.[94] Contrast results from interactions between the specimen with light. For opaque specimens (that absorb light), epi-illumination is used to illuminate the specimen from the same side of the objective. Transparent specimens (such as living cells and unstained specimens) are typically illuminated from the opposite side of the objective, or transmitted illumination. Using transmitted light, contrast of stained biological sections and histochemical reactions that yield colored end products arises from selective absorption of light in the visible spectrum (resulting in a change in color of the transmitted light). Contrast of transparent specimens can also be enhanced through use of monochromatic light, in particular green (550 nm, in the peak sensitivity range of the human visual perception system) that is well known to minimize chromatic and spherical aberrations in standard achromatic objectives.[94]

Diffraction results when an object with regularly repeating features produces an orderly redistribution of light (diffraction pattern). It can also be used to enhance contrast of transparent microscopic specimens, in particular accentuating borders.[94] In *phase-contrast*, the phase difference between the direct and diffracted rays (one-quarter wavelength out of phase), and their relative amplitudes, can be altered to produce conditions for interference and increased contrast.[94] Phase contrast is ideal for contrast enhancement of nonabsorbing, thin objects that have no large refraction differences (or halos will be introduced) (see Figure 15.2d). *Differential interference contrast* based on principles by Nomarski yields in-focus, high contrast, shadowcast images of phase details in which the direction of shadowing is opposite for phase-advancing and phase-retarding details. Because DIC is an optical technique to generate contrast, the image may not reflect actual topography and features of the cell, thereby being more qualitative than quantitative. *Hoffman modulation contrast* is another contrast-enhancement technique used to increase specimen visibility and contrast for unstained and living specimens, also creating a pseudo-three-dimensional effect. This technique is sensitive to gradients of optical path length and produces an asymmetrical, directional image with phase gradients in one direction always rendered bright and those in the opposite direction dark.[94] Interpretation of modulation contrast should be made with the same caveat as DIC. Phase contrast, DIC and modulation contrast are generally considered complementary techniques, with the latter more suitable for observation of relatively thick objects.[92] *Polarized light microscopy* is a contrast-enhancing technique that improves image quality of birefringent materials due to their anisotropic character.

15.3.2 Fluorescent Microscopy

15.3.2.1 Fluorophores

Fluorophores are molecules capable of absorbing and then reradiating secondary light (i.e., fluorescence). The latter continues as long as the excitation light is applied. When conjugated to antibodies, fluorophores bind specifically to targets and can be used for a variety of biological studies (e.g., identification of submicroscopic cellular components [see Figures 15.6 and 15.7], cell signaling, intracellular trafficking, gene reporter assays), as reviewed by Oksvold and co-workers.[100] Fluorescent probes can be used, for example, to monitor rapidly changing intracellular calcium levels real-time using the ratiometric dye fura-2AM (see Figure 15.5),[95,96] as well as to monitor cytoskeletal microtubule reorganization in living cells using green fluorescent protein (GFP)[97] (see Figure 15.6). Upon absorbing the excitation light, electrons are raised to a higher vibrational energy state and rapidly (~1 billionth of a second) undergo a loss of vibrational energy, returning to the ground state with a simultaneous emission of fluorescent light. Due to Stoke's shift, this emission wavelength is always of longer wavelength than the excitation wavelength (i.e., the emission spectrum is shifted to longer wavelengths than the excitation spectrum). Fluorophores have a peak excitation/fluorescence corresponding to a peak emission/fluorescence intensity, which can be applied in practice using a combination of appropriate excitation filters (that only permit specific excitation wavelengths to pass), dichromatic beamsplitters (or dichroic mirrors, designed to enhance or block transmission and reflectance at specific wavelengths), and barrier filters (designed to block or transmit fluorescence below and above a particular wavelength, respectively). The intensity of the fluorescence emission may be reduced (called fading) due to photobleaching or quenching. Irreversible decomposition of the fluorescent molecules due to light intensity in the presence of molecular oxygen is referred to as bleaching. Photobleaching gives rise to the technique fluorescence recovery after photobleaching (FRAP). Quenching results from transfer of energy to other so-called acceptor molecules (resonance energy transfer) in close proximity, and serves as the basis for fluorescence resonance energy transfer (FRET).

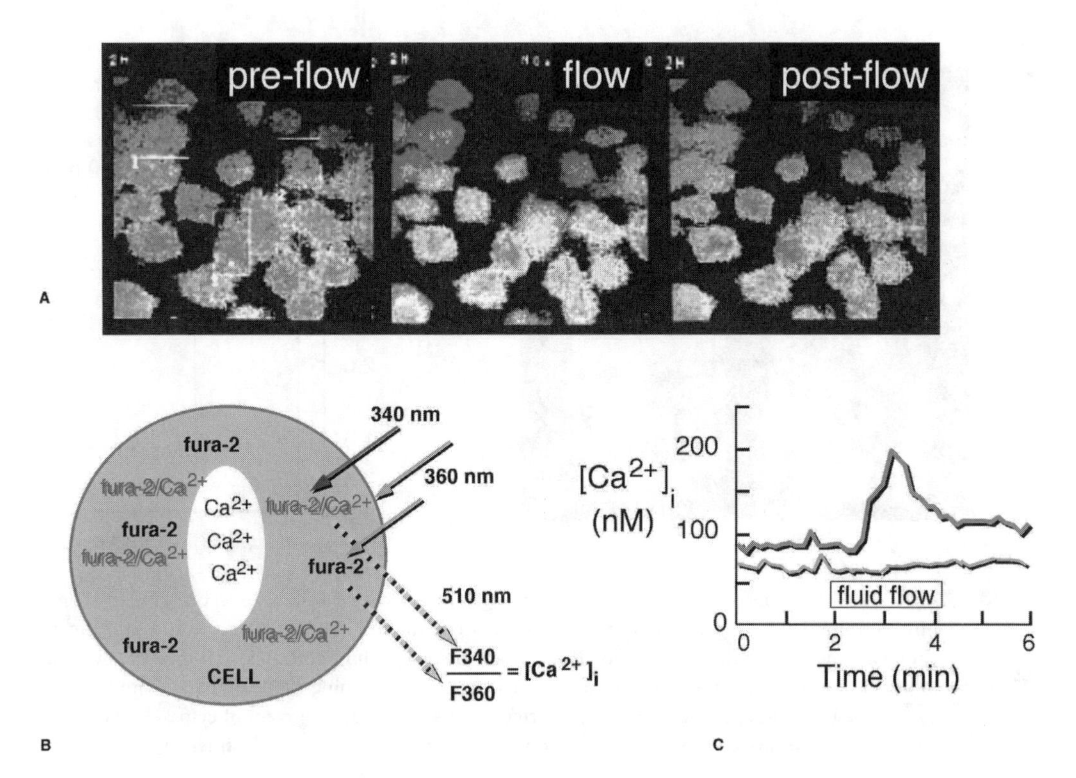

FIGURE 15.5 Real-time intracellular calcium response, $[Ca^{2+}]_i$, of primary bone cells (derived from rat calvaria) subjected to fluid-induced shear stress (35 dynes/cm^2), using the calcium indicator dye fura-2 and fluorescence microscopy, and a parallel-plate flow chamber.[232] (A) Light intensity was recorded with a CCD camera, and converted to pseudocolor (blue/green for low levels, orange/red for high levels) for visualization and analysis. Olympus software was used to subtract background noise and single cells selected for analysis by boxing or tracing of the cell contour. (B) The cell-permeant acetoxymethyl ester form of the dye, Fura-2 AM, was loaded into living cells using DMSO and Pluronic®-127 in a buffered saline solution. Upon entering, the AM tail is cleaved by endogenous esterase activity, trapping fura-2 within the cytoplasm.[95,96] (C) Fura-2 is a ratiometric dye, which has the advantage of minimizing artifacts of motion, uneven dye loading, and dye leakage. Rapidly alternating 340/360-nm excitation wavelengths are used to elicit 510-nm wavelength emissions from calcium-bound dye and the fura-2 isobestic point (calcium concentration insensitive),[20] respectively. The ratio of the 510-nm emissions from the R = 340/360 nm is compared to a calibration curve, providing a real-time measure to get $[Ca^{2+}]_i$.

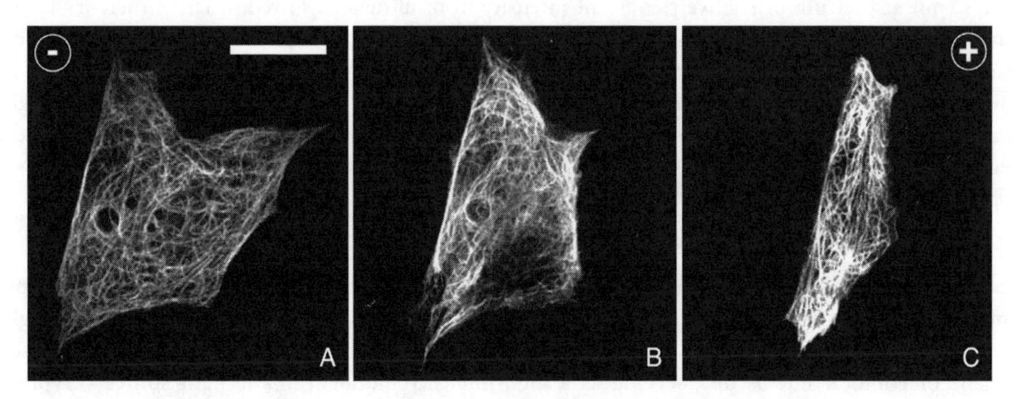

FIGURE 15.6 Confocal microscopy image of NIH3T3 fibroblasts[191] stably transfected with GFP labeled microtubule associating protein that enables real-time visualization of changes to microtubule organization. Microtubule reorganization of a single cell in response to direct current electric field, at a field strength of 6 V/cm, at (A) time = 0 h, (B) time = 1.5 h, and (C) time = 3 h. The (+) and (–) indicate direction of field. The scale bar represents 10 μm. (Courtesy of P.H. Grace Chao, Clark Hung, and Chloe Bulinski, Columbia University, New York.)

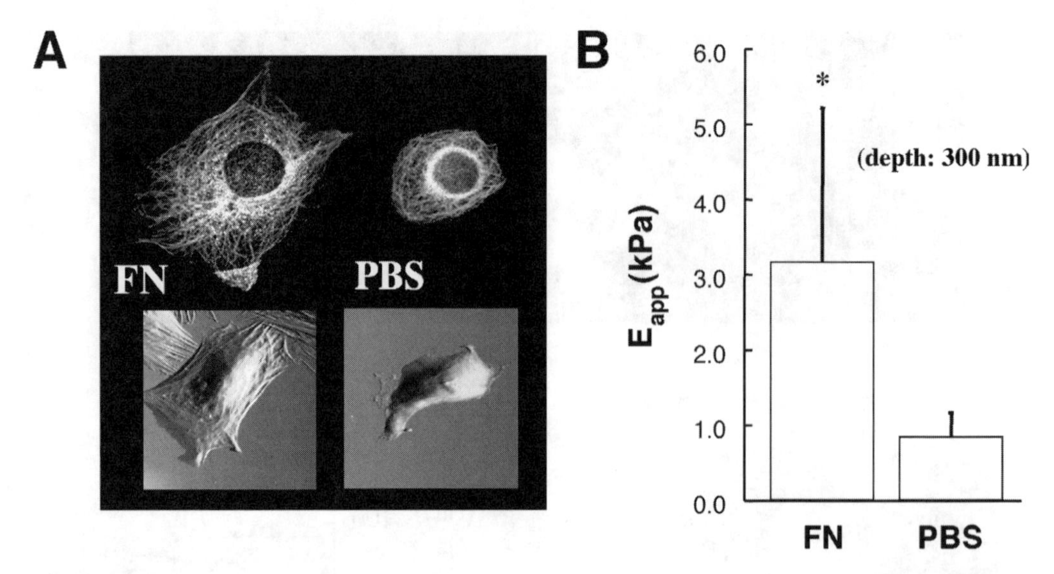

FIGURE 15.7 MC3T3-E1 osteoblast-like cell line cultured on glass slides coated with fibronectin (FN) and control phosphate buffered saline (PBS).[233] (A) Using confocal microscopy, double staining of actin and vinculin was performed to compare the cytoskeletal organization due to the different plating substrates. Cell topography images obtained from atomic force microscope (Digital Instruments) using the scanning mode and (B) complementary modulus data using the indentation mode were also performed.[140] A stronger development of cytoskeletal organization in the fibronectin-coated surface appears to correspond with increased spreading and stiffening of the cell.

15.3.2.2 Conventional Fluorescence Microscopy

In fluorescence microscopy with epifluorescence vs. transmitted illumination, excitation light is focused by the objective on to the microscope field, after which the same lens system collects the fluorescence emission light.[92] Because the brightness of the image in epifluorescence microscopy is proportional to the $(NA_{obj})^4/(magnification)^2$,[98] an objective with the lowest overall magnification having acceptable resolution and the highest light-gathering power yields the best results.[99] Observation of thick specimens yields an image that is the sum of the sharp in-focus image and the blurred image of regions that are out of focus (see advantages of confocal microscopy). A xenon or mercury lamp that produces a high-intensity illumination (arc discharge lamps have an average lifetime of 200 h) is usually used. Xenon lamps emit a spectrum of relatively constant intensity from ultraviolet to red, whereas mercury lamps have distinct peaks in the emission spectrum (360-ultraviolet, 405-violet, 546-green, and 578-yellow nm), making the latter generally more flexible with respect to usable fluorophores in fluorescence microscopy.[92] The choice of *fluorophores* should be based on the compatibility of the excitation maximum with light source (lamp or laser), resistance to photobleaching (when strong or prolonged excitation is needed), avoidance of overlapping emissions that can disrupt multistaining studies (see Figure 15.7a), and fluorophore size, which may impede staining penetration.[100]

15.3.2.3 Scanning Confocal Fluorescence Microscopy

Scanning "confocal" microscopy derives from the fact that the illumination spot on the microscopic object is exactly imaged on the detector.[92] The microscopic field is scanned by a small focused light spot that is directed across the microscopic object by computer-controlled mirrors. Lasers are used widely for confocal microscopy, serving as a high-intensity monochromatic light source (krypton, argon, neon, helium) (see Figures 15.4d, 15.6, 15.7a). Compared to conventional fluorescence microscopy, confocal microscopy offers increased resolution, ~1.4-fold,[100-102] and improved resolution for thicker specimens (5 to 15 μm) which are a greater source of out-of-focus, extraneous background fluorescence. Confocal microscopy achieves this enhanced resolution by providing a controllable depth of field, elimination of out-of-focus information (from outside the plane of focus) using a pair of pinhole apertures, and the ability to acquire serial optical sections from thick specimens. From serial optical sections, three-dimensional reconstruction using digital imaging tools of scans in the xz and xy plane provide spatial localization of molecules of interest in the z-direction that may not be discernible in horizontal (xy) scan or conventional microscopy (e.g., localization at the surface or just below). The confocal has superior horizontal resolution, however, compared to vertical resolution. For applications requiring real-time acquisition under low light conditions, a conventional fluorescence microscopy system with a digital camera may yield better results. Low light conditions necessitate a larger pinhole size that decreases the signal-to-noise ratio (permitting more background out-of-focus light) by reducing the resolution and increasing the thickness of optical sections. More recently, fiber-optic monitoring coupled with confocal microscopy (e.g., endoscope) has permitted imaging of gene expression *in vitro* and *in vivo* using GFP-labeled probes.[103]

15.3.2.4 Multiphoton Confocal Microscopy

Multiphoton confocal microscopy involves the integration of confocal scanning microscopy with near-infrared, long-wavelength multiphoton fluorescence excitation. In dual photon microscopy, as an example, excitation arises from the simultaneous absorption of two photons by the fluorophore.[102,104,105] This reflects the fact that the radiation energy is linearly proportional to the inverse of the wavelength (Planck's law), meaning that radiation from a short wavelength has a higher quantum energy than from long wavelengths.[92] As an illustration, one 350-nm absorption (ultraviolet) is equivalent to two simultaneously applied 700-nm absorptions (red). Pulsed lasers are used to increase the photon density necessary to achieve the latter with an average power that is only slightly higher than in confocal microscopy.[100] This technique is ideal for applications with living cells, and has several advantages over conventional confocal microscopy; it minimizes photobleaching and cell damage since two-photon excitation is restricted to only the focal point of the microscope. Additionally, sample penetration is increased (often two- to threefold). The resolution in multiphoton confocal microscopy, however, may be decreased due to the longer excitation wavelengths used.

15.3.2.5 Total Internal Reflection Fluorescence Microscopy (TIRFM)

Total internal reflection fluorescence microscopy is used to observe molecule-surface interactions.[106,107] The technique is based on Snell's law, the principle that when light hits a less dense medium beyond a certain angle it is reflected. Such interfaces exist at the culture dish/slide-cell interface or cell-culture medium interface. At a critical angle, the incident light is completely reflected. However, the reflection generates an electromagnetic field or evansescent wave (illuminating less than a few tenths of a micrometer) in the aqueous media that decays exponentially in magnitude with distance from the interface. For fluorescence applications, the exponential decay permits fluorophores beyond the surface (and out of the focus plane) from being excited. This effect gives rise to a powerful methodology to visualize interface events with an increased signal-to-background ratio over traditional widefield techniques. Applications include study of ligand-receptor interactions, cytoskeletal and membrane dynamics, and cell/stratum contacts.[100,108,109]

15.3.2.6 Fluorescence Recovery after Photobleaching (FRAP)

Fluorescence recovery after photobleaching is a technique to monitor the mobility and dynamics of fluorescent proteins (e.g., References 110–113). Fluorescent-tagged proteins are irreversibly photobleached in a small region of the specimen using maximal laser intensity. The redistribution of non-bleached fluorescent molecules to the photobleached region is then visualized in the microscope.

15.3.2.7 Fluorescence Correlation Microscopy (FCM)

Fluorescence correlation microscopy measures the emission fluctuations arising from diffusion of fluorescently labeled molecules in and out of a defined volume with a spatial resolution of fractions of femtoliters. These fluctuations reflect the average number of labeled molecules in the volume, as well as the characteristic diffusion time of each molecule across the defined volume (see review in References 114–116).

15.3.2.8 Fluorescence Resonance Energy Transfer (FRET)

Fluorescence resonance energy transfer is a technique to detect direct protein–protein interactions, and is made possible with fluorescent tags that have overlapping fluorescence spectra.[100,117,118] When two overlapping fluorophores are located within 5 nm of one another, the excitation of the lower wavelength fluorophore induces energy transfer to the neighboring higher wavelength fluorophore.[119] Alternatively, when energy is transferred to a nearby nonfluorescent molecule, an attenuation of the emission can be detected. Energy transfer also protects against fading, which can be exploited to detect protein interaction.

15.3.3 Atomic Force Microscopy

Since its invention nearly two decades ago,[120] the atomic force microscope (AFM) has become the most widely used tool for studying mechanical properties of living cells. Atomic force microscopy involves tracking the deflection of a small (200 to 300 μm long) cantilever probe as its tip (~50-nm radius of curvature) scans, indents, or otherwise probes the sample. In particular, nano-indentation with AFM is well suited for cell mechanics applications due to its high sensitivity (subnano-Newton), high spatial resolution (submicron), and the ability to be used for real-time measurements in an aqueous cell culture environment in conjunction with an inverted microscope (see Figures 15.4b and 15.7a). In recent years the AFM has been widely used to study the mechanical properties of cells and other soft samples. AFM has been used to monitor mechanical changes associated with platelet activation,[121,122] cell locomotion,[123] and myocyte contraction at the subcellular level,[124] and to examine the effects of chemical treatments that target specific cytoskeletal constituents.[125,126] Among these many studies, some findings have shown regional differences on the nucleus compared to the cytoplasm,[127-132] the actin cytoskeleton appears to be largely responsible for cell stiffness,[125,126,130,133,134] and in some cases regions of altered perinuclear stiffness have been identified but could not be correlated with a specific cytoskeletal structure.[132]

Only through computational methods can we accurately model the interaction between the AFM probe and the sample, and ultimately extract a correct mathematical representation of the material properties of living cells. There are limitations, however, in the predominant method of analyzing AFM indentation data (the so-called Hertz theory[135-137]) for studies of cells.[138,139] Costa and Yin[140] have recently published a new analysis method for AFM indentation data whereby accounting for the indenter geometry to compute an apparent elastic modulus as a function of indentation depth can reveal nonlinearity and heterogeneity of material properties from AFM indentation tests. An important advantage of AFM over other cell mechanics techniques is the ability to combine high-resolution scanning with microindentation, which allows direct correlation of local mechanical properties with underlying cytoskeletal structures[126,132] (see Figure 15.7). In addition, the geometry of the probe tip can be modified relatively easily to allow measurements over a range of length scales from submicron to tens of microns. This feature is especially useful for testing the applicability of continuum models for describing cellular mechanical properties.

15.3.4 Digital Microscopy

Digital imaging is the process of converting visual information into numeric form, which allows the study of cells and cellular events with quantitative temporal and spatial resolution.[98] Ultrasensitive spatial cameras divide captured fluorescent images into an array of discrete picture elements (pixels), converting fluorescence intensity in each pixel to a number (e.g., 256 grayscale). These detectors permit quantitative analysis of variations in two-dimensional intensity distributions in time.[98] The choice of electronic imaging detectors is a critical determinant in the range of light detection in fluorescence applications. Compared to traditional emulsion film, digital images can be acquired using a charge-coupled device (CCD) or video camera system. Another light-detecting device is the photomultiplier tube (PMT). PMTs are photoemissive devices in which the absorption of a photon results in electron emission. These devices offer high signal-to-noise ratio and are appropriate for weak signals and can be used for recording rapid events. During acquisition, frame averaging can further improve signal-to-noise ratio, boosting detection of weakly fluorescent specimens.

Post-processing of video or electronic image acquired through an optical microscope using various digital imaging techniques permits modification of the image that may enhance features as well as the information that is yielded. This post-processing permits reversible, essentially noise-free modification of the image as an ordered matrix of integers rather than a series of analog variations in color and intensity.[100] One such digital procedure is termed deconvolution,[141,142] which can further increase the resolution of the confocal system up to ~twofold.[100,105] In deconvolution, the point-spread function of the microscope optics is used to remove out-of-focus fluorescence when a series of images at variable depths is compared. In addition to improving image quality, digital tools can also be used to extract useful information about cell and tissue properties. For example, researchers have used cell nuclei[143] and cell borders as well as the material texture to obtain material properties of cells cultured in three-dimensional scaffolds[144] and tissues.[145,146] Confocal reflection microscopy has been used to determine the fiber organization and mechanical properties of type I collagen three-dimensional matrices[147] (see Figure 15.4c), whereas an optimized digital image correlation technique using both cell nuclei (epifluorescence microscopy) and material texture has been developed by Wang and co-workers for determination of local strain fields and material properties of tissues and tissue-engineered constructs[148,149] (see Figure 15.8).

15.4 Flow Cytometry

15.4.1 Technical Background

While the microscopic techniques outlined above have furthered our insight into single cells, the advent of flow cytometry has permitted the examination of a large population of cells. The basic flow cytometry system is composed of a light source (generally a laser) for illuminating particles, a flow cell (a microfluidics channel through which single cells pass in a sheath fluid), a lens (for focusing light), a series of filters for isolating emitted light of particular wavelengths, and sensors (photomultiplier tubes) for measuring the resulting output[150-152] (see Figure 15.9). Within the flow cell, individual cells or particles emerge from an injector tip and are maintained within the optical path of the laser by hydrodynamic focusing, in which a larger volume (the sheath fluid) is forced into a smaller volume.[152] Cells generally do not mix with the sheath fluid, and flow is maintained at laminar levels. This is accomplished by differential pressure or volume injection systems. Shear stresses cause cells to orient with long axes along the flow direction. As the suspension of single cells passes through the flow cell, each cell is exposed to the laser and a number of measures are collected from the resulting light (see Figure 15.9A). Flow cytometry offers a very high throughput, with upward of 1000 cells per second screened for a number of different parameters.[150,152]

The measured parameters are generally of two different kinds: light scatter and fluorescence emission.[150,152] Light scatter describes the manner in which light interacts with the passing cells, and is collected in two different ways. First, forward scatter light is collected in line with the direction of the laser, and is a measure of the size, shape, and optical homogeneity of the object scattering the light. Forward scatter light is sensitive to surface characteristics, and can be used to determine the difference between live and dead cells.[150,152] Side scatter light is collected in the direction perpendicular to the applied laser, and provides information about the granularity of the cell. Fluorescent light originates from the excitation at particular wavelengths of fluorophores bound to or internalized by cells.[151] Fluorescent emission (at a slightly higher wavelength) is in proportion to the amount of fluorescent dye active in the field of view, and the power of the laser. The side scatter light and fluorescent light generally are collected in the same direction. The increase in the utility of flow cytometry for cellular analysis has been proportional to the development of fluorescently labeled tags of cellular components (e.g., DNA, RNA, intracellular ions, proteins, phospholipids and membrane receptors).[151]

Data generated in a flow cytometry system is collected in the flow cytometry standard (FCS) format consisting of a text header followed by a sequential listing of the measured parameter values for each particle in order of occurrence. Display of data can take a number of forms, with the two most common displays being the histogram and the dot plot.[150,152] Histograms represent the number of events (cells with

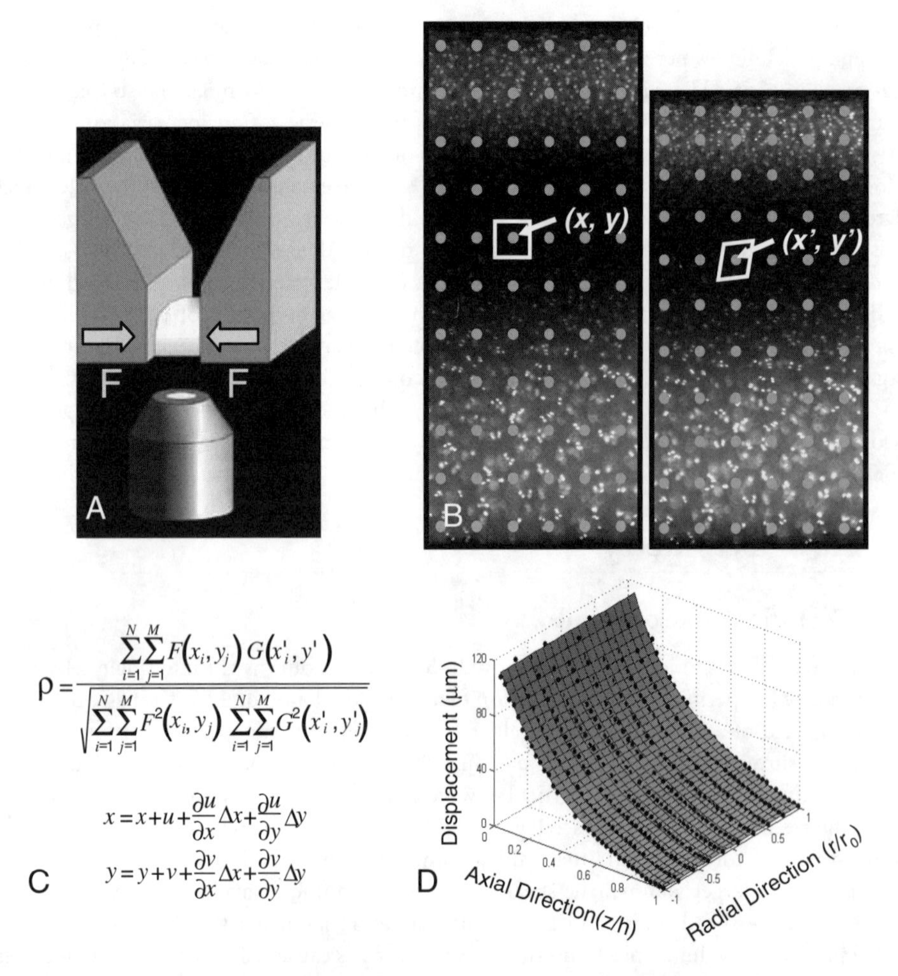

FIGURE 15.8 (A) Cell nuclei of chondrocytes in devitalized articular cartilage explant that have been labeled with Hoechst dye, which act as fiducial markers for determination of deformation fields within the tissue under applied axial loading using impermeable platens (arrows). (B) Epifluorescence microscopy (DAPI filter set) images of initially unloaded and then axially loaded cartilage specimen were obtained with a CCD camera. (C) Optimized digital image correlation was used to track the displacement of nuclei within the tissue, smoothed, and then strain fields determined.[148,149] The program automatically tracks displacements with subpixel resolution (4× objective, 1 pixel = 1.66 μm). (D) Measured displacement fields in the axial (direction of loading) and radial (perpendicular to loading) directions.

a particular measured value) vs. the magnitude of the measured values. Dot plots combine individual histograms for two separate parameters (e.g., forward scatter vs. side scatter) on one plot, with each dot indicating the occurrence of a measurement, and the position of the dot dictated by the magnitude of the measured parameters (see Figure 15.9B). This display method results in areas on the dot plot that indicate unique subsets of the whole cell population. Further information from dot plots can be gained by partitioning plots into regions to display the percentage of total cells within each grouping, giving an indication of the relative abundance of a subset of interest within the larger cell population.[150,152] With post-processing analysis, gates can be drawn around particular regions, and the cells within this gate analyzed more completely. Alternatively, gates can be used for cell sorting (commonly called fluorescent activated cell sorting, or FACS) in which a droplet containing a cell that meets the gate criteria breaks off from the stream, is given a net charge by a short burst of electricity, and then passes by charged plates as it falls, directing it into the correct sorting container.[152] Cell sorting can be further refined to identify rare cells with complex Boolean gate criteria based on the multiparameter values. These selected cells can then be used for further experiments, cultured, or stained with another dye/antibody and reanalyzed.

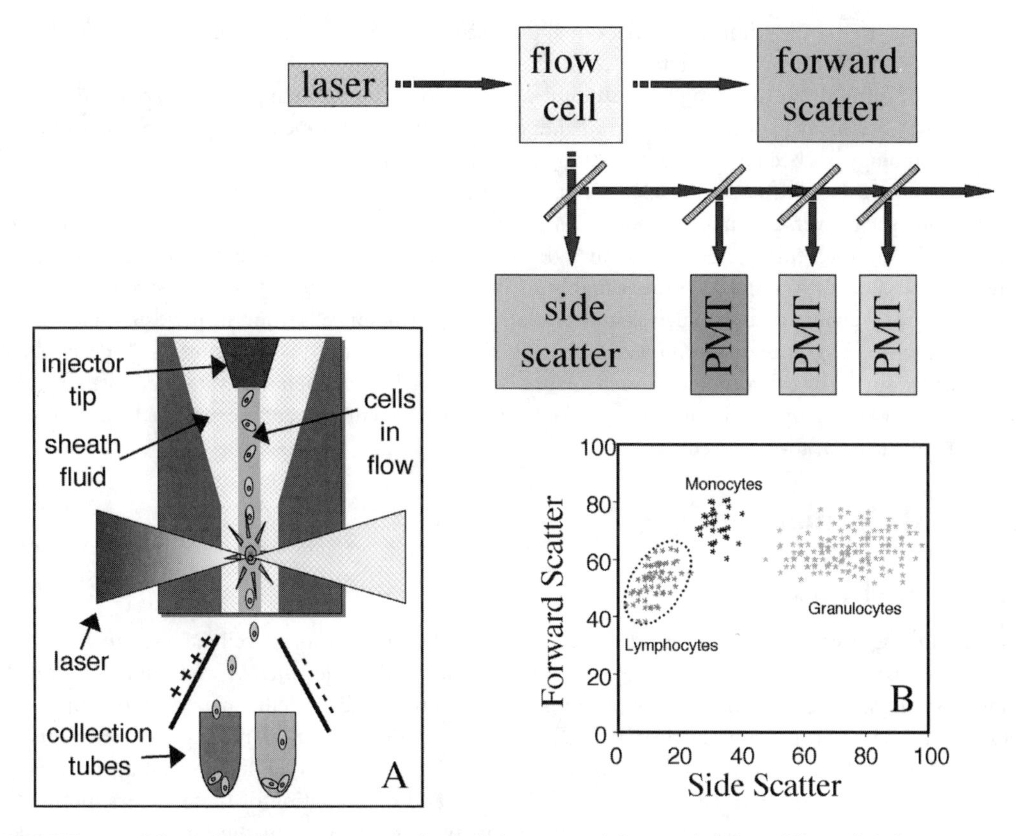

FIGURE 15.9 Schematic of flow cytometry and cell sorting system. (A) Expanded view of flow cell; (B) representative plot of scatter data for whole blood. (Adapted from Shapiro[150] and Carter and Meyer.[152])

15.4.2 Applications

Flow cytometry and cell sorting have found numerous applications in cell biology. One of the first applications of flow cytometry was determination of cell cycle by examining the ploidy of a cell population.[152] To determine ploidy, DNA amount is quantified using fluorescent nuclear binding dyes, such as propidium iodide or Hoechst, or by measuring the incorporation of BrdU in fixed samples. Such techniques are useful in the identification and prognosis of malignant cells within a larger population. Analysis of ploidy continues to find application in investigations of disease processes such as osteoarthritis,[153] as well as in the insurance of euploidy in tissue-engineered constructs that have been treated with high levels of growth factors.[154] Flow cytometry is also well suited for transient measurements of cell populations, and can effectively be used to monitor real-time intracellular changes in the pH, [Ca^{2+}], [Mg^{2+}], and membrane potential[151] of a population of cells. With increasing resolution, flow cytometry systems have become molecular flow analyzers, allowing for analysis of both full chromosomes and small DNA fragments.[155]

It was also noted early in its use that flow cytometry could identify the distinct populations of whole blood based on their distinct forward and side scatter profiles.[152] The inherent differences in populations and the characterization of a multitude of cluster of differentiation numbers (CD number) has allowed the process of "immunophenotyping" to be extended to a number of further applications. Immunophenotyping has been widely used to characterize leukemias and other cancers of the blood.[156] Additionally, immunophenotyping has been used to examine the phenotypic state of de- and redifferentiating cells, such as chondrocytes, expanded in monolayer culture or suspended within a three-dimensional hydrogel. Flow cytometry offers the advantage of observing not only the presence of redifferentiation signals but the quantification of the number of cells expressing cell-associated matrix proteins.[157] Flow cytometry can further be used to monitor the changes in abundance of these molecules with administration of or other variations of culture parameters.[158]

The use of immunophenotyping has naturally been extended to cell sorting methodologies, in which rare cells are both identified and sorted for further experimentation.[159] One of the principle uses of flow sorting technology has been in the identification of distinct populations of mesenchymal stem cells based on CD numbers (see http://130.189.200.66/AboutFlow/cd_table.html). Stem cells are now routinely sorted from such diverse sources as bone marrow aspirates,[160-162] periosteum,[163] liver,[164] muscle and dermis,[165,166] and the central nervous system.[167] In this process, one begins with a poorly characterized heterogeneous population, and sorts into a highly purified subset of stem cells. In some instances, intrinsic properties are taken into account, such as in the isolation of precursor cells from the periosteum in which small cells with low granularity exhibit distinct side scatter and forward scatter profiles.[163] Even when stem cells are sorted by other methods, such as simple adhesion[9] or magnetic-activated cell sorting,[168-170] flow cytometry offers a powerful tool for characterization of the enrichment, homogeneity, and reproducibility of the separation procedures.

15.5 Molecular Biology

15.5.1 Brief Background

The abundance, form, and function of the building blocks that comprise cellular architecture and activity originate in the genetic material contained in each cell nucleus. DNA, the double-stranded stable storehouse of cellular information, is transcribed in a regionally specific manner into temporary messages called heterogeneous nuclear RNA (hnRNA).[171-174] Production of these gene transcripts is controlled by a rich interplay of transcription factors and RNA polymerases interacting at the promoter region of a particular gene or set of genes.[171,175] The state and combination of these factors modulate the level to which transcription occurs. The transient message encoded in the hnRNA is processed into a final form, called messenger RNA (mRNA), which is transported from the nucleus to the cytoplasm (or into the lumen of the rough endoplasmic reticulum). Steady-state levels of mRNA are dictated by the rate of transcription, the rate of degradation, and the rate of transport of these molecules. In mammalian cells, the half-life of mRNA is on the order of hours to days, but can be modulated by alterations in cellular activity. Messenger RNA makes up 1 to 5% of the total RNA of a cell,[176] and is translated at ribosomes into proteins. Translation involves the reading of the message (or open reading frame) in each mRNA via the transient coupling of transfer RNA molecules (tRNA).[171,173,174] Transfer RNA molecules, each with a single amino acid in tow, arrive at the ribosome where the amino acid is covalently linked to its predecessor to sequentially form polypeptide structures, or proteins.

When a cell undergoes an alteration in its physical and/or chemical environment, short-term (minutes to hours) transduction cascades signal these changes to the nucleus, wherein the numerous signals are summed up, resulting in long-term (hours to days) changes to the resting level of mRNA within the cell. It is often of interest to understand the basal levels of gene expression, which define the cellular phenotype, and how expression levels are modulated by alterations in the mechanochemical environment. Most interesting is the control of gene expression at the promoter level, the amount and stability of mRNA produced, the sequence of these transcripts, and how changes in these parameters are affected by normal and disease processes. Using the ever-growing toolbox of molecular biology, one can assess the transcriptional state of both isolated cells, cells in their native tissue environment, or cells in tissue-engineered composites.

15.5.2 Isolation Techniques

To assay the state and sequence of genetic material, it must first be extracted from a population of cells. The protocol for extraction is dependent on the type of genetic material to be extracted (DNA or RNA), as well as the size of the molecule and the milieu from which it is to be extracted. Extraction of DNA and RNA from single cells tends to be the most straightforward, with complications arising when extracting from tissues and other structures. In addition, care must be taken to ensure that contaminating DNA or RNA is not intermingled with extracted material, and that the extraction protocol does not influence the hypothesis being tested.

15.5.2.1 DNA Isolation

The easiest method of extracting genomic DNA from a cluster of cells is by introducing a hypotonic media (i.e., distilled water) which causes the cell and nucleus to lyse, followed by boiling to free the genomic DNA.[177] Such preparations are crude but are suitable for PCR applications (see below). Where longer fragments of DNA are necessary, as in the case of making genomic libraries and cloning vectors, a number of techniques have been utilized that produce genomic fragments of varying sizes. To generate short stretches of DNA that are suitable for most PCR applications, cells or tissue can be extracted with guanidine HCl with sodium acetate followed by ethanol precipitation.[178] If longer stretches of genomic DNA are required, cells may first be digested with proteinase K in a buffer containing sodium dodecyl sulfate (SDS, to solubilize proteins), EDTA (to chelate Mg, which inhibits DNases), and RNase (to remove contaminating RNA).[178,179] After digestion, DNA is extracted with phenol and precipitated in ethanol. Once dry, DNA can be resuspended in TE buffer (tris-EDTA). This method generates genomic DNA strands ranging from 100 to 150 kb.[178] Finally, if even longer fragments are required, a similar procedure can be followed using a formamide-based denaturation buffer.

Another common requirement for DNA extraction involves the recovery of recombinant DNA vectors, such as plasmids, from host organisms. In this situation, it is critical that there be high yield of the fragment of interest with little contamination from the host organisms genomic DNA. The two most common methods for plasmid isolation are lithium chloride/Triton X-100 lysis and SDS-alkaline denaturation.[180] The lithium chloride/Triton X-100 method involves dissolving away part of the cell membrane, and then adding phenol/chloroform, which rapidly denatures proteins, and causes cells to shrink, forcing the lower molecular weight plasmids out of the cell membrane while retaining the larger nuclear DNA within the cell. Alternatively, with SDS-alkaline denaturation, both plasmid and chromosomal DNA is denatured (at pH 11) followed by rapid neutralization with a high salt buffer in the presence of SDS. Under these conditions, genomic DNA hybridizes in an intrastrand manner, forming insoluble aggregates, while plasmid DNA renatures and remains in solution. The resulting "cleared" supernatant from either method can be further purified by ethanol precipitation and/or adsorption to silica resin columns.[180]

15.5.2.2 RNA Isolation

While the aforementioned techniques are reliable for DNA extraction, isolation of mRNA poses a more formidable challenge. By design, mRNA is a transient molecule, meant to convey its message in a spatially and temporally specific manner.[176] Breakdown of mRNA occurs naturally in solution, due to hydrophilic attack of the 2′ hydroxyl group on the backbone. Additionally, endoribonucleases (RNases) that cleave the backbone are numerous (present in internal organelles as well as on skin) and extremely stable.[176] For this reason, RNase-free plastic ware and diethylpyrocarbonate (DEPC)-treated glassware and water should be used at all times. Due to the inherent instability of the molecule, most RNA extraction protocols begin with guanidine thiocyanate, a strong denaturant and RNase inhibitor.[176,181-183] After complete dissolution of cells in 4 *M* guanidinium thiocyanate at pH 4, RNA will preferentially partition into the aqueous phase after mixing with phenol and chloroform.[182] With centriguation ($13,000 \times g$), proteins segregate to the lower organic phase, DNA molecules remain at the interface region, and RNA remains soluble and partitions into the upper aqueous phase. Soluble RNA can then be washed and precipitated in isopropanol, pelleted, and resuspended in RNase-free DEPC-treated water. The purity and amount of RNA can then be measured by the absorbance at 260 nm, and the ratio of absorbance at 260 and 280 nm; pure RNA has a ratio of 1.8 to 2.0.[183] Alternatively, agarose-formaldehyde gels can be used to assess the amount and purity of RNA samples.[176] At this point, samples may be treated with RNase-free DNase to remove any contaminating genomic DNA, or further enriched for mRNA by a number of techniques (e.g., using oligo-dT affinity columns).[184]

15.5.2.3 First-Strand Synthesis

As RNA is quite unstable, even in DEPC-treated water, it is often useful to convert RNA to complementary DNA (cDNA), a much more stable molecule.[176] Complementary DNA is produced from RNA by a process called first-strand synthesis. In this process, reverse transcriptase (RT), a DNA polymerase that uses RNA as a template, creates complementary strands of DNA based on the sequence of the RNA transcript.[176] Choice of RT is critical in determining the length of the cDNA products and their fidelity to the original transcript. In addition to an RNA template and deoxynucleotide phosphates (dNTPs), RT requires a primer from which to initiate transcription, which can be of three forms.[176] Oligo-dT priming makes use of the fact that mRNA is poly-adenylated at the 3′ end of the molecule, and therefore sequences of 12 to 18 dTs can be used to prime from the 3′ tail. While oligo-dT priming selects for messenger RNA, many transcripts have long stretches of noncoding sequences at the 3′ end, and therefore cDNA products may lack open reading frames. Alternatively, random hexamers, as the name implies, use small random sequences to prime reverse transcription. This method generates a large cDNA library from a given RNA source, though nonmessenger RNA is transcribed as well. Finally, if the sequence of the gene of interest is well characterized, gene-specific primers (GSPs) can be designed to enrich the cDNA pool for a particular transcript.

15.5.2.4 Special Considerations

Extraction of mRNA from tissues can pose challenges not present during extraction from monolayer cultures. Extraction of mRNA from tissues with a low cellular density and high content of charged proteoglycans, such as articular cartilage, generally results in low yield. Furthermore, proteoglycans partition with mRNA and can interfere with later RT and PCR reactions.[184] To overcome these challenges, silica-based spin columns[184,185] have been reliably used to further purifiy extracted mRNA. In the case of tissue-engineered equivalents, the three-dimensional environment in which the cells were cultured can interfere with extraction techniques, especially in the case of hydrogels. In a recent paper,[186] a multiple step isolation technique involving both guanidinium hydrochloride and guanidinium isothiocyanate has been used to sequentially separate RNA, DNA, proteins, and other matrix molecules from both agarose and chitosan hydrogels. As is clear from this work, the extraction method used for different tissues and/or three-dimensional culture environments should be optimized prior to the testing of experimental hypotheses.

15.5.3 Measurement Basics

The measurement of gene regulation in cultured cells is largely dependent on the hypothesis to be tested and the level of characterization of the gene of interest. When the gene sequence is known and the objective is to evaluate the regulation of gene transcription in response to an applied stimulus, one can measure the amount and stability of mRNA levels (using the reverse transcriptase polymerase chain reaction, RT-PCR) or the regulation of promoter activity using reporter constructs. If the mechanism of interest is not well characterized and the molecular mechanism is unknown, more complicated analytical steps must be taken. Methods such as differential display RT-PCR (DDRT-PCR) and subtractive hybridization allow for the identification of genes whose regulation changes without any knowledge of the gene *a priori*. A newly emerging alternative to these methods involves the use of DNA microarrays, which allow many different genes to be monitored simultaneously, with the goal of finding genes whose regulation is clearly changed among a sea of other signals. In each of these situations, characterization must be done on multiple levels to ensure that the conclusions from any one technique are valid.

15.5.3.1 Promoter Studies

Functional maps of the promoter region of a particular gene can be constructed from multiple site-specific deletions in that region. In a cell line this process can be quite arduous, and in an isolated tissue, impossible. For this reason, studies of promoter regulation are often performed using reporter constructs, such as plasmids. Once established, studies of this sort offer the advantage over the laborious (and expensive) procedures of mRNA extraction and quantitative PCR in their repeatability, and the ease with which changes to and deletions of the construct can be made.[187] To carry out studies of promoter architecture, the promoter region is isolated and cloned into an expression vector such as a plasmid. In conjunction with the promoter is included a reporter gene. The reporter gene encodes an enzyme whose product is easily assayed (sensitive over several orders of magnitude), is not endogenous to the cell being tested, and does not interfere with the normal functioning of the cell.[187] One major assumption of this assay system is that the reporter mRNA is processed into protein in the same manner that the normal protein is processed (i.e., post-transcriptional control is not a major factor in gene regulation).

A number of enzymes exist that can effectively be used as reporter genes. Luciferase, the enzyme product of the *luc* gene in the firefly, catalyzes an ATP-dependent oxidation of its preferred substrate, luciferan.[188] This process generates a fluorescent emission that is in proportion to the amount of enzyme present and is detectable with a standard lumenometer.[189] β-Galactosidase is another common reporter gene, and its presence can be assayed in cell extracts as well as identified by histochemical analysis to determine the location of expressed products.[187] More recently a reporter gene called green fluorescent protein (GFP), isolated from the Pacific-Northwest jellyfish *Aequorea victoria*, has been developed for use in gene expression studies.[97] Exposure of this protein and other color-shifted family members to UV light results in autofluorescence, making these proteins good *in vivo* markers of transfection.[190] Another interesting application of GFP is that one can use the molecule to produce chimeric proteins that function normally and incorporate GFP, which allows one to monitor cellular dynamics in real-time[191] (as in Figure 15.6). Newer reporter molecules, called "fluorescent timers," are now commercially available that take advantage of time-dependent color shifts in fluorescent proteins to indicate not only the level of reporter expression, but also the lifetime of the molecule, allowing for a continuous monitoring of kinetic responses in gene expression in individual cells.[192,193]

After producing a plasmid containing the promoter of interest controlling a reporter gene, the construct must be amplified. Most plasmids for this purpose have origins of replication, as well as selectable markers. Competent cells are transformed with the plasmid, and expanded under selective conditions.[187] After growing a population of competent cells containing plasmid, stocks can be frozen down for future use or plasmid isolated and quantified directly.[180] Pure solutions of plasmids can then be transfected into primary cells or cell lines. Incorporation of plasmid is generally transient (lasting 2 to 3 days), and the plasmid becomes diluted through the process of cell division.[187] A subset of cells will randomly incorporate the plasmid into the genome, however, becoming stably transfected, and can be used for numerous generations and long-term studies. In stably transfected lines, a drug resistance gene is often incorporated into the plasmid for selection purposes.[187] Transfection is mediated by a number of techniques, ranging from electroporation to viral infection. Most common nonviral methods use cationic carrier molecules (including calcium phosphate and DEAE dextran) that form an insoluble complex of DNA and carrier that is brought in close contact with the cell membrane and is then taken up by an unknown mechanism. Alternative strategies use positively charged liposomes that bring plasmid DNA in close contact to the negatively charged cell membrane, and generally result in transfection at a higher efficiency.[194] Finally, plasmid DNA can be incorporated into retroviral or adenoviral delivery systems that transfect with very high efficiencies. As with any technique, adequate controls must be undertaken to ensure that the measured response is not artifactual. For this reason, transfection studies are often carried out with two plasmids, with one reporter gene under the control of the sequence of interest, while a second reporter is linked to a constituitively active promoter (as in Palmer et al.[195]).

Promoter studies have been carried out for the characterization of the regulatory elements of numerous genes. In our own laboratory, these techniques have been used to examine the functional composition of the aggrecan gene promoter region. By constructing a variety of promoter constructs with multiple deletions and rearrangements, Valhmu et al. examined the influence of the 3′ and 5′ untranslated regions (UTRs) on aggrecan gene expression.[196] Similar promoter constructs have been used to determine the regulatory regions of the promoter that respond to physical stimuli such as fluid-induced shear stress[19] and osmotic loading[195,197] in articular chondrocytes (see Figure 15.10).

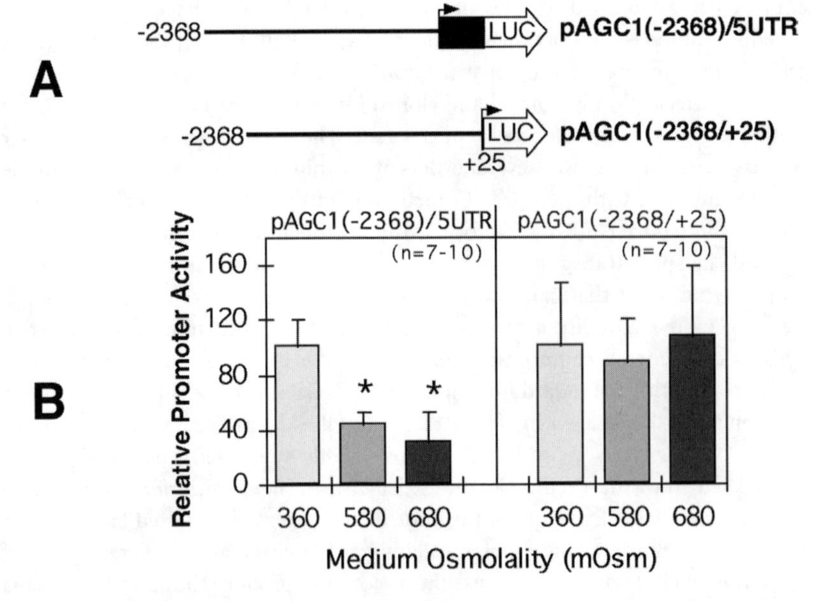

FIGURE 15.10 Promoter studies for aggrecan gene transcriptional regulation adapted from Palmer et al.[195] (A) A luciferase reporter construct containing a 2.4-kb fragment of the promoter region with exon 1 (5′UTR) of the human aggrecan gene, and a deletion construct in which exon 1 has been removed were transiently transfected in primary bovine chondrocytes. (B) Cultured chondrocytes exhibited decreased promoter activity in response to hypertonic loading (5 h with sucrose addition) that was dependent on exon 1 (which contains mechano-responsive elements).

15.5.3.2 Polymerase Chain Reaction (PCR)

Rather than measuring the rate of transcription, as is done with promoter studies, direct measures of mRNA levels can be undertaken with the polymerase chain reaction (PCR).[198,199] This reaction, first conceived of by Kary Mullis in the 1980s (for which he won a Nobel prize in 1993), is based on the amplification of specific regions of a DNA (or cDNA) template in a series of controlled reactions.[177] The PCR reaction mixture contains DNA (or cDNA), a pair of short sequence specific primers, dNTPs, and a thermostable DNA polymerase.[200] The DNA polymerase (Taq) uses one strand of DNA as a template and extends from primers in the 5′ to 3′ direction. Repeated temperature changes, from 95°C to 55–65°C to 72°C, leads to denaturing of DNA, annealing of primers, and extension of product. With each reaction, a doubling of product is accomplished, with up to a million-fold increase in amount of target sequence in a short period of time. The initial phase of amplification is exponential (linear on a log plot) followed by a plateau phase that results from the stoichiometric limitations of reaction components and the decreased enzyme activity due to repeated exposure to high temperatures.[199] For each PCR reaction, there are a number of parameters to be optimized, including the choice of polymerase, the size and specificity of primers, the size of amplified product, and the annealing temperature. Conditions can be optimized for small (~100 bp) or large (up to 20 kb) products (e.g., see http://www.in vitrogen.com/Content/Tech-Online/molecular_biology/manuals_pps/superscript_firststrand_man.pdf). Different Taq molecules offer different processivities, extension rates, and error rates, and should be chosen based on experimental needs. Furthermore, Taq can be kept separate from the reaction mixture until full denaturation has occurred, called "hot-start" PCR, to ensure that mispriming and amplification does not occur in early cycles.[199] Primers are designed to anneal to known complementary DNA sequences on the template, and are themselves generally 18 to 24 nucleotides in length to ensure appropriate specificity and binding temperature. Primer concentration should be maintained at low levels, and care should be taken to design intron-spanning primers where possible so as to differentiate mRNA from carryover genomic DNA. A number of web-based programs are available to aid in the design and selection of suitable primers, and for calculations of annealing temperature (http://www-genome.wi.mit.edu/cgi-bin/primer/primer3.cgi, http://alces.med.umn.edu/rawtm.html). The product resulting from any new primer set should be characterized by restriction enzyme analysis or DNA sequencing to ensure amplification of the correct target.

15.5.3.3 Quantitative PCR

While PCR is adept at demonstrating the presence of specific gene products, it is also of interest to quantify the relative amounts of these products with a change in experimental conditions. Originally, this was done by Northern blots or RNase protection assays, both of which are labor-intensive procedures that require a large amount of RNA.[199] More recent techniques utilize the PCR reaction to quantify the resting level of transcript starting from relatively small amounts of total RNA. Meaningful results require an internal standard by which to normalize to varying levels of starting material.[201] This can be accomplished by normalizing to the starting total RNA amounts (quantified with spectroscopy) or by using endogenous controls sequences that are constituitively expressed in all cells (such as GAPDH or actin). The drawback of such a method is that the use of different primers, the amplification of products of different lengths, and starting from drastically different copy numbers generally results in different amplification efficiencies.[199] In an alternative approach, both the sequence of interest and the normalizing sequence can be cloned into plasmids that are diluted to known concentrations, and then amplified alongside of experimental reactions to create a standard curve.[184] By making serial dilutions of sample mRNA, one can ensure that product intensities remain in the linear range of amplification (see Figure 15.11A).[202] Another method of normalizing is by using a complementary RNA sequence of known

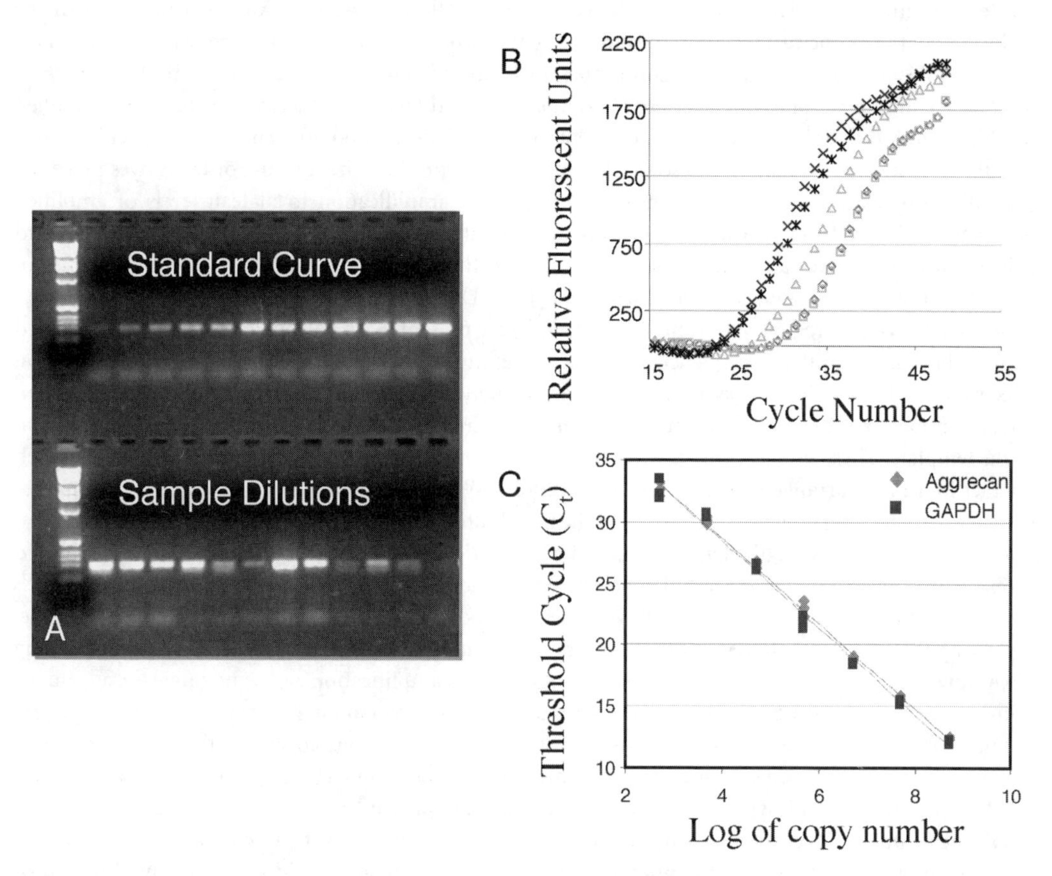

FIGURE 15.11 (A) Agarose gel electrophoresis of PCR products (aggrecan) with corresponding non-competitive quantitative standard curve. (B) Increasing relative fluorescence intensity with increasing cycle number for real-time PCR for aggrecan of five experimental aggrecan samples (curves generated with the Biorad iCycler). (C) Copy number for these samples can be determined from an existing standard curve for aggrecan (and GAPDH also shown) relating the threshold cycle to the log of the initial copy number. (Courtesy of Wilmot Valhmu, University of Wisconsin, Madison.)

concentration that differs from the native sequence by only a small insertion or deletion. Such vectors will generally have similar amplification efficiencies, and can be used noncompetitively (in parallel reactions) or competitively (added to the same reaction mixture).[203,204] The competitive method has the benefit of using the same primer set and reaction mixture, and the amplified products can be run on the same gel. More recently, the StaRT PCR method,[205] which incorporates competitive transcripts for as many as 40 genes at known concentrations (both absolute and relative), has been proposed as a standardized quantitative competitive RT-PCR for the simultaneous analysis of multiple genes.

15.5.3.4 Real-Time PCR

While standardization of traditional PCR techniques can minimize variations in quantitative RT-PCR results, significant errors may still occur between even experienced users within the same lab.[206] Kinetic or "real-time" PCR offers better control and is significantly less variable and more specific than conventional RT-PCR procedures because it does not rely on endpoint intensity measures of amplified product.[207,208] A number of fully automated machines are commercially available that can carry out many simultaneous reactions in a closed-tube environment, requiring no post-amplification manipulation for quantification of amplified product. This makes real-time PCR suited for high throughput screening applications. Furthermore, the amplified sequence is generally shorter than 100 bp, and for this reason, reactions can be carried out more rapidly than with traditional PCR reactions.

The basic real-time PCR system is composed of a thermocycler combined with a system for monitoring fluorescent emission.[208] The real-time PCR reaction is identical to the traditional reaction,[200] with the inclusion of at least one further fluorescent probe. These probes can be DNA-binding dyes (such as SYBR Green), molecular beacons, hybridization probes, or hydrolysis probes.[208] The simplest probe, the DNA-binding dye, fluoresces only when adhered to double-stranded DNA, and therefore increases in amplified product lead directly to an increase in fluorescent intensity. This method offers no further specificity over traditional PCR methods, and fluorescence is dependent on product size, but use of DNA dyes make the quantification easier with obvious transitions from linear amplification to plateau levels of amplified products (see Figure 15.11A). Molecular beacons are specially designed probes, used in addition to standard primers, which provides a further level of specificity to the RT-PCR reaction. These probes form stem loop structures in free solution, but unwind and bind DNA when specific complementary sequences (located in the central region of the amplified product) are present. Each hairpin loop structure is designed with a fluorescent emitter and quencher molecule that are in close spatial association. This association effectively blocks emission unless a complementary sequence is present. Hybridization probes are similar, but are composed of two individual probe sequences designed to line up head to tail on the central region of the template. These probes contain two dyes with overlapping emission and absorption spectra, which interact in a FRET arrangement (see previous section). When the sequences are lined up on a complementary sequence and excited, the emission of the first fluorophore excites the second, resulting at emission at an even higher wavelength that is detected by the device. Finally, hydrolysis probes are dual-labeled probes which quench one another and are designed to bind to the center of the amplified region. At each step of the amplification process, the 5′ exonuclease activity of the Taq DNA polymerase cleaves the probe, separating the two fluorophores from one another, allowing free emission.[208] The level of probe binding DNA can be measured in real time, or at the terminus of each amplification cycle, and offers the advantage of using more than one set of primers and probes at the same time (so long as they have distinct spectral characteristics). Many commercial systems include a software package to aid in the design of probe sequences (e.g., http://www.premierbiosoft.com/molecular_beacons/taqman_molecular_beacons.html and http://www.appliedbiosystems.com/support/tutorials/taqman/index.cfm).

Each real-time PCR reaction is characterized by a Ct value,[208] which is the fractional number of cycles at which the reporter fluorescent emission reaches a fixed threshold level in the exponential region of the amplification plot (see Figure 15.11A). This value can be correlated to the input mRNA amount, with larger starting amounts producing lower Ct values (Ct is inversely proportional to the log of the starting copy number).[208] This ensures that real-time PCR methods are not based on measurement of final amount of amplified product, and therefore do not have the same possibilities for error associated with standard PCR methods. In many systems, measurements are taken over the entire time course, and reactions can be halted before stoichiometric limitions of reaction components arise. As with standard PCR, relative measures compared to an internal control can be made (to actin, GAPDH, and/or ribosomal RNA), or standard curves can be constructed to determine the absolute copy number of a specific sequence (see Figure 15.11B). In most cases, the detection limit with real-time PCR is on the order of 50 to 500 copies of target mRNA.[208]

While the initial monetary investment in reagents and instrumentation for carrying out real-time PCR may at first seem prohibitive, the ease of use, specificity, and reproducibility of results may actually lead to savings in the long run by overcoming the need for the time-consuming and numerous duplications involved in traditional RT-PCR analysis. For this reason, real-time PCR has been widely adopted, quickly becoming the gold standard in the field. Recent studies have used real-time PCR to quantify mRNA expression in chondrocytes and intervertebral disc cells in response to osmotic loading, both in monolayer cultures and in three-dimensional hydrogels.[197,209] It has additionally been employed to examine the changes in gene expression that occur with the onset of osteoarthritis.[185] Even more interesting, real-time PCR can be used reliably for single cell analysis of mRNA in the cytoplasm of a single large cell,[210] or from individual tumor cells isolated with laser capture microdissection (LCM).[211]

15.5.3.5 Differential Display and Subtractive Hybridization

When less is known about the molecular mechanism involved in the response to an applied stimulus, other methodologies must be utilized. Two techniques can be used to identify gene transcripts present at different levels in different mRNA populations with no *a priori* knowledge of the sequence in question. Differential display reverse transcriptase PCR (DDRT-PCR) uses reverse transcription with oligo-dT primers directed to a subset of the RNA.[212,213] In this method oligo-dT primers, coupled with two additional dinucleotides (for example, AGTTTT), are used to generate cDNA in the presence of ^{32}P-dATP. The resulting radiolabeled products are then resolved on a gel, and differentially expressed bands excised. The purified cDNA is then reamplified with the same primer set, and the sequence determined by standard techniques. This reaction is carried out for all possible dinucleotide combinations to generate a full representation of the overall mRNA population. While the incidence of false positives can be high, DDRT-PCR offers one method for identifying genes that are differentially regulated, and is a starting point for further characterization of unknown molecular mechanisms.[199] Another method with similar properties is subtractive suppression hybridization (SSH).[214] This method combines cDNA normalization with selective PCR amplification to enrich differentially expressed gene transcripts. In this method, "tester" cDNA from the altered state and "driver" cDNA from control conditions are combined after a sequence of specific modifications.[199] After mRNA extraction and reverse transcription, two different pools of tester cDNA are digested to blunt ends, and then each population is annealed with a different primer adapter. Each pool is denatured separately and rapidly reassociated in the presence of excess driver cDNA. The two populations are then denatured a second time, combined, and again rapidly reassociated in presence of excess driver cDNA. The resultant mixture of cDNA contains commonly expressed sequences that are mixed (without a full set of unique primer ends) while unique sequences remain paired to one another (with their unique primer ends). All sequences are then amplified with one primer each directed at each of the unique ends, and only those sequences that contain one of each end are amplified.[214] This procedure, while difficult in practice, can reduce the amplification of commonly expressed genes while enriching the amplification of rare transcripts up to 100- to 1000-fold.[199]

These methods have found numerous applications in identifying unknown molecular mechanisms. In a recent study, traditional RT-PCR methods were used to characterize changes in known genes in an experimental model of osteoarthritis, while DDRT-PCR was carried out to identify other candidate genes involved in the disease process.[215] In another study, stem cells in micromass culture were converted to a chondrogenic phenotype in the presence of BMP-2, and the molecular mechanisms were monitored with subtractive hybridization.[216] This study identified a number of previously unknown genes that were up- or down-regulated in conjunction with the phenotype conversion process. Additionally, SSH can be combined with DNA microarray technology (see below) to profile differential expressed genes with transformation.[217]

15.5.3.6 DNA Microarrays

Given the observed changes in expression of so many genes in response to even the simplest chemical or mechanical stimulus, it is clear that a more global approach to expression profiling is warranted. Such a global approach will allow for a more complete picture to be taken at each experimental condition, enabling a better understanding of the underlying order of multiple gene regulation.[218] The recent development of DNA microarray technology has made this global analysis possible in an efficient and increasingly economical manner. DNA microarrays consist of many thousands of individual DNA (or cDNA) pieces affixed to a glass, silicon or plastic substrate.[219] A variety of competing technologies allow for the placing of up to one million test sequences on as little as 1 to 2 cm.[2] These DNA sequences can be accurately fixed in place (either covalently or noncovalently), and the position and corresponding sequence indexed. The two most widely used chip fabrication technologies today involve either the physical delivery of known sequences to specific sites with inkjet or microjet deposition technology,[219] or the combination of photolithography and solid phase oligonucleotide chemistry to build DNA sequences of up to 25 nucleotides from the solid substrate.[220] Target DNA (or cDNA) molecules from experimental conditions are fluorescently tagged and hybridized to the test sequences on the chip. Specificity of binding is controlled, and the position and intensity of fluorescence is measured across the chip surface and related back to the location of specific sequences. Alternatively, mass spectroscopy can be used to read the chip.

Due to the large amount of information contained in a single hybridized array, the construction of databases for the management of information is necessary. Mining and recognizing patterns within this data with bioinformatics may provide insight into the operation of genetic networks.[221] As with any new technology, however, care should be taken to ensure the correct design of studies.[222] One investigator likened the interpretation of DNA microarray results to "examining a battlefield and trying to infer the cause of war."[220] While the situation may not be so stark, care should be taken to ensure that studies are hypothesis-driven, with clear objectives, and an understanding of the variance in the system.[223] Additionally, as there might be different amounts of cDNA in any one sample, data should be normalized to constituitively expressed genes (as with PCR methods).

The development of microarray technology has mirrored that of the computer microchip, with higher levels of data analysis possible in less surface area, with concurrent increases in sensitivity and selectivity. As with real-time PCR, cost was at first prohibitive, but has slowly decreased, and many research institutions now have established core facilities.[218] More than a dozen companies[219] have some form of DNA microarray technology on the market, each with a niche application (e.g., high-density Gene Chips [www.affymetrix.com] and Atlas arrays [www.clontech.com] for expression profiling and genotyping, low-density microarrays from Orchid Biosciences, Inc. [www.orchid.com] for screening and diagnostics[219]). Chips can be used to sequence by hybridization (SBH), a procedure in which binding affinity is measured in the presence of single nucleotide changes in sequence (Hychip, www.hyseq.com). For analysis of gene expression profiles,[224,225] chips are commercially available that incorporate expressed sequence tags (ESTs) representing individual tissues to whole organisms (e.g., all 6200 ESTs from *S. cerevisiae*[226]). The chips can be probed with experimental cDNA transcribed from mRNA that has been fluorescently tagged to allow efficient visualization of hybridization. In such cases, the normal condition may be compared to pathologic conditions by using two separate fluorescent tags (one for each mRNA pool) and the relative expression levels viewed on the same chip.[226] Such approaches have been successfully employed to examine the changes in gene expression in human cancers[227,228] and in cells responding to applied stimuli (e.g., hydrostatic pressure[229]). Coupling this technology with unique single cell acquisition devices (i.e., laser capture microscopy) allows for the characterization of subtle differences in individual cancer cells.[230] Microarrays are finding further use in the mapping of single nucleotide polymorphisms (SNPs), in pharmacogenomic research,[231] and in forensic and genetic identification applications.[219]

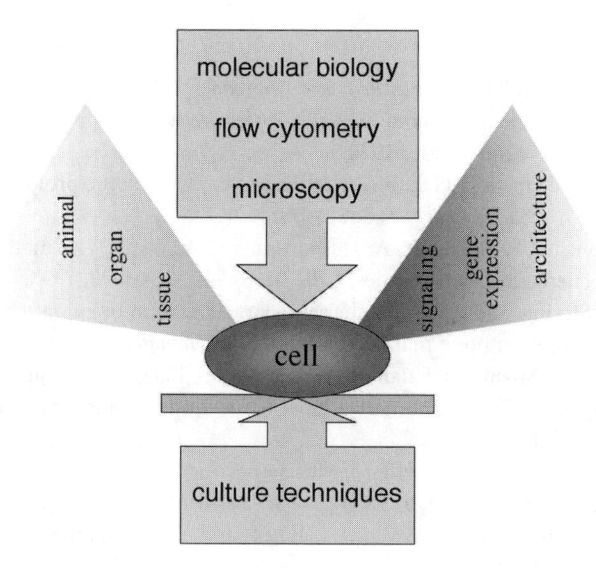

FIGURE 15.12 Paradigm for approaches to cellular level biological assays. From whole animal, organ, and tissue sources, tissue culture techniques form the foundation for the examination of cellular form and function. With microscopy, flow cytometry, and molecular biology techniques, new insights into cell signaling, gene expression pathways, and cell architecture can be gained.

15.6 Conclusions

For decades, significant efforts have focused on gaining a better understanding of the *in vivo* situation by focusing studies on the basic building block of life, the cell. With dynamic innovations in technology, it is becoming more permissible (and perhaps more routine) to extract greater volumes of data from smaller and smaller amounts of tissue and cells. Sophisticated culture techniques, spurred by interdisciplinary research efforts (e.g., biomaterials, bioengineering, molecular and cell biology), have permitted investigators to modulate cell phenotype and expression levels in a manner similar to their native environment *in vivo*. Microscopy techniques, further refined and optimized with the incorporation of advances from the acquisition side and post-processing side, enable noninvasive examination of structure, protein interactions, ion fluxes, expression, and material characteristics of cells, providing new insights to intracellular and extracellular phenomena with continually growing sensitivity and specificity. Similarly, flow cytometry allows for identification and sorting of mixed cell populations, permitting isolation of rare subsets of cells. Real-time PCR allows for transcripts from these isolated cells/tissues to be efficiently and reliably quantified. Finally, DNA microarrays allow for multiple genes to be monitored simultaneously. Just as technology and economies of scale spurred a revolution in the world of personal computing, so might DNA microarrays become commonplace in biological research and lead to a better understanding of the complexities of genetic regulation. Together, these tools represent a compendium of assays that permit researchers to examine questions regarding heterogeneity within populations (cells or molecules), instead of measuring attributes representing their average response. A new challenge that has emerged involves the interpretation of this plethora of information in the context of real physiologic situations, such as in development and the regulation of disease and pathology, as well as in efforts to engineer and grow replacement tissues.

Acknowledgments

This work was supported by the National Institutes of Health (R01 AR46568 and R21 AR48791), and a pre-doctoral fellowship and a Biomedical Engineering Research grant from the Whitaker Foundation.

References

1. J.M. Davis, Ed., *Basic Cell Culture: A Practical Approach*, Oxford University Press, Oxford, 1996.
2. A.I. Caplan, Effects of the nicotinamide-sensitive teratogen 3-acetylpyridine on chick limb cells in culture, *Exp. Cell Res.*, 62, 341–355, 1970.
3. T.M. Dexter, T.D. Allen, and L.G. Lajtha, Conditions controlling the proliferation of haemopoietic stem cells *in vitro*, *J. Cell. Physiol.*, 91, 335, 1977.
4. Z. Nevo, D. Robinson, S. Horowitz, A. Hasharoni, and A. Yayon, The manipulated mesenchymal stem cells in regenerated skeletal tissues, *Cell. Transplant.*, 7, 63–70, 1998.
5. F.E. Angela, A.I. Stering, and P.J. Quesenberry, Characterization of engraftable hematopoietic stem cells in murine long-term bone marrow cultures, *Exp. Hematol.*, 29, 643–652, 2001.
6. P.A. Zuk, M. Zhu, H. Mizuno, J. Huang, J. W. Futrell, A.J. Katz, P. Benhaim, H.P. Lorenz, and M.H. Hedrick, Multilineage cells from human adipose tissue: implications for cell-based therapies, *Tissue Eng.*, 7, 211–228, 2001.
7. R.J. Jankowski, B.M. Deasy, and J. Huard, Muscle-derived stem cells, *Gene Ther.*, 9, 642–647, 2002.
8. M.K. Majumdar, E. Wang, and E.A. Morris, BMP-2 and BMP-9 promotes chondrogenic differentiation of human multipotential mesenchymal cells and overcomes the inhibitory effect of IL-1, *J. Cell. Physiol.*, 189, 275–284, 2001.
9. M.F. Pittenger, A.M. Mackay, S.C. Beck, R.K. Jaiswal, R. Douglas, J.D. Mosca, M.A. Moorman, D.W. Simonetti, S. Craig, and D.R. Marshak, Multilineage potential of adult human mesenchymal stem cells, *Science*, 284, 143–147, 1999.
10. G.R. Erickson, J.M. Gimble, D.M. Franklin, H.E. Rice, H. Awad, and F. Guilak, Chondrogenic potential of adipose tissue-derived stromal cells *in vitro* and *in vivo*, *Biochem. Biophys. Res. Commun.*, 290, 763–769, 2002.
11. G.H. Altman, R.L. Horan, I. Martin, J. Farhadi, P.R.H. Stark, V. Volloch, J.C. Richmond, G. Vunjak-Novakovic, and D.L. Kaplan, Cell differentiation by mechanical stress, *FASEB J.*, 16, 270–272, 2002.
12. S.H. Elder, S.A. Goldstein, J.H. Kimura, L.J. Soslowsky, and D.M. Spengler, Chondrocyte differentiation is modulated by frequency and druation of cyclic compressive loading, *Ann. Biomed. Eng.*, 29, 476–482, 2001.
13. S.B. Nicoll, A. Wedrychowska, N.R. Smith, and R.S. Bhatnagar, Modulation of proteoglycan and collagen profiles in human dermal fibroblasts by high density micromass culture and treatment with lactic acid suggests change to a chondrogenic phenotype, *Connect. Tissue Res.*, 42, 59–69, 2001.
14. D. Chafik, D. Bear, P. Bui, A. Patel, N.F. Jones, B.T. Kim, C.T. Hung, and R. Gupta, Optimization of Schwann cell adhesion in response to shear stress in an *in vitro* model for peripheral nerve tissue engineering, *Tissue Eng.*, in press.
15. K.M. Haberstroh, M. Kaefer, N. DePaola, S.A. Frommer, and R. Bizios, A novel *in vitro* system for the simultaneous exposure of bladder smooth muscle cells to mechanical strain and sustained hydrostatic pressure, *J. Biomech. Eng.*, 124, 208–213, 2002.
16. L.M. Wilkins, S.R. Watson, S.J. Prosky, S.F. Meunier and N.L. Parenteau, Development of bilayered living skin construct for clinical applications, *Biotech Bioeng*, 43, 747–756, 1994.
17. M.J. Levesque and R.M. Nerem, Elongation and orientation of cultured endothelial cells in response to shear stress, *J. Biomech. Eng.*, 107, 341–347, 1985.
18. S.N. Bhatia, U.J. Balis, M.L. Yarmush, and M. Toner, Effect of cell-cell interactions in preservation of cellular phenotype. Cocultivation of hepatocytes and nonparenchymal cells, *FASEB J.*, 13, 1883–1900, 1999.
19. C. Hung, D. Henshaw, C. Wang, R. Mauck, F. Raia, G. Palmer, V. Mow, A. Ratcliffe, and W. Valhmu, Mitogen-activated protein kinase signaling in bovine articular chondrocytes in response to fluid flow does not require calcium mobilization, *J. Biomechanics*, 33, 73–80, 2000.
20. C.T. Hung, S.R. Pollack, T.M. Reilly, and C.T. Brighton, Real-time calcium response of cultured bone cells to fluid flow, *Clin. Orthop.*, 313, 256–269, 1995.

21. R.A. Luben, G.L. Wong, and D.V. Cohn, Biochemical characterization with parathormone and calcitonin of isolated bone cells: provisional identification of osteoclasts and osteoblasts, *Endocrinology*, 99, 526–534, 1976.
22. J.S. Brand and T.J. Hefley, Collagenase and the isolation of cells from bone, in *Cell Separation: Methods and Selected Applications*, T.G. Pretlow and T.P. Pretlow, Eds., Academic Press, Orlando, 1984, pp. 265–283.
23. G. Wong, Isolation and behavior of isolated bone-forming cells, in *The Osteoblast and Osteocyte, Volume 1*, B.K. Hall, Ed., Telford Press, Caldwell, 1990, pp. 494.
24. W.E. Modderman, A.F. Weidema, T. Vrijheid-Lammers, A.M. Wassenaar, and P.J. Nijweide, Permeabilization of cells of hemopoietic origin by extracellular ATP^{4-}: elimination of osteoclasts, macrophages, and their precursors from isolated bone cell populations and fetal bone rudiments, *Calcif. Tissue Int.*, 55, 141–150, 1994.
25. I. Martin, R.F. Padera, G. Vunjak-Novakovic, and L.E. Freed, In vitro differentiation of chick embryo bone marrow stromal cells into cartilaginous and bone-like tissues, *J. Orthop. Res.*, 16, 181–189, 1998.
26. M. Aydelotte and K. Kuettner, Differences between sub-populations of cultured bovine articular chondrocytes. I. Morphology and cartilage matrix production, *Connect. Tissue Res.*, 18, 205–222, 1988.
27. M.M. Knight, D.A. Lee, and D.L. Bader, The influence of elaborated pericellular matrix on the deformation of isolated articular chondrocytes cultured in agarose, *Biochem. Biophys. Acta*, 1405, 67–77, 1998.
28. C.A. Poole, Articular cartilage chondrons: form, function and failure, *J. Anat.*, 191, 1–13, 1997.
29. R.D. Graff, E.R. Lazarowski, A.J. Banes, and G.M. Lee, ATP release by mechanically loaded porcine chondrons in pellet culture, *Arthritis Rheum.*, 43, 1571–1579, 2000.
30. M.M. Knight, J.M. Ross, A.F. Sherwin, D.A. Lee, D.L. Bader, and C.A. Poole, Chondrocyte deformation within mechanically and enzymatically extracted chondrons compressed in agarose, *Biochim. Biophys. Acta*, 1526, 141–146, 2001.
31. S. Katzburg, M. Lieberherr, A. Ornoy, B.Y. Klein, D. Hendel, and D. Somjen, Isolation and hormonal responsiveness of primary cultures of human bone-derived cells: gender and age differences, *Bone*, 25, 667–673, 1999.
32. K.B. Jonsson, A. Frost, O. Nilsson, S. Ljunghall, and O. Ljunggren, Three isolation techniques for primary culture of human osteoblast-like cells: a comparison, *Acta Orthop. Scand.*, 70, 365–373, 1999.
33. T.J. Voegele, M. Voegele-Kadletz, V. Esposito, K. Macfelda, U. Oberndorfer, V. Vecsei, and R. Schabus, The effect of different isolation techniques on human osteoblast-like cell growth, *Anticancer Res.*, 20, 3575–3581, 2000.
34. K. Kobayashi, R.M. Healey, R.L. Sah, J. J. Clark, B.P. Tu, R.S. Goomer, W.H. Akeson, H. Moriya, and D. Amiel, Novel method for quantitative assessment of cell migration: a study on the motility of rabbit anterior cruciate (ACL) and medial collateral ligament (MCL) cells, *Tissue Eng.*, 6, 29–38, 2000.
35. C.N. Nagineni, D. Amiel, M.H. Green, M. Berchuck, and W.H. Akeson, Characterization of the intrinsic properties of the anterior cruciate and medial collateral ligament cells: an *in vitro* cell culture study, *J. Orthop. Res.*, 10, 465–475, 1992.
36. C.T. Hung, F.D. Allen, S.R. Pollack, E.T. Attia, J. A. Hannafin, and P.A. Torzilli, Intracellular calcium response of ACL and MCL ligament fibroblasts to fluid-induced shear stress, *Cell Signal.*, 9(8), 587–594, 1997.
37. J. Dumont, M. Ionescu, A. Reiner, A.R. Poole, N. Tran-Khanh, C.D. Hoemann, M.D. McKee, and M.D. Buschmann, Mature full-thickness articular cartilage explants attached to bone are physiologically stable over long-term culture in serum-free media, *Connect. Tissue Res.*, 40, 259–272, 2000.

38. J. Kisiday, M. Jin, B. Kurz, H. Hung, C. Semino, S. Zhang, and A.J. Grodzinsky, Self-assembling peptide hydrogel fosters chondrocyte extracellular matrix production and cell division: implications for cartilage tissue repair, *Proc. Natl. Acad. Sci.*, 99, 9996–10001, 2002.
39. C.T. Brighton, J.L. Schaffer, D.B. Shapiro, J.J.S. Tang, and C.C. Clark, Proliferation and macromolecular synthesis by rat calvarial bone cells grown in various oxygen tension, *J. Orthop. Res.*, 9, 847–854, 1991.
40. U. Hansen, M. Schunke, C. Domm, N. Ioannidis, J. Hassenpflug, T. Gehrke, and B. Kurz, Combination of reduced oxygen tension and intermittent hydrostatic pressure: a useful tool in articular cartilage tissue engineering, *J. Biomech.*, 34, 941–949, 2001.
41. C. Perka, O. Schultz, R.-S. Spitzer, and K. Lindenhayn, The influence of transforming growth factor B1 on mesenchymal cell repair of full-thickness cartilage defects, *J. Biomed. Mater. Res.*, 52, 543–552, 2000.
42. S. Einheber, M.J. Hannocks, C.N. Metz, D.B. Rifkin, and J.L. Salzer, Transforming growth factor-beta 1 regulates axon/Schwann cell interactions, *J. Cell. Biol.*, 129, 443–458, 1995.
43. E. Lucchinetti, C.S. Adams, W.E. Horton, Jr., and P.A. Torzilli, Cartilage viability after repetitive loading: a preliminary report, *Osteoarthritis Cartilage*, 10, 71–81, 2002.
44. C. Labarca and K. Paigen, A simple, rapid, and sensitive DNA assay procedure, *Analyt. Biochem.*, 102, 344–352, 1980.
45. Y.J. Kim, R.L. Sah, J.Y. Doong, and A.J. Grodzinsky, Fluorometric assay of DNA in cartilage explants using Hoecsht 33258, *Anal. Biochem.*, 174, 168–176, 1988.
46. V.L. Singer, L.J. Jones, S.T. Yue, and R.P. Haugland, Characterization of PicoGreen reagent and the development of a fluorescence-based solution assay for double stranded DNA quantitation, *Anal. Biochem.*, 249, 228–238, 1997.
47. J. Shyy and S. Chien, Role of integrins in cellular responses to mechanical stress and adhesion, *Curr. Opin. Cell Biol.*, 9, 707–713, 1997.
48. S. Takayama, J.C. McDonanld, E. Ostuni, M.N. Liang, P.J.A. Kenis, R.F. Ismagilov, and G.M. Whitesides, Patterning cells and their environments using multiple laminar fluid flows in capillary networks, *Proc. Natl. Acad. Sci.*, 96, 5545–5548, 1999.
49. S.N. Bhatia, M.L. Yarmush, and M. Toner, Controlling cell interactions by micropatterning in co-cultures. Hepatocyes and 3T3 fibroblasts, *J. Biomed. Mater.*, 34, 189–199, 1997.
50. C.S. Chen, M. Mrksich, S. Huang, G.M. Whitesides, and D.E. Ingber, Geometric control of cell life and death, *Science*, 276, 1425–1428, 1997.
51. R. Singhvi, A. Kumar, G.P. Lopez, G.N. Stephanopoulos, D.I. Wang, G.M. Whitesides, and D.E. Ingber, Engineering cell shape and function, *Science*, 264, 696–698, 1994.
52. C.H. Thomas, C.D. McFarland, A. Rezania, J.G. Steele, and K.E. Healy, The role of vitronectin in the attachment and spatial distribution of bone-derived cells on materials with patterned surface chemistry, *J. Biomed. Mater. Res.*, 37, 81–93, 1997.
53. V.A. Liu, W.E. Jastromb, and S.N. Bhatia, Engineering protein and cell adhesivity using PEO-terminated triblock polymers, *J. Biomed. Mater. Res.*, 60, 126–134, 2001.
54. K.K. Parker, A.L. Brock, C. Brangwynne, R.J. Mannix, N. Wang, E. Ostuni, N.A. Geisse, J.C. Adams, G.M. Whitesides, and D.E. Ingber, Directional control of lamellipodia extension by constraining cell shape and orienting cell tractional forces, *FASEB J.*, 16, 1195–1204, 2002.
55. E.F. Petersen, R.G.S. Spencer, and E.W. McFarland, Microengineering neocartilage scaffolds, *Biotechnol. Bioeng.*, 78, 802–805, 2002.
56. P.D. Benya and J.D. Shaffer, Dedifferentiated chondrocytes reexpress the differentiated collagen phenotype when cultured in agarose gels, *Cell*, 30, 215–224, 1982.
57. E. Kolettas, L. Buluwela, M.T. Bayliss, and H.I. Muir, Expression of cartilage-specific molecules is retained on long-term culture of human articular chondroctyes, *J. Cell Sci.*, 108, 1991–1999, 1995.
58. T. Linkhart and S. Mohan, Parathyroid hormone stimulates release of insulin-like growth factor (IGF-I) and IGF-II from neonatal mouse calvaria in organ culture, *Endocrinology*, 125(3), 1484–1491, 1989.

59. B. Morrison III, J.H. Eberwine, D.F. Meaney, and T.K. McIntosh, Traumatic injury induces differential expression of cell death genes in organotypic brain slice cultures determined by complementary DNA array hybridization, *Neuroscience*, 2000, 131–139, 2000.
60. R.L.Y. Sah, Y.J. Kim, J.-Y.H. Doong, A.J. Grodzinsky, A.H.K. Plaas, and J.D. Sandy, Biosynthetic response of cartilage explants to dynamic compression, *J. Orthop. Res.*, 7, 619–636, 1989.
61. A.J. Banes, G. Horesovsky, C. Larson, M. Tsuzaki, S. Judex, J. Archambault, R. Zernicke, W. Herzog, S. Kelley, and L. Miller, Mechanical load stimulates expression of novel genes *in vivo* and *in vitro* in avian flexor tendon cells, *Osteoarthritis Cartilage*, 7, 141–153, 1999.
62. A.E. Denker, S.B. Nicoll, and R.S. Tuan, Formation of cartilage-like spheroids by micromass cultures of murine C3H10T1/2 cells upon treatment with transforming growth factor-beta 1, *Differentiation*, 59, 25–34, 1995.
63. R.L. Mauck, M.A. Soltz, C.C.-B. Wang, D.D. Wong, P.-H.G. Chao, W.B. Valhmu, C.T. Hung, and G.A. Ateshian, Functional tissue engineering of articular cartilage through dynamic loading of chondrocyte-seeded agarose gels, *J. Biomech. Eng.*, 122, 252–260, 2000.
64. A.J. Nixon, L.A. Fortier, J. Williams, and H. Mohammed, Enhanced repair of extensive articular defects by insulin-like growth factor-I-laden fibrin composites, *J. Orthop. Res.*, 17, 475–487, 1999.
65. J.L. van Susante, P. Buma, G.N. Homminga, W.B. van den Berg, and R.P. Veth, Chondrocyte-seeded hydroxyapatite for repair of large articular cartilage defects. A pilot study in the goat, *Biomaterials*, 19, 2367–2374, 1998.
66. K. Kanda and T. Matsuda, Mechanical stress-induced orientation and ultrastructural change of smooth muscle cells cultured in three-dimensional collagen lattices, *Cell Transplant.*, 3, 481–492, 1994.
67. J.L. Andresen, T. Ledet, and N. Ehlers, Keratocyte migration and peptide growth factors: the effect of PDGF, bFGF,EGF,IGF-I,aFGF and TGF-beta on human keratocyte migration in a collagen gel, *Curr. Eye Res.*, 16(6), 605–613, 1997.
68. S.R. Pollack, D.F. Meaney, E.M. Levine, M. Litt, and E.D. Johnston, Numerical model and experimental validation of microcarrier motion in a rotating bioreactor, *Tissue Eng.*, 6, 519–530, 2000.
69. K.T. Paige and C.A. Vacanti, Engineering new tissue: formation of neo-cartilage, *Tissue Eng.*, 1, 97, 1995.
70. E.F. Petersen, K.W. Fishbein, E.W. McFarland, and R.G.S. Spencer, ^{31}P NMR spectroscopy of developing cartilage produced from chick chondrocytes in a hollow-fiber bioreactor, *Magnetic Resonance Med.*, 44, 367–372, 2000.
71. N.S. Dunkelman, M.P. Zimber, R.G. LeBaron, R. Pavelec, M. Kwan, and A.F. Purchio, Cartilage production by rabbit articular chondrocytes on polyglycolic acid scaffolds in a closed bioreactor system, *Biotech. Bioeng.*, 46, 299–305, 1995.
72. D. Pazzano, K.A. Mercier, J.M. Moran, S.S. Fong, D.D. DiBiasio, J.X. Rulfs, S.S. Kohles, and L.J. Bonassar, Comparison of chondrogensis in static and perfused bioreactor culture, *Biotechnol. Progr.*, 16, 893–896, 2000.
73. B.J. Klement and B.S. Spooner, Utilization of microgravity bioreactors for differentiation of mammalian skeletal tissue, *J. Cell Biochem.*, 51, 252–256, 1993.
74. L.E. Freed, G. Vunjak-Novakovic, and R. Langer, Cultivation of cell-polymer cartilage implants in bioreactors, *J. Cell Biochem.*, 51, 257–264, 1993.
75. G. Vunjak-Novakovic, L.E. Freed, R.J. Biron, and R. Langer, Effects of mixing on the composition and morphology of tissue-engineered cartilage, *AIChE*, 42, 850–860, 1996.
76. S.E. Carver and C.A. Heath, Influence of intermittent pressure, fluid flow, and mixing on the regenerative properties of articular chondrocytes, *Bitechnol. Bioeng.*, 65, 274–281, 1999.
77. K.J. Gooch, J.H. Kwon, T. Blunk, R. Langer, L.E. Freed, and G. Vunjak-Novakovic, Effects of mixing intensity on tissue-engineered cartilage, *Biotechnol. Bioeng.*, 72, 402–407, 2001.
78. T. Brown, Techniques for mechanical stimulation of cells *in vitro*: a review, *J. Biomechanics*, 33, 3–14, 2000.

79. A.N. Brown, B.S. Kim, E. Alsberg, and D.J. Mooney, Combining chondrocytes and smooth muscle cells to engineer hybrid soft tissue constructs, *Tissue Eng.*, 6, 297–305, 2000.
80. L.E. Niklason, J. Gao, W.M. Abbott, K.K. Hirschi, S. Houser, R. Marini, and R. Langer, Functional arteries grown *in vitro*, *Science*, 284, 489–493, 1999.
81. L.G. Braddon, D. Karoyli, D.G. Harrison, and R.M. Nerem, Maintenance of a functional endothelial cell monolayer on a fibroblast/polymer substrate under physiologically relevant shear stress conditions, *Tissue Eng.*, 8, 695–708, 2002.
82. P. Mazur, Freezing of living cells: mechanisms and implications, *Am. J. Physiol.*, 247, 125–142, 1984.
83. J.O.M. Karlsson and M. Toner, Long-term storage of tissues by cryopreservation: critical issues, *Biomaterials*, 17, 243–256, 1996.
84. Z.F. Cui, R.C. Dykhuizen, R.M. Nerem, and A. Sembanis, Modeling of cryopreservation of engineered tissues with one-dimensional geometery, *Biotechnol. Prog.*, 18, 354–361, 2002.
85. M.S. Simione, Cryopreservation Manual, American Type Culture Collection (ATCC)-Nalge Nunc International Corp., Rockville, MD, 1998.
86. P. Mazur, The role of cell membranes in the freezing of yeast and other single cells, *Ann. N.Y. Acad. Sci.*, 125, 658–676, 1965.
87. L.E. McGann, M. Stevenson, K. Muldrew, and N. Schachar, Kinetics of osmotic water movement in chondrocytes isolated from articular cartilage and applications to cryopreservation, *J. Orthop. Res.*, 6, 109–115, 1988.
88. E.E. Noiles, K.A. Thompson, and B.T. Storey, Water permeability, Lp, of the mouse sperm plasma membrane and its activation energy are strongly dependent on interaction of the plasma membrane with sperm cytoskeleton, *Cryobiology*, 35, 79–92, 1997.
89. I. Martinez de Maranon, P. Gervais, and P. Molin, Determination of cell's water membrane permeability: unexpected high osmotic permeability of *Saccharomyces cerevisiae*, *Biotechnol. Bioeng.*, 56, 62–70, 1997.
90. K.R. Diller, Engineering-based contributions in cryobiology, *Cryobiology*, 34, 304–314, 1997.
91. J.E. Lovelock, The denaturation of lipid-protein complexes as a cause of damage by freezing, *Proc. R. Soc. London Ser. B*, 147, 427–433, 1957.
92. J. James and H.J. Tanke, *Biomedical Light Microscopy*, Kluwer Academic, Dordrecht, 1991.
93. D.G. Weiss and W. Maile, Principles, practice, and applications of video-enhanced contrast microscopy, in *Electronic Light Microscopy*, D. Shotton, Ed., Wiley-Liss, New York, 1993, pp. 105–140.
94. S. Bradbury and P. Evennett, *Contrast Techniques in Light Microscopy*, BIOS Scientific, Oxford, 1996.
95. R.Y. Tsien, T.J. Rink, and M. Poenie, Measurement of cytosolic free Ca^{2+} in individual small cells using fluorescence microscopy with dual excitation wavelengths, *Cell Calcium*, 6, 145–157, 1985.
96. G. Grynkiewicz, M. Poenie, and R.Y. Tsien, A new generation of Ca^{2+} indicators with greatly improved fluorescence properties, *J. Biol. Chem.*, 280, 3440–3450, 1985.
97. M. Chalfie, Y. Tu, G. Euskirchen, W.W. Ward, and D.C. Prasher, Green fluorescent protein as a marker for gene expression, *Science*, 263, 802–805, 1994.
98. B. Herman, Fluorescence microscopy: state of the art, in *Fluorescence Microscopy and Fluorescent Probes*, J. Slavik, Ed., Plenum Press, New York, 1996.
99. D. Shotton, An introduction to the electronic acquistion of light microscope images, in *Electronic Light Microscopy*, D. Shotton, Ed., John Wiley & Sons, New York, 1993, pp. 355.
100. M.P. Oksvold, E. Skarpen, J. Widerberg and H.S. Huitfeldt, Fluorescent histochemical techniques for analysis of intracellular signaling, *J. Histochem. Cytochem.*, 50, 289–303, 2002.
101. J. G. White, W.B. Amos, and M. Fordham, An evaluation of confocal versus conventional imaging of biological structures by fluorescence light microscopy, *J. Cell Biol.*, 105, 41–48, 1987.
102. R. Yuste, F. Lanni, and A. Konnerth, Eds., *Imaging: A Laboratory Manual*, Cold Spring Harbor Press, Cold Spring Harbor, 1999.
103. S.E. Ilyin, M.C. Flynn, and C.R. Plata-Salaman, Fiber-optic monitoring coupled with confocal microscopy for imaging gene expression *in vitro* and *in vivo*, *J. Neurosc. Meth.*, 108, 91–96, 2001.

104. W. Denk, J.H. Strickler, and W. Webb, Two-photon laser scanning fluorescence microscopy, *Science*, 648, 73–76, 1990.
105. A. Majewska, G. Yiu, and R. Yuste, A custom-made two-photon microscope and deconvolution system, *Pflugers Arch-Eur. J. Physiol.*, 441, 398–408, 2000.
106. D. Axelrod, N.L. Thompson, and T.P. Burghardt, Total internal reflection fluorescence microscopy, *J. Microsc.*, 129, 19–28, 1982.
107. D. Toomre and D.J. Manstein, Lighting up the cell surface with evanescent wave microscopy, *Trend Cell Biol.*, 11, 298–303, 2001.
108. F. Lanni, A.S. Waggoner, and D.L. Taylor, Structural organization of interface 3T3 fibroblasts studied by total internal reflection fluorescence microscopy, *J. Cell Biol.*, 100, 1091–1102, 1985.
109. G.A. Truskey, J.S. Burmeister, E. Grapa, and W.M. Reichert, Total internal reflection microscopy (TIRFM), *J. Cell Sci.*, 103, 491–499, 1992.
110. D. Axelrod, D.E. Koppel, J. Schlessinger, E.L. Elson, and W.W. Webb, Mobility measurements by analysis of fluorescence photobleaching recovery kinetics, *Biophys. J.*, 16, 1055–1089, 1976.
111. P. Gribbon and T.E. Hardingham, Macromolecular diffusion of biological polymers measured by confocal fluorescence recovery after photobleaching, *Biophys. J.*, 75, 1032–1039, 1998.
112. R.K. Jain, R.J. Stock, S.R. Chary, and M. Rueter, Convection and diffusion measurements using fluorescence recovery after photobleaching and video image analysis: *in vitro* calibration and assessment, *Microvasc. Res.*, 39, 77–93, 1990.
113. E.A. Reits and J.J. Neefjes, From fixed to FRAP: measuring protein mobility and activity in living cells, *Nature Cell Biol.*, 3, E145–E147, 2001.
114. P. Schille, Fluorescence correlation spectroscopy and its potential for intracellular applications, *Cell Biochem. Biophys.*, 34, 383–408, 2001.
115. R. Brock and T.M. Jovin, Fluorescence correlation microscopy (FCM)-fluorescence correlation spectroscopy (FCS) taken into the cell, *Cell Mol. Biol.*, 44, 847–856, 1998.
116. R. Brock, G. Vamosi, G. Vereb, and T.M. Jovin, Rapid characterization of green fluorescent protein fusion proteins on the molecular and cellular level by fluorescence correlation microscopy, *Proc. Natl. Acad. Sci. U.S.A.*, 96, 10123–10128, 1999.
117. M. Sato, T. Ozawa, T. Yoshida, and Y. Umezawa, A fluorescent indicator for tyrosine phosphorylation-based insulin signaling pathways, *Anal. Chem.*, 71, 3948–3954, 1999.
118. A.G. Harpur, F.S. Wouters, and P.I.H. Bastiaens, Imaging FRET between spectrally similar GFP molecules in single cells, *Nature Biotechnol.*, 19, 167–169, 2001.
119. R.M. Clegg, Fluorescence resonance energy transfer, *Curr. Opin. Biotechnol.*, 6, 103–110, 1995.
120. G. Binnig, C.F. Quate, and C. Gerber, Atomic force microscope, *Phys. Rev. Lett.*, 56, 930–933, 1986.
121. M. Fritz, M. Radmacher, N. Peterson, and H.E. Gaub, Visualization and identification of intracellular structures by force modulation microscopy and drug induced degradation, *J. Vac. Sci. Technol. B*, 12, 1526–1529, 1994.
122. M. Walch, U. Ziegler, and P. Groscurth, Effect of streptolysin O on the microelasticity of human platelets analyzed by atomic force microscopy, *Ultramicroscopy*, 82, 259–267, 2000.
123. C. Rotsch, K. Jacobson, and M. Radmacher, Dimensional and mechanical dynamics of active and stable edges in motile fibroblasts investigated by using atomic force microscopy, *Proc. Natl. Acad. Sci. U.S.A.*, 96, 921–926, 1999.
124. J. Domke and M. Radmacher, Measuring the elastic properties of thin polymer films with the atomic force microscope, *Langmuir*, 14, 3320–3325, 1998.
125. H.W. Wu, T. Kuhn, and V.T. Moy, Mechanical properties of L929 cells measured by atomic force microscopy: effects of anticytoskeletal drugs and membrane crosslinking, *Scanning*, 20, 389–397, 1998.
126. C. Rotsch and M. Radmacher, Drug-induced changes of cytoskeletal structure and mechanics in fibroblasts: an atomic force microscopy study, *Biophys. J.*, 78, 520–535, 2000.

127. A.B. Mathur, G.A. Truskey, and W.M. Reichert, Atomic force and total internal reflection fluorescence microscopy for the study of force transmission in endothelial cells, *Biophys. J.*, 78, 1725–1735, 2000.
128. Y. Yamane, H. Shiga, H. Haga, K. Kawabata, K. Abe, and E. Ito, Quantitative analyses of topography and elasticity of living and fixed astrocytes, *J. Electron Microsc.*, 49, 463–471, 2000.
129. E. Nagao and J. A. Dvorak, Phase imaging by atomic force microscopy: analysis of living homoiothermic vertebrate cells, *Biophys. J.*, 76, 3289–3297, 1999.
130. M. Sato, K. Nagayama, N. Kataoka, M. Sasaki, and K. Hane, Local mechanical properties measured by atomic force microscopy for cultured bovine endothelial cells exposed to shear stress, *J. Biomech.*, 33, 127–135, 2000.
131. J.H. Hoh and C.-A. Schoenenberger, Surface morphology and mechanical properties of MDCK monolayers by atomic force microscopy, *J. Cell Sci.*, 107, 1105–1114, 1994.
132. E.A. Hassan, W.F. Heinz, M.D. Antonik, N.P. D'Costa, S. Nagaswaran, C.-A. Schoenenberger, and J. H. Hoh, Relative microelastic mapping of living cells by atomic force microscopy, *Biophys. J.*, 74, 1564–1578, 1998.
133. E. Henderson, P.G. Haydon, and D.S. Sakaguchi, Actin filament dynamics in living glial cells imaged by atomic force microscopy, *Science*, 257, 1944–1946, 1992.
134. J.H. Haga, A.J. Beaudoin, J. G. White, and J. Strony, Quantification of the passive mechanical properties of the resting platelet, *Ann. Biomed. Eng.*, 26, 268–277, 1998.
135. A.E.H. Love, Boussinesq's problem for a rigid cone, *Q. J. Math.*, 10, 161–175, 1939.
136. A.L. Weisenhorn, P. Maivald, H.-J. Butt, and P.K. Hansma, Measuring adhesion, attraction, and repulsion between surfaces in liquids with an atomic force microscope, *Phys. Rev. B*, 45, 11226–11232, 1992.
137. M. Radmacher, M. Fritz, and P.K. Hansma, Imaging soft samples with the atomic force microscope: gelatin in water and propanol, *Biophys. J.*, 69, 264–270, 1995.
138. J. Pourati, A. Maniotis, D. Spiegel, J.L. Schaffer, J.P. Butler, J.J. Fredberg, D.E. Ingber, D. Stamenovic, and N. Wang, Is cytoskeletal tension a major determinant of cell deformability in adherent endothelial cells?, *Am. J. Physiol.*, 247, C1283–C1289, 1998.
139. R.E. Mahaffy, C.K. Shih, F.C. MacKintosh, and J. Kas, Scanning probe-based frequency-dependent microrheology of polymer gels and biological cells, *Phys. Rev. Lett.*, 85, 880–883, 2000.
140. K.D. Costa and F.C. Yin, Analysis of indentation: implications for measuring mechanical properties with atomic force microscopy, *J. Biomech. Eng.*, 121, 462–471, 1999.
141. J.A. Conchello, J.J. Kim, and E.W. Hansen, Enhanced three-dimensional reconstruction from confocal scanning microscopy images. II. Depth discrimination versus signal-to-noise ratio in partically confocal images, *Appl. Opt.*, 33, 3740–3750, 1994.
142. Y.L. Wang, Digital deconvolution of fluorescence images for biologists, *Methods Cell Biol.*, 56, 305–315, 1998.
143. R.M. Schinagl, M.K. Ting, J.H. Price, and R.L. Sah, Video microscopy to quantitate the inhomogeneous equilibrium strain within articular cartilage during confined compression, *Ann. Biomed. Eng.*, 24, 500–512, 1996.
144. M.M. Knight, J. van de Breevaart Bravenboer, D.A. Lee, G.J.V.M. van Osch, H. Weinans, and D.L. Bader, Cell and nucleus deformation in compressed chondrocyte-alginate constructs: temporal changes and calculation of cell modulus, *Biochim. Biophys. Acta*, 1570, 1–8, 2002.
145. F. Guilak, Volume and surface area measurement of viable chondrocytes *in situ* using geometric modeling of serial confocal sections, *J. Microsc.*, 173, 245–256, 1994.
146. F. Guilak, A. Ratcliffe, and V.C. Mow, Chondrocyte deformation and local tissue strain in articular cartilage: a confocal microscopy study, *J. Orthop. Res.*, 13, 410–422, 1995.
147. B.A. Roeder, K. Kokini, J.E. Sturgis, J.P. Robinson, and S.L. Voytik-Harbin, Tensile mechanical properties of three-dimensional type I collagen extracellular matrices with varied microstructure, *J. Biomech. Eng.*, 124, 214–222, 2002.

148. C.C.-B. Wang, G.A. Ateshian, and C.T. Hung, An automated approach for direct measurement of strain distributions within articular cartilage under unconfined compression, *J. Biomech. Eng.*, 124, 557–567, 2002.
149. C.C.-B. Wang, X.E. Guo, D. Sun, V.C. Mow, G.A. Ateshian, and C.T. Hung, The functional environment of chondrocytes within cartilage subjected to compressive loading: theoretical and experimental approach, *Biorheology*, 39, 39–45, 2002.
150. H.M. Shapiro, *Practical Flow Cytometry*, Wiley-Liss, New York, 1995.
151. M.G. Ormerod, An introduction to fluorescent technology, in *Flow Cytometry: A Practical Approach*, M.G. Ormerod, Ed., Oxford University Press, Oxford, U.K., 1994, pp. 1–25.
152. N.P. Carter and E.W. Meyer, Introduction to the principles of flow cytometry, in *Flow Cytometry: A Practical Approach*, M.G. Ormerod, Ed., Oxford University Press, Oxford, U.K., 1994, pp. 1–25.
153. K. Kusuzaki, S. Sugimoto, H. Takeshita, H. Murata, S. Hashiguchi, T. Nozaki, K. Emoto, T. Ashihara, and Y. Hirasawa, DNA cytofluorometric analysis of chondrocytes in human articular cartilages under normal aging or arthritic conditions, *Osteoarthritis Cartilage*, 9, 664–670, 2001.
154. S.H. Kamil, B.S. Aminuddin, L.J. Bonassar, C.A. Arevalo Silva, Y. Weng, M. Woda, C.A. Vacanti, R.D. Eavey, and M.P. Vacanti, Tissue-engineered human auricular cartilage demonstrates euploidy by flow cytometry, *Tissue Eng.*, 8, 85–92, 2002.
155. R.C. Habbersett, J.H. Jett, and R.A. Keller, Single DNA fragment detection by flow cytometry, in *Emerging Tools for Single-Cell Analysis*, G. Durack and J.P. Robinson, Eds., Wiley-Liss, New York, 2000, pp. 73–93.
156. Y.O. Huh and S. Ibrahim, Immunophenotypes in adult acute lymphocytic leukemia. Role of flow cytometry in diagnosis and monitoring of disease, *Hematol. Oncol. Clin. North Am.*, 14, 1251–1265, 2000.
157. L. Wang, G. Verbruggen, K.F. Almqvist, D. Elewaut, C. Broddelez, and E.M. Veys, Flow cytometric analysis of the human articular chondrocyte phenotype *in vitro*, *Osteoarthritis Cartilage*, 9, 73–84, 2001.
158. L. Wang, K.F. Almqvist, C. Broddelez, E.M. Veys, and G. Verbruggen, Evaluation of chondrocyte cell-associated matrix metabolism by flow cytometry, *Osteoarthritis Cartilage*, 9, 454–462, 2001.
159. G. Durack, Cell-sorting technology, in *Emerging Tools for Single-Cell Analysis*, G. Durack and J.P. Robinson, Eds., Wiley-Liss, New York, 2000, pp. 73–93.
160. T. Leemhuis and D. Adams, Applications of high-speed sorting for CD34+ hematopoietic stem cells, in *Emerging Tools for Single-Cell Analysis*, G. Durack and J.P. Robinson, Eds., Wiley-Liss, New York, 2000, pp. 73–93.
161. G. Gaipa, E. Coustan-Smith, E. Todisco, O. Maglia, A. Biondi, and D. Campana, Characterization of CD34+, CD13+, CD33- cells, a rare subset of immature human hematopoietic cells, *Haematologica*, 87, 347–356, 2002.
162. C. Campagnoli, I.A. Roberts, S. Kumar, P.R. Bennett, I. Bellantuono, and N.M. Fisk, Identification of mesenchymal stem/progenitor cells in human first-trimester fetal blood, liver, and bone marrow, *Blood*, 98, 2396–2402, 2001.
163. R. Zohar, J. Sodek, and C.A.G. McCulloch, Characterization of stromal progenitor cells enriched by flow cytometry, *Blood*, 90, 3471–3481, 1997.
164. A. Suzuki, Y. Zheng, R. Kondo, M. Kusakabe, Y. Takada, K. Fukao, H. Nakauchi, and H. Taniguchi, Flow-cytometric separation and enrichment of hepatic progenitor cells in the developing mouse liver, *Hepatology*, 32, 1230–1239, 2000.
165. H.E. Young, T.A. Steele, R.A. Bray, J. Hudson, J.A. Floyd, K. Hawkins, K. Thomas, T. Austin, C. Edwards, J. Cuzzourt, M. Duenzl, P.A. Lucas, and A.C. Black, Human reserve pluripotent mesenchymal stem cells are present in the connective tissues of skeletal muscle and dermis derived from fetal, adult, and geriatric donors, *Anat. Rec.*, 264, 51–62, 2001.
166. R.J. Jankowski, C. Haluszczak, M. Trucco, and J. Huard, Flow cytometric characterization of myogenic cell populations obtained via the preplate technique: potential for rapid isolation of muscle-derived stem cells, *Hum. Gene Ther.*, 12, 619–628, 2001.

167. N. Uchida, D.W. Buck, D. He, M.J. Reitsma, M. Masek, T.V. Phan, A.S. Tsukamoto, F.H. Gage, and I.L. Weissman, Direct isolation of human central nervous system stem cells, *Proc. Natl. Acad. Sci. U.S.A.*, 97, 14720–14725, 2000.
168. J.E. Dennis, J.P. Carbillet, A.I. Caplan, and P. Charbord, The STRO-1+ marrow cell population is multipotential, *Cells Tissues Organs*, 170, 73–82, 2002.
169. M.K. Majumdar, V. Banks, D.P. Peluso, and E.A. Morris, Isolation, characterization, and chondrogenic potential of human bone marrow-derived multipotential stromal cells, *J. Cell Physiol.*, 185, 98–106, 2000.
170. C. Pafumi, P. Bosco, A. Cavallaro, M. Farina, I. Leonardi, G. Pernicone, S. Bandiera, A. Russo, P. Giardina, M. Chiarenza, and A.E. Calogero, Two CD34+ stem cells from umbilical cord blood enrichment methods, *Pediat. Hemat. Oncol.*, 19, 239–245, 2002.
171. B. Alberts, D. Bray, J. Lewis, M. Raff, K. Roberts, and J. D. Watson, Basic genetic mechanisms, *Mol. Biol. Cell*, Garland Publishing, New York, pp. 223–290, 1994.
172. R.L. Miesfeld, Biochemical basis of applied molecular genetics, in *Applied Molecular Genetics*, Wiley-Liss, New York, pp. 3–29, 1999.
173. W.K. Purves, G.H. Orians, and C.H. Heller, Nucleic acids as the genetic material, in *Life: The Science of Biology*, Sinauer Assoc., Sunderland, MA, pp. 236–266, 1992.
174. N.A. Cambell, From gene to protein, in *Biology*, Benjamin/Cummings, Redwood City, CA, 1993, pp. 316–343.
175. W.K. Purves, G.H. Orians, and C.H. Heller, Gene expression in eukaryotes, in *Life: The Science of Biology*, Sinauer Assoc., Inc., Sunderland, MA, 1992, pp. 288–305.
176. R.L. Miesfeld, Isolation and characterization of gene transcripts, in *Applied Molecular Genetics*, Wiley-Liss, New York, 1999, pp. 115–120.
177. M.A. Innis, D.H. Gelfand, and J.J. Sinsky, Amplification of genomic DNA, in *PCR Protocols: A Guide to Methods and Applications*, Academic Press, New York, 1990, pp. 13–20.
178. J. Sambrook, E.J. Fritsch, and T. Maniatis, Analysis and cloning of eukaryotic genomic DNA, in *Molecular Cloning: A Laboratory Manual*, Cold Springs Harbor Laboratory Press, New York, 1989, pp. 9.4–9.59.
179. M.A. Innis, D.H. Gelfand, and J.J. Sinsky, Sample preparation from blood, cells, and other fluids, in *PCR Protocols: A Guide to Methods and Applications*, Academic Press, New York, 1990, pp. 146–152.
180. K. Doyle, DNA purification, in *Promega Protocols and Applications Guide*, K. Doyle, Ed., Promega Corp., Madison, WI, 1996, pp. 75–90.
181. J. Sambrook, E.J. Fritsch, and T. Maniatis, Extraction, purification, and analysis of messenger RNA from eukaryotic cells, in *Molecular Cloning: A Laboratory Manual*, Cold Springs Harbor Laboratory Press, New York, 1989, pp. 7.3–7.87.
182. P. Chomczynski and N. Sacchi, Single-step method of RNA isolation by acid guanidinium thiocyanate-phenol-chloroform extraction, *Anal. Biochem.*, 162, 156–159, 1987.
183. K. Doyle, RNA purification and analysis, in *Promega Protocols and Applications Guide*, K. Doyle, Ed., 1996, pp. 93–111.
184. P. Re, W.B. Valhmu, M. Vostrejs, D.S. Howell, S.G. Fischer, and A. Ratcliffe, Quantitative polymerase chain reaction assay for Aggrecan and Link protein gene expression in cartilage, *Anal. Biochem.*, 225, 356–360, 1995.
185. I. Martin, M. Jakob, D. Schafer, W. Dick, G. Spagnoli, and M. Heberer, Quantitative analysis of gene expression in human articular cartilage from normal and osteoarthritic joints, *Osteoarthritis Cartilage*, 9, 112–118, 2001.
186. C.D. Hoemann, J. Sun, V. Chrzanowski, and M.D. Buschmann, A multivalent assay to detect glycosaminoglycan, protein, collagen, RNA, and DNA content of milligram samples of cartilage or hydrogel-based repair cartilage, *Anal. Biochem.*, 300, 1–10, 2002.
187. R.L. Miesfeld, Expression of cloned genes in cultured cells, in *Applied Molecular Genetics*, Wiley-Liss, New York, 1999, pp. 175–204.

188. J.R. De Wet, K.V. Wood, M. Deluca, D.R. Helinski, and S. Subramani, Firefly luciferase gene: structure and expression in mammalian cells, *Mol. Cell. Biol.*, 7, 725–737, 1987.
189. C.H. Contag and M.H. Bachman, Advances in in vivo bioluminescence imaging of gene expression, *Ann. Rev. Biomed. Eng.*, 4, 235–260, 2002.
190. P.M. Schenk, A.R. Elliot, and J.M. Manners, Assessment of transient gene expression in plant tissues using the green fluorescent protein as a reference, *Plant Mol. Biol. Rep.*, 16, 313–322, 1998.
191. K. Faire, C. Waterman-Storer, D. Gruber, D. Masson, E. Salmon, and J.C. Bulinski, E-MAP-115 (Ensconsin) associates dynamically with microtubules in vivo and is not a physiological modulator of microtubule dynamics, *J. Cell Sci.*, 112, 1999.
192. A. Terskikh, A. Fradkov, G. Ermakova, A. Zaraisky, P. Tan, A.V. Kajava, X. Zhao, S. Lukyanov, M. Matz, S. Kim, I.L. Weissman, and P. Siebert, Fluorescent timer: protein that changes color with time, *Science*, 290, 1585–1588, 2000.
193. P. van Roessel and A.H. Brand, Imaging into the future: visualizing gene expression and protein interactions with fluorescent proteins, *Nature Cell Biol.*, 4, E15–E20, 2002.
194. P.L. Felgner, T.R. Gadek, M. Holm, R. Roman, H.W. Chan, M. Wanz, J.P. Northrop, G.M. Ringold, and M. Danielson, Lipofectin: a highly efficient, lipid-mediated DNA/transfection procedure, *Proc. Natl. Acad. Sci. U.S.A.*, 84, 7413–7417, 1987.
195. G.D. Palmer, P.-H.G. Chao, F. Raia, R.L. Mauck, W.B. Valhmu, and C.T. Hung, Time dependent aggrecan gene expression of articular chondrocytes in response to hyperosmotic loading, *Osteoarthritis Cartilage*, 9, 761–770, 2001.
196. W.B. Valhmu, G.D. Palmer, J. Dobson, S.G. Fischer, and A. Ratcliffe, Regulatory activities of the 5′- and 3′- untranslated regions and promoter of the human aggrecan gene, *J. Biol. Chem.*, 273, 6196–6202, 1998.
197. C.T. Hung, M.A. LeRoux, G.D. Palmer, P.-H.G. Chao, S. Lo, and W.B. Valhmu, Disparate aggrecan gene expression in chondrocytes subjected to hypotonic and hypertonic loading in two-dimensional and three-dimensional culture, *Biorheology*, 40, 61–72, 2003.
198. B. Alberts, D. Bray, J. Lewis, M. Raff, K. Roberts, and J.D. Watson, Recombinant DNA technology, in *Molecular Biology of the Cell*, Garland Publishing, New York, 1994, pp. 291–334.
199. R.L. Miesfeld, The polymerase chain reaction, in *Applied Molecular Genetics*, Wiley-Liss, New York, 1999, pp. 143–172.
200. R.K. Saiki, D.H. Gelfand, S. Stoffel, S.J. Scharf, R. Higuchi, G.T. Horn, K.B. Mullis, and H.A. Erlich, Primer-directed enzymatic amplification of DNA with a thermostable DNA polymerase, *Science*, 239, 487–491, 1988.
201. F. Souaze, A. Ntodue-Thome, C.Y. Tran, W. Rostene, and P. Forgez, Quantitative PCR: limits and accuracy, *Biotechniques*, 21, 280–285, 1996.
202. W.B. Valhmu, E.J. Stazzone, N.M. Bachrach, F. Saed-Nejad, S.G. Fischer, V.C. Mow, and A. Ratcliffe, Load-controlled compression of articular cartilage induces a transient stimulation of aggrecan gene expression, *Arch. Biochem. Biophys.*, 353, 29–36, 1998.
203. M. Becher-Andre and K. Hahlbrock, Absolute mRNA quantitation using the polymerase chain reaction (PCR): a novel approach by a PCR aided transcript titration assay (PATTY), *Nucl. Acids Res.*, 17, 9437–9446, 1989.
204. P. Siebert and J. Larrick, Competitive PCR, *Nature*, 359, 557–558, 1992.
205. J. C. Willey, E.L. Crawford, C.M. Jackson, D.A. Weaver, J.C. Hoban, S.A. Khuder, and J. P. Demuth, Expression measurement of many genes simultaneously by quantitative PCR using standardized mixtures of competitive templates, *Am. J. Respir. Cell Mol. Biol.*, 19, 6–17, 1998.
206. S.A. Bustin, Quantification of mRNA using real-time reverse transcription PCR (RT-PCR): trends and problems, *J. Mol. Endocrinol.*, 29, 23–39, 2002.
207. U.E. Gibson, C.A. Heid, and P.M. Williams, A novel method for real time quantitative RT-PCR, *Gen. Res.*, 6, 995–1001, 1996.
208. S.A. Bustin, Absolute quantification of mRNA using real-time reverse transcription polymerase chain reaction assays, *J. Mol. Endocrinol.*, 25, 169–193, 2000.

209. J. Chen, A.E. Baer, P.Y. Paik, W. Yan, and L.A. Setton, Matrix protein gene expression in intervertebral disc cells subjected to altered osmolarity, *Biochem. Biophys. Res. Commun.*, 293, 932–938, 2002.
210. B. Liss, Improved quantitative real-time RT-PCR for expression profiling of individual cells, *Nucl. Acids Res.*, 30, e89, 2002.
211. M.R. Emmert-Buck, R.F. Bonner, P.D. Smith, R.F. Chuaqui, Z. Ahuang, S.R. Goldstein, R.A. Wiess, and L.A. Liotta, Laser capture microdissection, *Science*, 274, 998–1001, 1996.
212. P. Liang and A.B. Pardee, Differential display of eukaryotic messenger RNA by means of the polymerase chain reaction, *Science*, 257, 967–971, 1992.
213. P. Liang and A.B. Pardee, Differential display. A general protocol, *Mol. Biotechnol.*, 10, 261–267, 1998.
214. L. Diatchenko, Y. Lau, and A. Cambell, Suppression subtractive hybridization: a method for generating differentially regulated or tissue-specific cDNA probes and libraries, *Proc. Natl. Acad. Sci. U.S.A.*, 93, 6025–6030, 1996.
215. G. Bluteau, J. Gouttenoire, T. Conrozier, P. Mathieu, E. Vignon, M. Richard, D. Herbage, and F. Mallein-Gerin, Differential gene expression analysis in a rabbit model of osteoarthritis induced by anterior cruciate ligament (ACL) section, *Biorheology*, 39, 247–258, 2002.
216. M.W. Izzo, B. Pucci, R.S. Tuan, and D.J. Hall, Gene expression profiling following BMP-2 induction of mesenchymal chondrogenesis *in vitro*, *Osteoarthritis Cartilage*, 10, 23–33, 2002.
217. C. Sers, O.I. Tchernitsa, J. Zuber, L. Diatchenko, B. Zhumabayeva, S. Desai, S. Htun, K. Hyder, K. Wiechen, A. Agoulnik, K.M. Scharff, P. Siebert, and R. Schafer, Gene expression profiling in RAS oncogene-transformed cell lines and in solid tumors using subtractive suppression hybridization and cDNA arrays, *Adv. Enzyme Regul.*, 42, 63–82, 2002.
218. E.S. Lander, Arrays of hope, *Nature Genet.*, 21, 3–4, 1999.
219. M.J. Heller, DNA microarray technology: devices, systems, and applications, *Ann. Rev. Biomed. Eng.*, 4, 129–153, 2002.
220. D. Gerhold, T. Rushmore, and C.T. Caskey, DNA chips: promising toys have become powerful tools, *Trends Biol. Sci.*, 24, 168–173, 1999.
221. K.K. Jain, Biotechnological applications of lab-chips and microarrays, *Trends Biotechnol.*, 18, 278–280, 2000.
222. D.J. Graves, Powerful tools for genetic analysis come of age, *TIBTECH*, 17, 127–134, 1999.
223. R. Simon, M.D. Radmacher, and K. Dobbin, Design of studies using DNA microarrays, *Gen. Epidemiol.*, 23, 21–36, 2002.
224. P. Bucher, Regulatory elements and expression profiles, *Curr. Opin. Struct. Biol.*, 9, 400–407, 1999.
225. D.J. Duggan, M. Bittner, Y. Chen, P. Meltzer, and J.M. Trent, Expression profiling using cDNA microarrays, *Nature Genet.*, 21, 10–14, 1999.
226. P.O. Brown and D. Botstein, Exploring the new world of the genome with DNA microarrays, *Nature Genet.*, 21, 33–37, 1999.
227. J. Derisi, L. Penland, P.O. Brown, M. Bittner, P. Meltzer, M. Ray, Y. Chen, Y.A. Su, and J.M. Trent, Use of a cDNA microarray to analyze gene expression patterns in human cancer, *Nature Genet.*, 14, 457–460, 1996.
228. J. Hacia, L. Brody, M. Chee, S. Fodor, and F. Collins, Detection of heterozygous mutations in BRCA1 using high density arrays and two colour fluorescence analysis, *Nature Genet.*, 14, 441–447, 1996.
229. R.K. Sironen, H.M. Karjalainen, K. Torronen, M.A. Elo, K. Kaarniranta, M. Takigawa, H.J. Helminen, and M.J. Lammi, High pressure effects on cellular expression profile and mRNA stability. A cDNA array analysis, *Biorheology*, 39, 111–117, 2002.
230. C. Leethanakul, V. Patel, J. Gillespie, M. Pallente, J.F. Ensley, S. Koontongkaew, L.A. Liotta, M.R. Emmert-Buck, and J.S. Gutkind, Distinct pattern of expression of differentiation and growth-related genes in squamous cell carcinomas of the head and neck revealed by the use of laser capture microdissection and cDNA arrays, *Oncogene*, 19, 3220–3224, 2000.

231. C. Debouck and P.N. Goodfellow, DNA microarrays in drug discovery and development, *Nature Genet.*, 21, 48–50, 1999.
232. F.D. Allen, C.T. Hung, S.R. Pollack, and C.T. Brighton, Mechano-chemical coupling in the flow-induced activation of intracellular calcium signaling in primary cultured bone cells, *J. Biomech.*, 33, 1585–1591, 2000.
233. X.E. Guo, J. Shyu, E. Takai, K.D. Costa, and C.T. Hung, Substrates influence osteoblast elastic modulus measured by atomic force microscopy, *Trans. Orthop. Res. Soc.*, 521, 2002.

16

Histology and Staining

S.E. Greenwald
University of London

A.G. Brown
University of London

CONTENTS

16.1 Introduction

Histology is defined as "the science of organic tissue" although it is more commonly regarded as "that branch of biology or anatomy concerned with the minute structure of the tissues of plants or animals" (Shorter Oxford Dictionary, 1973). Although its origins have been ascribed to Aristotle, who distinguished between tissues and organs, histology as a modern science began with the invention of the compound microscope in about 1600 by Iansen and or Gallileo, and developed with the evolution of microscopy. Nevertheless, many important observations using a single magnifying lens continued to be reported until early in the 18th century, notably by van Leeuwenhoek (1791). Perhaps the first mention of tissue being composed of separate cells was by Robert Hooke (1665). For a detailed outline and chronology of the history of microscopy and histology see for instance (Kaiser, 1985).

Although it is possible to visualize microscopic structures in living tissue, the amount of information obtainable is limited by the inability of visible light to penetrate most organisms beyond a depth of a millimeter or so. Consequently, two of the three main aims of practical histology are the preservation of dead tissue and the cutting of it into slices thin enough to be transparent. Under these conditions, it is often difficult to distinguish different parts of the specimen because they will generally have closely similar refractive indices. Therefore, the third aim is the staining of the specimen to make its components and structure distinguishable.

The acquisition from a living tissue or organ of a magnified image in which the composite materials can be identified and from which a pathologist can make a diagnosis or scientist can derive structural and functional information usually follows a well-defined sequence of steps, summarized in Figure 16.1. The aim of this chapter is to expand briefly on the major steps of the sequence.

0-8493-1140-3/04/$0.00+$1.50

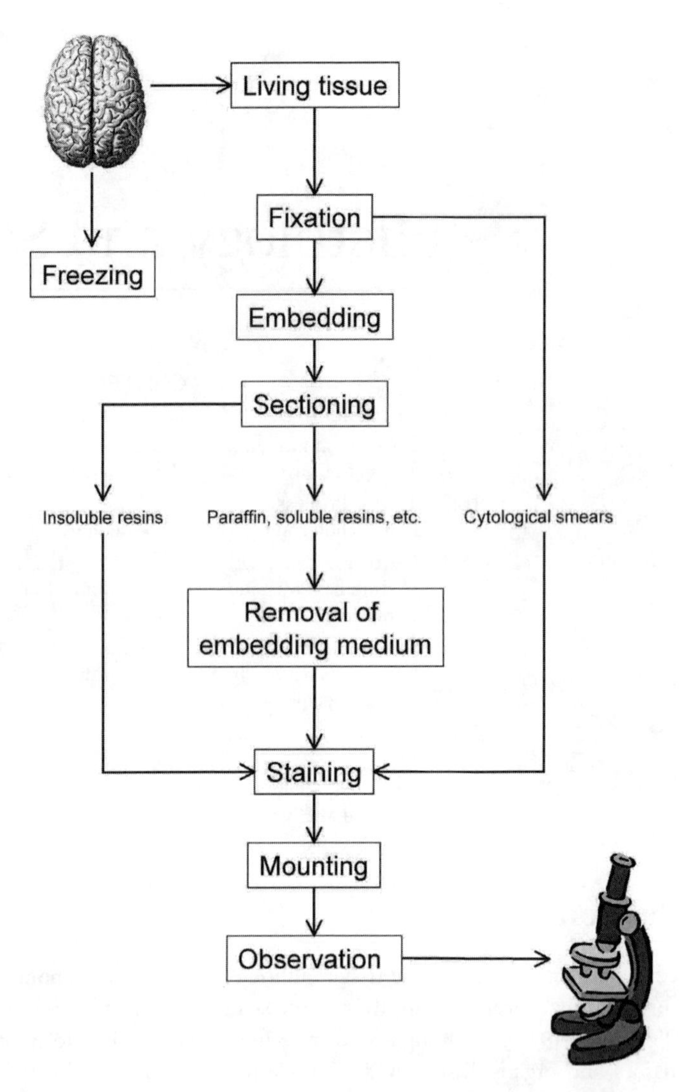

FIGURE 16.1 Summary of the basic steps in histological processing, from living tissue to a stained section suitable for light microscopy. (Redrawn from Horobin, R.W., *Histochemistry: An Explanatory Outline of Histochemistry and Biophysical Staining*, Gustav Fischer Verlag, Stuttgart; Butterworth's, London, 1982. With the permission of the author and publishers.)

Ideally, tissue would be examined in three dimensions. This obviously requires transparency which, for optical microscopy, limits specimen thickness to approximately 600 μm. To study opaque material or more deeply buried structures, the tissue must be sectioned and stained to produce the necessary contrast. Using tomographic software, digital images from contiguous or serial sections can be combined and a three-dimensional image reconstructed. In practice, however, three-dimensional reconstruction is not commonly performed because processing the large number of sections required to produce a high-resolution image is extremely time consuming. Furthermore, small but cumulative errors in aligning successive sections often result in distortion of the three-dimensional geometry and render measurements of length and volume unreliable. During the last 20 years or so, advances in confocal microscopy (see below) have greatly reduced these problems, although structures more than 600 μm below the specimen surface cannot currently be visualized.

As an alternative approach used in cytological screening, where the pathologist is primarily interested in changes in the internal structure of cells, a small sample obtained, for instance, by a needle biopsy is smeared into a thin layer onto a glass slide. After staining, these structures can be seen although information about the architecture of the tissue from which the cells are derived is lost.

16.2 Fixation

Unless it is to be examined very soon after death, nonliving tissue must be *fixed*. The aims of fixation and its effects are (Sanderson, 1994):

- To maintain geometry and dimension as close as possible to that of the living state.
- To prevent autolysis (destruction by enzymes released by dead or dying cells) and putrefaction (attack and digestion by microorganisms).
- To make tissue receptive to staining by changing its chemical composition. Unfixed tissue has little affinity for most histological stains. An additional benefit of the alteration in chemical structure is to produce differential changes in the refractive index of the tissue components thus improving contrast when examined unstained.
- To harden tissue sufficiently to make it more resistant to damage caused by subsequent processing, without making it difficult to cut.

Fixatives can be divided into a number of groups (see below) on the basis of their chemical structure and mode of action (Baker, 1958b), the most important of which stabilize proteins, usually by promoting chemical cross-linking between their molecules forming a gel or a harder polymer surrounding softer components. In this way the morphology of the tissue is stabilized making it easier to cut clean sections. Fixation is normally achieved by immersion in an aqueous solution or, for small fragile specimens, by exposure to vapor. The time taken to fix a tissue depends on the rate at which the fixative diffuses, the temperature and the nature of the tissue itself (Hopwood, 1990). The following empirical relationship between the distance penetrated by the fixative (d) and time (t) was derived by Medewar (1941) for noncoagulating fixatives and by Baker (cited in Baker (1958b)) for fixatives that coagulate protein (i.e., form cross-links).

$$d = kt^{0.5} \tag{16.1}$$

The value of k (at room temperature) for formaldehyde (Baker, 1958b) is 0.06 mm $sec^{-0.5}$ from which it follows that it will take approximately 5 min for this fixative to penetrate 1 mm into a homogenous piece of soft tissue and nearly 8 h to penetrate 10 mm.

In *phase partition* fixation the tissue is immersed in an aqueous solution of fixative in equilibrium with an organic solvent (Nettleton and McAuliffe, 1986) (e.g., 50% glutaraldehyde/water in heptane). It is suitable for delicate tissues and has been used to fix and study mucus on the surface of the trachea that would otherwise be dissolved by aqueous immersion (Sims et al., 1991).

To ensure rapid fixation of whole organs such as lung, heart, liver, etc., the fixative may be perfused through the vasculature (Rostgaard et al., 1993). For reliable morphometric analysis of blood vessels the mean pressure should be close to *in vivo* values (Berry et al., 1993).

16.2.1 Types of Fixative

16.2.1.1 Aldehydes

This group includes formaldehyde, the most commonly used fixative for light microscopy and glutaraldehyde, favored for electron microscopy. Formaldehyde is usually used as *formol saline*, a 4% solution of formaldehyde gas in water containing 0.9% sodium chloride. It reacts with protein by a condensation reaction thereby forming cross-links frequently between lysine residues on the exterior of the protein chains (see, for example, Baker (1958b) for a review of reaction mechanisms).

Fixation with glutaraldehyde often involving the formation of cross-links between pyridine residues (Hilger and Medan, 1987) greatly reduces the immunological activity of proteins, a process sometimes referred to as *denaturation*, thus rendering them unsuitable for immunohistochemical staining (see below). On the other hand it disturbs tissue morphology less severely than formaldehyde and is therefore preferred for investigations of cellular architecture. Acrolein, also an aldehyde, is often mixed with formaldehyde or glutaraldehyde. It has the advantage of rapid penetration and good preservation of morphology (Saito and Keino, 1976).

16.2.1.2 Oxidizing Agents

The most commonly used of this group, which includes potassium dichromate and potassium permanganate, is osmium tetroxide. The reactions of oxidizing agents with different types of tissue have been reviewed by Baker (1958b) and more recently by Kiernan (1990). With proteins, osmium tetroxide is thought to form cross-links. It is soluble in some lipids and is also reduced to the black dioxide by them, which then take on this color and become crumbly, making sections difficult to cut. In spite of these drawbacks and its slow rate of penetration (Baker, 1958a), osmium tetroxide "preserves the structure of the living cell better than any other primary or mixed fixative" (Baker, 1958b) and for this reason is used extensively both as a fixative and as a stain in electron microscopy. Dissolved in a nonaqueous fluorocarbon solvent (FC-72), osmium tetraoxide has been used to demonstrate the ultrastructure of the glycocalyx, the fragile coating of vascular endothelial cells (Sims and Horne, 1994), and used alone in perfused brain tissue for both light and electron microscopy (Branchereau et al., 1995).

16.2.1.3 Alcohols and Acetone

Wine has been used as a preservative since antiquity and, according to Baker (1958b), was first used as a preservative for anatomical purposes in 1663 by Robert Boyle. Alcohols and ketones displace water from protein and dehydrate the tissue as a whole, causing it to harden and shrink. Their main advantage is rapid penetration and, when used at low temperature, preservation of enzymatic and immunological activity (Sato et al., 1986). Ethanol, in particular, is the fixative of choice when transporting specimens by air, as the airlines have little objection to their customers carrying large quantities of this material while remaining suspicious of other toxic chemicals.

16.2.1.4 Other Cross-Linking Agents

This group includes the carbodiimides introduced in 1971 (Kendall et al., 1971) and is seeing increasing use in light and electron microscopy due to their speed of action and specificity (Tymianski et al., 1997), both as a mixture with glutaraldehyde (Willingham and Yamada, 1979) and alone (Panula et al., 1988). They have recently been shown to be suitable for denaturing heart valve tissue prior to implantation as they can easily be washed out and leave little or no toxic residues (Girardot and Girardot, 1996).

16.2.4.5 Heat

Heat alone will cause many proteins to coagulate. Microwaves usually in conjunction with fixatives allow rapid heating although the degree of fixation tends to be nonuniform with the center of the specimen less well fixed (Leong and Duncis, 1986). For large specimens such as whole organs, preliminary fixation by immersion in 0.9% saline and irradiation to a temperature of 68 to 74°C is recommended. The process is completed by irradiating 2- to 3-mm pieces to a temperature pf 50 to 68°C for about 2 min (Leong, 1994). In conjunction with formaldehyde or glutaraldehyde, fixation times as little as 10 sec can be achieved thus reducing the effects of autolysis, diffusion of cell contents, and retaining ultrastructural detail (Leong et al., 1985; Login and Dvorak, 1985). Among other applications in the histology laboratory, microwave irradiation has been used to preserve immunological activity (Leong et al., 1988), improve the quality of frozen sections, and enhance the staining of ultrathin sections for electron microscopy (EM). Technical details are discussed at some length by Leong (1994) and general reviews may be found in Leong (1988, 1993).

16.2.1.6 Unknown Mechanism

Although fixatives have been in use for many decades, the mode of action of several standard fixatives is not well understood. These include mercuric chloride which penetrates tissue rapidly and coagulates proteins by reacting with many different amino acid residues (Hopwood, 1990), and picric acid which, in conjunction with other fixatives such as ethanol or formalin, also coagulates protein while leaving the tissue soft (Leong, 1994).

16.2.2 Post-Fixation

It has been found that staining intensity can be improved by following a period of primary fixation in formalin, for example, by a few hours of additional treatment with mercuric chloride (Leong, 1994). Sections are said to be easier to cut and to flatten more readily when post-fixed (Hopwood, 1990). Staining of cell membranes in samples fixed in glutaraldehyde for electron microscopy is improved by post-fixation with osmium tetroxide. Blocks destined for both light and electron microscopic investigation can be post-fixed with 10% formalin following standard glutaraldehyde treatment, which has the additional advantage of retaining intracellular structure (Tandler, 1990).

16.2.3 Fixation Artifacts

Tissue volume may change during fixation although the effects are small compared to shrinkage during embedding. They are discussed in the next section. Specimens that have been stored in formalin for extended periods under acidic conditions become suffused with fine brown crystals of *formalin pigment*, which is thought to be formed by the reaction of formalin with hematin derived from the hemoglobin of ruptured red blood cells (Baker, 1958b). Its formation is inhibited by the addition of 2% phenol to formalin. If it has formed, it may be removed by brief treatment with a saturated solution of picric acid in ethanol followed by washing in water (Drury and Wallington, 1980).

Although fixation normally stiffens the tissue as well as removing water, highly mobile inorganic ions as well as large molecules such as hemoglobin (Reale and Luciano, 1970) may diffuse through the specimen toward its periphery as it fixes, giving a spurious view of their localization and distribution. In metabolic studies of living tissue, the uptake of radioactively labeled amino acids or sugars may be studied postmortem by assessing the distribution of the label in the tissue. However, glutaraldehyde binds strongly to many of these substances and therefore their distribution in fixed tissue assessed microscopically by autoradiography (see below) may be altered. Finally, some tissue components, for example, lipids and mucopolysaccharides, do not react with commonly used fixatives and may be lost from the tissue during subsequent processing.

16.3 Tissue Processing

16.3.1 Dehydration and Clearing

Following fixation, tissue must be *processed* to render it suitable for embedding and subsequent sectioning. Paraffin wax, the most common embedding medium, is hydrophobic, whereas most fixatives are aqueous. Therefore, the material must first be dehydrated and then infiltrated with a solvent that is miscible with the embedding medium. Typically, the specimen is soaked initially in an aqueous solution of an alcohol and transferred at intervals through successively more concentrated solutions until no more water remains. The processing continues with the replacement of the alcohol by a transfer agent or transition medium (most commonly xylene or toluene) which is both miscible with alcohol and a solvent for paraffin wax, the embedding agent. Finally, the xylene is replaced by molten wax resulting in complete infiltration of the tissue. Typically, the entire process under automatic control takes around 16 h (Gordon, 1990), although small specimens, e.g., needle biopsies, may be processed in 3 h. Dehydration with ethanol and treatment with xylene usually cause hardening, which may be reduced by using *n*-butanol; and loss of lipids, which is minimized by rapid treatment.

16.3.2 Embedding

Ideally, the embedding medium should be of approximately equal density and resilience to the tissue to allow cutting of sections with minimal damage. The most commonly used medium is paraffin wax because it is easy to cut, cheap, and widely available. Sections thinner than 2 μm, which are needed to examine details of intracellular structure, require a tougher medium such as a plastic resin (see below), from which sections as thin as 0.2 μm can be cut. However, this requires harder and sharper knives made of tungsten carbide or glass (Bennett et al., 1976).

The tissue permeated with embedding medium is placed in a mold, orientated for subsequent sectioning (Hilger and Medan, 1987; Arnolds, 1978). The mold is filled with the medium and allowed to cool, usually under automatic control.

Other embedding media with lower melting points, such as polyethylene glycol or polyester waxes, can be used when excessive heat may reduce immunological activity of proteins that are to be stained by antibodies (see below). For hard and tough specimens or those that contain tissues with differing degrees of hardness, cellulose nitrate has traditionally been used. However, this material is chemically hazardous and is not suitable for sections less than 10-μm thick.

During the last 50 years plastic resins have been developed for use as embedding media driven initially by the development of the electron microscope and the consequent need for a material which could produce sections no thicker than 80 nm and able to withstand temperatures to 200°C (Nunn, 1970). Plastic resins are tougher than paraffin wax and therefore make it possible to cut thinner sections and harder tissues with less damage to the section. They also cause less shrinkage during processing than waxes. The three main types are briefly compared in Table 16.1.

16.3.3 Tissue Shrinkage

Most fixatives cause tissue to shrink, largely due to their dehydrating effect, although acidic fixatives including formalin lead, at least initially, to swelling driven by osmotic pressure (Baker, 1958a). However, as fixation and dehydration proceed, shrinkage inevitably occurs, different tissues being affected to different extents. The early literature (reviewed by Baker [1958b]) reports quite variable results on the effects of dehydration on different tissues. More recent reviews (see, for example, Fox et al. [1985])and more modern studies agree that fixation and dehydration account for a reduction in volume of between 3 and 6% for whole organs (Iwadare et al., 1984) and up to 30% for individual cells (Ross, 1953). Removal of fixative by treatment with transition medium prior to embedding causes a further reduction of around 10% (with respect to the original volume). Finally, embedding in wax results in an overall reduction in volume of no less than 35%. Resin shrinks less than wax during the embedding process and, when sectioned and dried, may stretch. Overall, tissues in resin sections are nearer to their living dimensions

TABLE 16.1 Summary of the Properties of Embedding Resins

Material	Advantages	Drawbacks
Epoxy (Spurr, 1969)	Tough, thin sections possible Can be softened with plasticizers for easier sectioning Shrinkage ≈3%	Curing temperature 60°C, may cause tissue damage Hydrophobic, therefore compatible with limited range of stains
Acrylic (Murray, 1988; Litwin, 1985)	Low viscosity, easier processing Monomer water miscible; polymer water permeable; dehydration not necessary, compatible with many stains	Shrinkage ≈15%
Polyester	Low viscosity, easier processing Some can be polymerized at low temp with UV light, therefore suitable for immunological staining (Altman et al., 1984) Controllable hardness to match tissue; more water compatible than epoxy, less than acrylic Tolerant of electron beam; suitable for electron microscopy	Small specimens only due to limited penetration of UV for curing; non-UV-curable have curing temperature

than those embedded in wax, although factors such as temperature and section thickness affect the overall degree of volume change (Hanstede and Gerrits, 1983). In a study of arterial sections, Dobrin (1996) has shown that formalin fixation followed by dehydration and embedding in paraffin wax leads to a reduction in cross-sectional area of 19%. Fixation in McDowell's solution (recipe given in Dobrin [1996]) followed by embedding in glycol methacrylate (which avoids the need to further dehydrate the tissue) resulted in an overall increase in cross-sectional area as little as 4%. This procedure appears to be optimal at least for vascular histomorphometry. Clearly, when measuring absolute dimensions of cells or other tissue components careful assessment of shrinkage is essential.

16.4 Cutting

16.4.1 Microtomes

The purpose of the microtome is to cut sections of known and uniform thickness through tissue, which is surrounded by and infused with embedding medium, in the form of a cuboidal or cylindrical block. At its most basic, the microtome consists of a chuck to hold the tissue block near to a blade that is passed over the specimen and that removes thin slices in the manner of a carpenter's plane. A later development allows the specimen to advance toward the blade, as each slice is removed, by rotating a lead screw attached to the chuck (Figure 16.2a). This type of rocking blade device was introduced in 1881 (Kaiser, 1985). In its modern form, the base sledge microtome (Figure 16.2b), the chuck and lead screw assembly, in a heavy casting moving on runners within a massive frame, is passed repeatedly under a fixed blade. Each pass of the specimen causes the lead screw to advance by a preset amount. The inertia of the rocking mechanism, which is usually driven by hand, minimizes chattering between the blade and the block, and consequent tearing of the specimen. The base sledge microtome is largely confined to the cutting of wax embedded sections. As the sections are cut, they are pushed onto the upper surface of the blade where they collect as a delicate ribbon of crinkled sections. From time to time these are carefully picked up and floated onto water held at some 10°C below the melting point of the wax. The softened wax is stretched by surface tension and the flattened section is transferred to a glass slide by passing the slide underneath the section, to which it adheres by surface tension, and lifting it out of the water (Figure 16.3). Thin resin sections suitable for electron microscopy may be flattened by exposure to xylene or chloroform vapor and picked up onto a fine metal grid rather than a glass slide (Nunn, 1970). Slides with sections containing elastin such as blood vessels, skin and lung tissue, which retain some resilience even after prolonged fixation and which tend to curl at the edges, are placed on a hot plate that softens the wax further and allows greater stretching. These processes require considerable manual dexterity and training. The tricks of the trade may be found in practical texts such as Bancroft and Stevens (1990) and Sanderson (1994).

In the rotary microtome, the chuck and embedded specimen block are moved against a blade in a reciprocating motion by a crank connected to a motor or manually driven flywheel. These widely used devices can cut sections varying in thickness from 0.5 to 25 μm in wax and resins and lend themselves well to automated section cutting (Vincent, 1991).

Sections once picked up onto the slides are placed in an incubator at just below the melting point of the wax for about 30 min. This dries the slide and increases the adhesion between section and glass. Finally, they are soaked in xylene and, if they are to be stained with an aqueous dye, are rehydrated with aqueous ethanol and water. (If alcoholic dyes are to be used, the rehydration stage is omitted.)

Fixed or unfixed tissue can be hardened by freezing and cut in a *freezing microtome* designed or modified to maintain the specimen at a low temperature (–20 to –40°C). This allows the rapid assessment of biopsies obtained during a surgical procedure so that the surgeon's subsequent decisions may then be based on the pathologist's diagnosis. Frozen sections are also used for investigating tissues that are prone to rapid enzymatic degradation (e.g., liver, central nervous system), or that contain diffusible or soluble materials such as lipid.

In the vibrating blade microtome, or *vibratome*, a thin razor-like blade oscillating at main frequency is advanced across the specimen glued to a stub, held in a chuck, and immersed in water, saline, or fixative

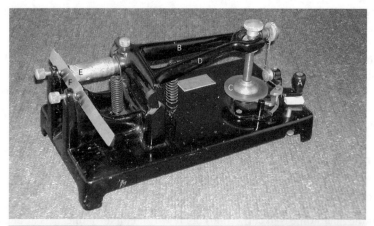

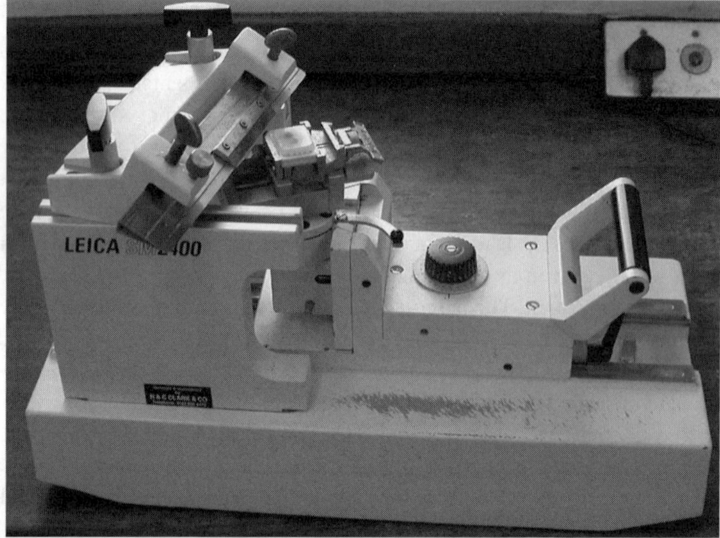

FIGURE 16.2 (Upper panel) "Cambridge Rocker" microtome. This instrument, built in the late 19th century, was in routine use until the 1930s. The spring-loaded handle (A) is pulled toward the operator causing arm (B) to lift the specimen embedded in a wax block (E) above the edge of the blade (F). At the same time a pawl engages in the toothed wheel causing and the attached threaded rod to rotate lifting arm (D) and advancing the specimen toward the blade by a set amount which determines the section thickness. On releasing the handle, the specimen is drawn down over the blade, thus producing a thin slice that rides up onto the blade. (Lower panel) Base sledge microtome.

to prevent undue heating. The amplitude of the vibration and the speed at which the blade advances through the specimen can be adjusted to suit different types of tissue (Zelander and Kirkeby, 1978; Sallee and Russell, 1993). The major advantage of these devices is that they will cut cleanly through unfixed and unembedded tissue at room temperature. Their major drawback is that unprocessed specimens less than 20-μm thick cannot be cut because they tend to disintegrate.

16.4.2 Microtome Blades

The profile and sharpness of the blade is of critical importance in maintaining a clean cut and uniform section thickness. In paraffin sections under optimal conditions, the thickness of adjacent sections can vary by 10% in a standard 5-μm section and by as much as 50% in 1-μm sections. In tests on typical sections of nominal thickness 5 μm, although the mean measured thickness was 4.8 μm (SD 0.14 μm), individual sections varied between 3 and 7 μm. In thinner sections (nominal thickness 1 μm), the variation

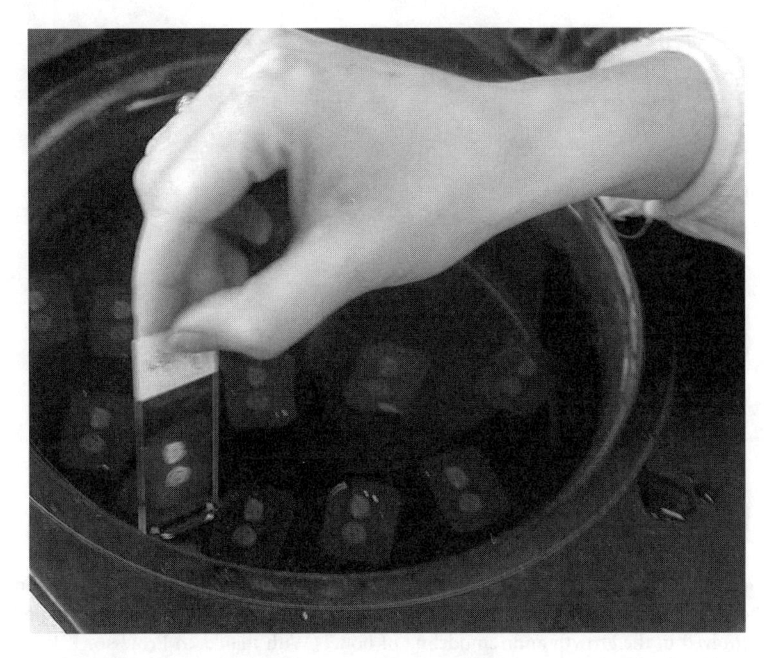

FIGURE 16.3 Sections cut from a wax block floating on water and flattened by surface tension. A single slice has been lifted onto a glass slide.

was as much as 50% (Merriam, 1957; Helander, 1983). Thickness variation in resin sections that are harder and more homogenous than wax is, however, considerably smaller (Helander, 1983). Nevertheless, thickness variation must be carefully assessed, especially in studies involving three-dimensional reconstruction from serial sections (Bibb et al., 1993).

Microtome blades are typically made of high carbon steel and commonly have a plane wedge-shaped profile with a raked edge, although other profiles are used for particularly hard or soft materials (Ellis, 1994). Sharpening is a highly skilled procedure, details of which may be found in standard practical histology texts (Ellis, 1994; Sanderson, 1994). For harder materials such as teeth and bone, a cutting edge of sintered tungsten carbide is bonded to a steel body.

For very thin sections of hard material, glass knives made by fracturing a glass block under controlled conditions (Reid and Beesley, 1991) are suitable. They can be used in a base sledge, rotating blade, or specialized power-driven microtomes (for example, the Ultramicrotome, Dupont Biomedical Products Division, Wilmington, Delaware) designed to cut sections from hard resin blocks as thin as 10 nm, suitable for electron microscopy. In this device, section thickness is controlled by advancing the block by a stepper motor under microprocessor control. Diamond knives may be used in place of glass with the advantage of increased sharpness and durability. The drawbacks are high cost and a cutting width limited to 4 mm.

16.4.3 Cutting Metal/Tissue Composites

When studying the pathology of the interaction between living tissue and metal implants such as joint prostheses or intravascular stents, it is frequently necessary to cut sections containing soft tissue in proximity to metals such as stainless steel or titanium (Figure 16.4). A standard technique developed to deal with these problems involves the following steps (Donath, 1985):

- Embed fixed specimen in resin to form a cylindrical block.
- Cut a disk (say, 5 mm in thickness) from the cylindrical block using a diamond-coated band saw.
- Glue disk to plastic base plate, typically with epoxy resin.
- Remove cutting marks by grinding one face of the disk flat using graded grinding paste and polish.

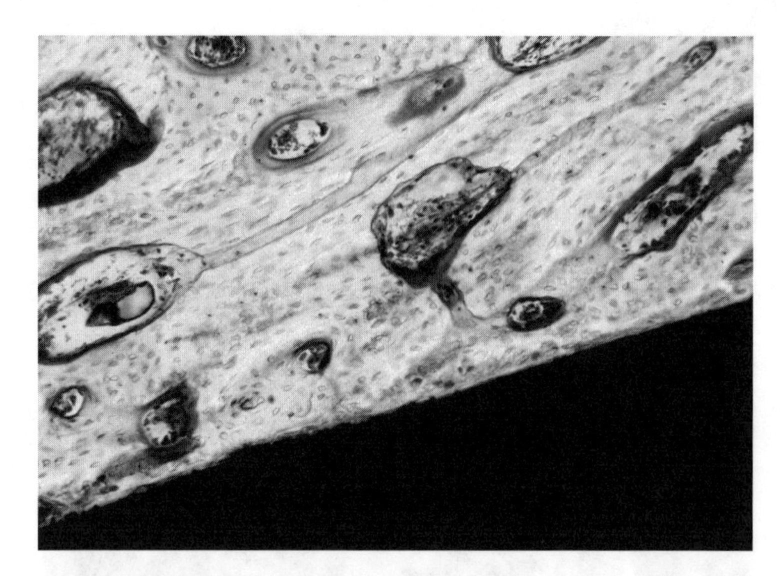

FIGURE 16.4 **(See color insert following page 14-10.)** Section of the femoral head and adjoining stainless steel implant. Note the "clean" interface between the tissue and the implant. Elliptical areas contain osteoclasts and osteoblasts, cells involved in the growth and remodeling of bone. (With thanks to Professor P. Revell.)

- Glue plastic slide to polished face of the disk.
- Cut the sandwich formed by the base plate, the disk, and the plastic slide with the band saw so that the distance between the plastic slide and the cut edge is slightly greater than the desired section thickness.
- Grind the cut face until the desired section thickness is achieved and polish.
- Glue cover slip over the exposed polished face of the disk.

This elaborate and time-consuming process minimizes the risk of crushing the soft tissue or tearing the metal out of the section while preserving its geometry and producing a section of known thickness and good optical quality. Sections as thin as 25 μm may be reliably produced.

16.5 Staining

A biological stain has been defined as "a dye for making biological objects more clearly visible than they would be unstained" (Lillie, 1969). Initially, all dyes were of natural origin, obtained by extraction from plants such as crocus (saffron) (Leeuwenhoek, 1791) cited in Baker (1958b), the tree *haemotoxylon campechianum* (hemotoxylin) (Waldeyer, 1863) and the cochineal beetle (carmine) (Goppert and Cohn, 1849), the latter being the first systematically to study dyed tissues with the microscope although, as mentioned above, von Leeuwenhoek certainly employed dyes. The early history of histological staining has been briefly reviewed by Conn (1969) and Baker (1958b) and in more detail by, for instance, Lewis (1942).

The term *staining* is generally used to include any method of coloring tissue. This may be achieved by using a dye containing a chemical group (or groups) that binds with reactive sites in the tissue. This process is sometimes referred to as *dyeing* (Kiernan, 1990). Alternatively, the tissue may be allowed to absorb a solution of a coloring agent that remains in the tissue when the solvent evaporates in the manner of a coffee stain on a tablecloth.

Baker (1958b) defines dyes as "aromatic, salt-like, crystalline solids, that dissolve in aqueous solutions in the form of coloured ions which can attach themselves chemically to tissue components. When the attachment takes place they do not lose or change colour." This raises two questions: What makes ions colored? And how do they attach to tissues?

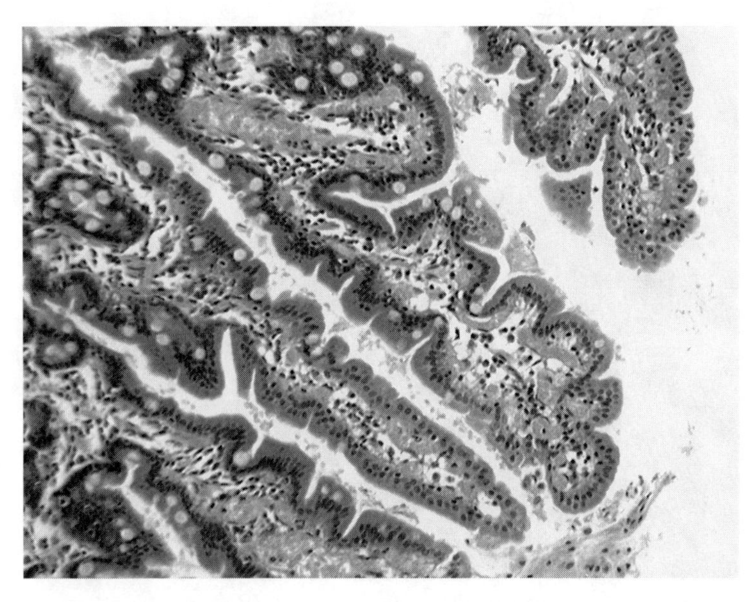

FIGURE 16.5 (**See color insert following page 14**-10.) Section through the lining of the small intestine stained with hematoxylin and eosin.

The majority of dyes used in histological staining are organic molecules containing conjugated double bonds consisting of electronic orbitals delocalized over several atoms (a chromogen) and polar residues which enable them to form ionic bonds with polar molecules in the tissue (auxochromes). The energy required to raise electrons in the delocalized orbitals to an excited state often corresponds to frequencies in the visible part of the EM spectrum, and most organic compounds with conjugated bonds (for instance, quinoids in which two of the hydrogen atoms on the benzene ring are replaced by an oxygen) are therefore colored.

There are many types of chemical bonds formed between dye and tissue. For instance, acidic dyes are commonly used to stain basic components in cellular cytoplasm and collagen in connective tissue; whereas basic dyes are more suitable for nucleic acids in the cell nucleus and other acidic moieties such as phospholipids or mucins. Neutral or amphoteric dyes such as hematoxylin require the presence of a *mordant*, usually a metal ion, which has the effect of making the amphoteric dye basic, thus strengthening the bond between dye and tissue. Mordants in general are able to bond chemically both with the tissue and the dye and are often used to ensure that the dye does not leach out during subsequent treatment such as using a second dye to stain another tissue component.

Perhaps the most frequently used coloring process in histology combines the dyes hematoxylin which, ideally, stains cell nuclei blue and eosin, the "counterstain," which is taken up by the cytoplasm, rendering it red or pink (Figure 16.5).

Polychrome stains result when three or more dyes are applied sequentially to the same section to give a multicolored preparation. The classic trichrome technique described by Masson (Masson, 1929) gives striking results, wherein the connective tissue protein collagen stains blue, while muscle cells are red (Figure 16.6), which also shows the results of the MSB stain. In Johansen's quadruple stain for plant tissue, for example, parasitic fungi stain green, cytoplasm stains orange, cellulose appears as a yellowish green, and lignin takes on a red color (Johansen, 1939). Polychrome stains have been reviewed by Culling et al. (1985).

The rubber-like protein elastin, which is unusually hydrophobic, is effectively stained by water-soluble dyes such as Orcein or acid fuchsin which contain hydrophobic groups surrounded by molecular clusters of water stabilized by hydrogen bonding. A similar process takes place when the dye congo red is used to demonstrate the presence of amyloid, a protein formed in the brain and other organs as a result of

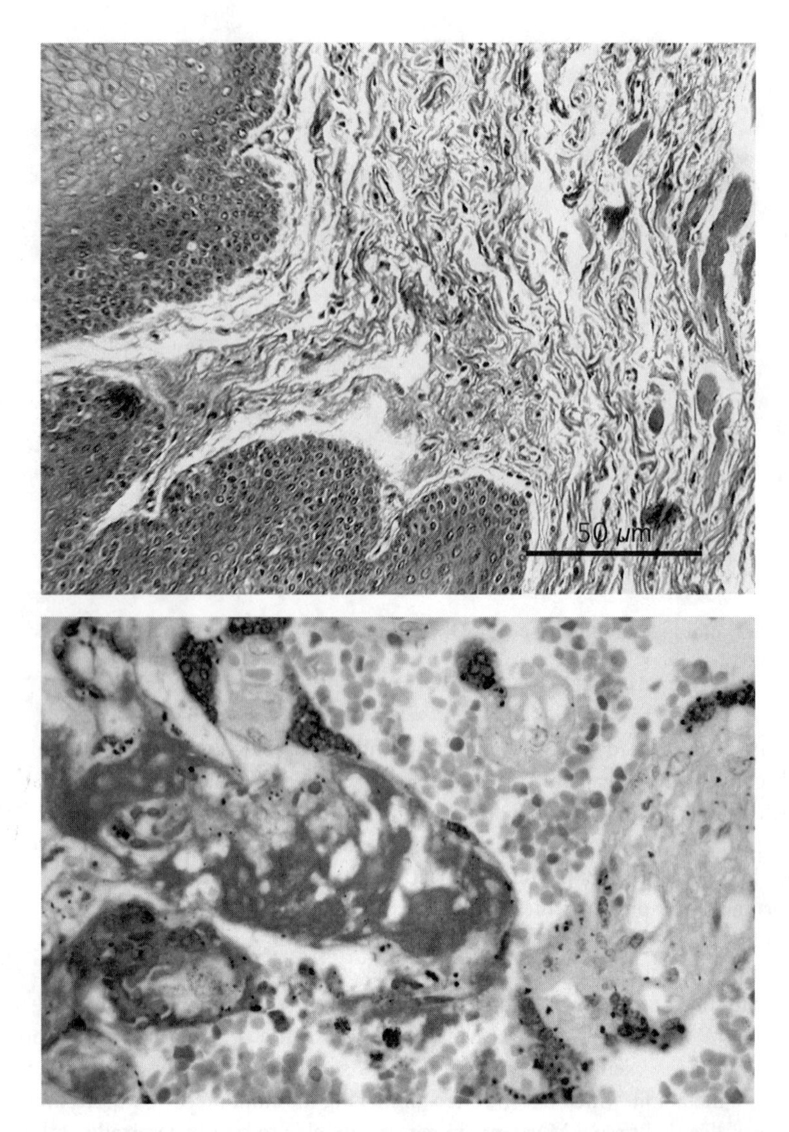

FIGURE 16.6 (See color insert following page 14-10.) (Upper panel) Transverse section of the tongue treated with Masson's trichrome stain, showing muscle in red, connective tissue in blue/green, and cell nuclei in purple. (Lower panel) Section of placenta stained with MSB. With this stain, fibrin is red, other connective tissue is blue, and red blood cells are yellow.

degenerative disease. When the hydrophobic groups in the dye and on the protein come together, the water clusters are destabilized and the entropy of the system is increased. This process has been termed hydrophobic bonding. It and other types of chemical bonding between dye and tissue are summarized in Horobin (1988, 1990).

In wax-embedded material, the wax is dissolved away after mounting the section on the slide and the tissue can then be exposed to a wide variety of aqueous or nonaqueous dye solutions. Resin-embedded material normally cannot be removed in this way, thus the variety of dyes is limited to those that are compatible with the resin used. Nevertheless, the number of resin-compatible dyes continues to increase and several polychrome varieties have been developed (see, for example, Johansen [1939] and Scala et al. [1993]). Acrylic resins on the other hand, being water soluble do not suffer from this incompatibility with aqueous dyes.

Other methods of coloring tissue include:

- The staining of lipid by nonpolar dyes such as Sudan Red dissolved in nonaqueous solvents (e.g., iso-propanol). The degree of uptake depends on the relative solubility of the dye in solvent and tissue.
- Metallic impregnation used in electron microscopy to increase electron density.
- The Gram stain (see, for example, Lillie [1965]) which exploits the difference between types of bacteria in the solubility of trapped dye molecules. Gram-positive bacteria retain the dye after treatment with iodine and appear blue, whereas Gram-negative organisms appear colorless and may then be visualized by treatment with a counterstain, usually neutral red, the background. The presence or absence of this stain together with the shape of the bacterium provides the pathologist with a simple method of classifying microorganisms found in infectious diseases and infected wounds.
- Vital staining in which a dye is taken up by living cells — for example, acridine orange stains intracellular DNA and connective tissue green, and intracellular RNA, red/orange. The dyes can be introduced via the vasculature, injected directly into muscle or, for freshly obtained biopsies, by immersion. Such stains are of particular value to the pathologist to demonstrate cell function in biopsies (Aschoff et al., 1982; Foskett and Grinstein, 1990).

16.5.1 Immunohistochemistry

A major problem with most staining techniques involving dyes is that staining intensity and even color are variable and interpretation depends on the knowledge and skill of the observer. The introduction of immunocytochemistry in the 1950s (Coons and Kaplan, 1950; Coons et al., 1955) largely overcame this, while at the same time introducing a different set of problems. In essence immunocytochemistry relies on the highly specific reaction between an applied antibody and the tissue constituent to which it binds (antigen). In order to visualize the point of reaction, the antibody must carry a molecule (label) that enables a colored end product to be formed. Originally, these labels were enzymes, which were then demonstrated by standard histochemical staining techniques already in use for the visualization of enzymes in tissue. Of those originally tried out, peroxidase and alkaline phosphatase have survived the test of time and are currently the most favored in routine use. In addition to enzymes, which remain the most commonly used labels for light microscopy, fluorescent dyes, colloidal metals or radioactive isotopes are used (Polak and Van Noorden, 1984).

Initially, a single labeled primary antibody was used in what has come to be known as the direct technique. This method had the advantage that it was quick to carry out, and nonspecific reactions were minimized as only the single antibody was used. However, it suffered from the fact that each antigenic site had only one colored molecule attached to it giving little signal amplification. Through a number of intermediate methods, the avidin-biotin complex (ABC) techniques most favored today were developed. These rely on the fact that avidin has four binding sites available for reaction with biotin with which it has a high affinity. Biotin can also be coupled to an antibody as well as an enzyme label such as peroxidase.

The first step in carrying out the ABC technique is to apply an unlabeled primary antibody to the antigen of interest. Step two is to apply a secondary antibody labeled with biotin that reacts with the primary. For example, if the first antibody was raised in a rabbit (rabbit anti-antigen), the second antibody could be biotinylated mouse anti-rabbit. The reason for using a secondary antibody rather than directly labeling the primary is that the general technique can then be applied to any antibody, no matter which animal it was raised in, simply by changing the secondary antibody species. The third step is to apply a preformed complex of avidin and peroxidase-labeled biotin. This is prepared such that not all of the biotin binding sites on the avidin are occupied. These free sites are able to join to the biotin of the secondary antibody and also to other avidin-biotin complex molecules. In this way the number of peroxidase molecules available for color formation is greatly increased providing the required signal amplification.

One of the major problems with the demonstration of antigenic sites is that they must be well preserved by the fixation process, but also be available for demonstration. This contradiction can be overcome by a number of poorly understood treatments grouped under the heading of antigen unmasking. Initially, enzymatic treatment was employed using enzymes such as trypsin and pronase. These are applied at the start of the technique under conditions that free the antigenic sites without destroying the structure of the remaining tissue. Enzymatic treatment has largely been replaced by heat-mediated antigen retrieval techniques where the sections are heated in the presence of heavy metal salts or, more often, buffers such as citrate at pH 6.0. Heating is carried out using microwaves or by boiling in a pressure cooker or autoclave. This would seem to be a very harsh treatment but it would appear that antigens survive better using these treatments than when unmasked by enzymes.

Great care must be taken when employing unmasking techniques as many antigens may be destroyed and larger proteins may be broken down to reveal molecules displaying antigenic sites leading to false negative and positive results, respectively. It is therefore very important when introducing a new antibody in to the laboratory that adequate tests are carried out using tissues known to contain the antigen for investigation and other tissues in which the antibody is lacking.

16.5.2 *In Situ* Hybridization

A further development of the principles of immunocytochemistry has been the introduction of *in situ* hybridization (ISH) for the demonstration of DNA and RNA. This technique relies upon the hybridization of labeled single-stranded fragments of nucleic acid (probes) to complementary strands of nucleic acid located within the tissue sample. This has the distinct advantage over other methods of nucleic acid demonstration in that it is the only technique that allows their localization to specific cells within tissues. As with immunocytochemistry, the major problem with this technique is that the nucleic acids are masked in a complex matrix of other tissue elements which have been cross-linked by the process of fixation. In addition, DNA is already masked by being double stranded, and one of these strands must be removed before hybridization can occur. As with immunocytochemistry, careful fixation preserves more of the nucleic acid of interest and gives better morphology, but also decreases the accessibility of the probe to the tissue. Similarly, mild protease treatment is employed, commonly proteinase K, and again the extent of this treatment must be determined in a series of trial runs.

Probe selection is an important step in carrying out successful hybridization and a number of different probes are available to suite particular circumstances. Double-stranded DNA probes are available that contain both complementary strands that have been labeled. As there is no way of controlling which of the two strands will be removed from the tissue by the pretreatment, double-stranded probes have the advantage that either will do. However, they suffer from the fact that the two strands of the probe will reanneal with themselves in solution thereby reducing their sensitivity. Single-stranded DNA and RNA probes are available, both providing greater sensitivity. However, it is the introduction of oligonucleotide probes that has allowed *in situ* hybridization to mature into a technique available for use in routine laboratories. These are readily synthesized short lengths (normally 20 to 30 bases) of nucleotide that have the label incorporated during the production process. Their synthesis allows the production of "designer" probes of known base sequence that can be used against specific regions on nucleic acid present in the tissue sample. They also have the advantage that their small size allows them easily to penetrate the spaces within the fixed tissue. However, because of their short length the choice of base sequence must be carefully controlled to avoid mismatches occurring with other similar regions on nucleic acid of the target tissue.

An important factor that has made *in situ* hybridization such a useful technique is that the specificity of reaction can be very accurately controlled by varying the conditions under which hybridization is carried out. Thus length and concentration of the probe, pH, temperature and buffer composition are all factors that affect the sensitivity and specificity of the reaction. The variation of these factors determines the "stringency" under which the reaction occurs. Reactions carried out at high stringency (high temperature, low salt, high formamide buffer concentrations) ensure that only reactions with high homology are stable. Under low stringency conditions (low temperature, high salt, low formamide) some degree of stable mismatching will occur giving nonspecific reactions. One might ask why high stringency conditions are not employed all of the time. The answer is that, to a large extent, they are incompatible with the aims of keeping tissue sections on the slide and maintaining adequate tissue morphology because, for sufficient hybridization to occur, prolonged periods under harsh conditions are required. It is therefore left to the user to decide the level of mismatching that can be tolerated and in most cases moderate conditions over 4 to 6 h are used, with mismatches being removed by subsequent washing in buffer of high stringency.

Visualization of the label is carried out using the same techniques employed for immunocytochemistry. Today probes are mainly labeled with bioton or digoxigenin. The former can be demonstrated by an ABC technique while the latter requires an antidigoxigenin antibody followed by ABC.

16.5.3 Autoradiography

Autoradiography, a method of locating small quantities of radioactivity in biological material, can trace its origins to the observation in 1896 by Henri Bequerel that uranium and its compounds are able to fog a nearby photographic plate (for an account of its early history see Rogers, [1973]). A radioactively labeled marker chosen for its ability to bind with the tissue or cell under investigation is administered to an experimental animal, a tissue culture or a cell culture system and is taken up by the target cells. The tissue is then fixed, embedded and sectioned after which the section is placed in close contact with a specially prepared photographic emulsion, consisting of a suspension of silver bromide (AgBr) in gelatine bonded to the surface of the section. Radioactivity from the section is absorbed by the emulsion, producing free bromine ions which, in turn, yield free electrons. These are trapped by defects in the AgBr crystal lattice where they react with silver ions to produce atomic silver. This process is analogous to the exposure to light of a conventional photographic film. The free silver atoms act as nuclei for the formation of more atomic silver and during the development process, grains of silver are formed that are large enough to be detected microscopically. After development, the emulsion is treated with a fixative that dissolves the unreacted AgBr, rendering the emulsion transparent.

In principle it is possible to measure the amount of radioactivity in the section by counting the silver grains although changes in pressure, temperature or the effects of additional chemical reactions can all change their size as well as the number formed. To ensure the accuracy and repeatability of quantitative work, great care must be taken to standardize the experimental conditions. Ideally, an internal standard of known activity is processed in tandem with the test tissue or, where possible, actually incorporated with the tissue itself (Flitney, 1991).

When used in conjunction with conventional staining for light or electron microscopy, sites within a tissue or cell where a particular metabolic or synthetic process occurs can be related to microscopic structure and calibration is not normally necessary.

16.5.3.1 Isotopes Used

Of the isotopes in common use, which include [^{14}C], [^{35}S], and [^{125}I], tritium [^{3}H] is the most widely used for three reasons. First, hydrogen is found in most molecules of biological interest. Second, [^{3}H] is a ß emitter of low energy and therefore low penetrating power, giving sharper and higher resolution images. Third, it has a half-life of approximately 12 years, so the radioactive intensity does not change appreciably during the course of a typical experiment.

16.5.3.2 Emulsions

There are two general methods of applying emulsion to slides. *Stripping* (Doniach and Pelc, 1950) involves the following steps:

- The section, cut in the normal way, is mounted in the normal way on a slide precoated with gelatine and allowed to dry.
- A piece of emulsion is cut from the glass plate on which it is supplied and floated onto water, where it is left to absorb water for a few minutes.
- The slide and section are dipped into the water and withdrawn so that the emulsion is lifted out and covers the section.
- After drying, the emulsion is bonded to the slide and remains in close contact with the radioactive tissue.

Dipping, introduced in 1955 (Joftes and Warren, 1955), involves dipping the slide and attached specimen into liquid emulsion, withdrawing it, allowing the excess liquid to drain off and drying the preparation by evaporation. The advantages of dipping over stripping (Flitney, 1991) are:

- Closer contact between section and emulsion
- Better control of AgBr crystal size and therefore resolution
- Easier to make thin emulsion layers and hence better staining
- Speed and ease of preparation lending itself to partial automation

The main drawback is the difficulty in producing an emulsion layer of uniform thickness, limiting the accuracy and repeatability of quantitative work.

For electron microscopy resin, sections are mounted on ultra-clean microscope slides, pretreated with a very thin layer of emulsion (Salpeter and Bachmann, 1964) and stored during exposure. Due to the thinness of the emulsion exposure times approximately 10 times longer than comparable preparations for light microscopy are necessary. The autoradiographs are developed and fixed on the slide and stained. Finally, they are transferred to electron microscope grids and coated with a 5-nm layer of carbon to minimize chemical reaction between tissue and emulsion.

16.5.3.3 Resolution

Resolution has been defined empirically as the distance in the plane of the section from the radioactive source at which the grain density is half its value directly above the source (Doniach and Pelc, 1950) or the radius of a circle centered on the source which contains half the grains produced by the source (Bachmann and Salpeter, 1965) or, similarly, as the distance from a linear source of a strip parallel to the source which contains half the grains associated with the source (Salpeter et al., 1969). Factors affecting resolution include the size of the AgBr crystals and the thickness of the emulsion as well as the energy of the radioactive particles that determines the distance they penetrate into the emulsion. [^{3}H], which emits ß particles with energies up to 18 keV, has, under optimal conditions, a resolution of 0.5 μm; whereas a higher energy emitter such as [^{14}C] or [^{35}S] will have a resolution of 2 to 5 μm (Flitney, 1991).

16.5.3.4 Sensitivity

Sensitivity depends on emulsion thickness and *efficiency*, the fraction of ß particles captured by the emulsion and giving rise to detectable grains (typically 60 to 80% of those traveling toward the emulsion). As the thickness of the emulsion increases, the probability of a particle hitting an AgBr molecule, and thus ultimately producing a silver grain, increases. In general, increased sensitivity implies decreased resolution so, in practice, a compromise must be sought for individual experiments. Under ideal conditions approximately 10^{-9} μCi can be detected. This is equivalent to around 1 disintegration of a [^{3}H] atom per day. At this rate however, exposure times of several weeks would be required, assuming that approximately 100 disintegrations are needed to produce a grain visible under the light microscope (Rogers, 1973).

16.5.3.5 Tissue Fixation

The aims of fixation, preservation of tissue structure and no interference with subsequent staining are similar to those of conventional histology with the additional need of maintaining the resolution and sensitivity of the emulsion. Formalin and glutaraldehyde desensitize the emulsion while fixatives that do not, such as methanol, tend to harden the tissue and disrupt its morphology (Flitney, 1991).

16.5.3.6 Staining

If staining is carried out before applying the photographic emulsion, care must be taken to compensate for loss of staining intensity during development and photographic fixation; whereas if the staining is performed after the autoradiography stains must be chosen so as not to affect the stability of the silver grains. Suitable stains for each alternative are listed in Flitney (1991).

The techniques of immunohistochemistry and *in situ* hybridization may be combined with autoradiography to map the distribution of a particular antigen (Beckman et al., 1983), rates of cellular proliferation (Lacy, 1991) or the phase of DNA replication (Lockwood, 1980). However, as the range of available antibodies increases and their specificity improves, purely immunological techniques are finding favor over the combined approach, a tendency that is encouraged by the technical complexity of autoradiography as well as radiation safety issues.

16.6 Mounting

Once the stained tissue has been picked up onto a slide, it must be dehydrated and cleared in much the same way as the aqueous fixative was removed before embedding. Thus, water remaining from the staining process is removed by treatment with successively more concentrated solution of a water-miscible organic solvent such as ethanol or acetone, taking care to do this rapidly to avoid leaching out those stains that are soluble in these agents. Finally, the ethanol or acetone is removed by treatment with a transition agent such as xylene after which the section on the slide is ready for the application of the mounting agent, followed by a protective glass coverslip. Most resins used for embedding are only sparingly soluble in noncorrosive solvents in which case clearing is not attempted and the mounting agent is applied to the intact section.

The purpose of the mounting agent is to seal the space between the slide and the coverslip, keeping out air and moisture, and to "fine-tune" the optical properties of the entire preparation. With stained tissue, spherical aberration is minimized if the refractive index of the mounting agent is close to that of glass. For unstained tissue, on the other hand, contrast is enhanced by choosing a mounting agent with a refractive index different to that of glass. The most common mounting agents for stained tissue are Canada Balsam and DPX, an artificial resin introduced in 1941 (Kirkpatrick and Lendrum, 1941) with refractive indices (RIs) of 1.52, close to that of glass. More recently, methacrylate mounting resins have been introduced that polymerize on exposure to light, do not undergo shrinkage and do not cause fading of the stain with time (Silverman, 1986).

Aqueous mounting agents include Apathy's medium (RI 1.52), Farrant's medium (RI 1.42), and glycerol jelly (RI 1.4–1.47). Details of their composition and preparation are given in Sanderson (1994).

Figure 16.7 (left-hand side) shows that the presence of the coverslip between the section and the objective lens of the microscope can cause additional refraction at the glass/air interface. The resulting

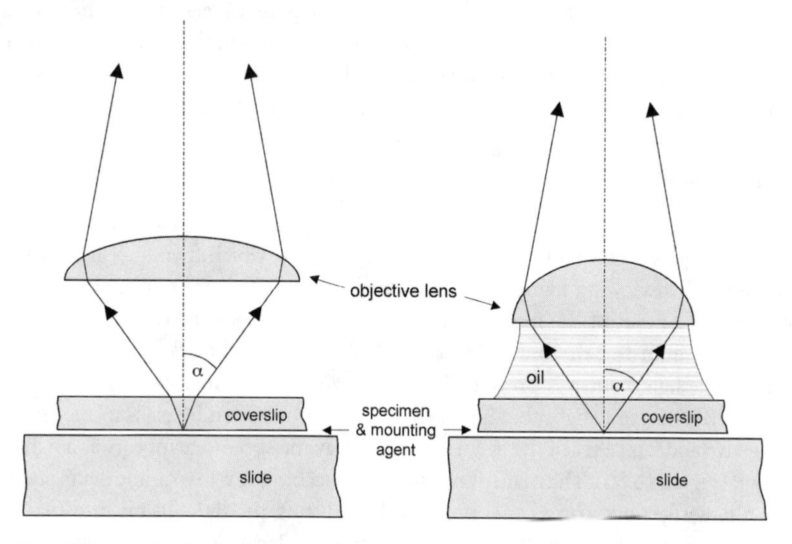

FIGURE 16.7 Ray diagrams for dry and oil immersion objectives showing how the oil (of refractive index similar to that of the glass coverslip) increases the "half-angle of acceptance" (α) and hence the resolving power of the lens.

spherical aberration is only a significant problem for lenses with a numerical aperture greater than 0.5 (see below). These lenses are normally designed for use with coverslips of a standard thickness (0.17 mm). The effect of deviations from these standard conditions has been investigated by Rawlins (1992) and Pluta (1988). Objective lenses fitted with an adjustable *correction collar* in which the spacing between the component lenses is adjustable may also be used to compensate for variations in coverslip thickness or depth of the mounting medium (White, 1974).

16.7 Microscopy

16.7.1 Resolution

The most obvious function of microscopy is to produce a *magnified* image of a specimen. Of equal importance is the ability to resolve two closely spaced objects. Resolution or minimum resolved distance is "the least separation between two points at which they may be distinguished as separate" (Bradbury and Bracegirdle, 1998). The healthy human eye with a near point of 250 mm can resolve two objects 70 μm apart. To achieve higher resolution, a lens or lenses are required to reduce the near point. The resolution (r) of a lens that is restricted by interference between the light diffracted by two closely separated points on the object is expressed by:

$$r = \frac{\lambda}{2NA} \tag{16.2}$$

where λ is the wavelength of the illumination and NA, the numerical aperture of the lens is given by the expression:

$$NA = n \sin \alpha \tag{16.3}$$

where n is the refractive index of the medium between the object and the lens, and α is the half angle of acceptance of the lens (Figure 16.7). Thus, resolving power may be increased by using shorter wavelength illumination or by increasing the numerical aperture of the lens. Modern high power objective lenses designed for use in air have an acceptance angle approaching 90° and numerical apertures up to 0.95. In practice, the diffraction of light passing through the glass coverslip over the specimen into the air above reduces the acceptance angle. This effect can be reduced and the resolution increased by using an *immersion lens* (Figure 16.7, right-hand side) in which the space between the cover slip and the lens is filled with a medium such as oil whose refractive index matches that of the coverslip (≈1.5).

16.7.2 Illumination

Most histological specimens viewed through the light microscope are illuminated by transmitted light, some of which is absorbed by dyes chosen to stain particular structures, which then appear as dark areas against a light background. When viewing living tissues or other materials that cannot be stained and that have a refractive index similar to that of the medium in which they are suspended or embedded, the structure is difficult to visualize (Figure 16.8a). To avoid this problem *dark ground* or *dark field* illumination must be used. In this mode the light source is prevented from entering the microscope objective lens directly by a suitably shaped mask. Thus, only light that has been reflected or refracted by parts of the specimen can pass through the objective and hence reach the eyepiece. In this way the specimen appears as a light image against a dark background (Figure 16.8b). The main drawback of this technique is loss of fine detail and poor contrast.

Interference microscopy overcomes this problem by splitting the light beam into two different path lengths arranged so that the observed field in the absence of a specimen consists of closely spaced interference fringes. The presence of the specimen in the beam path will cause slight shifts in the phase of one or both beams, and the interference pattern is correspondingly changed.

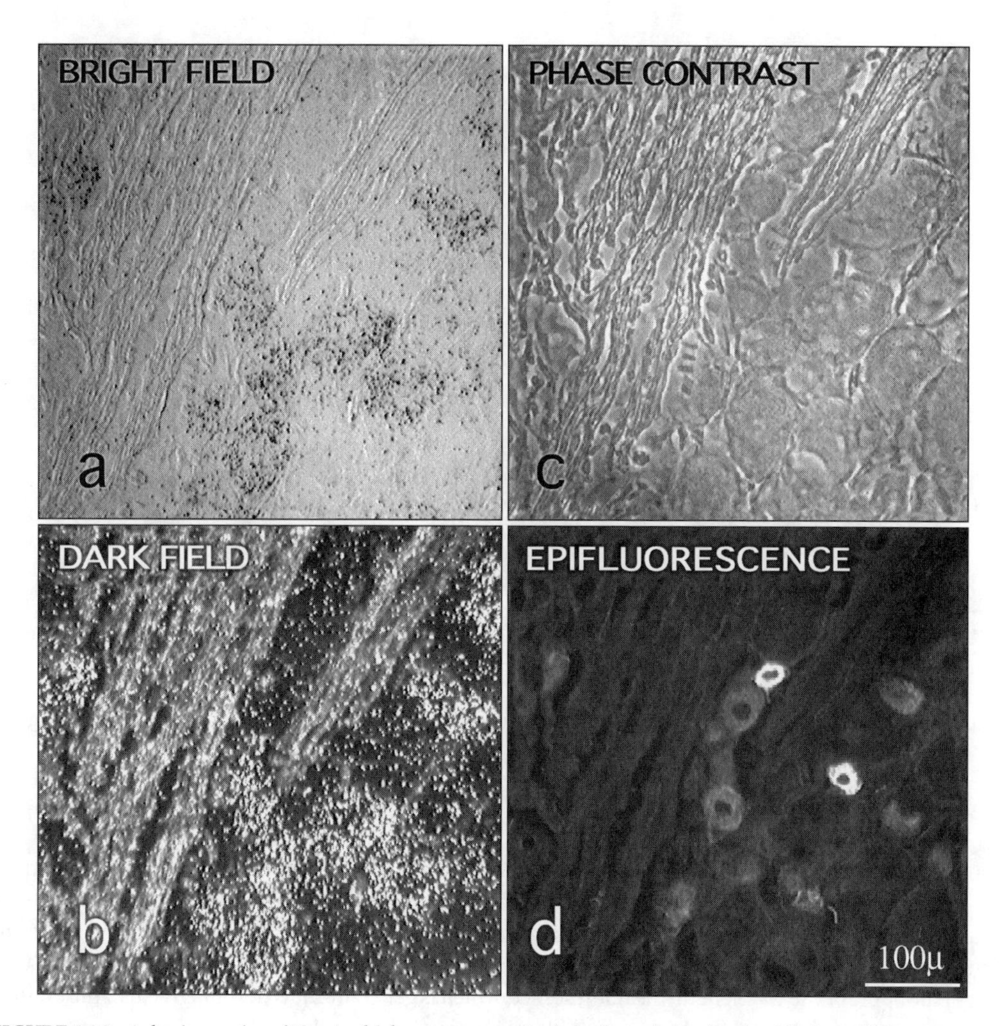

FIGURE 16.8 A brain section (10-µm-thick cryostat section) is shown visualized with four different types of illumination. The section contains neuronal cell bodies and myelinated fiber tracts, and the neurons have been marked with two different specialized histochemical stains. One is an immunofluorescence marker that identifies a neuropeptide and the other is a radiolabeled oligonucleotide probe that identifies a receptor mRNA. The probe is revealed using the technique of autoradiography (see text). Under normal bright field illumination (a), the tissue is difficult to see and the silver grains are just visible as faint dots. Dark field illumination (b) reveals the silver grains as bright white dots against a dark background (it also reveals the myelinated fiber tracts), and phase contrast illumination (c) reveals the tissue. Epifluorescence (d) illumination reveals the immunofluorescence marker. (With thanks to Professor J.V. Priestley.)

Phase contrast microscopes achieve a similar effect by passing an annular light beam through the specimen which is then shifted in phase by a similarly shaped *phase plate* in the objective lens system. Light that has been refracted by the specimen does not pass through the phase plate and when combined with the phase-shifted beam produces an interference pattern which corresponds to the shape and structure of the specimen (Figure 16.8c).

In polarized light microscopy, the birefringent properties of materials such as protein, bone and lipid are exploited to enhance contrast with or without staining. A plain polarizing filter is positioned between the light source and the specimen, and a similar filter is placed between the objective and eyepiece lenses. One of the filters is rotated so that its plane of polarization is nearly at right angles to the other, giving a dark background in the field of view. The birefringent components of the specimen, having rotated the plane of polarization, will therefore appear lighter than the background (Figure 16.9). Both phase

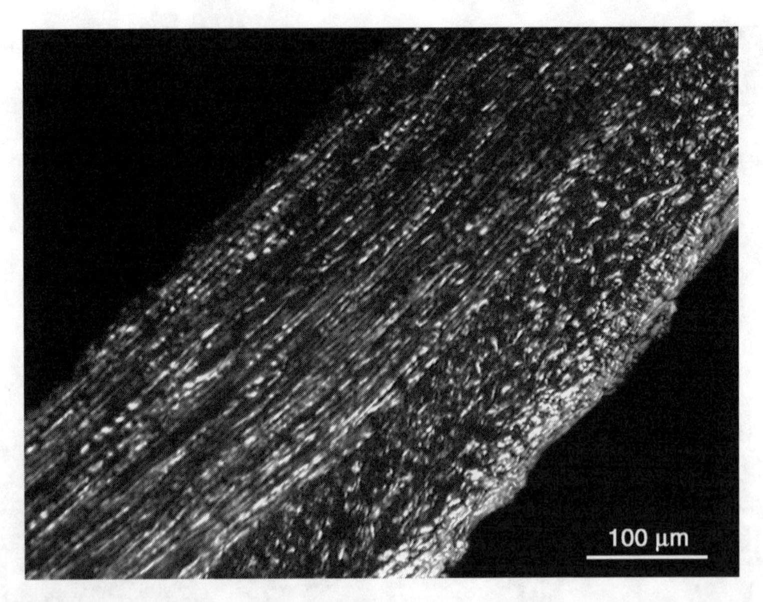

FIGURE 16.9 **(See color insert following page 14-10.)** Transverse section of a porcine carotid artery viewed under polarized light. The birefringent collagen fibers appear bright against a dark background.

contrast and polarized light techniques allow visualization of unstained and or living tissue, although at the expense of high contrast images.

16.7.3 Fluorescence Microscopy

Fluorescence is defined as the absorption of electromagnetic radiation of a specific wavelength (excitation) and its reemission at a longer wavelength. When a specimen containing naturally fluorescent material (e.g., vitamin A, chlorophyll, collagen), or one stained with a fluorescent compound having a specific affinity for a component of interest (i.e., a *fluorochrome)*, is illuminated by visible or ultraviolet (UV) light of the appropriate wavelength, the fluorescence, which is generally much less intense than the exciting light, is normally masked by the background illumination. Common fluorochromes such as rhodamine or fluoroscein are excited by UV light and emit in the visible part of the EM spectrum. The shorter wavelength of UV light improves the resolving power of the system (Equation 16.2). In early fluorescence microscopes the specimen was illuminated by transmission in the conventional manner and the exciting light as well as background illumination was attenuated by suitable bandpass filters. In modern fluorescence microscopes the specimen is normally visualized by incident light or *epi-illumination* (Figure 16.8d). In such instruments the light is directed via a filter and a dichroic mirror (a mirror that reflects light of some wavelengths and transmits at others) through the objective and the fluorescence returns via a second filter through the mirror and into the eyepiece. By careful choice of filter and mirror, it is possible to visualize low intensity fluorescence at a wavelength close to that of the exciting light.

In the technique of immunofluorescence originally reported in 1941 (Coons et al., 1941; Weller and Coons, 1954), a fluorescent stain is combined with an antibody having an affinity for an antigen in the specimen. The advantages of immunological specificity, fluorescent sensitivity and short wavelength resolving power are thus combined.

16.7.4 Confocal Microscopy

A major drawback of optical microscopy, especially at high magnification, is the low depth of focus and the difficulty of visualizing objects below the surface of the section. For instance, at an overall magnification sufficient to examine a cell nucleus, say, 300×, objects more than a few microns from the focal point will not be clearly resolved. In 1961 Minsky (1961) patented a device in which a pinhole is placed between the objective and the eyepiece, and the object is illuminated by a point source produced by a second pinhole in the light path. The pinholes allow light originating from object lying within or close to the focal plane to pass through, while blocking light from points remote from this plane. An image is then synthesized by moving the specimen in a raster pattern or by tandem scanning of the pinholes. The first successful use of such a system was reported by Egger and Petran (1967) who were able to examine unstained neural tissue; since then, neuroscientists have remained the most frequent and enthusiastic users of confocal microscopy (Fine et al., 1988). Commercial development was encouraged by the availability of compact and relatively low cost lasers that provided a source of light sufficiently intense and compact to overcome the low image brightness inherent in any pinhole device. In modern instruments, which usually incorporate epi-illumination suitable for fluorescence techniques, the laser beam is scanned over the object (Carlsson et al., 1985) and the final image is captured by a high definition video camera interfaced to a PC equipped with copious video memory. By moving the pinhole along the optical axis of the microscope, the position of the focal plane can be changed and a three-dimensional tomographic image can be constructed. Integral software allows these images to be reconstructed, displayed from different viewpoints and animated. With a combination of fluorescence induced by high intensity excitation and high sensitivity CCD cameras, objects as much as 600 μm below the surface of a specimen can be visualized.

Recently it has been reported that by using a modified form of confocal fluorescence microscopy, structures smaller than the resolution limit imposed by Equation 16.3 may be resolved (Dyba and Hell, 2002), although this claim has been questioned (Stelzer, 2002). Nevertheless, there is little doubt that technical improvements will continue to extend the scope and utility of confocal microscopy for the foreseeable future.

16.7.5 Electron Microscopy

By the end of the 19th century, the resolving power of the light microscope was approaching its theoretical limit, i.e., half the wavelength of blue light or approximately 0.2 μm (Equation 16.2). In 1931 (Kaiser, 1985) the introduction of the electron beam as a source of "illumination" led to the development of transmission electron microscopes (TEMs) with a resolution approaching 0.1 nm, with which it is possible to resolve the structure of intracellular organelles and even that of large molecules. In the TEM, electron-dense regions of the specimen scatter the electron beam, whereas electrons passing through the specimen are focused onto a fluorescent screen or photographic plate. The electron-dense regions thus appear dark against a light background. The degree of scatter depends on the energy of the electron beam, the atomic number of the scattering atoms and the thickness of the specimen. In the scanning electron microscope (Oatley, 1972), which has a lower resolution (5 to 10 nm) but a greater depth of focus, the specimen is scanned by the beam in a raster pattern and information is obtained primarily from scattered electrons and those produced by secondary emission. Thus it is possible to study surface details of a solid specimen whatever its thickness and to construct a pseudo-three-dimensional image of the surface. In addition to the scattered and secondary emission electrons, the primary beam gives rise to x-rays, the spectra of which are characteristic of the atoms from which they are emitted. By combining this information with the scattered electron signal, the spatial distribution of specific elements in the specimen may be mapped.

Due to their expense, electron microscopes are not widely used in diagnostic histopathology, although they are increasingly being called upon to provide specialist diagnostic information.

References

Shorter Oxford Dictionary, 3rd ed., Oxford University Press, Oxford, 1973.

Altman, L.G., Schneider, B.G., and Papermaster, D.S., Rapid embedding of tissues in Lowicryl K4M for immunoelectron microscopy, *J. Histochem. Cytochem.*, 32, 1217–1223, 1984.

Arnolds, W.J., Oriented embedding of small objects in agar-paraffin, with reference marks for serial section reconstruction, *Stain Technol.*, 53, 287–288, 1978.

Aschoff, A., Fritz, N., and Ilert, M., Axonal transport of fluorescent compounds in the brain and spinal cord of cat and rat, in *Axonal Transport in Physiology and Pathology*, Weiss, D.G. and Gorio, A., Eds., Springer, Berlin, 1982, p. 177.

Bachmann, L. and Salpeter, E.E., Autoradiography with the electron microscope. A quantitative investigation, *Lab. Invest.*, 14, 1041–1051, 1965.

Baker, J.R., Experiments on fixation, Unpublished observations, 1958a.

Baker, J.R., *Principles of Biological Microtechnique*, 1st ed., Methuen & Co. Ltd., London, 1958b.

Bancroft, J.D. and Stevens, A., *Theory and Practice of Histological Techniques*, Churchill Livingstone, Edinburgh, 1990.

Beckman, W.C.J., Stumpf, W.E., and Sar, M., Localisation of steroid hormones and their receptors. A comparison of autoradiographic and immunocytochemical techniques, in *Techniques in Imunocytochemistry*, Bullock, G.R. and Petrusz, P., Eds., 1983, Academic Press, London.

Bennett, H.S., Wyrick, A.D., Lee, S.W., and McNeil, J.H., Science and art in preparing tissues embedded in plastic for light microscopy, with special reference to glycol methacrylate, glass knives and simple stains, *Stain Technol.*, 51, 71–97, 1976.

Berry, C.L., Sosa-Melgarejo, J.A., and Greenwald, S.E., The relationship between wall tension, lamellar thickness and intercellular junctions in the fetal and adult aorta: its relevance to the pathology of dissecting aneurysm, *J. Pathol.*, 169, 15–20, 1993.

Bibb, C.A., Pullinger, A.G., and Baldioceda, F., Serial variation in histological character of articular soft tissue in young human adult temporomandibular joint condyles, *Arch. Oral Biol.*, 38, 343–352, 1993.

Bradbury, S. and Bracegirdle, B., *Introduction to Light Microsocopy*, Royal Microscopical Society Handbooks, Vol. 42, BIOS Scientific Publishers, Oxford, 1998.

Branchereau, P., Van Bockstaele, E.J., Chan, J., and Pickel, V.M., Ultrastructural characterization of neurons recorded intracellularly in vivo and injected with lucifer yellow: advantages of immunogold-silver vs. immunoperoxidase labeling, *Microsc. Res. Tech.*, 30, 427–436, 1995.

Carlsson, K., Danielsson, P.E., Lenz, R., Liljeborg, A., Majlof, L., and Aslund, N., Three-dimensional microscopy using a confocal laser scanning microscope, *Opt. Lett.*, 10, 53–55, 1985.

Coons, A.H. and Kaplan, M.H., Localization of antigen in tissue cells, *J. Exp. Med.*, 91, 1–13, 1950.

Coons, A.H., Creech, H.J., and Jones, R.N., Immunological properties of an antibody containing fluorescent groups, *Proc. Soc. Exp. Biol. Med.*, 47, 200, 1941.

Coons, A.H., Leduce, E.H., and Connolly, J.M., Studies on antibody production. I. A method for the histochemical demonstration of specific antibody and its application to a study of the hyperimmune rabbit, *J. Exp. Med.*, 102, 49–60, 1955.

Culling, C.F.A., Allison, R.T., and Barr, W.T., *Cellular Pathology Technique*, 4th ed., London, Butterworths, London, 1985.

Dobrin, P.B., Effect of histologic preparation on the cross-sectional area of arterial rings, *J. Surg. Res.*, 61, 413–415, 1996.

Donath, K., The diagnostic value of the new method for the study of undecalcified bones and teeth with attached soft tissue (Sage-Schliff (sawing and grinding) technique), *Pathol. Res. Pract.*, 179, 631–633, 1985.

Doniach, I. and Pelc, S.R., Autoradiographic technique, *Br. J. Radiogr.*, 23, 184–192, 1950.

Drury, R.A.B. and Wallington, E.A., *Carleton's Histological Technique*, 5th ed., Oxford University Press, Oxford, 1980.

Dyba, M. and Hell, S.W., Focal spots of size lambda/23 open up far-field fluorescence microscopy at 33 nm axial resolution, *Phys. Rev. Lett.*, 88, 163901-1–163901-4, 2002.

Egger, M.D. and Petran, M., New reflected-light microscope for viewing unstained brain and ganglion cells, *Science*, 157, 305–307, 1967.

Ellis, R.C., The microtome: function and design, in *Laboratory Histopathology A complete reference*, Woods, A.E. and Ellis, R.C., Eds., Churchill Livingstone, New York, 1994, pp. 4.4.1–4.4.23.

Fine, A., Amos, W.B., Durbin, R.M., and McNaughton, P.A., Confocal microscopy: applications in neurobiology, *Trends Neurosci.*, 11, 346–351, 1988.

Flitney, E., Autoradiography, in *Theory and Practice of Histological Techniques*, Bancroft, J.D. and Stevens, A., Ed., Churchill Livingstone, Edinburgh, 1991, pp. 645–665.

Foskett, J.K. and Grinstein, S., *Non Invasive Techniques in Molecular Biology*, Wiley-Liss, New York, 1990.

Fox, C.H., Johnson, F.B., Whiting, J., and Roller, P.P., Formaldehyde fixation, *J. Histochem. Cytochem.*, 33, 845–853, 1985.

Girardot, J.M. and Girardot, M.N., Amide cross-linking: an alternative to glutaraldehyde fixation, *J. Heart Valve Dis.*, 5, 518–525, 1996.

Goppert, H.R. and Cohn, F., Uber die Rotation des Zellinhaltes von Nitella fiexilis, *Bot. Ztg.*, 7, 665–719, 1849.

Gordon, K.C., Tissue processing, in *The Theory and Practice of Histological Techniques*, Bancroft, J.D. and Stevens, A., Eds., Churchill Livingstone, Edinburgh, 1990, pp. 44–59.

Hanstede, J.G. and Gerrits, P.O., The effects of embedding in water-soluble plastics on the final dimensions of liver sections, *J. Microsc.*, 131, 79–86, 1983.

Hardy, P.M., Nicholls, A.C., and Rydon, H., The nature of the cross linking of proteins with glutaraldehyde, *J. Chem. Soc.*, 1, 958–962, 1976.

Helander, K.G., Thickness variations within individual paraffin and glycol methacrylate sections, *J. Microsc.*, 132, 223–227, 1983.

Hilger, H.H. and Medan, D., A simple method for exact alignment of small paraffin embedded specimens to the cutting plane, *Stain Technol.*, 62, 282–283, 1987.

Hooke, R., *Micrographia* (facsimile edition), Royal Society London (1665), Dover, New York, 1961.

Hopwood, D., Fixation and fixatives, in *Theory and Practice of Histological Techniques*, Bancroft, J.D. and Stevens, A., Eds., Churchill Livingstone, Edinburgh, 1990, pp. 21–42.

Horobin, R.W., *Understanding Histochemistry: Evaluation and Design of Biological Stains*, Ellis Horwood, Chichester, 1988.

Horobin, R.W., An overview of the theory of staining, in *Theory and Practice of Histological Techniques*, Bancroft, J.D. and Stevens, A., Eds., Churchill Livingstone, Edinburgh, 1990, pp. 93–105.

Iwadare, T., Mori, H., Ishiguro, K., and Takeishi, M., Dimensional changes of tissues in the course of processing, *J. Microsc.*, 136, 323–327, 1984.

Joftes, D.L. and Warren, S., Simplified liquid emulsion radioautography, *J. Biol. Photogr. Assoc.*, 23, 145–151, 1955.

Johansen, D.A., A quadruple stain combination for plant tissues, *Stain Technol.*, 14, 125–128, 1939.

Kaiser, H.E., Functional comparative histology, *Gegenbaurs Morph Jahrb Lepzig*, 131, 815–862, 1985.

Kendall, P.A., Polak, J.M., and Pearse, A.G., Carbodiimide fixation for immunohistochemistry: observations on the fixation of polypeptide hormones, *Experientia*, 27, 1104–1106, 1971.

Kiernan, J.A., *Histological and Histochemical Methods: Theory and Practice*, 2nd ed., Pergamon Press, Oxford, 1990.

Kirkpatrick, J. and Lendrum, A.C., Further observations on the use of synthetic resin as a substitute for Canada balsam; precipitation of paraffin wax in medium and an improved plasticizer, *J. Pathol. Bacteriol.*, 53, 441–443, 1941.

Lacy, E.R., Kuwayama, H., Cowart, K.S., King, J.S., Deutz, A.H., and Sistrunk, S., A rapid, accurate, immunohistochemical method to label proliferating cells in the digestive tract. A comparison with tritiated thymidine, *Gastroenterology*, 100, 259–262, 1991.

Leeuwenhoek, A., Epistolae Physiologicae Super Compluribus Naturae Arcanis, Beman, Delft, 1791.

Leong, A.S., Microwave irradiation in histopathology, *Pathol Annu.*, 23, 213–234, 1988.

Leong, A.S., Microwave techniques for diagnostic laboratories, *Scanning*, 15, 88–98, 1993.

Leong, A.S., Tissue and section preparation, in *Laboratory Histopathology A Complete Reference*, Woods, A.E. and Ellis, R.C., Eds., Churchill Livingstone, New York, 1994, pp. 4.1.1–4.1.26.

Leong, A.S., Daymon, M.E., and Milios, J., Microwave irradiation as a form of fixation for light and electron microscopy, *J. Pathol.*, 146, 313–321, 1985.

Leong, A.S. and Duncis, C.G., A method of rapid fixation of large biopsy specimens using microwave irradiation, *Pathology*, 18, 222–225, 1986.

Leong, A.S., Milios, J., and Duncis, C.G., Antigen preservation in microwave-irradiated tissues: a comparison with formaldehyde fixation, *J. Pathol.*, 156, 275–282, 1988.

Lewis, F.T., The introduction of biological stains: employment of Saffron by Vieussens and van Leeuwenhoek, *Anat. Rec.*, 83, 229–253, 1942.

Lillie, R.D., *Histopathologic Technic and Modern Histochemistry*, 2nd ed., McGraw-Hill, New York, 1965.

Lillie, R.D., *H.J. Conn's Biological Stains*, 8th ed., Williams & Wilkins, Baltimore, 1969.

Litwin, J.A., Light microscopic histochemistry on plastic sections, *Prog. Histochem.Cytochem.*, 16, 1–84, 1985.

Lockwood, A.H., Immunofluorescence radioautography. Simultaneous visualization of DNA replication and supramolecular antigens in individual cells, *Exp. Cell Res.*, 128, 383–394, 1980.

Login, G.R. and Dvorak, A.M., Microwave energy fixation for electron microscopy, *Am. J. Pathol.*, 120, 230–243, 1985.

Masson, P., Some histological methods. Trichrome stainings and their preliminary technique, *Bull. Int. Assoc. Med.*, 12, 75–90, 1929.

Medewar, P.B., The rate of penetration of fixatives, *J. R. Microsc. Soc.*, 61, 46–57, 1941.

Merriam, R.W., Determination of section thickness in quantitative microspectrophotometry, *Lab. Invest.*, 6, 28–43, 1957.

Minsky, M., Microscopy Apparatus, U.S. Patent No. 3013467, 1961.

Murray, G.I., Is wax on the wane? *J. Pathol.*, 156, 187–188, 1988.

Nettleton, G.S. and McAuliffe, W.G., A histological comparison of phase-partition fixation with fixation in aqueous solutions, *J. Histochem. Cytochem.*, 34, 795–800, 1986.

Nunn, R.E., *Electron Microscopy: Microtomy, Staining and Specialized Techniques*, Butterworths Laboratory Aids, Baker, F.J., Ed., Butterworths, London, 1970.

Nunn, R.E., Electron Microscopy: Preparation of Biological Specimens, Butterworths Laboratory Aids, Baker, F.J., Ed., Butterworths, London, 1970.

Oatley, C.W., *The Scanning Electron Microscope*, Cambridge University Press, London, 1972.

Panula, P., Happola, O., Airaksinen, M.S., Auvinen, S., and Virkamaki, A., Carbodiimide as a tissue fixative in histamine immunohistochemistry and its application in developmental neurobiology, *J. Histochem. Cytochem.*, 36, 259–269, 1988.

Pearse, A.G.E., *Histochemistry, Theoretical and Applied*, 4th ed., Vol. 1, Churchill Livingstone, Edinburgh, 1980.

Pluta, M., *Advanced Light Microscopy. Principles and Basic Properties*, Vol.1, Elsevier, Amsterdam, 1988.

Polak, J.M. and Van Noorden, S., An introduction to immunocytochemistry: current techniques and problems, in *Royal Microscopy Society Handbook*, Vol. 111, Oxford University Press, Oxford, 1984.

Rawlins, D.J., *Light Microscopy*, Bios Scientific, Oxford, 1992.

Reale, E. and Luciano, L., Fixation with aldehydes. Their usefulness for histological and histochemical studies in light and electron microscopy, *Histochemie*, 23, 144–170, 1970.

Reid, N. and Beesley, J.E., Sectioning and cryosectioning for electron microscopy, in *Methods in Electron Microscopy*, Glauert, A.M., Ed., Elsevier, Amsterdam, 1991.

Rogers, A.W., *Techniques of Autoradiography*, Elsevier, London, 1973.

Ross, K.F.A., Cell shrinkage caused by fixatives and paraffin wax embedding in ordinary cytological preparations, *Q. J. Microsc.*, 94, 125–139, 1953.

Rostgaard, J., Qvortrup, K., and Poulsen, S.S., Improvements in the technique of vascular perfusion-fixation employing a fluorocarbon-containing perfusate and a peristaltic pump controlled by pressure feedback, *J. Microsc.*, 172, 137–151, 1993.

Saito, T. and Keino, H., Acrolein as a fixative for enzyme cytochemistry, *J. Histochem Cytochem.*, 24, 1258–1269, 1976.

Sallee, C.J. and Russell, D.F., Embedding of neural tissue in agarose or glyoxyl agarose for vibratome sectioning, *Biotechnol. Histochem.*, 68, 360–368, 1993.

Salpeter, E.E. and Bachmann, L., Autoradiography with the electron microscope, *J. Cell. Biol.*, 22, 469–474, 1964.

Salpeter, M.M., Bachmann, L., and Salpeter, E.E., Resolution in electron microscope radioautography, *J. Cell. Biol.*, 41, 1–32, 1969.

Sanderson, J.B., *Biological Microtechnique*, Royal Microscopical Society, Microscopical Handbooks, Vol. 28, Bradbury, S., Ed., BIOS Scientific Publ., Oxford, 1994.

Sato, Y., Mukai, K., Watanabe, S., Goto, M., and Shimosato, Y., The AMeX method. A simplified technique of tissue processing and paraffin embedding with improved preservation of antigens for immunostaining, *Am. J. Pathol.*, 125, 431–435, 1986.

Scala, C., Preda, P., Cennacchi, G., Martinelli, G.N., Manara, G.C., and Pasquinelli, G., A new polychrome stain and simultaneous methods of histological, histochemical and immunohistochemical stainings performed on semithin sections of Bioacryl-embedded human tissues, *Histochem. J.*, 25, 670–677, 1993.

Silverman, M., Light-polymerizing plastics as slide mounting media, *Stain Technol.*, 61, 135–137, 1986.

Sims, D.E. and Horne, M.M., Non-aqueous fixative preserves macromolecules on the endothelial cell surface: an in situ study, *Eur. J. Morphol.*, 32, 59–64, 1994.

Sims, D.E., Westfall, J.A., Kiorpes, A.L., and Horne, M.M., Preservation of tracheal mucus by nonaqueous fixative, *Biotechnol. Histochem.*, 66, 173–180, 1991.

Spurr, A.R., A low-viscosity epoxy resin embedding medium for electron microscopy, *J. Ultrastruct. Res.*, 26, 31–43, 1969.

Stelzer, E.H., Beyond the diffraction limit? *Nature*, 417, 806–807, 2002.

Tandler, B., Improved slides of semithin sections, *J. Electron. Microsc. Tech.*, 14, 285–286, 1990.

Tymianski, M., Bernstein, G.M., Abdel-Hamid, K.M., Sattler, R., Velumian, A., Carlen, P.L., Razavi, H., and Jones, O.T., A novel use for a carbodiimide compound for the fixation of fluorescent and non-fluorescent calcium indicators in situ following physiological experiments, *Cell Calcium*, 21, 175–183, 1997.

Vincent, J.F.V., Automating the microtome, *Microsc. Anal.*, 23, 19–21, 1991.

Waldeyer, R., Untersuchungen uber den Ursprung und den Verlauf des Axencylinders bei Wirbellosen und Wirbelthieren sowie uber dessen Endverhalten in der querdestreiften Muskelfaser, *Henle Pfeiffer Ztg Ration Med.*, 20, 193–256, 1863.

Weller, T.H. and Coons, A.H., Fluorescent antibody studies with agents of varicella and Herpes Zoster, *Proc. Soc. Exp. Biol. Med.*, 86, 789, 1954.

White, G.W., The correction of tube length to compensate for coverglass thickness variations, *Microscopy*, 32, 411–420, 1974.

Willingham, M.C. and Yamada, S.S., Development of a new primary fixative for electron microscopic immunocytochemical localization of intracellular antigens in cultured cells, *J. Histochem. Cytochem.*, 27, 947–960, 1979.

Zelander, T. and Kirkeby, S., Vibratome sections of difficult tissues, *Stain Technol.*, 53, 251–255, 1978.

17

Radioimmunoassay: Technical Background

Eiji Kawasaki
Nagasaki University School of Medicine

CONTENTS

17.1 Introduction

The technique of radioimmunoassay (RIA), first developed in 1960 by Berson and Yalow for the measurement of insulin, has expanded to include the detection of other biological agents.[1-8] Radioimmunosassays are based on the ability of an unlabeled antigen (Ag) to inhibit the binding of labeled antigen (Ag*) by antibody (Ab).

$$Ag - Ab \overset{Ag}{\rightleftharpoons} Ab \overset{Ag^*}{\rightleftharpoons} Ag^* \cdot Ab$$

The process may be viewed as a simple competition in which Ag reduces the amount of free Ab, decreasing the availability of Ab to Ag*. When the assay is performed, Ag* and Ab are incubated together in the presence and absence of samples containing unlabeled Ag. After equilibration, free Ag* and Ag*•Ab are separated. Commonly used separation procedures include solid-phase absorption, precipitation of Ag*Ab complexes with either a second antibody or a salt, and chromato-electrophoresis. Ag*•Ab (or free Ag*) is then determined by comparing the diminished Ag* binding of the sample to that of a standard curve obtained by adding graded, known amounts of Ag to Ag* and Ab. A new standard curve is determined in each assay to allow for variation in antigen binding from assay to assay. Radioimmunological methods combine the extreme sensitivity of detection of isotopically labeled compounds with the high specificity of immunological reactions. Thus, upon use of radioisotopes the detection limit is improved up to 10^7-fold over physicochemical analytical methods. Recently, in some fields of internal medicine, especially in autoimmune disease, radioimmunoassay to measure autoantibodies associated with disease prediction, diagnosis, and progression has been improved and simplified using a small amount of serum.[9,10]

17.2 Principle

Radioimmunoassay is a general method by which the concentration of virtually any substance can be determined. The principle on which it is based is summarized in the competing reactions shown in Figure

0-8493-1140-3/04/$0.00+$1.50

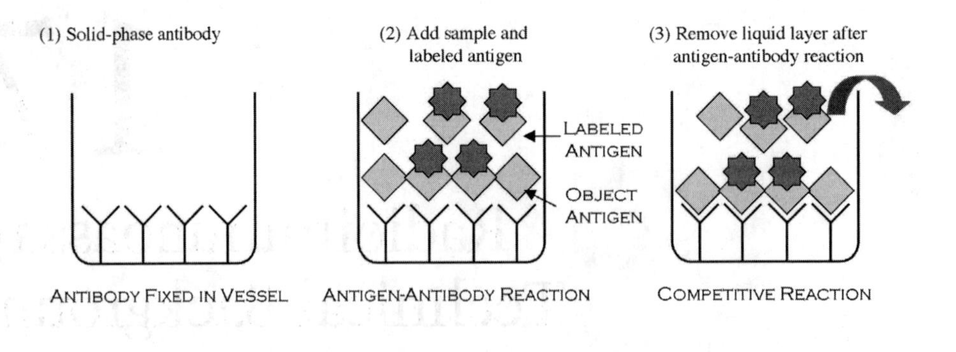

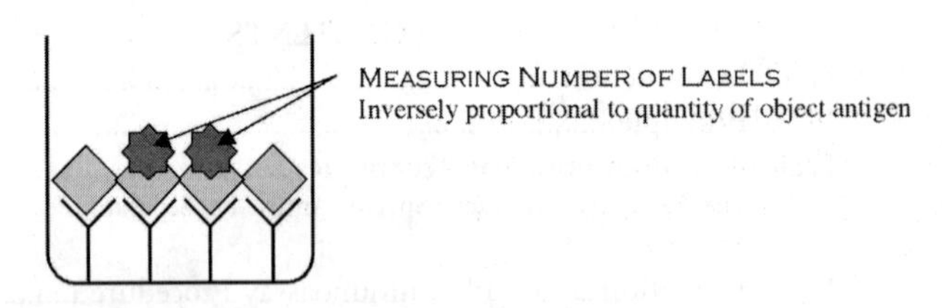

FIGURE 17.1 Principles of radioimmunoassay.

17.1. The concentration of unlabeled antigen in the unknown sample is obtained by comparing its inhibitory effect on the binding of labeled antigen to a limited amount of antibody with the inhibitory effect of known standards. A typical RIA is performed by the simultaneous preparation of standard and unknown mixtures in test tubes. To these tubes are added a fixed amount of labeled antigen and a fixed amount of antiserum. After an appropriate reaction time, the antibody-bound (B) and free (F) fractions of the labeled antigen are separated by one of many different techniques. The B/F ratios in the standards are plotted as a function of the concentration of unlabeled antigen ("standard curve"), and the concentration of antigen in the unknown sample is determined by comparing the observed B/F ratio with the standard curve (Figure 17.2). Radioactive isotopes most frequently used for labeling are ^{3}H, ^{14}C, ^{35}S, ^{57}Co, ^{75}Se, ^{125}I, and ^{131}I (Table 17.1). Of these, ^{125}I offers useful characteristics for labeling and is very widely used.

The RIA principle is not limited to immune systems, but can be extended to systems in which in place of the specific antibody there is a specific reactor (that is, a binding substance) that might be, for instance, a specific binding protein in plasma,[11] an autoantibody,[12] an enzyme,[13] or a tissue receptor site.[14] For

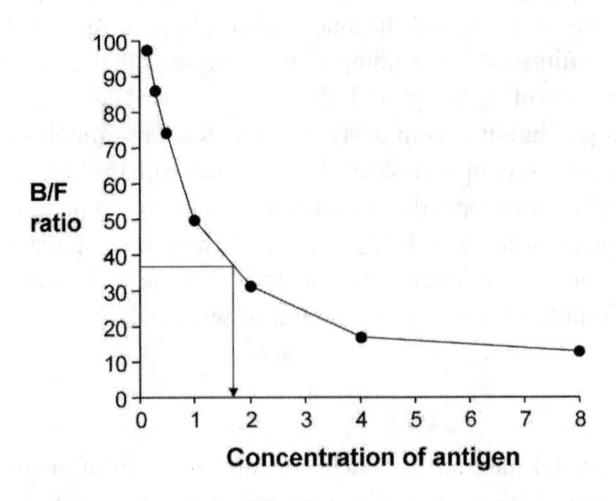

FIGURE 17.2 Standard curve for the assay of antigen. Concentration of antigen in unknown sample is determined by comparing the observed B/F ratio as shown.

TABLE 17.1 Radioactive Isotopes Used for Labeling in Radioimunoassay

Radioisotope	Half-life	Energy	Detection Method
^{3}H	12.3 years	β	Liquid scintillation
^{14}C	5730 years	β	Liquid scintillation
^{35}S	87.4 days	β	Liquid scintillation
^{57}Co	270 days	γ	Scintillation crystal
^{75}Se	120.4 days	γ	Scintillation crystal
^{125}I	60 days	γ	Scintillation crystal
^{131}I	8 days	β, γ	Scintillation crystal

example, concentration of antibody in an unknown sample can be obtained by measuring the binding to an appropriate labeled antigen. Recently, for *in vitro* assays, the quantity of samples and the number of items to be measured are rapidly increasing. To meet this trend, the equipment for radioimmunoassay has been semiautomated or automated.

17.3 Radioimmunoassay Techniques

The essential requirements for RIA include suitable reactants (labeled antigen and specific antibody) and some technique for separating the antibody-bound antigen from the free-labeled antigen, since under the usual conditions of assay, the antigen-antibody complexes do not spontaneously precipitate.

17.3.1 The Radioactive Marker

17.3.1.1 Radiolabeled Antigen

The first requirement for a radioimmunoassay is the preparation of a highly purified antigen that can be radiolabeled or "tagged" without producing any loss of immunoreactivity. Since most polypeptide hormones contain at least one tyrosine residue, they can be labeled with a radioisotope of iodine (e.g., ^{125}I or ^{131}I). The radioiodine usually substitutes onto a tyrosine residue. The radioisotopes of iodine have the advantage of higher specific activities than can be found with ^{3}H or ^{14}C. Because the isotopic abundance of ^{125}I is close to 100%, and the isotopic abundance of ^{131}I is not more than 15 to 30% at the time of receipt into the laboratory,[15] the shorter half-life of ^{131}I confers no advantage, and ^{125}I has been the radioiodine isotope of choice. The specific activity of a ^{125}I-labeled hormone may be increased by increasing the number of radioiodine substitutions. However, it has been shown that the more highly iodinated molecules have diminished immunoreactivity as well as increased susceptibility to damage.[16,17] The latter appears to arise from radiation self-damage within the molecule. Isotopes ^{3}H and ^{14}C can be used for labeling; however, because they emit extremely low-energy β rays, a liquid scintillation counter is used to make measurements with these two isotopes.

Recent advances of molecular biology techniques allow developing the cell-free protein synthesizing and labeling system.[18] With an *in vitro* transcription/translation system using reticulocyte lysate, wheat germ extract, or *E. coli* extract, one can directly prepare the labeled antigen from the plasmid-containing antigen cDNA using a radioactive amino acid (e.g., ^{35}S-methionine, ^{3}H-leucine).

Labeled antigen often needs to be purified for separating from the free isotope. There are various techniques available for purification. Adsorption column chromatography on powdered cellulose is a rapid assay.[6,19] For more extensive purification, one must resort to a separation involving dialysis, gel filtration (using a molecular sieve), or ion-exchange chromatography.[20-22] Inorganic iodine resin has also been used to absorb the unreacted ^{131}I.[23] After purification, one should determine the absolute quality of antigen required in a particular assay for high sensitivity. It is important that this quantity be kept at a minimum. Therefore, it is desirable to produce high specific activity of the radiolabeled antigen. If the labeled antigen is to be stored for a considerable time, it is usually kept at 2 to 4°C (e.g., steroids) or it may be quickly frozen for storage at –20°C (e.g., polypeptides). After storage, the antigen must be checked for changes in immunoreactivity before use in an assay. The actual conditions for storing the labeled antigen depend on the particular antigen.

17.3.1.2 Radiolabeled Antibody

Wide and co-workers[24] and Miles and Hales[25,26] have pointed out the possible advantage of radioiodinating the antibody instead of antigen. The larger molecular weight of immunoglubulin and the presence of multiple tyrosines on the molecule permit the introduction of multiple-radioiodine molecules without detrimental effects on antibody activity. Iodination of antibody rather than antigen may be especially advantageous if the antigen is easily damaged during iodination or lacks readily iodinatable tyrosines. The major difficulty of the radioimmunoassay using radioiodinated antibody is likely to come in the strong propensity of iodinated antibodies to adhere nonspecifically to glassware and insoluble resin. Thus, the selection of the immunoadsorbent is likely to be critical if this method is to be made to work. Nonspecific binding of the iodinated antibody to the resin can be diminished by preparing Fab fragments of the labeled antibody,[27] but this will reduce the functional avidity of the antibody for the resin and may adversely affect assay sensitivity. Another problem is the requirement for substantial amounts of antigen to prepare the resin, which includes the use of this approach for antigens that are in short supply.

17.3.2 Specific Antibody

The second prerequisite for a radioimmunoassay is the production of a suitable antiserum. The antibodies are a group of serum proteins that are also referred to as γ-globulins or immunoglobulins. Most of these immunoglobulins belong to the IgG class, while the other classes are termed IgA, IgM, IgD, and IgE. Because these immunoglobulins possess not only antibody-reaction sites, but also antigenic determinant sites, the immunoglubulins themselves can serve as antigens when injected into a "foreign" animal. The labeled antigen must, of course, be highly purified to avoid interaction of labeled contaminants with nonspecific antibody. The antigen-binding sites appear to reside on the H and L chains of the IgG molecule. While the titer, or concentration of the antibody is important, the main criterion for establishing a suitable antiserum is the energy of interaction between the antigen and antibody, or the specificity and affinity for the antigen being assayed. For most clinical chemists who are interested in performing radioimmunoassay procedures, it would be more advantageous to procure the specific antiserum from a laboratory or commercial supplier that has the facilities required for the generation and evaluation of antibodies.

The important limiting factors for the development of highly sensitive radioimmunoassays are antibody affinity, avidity, specificity, and cross reactivity. Antibody affinity is the strength of the reaction between a single antigenic determinant and a single combining site on the antibody. It is the sum of the attractive and repulsive forces operating between the antigenic determinant and the combining site of the antibody. Affinity is the equilibrium constant that describes the Ag-Ab reaction as illustrated below. Most antibodies have a high affinity for their antigens.

$$K_{eq} = \frac{[Ag - Ab]}{[Ag] \times [Ab]}$$

Avidity is a measure of the overall strength of binding of an antigen with many antigenic determinants and multivalent antibodies. Avidity is influenced by both the valence of the antibody and the valence of the antigen. Avidity is more than the sum of the individual affinities. Specificity refers to the ability of an individual antibody combining site to react with only one antigenic determinant or the ability of a population of antibody molecules to react with only one antigen. In general, there is a high degree of specificity in Ag-Ab reactions. Antibodies can distinguish differences in (1) the primary structure of an antigen, (2) isomeric forms of an antigen, and (3) secondary and tertiary structure of an antigen. Cross reactivity refers to the ability of an individual antibody combining site to react with more than one antigenic determinant or the ability of a population of antibody molecules to react with more than one antigen. Cross reactions arise because the cross-reacting antigen shares an epitope in common with the immunizing antigen or because it has an epitope that is structurally similar to one on the immunizing antigen (multispecificity).

The general method of inducing antibody formation is to inject into a number of animals the pure antigen mixed with "Freund's adjuvant."[28,29] Freund's adjuvant is a mixture of mineral oil, waxes, and killed bacilli that enhances and prolongs the antigenic response. Small peptides (mol wt 1000 to 5000) or nonpeptidal substances which are not of themselves antigenic may be rendered so by coupling to a large protein. A variety of methods may be employed to bind the small molecules to immunogenic carriers.[30-32] The antisera can be stored for long periods of time under proper conditions. Repeated freezing and thawing should be avoided and all antisera should be stored properly diluted. Reports vary as to the best temperature for antiserum storage; some researchers prefer –80°C, others prefer –20 or –15°C.[33] Once thawed, the sera are best kept at 4°C.

17.3.3 Separation Methods

The third requirement for a radioimmunoassay is a suitable method for complete and rapid separation of the bound antigen from the free antigen. In addition, a separation procedure that permits further association and dissociation of the reactants will seriously impair the effectiveness of the assay. Regardless of the method of separation chosen, it must be reproducible, simple to perform, and economically feasible. Table 17.2 lists a variety of techniques that have been used for separation of antibody-bound and free-labeled antigens. The use of so many methods is a tribute to the imagination and versatility of investigators in the field, and is also due to the recognition that no single method has proved completely satisfactory for all antigens. Following are some examples of the separation method.

17.3.3.1 Precipitation with Ammonium Sulfate

Ammonium sulfate (33 to 50% final concentration) will precipitate immunoglobulins, but not many antigens. Thus, this can be used to separate the immune complexes from free antigen. This has been called the Farr technique.

TABLE 17.2 Methods and Materials for the Separation of Antibody-Bound and Free Antigen

Separating Action	Method/Material
Precipitation of the Ag-Ab complex	Ammonium sulfate
	Sodium hydrogen sulfate
	Zirconyl phosphate
	Ethanol
	2-Propanol
	Dioxane
	Polyethylene glycol (PEG)
Partition of the components due to their different mobility and molecular size	Chromatography
	Electrophoresis
	Gel filtration
	Ultracentrifugation
Adsorption of free antigen to solid-phase materials	Charcoal (also bound to dextran or albumin)
	Cellulose
	Sephadex (Cross-linked dextrans)
	Sepharose (Beaded agarose)
	Silicates
	Iron-exchange resins
	Polymerized antibodies
Binding of the antibody to a solid phase	Antibody chemically bound to polymer carrier
	Coated tubes or beads
Immunological complex formation with a second antibody	Double-antibody technique
	Second antibody chemically bound, e.g., to activated cellulose

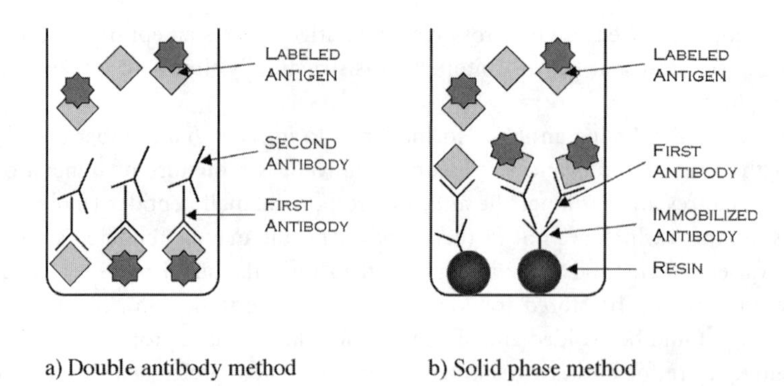

FIGURE 17.3 Separation of antibody-bound and free antigen.

17.3.3.2 Anti-Immunoglobulin Antibody

The addition of a second antibody directed against the first antibody can result in the precipitation of the immune complexes and thus the separation of the complexes from free antigens. This has been called the double antibody method (Figure 17.3). This method is widely applicable and gives highly satisfactory results provided careful attention is given to possible pitfalls. The diluted antiserum containing the first antibody must contain sufficient γ-globulin to give a macroscopic precipitate with an excess of second antibody (usually 2 to 5 μg/ml). To minimize the unnecessary expenditure of second antibody and to avoid nonspecific binding of radiolabeled antigen to bulky precipitate, the quantity of precipitate is adjusted just enough to give good precipitation of radioactivity. In the event that the first antibody has a low titer, the expenditure of the second antibody will be prohibitive and other methods must be used.

17.3.3.3 Immobilization of the Antibody

The antibody can be immobilized onto the surface of a plastic bead or coated onto the surface of a plastic plate, and thus the immune complexes can easily be separated from the other components by simply washing the beads or plate.[34] This is the most common method used today and is referred to as solid-phase RIA (Figure 17.3). A number of methods have been used for attaching antibody to the solid phase. Formation of a stable resin-protein complex may require an initial chemical reaction to activate the resin followed by exposure to the antibody. In conjunctions involving antibodies, ideally γ-globulin fractions rather than whole serum are used in the second step in order to minimize binding of extraneous proteins to the resin. Activation of the resin is commonly accomplished with bromoacetyl bromide or cyanogens bromide.[35] Alternatively, stable azide or aromatic amine residues can be introduced into a resin and the activation accomplished just prior to the introduction of the protein. Resins containing primary aliphatic amino or carboxyl groups combine with antibody in the presence of carboxyl activating reagents. Commonly used resins include agarose, Sephadex, and cellulose.

Solid phase systems have the advantage of simplicity and rapidity. However, specific problems may arise, such as difficulties in dispension of the resin. The establishment of equilibrium, although rapid in some systems, may require continuous mixing over a period of many hours in others.

17.4 Validation of a Radioimmunoassay Procedure

The radioimmunoassay differs from the traditional bioassay in that it is an immunochemical procedure, which is not affected by biological variability of the test system. The measurement depends only upon the interaction of chemical reagents in accordance with the low of mass action. However, nonspecific factors do interfere in chemical reactions, and cross-reacting prohormones, molecular fragments, and related hormonal antigens can alter the specificity of the immune reaction.

In order to ensure reliability and the results obtained, and thus to guarantee the quality of a radioimmunoassay, it is necessary to know a number of characteristic data. These include the specificity and sensitivity, and above all, the accuracy, reproducibility, and precision of an assay. The specificity of a radioimmunoassay is essentially determined by the antibody. It can be impaired by cross reactions with similar substances and fragments thereof, and also by the separating step. Serum factors, pH value, and additives such as albumin, buffer, heparin, or preservatives can also lower the specificity. The sensitivity depends on the specificity of the antibody and the adequate specific radioactivity of the tracer. The sensitivity can be regarded as the special case of the accuracy at zero concentration. The sensitivity of assays in which the immunological reaction is irreversible or measurement is performed at nonequilibrium can occasionally be raised by delayed addition of the radioactively labeled substance.[36]

The accuracy attainable in a determination depends on three errors of various magnitudes. Apart from experimental errors arising in several pipetting steps and interference of the reaction, errors also occur in measuring the radioactivity and on evaluation of the various samples. Owing to the different nature of these errors, it is clear that the accuracy cannot be the same in each portion of the curve. However, multiple determinations and long counting time can do much to reduce random errors and thus lead to a more accurate result.

Reproducibility is another criterion of quality, including intra- and interassay reproducibility. Duplicate or multiple determinations on samples of an assay and the resulting deviations from the average value yield the intraassay reproducibility. It normally lies below 5%. The interassay reproducibility is the coefficient of variation obtained on determination of the same sample in several different assay runs using different reagents. Its value lies below 10% for accurate and reproducible radioimmunoassay.[37]

17.5 Applications

In the years since the development of radioimmunoassay, the application of the technique has brought profound changes to medicine and biology. Figure 17.4 shows the schematic methods for radioligand binding assay currently used to detect autoantibodies against recombinant antigen in sera.[38] In the measurement of autoantibodies, the cDNA of autoantigens are required to prepare the radiolabeled autoantigens. Such cDNA are usually obtained from an appropriate cDNA library using plaque hybridization techniques or appropriate mRNA using the reverse-transcriptase (RT)-PCR method. The cloned cDNA are then subcloned into the plasmid vectors suitable for an *in vitro* transcription/translation system. Radiolabeled autoantigens are prepared using the *in vitro* transcription/translation system with reticu-

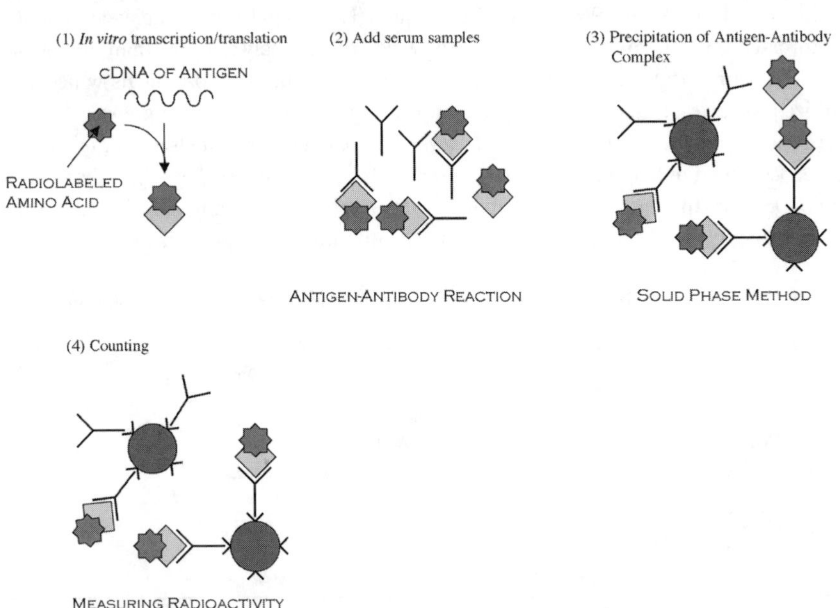

FIGURE 17.4 Schematic methods for radioligand binding assay.

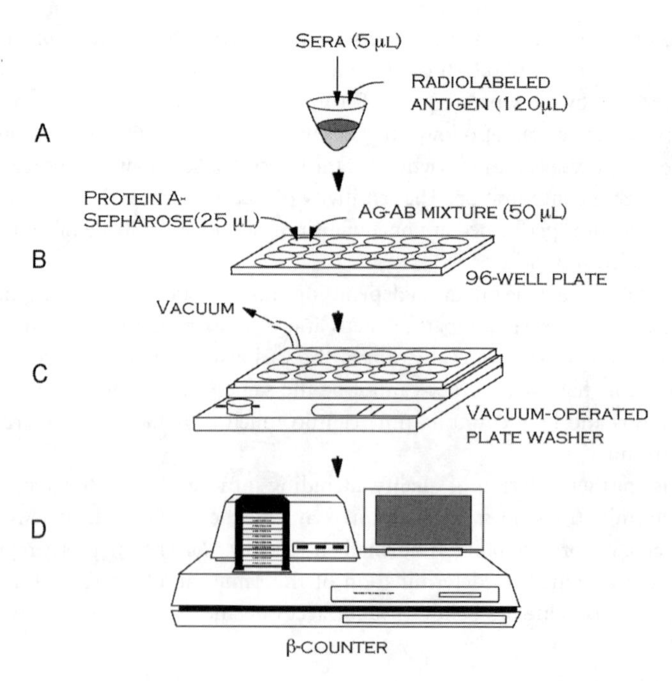

FIGURE 17.5 High-throughput radioimmunoassay for autoantibodies to recombinant autoantigens. (From Kawasaki, E. and Eisenbarth, G. S., *Front. Biosci.*, 5, E181, 2000. With permission.)

locyte lysates and a radioactive amino acid (e.g., ^{35}S-methionine, ^{3}H-leucine). For detection of autoantibodies to recombinat autoantigens, we use a 96-well plate filtration technology and a microplate direct β counter (Figure 17.5).[10,38] After determining the incorporation rate of radioisotope by trichloroacetic acid (TCA) precipitation method, *in vitro*-translated radiolabeled protein (20,000 cpm of TCA precipitable protein) is incubated with patients' sera (5 µl for duplicate) at a 1:25 dilution overnight at 4°C, and the resulting immunocomplexes are precipitated with 25 µl of protein A-Sepharose in the 96-well plate. After a washing step utilizing a vacuum-operated 96-well plate washer, radioactivity is determined directly in the 96-well plate with 96-well plate β counter. The adaptation of the assay to a 96-well plate and semiautomated 96-well counting allows a single person to analyze more than 40,000 samples per year. Table 17.3 lists *in vitro* transcribed and translated recombinant autoantigens which we have successfully utilized for disease diagnosis and prediction using radioligand binding assay.

A similar assay format can be used to measure several autoantibodies at the same time using recombinat autoantigens labeled with different radioisotopes. Eisenbarth and co-workers have recently developed a combined IA-2-GAD65 autoantibody radioassay utilizing [^{3}H]-labeled GAD65 and [^{35}S]-labeled IA-2 that allows simultaneous detection and discrimination of both autoantibody specificities.[39] *In vitro*-translated

TABLE 17.3 Autoantibody Radioassays Based on the *In Vitro* Transcription/Translation of Autoantigens

Worked	Didn't work
GAD65	Proinsulin
ICA512/IA-2	ICA69
Phogrin/IA-2β	H^+, K^+-ATPase
Carboxypeptidase H	
21-hydroxylase	
CYP2D6	
Transglutaminase	

Source: Kawasaki, E. and Eisenbarth, G.S., High-throughput radioassays for autoantibodies to recombinant autoantigens, *Front. Biosci.*, 5, E181, 2000. With permission.

[^{3}H]-GAD65 and [^{35}S]-IA-2 were mixed and incubated with serum in a tube and the radioactivity was counted in a 96-well plate with channel windows set for each radionucleotide after protein-A Sepharose precipitation. The combined assay gave essentially identical results to those obtained in the single radioassays. The simplicity of this assay with dual determination of the two antibodies utilizing 5 μl of sera, 96-well membrane separation of autoantibody-bound labeled autoantigen, and 96-well β counting facilitates the rapid screening of thousands of samples.

References

1. Berson, S.A. et al., Insulin-I^{131} metabolism in human subjects: demonstration of insulin binding globulin in the circulation of insulin treated subjects, *J. Clin. Invest.*, 35, 170, 1956.
2. Berson, S.A. and Yalow, R.S., Kinetics of reaction between insulin and insulin-binding antibody, *J. Clin. Invest.*, 36(Abstr.), 873, 1957.
3. Berson, S.A. and Yalow, R.S., Isotopic tracers in the study of diabetes, *Adv. Biol. Med. Phys.*, 6, 349, 1958.
4. Berson, S.A. and Yalow, R.S., Recent studies on insulin-binding antibodies, *Ann. N.Y. Acad. Sci.*, 82, 338, 1959.
5. Yalow, R.S. and Berson, S.A., Assay of plasma insulin in human subjects by immunological methods, *Nature*, 184, 1648, 1959.
6. Yalow, R.S. and Berson, S.A., Immunoassay of endogenous plasma insulin in man, *J. Clin. Invest.*, 39, 1157, 1960.
7. Yalow, R.S. and Berson, S.A., *Introduction and General Considerations*, J.B. Lippincott, Philadelphia, 1971, 1.
8. Yalow, R.S. and Berson, S.A., *Fundamental Principles of Radioimmunoassay Techniques in Measurement of Hormones*, Excepta Medica, Amsterdam, 1971, 16.
9. Kawasaki, E. and Eisenbarth, G.S., Multiple autoantigens in the prediction and pathogenesis of type I diabetes, *Diab. Nutr. Metab.*, 9, 188, 1996.
10. Kawasaki, E. and Eisenbarth, G.S., High-throughput radioassays for autoantibodies to recombinant autoantigens, *Front. Biosci.*, 5, E181, 2000.
11. Murphy, B.E.P., Engelberg, W., and Pattee, C.J., Simple method for the determination of plasma corticoids, *J. Clin. Endocr.*, 23, 293, 1963.
12. Carr, R.I., Wold, R.T., and Farr, R.S., Antibodies to bovine gamma globulin (BGG) and the occurrence of a BGG-like substance in systemic lupus erythematosus sera, *J. Allergy Clin. Immunol.*, 50, 18, 1972.
13. Rothenberg, S.P., A radio-enzymatic assay for folic acid, *Nature*, 206, 1154, 1965.
14. Lefkowitz, R.J. et al., ACTH receptors in the adrenal: specific binding of ACTH-^{125}I and its relation to adenyl cyclase, *Proc. Natl. Acad. Sci. U.S.A.*, 65, 745, 1970.
15. Yalow, R.S. and Berson, S.A., Labelling of proteins-problems and practices, *Trans. N.Y. Acad. Sci.*, 28, 1033, 1966.
16. Berson, S.A. and Yalow, R.S., *Recent Advances in Immunoassay of Peptide Hormones in Plasma*, Excepta Medica, Amsterdam, 1969, 50.
17. Berson, S.A. and Yalow, R.S., Iodoinsulin used to determine specific activity of iodine-131, *Science*, 152, 205, 1966.
18. Jackson, R.J. and Hunt, T., Preparation and use of nuclease-treated rabbit reticulocyte lysates for the translation of eukaryotic messenger RNA, *Methods Enzymol.*, 96, 50, 1983.
19. Berson, S.A. and Yalow, R.S., Preparation and purification of human insulin-I131; binding to human insulin-binding antibodies, *J. Clin. Invest.*, 40, 1803, 1961.
20. Desranleau, R., Gilardeau, C., and Chretien, M., Radioimmunoassay of ovine beta-lipotropic hormone, *Endocrinology*, 91, 1004, 1972.
21. Catt, K.J. and Cain, M.C., Measurement of angiotensin II in blood, *Lancet*, 2, 1005, 1967.

22. Midgley, A.R., Jr., Radioimmunoassay: a method for human chorionic gonadotropin and human luteinizing hormone, *Endocrinology,* 79, 10, 1966.
23. Saxena, B.B. et al., Radioimmunoassay of human follicle stimulating and luteinizing hormones in plasma, *J. Clin. Endocrinol. Metab.,* 28, 519, 1968.
24. Wide, L., Bennich, H., and Johansson, S.G., Diagnosis of allergy by an *in vitro* test for allergen antibodies, *Lancet,* 2, 1105, 1967.
25. Miles, L.E. and Hales, C.N., Labelled antibodies and immunological assay systems, *Nature,* 219, 186, 1968.
26. Miles, L.E. and Hales, C.N., The preparation and properties of purified 125-I-labelled antibodies to insulin, *Biochem. J.,* 108, 611, 1968.
27. Hubacek, J., Kubicek, R., and Vojacek, K., Immunoassay of human luteinizing hormone using univalent radioactive antibodies, *J. Endocrinol.,* 51, 91, 1971.
28. Freund, J., The effect of peraffin oil and mycobacteria on antibody formation and sensitization, *Am. J. Clin. Pathol.,* 21, 645, 1951.
29. Freund, J., Some aspects of active immunization, *Annu. Rev. Microbiol.,* 1, 291, 1947.
30. Erlanger, B.F. and Beiser, S., Antibodies specific for ribonucleosides and ribonucleotides and their reaction with DNA, *Proc. Natl. Acad. Sci. U.S.A.,* 52, 68, 1964.
31. Talamo, R.C., Haber, E., and Austen, K.F., Antibody to bradykinin: effect of carrier and method of coupling on specificity and affinity, *J. Immunol.,* 101, 333, 1968.
32. Richards, F.M. and Knowles, J.R., Glutaraldehyde as a protein cross-linkage reagent, *J. Mol. Biol.,* 37, 231, 1968.
33. Thoeneycroft, I.H. et al., *Preparation and Purification of Antibodies to Steroids,* Appleton-Century-Crofts, New York, 1970, 63.
34. Wide, L., Radioimmunoassays employing immunosorbents, *Acta Endocrinol. Suppl. (Copenhagen),* 142, 207, 1969.
35. Robbins, J.B., Haimovich, J., and Sela, M., Purification of antibodies with immunoadsorbents prepared using bromoacetyl cellulose, *Immunochemistry,* 4, 11, 1967.
36. Rodbard, D. et al., Mathematical analysis of kinetics of radioligand assays: improved sensitivity obtained by delayed addition of labeled ligand, *J. Clin. Endocrinol. Metab.,* 33, 343, 1971.
37. Rodbard, D., Statistical quality control and routine data processing for radioimmunoassays and immunoradiometric assays, *Clin. Chem.,* 20, 1255, 1974.
38. Sera, Y. et al., Autoantibodies to multiple islet autoantigens in patients with abrupt onset type 1 diabetes and diabetes diagnosed with urinary glucose screening, *J. Autoimmun.,* 13, 257, 1999.
39. Kawasaki, E. et al., Evaluation of islet cell antigen (ICA) 512/IA-2 autoantibody radioassays using overlapping ICA512/IA-2 constructs, *J. Clin. Endocrinol. Metab.,* 82, 375, 1997.

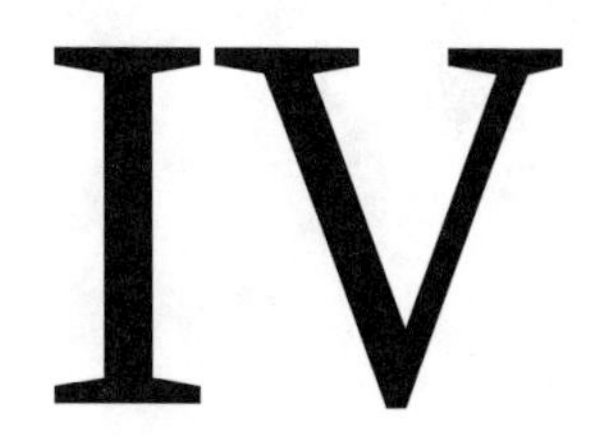

Genetic and Tissue Engineering

Role of Technology in Biomolecular Revolution

The information revealed by revolutionary undertakings, such as the human genome project, has provided unprecedented insight into the inner workings of the most basic structures of living tissues. With much of the molecular architecture defined, attention has turned to manipulating these structures for therapeutic purposes.

Techniques have been developed to transplant genetic material into a variety of living tissues. The reliability of animal models for human disease conditions has been enhanced by genetic manipulation. Disease treatment strategies can be more directly developed for maximum effectiveness.

While there are significant ethical issues involved, the potential to grow entire organs for implantation is exciting. The future of many areas of disease treatment will be affected by developments in the field of tissue engineering. As clinicians and patients alike realize the potential of such therapies, technologies will be developed that provide effective disease treatment.

This section includes the following chapters:

VI

Genetic and Tissue Engineering

[illegible]

18

Genetic Engineering of Animals

CONTENTS

Carl A. Pinkert
University of Rochester Medical Center

Our ability to manipulate the genome of whole animals has influenced the biological sciences in a most remarkable fashion. In two decades, manipulations of the genetic composition of transgenic animals have allowed researchers to address fundamental questions in fields ranging from production agriculture to biomedical research. In a host of transgenic animal models, basic research into the regulation and function of specific genes forged the way to *in vivo* genetic modifications that resulted in either the gain-of-function of a transferred gene or the ablation of an endogenous gene product. Pioneering efforts in transgenic animal technology have markedly influenced our appreciation of the factors that govern gene regulation and expression, and have contributed significantly to our understanding of the genetic bases of human development and disease.

18.1 Introduction

Animal modeling and technologies for genetic modification of animals have experienced a tremendous growth rate and garnered a broad presence in the life sciences over the last 25 years. From the first transgenic mouse models reported in the early 1980s, to the use of gene targeting and cloning technologies, to functional genomics and bioinformatics groundwork — science has and will continue to witness growth and dynamic use of animal modeling systems at an ever-increasing pace.

Production of genetically modified or "transgenic" animals marked the convergence of previous advances in the areas of recombinant DNA technology and the manipulation and culture of animal

0-8493-1140-3/04/$0.00+$1.50

germplasm. Transgenic mice provide powerful models to explore the regulation of gene expression as well as the regulation of cellular and physiological processes. Experimental designs have taken advantage of our ability to direct specific (e.g., cell-, tissue-, organ-specificity) as well as ubiquitous (whole-body) expression *in vivo*. From embryology to virology, transgenic technology provides unique animal models for studies in various disciplines that would otherwise be all but impossible to develop spontaneously (see Hogan et al., 1994; Pinkert, 1994, 2002; Monastersky and Robl, 1995; Houdebine, 1997; Pinkert et al., 1997b, 2002; Pinkert and Murray, 1998; Nagy et al., 2003).

18.1.1 Development of Transgenic Animals

The ability to introduce functional genes into animals provides a very powerful tool for dissecting complex biological processes and systems. Transgenic animals represent unique models that are custom tailored to address specific biological questions. Furthermore, classical genetic selection cannot engineer a specific genetic trait in a directed fashion. Thus, gene transfer in farm animals can surpass classical breeding practices where long life cycles slow the rate of genetic improvement.

Although the entire procedure for microinjection into living cells was described in the late 1960s, it took more than a decade before transgenic animals were actually created (Lin, 1966). Following the description of a microinjection process, the first technological hurdle was surpassed in 1977 when Gurdon transferred mRNA and DNA into *Xenopus laevis* embryos and observed that the transferred nucleic acids were indeed functional. Then, in 1980, Brinster and his colleagues reported on parallel studies using a mammalian model — the mouse. Sequentially, these studies laid the groundwork for the development of the first transgenic animals. From late 1980 through 1981, six research groups reported success at gene transfer and the development of transgenic mice. In gene transfer, animals harboring new genes (foreign DNA sequences integrated into their genome) are referred to as transgenic, a term first coined by Gordon and Ruddle in 1981. As such, transgenic animals are recognized as independent strains or even species variants, following the introduction and integration of new genetic material into their genetic composition. More recently, the term "transgenic" has been adapted to include chimeric and knock-out mice in which gene(s) have been selectively ablated from the host genome (Figure 18.1; Pinkert et al., 1995; Beardmore, 1997).

A few key terms will aid in understanding some of the underlying technologies associated with genetic engineering technologies (outlined in greater detail in Pinkert, 2002). *Gene transfer* is defined as one of a set of techniques directed toward manipulating biological function via the introduction of foreign DNA sequences (genes) into living cells. *DNA microinjection* is a gene transfer technique where DNA constructs (transgenes) are microinjected directly into pronuclei or nuclei of fertilized ova (zygotes). In contrast, *embryonic stem (ES) cell transfer* involves the transfer and incorporation of pluripotent embryonic stem cells into developing embryos. ES cell transfer also provides for gene targeting capability (allowing for creation of *knock-out* or *knock-in* modeling, where endogenous genes are selectively ablated or replaced by modified sequences, respectively). *Cloning* is generally associated with *nuclear transfer* whereby a nucleus provided by a donor cell is introduced into an enucleated oocyte (unfertilized ovum) or zygote allowing for reprogramming of the developing embryo. Today, a *transgenic animal* can be represented by animals integrating foreign DNA sequences into its genome following gene transfer, or resulting from the molecular manipulation of endogenous genomic DNA (hence, not only gain-of-function models are represented in the definition, but ablation or loss-of-function models are included as well). In defining a *transgenic line*, all animals in a direct familial lineage derived from one or more transgenic founders are included where the genetic modification is transmitted in successive generations as a stable genetic element or variant. The line includes the founder and any subsequent offspring inheriting the specific germ-line manipulation. Last, in addition to nuclear gene modifications, mitochondrial populations and mitochondrial DNA (mtDNA) genes can now be altered. *Mitochondria* are found in the cytoplasm of eukaryotic cells and serve as centers of intracellular enzyme activity, producing the energy needed for cellular metabolism. In turn, *heteroplasmy* refers to the coexistence of more than one mitochondrial population within a single cell or within cells that comprise an individual organism.

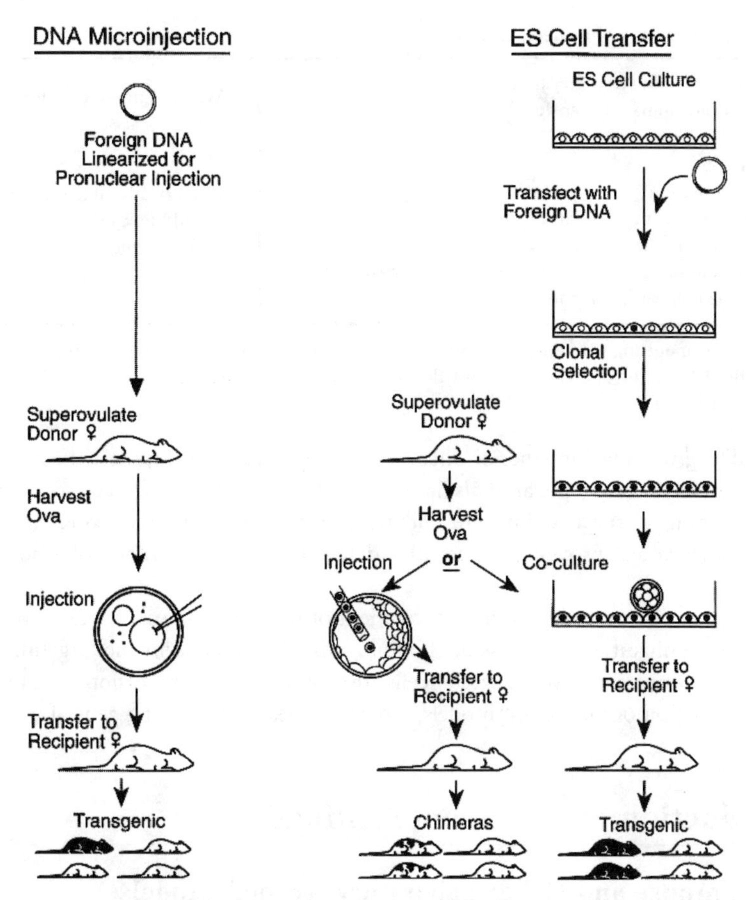

FIGURE 18.1 DNA microinjection and ES cell transfer in mice. For DNA microinjection, an *in vitro* culture step is not required (left). DNA is injected directly into the male pronucleus of a zygote. Generally, when transgenic mice (represented by black mouse) are created by DNA microinjection, all of their cells contain the new transgene(s). On the right, after clonal selection of transfected ES cells, either embryo injection or co-culture is employed. As such, ES cells are either injected directly into a host blastocyst or co-cultured with eight-cell to morula stage embryos. With blastocyst injection, transgenic offspring are termed "chimeric," as some of their cells are derived from the host blastocyst and some from the transfected ES cells (denoted by mice with black patches). Using co-culture and tetraploid embryos, one can obtain first generation founder mice derived completely from the transfected ES cells (denoted as solid black mice). (Reprinted from Pinkert, C.A., Irwin, M.H., and Moffatt, R.J., *Encyclopedia of Molecular Biology and Molecular Medicine*, Vol. 6, Meyers, R.A., Ed., VCH, New York, 1997b, pp. 63–74. With permission.)

18.1.2 Applications of Transgenic Animals

A number of methods exist for gene transfer in mammalian species (Table 18.1). Transgenic technology was reported in a variety of animal species including mice, rats, rabbits, swine, ruminants (including sheep, goats, and cattle), poultry, and fish. With advances in the characterization of factors that control gene expression (including promoter-enhancer elements and transcription-regulatory proteins), gene transfer technology has become a proven asset as a means of dissecting gene regulation and developmental pathways *in vivo.*

Normally, endogenous gene function is regulated by both *cis*-acting elements and *trans*-acting factors. For transferred genes, such regulators in conjunction with the gene integration/insertion event within the host genome act in concert to control gene function. Using genes that code for reporter proteins (e.g., fluorophores such as those encoded by luciferase or fluorescent protein genes, or growth

TABLE 18.1 Gene Transfer Methods[a]

Method	
Blastomere/embryo aggregation	Whole genome transfer only
Teratocarcinoma cell transfer	
Retroviral infection	Primary advantage allowing for addition or modification of discrete gene sequences
Electrofusion	
Microinjection	
Embryonic stem (ES) cell transfer	
Nuclear transplantation	
Spermatozoa- and spermatogonial cell-mediated transfer	
Particle bombardment and jet injection	

[a] Mouse modeling techniques evolved from procedures for nonspecific (whole genome) transfer to the transfer of discrete genes and the modification of endogenous genes (adapted from Pinkert, 1997).

factors encoded by growth factor genes or oncogenes that generate developmental consequences [gross phenotype]), analysis of transgenic animals has revealed the importance of such factors in determining developmental timing, tissue distribution, and relative efficiency of gene expression. Additionally, transgenic animals have also proven quite useful in determining *in vivo* artifacts of other model systems or techniques.

There are a number of strategies in the development of transgenic mouse models, including systems designed to study dominant gene expression, homologous recombination/gene targeting and the use of ES cells, efficiency of transformation of eggs or cells, disruption of gene expression by antisense transgene constructs, gene ablation or knock-out models, reporter genes, and marking genes for identification of developmental lineages.

18.2 Production of Transgenic Animals

18.2.1 The Mouse and Other Laboratory Animal Models

The relative importance of using particular strains or breeds of animals in gene transfer experimentation will vary dramatically according to the species under consideration. Probably the most complex system is encountered in the production of transgenic mice, simply because so much work has been done with this species. Well-documented differences in reproductive productivity, behavior, related husbandry requirements, and responses to various experimental procedures influence the efficiency and degree of effort associated with production of transgenic founder animals. A general discussion of these factors therefore serves as an appropriate starting point for understanding the many processes and procedures that must be evaluated and monitored when considering production of transgenic animals.

DNA microinjection, prior to nuclear transfer in domestic animals, was the most direct and reproducible method for producing transgenic animals (Figure 18.1). Beyond the mouse model, other laboratory animal species may be necessary to study a particular biological phenomenon. The significance and critical importance of optimized protocols cannot be underestimated. In any given species, selection and management of donor females that respond well to hormonal synchronization and superovulation, embryo transfer recipients that are able to carry fetuses to term and then care for neonates appropriately, and the effective use of males in a breeding regimen will all add to the relative experimental efficiency that one might encounter. In turn, transgenic animal protocols developed in mice have been modified to accommodate production of other transgenic species.

18.2.2 DNA Microinjection

DNA microinjection generally involves physical injection of a DNA construct solution into embryos (Polites and Pinkert, 2002). Virtually any cloned DNA construct can be used. With few exceptions, microinjected gene constructs integrate randomly throughout the host's genome. Yet, multiple integration sites per founder are rarely observed, with a single chromosomal "integration site" the general rule. Therefore, the integration phenomenon can be exploited to simultaneously co-inject more than one DNA construct into a zygote; where two or more constructs co-integrate together at a single, randomly located integration site. The integration process itself is still poorly understood, but it apparently does not involve homologous recombination. During integration, a single copy or multiple copies of a transgene (actually as many as a few hundred copies of the particular sequence) are incorporated into the genomic DNA, predominantly as a number of copies in head-to-tail concatemers. Regulatory elements in the host DNA near the site of integration, and the general availability of this region for transcription appear to play major roles in affecting the level of transgene expression. This "positional effect" is presumed to explain why the levels of expression of the same transgene may vary dramatically between individual founder animals as well as their offspring. It is therefore prudent to examine transgene expression in offspring from at least three or four founder animals in order to determine what might be a result of the integration location, and what might reflect the activity of the transgene.

Host DNA near the site of integration frequently undergoes various forms of sequence duplication, deletion, or rearrangement as a result of transgene incorporation. Such alterations, if sufficiently drastic, may disrupt the function of normally active host genes at the integration site and constitute insertional mutagenesis, wherein an aberrant phenotype may result. Such events are generally not purposefully designed, but have led to the serendipitous discovery of previously unsuspected genes and gene functions. Because DNA microinjection is usually accomplished in unicellular zygotes, transgene incorporation occurs in essentially every cell that contributes to the developing embryo. Incorporation of the transgene into cells that will eventually contribute to development of germ cells (sperm or ova) is a common occurrence with this method, and makes heritability of the transgene by offspring of founder animals likely within one generation. In such cases, the transgene has been said to be germ-line or the animals are referred to as germ-line competent. However, integration of the microinjected DNA construct into the host's genome occasionally may be inexplicably delayed. In such a case, if cells of the early embryo (blastomeres) undergo mitosis before the transgene-integration event occurs, some but not all of the cells will contain the transgene, and the founder animal, although still considered to be transgenic, will be classified as a mosaic or chimera.

18.2.3 Retrovirus-Mediated Gene Transfer

Transfer of foreign genes into animal genomes has also been accomplished using retroviruses (Chan et al., 1998). Although embryos can be infected with retroviruses up to midgestation, oocytes to 16-cell stage ova are generally used for infection with one or more recombinant retroviruses containing a foreign gene of interest. Immediately following infection, the retrovirus produces a DNA copy of its RNA genome using the viral enzyme, reverse transcriptase. Completion of this process requires that the host cell undergoes the S phase of the cell cycle. Therefore, retroviruses effectively transduce only mitotically active cells. Modifications to the retrovirus frequently consist of removal of structural genes, such as gag, pol, and env, which support viral particle formation. Additionally, most retroviruses and complementary lines are ecotropic in that they infect species-specific cell lines, limiting risk to humans in animal experimentation.

18.2.4 Embryonic Stem (ES) Cell Technology

Gene transfer has been used to produce both random and targeted insertion or ablation of discrete DNA fragments into the mouse genome (Figure 18.1). For targeted insertions (via homologous recombination — with insertion and integration of a gene sequence with a specific homology to an endogenous gene or gene sequences), the efficiency using DNA microinjection is extremely low (Brinster et al., 1989a). In contrast, the use of ES cells in gene targeting has been quite effective in utilizing *in vitro* selection of a specific chromosomal integration via homologous recombination in ES cell cultures. The transfected ES cell lineage is then clonally expanded for subsequent transfer into mouse embryos (Capecchi, 1989). The ability to screen ES cell clones *in vitro* has led to the production of mice that (1) incorporate novel foreign genes into their genome, (2) carry modified endogenous genes (knock-in models), and (3) lack specific endogenous genes following gene deletion or knock-out procedures. As such, technologies involving ES cells, and more recently primordial germ cells, have been used to produce a host of mouse models.

Pluripotential ES cells are for the most part derived from early pre-implantation embryos and maintained in culture for a sufficient period for one to perform various *in vitro* manipulations. The cells may then be injected directly into the blastocoel cavity of a host blastocyst (or into earlier stage embryos), or incubated in association with zona-free morulae. The host embryos are then transferred into intermediate hosts or surrogate females for continued development. The use of ES cells to produce transgenic mice faced a number of procedural obstacles before becoming competitive with DNA microinjection as a standard technique in mouse modeling. Additionally, the use of co-culture techniques involving tetraploid host embryos (8-cell stage to morulae) has resulted in first generation models derived completely from the co-cultured ES cells (Wood et al., 1993; Figure 18.1).

Yet, while ES cell lines have been identified for species other than the mouse, the production of germ-line-competent ES cell-derived/chimeric farm animals has not been reported. With the advent of nuclear transfer-related technologies, the need to identify and use ES or primordial germ cells (PGCs) to effect genetic change has in turn become of lesser consequence.

18.2.5 Production of Transgenic Domestic Animals

The success of transgenic mouse experiments led a number of research groups to study the transfer of similar gene constructs into the germ-line of domestic animal species. These efforts have been directed primarily toward three general endpoints: improving the productivity traits of domestic food animal species, development of transgenic animals for use as bioreactors (i.e., producers of recoverable quantities of medically or biologically important proteins), and in transplantation-related modeling efforts. Since 1985, numerous studies have focused on transgenic farm animals created using growth-related gene constructs. Unfortunately, for the most part, ideal growth phenotypes were not achieved because of an inability to coordinately regulate gene expression and the ensuing cascade of endocrine events that unfolded.

Today, DNA microinjection, retroviral transfection, and nuclear transfer procedures are the only methods used to successfully produce transgenic livestock (see Figures 18.2 and 18.3). Although involved and at times quite tedious, the steps in the development of transgenic models are relatively straightforward. For either DNA microinjection or nuclear transfer, once a specific fusion gene is cloned and characterized, sufficient quantities are isolated, purified, and tested in cell culture. If *in vitro* mRNA expression of the gene is identified, the appropriate fragment is linearized, purified, and readied for preliminary mammalian gene transfer experiments. In contrast to nuclear transfer studies, DNA microinjection experiments are first performed in the mouse. While the transgenic mouse model will not always identify likely phenotypic expression patterns in domestic animals, we have not observed any gene constructs that would function in a farm animal when there had been no evidence of transgene-encoded expression in a pilot mouse model.

In 1997, the successful cloning of a sheep captured the imagination of researchers around the world, and was rapidly followed by the use of nuclear transfer to produce transgenic domestic animals (Wilmut et al., 1997; Paterson et al., 2002; Godke et al., 2002). Within the next few years, nuclear transfer and subsequent technological breakthroughs should play a significant role in the development of new procedures for genetic engineering in a number of mammalian species. It should be noted that nuclear transfer, with nuclei obtained from either mammalian stem cells or differentiated adult cells, is an especially important development in species beyond the mouse model. This is because a technological barrier was surpassed that allowed for specific *in vitro* manipulations that lead to targeted genetic modifications in first generation founder animals. Previously, it was not possible to produce germ-line-competent transgenics in mammalian species (other than in mice), using any technique other than DNA microinjection (that only allowed for random and imprecise integration of transgenes in founder animals). Unfortunately, relative efficiencies for nuclear transfer experimentation still pale in comparison

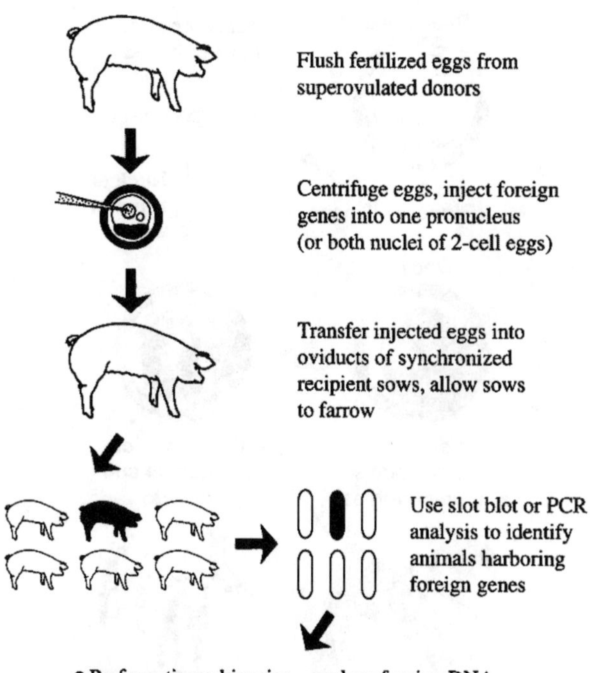
Flush fertilized eggs from superovulated donors
Centrifuge eggs, inject foreign genes into one pronucleus (or both nuclei of 2-cell eggs)
Transfer injected eggs into oviducts of synchronized recipient sows, allow sows to farrow
Use slot blot or PCR analysis to identify animals harboring foreign genes
• Perform tissue biopsies – analyze foreign DNA integration, mRNA transcription, and protein production
• Establish transgenic lines to study gene regulation in progeny

FIGURE 18.2 Transgenic pig production by DNA microinjection. In contrast to mouse modeling, visualization of the pronuclei (or nuclei) is necessary for microinjection into zygotes (or later-stage ova) for most domestic animal species. This is accomplished by centrifugation of the ova to stratify the opaque lipids (Wall et al., 1985), making pronuclei or nuclei readily visible. (Reprinted from Pinkert, C.A., Dyer, T.J., Kooyman, D.L., and Kiehm, D.J., *Dom. Anim. Endocrinol.*, 7, 1–18, 1990. With permission.)

to conventional DNA microinjection. However, while nuclear transfer might be considered inefficient in its current form, major strides in enhancing experimental protocols within the next few years are envisioned, comparable perhaps to the early advances in DNA microinjection technology.

In contrast to gene transfer in mice, the efficiency associated with the production of transgenic livestock, including swine, remains low (Martin and Pinkert, 2002). However, two advantages offered by swine over other domestic species are a favorable response to hormonal superovulation protocols (20 to 30 ova can be collected on average) and, as a polytocous species, they have a uterine capacity to nurture more offspring to term.

For studies where the pig may be the desired model, the use of outbred domestic pigs is the most practical way to produce transgenic founders. However, miniature or laboratory swine are now used with increasing frequency in biomedical research, where their well-characterized background genetics make them more suitable for human modeling studies (e.g., xenotransplantation research). Reproductive efficiency in miniature swine is low compared to commercial swine and is characterized by a low ovulation rate, low birth weight, and small litter size. Estrous cycles and gestation length are similar to standard commercial swine; however, sexual maturity in males and females actually occurs between 4 and 6 months of age in some breeds, which is sooner than observed in commercial swine, thereby hastening the generational interval.

In comparison to swine modeling, the relative experimental efficiencies associated with the production of transgenic ruminants (including goats, sheep, and cattle) are even lower (Rexroad and Hawk, 1994;

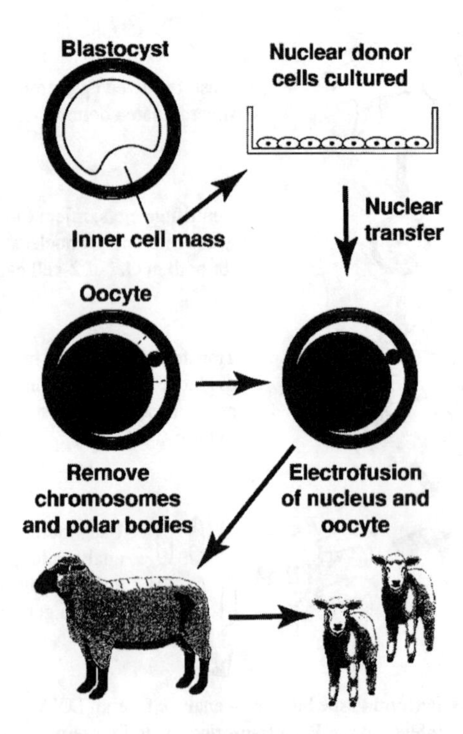

FIGURE 18.3 Cloning by nuclear transfer using sheep. Cells from blastocysts (e.g., inner cell mass cells) or other somatic tissues are obtained and propagated in culture. These cells are used as nucleus donors for transfer into enucleated oocytes. In contrast to DNA microinjection, a fusion step is generally employed to fuse the transferred nuclei and enucleated oocytes. Here, electrofusion is used to fuse couplets (transferred nucleus plus oocyte) that are transferred to recipients for the remainder of gestation. (Reprinted from Pinkert, C.A., *Reproduction in Farm Animals*, 7th ed., Hafez, E.S.E. and Hafez, B., Eds., Williams & Wilkins, Baltimore, 2000, Chap. 21, pp. 318–330. With permission.)

Niemann et al., 2002). While the different techniques from DNA microinjection to nuclear transfer require a large number of embryos to ensure varying levels of success, there are a number of pertinent considerations that will influence experimental yields. Such factors include the rate of embryo survival following manipulation, uterine capacity (generally these species are monotocous), generational interval, and animal maintenance, all impacting on experimental costs and efficiencies. In many laboratories, *in vitro* maturation (IVM), *in vitro* fertilization (IVF), and culture of ova (in surrogate hosts or incubators, although culture conditions are not optimal for embryo survival at this time) prior to final transfer aid in maximizing resources for production of genetically engineered ruminants. Many of these steps are timely, as is the ability to biopsy individual blastomeres for analysis of specific genetic modifications, which can minimize the number of animals used and maintained in such endeavors.

18.3 Evolving Technologies

18.3.1 From Spermatozoa to Cloning

In contrast to progress in embryo manipulation, a completely different avenue was taken with the advent of sperm-related transfer procedures. In 1989, sperm-mediated gene transfer was reported but hotly disputed when many laboratories around the world were unable to duplicate the outlined procedures (Brinster et al., 1989b). Yet, by 1994, the sperm-mediated story generated interest that resulted in the development of spermatogonial cell transplantation procedures as feasible alternatives for *in vivo* gene transfer (Brinster and Avarbock, 1994; Nagano et al., 2001). However, whole-animal and somatic-cell techniques (including liposome-mediated gene transfer, jet injection, and particle bombardment), coupled with novel vector systems and innovative use of bioinformatics data, will continue to evolve in order to genetically engineer animals in an efficient and effective manner.

18.3.2 From the Nucleus to the Mitochondrion

Until recently, *in vivo* mitochondrial transfer remained a technological hurdle in the development of mitochondrial-based gene transfer and therapies. The field of mitochondrial medicine is now just emerging. The first published accounts of diseases caused by mutations of mtDNA were reported in 1988 and there are now scores of characterized mutations within the mitochondrial genome in addition to nuclear gene defects influencing mitochondrial function that are known to be the underlying causes of various degenerative disorders (Clayton, 1991, 1992; Wallace, 1992a, 1992b, 2001; Larsson and Clayton, 1995; Luft, 1995; Graff et al., 1999; Pinkert and Trounce, 2002). In humans, metabolic and cellular pathologies exist due to mutations arising exclusively within the mitochondrial genome (Wallace, 2001). Various diseases have been associated with mtDNA point mutations, deletions, and duplications as well as age-associated changes in the functional integrity of mitochondria. In addition, mitochondrial DNA polymorphisms were identified and associated with specific developmental characteristics in domestic species (Brown et al., 1989; Koehler et al., 1991). Therefore, for a host of applications, the ability to manipulate the mitochondrial genome and to regulate mitochondrial gene function would provide an additional target in modifying mammalian development.

We and others have initiated studies revolving around mitochondrial transfer and techniques to produce animals harboring foreign mitochondrial genomes (Pinkert et al., 1997a; Irwin et al., 1999, 2001; Levy et al., 1999; Marchington et al., 1999; Inoue et al., 1999; Sligh et al., 2000; Pinkert and Trounce, 2002). The creation of transmitochondrial animals represents a new model system that will provide a greater understanding of mitochondrial dynamics, leading to the development of genetically engineered production animals, and therapeutic strategies for human metabolic diseases affected by aberrations in mitochondrial function.

18.4 Conclusions and Future Directions

18.4.1 Gene Transfer and Genetic Engineering Today

The expertise and effort associated with gene transfer experimentation in animal biology are quite significant and challenging. Innovative technologies to enhance experimental gene transfer efficiency in different species are desperately needed. Such enabling techniques would not only bring the cost of individual projects into a reasonable realm, but would also increase the likelihood of new innovations in many disciplines. The outlined methodology for transgenic animal production represents what is considered current state-of-the-art technology. It is envisioned that procedures will continue to evolve, particularly with the data mining efforts associated with microarray analyses and bioinformatics management. In this regard, microarray technologies coupled with developments at bioinformatics and access to the wealth of data being generated on genomic, proteomic, and metabonomic platforms will provide significant inroads and direction to gene discovery in the near-term. Until recently, gene discovery was performed studying individual genes, one gene at a time. With microarray technologies, standard molecular biological principles are employed on an industrial scale, allowing generation of quantitative gene expression profiles for thousands of genes simultaneously. Such gene expression profiles are then used to decipher molecular mechanisms that underlie targeted biological perturbations, as well as comparative development in various biological systems.

18.4.2 Future Directions

Much has been learned about various physiological processes in transgenic models created to date. Transgenic animals have provided far-reaching insights in medicine, helping to redefine many regulatory and developmental processes in mammalian species. While studies of genetically modified animal models may not always correlate exactly to human biology and disease pathogenesis, the utility of transgenic animal models to scientific discovery cannot be underestimated. The systematic achievements envisioned through such model efforts will continue to provide stimulating challenges in the 21st century.

Acknowledgments

I gratefully acknowledge R.L. Howell, C.A. Cassar, C.A. Ingraham, and D.A. Dunn for their helpful comments and suggestions. Current studies are supported by NCRR, NIDCR, and the University of Rochester Medical Center.

References

Beardmore, J.A., Transgenics: autotransgenics and allotransgenics, *Transgenic Res.*, 6, 107–108, 1997.

Brinster, R.L., Stem cells and transgenic mice in the study of development, *Intl. J. Devel. Biol.*, 3, 89–99, 1993.

Brinster, R.L. and Avarbock, M.R., Germline transmission of donor haplotype following spermatogonial transplantation, *Proc. Natl. Acad. Sci. U.S.A.*, 91, 11303–11307, 1994.

Brinster, R.L., Chen, H.Y., Trumbauer, M.E. and Avarbock, M.R., Translation of globin messenger RNA by the mouse ovum, *Nature,* 283, 499–501, 1980.

Brinster, R.L., Braun, R.E., Lo, D., Avarbock, M.R., Oram, F., and Palmiter, R.D., Targeted correction of a major histocompatibility class II Eα gene by DNA microinjected into mouse eggs, *Proc. Natl. Acad. Sci. U.S.A.*, 86, 7087–7091, 1989a.

Brinster, R.L., Sandgren, E.P., Behringer, R.R., and Palmiter, R.D., No simple solution for making transgenic mice, *Cell,* 59, 239–241, 1989b.

Brown, D.R., Koehler, C.M., Lindberg, G.L., Freeman, A.E., Mayfield, J.E., Myers, A.M., Schutz, M.M., and Beitz, D.C., Molecular analysis of cytoplasmic genetic variation in Holstein cows, *J. Anim. Sci.*, 67, 1926–1932, 1989.

Cappechi, M.R., Altering the genome by homologous recombination, *Science*, 244, 1288–1292, 1989.

Chan, A.W.S., Homan, E.J., Ballou, L.B., Burns, J.C., and Bremel, R.D., Transgenic cattle produced by reverse-transcribed gene transfer in oocytes, *Proc. Natl. Acad. Sci. U.S.A.*, 95, 14028–14033, 1998.

Clayton, D.A., Replication and transcription of vertebrate mitochondrial DNA, *Annu. Rev. Cell Biol.*, 7, 453–478, 1991.

Clayton, D.A., Structure and function of the mitochondrial genome, *J. Inher. Metab. Dis.*, 15, 439–447, 1992.

Godke, R.A., Sansinena, M., and Youngs, C., Assisted reproductive technologies and embryo culture methods for farm animals, in *Transgenic Animal Technology: A Laboratory Handbook*, 2nd ed., Pinkert, C.A., Ed., Academic Press, New York, 2002, pp. 513–568.

Gordon, J.W. and Ruddle, F.H., Integration and stable germ line transmission of genes injected into mouse pronuclei, *Science*, 214, 1244–1246, 1981.

Graff, C., Clayton, D.A., and Larsson, N.-G., Mitochondrial medicine — recent advances, *J. Int. Med.*, 246, 11–23, 1999.

Gurdon, J.B., Egg cytoplasm and gene control in development, *Proc. R. Soc. London B*, 198, 211–247, 1977.

Hogan, B., Beddington, R., Costantini, F., and Lacy, E., *Manipulating the Mouse Embryo: A Laboratory Manual*, Cold Spring Harbor Laboratory, Cold Spring Harbor, NY, 1994.

Houdebine, L.M., *Transgenic Animals: Generation and Use*, Harwood Academic Publishers, Amsterdam, 1997.

Inoue, K., Nakada, K., Ogura, A., Isobe, K., Goto, Y.-I., Nonaka, I., and Hayashi, J.-I., Generation of mice with mitochondrial dysfunction by introducing mouse mtDNA carrying a deletion into zygotes, *Nature Genet.*, 26, 176–181, 1999.

Irwin, M.H., Johnson, L.W., and Pinkert, C.A., Isolation and microinjection of somatic cell-derived mitochondria and germline heteroplasmy in transmitochondrial mice, *Transgenic Res.*, 8, 119–123, 1999.

Irwin, M.H., Parrino, V., and Pinkert, C.A., Construction of a mutated mtDNA genome and transfection into isolated mitochondria by electroporation. *Adv. Reprod.*, 5, 59–66, 2001.

Irwin, M.H., Pogozelski, W.K., and Pinkert, C.A., PCR optimization for detection of transgenic integration, in *Transgenic Animal Technology: A Laboratory Handbook*, 2nd ed., Pinkert, C.A., Ed., Academic Press, New York, 2002, pp. 475–484.

Koehler, C.M., Lindberg, G.L., Brown, D.R., Beitz, D.C., Freeman, A.E., Mayfield, J.E., and Myers, A.M., Replacement of bovine mitochondrial DNA by a sequence variant within one generation, *Genetics*, 129, 247–255, 1991.

Larsson, N.-G. and Clayton, D.A., Molecular genetic aspects of human mitochondrial disorders, *Annu. Rev. Genet.*, 29, 151–178, 1995.

Levy, S.E., Waymire, K.G., Kim, Y.L., MacGregor, G.R., and Wallace, D.C., Transfer of chloramphenicol-resistant mitochondrial DNA into the chimeric mouse, *Transgenic Res.*, 8, 137–145, 1999.

Lin, T.P., Microinjection of mouse eggs, *Science*, 151, 333–337, 1966.

Luft, R., The development of mitochondrial medicine, *Biochim. Biophys. Acta*, 1271, 1–6, 1995.

Marchington, D.R., Barlow, D., and Poulton, J., Transmitochondrial mice carrying resistance to chloramphenicol on mitochondrial DNA: developing the first mouse model of mitochondrial DNA disease, *Nature Med.*, 5, 957–960, 1999.

Martin, M.J. and Pinkert, C.A., Production of transgenic swine by DNA microinjection, in *Transgenic Animal Technology: A Laboratory Handbook*, 2nd ed., Pinkert, C.A., Ed., Academic Press, New York, 2002, pp. 307–336.

Matsui, Y., Zsebo, K., and Hogan, B.L., Derivation of pluripotential embryonic stem cells from murine primordial germ cells in culture, *Cell*, 70, 841–847, 1992.

Monastersky, G.M. and Robl, J.M., *Strategies in Transgenic Animal Science*, American Society of Microbiology Press, Washington, D.C., 1995.

Nagano, M., Brinster, C.J., Orwig, K.E., Rye, B.-Y., Avarbock, M.R., and Brinster, R.L., Transgenic mice produced by retroviral transduction of male germ-line stem cells, *Proc. Natl. Acad. Sci. U.S.A.*, 98, 13090–13095, 2001.

Nagy, A., Gertsenstein, M., Vintersten, K., and Behringer, R., *Manipulating the Mouse Embryo: A Laboratory Manual*, Cold Spring Harber Laboratory, Cold Spring Harbor, New York, 2003.

Niemann, H., Dopke, H.H., and Hadeler, K.G., Production of transgenic ruminants by DNA microinjection, in *Transgenic Animal Technology: A Laboratory Handbook*, 2nd ed., Pinkert, C.A., Ed., Academic Press, New York, 2002, pp. 337–357.

Palmiter, R.D., Brinster, L., Hammer, R.E., Trumbauer, M.E., Rosenfeld, M.G., Birnberg, N.C., and Evans, R.M., Dramatic growth of mice that develop from eggs microinjected with metallothionein-growth hormone fusion genes, *Nature*, 300, 611–615, 1982.

Paterson, L., Ritchie, W., and Wilmut, I., Nuclear transfer technology in cattle, sheep and swine, in *Transgenic Animal Technology: A Laboratory Handbook*, 2nd ed., Pinkert, C.A., Ed., Academic Press, New York, 2002, pp. 395–416.

Pinkert, C.A., Gene transfer and the production of transgenic livestock, *Proc. U.S. Anim. Health Assn.*, 91, 129–141, 1987.

Pinkert, C.A., Transgenic swine models for xenotransplantation, *Xeno*, 2, 10–15, 1994.

Pinkert, C.A., The history and theory of transgenic animals, *Lab. Anim.*, 26, 29–34, 1997.

Pinkert, C.A., Genetic engineering of farm mammals, in *Reproduction in Farm Animals*, 7th ed., Hafez, E.S.E. and Hafez, B., Eds., Williams & Wilkins, Baltimore, 2000, Chap. 21, pp. 318–330.

Pinkert, C.A., *Transgenic Animal Technology: A Laboratory Handbook*, Academic Press, New York, 2002.

Pinkert, C.A. and Murray, J.D., Transgenic farm animals, in *Transgenic Animals in Agriculture*, Murray, J.D., Anderson, G.B., McGloughlin, M.M., and Oberbauer, A.M., Eds., CAB International, Wallingford, U.K., 1998.

Pinkert, C.A. and Trounce, I.A., Production of transmitochondrial mice, *Methods*, 26, 348–357, 2002.

Pinkert, C.A., Dyer, T.J., Kooyman, D.L., and Kiehm, D.J., Characterization of transgenic livestock production, *Dom. Anim. Endocrinol.*, 7, 1–18, 1990.

Pinkert, C.A., Irwin, M.H., and Moffatt, R.J., Transgenic animal modeling, in *Molecular Biology and Biotechnology*, Meyers, R.A., Ed., VCH, New York, 1995, 901–907.

Pinkert, C.A., Irwin, M.H., Johnson, L.W., and Moffatt, R.J., Mitochondria transfer into mouse ova by microinjection, *Transgenic Res.*, 6, 379–383, 1997a.

Pinkert, C.A., Irwin, M.H., and Moffatt, R.J., Transgenic animal modeling, in *Encyclopedia of Molecular Biology and Molecular Medicine*, Vol. 6, Meyers, R.A., Ed., VCH, New York, 1997b, pp. 63–74.

Pinkert, C.A., Kooyman, D.L., and Martin, M.J., Genetic engineering of farm animals: from transgenesis to gene mapping, what does the future hold? KRMIVA 2002 Conference, Opatija, Croatia, *Proc.*, 9, 18–34, 2002.

Polites, H.G. and Pinkert, C.A., DNA microinjection and transgenic animal production, in *Transgenic Animal Technology: A Laboratory Handbook*, 2nd ed., Pinkert, C.A., Ed., Academic Press, New York, 2002, pp. 15–70.

Pursel, V.G. and Rexroad, C.E., Jr., Status of research with transgenic farm animals, *J. Anim. Sci.*, 71(Suppl. 3), 10–19, 1993.

Rexroad, C.E., Jr. and Hawk, H.W., Production of transgenic ruminants, in *Transgenic Animal Technology: A Laboratory Handbook*, Pinkert, C.A., Ed., Academic Press, San Diego, 1994, pp. 339–355.

Sligh, J.E., Levy, S.E., Waymire, K.G., Allard, P., Dillehay, D.L., Heckenlively, J.R., MacGregor, G.R., and Wallace, D.C., Maternal germ-line transmission of mutant mtDNAs from embryonic stem cell-derived chimeric mice, *Proc. Natl. Acad. Sci. U.S.A.*, 97, 14461–14466, 2000.

Wall, R.J., Pursel, V.G., Hammer, R.E., and Brinster, R.L., Development of porcine ova that were centrifuged to permit visualization of pronuclei and nuclei, *Biol. Reprod.*, 32, 645–651, 1985.

Wall, R.J., Hawk, H.W., and Nel, N., Making transgenic livestock: genetic engineering on a large scale, *J. Cell. Biochem.*, 49, 113–120, 1992.

Wallace, D.C., Diseases of the mitochondrial DNA, *Annu. Rev. Biochem.*, 61, 1175–1212, 1992a.

Wallace, D.C., Mitochondria genetics: a paradigm for aging and degenerative diseases? *Science*, 256, 628–632, 1992b.

Wallace, D.C., Mouse models for mitochondrial disease, *Am. J. Med. Genet.*, 106, 71–93, 2001.

Wilmut, I., Schnieke, A.E., McWhir, J., Kind, A.J., and Campbell, K.H., Viable offspring derived from fetal and adult mammalian cells, *Nature*, 385, 810–813, 1997.

Wood, S.A., Allen, N.D., Rossant, J., Auerbach, A., and Nagy, A., Non-injection methods for the production of embryonic stem cell-embryo chimaeras, *Nature*, 365, 87–89, 1993.

19

Gene-Enhanced Tissue Engineering

CONTENTS

Stelios T. Andreadis
State University of New York at Buffalo

19.1 Introduction

Tissue engineering applies the principles and methods of engineering and the life sciences toward the development of tissue substitutes to restore, maintain or improve tissue function.[1-3] The field of tissue engineering is motivated by the tremendous need for transplantation of human tissue. Engineered tissues can also be used as realistic biological models to obtain fundamental understanding of the structure–function relationships under normal and disease conditions and as toxicological models to facilitate drug development and testing.

In order to engineer tissues in the laboratory, cells must grow on three-dimensional scaffolds that provide the right geometric configuration, mechanical support and bioactive signals that promote tissue growth and differentiation. The cells may come from the patient (autologous), another individual (allogeneic) or a different species (xenogeneic). Cell sourcing may be overcome by use of adult or embryonic stem cells that have the capacity for self-renewal and can differentiate into multiple cell types, thus providing an unlimited supply of cells for tissue and cellular therapies. Application of stem cells in tissue engineering requires control of their differentiation into specific cell types, which in turn depends on fundamental understanding of the factors that affect stem cell self-renewal and lineage commitment.[4,5]

Alternatively, implantation of biomaterials at the site of tissue injury may be used to stimulate the surrounding cells to regenerate the severed tissue. Examples include induction of nerve regeneration, dermal wound healing and neovascularization (i.e., formation of new blood vessels) of implanted tissues. The main challenge in this approach is to recreate the conditions that induce tissue regeneration instead of repair. Since embryonic tissues heal without scaring, understanding the molecular differences between fetal and adult wound healing and cell–cell interactions during embryological development could lead to significant advances in engineering of a regenerative environment for successful healing.

0-8493-1140-3/04/$0.00+$1.50

TABLE 19.1 Current Gene Therapy Clinical Trials and Disease Targets

	Clinical Trials		Patients	
Disease	Number	%	Number	%
Cancer	378	63	2392	68.5
Monogenic	75	12.5	309	8.8
Infectious	38	6.3	408	11.7
Vascular	48	8	86	2.5
Other diseases	13	2.1	25	0.7
Gene marking	48	8	274	7.8
Total	600		3494	

Taken from the Web site of the *Journal of Gene Medicine* (http://www.wiley.co.uk/genetherapy/clinical/).

The challenge in engineering living tissues lies in creating the right macroscopic (tissue) architecture and function starting from microscopic components (cells and molecules). Part of the challenge may be addressed by appropriate design of bioactive scaffolds that provide the appropriate molecular signals and mechanical environment to guide cellular function.

Alternatively, cellular function may be directed by molecular engineering at the most fundamental level, the genome. Gene delivery can be applied in tissue engineering in order to impart new functions or enhance existing cellular activities in tissue substitutes.[6] This is achieved by genetic modification of cells that will be part of the implant or gene transfer to the site of injury to facilitate *in situ* tissue regeneration. Cells can be genetically engineered to express a variety of molecules including growth factors that induce cell growth/differentiation or cytokines that prevent an immunologic reaction to the implant. Therefore, gene delivery has the potential to improve the quality of tissue substitutes by altering the genetic basis of the cells that make up the tissues.

19.2 Gene Therapeutics

Gene therapy is the transfer of genes into cells to achieve a therapeutic effect. Expression of the transferred gene(s) can result in the synthesis of therapeutic proteins and potentially the correction of biochemical defects. Although gene therapy was initially developed for the treatment of genetic diseases, the majority of ongoing clinical trials involve various gene transfer technologies for the treatment of a wide variety of cancers and infectious diseases (Table 19.1).

In general, two classes of methods are employed to deliver genes into target cells. They are broadly classified as viral and nonviral.[7,8] Viral methods, which use recombinant viruses as gene delivery vehicles, are used in the majority of clinical trials (Table 19.2). The genome of recombinant viruses has been

TABLE 19.2 Current Gene Therapy Clinical Trials and Disease Targets

Disease	RT	AV	AAV	Naked DNA	LP	Other
Cancer	96	118	1	33	62	68
Monogenic	32	17	11	1	12	2
Infectious	36					2
Vascular		26		19	3	
Gene marking	45	1		1		1
Other diseases	3	2	1	5		2
Total	212	164	13	59	77	75
% of all trials	35.3	27.3	2.2	9.8	12.8	12.5

RT = retrovirus; AV = adenovirus; AAV = adeno-associated virus; LP = lipofection; Other = Herpes simplex virus, poxvirus, vaccinia virus, salmonella typhimurium, RNA and gene gun.

The information was compiled from the Web site of the *Journal of Gene Medicine* (http://www.wiley.co.uk/genetherapy/clinical/).

TABLE 19.3 Characteristics of the Most Common Gene Transfer Vehicles

Properties	RT	LT	AV	AAV	Plasmid DNA
Titer	10^5–10^7	10^5–10^7	10^7	10^{12}	10^7
Integrates into host genome?	Yes	Yes	No	Yes	No
Persistence of gene expression	Years	Years	Months	Years	Weeks
Stability	No	No	Yes	Yes	Yes
Maximum transgene size	7–8	7–8	36	4–5	Unlimited
Immunogenicity	No	No	Yes	Yes	No
Gene transfer to non-dividing cells	No	Yes	Yes	Yes	Yes
Potential for gene transfer to stem cells	Yes	Yes	No	Yes	No

RT = retrovirus; LT = lentivirus; AV = adenovirus; AAV = adeno-associated virus.

modified by deletion of some or all viral genes and replacement with foreign therapeutic or marker genes. Recombinant viruses that are currently used in gene therapy include retrovirus, lentivirus (HIV-based), adenovirus and adeno-associated virus.

Nonviral methods include delivery of DNA using physical and chemical means. Physical methods such as electroporation and particle acceleration (gene gun) facilitate entry into target cells, but compromise cell viability and therefore may not be appropriate for use in tissue engineering. On the other hand, delivery of DNA complexed with lipids or polymers has met with some success *in vitro* and is employed in a significant fraction of current clinical trials (Table 19.2). More recently, natural and synthetic polymeric materials were used as scaffolds for DNA delivery *in vivo* to promote tissue regeneration. Here we review the most commonly used viral and nonviral gene transfer vehicles, their use in tissue engineering and the major limitations that need to be overcome to realize the potential of gene therapy in regenerative medicine. A comparison of the main characteristics of viral and nonviral technologies is given in Table 19.3.

19.2.1 Viral Gene Delivery

19.2.1.1 Recombinant Retroviruses

Retroviruses are enveloped particles with a diameter of approximately 100 nm. The lipid bilayer contains the envelope glycoproteins that confer the host range of the virus by interacting with receptors on the surface of target cells.[9] The bilayer surrounds a nucleocapsid that contains two single-stranded RNA molecules and enzymes necessary for virus replication. The genome of retroviruses has three genes: *gag*, which encodes the major capsid protein; *pol*, which encodes the enzymes reverse transcriptase and integrase that participate in early events in viral replication, as well as a protease that is used in the processing of viral proteins; and *env*, which encodes the envelope glycoprotein. In addition, the viral genome contains regulatory sequences that are necessary for transcription (LTRs: long terminal repeats) and a *cis*-acting sequence (Ψ) that mediates packaging of the RNA into the viral capsid.

Recombinant retroviruses are produced by a two-part system: a retroviral vector and a packaging cell line (Figure 19.1).[10] The recombinant vector is derived from a provirus, usually the Moloney Murine Leukemia Virus (MMuLV), in which a therapeutic or marker gene has replaced the *env*, *pol* and *gag* sequences. The latter are provided by the packaging cells to enable the formation of the viral particle. The recombinant vector is transfected into the packaging cells, where it is transcribed and the resulting RNA is recognized by viral proteins and incorporated into the viral capsid. The capsid containing the RNA genome and all the enzymatic activities of the virus buds from the cell surface acquiring its plasma membrane and envelope glycoproteins. Recombinant retroviruses are able to transfer genes to target cells, but they cannot replicate because they lack the genes that encode for the structural proteins.

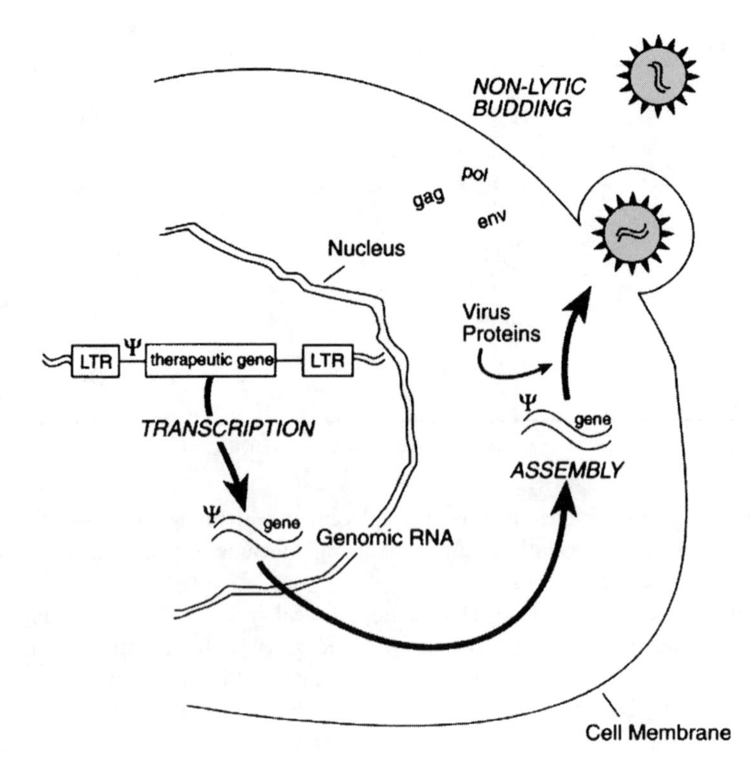

FIGURE 19.1 Schematic of retrovirus production from a packaging cell. (From Andreadis et al., *Biotechnol. Prog.*, 15, 1, 1999. With permission.)

Gene transfer is a multistep process that begins with diffusion of the virus particle to the cell surface, binding of the virus to specific cell surface receptors and internalization into the cell cytoplasm (Figure 19.2). Following entry into the cell, the RNA genome is reverse transcribed into a double-stranded DNA molecule, by the combined action of reverse transcriptase and RNase H. The newly synthesized viral DNA is transported to the nucleus where it is covalently joined to the genomic DNA of the host cell to form an integrated provirus.[11] Once integrated, the provirus is stable and inherited by daughter cells as any other autosomal gene. The newly integrated gene serves as a template for synthesis of mRNA and protein that the target cells may not normally express.

Recombinant retroviruses are ideal vehicles for gene delivery, as they have several advantages over other gene transfer technologies: (1) they have a broad host range; (2) the transferred genes are stably integrated into the chromosomes of the host, resulting in permanent modification of the transduced cells; and (3) the transferred gene is transmitted without rearrangements. The disadvantages of recombinant retroviruses include: (1) limited size of the genes that they can accommodate (7 to 8 kb); (2) low transduction efficiencies; and (3) requirement for cell division for integration into the genome of the target cell. Recently, recombinant retroviruses based on lentiviruses have been developed that are capable of introducing genes into nondividing cells.[12-16]

19.2.1.2 Recombinant Lentivirus

Lentiviruses belong to a family of complex pathogenic retroviruses that include members such as human immunodeficiency virus (HIV-1). Lentiviruses have a complex genome which, in addition to the structural genes *gag*, *pol* and *env*, contain other regulatory (*rev, tat*) and accessory genes (*vif, vpr, vpu, nef*). The regulatory genes are essential for virus replication. *Tat* encodes for a protein, which binds to the viral LTR and promotes RNA synthesis. *Rev* encodes for a protein, which binds a region of the viral RNA known as rev-responsive element (RRE) and promotes transport of the RNA from the nucleus to the cytoplasm.[17] The accessory genes are essential for pathogenesis but not for virus replication.[18]

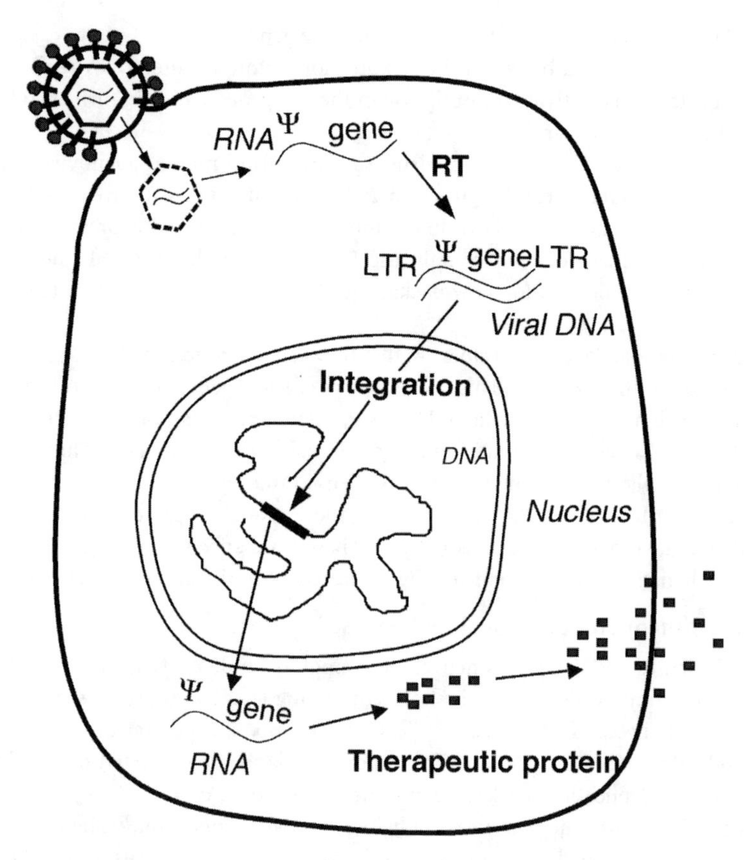

FIGURE 19.2 Schematic of the steps involved in retroviral gene transfer to a target cell.

First generation recombinant lentivirus is produced by co-transfection of three plasmids.[14] The first plasmid contains all viral genes except for the gene that encodes for the envelope glycoprotein, *env*, which is provided by a separate plasmid. *Env* may encode for the envelope glycoprotein of the amphotropic retrovirus, the vesicular stomatitis virus (VSV-G) or some other protein that may confer targeting specificity. The third plasmid encodes for the therapeutic gene and contains sequences necessary for packaging, reverse transcription and integration into the genome of the target cells.

The first plasmid has been modified to reduce the probability of recombination and increase the safety of lentiviral vectors. These modifications have led to the development of the second generation recombinant lentivirus in which all accessory genes were deleted to eliminate the virulence of any replication-competent virus that may be present in the viral preparations.[19] Further gains in safety were afforded by the third-generation constructs, in which the sequences encoding for *tat* and *rev* were also deleted and *rev* was provided by a fourth plasmid under the control of the rous sarcoma virus (RSV) promoter. The elimination of six genes that are essential for replication and pathogenesis significantly reduced the risk associated with the use of recombinant lentivirus as a tool for gene transfer and for treatment of disease.

The main advantage of recombinant lentivirus is the ability to transfer genes to nondividing, quiescent target cells including neurons and hematopoietic stem cells. Similar to murine retrovirus, lentivirus integrates stably into the genome of the target cells. But unlike murine retrovirus, there is no evidence for lentivirus promoter shut-off *in vivo*.[18] However, the efficiency of lentiviral gene transfer remains low and its efficacy has not as yet been evaluated in clinical trials due to safety concerns.

19.2.1.3 Recombinant Adenoviruses

Adenoviruses are icosahedral, nonenveloped viral particles with a diameter of 70 to 100 nm. Their genetic material is double-stranded DNA that is 36-kb pairs long. Two short inverted terminal repeats (ITR) at each end of the DNA are necessary for viral replication. The genome consists of five early (E1 to E5) and five late genes (L1 to L5) named based on their expression before or after DNA replication. The early genes encode for proteins that activate transcription of the late genes, which in turn encode for structural proteins that make up the viral capsid.[20]

The first generation of recombinant adenovirus is derived from mutant adenovirus in which the E1 gene is deleted. The $E1^-$ mutants can be grown in 293 cells that express the E1 gene that provides the lost function. The resulting adenovirus can infect multiple cell types and express the transgene but it cannot replicate in a cell that does not contain the E1 gene. In addition to E1, the E3 region of the adenoviral genome is often deleted to allow packaging of approximately 8 kb of foreign DNA without affecting the viral titer.[21]

The major advantages of adenoviral vectors are that they can infect nondividing cells and can be grown to very high titers (10^{10} to 10^{12} CFU/ml). This results in very efficient gene transfer in tissues with terminally differentiated cells, such as the brain or lung. However, these vectors can only transfer small genes (less than 7 kb) and their DNA does not integrate, resulting in transient gene expression. The major disadvantage that hinders clinical application of adenoviruses is their immunogenicity. Unfortunately, the immune response is raised not only against the virus but also the therapeutic protein, possibly due to marked elevation of inflammatory cytokines such as IL-6.[22,23] These toxic effects may limit the use of adenovirus *in vivo*, especially when efficient treatment requires repeated administration of the virus.[24-26]

19.2.1.4 Recombinant Adeno-Associated Viruses

Adeno-associated viruses (AAVs) are nonenveloped, single-stranded DNA viruses that do not cause disease in humans or animals. Their DNA is short, containing less than 5-kb pairs, and encodes for two proteins: *Rep*, which is necessary for virus replication and *cap*, a structural protein, which forms the icosahedral capsid that houses the genome. The genome is flanked by inverted terminal repeats, ITRs, which are necessary for replication, packaging and integration of AAV.

Production of AAV requires the presence of a helper virus for replication.[27] The helper function may be provided by other viruses including adenovirus, herpes and vaccinia virus. Production involves co-transfection of 293 or HeLa cells with two plasmids. One plasmid contains the therapeutic gene flanked by the viral ITRs, and the other contains the *rep* and *cap* genes but lacks the packaging sequences. Subsequently, the transfected cells are infected with wild-type adenovirus that provides the helper functions. Two days later the cells are lysed, the wild type adenovirus is heat-inactivated and AAV viral particles are purified with density gradient centrifugation or column chromatography, yielding highly concentrated viral preparations (10^{12} to 10^{13} AAV particles from $\sim 10^9$ cells[27]).

The major drawback of AAV is the potential of contamination of the final product by wild type adenovirus. Other disadvantages of this system include the short foreign DNA (4 to 5 kb) that can be incorporated in these vectors, and the imprecise integration that often results in tandem repeats of the transferred gene. However, these vectors have certain characteristics that make them particularly attractive, namely, stable integration in a specific location in the cellular genome (chromosome 19) and the ability to transfer genes to nondividing cells.

19.2.2 Nonviral Gene Delivery

The second class of gene delivery methods is nonviral. These methods include use of naked DNA or DNA complexed with cations, cationic polymers, liposomes or combinations of lipids and polymers to enhance the efficiency of gene transfer.[28] Physical methods such as electroporation and particle acceleration are also employed to facilitate DNA transport into cells and tissues.[29]

Cationic polymers that are employed as DNA carriers include peptides,[30-33] poly(ethyleneimine),[34-38] poly-L-lysine,[39] modified poly-L-lysine with histidine[40-43] or imidazole,[44] and dendrimers.[45-47] The positively charged polymers interact with the negatively charged DNA and form a complex. The DNA-polymer complex has a net positive charge facilitating the interaction of DNA with the target cells. Additional modification such as conjugation of cationic polymers with ligands endows the complex with targeting specificity. Several ligands have been used to achieve targeting including asialoglycoprotein,[39,48] transferrin,[49,50] antibodies,[51,52] fibroblast growth factor[53] and epidermal growth factor.[54]

Cationic lipids are also used as DNA carriers.[55,56] Cationic lipids (e.g., DOTAP) contain a hydrophobic group that ensures their assembly into bilayer vesicles and a charged group (e.g., amine) that mediates the electrostatic interactions with the negatively charged DNA. Addition of neutral lipids (e.g., DOPE) has been shown to increase the transfection efficiency possibly by facilitating endosomal escape.[57] Liposome-mediated gene transfer, better known as lipofection, has enjoyed wide use resulting in commercial production of gene delivery kits and initiation of several clinical trials (Table 19.2). More recently, the use of natural and synthetic biomaterials for delivery of DNA *in vivo* has met with some success. This approach, which pertains to *in situ* tissue regeneration, is reviewed in detail below (see Section 19.3.2, "*In Situ* Gene Delivery for Tissue Regeneration").

The nonviral gene delivery systems are prepared by mixing the solution of plasmid DNA with the solution of polymers, lipids or both resulting in complexes of colloidal size (50 to 1000 nm) and positive charge.[28] Gene transfer is initiated by incubation of these complexes with the target cells.

The main advantages of nonviral technologies include: (1) unlimited size of DNA that can be transferred; (2) lack of immune response (unless proteins are inserted into the lipids to convey specificity); and (3) safety due to their inability to replicate or recombine to produce infectious particles.[58] The main disadvantages include: (1) very low efficiencies of gene transfer, especially *in vivo*; (2) short-lived transgene expression; and (3) cytotoxicity.[34,59,60] These shortcomings may hinder the use of nonviral technologies in gene therapy of stem cells and tissue engineering applications that require sustained gene expression.

19.3 Genetic Modification for Tissue Engineering

Gene transfer can be used in tissue engineering in two settings. First, genes can be introduced into cells that are subsequently used to prepare three-dimensional tissue substitutes, such as skin, cartilage and bone. Alternatively, genes can be delivered *in vivo* to enhance *in situ* tissue regeneration. The first approach is useful when tissues must be replaced to restore or improve function. Interestingly, genetically modified tissues may also be used as biological models for studying the role of effector molecules on organ/tissue development. The second approach can be used when the defects are relatively small or engineered tissues are not yet available (e.g., peripheral nerve injury).

19.3.1 Genetically Engineered Tissues

In this setting, cells are genetically modified using one of the viral or nonviral methods described above and then used to engineer tissue substitutes. Genetic modification of tissues may be used to enhance tissue function or improve existing cellular activities for treatment of genetic diseases. Interestingly, genetically modified tissues may also be used as ectopic sites for protein production and delivery into the systemic circulation. In this case, *permanent* genetic modification is required to provide long lasting effects. Consequently, the most suitable vectors are the recombinant viruses that can mediate permanent gene transfer such as retrovirus, lentivirus and adeno-associated virus.

In other cases, genetic modification of the engineered tissue may be used to increase the rate of graft survival by inducing ingrowth of new vessels (angiogenesis) or suppressing immune rejection. These applications may require *transient* gene expression until the transplant integrates with the surrounding tissue or until wound healing is complete. Therefore, adenoviruses or nonviral technologies of gene delivery may be more appropriate.

19.3.1.1 Genetically Engineered Skin

The epidermis is an attractive target for gene therapy because it is easily accessible and shows great potential as an ectopic site for protein delivery *in vivo*. The cells that are primarily used to recreate skin substitutes are epidermal keratinocytes and/or dermal fibroblasts, which can be genetically modified with viral or nonviral vectors.[6,61] Genetically modified cells are then used to prepare three-dimensional skin equivalents which, when transplanted into animals, act as *in vivo* "bioreactors" that produce and deliver the desired therapeutic proteins either locally or systemically. Local delivery of proteins may be used for treatment of genetic diseases of the skin or wound healing of burns or injuries, while systemic delivery may be used for correction of systemic diseases like hemophilia or diabetes.

Retroviral gene transfer to epidermal cells has been used for correction of genetic diseases of the skin such as epidermolysis bullosa and lamellar ichthyosis.[62-65] The same technology has been used to genetically modify keratinocytes to express wound-healing factors such as PDGF-A,[66] IGF-I[67] and keratinocyte growth factor (KGF)[68] to examine their potential in enhancing wound healing. Gene transfer of angiogenic factors using retroviral[69,70] and nonviral approaches[71] has also been used to increase vascularization of transplanted skin substitutes *in vivo*.

Genetically modified tissues may also be used as "bioreactors" to deliver proteins to the systemic circulation. The main property that makes skin an ideal target for gene delivery is the ease of accessibility for transplantation or tissue removal if adverse effects occur. Some of the first studies have used recombinant retroviruses to genetically modify human keratinocytes with genes encoding for human growth hormone (hGH),[72] apoE[73] and clotting factor.[74] In all these cases, genetically modified cells expressed the transgenes and secreted functional proteins to the systemic circulation of grafted animals. Since then, other investigators have used recombinant retroviruses to introduce genes into human keratinocytes for the correction of metabolic[75,76] and systemic diseases.[77,78]

Genetically engineered tissues can also be employed as models for studying tissue development and physiology. We prepared skin equivalents that were genetically modified to express keratinocyte growth factor (KGF),[68] a protein that plays an important role in tissue morphogenesis and wound healing.[79,80] The modified tissues showed dramatic changes in the three-dimensional organization of the epidermis including hyperthickening and flattening of the corrugations of the dermo-epidermal junction (rete-ridges) (Figure 19.3A and D). KGF increased proliferation of basal cells, induced proliferation in the suprabasal cell compartment which is normally quiescent (Figure 19.3B and E) and delayed differentiation (Figure 19.3C and F). This study demonstrated that expression of a single growth factor is able to mediate many of the events associated with epidermal growth and differentiation.[68] It also demonstrated the usefulness of "transgenic" engineered tissues in studying the effects of a single gene in tissue development. Although transgenic animal models have been successfully employed for many years, "transgenic" engineered tissues may provide an alternative approach for better-controlled and quantitative studies. Furthermore, deletion of some genes may be lethal for animal embryos but it may still be possible to study gene knockouts using "transgenic" tissue equivalents.

19.3.1.2 Genetically Engineered Cartilage

Articular cartilage, the tissue that forms the surface of the joints has limited regenerative capacity. As a result, tissue-engineering approaches may be very useful in restoring loss of cartilage due to trauma, osteoarthritis or inflammatory diseases such as rheumatoid arthritis. Genetic modification may be used to reduce inflammation or increase the regenerative capacity of engineered cartilage ultimately restoring function and reducing pain.

Interleukin-1 (IL-1) is a key mediator of degradation of the extracellular matrix of cartilage associated with osteoarthritis. In one study, chondrocytes that were genetically modified with adenovirus to express IL-1 receptor antagonist (IL-1RA) were able to protect osteoarthritic cartilage by blocking IL-1.[81] In another study, synovial cells that were transduced with a retrovirus encoding IL-1RA were also able to protect the joint from IL-1–mediated degradation.[82]

Other studies used nonviral technologies to transfer genes that promote the chondrocytic phenotype, such as TGF-β1 or parathyroid hormone-related protein (PTHrP). When the modified chondrocytes were seeded into PLA scaffolds and placed into rabbit femoral defects, they expressed the transgenes for at least 2 weeks.[83] Similarly, cartilage cells transfected with a plasmid encoding for IGF-1 synthesized proteoglycan and type II collagen, two extracellular matrix proteins indicative of mature chondrocytes. IGF-I overexpressing chondrocytes also exhibited higher levels of proliferation and proteoglycan synthesis following transplantation *in vivo*.[84] These studies suggest that gene transfer may enhance the function of engineered cartilage and ultimately reduce inflammation and promote tissue regeneration.

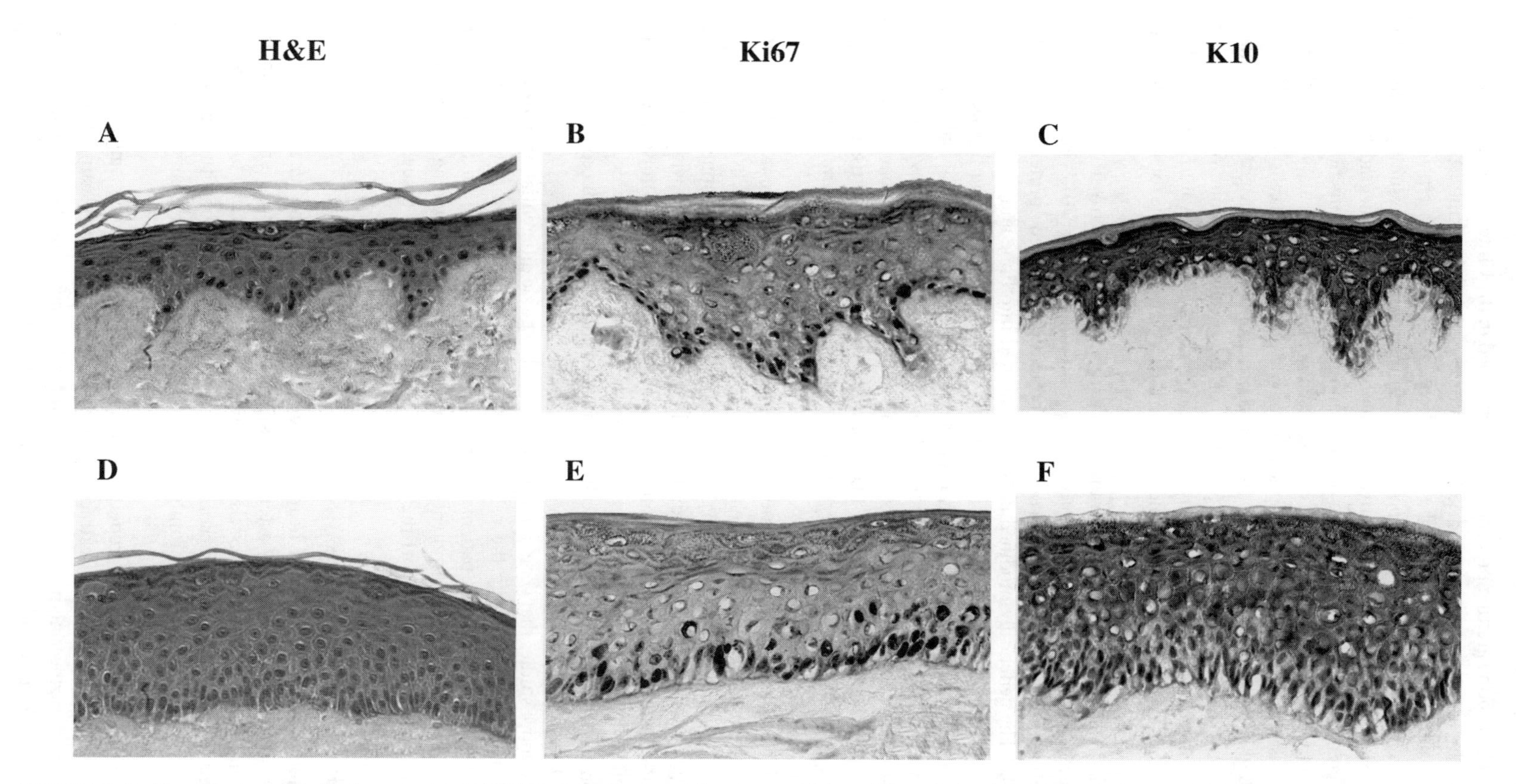

FIGURE 19.3 (**See color insert following page 14**-10.) KGF induces hyperproliferation and delays differentiation in a skin equivalent model system. Sections of skin equivalents unmodified (A, B, C) and genetically modified to express KGF (D, E, F) were cultured for 7 days at the air/liquid interface. Cryosections were stained with hematoxylin and eosin (H&E; A, D), a nuclear proliferation antigen (Ki67; brown; B, E), and the differentiation marker keratin 10 (K10; brown; C, F). Ki67 and K10 sections were counterstained with hematoxylin (blue) (magnification 40×). Note the increased thickness and basal cell density of the KGF-modified tissues. Also note that in unmodified tissues proliferation is confined to the basal layer, while in KGF-modified tissues proliferating cells extend up to three to four suprabasal layers. The same suprabasal layers that contain proliferating cells are also negative for the differentiation marker K10, suggesting that KGF alters the spatial control of proliferation and differentiation in the genetically modified tissues.[68]

19.3.1.3 Genetically Engineered Bone

Every year more than 800,000 bone grafting procedures are performed in the United States to reconstruct or replace bone affected by trauma, pathological degeneration or congenital deformity. Although many synthetic and natural materials, e.g., ceramics, polymers and collagen, are used to replace bone, these materials have markedly different mechanical properties than human bone often resulting in implant failure.[85] Tissue engineering may provide an alternative treatment by combining biodegradable materials with cells that can differentiate along the osteogenic pathway and provide the lost function.

Human bone marrow-derived mesenchymal stem cells represent a pluripotent population of cells that serve as precursors for osteoprogenitor cells.[86] The potential of mesenchymal stem cells as a source in tissue engineering is highly augmented by the lack immunogenicity and their high growth potential. Gene therapy can serve as a means to guide differentiation of these cells into bone or cartilage by expression of signaling molecules such as bone morphogenetic proteins (BMPs). A number of studies have recently demonstrated that delivery of genes encoding for BMPs promotes bone formation *in vitro* and *in vivo*.

Human mesenchymal stem cells were effectively transduced with recombinant retrovirus encoding for green fluorescence protein[87] as well as functional proteins such as human factor VIII.[88] Recent studies used recombinant adenovirus to transfer genes encoding for bone morphogenetic protein (BMP-2) to mesenchymal stem cells. The genetically modified cells differentiated into bone and cartilage cells and corrected a bone defect after implantation *in vivo*. In contrast, control cells expressing β-galactosidase differentiated into fibrous tissue. Most importantly, expression of BMP-2 by mesenchymal stem cells derived from an aged osteoporotic patient formed bone ectopically in subcutaneous sites similar to cells derived from young healthy patients.[89] In another study, genetically modified bone marrow osteoprogenitor cells expressing BMP-2 were seeded onto PLGA scaffolds to engineer bone tissue. Although engineered cells secreted BMP-2 for 8 days only, they differentiated into osteoblasts *in vitro* and produced bone tissue after implantation *in vivo*.[90]

Periosteal cells, which contain osteoprogenitor and chondroprogenitor cells, were also transduced with a retrovirus encoding for bone morphogenetic protein 7 (BMP-7). When the modified cells were delivered into rabbit cranial defects using polyglycolic acid (PGA) as a scaffold, they promoted bone healing in 12 weeks.[91] Likewise, W-20 stromal cells (a marrow-derived cell-line) were transduced with a retrovirus encoding for the BMP-2 gene and transplanted into the pocket of the quadriceps muscles of severe combined immune deficient (SCID) mice using polymer-ceramic scaffolds (poly[lactide-co-glycolide]-hydroxyapatite). In contrast to unmodified control cells, genetically modified cells induced ectopic bone formation around the implant.[92]

It is evident from the above studies that gene transfer may be used to guide differentiation of osteoprogenitor and mesenchymal stem cells along the osteogenic pathway and even restore the osteogenic potential of cells derived from osteoporotic patients. Delivery of genes encoding for angiogenic factors (e.g., FGF, VEGF) may further enhance the potential of engineered bone by providing the necessary blood supply to maintain viability and support the function of the newly formed tissue, especially for treatment of large size defects.

19.3.1.4 Genetically Engineered Vessels

One the most common and severe forms of heart disease is atherosclerosis, the narrowing of the vessels.[93] Current treatment involves coronary artery bypass graft surgery using a patient's mammary artery or sephanous vein. Tissue-engineered vessels may provide an alternative source to the currently employed native vessels in bypass surgery. To accomplish this goal, blood vessel substitutes must meet certain performance criteria including nonthrombogenicity, vasoactivity and mechanical properties that match those of native vessels.[93]

Gene therapy can be used to improve the properties of engineered vessels by enhancing secretion of nonthrombogenic compounds, expression of extracellular matrix molecules (e.g., elastin) that provide strength and elasticity or by engineering immune acceptance into allogeneic cells.[93] In one study, endothelial cells were genetically modified with a recombinant retrovirus to express an antithrombotic protein, tissue plasminogen activator (TPA). The genetically modified cells were seeded onto 4-mm Dacron grafts and either exposed to a nonpulsatile flow system *in vitro* or transplanted as femoral and carotid interposition grafts *in vivo*. In both cases, genetically modified cells showed decreased adherence, suggesting that gene therapy strategies for decreasing thrombosis of engineered vessels may require expression of molecules that lack proteolytic activity.[94]

Viral and nonviral vehicles have also been used to transfer genes into large and small vessels *in vivo*. A number of studies showed that gene transfer of NO-synthase (eNOS) increased NO bioavailability and improved vascular reactivity of surgically removed vessels from several animal models including hypertensive rats and hypercholesterolimic rabbits.[95-98] However, gene transfer is restricted to the endothelial cell layer unless the vessel wall is damaged.[99]

To improve the efficiency of gene transfer to the underlying smooth muscle cells standard angioplasty was used to increase the pressure in the lumen of the vessel resulting in significant enhancement of plasmid DNA and oligonucleotide delivery.[100] In addition to pressure, application of electric fields has been used to facilitate gene transfer by creating transient pores in cell membranes to allow macromolecules into the cell cytoplasm. Electroporation increased DNA delivery to large[101] and small vessels,[102] with peak gene transfer achieved at a field strength of 200 V/cm. In particular, in small vessels gene expression was observed in all cell layers including endothelial, smooth muscle and adventitial cells.[102] However, gene expression was short-lived, declining to background levels by 5 days after treatment.

19.3.1.4.1 Gene Transfer to Modulate Angiogenesis

Gene transfer to small vessels has been used to inhibit angiogenesis as a means to hinder tumor growth or increase vascularization to treat ischemia and promote wound healing. For example, gene transfer of VEGF and fibroblast growth factor (FGF) receptors inhibited angiogenesis in pancreatic tumors.[103] On the other hand, adenoviral gene transfer of angiogenic factors such as FGF and VEGF increased angiogenesis in several tissues including skeletal muscle,[104] ischemic rabbit hindlimbs[105] and adipose tissue.[106]

One of the most important challenges facing tissue engineering is vascularization of engineered tissues after implantation *in vivo*. Since oxygen diffuses only a few hundred microns before it is consumed,[107] new vessels must form quickly to supply oxygen and nutrients to transplanted tissues. One way to promote new vessel formation is to genetically modify the engineered tissue to express angiogenic factors. Recent studies demonstrated that overexpression of vascular endothelial growth factor (VEGF) by genetically modified skin substitutes promoted early vascularization following transplantation onto athymic mice.[69-71] Similarly, meniscal cells were genetically modified to express hepatocyte growth factor (HGF) using recombinant adenovirus. When the genetically modified cells were seeded onto PLGA scaffolds and transplanted into athymic mice, angiogenesis increased significantly.[108] These studies suggest that gene therapy can be used to promote vascularization of engineered tissues ultimately improving the clinical outcome of tissue replacement therapy.

19.3.2 *In Situ* Gene Delivery for Tissue Regeneration

In this setting biomaterials are directly applied to the site of injury in order to promote and guide tissue regeneration. The biomaterials may be decorated by signals that promote a cellular response such as adhesion peptides, enzymatic recognition sites or growth factors.[109] In general, it has been difficult to maintain full bioactivity of the proteins released from controlled delivery systems mainly due to protein instability. Gene delivery may overcome this problem, as infiltrating cells may uptake the genes and produce the therapeutic protein(s) continuously. However, gene delivery by injection may result in loss of the genes from the site of administration and subsequent degradation by nucleases.[110,111] Alternatively, bioactive materials may be employed as gene delivery vehicles and at the same time serve as scaffolds to promote tissue regeneration.[112] Biomaterials that have been used to deliver plasmid DNA include gelatin nanospheres,[113] collagen,[114,115] poly(ethylene-co-vinyl acetate) (EVAc)[116] and poly(lactide-co-glycolide).[117]

Efficient gene delivery has been demonstrated using natural and synthetic biomaterials. Plasmid DNA encoding for human parathyroid hormone was delivered to a canine bone defect in a collagen sponge yielding significant bone regeneration in a dose and time-dependent manner.[114] Similarly, collagen embedded DNA encoding for platelet-derived growth factor (PDGF-A or -B) increased granulation tissue, epithelialization and wound closure in an ischemic rabbit ear model.[118] In another study, gelatin/alginate nanospheres conjugated with human transferring-enhanced gene transfer to mouse tibialis muscle as compared to naked DNA.[113]

Synthetic biomaterials have also been used as DNA carriers. Synthetic sutures coated with DNA were used to deliver the alkaline phosphatase gene to rat skeletal muscle and canine myocardium.[119] Poly(lactide-co-glycolide) matrices were also used to deliver the PDGF gene into skin wounds resulting in significantly increased vascularization and granulation tissue formation up to 4 weeks post-wounding.[117] Similarly, PLGA nanoparticles were shown to encapsulate DNA efficiently and exhibited sustained release over a period of 4 weeks.[120] These examples are encouraging as they demonstrate the feasibility of *in vivo* gene delivery using bioactive materials. Further advances in biomaterial and vector design are required to achieve controlled release for prolonged periods of time, protection of DNA from nuclease degradation and targeting of the plasmid to specific cell types of the wound. Strategies that employ liposomes or DNA condensing agents may be integrated into this approach to release the DNA from the endosomes or target it to the nucleus.[121]

Bioactive matrix may also be used to deliver recombinant viruses to the site of injury. Encapsulation of viral particles in biomaterials may increase viral stability, reduce immunogenicity and achieve targeted gene transfer only to the cells that infiltrate the wound bed. Indeed, encapsulation in gelatin/alginate microspheres protected adenovirus particles from degradation and the release kinetics could be controlled by changes in microsphere formulation.[122] Delivery of a PDGF-BB encoding adenovirus increased granulation tissue formation and neovascularization of full thickness wounds. Conjugation of adenoviral particles with fibroblast growth factor (FGF2) further increased the potency of the preparation by targeting cellular uptake through the FGF receptor.[123,124] Additionally, encapsulation of adenovirus in PLGA matrices reduced immunogenicity and decreased inactivation by neutralizing antibodies, thus facilitating repeating virus administrations that may be required for a therapeutic effect.[125-127]

Although temporary genetic modification (adenovirus) may be required in most cases to ensure no transgene expression after the healing is complete, permanent genetic modification (retrovirus, adeno-associated virus) may be advantageous in the treatment of chronic wounds such as diabetic ulcers.[128] In the environment of the wound, retroviral gene transfer may be facilitated by the natural propensity of the wound-infiltrating cells to divide. More studies are required to establish matrix-assisted retroviral delivery as an efficient strategy to enhance tissue regeneration especially in chronic wounds.

19.4 Challenges Facing Gene Delivery

19.4.1 Low Efficiency of Gene Transfer

The major challenges of gene transfer are to deliver therapeutic levels of genes to specific target cells and to control the level and the length of time of transgene expression. While each gene transfer technology has its own idiosyncrasies, they all have to undergo a series of physicochemical steps to deliver their cargo successfully. These steps include transport to the target cells, binding to the cell surface, internalization into the cell cytoplasm, entry into the nucleus and for some viral vectors (retrovirus, lentivirus, adeno-associated virus) integration of the transgene into the genome of the target cells. Each one of these steps can potentially limit the efficiency of gene transfer. Here we will briefly discuss the physicochemical factors that govern gene transfer. For a more detailed review on the subject see Palsson and Andreadis.[129]

19.4.1.1 Transport to the Target Cells

The first step in gene transfer is transport of viral or nonviral vectors to the cell surface. The size of viral particles and many complexes of DNA with cationic lipids and polymers are on the order of 100 nm yielding diffusion coefficients on the order of 10^{-8} cm^2/sec.[130,131] As a result, transport to the cell surface is limited by Brownian motion.[131,132] The slow diffusion in conjunction with the short half-life (5 to 7 h[131-133]) limits the distance that retroviral particles can diffuse before they lose biological activity. Mathematical modeling and experiments showed that only particles in close proximity to the target cells (within 500 μm) contribute to gene transfer. Increasing the depth of retroviral supernatant beyond 500 μm did not increase the efficiency of gene transfer further.[131] Therefore, methods to overcome the diffusion limitation and increase the probability of virus–cell encounter may increase the efficiency of gene transfer. Methods such as centrifugation of viral particles onto target cells[134] and convective flow of the virus past a monolayer of target cells have shown considerable promise for gene delivery to some cell types.[135-137]

More recently, fibronectin was used to immobilize retroviral particles and increase their surface concentration facilitating virus–cell interactions.[138,139] Using mathematical modeling and experiments, we optimized the time, temperature and virus adsorption to FN yielding tenfold enhancement of the gene transfer efficiency.[140] We have also identified the mechanism of retrovirus binding to FN. Our results indicate that retrovirus binds FN through virus-associated heparan sulfate (HS) and that gene transfer with immobilized retrovirus does not depend on polycations, e.g., polybrene.[141] A better understanding of these interactions may provide insight into virus-cell interactions and lead to a more rational design of transduction protocols.

19.4.1.2 Binding to the Cell Surface

Several physicochemical forces including electrostatic, van der Waals, osmotic and steric mediate the initial interaction viral and nonviral vectors with the cell surface.[129] Electrostatic forces play an important role since polycations such as polybrene (PB), protamine sulfate (PS), poly-L-lysine (PLL) and polyethyleneimine (PEI) are necessary for viral and nonviral gene transfer. These positively charged polymers screen the electrostatic repulsion between the negatively charged virus or DNA and the target cells ultimately promoting binding and gene transfer. On the other hand, negatively charged proteoglycans (e.g., chondroitin sulfate) were found to inhibit retroviral gene transfer.[142]

Following an initial nonspecific interaction, viruses have evolved to bind to receptor(s) that are ubiquitously expressed on the cell surface. For instance, amphotropic retrovirus binds to a phosphate symporter,[143,144] adeno-associated virus binds integrin αvβ5,[145] and adenovirus binds several integrins including αvβ5, αvβ3 and αvβ1.[146-149] On the other hand, plasmid DNA and liposomes bind nonspecifically unless engineered to possess a ligand, e.g., transferrin that mediates binding to a specific receptor.[49,50]

Molecular engineering has been used to increase gene transfer and to target viruses and nonviral vectors to specific cell types. Retroviruses pseudotyped with gibbon-ape leukemia virus envelope protein,[150] T-cell leukemia virus envelope protein[151] and parts of the erythropoietin molecule (Epo)[152] have shown altered host range. Interestingly, retrovirus pseudotyped with the G glycoprotein of vesicular stomatitis virus (VSV-G)[153] showed resistance to shear when concentrated by ultracentrifugation, yielding preparations of $>10^9$ infectious particles per milliliter. In another approach, an antibody to melanoma-associated antigen was fused to the amphotropic murine leukemia virus envelope and was used to target recombinant retroviruses to melanoma cells.[154] Similarly, a bispecific antibody targeted adeno-associated virus to megakaryocytes.[155] Ultimately, a combination of physical methods and molecular engineering may be necessary to increase adsorption to the cell surface, promote internalization and achieve targeting specificity.

19.4.1.3 Intracellular Trafficking and Transgene Expression

Once in the cell, viral and nonviral vectors undergo a series of steps that eventually lead to gene expression. In general, there are two pathways of entry into the cell cytoplasm: fusion with the plasma membrane and endocytosis. Amphotropic retrovirus follows the first, while adenovirus, adeno-associated virus and plasmid DNA follow the second route.

Retrovirus internalization into the cell is followed by uncoating, reverse transcription, nuclear entry and integration of the newly synthesized DNA into the genome of the target cells. Entry into the nucleus depends on the position of the cell in the cell cycle[156,157] leading to complicating dynamics that have been described by a mathematical model that accounts for the intracellular retrovirus trafficking and the kinetics of the cell cycle.[158] This model identified intracellular decay as the rate-limiting step and was very useful in the design of experiments to determine the intracellular half-life of recombinant retrovirus.[158,159] These studies suggested that strategies to induce cells into cell cycle or increase nuclear entry would increase the efficiency of gene transfer. Indeed lentiviruses, which contain nuclear localization signals in several of their proteins (e.g., matrix, integrase and vpr proteins), exhibit efficient entry into the nucleus.[160] As a result they can transduce slowly dividing hematopoietic stem cells[161,162] and even nondividing neurons.[14,15]

Mathematical models have been proposed to describe the process of binding, internalization and intracellular trafficking for several other viruses. These models were used to determine the mode of binding — monovalent vs. multivalent — and extract key physical parameters such as receptor number and affinity.[163,164] Others have also included postbinding steps such as endocytosis, lysosomal routing and nuclear accumulation in order to identify rate-limiting steps and predict kinetic parameters of the infection process.[165,166] This approach may prove useful in understanding the overall dynamics of the gene transfer process and identifying key targets for intervention to overcome the bottlenecks and increase the efficiency of gene transfer.

Adenoviruses, adeno-associated viruses and nonviral vectors internalize through endocytosis. Entry of adenovirus and adeno-associated virus is facilitated by further interactions with several integrins on the cell surface[145-149,167] and requires activation of intracellular mediators such as phosphatidylinositol-3-kinases (PI3K).[167] Escape from the endosome, which is induced by the low endosomal pH, is a major resistance to successful gene transfer. Indeed, fusogenic lipids such as DOPE,[168] polycations, e.g., PEI[34,169] and fusogenic peptides,[170,171]enhance endosomal escape and transgene expression.

Entry into the nucleus is a major resistance to gene transfer, not only for retrovirus but also for plasmid DNA. Sequences that contain nuclear localization signals (NLS) were shown to promote entry of the DNA into the nucleus and transgene expression.[31,172,173] Others used DNA sequences (e.g., portions of the SV40 enhancer) that bind transcription factors, which harbor nuclear localization signals and facilitate entry of the plasmid DNA into the nucleus.[174] Sequences with binding sites for cell-specific transcription factors were also used to afford target cell specificity. In one study, plasmids containing portions of the smooth muscle gamma actin promoter entered the nucleus and increased gene expression in smooth muscle cells, but not in fibroblasts or CV1 cells.[175]

These studies suggest that understanding the rate-limiting steps of gene transfer may facilitate the development of strategies that improve the transduction efficiency and promote targeted and controlled delivery. One of the most important targets of gene therapy is the population of cells with the highest potential for tissue regeneration, namely, the stem cells.

19.4.2 Gene Therapy to Stem Cells

Continuously renewing tissues like skin, blood and bone contain cells with different growth potential and at different stages of differentiation: slowly dividing stem cells that continue to proliferate for the lifetime of the tissue; progenitor cells that divide fast but are limited to a finite number of cell divisions before their progeny must commit to differentiate; and cells that are committed to differentiation along a certain lineage, which will eventually reach full maturity and die. Although certain gene transfer technologies, such as retroviruses, allow for permanent genetic modification of target cells, differentiation and eventually loss of the transduced cells from the engineered tissue may result in temporary transgene expression (Figure 19.4). Therefore, to achieve stable long-term gene expression, it is critical that stem cells are transduced with high efficiency. Additionally, recent studies suggest that stem cells do not express molecules that are recognized by the immune system and therefore appear to be immunoprivileged.[176] The potential of stem cells to establish universal donor cells makes them ideal targets for both gene therapy and tissue engineering.

Retrovirus is the most appropriate vector for gene delivery into stem cells due to its ability to integrate into the genome of the target cells and thus be part of the genome of daughter cells for all future generations. However, retroviral gene transfer depends on cell cycle[156,177] and the intracellular half-life of retroviruses results in low efficiency of gene transfer to the slowly dividing stem cells.[157-159] Although lentiviruses also integrate and can transduce even nondividing stem cells, difficulties with safety make their use problematic. Safety may also be a problem with preparations of adeno-associated virus that

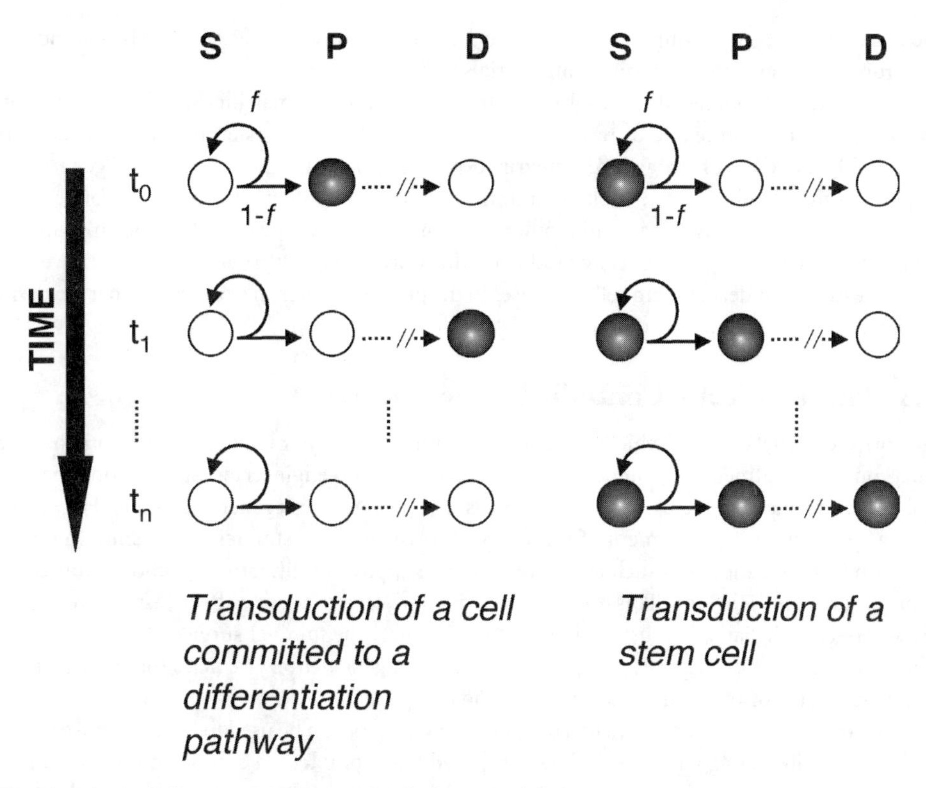

FIGURE 19.4 Retroviral gene transfer to stem cells is required in long-term transgene expression. Stem cells (S) give rise to other stem cells with probability, f, and to progenitor cells (P) with probability, 1-f. In turn, progenitor cells give rise to cells that are committed to terminal differentiation (D). Retroviral gene transfer may result in permanent genetic modification as the transgene integrates into the genome of transduced cells (filled circles) and is inherited by daughter cells as any other autosomal gene. However, differentiated cells have a finite life span resulting in loss of the transgene(s) from the lineage and temporary genetic modification. In contrast, when stem cells are transduced, the pool of genetically modified stem cells is maintained through self-renewal. The modified stem cells give rise to modified progenitor and differentiated cells sustaining long-term transgene expression. Filled and open circles represent genetically modified and non-modified cells, respectively.

may contain infectious adenovirus. Therefore, efforts to increase the efficiency of retroviral gene transfer to stem cells is needed to provide a clinically acceptable means of stem cell gene therapy.

Gene transfer to stem cells can be achieved by either isolation and expansion of stem cells that are subsequently genetically modified or by targeting stem cells in cultures containing stem and differentiated cells. The first approach requires knowledge of specific stem cell markers (e.g., hematopoietic stem cells may be enriched 100- to 1000-fold by selecting cells that express CD34 but not CD38 and major histocompatibility class II [HLA-DR][178]) that can be used to obtain pure stem cells from tissues or heterogeneous cultures. Even more important is maintenance and expansion of the genetically modified stem cells to large numbers necessary for clinical applications. This is a major challenge facing the field of tissue engineering since for most tissues including the skin and the hematopoietic system, it is still not clear how to maintain and expand the stem cell pool *in vitro*.[4] Despite limited knowledge in stem cell maintenance and expansion, use of combinations of growth factors and cytokines increased gene transfer by promoting proliferation of the slowly growing stem cells.[178] Interestingly, the presence of stroma improved the efficiency of retroviral gene transfer into hematopoietic progenitor and stem cells as compared to the use of growth factors alone.[179-181]

Another promising way to transduce stem cells is by use of extracellular matrix molecules to maintain the stem cell phenotype and at the same time co-localize stem cells and retroviral particles. Recombinant retroviruses have been shown to bind to the heparin-binding domain of fibronectin (FN)[138,139] and promote gene transfer to T-lymphocytes[182,183] and hematopoietic stem cells.[184-187] This method has also shown promising results in two recent clinical trials.[188,189]

More recently, we hypothesized that retroviral transduction on FN may increase the efficiency of gene transfer to epidermal stem cells. Our results show that retroviral gene transfer to epidermal keratinocytes correlates with the levels of $\alpha5$ and $\beta1$ integrin expression and that the efficiency of gene transfer is significantly higher on fibronectin.[190] These findings are novel and potentially important for gene therapy since integrins have been associated with epidermal stem cell phenotype.[191-193] Long term growth assays and *in vivo* transplantation of genetically modified skin equivalents may provide more definitive evidence that gene transfer to epidermal stem cells increases in the presence of fibronectin. Preliminary experiments in our laboratory support this hypothesis.[194]

19.4.3 Physiologically Controlled Gene Therapy

The majority of gene transfer vehicles provide constitutive (always on) gene expression that may be advantageous for treatment of genetic diseases. However, tissue-engineering applications may require physiologically regulated gene expression by a subset of cells in the regenerated tissue. For example, a promising approach for the treatment of intimal hyperplasia involves suppression of smooth muscle cell proliferation.[195] Cytostatic genes such as p21 or p27 can suppress proliferation of smooth muscle as well as the neighboring endothelium. This nonspecific action may lead to adverse effects, especially in damaged vessels, where endothelial cells must proliferate to repopulate the luminal surface. Spatial and temporal control of gene expression requires design of a new class of gene delivery vehicles that may be regulated by host mechanisms or by administration of secondary agents.

Tissue specific transcriptional elements, promoters/enhancers, can be used to restrict transgene expression in specific cells. Young and Dean[195] have proposed the promoters of smooth muscle myosin heavy chain,[196] smooth muscle alpha-actin,[197] gamma actin[198] and calponin[199] as potential candidates for this approach. On the other hand, endothelial-specific promoters for genes such as von Willebrand factor,[200] flk-1/KDR[201] or endothelin-1[202] may be used to restrict gene expression in the lumen of the vessels. Others have inserted the liver-specific promoters human alpha1-antitrypsin (hAAT) and murine albumin (mAIb) into retroviral vectors. *In vivo* gene delivery resulted in highly up-regulated and long-term transgene expression as compared to expression driven by a constitutive Pol-II promoter.[203] Similarly, hybrid promoters have been used for gene transfer into epidermal keratinocytes. One such promoter, containing the cytomegalovirus (CMV) immediate early enhancer/promoter and regulatory elements of the human keratin 5 (hK5), was inserted into the backbone of a retroviral vector encoding for Factor IX. This hybrid promoter increased the levels of Factor IX in the plasma of mice by two- to threefold as compared to a CMV promoter alone.[204]

Synthetic promoters that can be regulated by administration of exogenous agents show much promise for controlled gene expression. For example, a tetracycline-dependent promoter has been constructed by two regulatory elements: the tetracycline resistance *tet* operon embedded in a cytomegalovirus promoter and a hybrid activator protein (tTA). Using this system, it was shown that gene expression could be tightly regulated by addition of tetracycline in a dose-dependent way.[205-208] Such promoters have been incorporated into retroviral[209] and adenoviral vectors[210,211] to achieve tetracycline-dependent regulated transgene expression *in vitro* and *in vivo*. These genetic switches could control the temporal and spatial expression of the transgene quantitatively and reversibly,[207] ultimately providing physiological control of transgene expression.

19.5 Summary

In summary, gene therapy is currently used in the field of tissue engineering as a means to enhance the clinical performance of tissue substitutes. Delivery of genes can be used to guide differentiation along a specific lineage, improve the properties of the engineered tissue, reduce or eliminate immune reaction to transplanted tissues, treat genetic diseases, promote tissue regeneration or transform engineered tissues into "bioreactors" for systemic delivery of therapeutic proteins *in vivo*. As a result, genetically modified tissues can be thought of as the next generation of tissue substitutes.

Viral and nonviral vehicles are currently used in gene therapy. Although several studies have demonstrated the usefulness of these vectors, many challenges facing gene therapy must be overcome in order to achieve clinically relevant results. Understanding the rate-limiting steps of the gene transfer process will certainly facilitate production of improved vectors and engineering of more efficient physicochemical strategies to deliver genes.

Finally, genetically engineered tissue substitutes will have a tremendous impact as biological models of tissue physiology and disease states. They can serve as realistic models to understand the molecular and cellular mechanisms of biological processes such as differentiation,[68] three-dimensional migration[212] and tumor metastasis. They may also be employed as toxicological models for testing of molecular and gene therapeutics. In combination with the new technologies of genomics, proteomics and bioinformatics, they have an enormous potential to impact biology, medicine and bioengineering by integrating global molecular information with three-dimensional cellular organization and tissue architecture.

References

1. Langer, R. and Vacanti, J.P., Tissue engineering, *Science*, 260, 920, 1993.
2. Berthiaume, F. and Yarmush, M.L., Tissue engineering, in *Biomedical Engineering Handbook*, Bronzino, G.J., Ed., CRC Press, New York, 1995.
3. Griffith, L.G. and Naughton, G., Tissue engineering — current challenges and expanding opportunities, *Science*, 295, 1009, 2002.
4. Zandstra, P.W. and Nagy, A., Stem cell bioengineering, *Annu. Rev. Biomed. Eng.*, 3, 275, 2001.
5. Watt, F.M. and Hogan, B.L., Out of Eden: stem cells and their niches, *Science*, 287, 1427, 2000.
6. Morgan, J.R. and Yarmush, M.L., Gene therapy in tissue engineering, in *Frontiers in Tissue Engineering*, Patrick, C.W. J., Mikos, A.G., and McIntire, L.V., Eds., Pergamon Press, New York, 1998, 278.
7. Anderson, W.F., Human gene therapy, *Science*, 256, 808, 1992.
8. Mulligan, R.C., The basic science of gene therapy, *Science*, 260, 926, 1993.
9. Hunter, E., Viral entry and receptors, in *Retroviruses*, Coffin, J.M., Hughes, S.H., and Varmus, H.E., Eds., Cold Spring Harbor Laboratory Press, Cold Spring Harbor, New York, 1997, 71.
10. Andreadis, S.T., Roth, C.M., Le Doux, J.M., Morgan, J.R., and Yarmush, M.L., Large-scale processing of recombinant retroviruses for gene therapy, *Biotechnol. Prog.*, 15, 1, 1999.
11. Goff, S.P., Intracellular trafficking of retroviral genomes during the early phase of infection: viral exploitation of cellular pathways, *J. Gene Med.*, 3, 517, 2001.
12. Kafri, T., Blomer, U., Peterson, D.A., Gage, F.H., and Verma, I.M., Sustained expression of genes delivered directly into liver and muscle by lentiviral vectors, *Nat. Genet.*, 17, 314, 1997.
13. Miyoshi, H., Takahashi, M., Gage, F.H., and Verma, I.M., Stable and efficient gene transfer into the retina using an HIV-based lentiviral vector, *Proc. Natl. Acad. Sci. U.S.A.*, 94, 10319, 1997.
14. Naldini, L., Blomer, U., Gage, F.H., Trono, D., and Verma, I.M., Efficient transfer, integration, and sustained long-term expression of the transgene in adult rat brains injected with a lentiviral vector, *Proc. Natl. Acad. Sci. U.S.A.*, 93, 11382, 1996.
15. Naldini, L., Blomer, U., Gallay, P., Ory, D., Mulligan, R., Gage, F.H., Verma, I.M., and Trono, D., In vivo gene delivery and stable transduction of nondividing cells by a lentiviral vector [see comments], *Science*, 272, 263, 1996.
16. Reiser, J., Harmison, G., Kluepfel-Stahl, S., Brady, R.O., Karlsson, S., and Schubert, M., Transduction of nondividing cells using pseudotyped defective high-titer HIV type 1 particles, *Proc. Natl. Acad. Sci. U.S.A.*, 93, 15266, 1996.
17. Buchschacher, G.L., Jr. and Wong-Staal, F., Development of lentiviral vectors for gene therapy for human diseases, *Blood*, 95, 2499, 2000.

18. Vigna, E. and Naldini, L., Lentiviral vectors: excellent tools for experimental gene transfer and promising candidates for gene therapy, *J. Gene Med.*, 2, 308, 2000.
19. Zufferey, R., Nagy, D., Mandel, R.J., Naldini, L., and Trono, D., Multiply attenuated lentiviral vector achieves efficient gene delivery in vivo, *Nat. Biotechnol.*, 15, 871, 1997.
20. Wilson, J.M., Adenovirus-mediated gene transfer to liver, *Adv. Drug Deliv. Rev.*, 46, 205, 2001.
21. Mizuguchi, H., Kay, M.A., and Hayakawa, T., Approaches for generating recombinant adenovirus vectors, *Adv. Drug Deliv. Rev.*, 52, 165, 2001.
22. Lozier, J.N., Metzger, M.E., Donahue, R.E., and Morgan, R.A., Adenovirus-mediated expression of human coagulation factor IX in the rhesus macaque is associated with dose-limiting toxicity, *Blood*, 94, 3968, 1999.
23. Lozier, J.N., Csako, G., Mondoro, T.H., Krizek, D.M., Metzger, M.E., Costello, R., Vostal, J.G., Rick, M.E., Donahue, R.E., and Morgan, R.A., Toxicity of a first-generation adenoviral vector in rhesus macaques, *Hum. Gene Ther.*, 13, 113, 2002.
24. Yang, Y., Su, Q., and Wilson, J.M., Role of viral antigens in destructive cellular immune responses to adenovirus vector-transduced cells in mouse lungs, *J. Virol.*, 70, 7209, 1996.
25. Kaplan, J.M., St. George, J.A., Pennington, S.E., Keyes, L.D., Johnson, R.P., Wadsworth, S.C., and Smith, A.E., Humoral and cellular immune responses of nonhuman primates to long-term repeated lung exposure to Ad2/CFTR-2, *Gene Ther.*, 3, 117, 1996.
26. Chirmule, N., Raper, S.E., Burkly, L., Thomas, D., Tazelaar, J., Hughes, J.V., and Wilson, J.M., Readministration of adenovirus vector in nonhuman primate lungs by blockade of CD40–CD40 ligand interactions, *J. Virol.*, 74, 3345, 2000.
27. Ponnazhagan, S., Curiel, D.T., Shaw, D.R., Alvarez, R.D., and Siegal, G.P., Adeno-associated virus for cancer gene therapy, *Cancer Res.*, 61, 6313, 2001.
28. Brown, M.D., Schatzlein, A.G., and Uchegbu, I.F., Gene delivery with synthetic (non viral) carriers, *Int. J. Pharm.*, 229, 1, 2001.
29. Hodgson, C.P., The vector void in gene therapy, *Bio/Technology*, 13, 222, 1995.
30. Mahat, R.I., Monera, O.D., Smith, L.C., and Rolland, A., Peptide-based gene delivery, *Curr. Opin. Mol. Ther.*, 1, 226, 1999.
31. Subramanian, A., Ranganathan, P., and Diamond, S.L., Nuclear targeting peptide scaffolds for lipofection of nondividing mammalian cells, *Nat. Biotechnol.*, 17, 873, 1999.
32. Vaysse, L., Guillaume, C., Burgelin, I., Gorry, P., Ferec, C., and Arveiler, B., Proteolipidic vectors for gene transfer to the lung, *Biochem. Biophys. Res. Commun.*, 290, 1489, 2002.
33. Vaysse, L., Burgelin, I., Merlio, J.P., and Arveiler, B., Improved transfection using epithelial cell line-selected ligands and fusogenic peptides, *Biochim. Biophys. Acta*, 1475, 369, 2000.
34. Boussif, O., Lezoualc'h, F., Zanta, M.A., Mergny, M.D., Scherman, D., Demeneix, B., and Behr, J.P., A versatile vector for gene and oligonucleotide transfer into cells in culture and in vivo: polyethylenimine, *Proc. Natl. Acad. Sci. U.S.A.*, 92, 7297, 1995.
35. Ferrari, S., Pettenazzo, A., Garbati, N., Zacchello, F., Behr, J.P., and Scarpa, M., Polyethylenimine shows properties of interest for cystic fibrosis gene therapy, *Biochim. Biophys. Acta*, 1447, 219, 1999.
36. Godbey, W.T., Wu, K.K., Hirasaki, G.J., and Mikos, A.G., Improved packing of poly(ethylenimine)/DNA complexes increases transfection efficiency, *Gene Ther.*, 6, 1380, 1999.
37. Godbey, W.T., Wu, K.K., and Mikos, A.G., Tracking the intracellular path of poly(ethylenimine)/DNA complexes for gene delivery, *Proc. Natl. Acad. Sci. U.S.A.*, 96, 5177, 1999.
38. Erbacher, P., Bettinger, T., Belguise-Valladier, P., Zou, S., Coll, J.L., Behr, J.P., and Remy, J.S., Transfection and physical properties of various saccharide, poly(ethylene glycol), and antibody-derivatized polyethylenimines (PEI), *J. Gene Med.*, 1, 210, 1999.
39. Wu, G.Y. and Wu, C.H., Receptor-mediated *in vitro* gene transformation by a soluble DNA carrier system, *J. Biol. Chem.*, 262, 4429, 1987.
40. Midoux, P. and Monsigny, M., Efficient gene transfer by histidylated polylysine/pDNA complexes, *Bioconjug. Chem.*, 10, 406, 1999.

41. Chen, Q.R., Zhang, L., Stass, S.A., and Mixson, A.J., Co-polymer of histidine and lysine markedly enhances transfection efficiency of liposomes, *Gene Ther.*, 7, 1698, 2000.
42. Benns, J.M., Choi, J.S., Mahato, R.I., Park, J.S., and Kim, S.W., pH-sensitive cationic polymer gene delivery vehicle: N-Ac-poly(L-histidine)-graft-poly(L-lysine) comb shaped polymer, *Bioconjug. Chem.*, 11, 637, 2000.
43. Chen, Q.R., Zhang, L., Stass, S.A., and Mixson, A.J., Branched co-polymers of histidine and lysine are efficient carriers of plasmids, *Nucleic Acids Res.*, 29, 1334, 2001.
44. Putnam, D., Gentry, C.A., Pack, D.W., and Langer, R., Polymer-based gene delivery with low cytotoxicity by a unique balance of side-chain termini, *Proc. Natl. Acad. Sci. U.S.A.*, 98, 1200, 2001.
45. Kukowska-Latallo, J.F., Bielinska, A.U., Johnson, J., Spindler, R., Tomalia, D.A., and Baker, J.R., Jr., Efficient transfer of genetic material into mammalian cells using Starburst polyamidoamine dendrimers, *Proc. Natl. Acad. Sci. U.S.A.*, 93, 4897, 1996.
46. Bielinska, A.U., Chen, C., Johnson, J., and Baker, J.R., Jr., DNA complexing with polyamidoamine dendrimers: implications for transfection, *Bioconjug. Chem.*, 10, 843, 1999.
47. Hudde, T., Rayner, S.A., Comer, R.M., Weber, M., Isaacs, J.D., Waldmann, H., Larkin, D.F., and George, A.J., Activated polyamidoamine dendrimers, a nonviral vector for gene transfer to the corneal endothelium, *Gene Ther.*, 6, 939, 1999.
48. Wu, G.Y., Wilson, J.M., Shalaby, F., Grossman, M., Shafritz, D.A., and Wu, C.H., Receptor-mediated gene delivery in vivo. Partial correction of genetic analbuminemia in Nagase rats, *J. Biol. Chem.*, 266, 14338, 1991.
49. Zenke, M., Steinlein, P., Wagner, E., Cotten, M., Beug, H., and Birnstiel, M.L., Receptor-mediated endocytosis of transferrin-polycation conjugates: an efficient way to introduce DNA into hematopoietic cells, *Proc. Natl. Acad. Sci. U.S.A.*, 87, 3655, 1990.
50. Wagner, E., Zenke, M., Cotten, M., Beug, H., and Birnstiel, M.L., Transferrin-polycation conjugates as carriers for DNA uptake into cells, *Proc. Natl. Acad. Sci. U.S.A.*, 87, 3410, 1990.
51. Shimizu, N., Chen, J., Gamou, S., and Takayanagi, A., Immunogene approach toward cancer therapy using erythrocyte growth factor receptor-mediated gene delivery, *Cancer Gene Ther.*, 3, 113, 1996.
52. Chen, J., Gamou, S., Takayanagi, A., Ohtake, Y., Ohtsubo, M., and Shimizu, N., Targeted in vivo delivery of therapeutic gene into experimental squamous cell carcinomas using anti-epidermal growth factor receptor antibody: immunogene approach, *Hum. Gene Ther.*, 9, 2673, 1998.
53. Sosnowski, B.A., Gonzalez, A.M., Chandler, L.A., Buechler, Y.J., Pierce, G.F., and Baird, A., Targeting DNA to cells with basic fibroblast growth factor (FGF2), *J. Biol. Chem.*, 271, 33647, 1996.
54. Schaffer, D.V. and Lauffenburger, D.A., Optimization of cell surface binding enhances efficiency and specificity of molecular conjugate gene delivery, *J. Biol. Chem.*, 273, 28004, 1998.
55. Felgner, P.L. and Ringold, G.M., Cationic liposome-mediated transfection, *Nature*, 337, 387, 1989.
56. Felgner, P.L., Gadek, T.R., Holm, M., Roman, R., Chan, H.W., Wenz, M., Northrop, J.P., Ringold, G.M., and Danielsen, M., Lipofection: a highly efficient, lipid-mediated DNA-transfection procedure, *Proc. Natl. Acad. Sci. U.S.A.*, 84, 7413, 1987.
57. Farhood, H., Serbina, N., and Huang, L., The role of dioleoyl phosphatidylethanolamine in cationic liposome mediated gene transfer, *Biochim. Biophys. Acta*, 1235, 289, 1995.
58. Crystal, R.G., Transfer of genes to humans: early lessons and obstacles to success, *Science*, 270, 404, 1995.
59. Filion, M.C. and Phillips, N.C., Toxicity and immunomodulatory activity of liposomal vectors formulated with cationic lipids toward immune effector cells, *Biochim. Biophys. Acta*, 1329, 345, 1997.
60. Godbey, W.T., Wu, K.K., and Mikos, A.G., Poly(ethylenimine)-mediated gene delivery affects endothelial cell function and viability, *Biomaterials*, 22, 471, 2001.
61. De Luca, M. and Pellegrini, G., The importance of epidermal stem cells in keratinocyte-mediated gene therapy [editorial], *Gene Ther.*, 4, 381, 1997.

62. Choate, K.A., Medalie, D.A., Morgan, J.R., and Khavari, P.A., Corrective gene transfer in the human skin disorder lamellar ichthyosis, *Nat. Med.*, 2, 1263, 1996.
63. Freiberg, R.A., Choate, K.A., Deng, H., Alperin, E.S., Shapiro, L.J., and Khavari, P.A., A model of corrective gene transfer in X-linked ichthyosis, *Hum. Mol. Genet.*, 6, 927, 1997.
64. Page, S.M. and Brownlee, G.G., An ex vivo keratinocyte model for gene therapy of hemophilia B, *J. Invest. Dermatol.*, 109, 139, 1997.
65. Dellambra, E., Vailly, J., Pellegrini, G., Bondanza, S., Golisano, O., Macchia, C., Zambruno, G., Meneguzzi, G., and De Luca, M., Corrective transduction of human epidermal stem cells in laminin-5-dependent junctional epidermolysis bullosa, *Hum. Gene Ther.*, 9, 1359, 1998.
66. Eming, S.A., Lee, J., Snow, R.G., Tompkins, R.G., Yarmush, M.L., and Morgan, J.R., Genetically modified human epidermis overexpressing PDGF-A directs the development of a cellular and vascular connective tissue stroma when transplanted to athymic mice — implications for the use of genetically modified keratinocytes to modulate dermal regeneration, *J. Invest. Dermatol.*, 105, 756, 1995.
67. Eming, S.A., Snow, R.G., Yarmush, M.L., and Morgan, J.R., Targeted expression of insulin-like growth factor to human keratinocytes: modification of the autocrine control of keratinocyte proliferation, *J. Invest. Dermatol.*, 107, 113, 1996.
68. Andreadis, S.T., Hamoen, K.E., Yarmush, M.L., and Morgan, J.R., Keratinocyte growth factor induces hyperproliferation and delays differentiation in a skin equivalent model system, *FASEB J.*, 15, 898, 2001.
69. Supp, D.M., Supp, A.P., Bell, S.M., and Boyce, S.T., Enhanced vascularization of cultured skin substitutes genetically modified to overexpress vascular endothelial growth factor, *J. Invest. Dermatol.*, 114, 5, 2000.
70. Supp, D.M. and Boyce, S.T., Overexpression of vascular endothelial growth factor accelerates early vascularization and improves healing of genetically modified cultured skin substitutes, *J. Burn Care Rehabil.*, 23, 10, 2002.
71. Rio, M.D., Larcher, F., Meana, A., Segovia, J., Alvarez, A., and Jorcano, J., Nonviral transfer of genes to pig primary keratinocytes. Induction of angiogenesis by composite grafts of modified keratinocytes overexpressing VEGF driven by a keratin promoter, *Gene Ther.*, 6, 1734, 1999.
72. Morgan, J.R., Barrandon, Y., Green, H., and Mulligan, R.C., Expression of an exogenous growth hormone gene by transplantable human epidermal cells, *Science*, 237, 1476, 1987.
73. Fenjves, E.S., Smith, J., Zaradic, S., and Taichman, L.B., Systemic delivery of secreted protein by grafts of epidermal keratinocytes: prospects for keratinocyte gene therapy, *Hum. Gene Ther.*, 5, 1241, 1994.
74. Gerrard, A.J., Hudson, D.L., Brownlee, G.G., and Watt, F.M., Towards gene therapy for haemophilia B using primary human keratinocytes, *Nat. Genet.*, 3, 180, 1993.
75. Fenjves, E.S., Schwartz, P.M., Blaese, R.M., and Taichman, L.B., Keratinocyte gene therapy for adenosine deaminase deficiency: a model approach for inherited metabolic disorders, *Hum. Gene Ther.*, 8, 911, 1997.
76. Sullivan, D.M., Jensen, T.G., Taichman, L.B., and Csaky, K.G., Ornithine-delta-aminotransferase expression and ornithine metabolism in cultured epidermal keratinocytes: toward metabolic sink therapy for gyrate atrophy, *Gene Ther.*, 4, 1036, 1997.
77. Fenjves, E.S., Yao, S.N., Kurachi, K., and Taichman, L.B., Loss of expression of a retrovirus-transduced gene in human keratinocytes, *J. Invest. Dermatol.*, 106, 576, 1996.
78. Meng, X., Sawamura, D., Tamai, K., Hanada, K., Ishida, H., and Hashimoto, I., Keratinocyte gene therapy for systemic diseases. Circulating interleukin 10 released from gene-transferred keratinocytes inhibits contact hypersensitivity at distant areas of the skin, *J. Clin. Invest.*, 101, 1462, 1998.
79. Werner, S., Smola, H., Liao, X., Longaker, M.T., Krieg, T., Hofschneider, P.H., and Williams, L.T., The function of KGF in morphogenesis of epithelium and reepithelialization of wounds, *Science*, 266, 819, 1994.

80. Finch, P.W., Cunha, G.R., Rubin, J.S., Wong, J., and Ron, D., Pattern of keratinocyte growth factor and keratinocyte growth factor receptor expression during mouse fetal development suggests a role in mediating morphogenetic mesenchymal-epithelial interactions, *Dev. Dyn.*, 203, 223, 1995.
81. Baragi, V.M., Renkiewicz, R.R., Jordan, H., Bonadio, J., Hartman, J.W., and Roessler, B.J., Transplantation of transduced chondrocytes protects articular cartilage from interleukin 1-induced extracellular matrix degradation, *J. Clin. Invest.*, 96, 2454, 1995.
82. Bandara, G., Mueller, G.M., Galea-Lauri, J., Tindal, M.H., Georgescu, H.I., Suchanek, M.K., Hung, G.L., Glorioso, J.C., Robbins, P.D., and Evans, C.H., Intraarticular expression of biologically active interleukin 1-receptor-antagonist protein by ex vivo gene transfer, *Proc. Natl. Acad. Sci. U.S.A.*, 90, 10764, 1993.
83. Goomer, R.S., Deftos, L.J., Terkeltaub, R., Maris, T., Lee, M.C., Harwood, F.L., and Amiel, D., High-efficiency nonviral transfection of primary chondrocytes and perichondrial cells for ex-vivo gene therapy to repair articular cartilage defects, *Osteoarthritis Cartilage*, 9, 248, 2001.
84. Madry, H., Zurakowski, D., and Trippel, S.B., Overexpression of human insulin-like growth factor-I promotes new tissue formation in an ex vivo model of articular chondrocyte transplantation, *Gene Ther.*, 8, 1443, 2001.
85. Laurencin, C.T., Ambrosio, A.M., Borden, M.D., and Cooper, J.A., Jr., Tissue engineering: orthopedic applications, *Annu. Rev. Biomed. Eng.*, 1, 19, 1999.
86. Rose, F.R. and Oreffo, R.O., Bone tissue engineering: hope vs hype, *Biochem. Biophys. Res. Commun.*, 292, 1, 2002.
87. Marx, J.C., Allay, J.A., Persons, D.A., Nooner, S.A., Hargrove, P.W., Kelly, P.F., Vanin, E.F., and Horwitz, E.M., High-efficiency transduction and long-term gene expression with a murine stem cell retroviral vector encoding the green fluorescent protein in human marrow stromal cells, *Hum. Gene Ther.*, 10, 1163, 1999.
88. Chuah, M.K., Brems, H., Vanslembrouck, V., Collen, D., and Vandendriessche, T., Bone marrow stromal cells as targets for gene therapy of hemophilia A, *Hum. Gene Ther.*, 9, 353, 1998.
89. Turgeman, G., Pittman, D.D., Muller, R., Kurkalli, B.G., Zhou, S., Pelled, G., Peyser, A., Zilberman, Y., Moutsatsos, I.K., and Gazit, D., Engineered human mesenchymal stem cells: a novel platform for skeletal cell mediated gene therapy, *J. Gene Med.*, 3, 240, 2001.
90. Partridge, K., Yang, X., Clarke, N.M., Okubo, Y., Bessho, K., Sebald, W., Howdle, S.M., Shakesheff, K.M., and Oreffo, R.O., Adenoviral BMP-2 gene transfer in mesenchymal stem cells: in vitro and in vivo bone formation on biodegradable polymer scaffolds, *Biochem. Biophys. Res. Commun.*, 292, 144, 2002.
91. Breitbart, A.S., Grande, D.A., Mason, J.M., Barcia, M., James, T., and Grant, R.T., Gene-enhanced tissue engineering: applications for bone healing using cultured periosteal cells transduced retrovirally with the BMP-7 gene, *Ann. Plast. Surg.*, 42, 488, 1999.
92. Laurencin, C.T., Attawia, M.A., Lu, L.Q., Borden, M.D., Lu, H.H., Gorum, W.J., and Lieberman, J.R., Poly(lactide-co-glycolide)/hydroxyapatite delivery of BMP-2-producing cells: a regional gene therapy approach to bone regeneration, *Biomaterials*, 22, 1271, 2001.
93. Nerem, R.M. and Seliktar, D., Vascular tissue engineering, *Annu. Rev. Biomed. Eng.*, 3, 225, 2001.
94. Dunn, P.F., Newman, K.D., Jones, M., Yamada, I., Shayani, V., Virmani, R., and Dichek, D.A., Seeding of vascular grafts with genetically modified endothelial cells. Secretion of recombinant TPA results in decreased seeded cell retention *in vitro* and *in vivo*, *Circulation*, 93, 1439, 1996.
95. Kullo, I.J., Mozes, G., Schwartz, R.S., Gloviczki, P., Crotty, T.B., Barber, D.A., Katusic, Z.S., and O'Brien, T., Adventitial gene transfer of recombinant endothelial nitric oxide synthase to rabbit carotid arteries alters vascular reactivity, *Circulation*, 96, 2254, 1997.
96. Mozes, G., Kullo, I.J., Mohacsi, T.G., Cable, D.G., Spector, D.J., Crotty, T.B., Gloviczki, P., Katusic, Z.S., and O'Brien, T., Ex vivo gene transfer of endothelial nitric oxide synthase to atherosclerotic rabbit aortic rings improves relaxations to acetylcholine, *Atherosclerosis*, 141, 265, 1998.

97. Alexander, M.Y., Brosnan, M.J., Hamilton, C.A., Fennell, J.P., Beattie, E.C., Jardine, E., Heistad, D.D., and Dominiczak, A.F., Gene transfer of endothelial nitric oxide synthase but not Cu/Zn superoxide dismutase restores nitric oxide availability in the SHRSP, *Cardiovasc. Res.*, 47, 609, 2000.
98. Sato, J., Mohacsi, T., Noel, A., Jost, C., Gloviczki, P., Mozes, G., Katusic, Z.S., O'Brien, T., and Mayhan, W.G., In vivo gene transfer of endothelial nitric oxide synthase to carotid arteries from hypercholesterolemic rabbits enhances endothelium-dependent relaxations, *Stroke*, 31, 968, 2000.
99. Armeanu, S., Pelisek, J., Krausz, E., Fuchs, A., Groth, D., Curth, R., Keil, O., Quilici, J., Rolland, P.H., Reszka, R., and Nikol, S., Optimization of nonviral gene transfer of vascular smooth muscle cells *in vitro* and *in vivo*, *Mol. Ther.*, 1, 366, 2000.
100. von der Leyen, H.E., Braun-Dullaeus, R., Mann, M.J., Zhang, L., Niebauer, J., and Dzau, V.J., A pressure-mediated nonviral method for efficient arterial gene and oligonucleotide transfer, *Hum. Gene Ther.*, 10, 2355, 1999.
101. Matsumoto, T., Komori, K., Shoji, T., Kuma, S., Kume, M., Yamaoka, T., Mori, E., Furuyama, T., Yonemitsu, Y., and Sugimachi, K., Successful and optimized in vivo gene transfer to rabbit carotid artery mediated by electronic pulse, *Gene Ther.*, 8, 1174, 2001.
102. Martin, J.B., Young, J.L., Benoit, J.N., and Dean, D.A., Gene transfer to intact mesenteric arteries by electroporation, *J. Vasc. Res.*, 37, 372, 2000.
103. Compagni, A., Wilgenbus, P., Impagnatiello, M.A., Cotten, M., and Christofori, G., Fibroblast growth factors are required for efficient tumor angiogenesis, *Cancer Res.*, 60, 7163, 2000.
104. Gowdak, L.H., Poliakova, L., Wang, X., Kovesdi, I., Fishbein, K.W., Zacheo, A., Palumbo, R., Straino, S., Emanueli, C., Marrocco-Trischitta, M., Lakatta, E.G., Anversa, P., Spencer, R.G., Talan, M., and Capogrossi, M.C., Adenovirus-mediated VEGF(121) gene transfer stimulates angiogenesis in normoperfused skeletal muscle and preserves tissue perfusion after induction of ischemia, *Circulation*, 102, 565, 2000.
105. Gowdak, L.H., Poliakova, L., Li, Z., Grove, R., Lakatta, E.G., and Talan, M., Induction of angiogenesis by cationic lipid-mediated VEGF165 gene transfer in the rabbit ischemic hindlimb model, *J. Vasc. Surg.*, 32, 343, 2000.
106. Magovern, C.J., Mack, C.A., Zhang, J., Rosengart, T.K., Isom, O.W., and Crystal, R.G., Regional angiogenesis induced in nonischemic tissue by an adenoviral vector expressing vascular endothelial growth factor, *Hum. Gene Ther.*, 8, 215, 1997.
107. Avgoustiniatos, E.S. and Colton, C.K., Effect of external oxygen mass transfer resistances on viability of immunoisolated tissue, *Ann. N.Y. Acad. Sci.*, 831, 145, 1997.
108. Hidaka, C., Ibarra, C., Hannafin, J.A., Torzilli, P.A., Quitoriano, M., Jen, S.S., Warren, R.F., and Crystal, R.G., Formation of vascularized meniscal tissue by combining gene therapy with tissue engineering, *Tissue Eng.*, 8, 93, 2002.
109. Hubbell, J.A., Bioactive biomaterials, *Curr. Opin. Biotechnol.*, 10, 123, 1999.
110. Choate, K.A. and Khavari, P.A., Direct cutaneous gene delivery in a human genetic skin disease, *Hum. Gene Ther.*, 8, 1659, 1997.
111. Levy, M.Y., Barron, L.G., Meyer, K.B., and Szoka, F.C., Jr., Characterization of plasmid DNA transfer into mouse skeletal muscle: evaluation of uptake mechanism, expression and secretion of gene products into blood, *Gene Ther.*, 3, 201, 1996.
112. Bonadio, J., Tissue engineering via local gene delivery: update and future prospects for enhancing the technology, *Adv. Drug Deliv. Rev.*, 44, 185, 2000.
113. Truong-Le, V.L., August, J.T., and Leong, K.W., Controlled gene delivery by DNA-gelatin nanospheres, *Hum. Gene Ther.*, 9, 1709, 1998.
114. Bonadio, J., Smiley, E., Patil, P., and Goldstein, S., Localized, direct plasmid gene delivery in vivo: prolonged therapy results in reproducible tissue regeneration [see comments], *Nat. Med.*, 5, 753, 1999.
115. Fang, J., Zhu, Y.Y., Smiley, E., Bonadio, J., Rouleau, J.P., Goldstein, S.A., McCauley, L.K., Davidson, B.L., and Roessler, B.J., Stimulation of new bone formation by direct transfer of osteogenic plasmid genes, *Proc. Natl. Acad. Sci. U.S.A.*, 93, 5753, 1996.

116. Luo, D., Woodrow-Mumford, K., Belcheva, N., and Saltzman, W.M., Controlled DNA delivery systems, *Pharm. Res.*, 16, 1300, 1999.
117. Shea, L.D., Smiley, E., Bonadio, J., and Mooney, D.J., DNA delivery from polymer matrices for tissue engineering, *Nat. Biotechnol.*, 17, 551, 1999.
118. Tyrone, J.W., Mogford, J.E., Chandler, L.A., Ma, C., Xia, Y., Pierce, G.F., and Mustoe, T.A., Collagen-embedded platelet-derived growth factor DNA plasmid promotes wound healing in a dermal ulcer model, *J. Surg. Res.*, 93, 230, 2000.
119. Labhasetwar, V., Bonadio, J., Goldstein, S., Chen, W., and Levy, R.J., A DNA controlled-release coating for gene transfer: transfection in skeletal and cardiac muscle, *J. Pharm. Sci.*, 87, 1347, 1998.
120. Cohen, H., Levy, R.J., Gao, J., Fishbein, I., Kousaev, V., Sosnowski, S., Slomkowski, S., and Golomb, G., Sustained delivery and expression of DNA encapsulated in polymeric nanoparticles, *Gene Ther.*, 7, 1896, 2000.
121. Madsen, S. and Mooney, D.J., Delivering DNA with polymer matrices: applications in tissue engineering and gene therapy, *Pharm. Sci. Technol. Today*, 3, 381, 2000.
122. Kalyanasundaram, S., Feinstein, S., Nicholson, J.P., Leong, K.W., and Garver, R.I., Jr., Coacervate microspheres as carriers of recombinant adenoviruses, *Cancer Gene Ther.*, 6, 107, 1999.
123. Chandler, L.A., Gu, D.L., Ma, C., Gonzalez, A.M., Doukas, J., Nguyen, T., Pierce, G.F., and Phillips, M.L., Matrix-enabled gene transfer for cutaneous wound repair, *Wound Repair Regen.*, 8, 473, 2000.
124. Chandler, L.A., Doukas, J., Gonzalez, A.M., Hoganson, D.K., Gu, D.L., Ma, C., Nesbit, M., Crombleholme, T.M., Herlyn, M., Sosnowski, B.A., and Pierce, G.F., FGF2-Targeted adenovirus encoding platelet-derived growth factor-B enhances de novo tissue formation, *Mol. Ther.*, 2, 153, 2000.
125. Beer, S.J., Matthews, C.B., Stein, C.S., Ross, B.D., Hilfinger, J.M., and Davidson, B.L., Poly (lactic-glycolic) acid copolymer encapsulation of recombinant adenovirus reduces immunogenicity in vivo, *Gene Ther.*, 5, 740, 1998.
126. Chillon, M., Lee, J.H., Fasbender, A., and Welsh, M.J., Adenovirus complexed with polyethylene glycol and cationic lipid is shielded from neutralizing antibodies *in vitro*, *Gene Ther.*, 5, 995, 1998.
127. Matthews, C., Jenkins, G., Hilfinger, J., and Davidson, B., Poly-L-lysine improves gene transfer with adenovirus formulated in PLGA microspheres, *Gene Ther.*, 6, 1558, 1999.
128. Falanga, V., Wound healing and chronic wounds, *J. Cutan. Med. Surg.*, 3, S1, 1998.
129. Palsson, B.O. and Andreadis, S., The physico-chemical factors that govern retrovirus-mediated gene transfer, *Exp. Hematol.*, 25, 94, 1997.
130. Salmeen, I., Rimai, L., Luftig, R.B., Liebes, L., Retzer, E., Rich, M., and McCormick, J.J., Hydrodynamic diameters of murine mammary, rous sarcoma and feline leukemia RNA tumor viruses: studies by laser beat frequency light-scattering spectroscopy and electron microscopy, *J. Virol.*, 17, 584, 1976.
131. Andreadis, S., Lavery, T., Davis, H.E., Le Doux, J.M., Yarmush, M.L., and Morgan, J.R., Toward a more accurate quantitation of the activity of recombinant retroviruses: alternatives to titer and multiplicity of infection, *J. Virol.*, 74, 3431, 2000.
132. Chuck, A.C., Clarke, M.F., and Palsson, B.O., Retroviral infection is limited by Brownian motion, *Hum. Gene Ther.*. 7, 1527, 1996.
133. LeDoux, J.M., Davis, H.E., Yarmush, M.L., and Morgan, J.R., Kinetics of retrovirus production and decay, *Biotech. Bioeng.*, 63, 654, 1999.
134. Bunnell, B.A., Muul, L.M., Donahue, R.E., Blaese, R.M., and Morgan, R.A., High-efficiency retroviral-mediated gene transfer into human and nonhuman primate peripheral blood lymphocytes, *Proc. Natl. Acad. Sci. U.S.A.*, 92, 7739, 1995.
135. Chuck, A.S. and Palsson, B.O., Consistent and high rates of gene transfer can be obtained using flow-through transduction over a wide range of retroviral titers, *Hum. Gene Ther.*. 7, 743, 1996.
136. Chuck, A.S. and Palsson, B.O., Membrane adsorption characteristics determine the kinetics of flow-through transductions, *Biotech. Bioeng.*, 51, 260, 1996.

137. Bertolini, F., Battaglia, M., Corsini, C., Lazzari, L., Soligo, D., Zibera, C., and Thalmeier, K., Engineered stromal layers and continuous flow culture enhance multidrug resistance gene transfer in hematopoietic progenitors, *Cancer Res.*, 56, 2566, 1996.
138. Hanenberg, H., Xiao, X.L., Dilloo, D., Hashino, K., Kato, I., and Williams, D.A., Colocalization of retrovirus and target cells on specific fibronectin fragments increases genetic transduction of mammalian cells, *Nat. Med.*, 2, 876, 1996.
139. Hanenberg, H., Hashino, K., Konishi, H., Hock, R.A., Kato, I., and Williams, D.A., Optimization of fibronectin-assisted retroviral gene transfer into human CD34+ hematopoietic cells, *Hum. Gene Ther.*, 8, 2193, 1997.
140. Bajaj, B., Lei, P., and Andreadis, S.T., High efficiencies of gene transfer with immobilized recombinant retrovirus: kinetics and optimization, *Biotechnol. Prog.*, 17, 587, 2001.
141. Lei, P., Bajaj, B., and Andreadis, S.T., Retrovirus-associated heparan sulfate mediates immobilization and gene transfer on recombinant fibronectin, *J. Virol.*, 76(17), 8722, 2002.
142. LeDoux, J.M., Morgan, J.R., and Yarmush, M.L., Proteoglycans secreted by packaging cell lines inhibit retrovirus infection, *J. Virol.*, 70, 6468, 1996.
143. Kavanaugh, M.P., Miller, D.G., Zhang, W., Law, W., Kozak, S.L., Kabat, D., and Miller, A.D., Cell-surface receptors for gibbon ape leukemia virus and amphotropic murine retrovirus are inducible sodium-dependent phosphate symporters, *Proc. Natl. Acad. Sci. U.S.A.*, 91, 7071, 1994.
144. Kozak, S.L., Siess, D.C., Kavanaugh, M.P., Miller, A.D., and Kabat, D., The envelope glycoprotein of an amphotropic murine retrovirus binds specifically to the cellular receptor/phosphate transporter of susceptible species, *J. Virol.*, 69, 3433, 1995.
145. Summerford, C., Bartlett, J.S., and Samulski, R.J., AlphaVbeta5 integrin: a co-receptor for adeno-associated virus type 2 infection., *Nat. Med.*, 5, 78, 1999.
146. Wickham, T.J., Mathias, P., Cheresh, D.A., and Nemerow, G.R., Integrins alpha v beta 3 and alpha v beta 5 promote adenovirus internalization but not virus attachment, *Cell*, 73, 309, 1993.
147. Wickham, T.J., Filardo, E.J., Cheresh, D.A., and Nemerow, G.R., Integrin alpha v beta 5 selectively promotes adenovirus mediated cell membrane permeabilization, *J. Cell Biol.*, 127, 257, 1994.
148. Davison, E., Diaz, R.M., Hart, I.R., Santis, G., and Marshall, J.F., Integrin alpha5beta1-mediated adenovirus infection is enhanced by the integrin-activating antibody TS2/16, *J. Virol.*, 71, 6204, 1997.
149. Li, E., Brown, S.L., Stupack, D.G., Puente, X.S., Cheresh, D.A., and Nemerow, G.R., Integrin alphavbeta1 is an adenovirus coreceptor, *J. Virol.*, 75, 5405, 2001.
150. Miller, A.D., Garcia, J.V., von Suhr, N., Lynch, C.M., Wilson, C., and Eiden, M.V., Construction and properties of retrovirus packaging cells based on gibbon ape leukemia virus, *J. Virol.*, 65, 2220, 1991.
151. Wilson, C., Reitz, M.S., Okayama, H., and Eiden, M.V., Formation of infectious hybrid virions with gibbon ape leukemia virus and human T-cell leukemia virus retroviral envelope glycoproteins and the *gag* and *pol* proteins of Moloney murine leukemia virus, *J. Virol.*, 63, 2374, 1989.
152. Kasahara, N., Dozy, A.M., and Kan, Y.W., Tissue-specific targeting of retroviral vectors through ligand-receptor interactions, *Science*, 266, 1373, 1994.
153. Burns, J.C., Friedmann, T., Driever, W., Burrascano, M., and Yee, J.K., Vesicular stomatitis virus G glycoprotein pseudotyped retroviral vectors: Concentration to very high titer and efficient gene transfer into mammalian and non-mammalian cells, *Proc. Natl.. Acad.. Sci. U.S.A.*, 90, 8033, 1993.
154. Martin, F., Neil, S., Kupsch, J., Maurice, M., Cosset, F., and Collins, M., Retrovirus targeting by tropism restriction to melanoma cells, *J. Virol.*, 73, 6923, 1999.
155. Bartlett, J.S., Kleinschmidt, J., Boucher, R.C., and Samulski, R.J., Targeted adeno-associated virus vector transduction of nonpermissive cells mediated by a bispecific F(ab′gamma)2 antibody, *Nat. Biotechnol.*, 17, 181, 1999.
156. Andreadis, S., Fuller, A.O., and Palsson, B.O., Cell cycle dependence of retroviral transduction: An issue of overlapping time scales, *Biotechnol. Bioeng.*, 58, 272, 1998.

157. Roe, T., Reynolds, T.C., Yu, G., and Brown, P.O., Integration of murine leukemia virus DNA depends on mitosis, *EMBO J.*, 12, 2099, 1993.
158. Andreadis, S. and Palsson, B.O., Kinetics of retrovirus mediated gene transfer: the importance of the intracellular half-life of retroviruses, *J. Theor. Biol.*, 182, 1, 1996.
159. Andreadis, S., Brott, D.A., Fuller, A.O., and Palsson, B.O., Moloney murine leukemia virus-derived retroviral vectors decay intracellularly with a half-life in the range of 5.5 to 7.5 hours, *J. Virol.*, 71, 7541, 1997.
160. Lewis, P.F. and Emerman, M., Passage through mitosis is required for oncoretroviruses but not for the human immunodeficiency virus, *J. Virol.*, 68, 510, 1994.
161. Case, S.S., Price, M.A., Jordan, C.T., Yu, X.J., Wang, L., Bauer, G., Haas, D.L., Xu, D., Stripecke, R., Naldini, L., Kohn, D.B., and Crooks, G.M., Stable transduction of quiescent CD34(+)CD38(−) human hematopoietic cells by HIV-1-based lentiviral vectors, *Proc. Natl. Acad. Sci. U.S.A.*, 96, 2988, 1999.
162. Guenechea, G., Gan, O.I., Inamitsu, T., Dorrell, C., Pereira, D.S., Kelly, M., Naldini, L., and Dick, J.E., Transduction of human CD34+ CD38– bone marrow and cord blood-derived SCID-repopulating cells with third-generation lentiviral vectors, *Mol. Ther.*, 1, 566, 2000.
163. Wickham, T.J., Granados, R.R., Wood, H.A., Hammer, D.A., and Shuler, M.L., General analysis of receptor-mediated viral attachment to cell surfaces, *Biophys. J.*, 58, 1501, 1990.
164. Wickham, T.J., Shuler, M.L., Hammer, D.A., Granados, R.R., and Wood, H.A., Equilibrium and kinetic analysis of Autographa californica nuclear polyhedrosis virus attachment to different insect cell lines, *J. Gen. Virol.*, 73, 3185, 1992.
165. Dee, K.U., Hammer, D.A., and Shuler, M.L., A model of the binding, entry, uncoating, and RNA synthesis of Semliki Forest virus in baby hamster kidney (BHK-21) cells, *Biotechnol. Bioeng.*, 46, 485, 1995.
166. Dee, K.U. and Shuler, M.L., A mathematical model of the trafficking of acid-dependent enveloped viruses: application to the binding, uptake, and nuclear accumulation of baculovirus, *Biotechnol. Bioeng.*, 54, 1997.
167. Sanlioglu, S., Benson, P.K., Yang, J., Atkinson, E.M., Reynolds, T., and Engelhardt, J.F., Endocytosis and nuclear trafficking of adeno-associated virus type 2 are controlled by rac1 and phosphatidylinositol-3 kinase activation, *J. Virol.*, 74, 9184, 2000.
168. Xu, Y. and Szoka, F.C., Jr., Mechanism of DNA release from cationic liposome/DNA complexes used in cell transfection, *Biochemistry*, 35, 5616, 1996.
169. Godbey, W.T., Wu, K.K., and Mikos, A.G., Poly(ethylenimine) and its role in gene delivery, *J. Controlled Release*, 60, 149, 1999.
170. Plank, C., Oberhauser, B., Mechtler, K., Koch, C., and Wagner, E., The influence of endosome-disruptive peptides on gene transfer using synthetic virus-like gene transfer systems, *J. Biol. Chem.*, 269, 12918, 1994.
171. Nishikawa, M., Yamauchi, M., Morimoto, K., Ishida, E., Takakura, Y., and Hashida, M., Hepatocyte-targeted in vivo gene expression by intravenous injection of plasmid DNA complexed with synthetic multi-functional gene delivery system, *Gene Ther.*, 7, 548, 2000.
172. Zanta, M.A., Belguise-Valladier, P., and Behr, J.P., Gene delivery: a single nuclear localization signal peptide is sufficient to carry DNA to the cell nucleus, *Proc. Natl. Acad. Sci. U.S.A.*, 96, 91, 1999.
173. Branden, L.J., Mohamed, A.J., and Smith, C.I., A peptide nucleic acid-nuclear localization signal fusion that mediates nuclear transport of DNA, *Nat. Biotechnol.*, 17, 784, 1999.
174. Dean, D.A., Dean, B.S., Muller, S., and Smith, L.C., Sequence requirements for plasmid nuclear import, *Exp. Cell Res.*, 253, 713, 1999.
175. Vacik, J., Dean, B.S., Zimmer, W.E., and Dean, D.A., Cell-specific nuclear import of plasmid DNA, *Gene Ther.*, 6, 1006, 1999.
176. Caplan, A.I., and Bruder, S.P., Mesenchymal stem cells: building blocks for molecular medicine in the 21st century, *Trends Mol. Med.*, 7, 259, 2001.

177. Miller, D.G., Adam, M.A., and Miller, A.D., Gene transfer by retrovirus vectors occurs only in cells that are actively replicating at the time of infection, *Mol. Cell. Biol.*, 10, 4239, 1990.
178. Lutzko, C., Dube, I.D., and Stewart, A.K., Recent progress in gene transfer into hematopoietic stem cells, *Crit. Rev. Oncol. Hematol.*, 30, 143, 1999.
179. Moore, K.A., Deisseroth, A.B., Reading, C.L., Williams, D.E., and Belmont, J.W., Stromal support enhances cell-free retroviral vector transduction of human bone marrow long-term culture-initiating cells, *Blood*, 79, 1393, 1992.
180. Bienzle, D., Abrams-Ogg, A.C., Kruth, S.A., Ackland-Snow, J., Carter, R.F., Dick, J.E., Jacobs, R.M., Kamel-Reid, S., and Dube, I.D., Gene transfer into hematopoietic stem cells: long-term maintenance of *in vitro* activated progenitors without marrow ablation, *Proc. Natl. Acad. Sci. U.S.A.*, 91, 350, 1994.
181. Xu, L.C., Kluepfel-Stahl, S., Blanco, M., Schiffmann, R., Dunbar, C., and Karlsson, S., Growth factors and stromal support generate very efficient retroviral transduction of peripheral blood CD34+ cells from Gaucher patients, *Blood*, 86, 141, 1995.
182. Pollok, K.E., Hanenberg, H., Noblitt, T.W., Schroeder, W.L., Kato, I., Emanuel, D., and Williams, D.A., High-efficiency gene transfer into normal and adenosine deaminase-deficient T lymphocytes is mediated by transduction on recombinant fibronectin fragments, *J. Virol.*, 72, 4882, 1998.
183. Dardalhon, V., Noraz, N., Pollok, K., Rebouissou, C., Boyer, M., Bakker, A.Q., Spits, H., and Taylor, N., Green fluorescent protein as a selectable marker of fibronectin-facilitated retroviral gene transfer in primary human T lymphocytes, *Hum. Gene Ther.*, 10, 5, 1999.
184. Moritz, T., Dutt, P., Xiao, X., Carstanjen, D., Vik, T., Hanenberg, H., and Williams, D.A., Fibronectin improves transduction of reconstituting hematopoietic stem cells by retroviral vectors: evidence of direct viral binding to chymotryptic carboxy-terminal fragments, *Blood*, 88, 855, 1996.
185. Conneally, E., Eaves, C.J., and Humphries, R.K., Efficient retroviral-mediated gene transfer to human cord blood stem cells with in vivo repopulating potential, *Blood*, 91, 3487, 1998.
186. Dao, M.A., Hashino, K., Kato, I., and Nolta, J.A., Adhesion to fibronectin maintains regenerative capacity during ex vivo culture and transduction of human hematopoietic stem and progenitor cells, *Blood*, 92, 4612, 1998.
187. Kiem, H.P., Andrews, R.G., Morris, J., Peterson, L., Heyward, S., Allen, J.M., Rasko, J.E., Potter, J., and Miller, A.D., Improved gene transfer into baboon marrow repopulating cells using recombinant human fibronectin fragment CH-296 in combination with interleukin-6, stem cell factor, FLT-3 ligand, and megakaryocyte growth and development factor, *Blood*, 92, 1878, 1998.
188. Cavazzana-Calvo, M., Hacein-Bey, S., de Saint Basile, G., Gross, F., Yvon, E., Nusbaum, P., Selz, F., Hue, C., Certain, S., Casanova, J.L., Bousso, P., Deist, F.L., and Fischer, A., Gene therapy of human severe combined immunodeficiency (SCID)-X1 disease, *Science*, 288, 669, 2000.
189. Abonour, R., Williams, D.A., Einhorn, L., Hall, K.M., Chen, J., Coffman, J., Traycoff, C.M., Bank, A., Kato, I., Ward, M., Williams, S.D., Hromas, R., Robertson, M.J., Smith, F.O., Woo, D., Mills, B., Srour, E.F., and Cornetta, K., Efficient retrovirus-mediated transfer of the multidrug resistance 1 gene into autologous human long-term repopulating hematopoietic stem cells, *Nat. Med.*, 6, 652, 2000.
190. Bajaj, B., Behshad, S., and Andreadis, S.T., Retroviral gene transfer to human epidermal keratinocytes correlates with integrin expression and is significantly enhanced on fibronectin, *Hum. Gene Ther.*, 13(15), 1821, 2002.
191. Jones, P.H. and Watt, F.M., Separation of human epidermal stem cells from transit amplifying cells on the basis of differences in integrin function and expression, *Cell*, 73, 713, 1993.
192. Jones, P.H., Harper, S., and Watt, F.M., Stem cell patterning and fate in human epidermis, *Cell*, 80, 83, 1995.
193. Zhu, A.J., Haase, I., and Watt, F.M., Signaling via beta1 integrins and mitogen-activated protein kinase determines human epidermal stem cell fate *in vitro*, *Proc. Natl. Acad. Sci. U.S.A.*, 96, 6728, 1999.
194. Bajaj, B. and Andreadis, S.T., Retroviral gene transfer to epidermal stem cells, in preparation.

195. Young, J.L. and Dean, D.A., Nonviral gene transfer strategies for the vasculature, *Microcirculation*, 9, 35, 2002.
196. Manabe, I. and Owens, G.K., CArG elements control smooth muscle subtype-specific expression of smooth muscle myosin in vivo, *J. Clin. Invest.*, 107, 823, 2001.
197. Owens, G.K., Loeb, A., Gordon, D., and Thompson, M.M., Expression of smooth muscle-specific alpha-isoactin in cultured vascular smooth muscle cells: relationship between growth and cyto-differentiation. *J. Cell Biol.*, 102, 343, 1986.
198. Kovacs, A.M. and Zimmer, W.E., Molecular cloning and expression of the chicken smooth muscle gamma-actin mRNA, *Cell Motil. Cytoskeleton*, 24, 67, 1993.
199. Samaha, F.F., Ip, H.S., Morrisey, E.E., Seltzer, J., Tang, Z., Solway, J., and Parmacek, M.S., Developmental pattern of expression and genomic organization of the calponin-h1 gene. A contractile smooth muscle cell marker, *J. Biol. Chem.*, 271, 395, 1996.
200. Ferreira, V., Assouline, Z., Schwachtgen, J.L., Bahnak, B.R., Meyer, D., and Kerbiriou-Nabias, D., The role of the 5′-flanking region in the cell-specific transcription of the human von Willebrand factor gene, *Biochem. J.*, 293, 641, 1993.
201. Patterson, C., Perrella, M.A., Hsieh, C.M., Yoshizumi, M., Lee, M.E., and Haber, E., Cloning and functional analysis of the promoter for KDR/flk-1, a receptor for vascular endothelial growth factor, *J. Biol. Chem.*, 270, 23111, 1995.
202. Lee, M.E., Bloch, K.D., Clifford, J.A., and Quertermous, T., Functional analysis of the endothelin-1 gene promoter. Evidence for an endothelial cell-specific cis-acting sequence, *J. Biol. Chem.*, 265, 10446, 1990.
203. Hafenrichter, D.G., Wu, X., Rettinger, S.D., Kennedy, S.C., Flye, M.W., and Ponder, K.P., Quantitative evaluation of liver-specific promoters from retroviral vectors after in vivo transduction of hepatocytes, *Blood*, 84, 3394, 1994.
204. Page, S.M. and Brownlee, G.G., Differentiation-specific enhancer activity in transduced keratinocytes: a model for epidermal gene therapy, *Gene Ther.*, 5, 394, 1998.
205. Gossen, M. and Bujard, H., Tight control of gene expression in mammalian cells by tetracycline-responsive promoters, *Proc. Natl. Acad. Sci. U.S.A.*, 89, 5547, 1992.
206. Furth, P.A., St Onge, L., Boger, H., Gruss, P., Gossen, M., Kistner, A., Bujard, H., and Hennighausen, L., Temporal control of gene expression in transgenic mice by a tetracycline-responsive promoter, *Proc. Natl. Acad. Sci. U.S.A.*, 91, 9302, 1994.
207. Kistner, A., Gossen, M., Zimmermann, F., Jerecic, J., Ullmer, C., Lubbert, H., and Bujard, H., Doxycycline-mediated quantitative and tissue-specific control of gene expression in transgenic mice, *Proc. Natl. Acad. Sci. U.S.A.*, 93, 10933, 1996.
208. Baron, U., Gossen, M., and Bujard, H., Tetracycline-controlled transcription in eukaryotes: novel transactivators with graded transactivation potential, *Nucleic Acids Res.*, 25, 2723, 1997.
209. Paulus, W., Baur, I., Boyce, F.M., Breakefield, X.O., and Reeves, S.A., Self-contained, tetracycline-regulated retroviral vector system for gene delivery to mammalian cells, *J. Virol.*, 70, 62, 1996.
210. Harding, T.C., Geddes, B.J., Noel, J.D., Murphy, D., and Uney, J.B., Tetracycline-regulated transgene expression in hippocampal neurones following transfection with adenoviral vectors, *J. Neurochem.*, 69, 2620, 1997.
211. Harding, T.C., Geddes, B.J., Murphy, D., Knight, D., and Uney, J.B., Switching transgene expression in the brain using an adenoviral tetracycline-regulatable system [see comments], *Nat. Biotechnol.*, 16, 553, 1998.
212. Geer, D.J., Swartz, D.D., and Andreadis, S.T., Fibrin promotes migration in a three-dimensional *in vitro* model of wound regeneration, *Tissue Eng.*, 8(5), 787, 2002.

20

Shear Stress and Chondrocytes

C. Corey Scott
Rice University

Kyriacos A. Athanasiou
Rice University

CONTENTS

20.1 Introduction

20.1.1 Significance

Articular cartilage failure is currently a cause of much morbidity and patient suffering, and few solutions currently exist for any but the smallest defects. Though articular cartilage is relatively thin, avascular, and aneural,[1] replacement through tissue engineering still remains elusive. However, the field of tissue engineering has entered an exponential phase of growth and discovery, in particular in terms of elucidating the effects of the mechanical and biochemical environment on chondrocytes, as well as the synergy of the two.[2]

Osteoarthritis (OA), while affecting millions, is not fully understood. OA affects over a fifth of Americans over age 45, almost half of Americans over age 65, and affects women more often than men.[3] Predisposing factors include previous injury, fracture, ligament tear, and many other causes of misaligned or abnormal force transduction across a joint.[4] Also, heavily trained horses showed increased cartilage fibrillation and decreased stiffness compared to lightly trained horses.[5] Thus, mechanical forces are critical in cartilage pathology. Patients who have had their joints immobilized, resulting in much lower mechanical loading, eventually experienced cartilage thinning and alteration in composition in addition to bone loss.[6-8] These studies illustrate the critical importance of mechanical loading to normal cartilage maintenance as well as pathology.

0-8493-1140-3/04/$0.00+$1.50

Applying different forces to cartilage or chondrocytes has been shown to result in diverse genetic and metabolic effects. Compressive forces and hydrostatic pressure on cartilage and chondrocytes are known to be beneficial in certain amounts at certain frequencies and can be synergistic with particular growth factors, although some specifics are still unknown.[9-12] Shear stress, another form of mechanical loading on chondrocytes and cartilage, is not as fully understood.

20.1.2 Shear Stress

Shear stress has been shown to have diverse effects on chondrocytes through mechanotransductive mechanisms and cell adhesion studies. The difficulty of applying a known and uniform shear stress to cells adds complexity to the issue of shear and chondrocytes.

One method of exploring the effect of shear stress on chondrocytes involves cell adhesion or the force of detaching a cell from a substrate, particularly if detached by fluid flow or a force parallel to the substrate surface.[13-17] Also, cell adhesion is vital for cells and tissues to function, particularly for connective tissues.[18] Many techniques have been used to measure the detachment force or strength of cells on different surfaces, either individually, or in monolayer culture. In addition to knowing the adhesive strength of cells on various materials in different media, these experiments have led to some understanding of the surface characteristics and cytoskeletal behavior of chondrocytes with respect to resisting shear stress. The same techniques used for cell adhesion can be employed to apply a known amount of shear to chondrocytes, gauge the genetic and phenotypic response, and gather the mechanical properties. Cell adhesion techniques are used to understand chondrocyte metabolism and mechanotransduction, but the material properties must be known for the cell's mechanical environment to be characterized.

To obtain the shear mechanical environment experienced by the cell, the material properties of the chondrocyte must be identified.[19] Many models of the techniques used to study cell adhesion, such as micropipette adhesion[20,21] and microplates,[22] allow the material properties of the chondrocytes to be calculated. Other techniques, such as cytoindentation,[23] magnetic microbeads,[24-26] or atomic force microscopy[27,28] are also used to attain the mechanical properties of the whole cell or a locality of the cell.

The mechanotransduction of chondrocytes in response to shear stress has mostly been studied through fluid-induced shear. These studies have shown an array of effects in response to shear, some regenerative and some degenerative. Several investigations explore the changes in morphology and gene expression of chondrocytes under shear by applying a uniform average shear or simple shear to cartilage explants, while others explore cartilage tissue constructs in bioreactors. Many bioreactor studies compare static versus perfused culture[29-35] or attempt to tissue engineer cartilage constructs in a low shear or simulated microgravity environment.[36-39] Static versus perfused versus rotating-wall bioreactor comparisons allow conjecture as to the relative shear levels experienced by the cells and their phenotypic and genotypic response.

Consequently, biomechanical shear forces are important and integral in OA and tissue engineering of cartilage. While compressive, cyclical forces of a certain level are beneficial to chondrocytes, the effects of shear stress are largely unknown. One particularly difficult task is separating out the effects of shear stress from mass transit effects, while another intricacy entails knowledge of the forces transduced to the cell from the extracellular or pericellular matrix. Therefore, shear stress plays a vital and as yet not fully recognized function for chondrocytes.

20.2 Chondrocytes and Cell Adhesion

Cell adhesion, which is important to tissue formation, growth, and maturation, involves straightforward attempts to understand how well chondrocytes adhere to a material, which can indicate the level of biocompatibility or the receptors present in the membrane. Generally, a method is devised to remove cells from a substrate and measure the force or pressure of removal. The substrate may be coated with an extracellular matrix or basement membrane protein, such as fibronectin or laminin. Many studies were performed demonstrating how certain cells adhered better to certain substrates. The methods utilized included micropipette aspiration,[14,40-42] cytodetachment,[13,17] fluid-induced shear and cone viscometry,[15,43-45] and could include microplates.[46] The techniques used for cell detachment are not only important for adhesion studies, but they can also be modified to examine the effect of shear on genetic response.

20.2.1 Micropipette Aspiration

Micropipette aspiration uses a glass pipette with a micron scale tip combined with controlled negative pressure to pluck cells off of a surface (Figure 20.1a).[14,40-42,47] The pressure is increased in small steps until the cell is detached from the substrate. Moussy et al.[40] investigated the adhesion strength of endothelial cells on four different surfaces in either phosphate buffer solution (PBS) or culture medium, finding that the force of adhesion on both surfaces increased with time. In PBS, the force of detachment increased with surface tension, while in culture medium the opposite occurred.

Other experiments utilized chondrocytes or connective tissue cells. Lee and associates[14] performed experiments that measured the pressure necessary to pull chondrocytes off of the surface of cut cartilage that was treated with different amounts of chondroitinase ABC. Chondrocytes were seeded onto different zones of the transversely cut cartilage. Adhesion pressure increased with the duration of seeding four to six times and with chondroitinase treatment, though to a lesser extent. Sung and associates,[41,42,47] in three different studies, used micropipette aspiration to explore differences in adhesion of fibroblasts from two ligaments of the knee, the anterior cruciate ligament (ACL) and the posterior cruciate ligament (PCL). These studies are analogous to using chondrocytes from different zones, as the fibroblasts are two populations of the same cell type. The ACL fibroblasts adhered better to laminin,[41] while the MCL fibroblasts adhered better to fibronectin.[47] These results are thought to be due to the different receptor types present in different densities on the fibroblasts.

The micropipette studies demonstrate how cell adhesion studies extract detailed information about cell behavior and allow inferences as to cell membrane composition and organization. Using micropipette aspiration for cell adhesion studies does not measure shear, as the pipette pulls the cell perpendicular to the surface. The complex mechanical environment complicates attempts to compare this technique to others.

20.2.2 Cytodetachment

Cytodetachment is a method that measures the adhesion force by applying shear through a thin cantilever probe under microscopy.[13] A similar method also allows measuring cell adhesion.[49] The force is measured

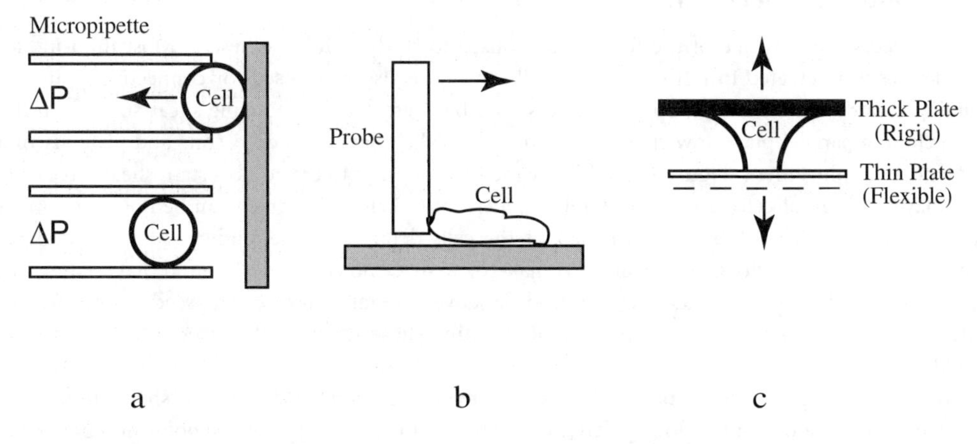

FIGURE 20.1 Techniques for cell adhesion experiments. (a) Micropipette aspiration — the pressure is recorded at the time the cell detaches; (b) cytodetachment — the deflection of the probe is recorded and calculated into the applied force at the time of detachment; (c) microplate adhesion rupture — the deflection of the flexible plate can be recorded and calculated into the applied force at the time of detachment.

through the deflection of the probe by a fiber optic sensor[48] or a photodiode (Figure 20.1b).[13] Athanasiou and associates[13] found that chondrocytes adhered to fibronectin-coated glass better than plain glass and bovine serum albumin-coated glass. This study also examined the cytoskeletal organization of chondrocytes on the different substrata, finding that the cytoskeleton was more organized on fibronectin than glass or bovine serum albumin. Hoben and associates[17] used cytodetachment and found fixed cells had more adhesiveness than living cells and that seeding time increased the adhesiveness. Using the cytodetacher, a study by Huang et al.[49] showed adhesion forces increased and cell height decreased with seeding time. Yamamoto et al.[48, 50] used fibroblasts and calculated the shear strength and adhesive energy by using the force to detach the cell and the projected area of the cell. The adhesion shear strength and detachment surface energy found necessary to detach the fibroblasts were 1.5 kPa and 29 pJ on collagen-coated polystyrene and 1 kPa and 16 pJ on fibronectin polystyrene, while these values were approximately 420 to 670 kPa and 7 to 11 pJ for both glass and uncoated polystyrene. These studies were able to find the shearing force of detachment, which allows inference as to the surface composition and binding site density. These methods also lend themselves to mechanical modeling. Further, cytodetachment could be used to explore the mechanical properties of single chondrocytes and combined with reverse transcriptase polymerase chain reaction (RT-PCR) to investigate the genetic and phylogenic response to shear stress.

20.2.3 Microplates

Microplates are glass beams of micron-scale thickness pulled from rectangular glass that are used to apply forces to single cells.[22,51] The microplates are coated with fibronectin or laminin to allow the cells to adhere more firmly and specifically. One of the plates is rigid, while the other plate is flexible and of known elastic moduli (Figure 20.1c). A cell is attached to the rigid plate, and then to the flexible plate. For testing cell adhesion, the rigid plate applies a force pulling the cell away from the flexible plate. The flexible plate's deflection allows the calculation of the force, from 1 to 1000 nN, exerted upon the cell using beam theory since its modulus and thickness is known.[51]

Thoumine and Ott[22] tested chick embryonic cardiac fibroblasts in tension and compression, defining three regimens of mechanical behavior delineated by time scale. During the initial seconds of deformation, the cells behaved elastically, while on the scale of several minutes, the cells behaved viscoelastically. After 10 min, the cells were found to have contractile forces dependent upon the actin cytoskeleton. The behavior of the cell was modeled using a three-element standard linear solid model. The cells' two elastic moduli were found to be from 0.6 to 1.0 kPa with an apparent viscosity of 10^4 Pa-s.

20.2.4 Fluid-Induced Shear

Fluid-induced shear was one of the first methods used to study cellular adhesion. Most fluid-induced shear devices were created to test endothelial cells, but have also been used for connective tissue cells, including chondrocytes. Several types of devices have been created for inducing shear stress with fluid flow, including parallel plate flow chambers,[15] coaxial parallel plate rotation,[52] cone and plate viscometers,[43] and jet impingement (Figure 20.2).[53] These methods attempt to create a constant shear force across a monolayer culture of cells. To test adhesion, the percent of cells that detach can be noted, a standard number being the shear stress at which half of the cells detach.[15] Some studies indirectly study cell adhesion through bioreactors. For instance, Vunjak-Novakovic and colleagues[54] found that seeding thick scaffolds uniformly requires fluid-flow in mixed flasks versus static culture. The seeding kinetics were modeled with fluid flow, though the role of the resulting shear stress in chondrocyte adhesion to the scaffold is unclear.

Bussolari et al.[43] described a cone and plate viscometer that applies a constant shear stress over a surface, including modeling the flow, which must be maintained at a very low Reynolds number (Figure 20.2a). Blackman and colleagues[44] described an advanced design of a cone and plate viscometer that includes a microstepper motor to allow close control of the rotation of the cone and the ensuing shear stress. The modeling of this device includes a nonsteady-state startup three-dimensional flow solution,

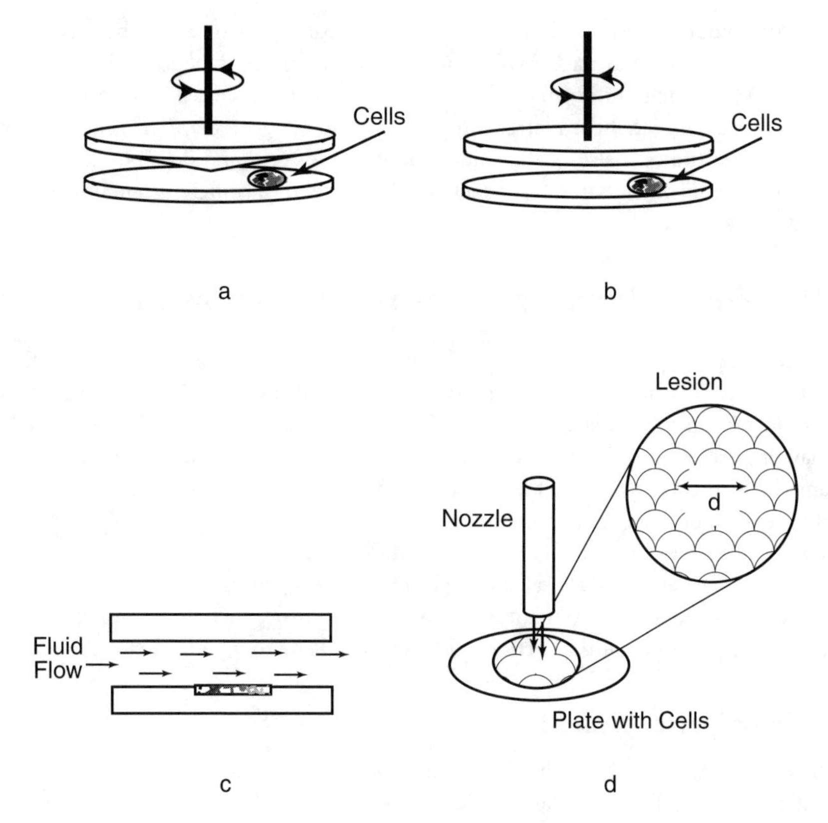

FIGURE 20.2 Techniques to apply fluid-induced shear stress over a population of cells. (a) Cone and plate viscometer; (b) coaxial plate viscometer; (c) parallel plate flow chamber; (d) jet impingement and lesion size.

as well as the steady-state solution. Wendl[52] described a model of a parallel coaxial disk device that simulates shear loading, solving for oscillatory flow conditions in addition to steady state (Figure 20.2b). The models of these devices have increased in complexity over time, demonstrating the difficulty of achieving a steady shear stress over groups of cells. Schnittler et al.[45] developed a cone plate viscometer for specifically measuring shear detachment force and showed endothelial cell adhesion increased with laminin and that stress fiber formation occurred under fluid-induced shear.

Schinagl and associates[15] used a parallel plate shear flow chamber, seeding chondrocytes onto a cartilage surface for between 5 and 40 min, inverting the chamber to count the percentage of cells still adherent, and then applying between 6 and 90 Pa of shear stress through fluid flow (Figure 20.2c). The fraction of detached cells was then measured. At 9 min of seeding time, half of the cells were detached due to the inversion and gravity. At 40 min of seeding time, half of the cells were detached by 26 Pa of shear stress. The study also found that increasing seeding time increased adhesion.

Bundy and colleagues[53] used jet impingement to measure adhesion forces of fibroblasts and the bacteria *Staphylococcus aureus* (Figure 20.2d). This technique uses a submerged jet of fluid to apply shear to a surface. The jet of fluid causes peak shear around its diameter and a gradient of less shear farther away from the stream. The jet detaches cells within a certain area on a plate, the diameter of which is fit with a computer. By modeling the shear stress as a function of radius and noting the greatest average diameter at which cells are detached, the approximate detachment force is calculated. This study found fibroblasts tend to detach due to shear, while the bacteria detached more due to pressure. Further, fibroblasts adhered to titanium and tissue culture plastic approximately the same, likely due to adsorbed proteins. The adhesion strength of bacteria was not as dependent on seeding time as fibroblasts, possibly due to fibroblasts' more complex cytoskeleton organization.

All of the fluid-induced shear studies of cell adhesion test groups of cells. The fluid-induced shear stress is an overall calculated average. While these studies are important to understanding how cells behave under shear, applying a uniform mechanical environment to each cell is not possible, due to small differences in adhesion, extracellular matrix composition, and cell geometry. The genetic response of the cells gauged by these studies is also of the whole population of cells and does not account for possible differences between cells of the same type, such as fibroblasts from different tendons or chondrocytes from different zones.

20.3 Mechanical Property Measurement of Single Cells

Cell mechanical properties must be obtained to understand the stress environment of the cell. Cells exhibit a wide array of mechanical properties. For example, while neutrophils tend to behave as a fluid,[55] the chondrocyte exhibits viscoelastic behavior.[56] Koay and colleagues[57] demonstrated viscoelastic chondrocyte behavior in response to a step load using cytoindentation. The material properties of the chondrocyte were obtained using a standard linear solid model. As the chondrocyte and its cytoskeleton are complex, different models are used depending on the type of loading and properties desired. Thus, different cells and different loading regimes require different models. Many of the techniques used for cell adhesion strength are also used for calculating mechanical properties. Once cell mechanical properties are known, the stress and strain profile of a cell undergoing a specific deformation can be interpreted and compared to other mechanical, genetic, and biochemical environmental factors.

20.3.1 Micropipette Aspiration

Micropipette aspiration to obtain mechanical, viscoelastic properties of chondrocytes has used a homogeneous elastic solid model[56,58] or a standard linear solid model,[20,59-61] which assumes an axisymmetric half-space and incompressibility (Figure 20.3a). The differences between using this technique for detachment and using it for measuring cell properties include a pipette tip diameter that is smaller than the cell and recording time displacement curves for the displacement of the cell membrane in the center of the pipette, L. Using an elastic solid model, the chondrocyte was found to behave as a viscoelastic solid; the Young's modulus of both osteoarthritic and nonosteoarthritic chondrocytes was calculated to be 0.67 and 0.65 kPa, respectively, and not significantly different.[56] The volume change after aspiration was greater in osteoarthritic chondrocytes. Trickey and colleagues[20] employed a more complex standard linear solid model with three parameters to characterize normal and osteoarthritic chondrocytes, finding that osteoarthritic chondrocytes displayed an increased instantaneous and equilibrium modulus, as well as a higher apparent viscosity. This model employs a Kelvin body to model the chondrocytes' viscoelasticity phenomenologically (Figure 20.4a).[20] Another study found decreasing osmolarity led to decreased moduli and apparent viscosity concurrently with dissociation of actin, though no change to hyperosmotic stress.[59] A study of the pericellular matrix with a chondrocyte found that the pericellular matrix was twice as stiff as the chondrocyte.[62] These models demonstrate viscoelastic solid behavior by the chondrocyte and alterations in mechanical properties that were due to loading, osmotic environment, and disease states. Further, the surrounding pericellular matrix was found to be stiffer than the cell and thought to be less stiff than the extracellular matrix. These results have implications for the transduction of force from the tissue to the cell and may be used in future modeling.

20.3.2 Single-Cell Cantilever Techniques

Another method of obtaining the material properties of a cell involves applying a force to the cell via a cantilever beam. Cytoindentation uses a thin probe to compress the cell (Figure 20.3b).[23] Modeling the cell with two continuum mechanics models, including a mixed-boundary value, linear elastic solid with Bousinesq-Papkovitch potential functions and a linear biphasic model, the compressive modulus of a cell line was found. This apparatus allows a prescribed displacement and force profile on a single cell.

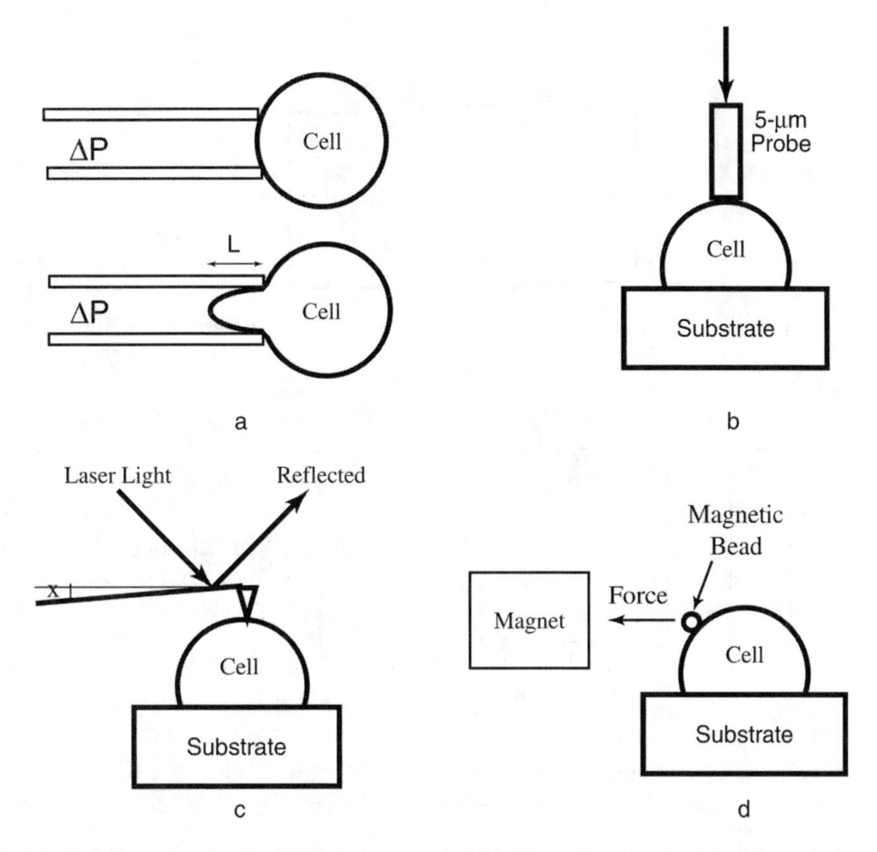

FIGURE 20.3 Techniques to obtain mechanical properties. (a) Micropipette aspiration; (b) cytoindentation; (c) atomic force microscopy; (d) magnetic bead microrheometry.

Another indentation technique used a glass probe to indent the surface of mouse embryonic carcinoma cells, looking at differences between cells with and without vinculin.[63] Vinculin-deficient cells were less resistant to indentation, indicating that vinculin is an important part of the cytoskeleton. Similar cantilever techniques, such as microplates,[22] have also been used to obtain cell mechanical properties, while other cantilever techniques could be modeled to obtain properties. Cytodetachment, discussed earlier, could be modeled to further understand how a single cell behaves under shear.[13]

20.3.3 Atomic Force Microscopy

Atomic force microscopy has been used to investigate the differences in mechanical properties of various cells, including endothelial, cardiac and skeletal muscle,[64] liver endothelial cells and fibroblasts,[27] aortic endothelial cells,[28] osteoblasts,[65] and a fibroblast cell line (Figure 20.3c).[66] The Hertz model is often used and assumes a pointed or spherical tip indentation probe and an elastic, homogenous material. The deflection of the probe is measured, and the applied force can be calculated using beam theory. The deformations are infinitesimal. Sato and colleagues[28] looked at the changes in local cell properties in endothelial cells exposed to fluid-induced shear stress, similar to studies of chondrocyte metabolism. Comparison of cardiac and skeletal muscle viscoelastic properties is similar to ascertaining the differences between zonal chondrocytes or between fibroblasts from two similar ligaments.[64]

20.3.4 Laser Tracking Microrheology

The procedure of using laser tracking microrheology involves implanting small spheres into the cytoskeleton and recording their micromotion.[67] Yamada and colleagues tracked polystyrene particles in

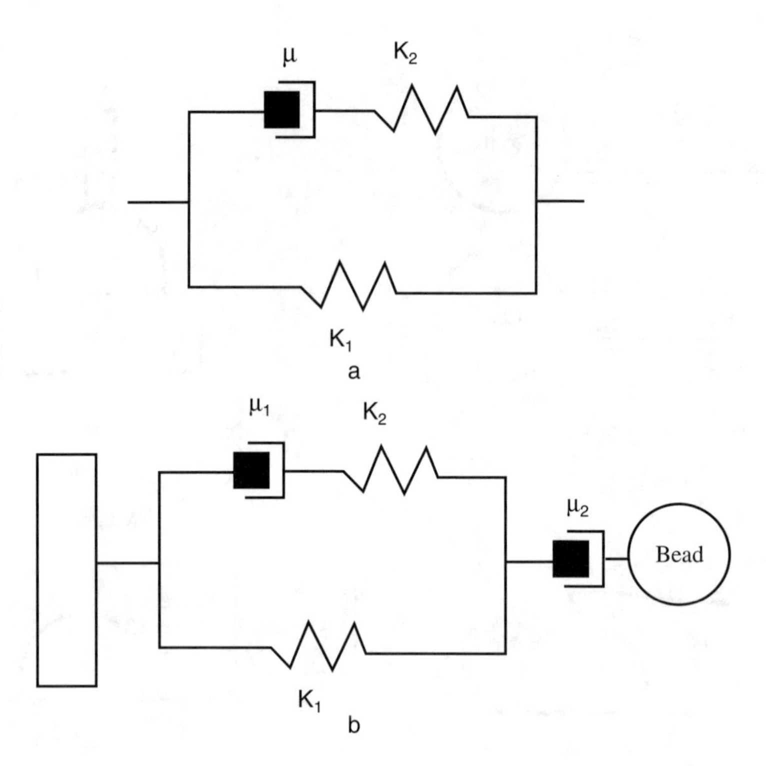

FIGURE 20.4 Phenomenological models of viscoelastic behavior. (a) Kelvin body with a spring in parallel with a series of a dashpot and a spring; (b) Kelvin body in series with a dashpot.

polymerized actin and COS-7 cell cytoplasm without applying any forces. The Brownian motion of the particles is indicative of the local mechanical properties. The technique demonstrated the viscoelastic nature of cytoplasm and measured local differences in the cytoplasm.

20.3.5 Magnetic Beads

One method that can test local membrane mechanical properties is called magnetic bead microrheometry.[26,68] A 4.5-μm magnetic bead is coated with a molecule that will bind a specific receptor and a magnetic field is applied to the bead, which applies a force to the membrane (Figure 20.3d). Those beads transmitting force onto the cells are tracked versus time, allowing force response curves to be generated. The viscoelastic behavior is modeled as a dashpot in series with a Kelvin body (Figure 20.4). The data are curve fit and an effective modulus, relaxation time, and viscosity are calculated. A similar study utilized the same size beads and applied tension on part of the cell membrane, but did not include modeling.[24] Force-displacement curves were compared between different cells with and without vinculin.

20.4 Effect of Shear Stress on Chondrocytes

While compressive or hydrostatic forces have been studied and shown to be beneficial at specific frequencies and levels, the effect of shear stress on chondrocytes remains controversial. While shear has been shown to increase proliferation,[69] glycosaminoglycan (GAG) size and amount,[70] proteoglycan size, and protein amount,[71] other effects of shear appear injurious to chondrocytes. Fluid-induced shear has been shown to increase pro-inflammatory mediators such as interleukin-6,[72] nitric oxide, and prostaglandin E2.[73] Protective molecules such as tissue inhibitor of metalloproteinase (TIMP-1)[70] and interleukin-4[74] are also induced by shear, possibly indictating activation of protective mechanisms.[70,72,73,75] The effects

TABLE 20.1 Effect of Shear Stress on Metabolism and Proliferation of Chondrocytes

Authors	Parameter	Change from Baseline	Shear Stress	Time
Smith et al., 1995	Cell orientation, peak angle	35–45° and 125–135°	1.6 Pa	48 h
	Glycosaminoglycans	Increased twofold	1.6 Pa	24, 48 h
	Glycosaminoglycan size	Increased	1.6 Pa	48 h
	Proteoglycan size	Increased	1.6 Pa	48 h
	TIMP-1	Increased ninefold	1.6 Pa	48 h
	Prostaglandin E2	Increased tenfold	1.6 Pa	48 h
Mohtai et al., 1996	Interleukin-6, protein	Increased 11-fold	1.6 Pa	48 h
	Interleukin-6, mRNA	Increased 10- to 15-fold	1.6 Pa	48 h
	Interleukin-1α	Not detected	1.6 Pa	48 h
	Interleukin-1β	Not detected	1.6 Pa	48 h
	Tumor necrosis factor-α	Not detected	1.6 Pa	48 h
	Transforming growth factor-β	Not detected	1.6 Pa	48 h
Das et al., 1997	Nitric oxide (NO)	Increased twofold	0.41 Pa	24 h
		Increased sixfold	0.82 Pa	24 h
		Increased fivefold	1.6 Pa	4 h
		Increased 18-fold	1.6 Pa	24 h
Malaviya et al., 1999	Proliferation	Increased 44%	3.5 Pa	4 days
Jin et al., 2001	Protein	Increased 50%	1–3% strain	24 h
	Proteoglycans	Increased 25%	1–3% strain	24 h

of shear on metabolism and proliferation are summarized in Table 20.1. Further adding to confusion, many studies compare static to perfused to rotating wall bioreactors. Rotating wall constructs attain the best results, yet the level of shear stress in these reactors is an average over a population and not always characterized.[29-32,35] Furthermore, mass transport effects cannot be separated from the mechanical effects of the shear using fluid-induced shear in a viscometer or bioreactor.

20.4.1 Metabolism and Proliferation

The metabolism of chondrocytes in response to shear appears increased and reflective of an injurious state. Smith and colleagues[70] found 1.6 Pa of fluid-induced shear in a cone viscometer caused bovine chondrocytes to align along the axis of flow and doubled GAG synthesis. Proteoglycan molecule size was increased, while prostaglandin E2 (PGE2) increased by a factor of nine. Other pro-inflammatory mediators were not increased, including matrix metalloproteinase-3 (MMP-3), collagenase, and stromolyesin, but an inhibitor of MMP-3, tissue inhibitor of metalloproteinase 1 (TIMP-1), was increased by a factor of 10. Archambault et al.[76] found that rabbit fibroblasts produce MMP-1, MMP-3, and cyclooxygenase-2 under fluid-induced shear. Das and colleagues[73] found that GAG and nitric oxide synthesis was increased in response to fluid-induced shear. Nitric oxide increased in proportion to the magnitude and duration of the shear stress. Mohtai et al.[72] explored the expression of the pro-inflammatory cytokine interleukin 6 (Il-6) in chondrocytes. Osteoarthritic chondrocytes produce Il-6, while normal chondrocytes do not. When fluid-induced shear was applied at 1.6 Pa for 48 h, Il-6 mRNA and protein increased approximately tenfold. Signals for mRNA from interferon-1α and 1β, tumor necrosis factor-α, and transforming growth factor-β were not affected by shear. Il-6 mRNA was increased within 1 h of applied shear, indicating a possible role in mechanotransduction. Under 1.64 Pa of fluid-induced shear stress, chondrocytes augmented the production of the nitric oxide synthase gene and increased nitric oxide delivery by the cells up to 3.5-fold at 24 h.[77] Collagen type II mRNA and aggrecan mRNA were both inhibited by shear stress, but inhibiting nitric oxide production increased both mRNA levels. Based on these studies and others, Smith and colleagues[75] put forth a model where shear stress causes chondrocytes to convert to an injurious state characterized by certain metabolic products, such as Il-6, PGE2, and TIMP-1.

Other studies confirmed the increase in GAG synthesis and showed other beneficial effects of shear. Gooch et al.[32] explored static versus mixed flasks and rotating bioreactors with and without IGF-I. The mixing in bioreactors causes fluid-induced shear; the rotating bioreactor likely has less shear stress than the mixed flasks. The mixed flask constructs proliferated more than the static, though not significantly different from the rotating bioreactor. IGF-I caused an increase in cell count in all conditions and an increased amount of GAGs in the rotating bioreactor. Interestingly, a decrease in GAG content was seen in the mixed flask versus static when IGF-I was not present. Collagen was increased in the mixed flasks and rotating bioreactors, while GAG was increased the most in the rotating bioreactors with added IGF-I. This study found a nonlinear correlation between GAG content and equilibrium compressive modulus. Although these results were rigorously obtained, comparison of these results with other studies on chondrocyte metabolism is confounded due to the uncharacterized nature of the flow and stress fields within each bioreactor. Millward-Sadler et al.[78] studied the effect of Il-4 on chondrocytes, which induces hyperpolarization of the membrane under hydrostatic pressure. Antibodies to Il-4 blocked the mechanical-induced hyperpolarization, and Il-4 knock-out mice did not exhibit hyperpolarization. These results indicate a role in mechanotransduction for Il-4, but do not indicate a mechanism. In another study, normal, but not osteoarthritic, chondrocytes under intermittent hydrostatic pressure decreased the amount of MMP-3 and increased the amount of aggrecan.[74] These changes in metabolism for normal chondrocytes were found to be coupled to mechanotransduction through Il-4. Malaviya and Nerem[69] found an increase in proliferation of chondrocytes under shear of 3.5 Pa (35 dynes/cm^2) after 4 days. Jin et al.[71] applied 1 to 3% simple shear strain at frequencies of 0.01 to 1.0 Hz to cartilage explant disks, illustrating an increase of protein and proteoglycans of approximately 50 and 25%, respectively. The only significant difference was between the static culture and shear; no significant differences were found based on the level of shear stress or frequency. These increases only occurred with fetal bovine serum, not in serum-free media. Jin and colleagues[71] concluded that the stimulatory effect of shear is mostly due to deformation, not fluid flow.

These studies demonstrate that shear stress, fluid-induced or not, has a dramatic effect on the metabolism and gene expression of chondrocytes. Somewhat contradictory data are also present in these studies; for example, one found MMP-3 mRNA levels change with intermittent hydrostatic pressure and another found no MMP-3.[70,74] The experiments involving fluid flow pose the problem of delineating the effects of mass transport and mechanical shear. Though mechanically induced shear stress did not exhibit a dose-dependent effect, the range of shear stresses was small, and the force transmission to the cells in matrix is not wholly known. So, a dose-dependence of cartilage gene expression and shear stress is possible. The pro-inflammatory and cytoprotective cytokines produced by chondrocytes in response to shear stress can be interpreted as a response to damage.[75] The increase in ECM production likewise may be a consequence of attempts at repair. However, the differential effects of fluid-induced shear, mechanical shear, and mass transport remain unidentified.

20.4.2 Bioreactors

A major thrust of tissue engineering involves developing cartilage constructs in bioreactors. Cartilage develops better in bioreactors that have some perfusion or flow vs. static conditions, and fluid flow induces shear stress. These observations can indirectly aid in understanding the effect of shear stress on chondrocytes, though the exact levels of shear are unknown for each cell and mass transport effects are again inseparable. Two major classes of bioreactor studies involve comparing static to perfused to rotating wall bioreactors[29-35] and simulated microgravity bioreactors.[36-39]

20.4.2.1 Static vs. Mixed vs. Rotating Bioreactors

Comparative studies between static culture, mixed flasks, and rotating bioreactors have shown that rotating bioreactors tend to produce the best constructs, followed by mixed flasks. Pazzano et al.[29] compared static to perfused bioreactors, finding that the perfusion of 1 μm/sec of flow increased DNA content, GAGs, and hydroxyproline by 118, 184, and 155%, respectively. Dunkelman et al.[80] built a bioreactor with a continuous flow rate of 50 μm/min (0.83 μm/sec), achieving 15 and 25% dry weights of collagen and GAG, respectively. Freed and colleagues[33] demonstrated that doubling time decreases approximately 60% with mixing vs. static, which was attributed to increased mass transport. Freed and colleagues[34] attempted to recapitulate native cartilage in a rotating wall bioreactor using bovine chondrocytes on PGA for 40 days, finding comparable cellularity, 68% GAG, and 33% collagen of native cartilage. Gooch et al.,[32] also using PGA and bovine chondrocytes, compared static culture to mixed petri dishes and flasks and a rotating wall bioreactor with and without IGF-I. In all cases, IGF-I increased wet weight. IGF-I also increased GAG content 1.7-fold in mixed flask and 2.9-fold in the rotating bioreactor and increased collagen 1.6-fold in the rotating bioreactor, while decreasing collagen in static culture. GAG content was found to be correlated to the equilibrium modulus. Mizuno et al.[30] used bovine chondrocytes on collagen sponges with and without perfusion. In contrast to other studies, the static cultures were found to have 3.5- and 2.4-fold increases in aggrecan and collagen type II compared to perfused cultures, respectively. Martin et al.[31] compared the mechanical properties of PGA-bovine chondrocyte constructs cultured in static vs. mixed flask vs. rotating bioreactors. Grossly, the rotating bioreactor construct was the most like native cartilage with 75% of the GAG, 39% of the collagen, and 20% of the equilibrium modulus. The study also included up to 7 months of culture in a rotating bioreactor and achieved the equilibrium modulus and GAG content of native cartilage, though not the stiffness or collagen content. While these studies have some conflicting results, rotating bioreactors seem to produce the best constructs. However, the particular combination of increasing mass transport and adding mechanical stimulation that will optimize cartilage tissue engineering is not fully known.

One other study that may shed light upon the issue of shear's effect on chondrocytes combines different bioreactors for the same culture. Carver and Heath[35] used five experimental groups with different combinations of spinner flasks (s), intermittent compression/perfusion system (p), and a control without the intermittent compression (c). The fluid flow in the spinner flasks was turbulent, while the rotating bioreactor likely had less fluid-induced shear, though neither was modeled. The five groups were noted by 1s5c, 1s5p, 2s4p, 4s2p, and 6s. The 2s4p experimental group outperformed the others in collagen and GAG content, though the 4s2p group was next best. This study, though the mechanics and mass transport are uncharacterized, put the chondrocytes in a higher-shear environment initially and switched to a lower shear environment, producing better constructs.

20.4.2.2 Bioreactors and Microgravity

Mathematical models of bioreactors attempt to characterize the mechanical and mass transport environment due to fluid flow, though this characterization is not always included in bioreactor studies. Much of the mathematical modeling of bioreactors explores simulated microgravity. The rotating wall bioreactor was designed to minimize shear stress and still provide mass transport. While several bioreactors have been designed to simulate microgravity for cells or aggregates of cells, some mechanical stresses are present.

The simplest model of the rotating wall bioreactor involves a force balance on a PGA construct.[37] The forces balanced were the gravitational, hydrodynamic, and centrifugal, resulting in a hydrodynamic force due to drag of 0.15 Pa (1.5 dyne/cm^2). This study assumed two-dimensional flow and that the constructs did not interrupt the fluid flow. The model also assumes a consistent construct size. Another early model of the rotating wall bioreactor by Tsao and colleagues[81] assumed steady, Couette flow (flow between two parallel plates), modeled with Navier-Stokes equations. This model showed a shear stress component in unit gravity up to approximately 0.1 Pa (1 dyne/cm^2), especially as the particle size increased. In the model, space-based operation of the bioreactor substantially decreased the shear stress component. Begley and Kleis[36] modeled the rotating wall bioreactor only assuming axisymmetric flow and validated the model with laser velocimetry. Their model also found large differences between space-based operation and simulated microgravity and used the inner and outer rotation regimes normal for space (inner rotation slower) or earth-based (inner and outer rotation equal) operation. Mean shear was found to be increased two- to threefold in earth-based operation. Though the shear levels were still low, the mass transport effects cannot be separated from the hydrodyamically imposed shear effects.

A new design for a bioreactor, the hydrodynamic focusing bioreactor designed for NASA, was modeled with results showing even less shear stress on constructs than the rotating wall bioreactor.[39]

This model assumed that mean shear stress is the same in space- and earth-based applications, which was shown not to be the case for the rotating wall bioreactor. Using FLUENT, software to model fluid-mechanics, the model of the dome-shaped bioreactor was calculated to have a maximum shear of 0.001 Pa (0.01 dyne/cm^2).

The bioreactor studies show promising results for tissue culture of cartilage, but the mass transport and mechanical environment, even if well characterized, are only averages over a population of cells. The genetic and phenotypic response of cell subpopulations, for example, different zones of chondrocytes, would be masked in these experiments. In both the bioreactor and metabolism studies, the reaction of a single chondrocyte to a particular level of shear is unknown and inseparable from the different levels of mass transport.

20.4.3 Mechanotransduction

The surface and cytoskeleton of the chondrocyte interact with each other and their environment to transduce mechanical signals into genetic expression and biochemical states. Schmidt et al.[82] found that stressing $\beta 1$ or $\alpha 2$ integrins on osteoblast membranes caused an increase in tyrosine phosphorylation, as well as increased phosphorylation of mitogen-activated kinases. The stresses were induced magnetically and nonspecifically. Das et al.[73] established that nitric oxide increases in response to shear 18-fold in 2 hours. By utilizing inhibitors of cellular cascade pathways, the investigators discovered that G-proteins, nitric oxide, and phospholipase C are involved in the transduction of GAGs. Calcium and potassium channel blockers did not inhibit GAG synthesis.

While studies revealed that ion channel blockers did not inhibit GAG synthesis, several studies do implicate ion transients as a method of mechanotransduction.[59,83,84] Guilak and colleagues[59] found changes in the viscoelastic moduli with osmotic stress. Hypo-osmotic stress generated decreased instantaneous and equilibrium moduli, as well as apparent viscosity. Hypo-osmotic stress also caused actin cytoskeleton dissociation. Erickson et al.[83] illustrated that hyper-osmotic stress increased calcium in the cell and decreased cell volume.

Mobasheri et al.[84] put forth a mechanoreceptor model involving integrins, ion channels, extracellular matrix (ECM), and cytoskeleton based on the co-localization of the ion channels and integrins. These mechanoreceptor complexes are thought to respond to deformation, changes in ion concentration, and possibly streaming potentials. The specific configuration or operation of these complexes is still unknown. Much of the chondrocyte mechanotransduction apparatus remains to be deciphered.

20.5 Conclusions

The relationship between shear and chondrocytes is not fully elucidated, though some aspects are more explicitly grasped than others. Cell adhesion studies result in information about chondrocyte mechanotransduction. The same techniques, accompanied by appropriate continuum mechanics models, furnish viscoelastic cell mechanical properties. Knowledge of these properties permits acquisition of the amount of shear stress the cell experiences when loaded in a certain way. Understanding the mechanical properties and the mechanical environment of the chondrocytes allows detailed study of how shear affects chondroctyes.

The metabolism, gene expression, proliferation, and phenotype of the chondrocyte in response to shear loading has been demonstrated to have various results. While pro-inflammatory cytokines increase in response to fluid-induced shear stress, proliferation, and extracellular matrix products have also been found to increase.[69-72,74,75,77] From the perspective of tissue engineering, increasing proliferation and extracellular matrix is beneficial, possibly decreasing the currently lengthy culture times for chondrocytes. However, the increase in pro-inflammatory cytokines due to shear stress is likely unsuitable for chondrocyte culture. Bioreactor studies have also had mixed results, demonstrating that static culture is not as suitable as perfusion or rotating wall bioreactor cultures, but the studies are unable to differentiate mechanical and mass transport effects on the culture. Simulated microgravity bioreactor studies have had success in improving tissue constructs, but have not reached native cartilage levels and cannot separate out effects of mass transport and mechanical environment. Further, earth- and space-based operation of the same bioreactor results in different mechanical and flow environments, which also depend on the particle or construct size. While shear stress has both regenerative and degenerative effects on chondrocytes, the amount of stress and the effects of mass transport on the cells to achieve these effects remain unknown.

Future work in the form of a single cell approach[19] to shear stress and chondrocytes is needed to be able to fully understand effects of shear in regenerative and degenerative processes. The single cell approach involves applying a known shear stress to a single chondrocyte with known cell material properties and measuring its genetic and phenotypic response. Using reverse transcriptase polymerase chain reaction (RT-PCR), the mRNA levels of degenerative and regenerative genes can be attained in chondrocytes that experience different shear stress regimes. By understanding what levels of shear induce particular cytokines and at what level, inhibitors of injurious cytokines at specific concentrations can be used to counteract negative effects. Knowledge of the intensity and duration of shear stress that induces proliferation and extracellular matrix permits shorter culture time and improved constructs. Combining current studies with a single cell approach will result in more comprehensive strategies for tissue engineering cartilage.

Acknowledgments

We gratefully acknowledge the support of The Whitaker Foundation and The Arthritis Foundation.

References

1. Junquiera, L.C., Carneiro, J., and Kelley, R.O., *Basic Histology*, 9th ed., Appleton and Lange, Stamford, CT, 1998, p. 494.
2. Athanasiou, K.A., Shah, A.R., Hernandez, R.J., and LeBaron, R.G., Basic science of articular cartilage repair, *Clin. Sports Med.*, 20(2), 223–247, 2001.
3. Hart, D.J., Doyle, D.V., and Spector, T.D., Incidence and risk factors for radiographic knee osteoarthritis in middle-aged women: the Chingford Study, *Arthritis Rheum.*, 42(1), 17–24, 1999.
4. Birchfield, P.C., Osteoarthritis overview, *Geriatr. Nurs.*, 22(3), 124–130; quiz 130–131, 2001.
5. Murray, R.C., Zhu, C.F., Goodship, A.E., Lakhani, K.H., Agrawal, C.M., and Athanasiou, K.A., Exercise affects the mechanical properties and histological appearance of equine articular cartilage, *J. Orthop Res.*, 17(5), 725–731, 1999.
6. Akeson, W.H., Amiel, D., Abel, M.F., Garfin, S.R., and Woo, S.L., Effects of immobilization on joints, *Clin. Orthop.*, 219, 28–37, 1987.
7. Smith, R.L., Thomas, K.D., Schurman, D.J., Carter, D.R., Wong, M., and van der Meulen, M.C., Rabbit knee immobilization: bone remodeling precedes cartilage degradation, *J. Orthop. Res.*, 10(1), 88–95, 1992.
8. Vanwanseele, B., Lucchinetti, E., and Stussi, E., The effects of immobilization on the characteristics of articular cartilage: current concepts and future directions, *Osteoarthritis Cartilage*, 10(5), 408–419, 2002.
9. Smith, R.L., Rusk, S.F., Ellison, B.E., Wessells, P., Tsuchiya, K., Carter, D.R., Caler, W.E., Sandell, L.J., and Schurman, D.J., In vitro stimulation of articular chondrocyte mRNA and extracellular matrix synthesis by hydrostatic pressure, *J. Orthop. Res.*, 14(1), 53–60, 1996.
10. Smith, R.L., Lin, J., Trindade, M.C., Shida, J., Kajiyama, G., Vu, T., Hoffman, A.R., van der Meulen, M.C., Goodman, S.B., Schurman, D.J., and Carter, D.R., Time-dependent effects of intermittent hydrostatic pressure on articular chondrocyte type II collagen and aggrecan mRNA expression, *J. Rehabil. Res. Dev.*, 37(2), 153–161, 2000.

11. Quinn, T.M., Grodzinsky, A.J., Buschmann, M.D., Kim, Y.J., and Hunziker, E.B., Mechanical compression alters proteoglycan deposition and matrix deformation around individual cells in cartilage explants, *J. Cell Sci.*, 111(Pt. 5), 573–583, 1998.
12. Sah, R.L., Kim, Y.J., Doong, J.Y., Grodzinsky, A.J., Plaas, A.H., and Sandy, J.D., Biosynthetic response of cartilage explants to dynamic compression, *J. Orthop. Res.*, 7(5), 619–636, 1989.
13. Athanasiou, K.A., Thoma, B.S., Lanctot, D.R., Shin, D., Agrawal, C.M., and LeBaron, R.G., Development of the cytodetachment technique to quantify mechanical adhesiveness of the single cell, *Biomaterials*, 20(23-24), 2405–2415, 1999.
14. Lee, M.C., Sung, K.L., Kurtis, M.S., Akeson, W.H., and Sah, R.L., Adhesive force of chondrocytes to cartilage. Effects of chondroitinase ABC, *Clin. Orthop.*, 370, 286–294, 2000.
15. Schinagl, R.M., Kurtis, M.S., Ellis, K.D., Chien, S., and Sah, R.L., Effect of seeding duration on the strength of chondrocyte adhesion to articular cartilage, *J. Orthop. Res.*, 17(1), 121–129, 1999.
16. van Kooten, T.G., Schakenraad, J.M., Van der Mei, H.C., and Busscher, H.J., Development and use of a parallel-plate flow chamber for studying cellular adhesion to solid surfaces, *J. Biomed. Mater. Res.*, 26(6), 725–738, 1992.
17. Hoben, G., Huang, W., Thoma, B.S., LeBaron, R.G., and Athanasiou, K.A., Quantification of varying adhesion levels in chondrocytes using the cytodetacher, *Ann. Biomed. Eng.*, 30(5), 703–712, 2002.
18. LeBaron, R.G. and Athanasiou, K.A., Extracellular matrix cell adhesion peptides: functional applications in orthopedic materials, *Tissue Eng.*, 6(2), 85–103, 2000.
19. Shieh, A.C. and Athanasiou, K.A., Biomechanics of single chondrocytes and osteoarthritis, *Crit. Rev. Biomed. Eng.*, in press.
20. Trickey, T.R., Lee, M., and Guilak, T., Viscoelastic properties of chondrocytes from normal and osteoarthritic human cartilage, *J. Orthop. Res.*, 18(6), 891–898, 2000.
21. Guilak, F., The deformation behavior and viscoelastic properties of chondrocytes in articular cartilage, *Biorheology*, 37(1-2), 27–44, 2000.
22. Thoumine, O. and Ott, A., Time scale dependent viscoelastic and contractile regimes in fibroblasts probed by microplate manipulation, *J. Cell Sci.*, 110 (Pt. 17), 2109–2116, 1997.
23. Shin, D. and Athanasiou, K., Cytoindentation for obtaining cell biomechanical properties, *J. Orthop. Res.*, 17(6), 880–890, 1999.
24. Alenghat, F.J., Fabry, B., Tsai, K.Y., Goldmann, W.H., and Ingber, D.E., Analysis of cell mechanics in single vinculin-deficient cells using a magnetic tweezer, *Biochem. Biophys. Res. Commun.*, 277(1), 93–99, 2000.
25. Bausch, A.R., Moller, W., and Sackmann, E., Measurement of local viscoelasticity and forces in living cells by magnetic tweezers, *Biophys. J.*, 76(Pt. 1), 573–579, 1999.
26. Bausch, A.R., Ziemann, F., Boulbitch, A.A., Jacobson, K., and Sackmann, E., Local measurements of viscoelastic parameters of adherent cell surfaces by magnetic bead microrheometry, *Biophys. J.*, 75(4), 2038–2049, 1998.
27. Braet, F., de Zanger, R., Seynaeve, C., Baekeland, M., and Wisse, E., A comparative atomic force microscopy study on living skin fibroblasts and liver endothelial cells, *J. Electron. Microsc. (Tokyo)*, 50(4), 283–290, 2001.
28. Sato, M., Nagayama, K., Kataoka, N., Sasaki, M., and Hane, K., Local mechanical properties measured by atomic force microscopy for cultured bovine endothelial cells exposed to shear stress, *J. Biomech.*, 33(1), 127–135, 2000.
29. Pazzano, D., Mercier, K.A., Moran, J.M., Fong, S.S., DiBiasio, D.D., Rulfs, J.X., Kohles, S.S., and Bonassar, L.J., Comparison of chondrogenesis in static and perfused bioreactor culture, *Biotechnol. Prog.*, 16(5), 893–896, 2000.
30. Mizuno, S., Allemann, F., and Glowacki, J., Effects of medium perfusion on matrix production by bovine chondrocytes in three-dimensional collagen sponges, *J. Biomed. Mater. Res.*, 56(3), 368–375, 2001.

31. Martin, I., Obradovic, B., Treppo, S., Grodzinsky, A.J., Langer, R., Freed, L.E., and Vunjak-Novakovic, G., Modulation of the mechanical properties of tissue engineered cartilage, *Biorheology*, 37(1-2), 141–147, 2000.
32. Gooch, K.J., Blunk, T., Courter, D.L., Sieminski, A.L., Bursac, P.M., Vunjak-Novakovic, G., and Freed, L.E., IGF-I and mechanical environment interact to modulate engineered cartilage development, *Biochem. Biophys. Res. Commun.*, 286(5), 909–915, 2001.
33. Freed, L.E., Vunjak-Novakovic, G., and Langer, R., Cultivation of cell-polymer cartilage implants in bioreactors, *J. Cell Biochem.*, 51(3), 257–264, 1993.
34. Freed, L.E., Hollander, A.P., Martin, I., Barry, J.R., Langer, R., and Vunjak-Novakovic, G., Chondrogenesis in a cell-polymer-bioreactor system, *Exp. Cell Res.*, 240(1), 58–65, 1998.
35. Carver, S.E. and Heath, C.A., Influence of intermittent pressure, fluid flow, and mixing on the regenerative properties of articular chondrocytes, *Biotechnol. Bioeng.*, 65(3), 274–281, 1999.
36. Begley, C.M. and Kleis, S.J., The fluid dynamic and shear environment in the NASA/JSC rotating-wall perfused-vessel bioreactor, *Biotechnol. Bioeng.*, 70(1), 32–40, 2000.
37. Freed, L.E. and Vunjak-Novakovic, G., Cultivation of cell-polymer tissue constructs in simulated microgravity, *Biotechnol. Bioeng.*, 46(4), 306–313, 1995.
38. Freed, L.E., Pellis, N., Searby, N., de Luis, J., Preda, C., Bordonaro, J., and Vunjak-Novakovic, G., Microgravity cultivation of cells and tissues, *Gravit. Space Biol. Bull.*, 12(2), 57–66, 1999.
39. Tsao, Y.-M.D. and Gonda, S.R., A new technology for three-dimensional cell culture: the hydrodynamic focusing bioreactor, *Biotechnol. Bioeng.*, 70(1), 39–40, 2000.
40. Moussy, F., Neumann, A.W., and Zingg, W., The force of detachment of endothelial cells from different solid surfaces, *ASAIO Trans.*, 36(3), M568–M572, 1990.
41. Sung, K.L., Steele, L.L., Whittermore, D., Hagan, J., and Akeson, W.H., Adhesiveness of human ligament fibroblasts to laminin, *J. Orthop. Res.*, 13(2), 166–173, 1995.
42. Sung, K.L., Yang, L., Whittemore, D.E., Shi, Y., Jin, G., Hsieh, A.H., Akeson, W.H., and Sung, L.A., The differential adhesion forces of anterior cruciate and medial collateral ligament fibroblasts: effects of tropomodulin, talin, vinculin, and alpha-actinin, *Proc. Natl. Acad. Sci. U.S.A.*, 93(17), 9182–9187, 1996.
43. Bussolari, S.R., Dewey, C.F., Jr., and Gimbrone, M.A., Jr., Apparatus for subjecting living cells to fluid shear stress, *Rev. Sci. Instrum.*, 53(12), 1851–1854, 1982.
44. Blackman, B.R., Barbee, K.A., and Thibault, L.E., In vitro cell shearing device to investigate the dynamic response of cells in a controlled hydrodynamic environment, *Ann. Biomed. Eng.*, 28(4), 363–372, 2000.
45. Schnittler, H.J., Franke, R.P., Akbay, U., Mrowietz, C., and Drenckhahn, D., Improved in vitro rheological system for studying the effect of fluid shear stress on cultured cells, *Am. J. Physiol.*, 265(Pt. 1), C289–298, 1993.
46. Thoumine, O., Cardoso, O., and Meister, J.J., Changes in the mechanical properties of fibroblasts during spreading: a micromanipulation study, *Eur. Biophys. J.*, 28(3), 222–234, 1999.
47. Sung, K.L., Kwan, M.K., Maldonado, F., and Akeson, W.H., Adhesion strength of human ligament fibroblasts, *J. Biomech. Eng.*, 116(3), 237–242, 1994.
48. Yamamoto, A., Mishima, S., Maruyama, N., and Sumita, M., A new technique for direct measurement of the shear force necessary to detach a cell from a material, *Biomaterials*, 19(7-9), 871–879, 1998.
49. Huang, W., Anvari, B., Torres, J.H., LeBaron, R.G., and Athanasiou, K.A., Temporal effects of cell adhesion on mechanical characteristics of the single chondrocyte, *J. Orthop. Res.*, in press.
50. Yamamoto, A., Mishima, S., Maruyama, N., and Sumita, M., Quantitative evaluation of cell attachment to glass, polystyrene, and fibronectin- or collagen-coated polystyrene by measurement of cell adhesive shear force and cell detachment energy, *J. Biomed. Mater. Res.*, 50(2), 114–124, 2000.
51. Thoumine, O., Ott, A., Cardoso, O., and Meister, J.J., Microplates: a new tool for manipulation and mechanical perturbation of individual cells, *J. Biochem. Biophys. Methods*, 39(1-2), 47–62, 1999.

52. Wendl, M.C., Mathematical analysis of coaxial disk cellular shear loading devices, *Rev. Sci. Instrum.*, 72(11), 4212–4217, 2001.
53. Bundy, K.J., Harris, L.G., Rahn, B.A., and Richards, R.G., Measurement of fibroblast and bacterial detachment from biomaterials using jet impingement, *Cell Biol. Int.*, 25(4), 289–307, 2001.
54. Vunjak-Novakovic, G., Obradovic, B., Martin, I., Bursac, P.M., Langer, R., and Freed, L.E., Dynamic cell seeding of polymer scaffolds for cartilage tissue engineering, *Biotechnol. Prog.*, 14(2), 193–202, 1998.
55. Ting-Beall, H.P., Needham, D., and Hochmuth, R.M., Volume and osmotic properties of human neutrophils, *Blood*, 81(10), 2774–2780, 1993.
56. Jones, W.R., Ting-Beall, H.P., Lee, G.M., Kelley, S.S., Hochmuth, R.M., and Guilak, F., Alterations in the Young's modulus and volumetric properties of chondrocytes isolated from normal and osteoarthritic human cartilage, *J. Biomech.*, 32(2), 119–127, 1999.
57. Koay, E.J., Shieh, A.C., and Athanasiou, K., Creep indentation of single cells, *ASME J. Biomech. Eng.*, submitted.
58. Theret, D.P., Levesque, M.J., Sato, M., Nerem, R.M., and Wheeler, L.T., The application of a homogeneous half-space model in the analysis of endothelial cell micropipette measurements, *J. Biomech. Eng.*, 110(3), 190–199, 1988.
59. Guilak, F., Erickson, G.R., and Ting-Beall, H.P., The effects of osmotic stress on the viscoelastic and physical properties of articular chondrocytes, *Biophys. J.*, 82(2), 720–727, 2002.
60. Hochmuth, R.M., Micropipette aspiration of living cells, *J. Biomech.*, 33(1), 15–22, 2000.
61. Haider, M.A. and Guilak, F., An axisymmetric boundary integral model for incompressible linear viscoelasticity: application to the micropipette aspiration contact problem, *J. Biomech. Eng.*, 122(3), 236–244, 2000.
62. Guilak, F., Alexopoulos, L., Nielsen, R., Ting-Beall, H.P., and Haider, M.A., 0405–The biomechanical properties of the chondrocyte pericellular matrix: micropipette aspiration of mechanically isolated chondrons, in 48th Annual Meeting of the Orthopaedic Research Society, Dallas, 2002.
63. Goldmann, W.H., Galneder, R., Ludwig, M., Kromm, A., and Ezzell, R.M., Differences in F9 and 5.51 cell elasticity determined by cell poking and atomic force microscopy, *FEBS Lett.*, 424(3), 139–142, 1998.
64. Mathur, A.B., Collinsworth, A.M., Reichert, W.M., Kraus, W.E., and Truskey, G.A., Endothelial, cardiac muscle and skeletal muscle exhibit different viscous and elastic properties as determined by atomic force microscopy, *J. Biomech.*, 34(12), 1545–1553, 2001.
65. Charras, G.T., Lehenkari, P.P., and Horton, M.A., Atomic force microscopy can be used to mechanically stimulate osteoblasts and evaluate cellular strain distributions, *Ultramicroscopy*, 86(1-2), 85–95, 2001.
66. Wu, H.W., Kuhn, T., and Moy, V.T., Mechanical properties of L929 cells measured by atomic force microscopy: effects of anticytoskeletal drugs and membrane crosslinking, *Scanning*, 20(5), 389–397, 1998.
67. Yamada, S., Wirtz, D., and Kuo, S.C., Mechanics of living cells measured by laser tracking microrheology, *Biophys. J.*, 78(4), 1736–1747, 2000.
68. Bausch, A.R., Hellerer, U., Essler, M., Aepfelbacher, M., and Sackmann, E., Rapid stiffening of integrin receptor-actin linkages in endothelial cells stimulated with thrombin: a magnetic bead microrheology study, *Biophys. J.*, 80(6), 2649–2657, 2001.
69. Malaviya, P. and Nerem, R.M., Steady shear stress stimulates bovine chondrocyte proliferation in monolayer cultures, in *Proc. 45th Ortho. Res. Soc.*, 1999.
70. Smith, R.L., Donlon, B.S., Gupta, M.K., Mohtai, M., Das, P., Carter, D.R., Cooke, J., Gibbons, G., Hutchinson, N., and Schurman, D.J., Effects of fluid-induced shear on articular chondrocyte morphology and metabolism in vitro, *J. Orthop. Res.*, 13(6), 824–831, 1995.
71. Jin, M., Frank, E.H., Quinn, T.M., Hunziker, E.B., and Grodzinsky, A.J., Tissue shear deformation stimulates proteoglycan and protein biosynthesis in bovine cartilage explants, *Arch. Biochem. Biophys.*, 395(1), 41–48, 2001.

72. Mohtai, M., Gupta, M.K., Donlon, B., Ellison, B., Cooke, J., Gibbons, G., Schurman, D.J., and Smith, R.L., Expression of interleukin-6 in osteoarthritic chondrocytes and effects of fluid-induced shear on this expression in normal human chondrocytes in vitro, *J. Orthop. Res.*, 14(1), 67–73, 1996.
73. Das, P., Schurman, D.J., and Smith, R.L., Nitric oxide and G proteins mediate the response of bovine articular chondrocytes to fluid-induced shear, *J. Orthop. Res.*, 15(1), 87–93, 1997.
74. Millward-Sadler, S.J., Wright, M.O., Davies, L.W., Nuki, G., and Salter, D.M., Mechanotransduction via integrins and interleukin-4 results in altered aggrecan and matrix metalloproteinase 3 gene expression in normal, but not osteoarthritic, human articular chondrocytes, *Arthritis Rheum.*, 43(9), 2091–2099, 2000.
75. Smith, R.L., Trindade, M.C., Ikenoue, T., Mohtai, M., Das, P., Carter, D.R., Goodman, S.B., and Schurman, D.J., Effects of shear stress on articular chondrocyte metabolism, *Biorheology*, 37(1-2), 95–107, 2000.
76. Archambault, J.M., Elfervig-Wall, M.K., Tsuzaki, M., Herzog, W., and Banes, A.J., Rabbit tendon cells produce MMP-3 in response to fluid flow without significant calcium transients, *J. Biomech.*, 35(3), 303–309, 2002.
77. Lee, M.S., Trindade, M.C., Ikenoue, T., Schurman, D.J., Goodman, S.B., and Smith, R.L., Effects of shear stress on nitric oxide and matrix protein gene expression in human osteoarthritic chondrocytes in vitro, *J. Orthop. Res.*, 20(3), 556–561, 2002.
78. Millward-Sadler, S.J., Wright, M.O., Lee, H., Caldwell, H., Nuki, G., and Salter, D.M., Altered electrophysiological responses to mechanical stimulation and abnormal signalling through alpha5beta1 integrin in chondrocytes from osteoarthritic cartilage, *Osteoarthritis Cartilage*, 8(4), 272–278, 2000.
79. Kwon, S.Y., Takei, H., Pioletti, D.P., Lin, T., Ma, Q.J., Akeson, W.H., Wood, D.J., and Sung, K.L., Titanium particles inhibit osteoblast adhesion to fibronectin-coated substrates, *J. Orthop. Res.*, 18(2), 203–211, 2000.
80. Dunkelman, N.S., Zimber, M.P., LeBaron, R.G., Pavelec, R., Kwan, M., and Purchio, A.F., Cartilage production by rabbit articular chondrocytes on polyglycolic acid scaffolds in a closed bioreactor system, *Biotechnol. Bioeng.*, 46(4), 299–305, 1995.
81. Tsao, Y., Boyd, E., Wolf, D.A., and Spaulding, G., Fluid dynamics within a rotating bioreactor in space and earth environments, *J. Spacecraft Rockets*, 31(6), 937–943, 1994.
82. Schmidt, C., Pommerenke, H., Durr, F., Nebe, B., and Rychly, J., Mechanical stressing of integrin receptors induces enhanced tyrosine phosphorylation of cytoskeletally anchored proteins, *J. Biol. Chem.*, 273(9), 5081–5085, 1998.
83. Erickson, G.R., Alexopoulos, L.G., and Guilak, F., Hyper-osmotic stress induces volume change and calcium transients in chondrocytes by transmembrane, phospholipid, and G-protein pathways, *J. Biomech.*, 34(12), 1527–1535, 2001.
84. Mobasheri, A., Carter, S.D., Martin-Vasallo, P., and Shakibaei, M., Integrins and stretch activated ion channels; putative components of functional cell surface mechanoreceptors in articular chondrocytes, *Cell Biol. Int.*, 26(1), 1–18, 2002.

21

Bioactive Scaffold Design for Articular Cartilage Engineering

Eric M. Darling
Rice University

Kyriacos A. Athanasiou
Rice University

CONTENTS

21.1 Introduction

Tissue engineering is increasingly poised to provide more viable alternatives to surgical procedures for the repair of orthopedic defects, such as focal articular cartilage lesions. Cartilage appears to be a relatively simple tissue, yet it is not amenable to regeneration with the techniques available to date. It is alymphatic and aneural, has no contact with blood, and exhibits low cellularity. The main constituents of cartilage are proteoglycans and type II collagen. Many researchers are currently pursuing the goal of creating functional cartilage, both *in vitro* and *in vivo*. By creating a tissue *in vitro*, the time required for healing is decreased, while the probability of a successful recovery is increased. Scaffolds that are designed to be used *in vivo* have the ability to reduce healing time even more dramatically because surgery can be done arthroscopically. However, current injectable materials do not fulfill all the structural and biological conditions needed to function in a mechanically loaded environment.

The physiological loading environment of cartilage in a diarthrodial joint is quite complicated, but one can consider it as consisting primarily of direct compression. As stated in a review by Darling and Athanasiou,[1] loads in the human knee range from 5 to 15 MPa. An implanted scaffold or tissue engineered construct has to be able to withstand these forces until the new tissue is able to support itself. For *in vitro* tissue engineering approaches, the scaffold has to be able to withstand the mechanical environment in which it is cultured, whether that be hydrostatic pressure, direct compression, or just a static environment. In addition to the mechanical constraints, the scaffold has to degrade in such a way that it transfers the load onto the newly formed tissue gradually. This is especially important for *in vivo* applications. The degradation properties as well as the biocompatibility of the degradation products are an important concern when choosing an implant material.

0-8493-1140-3/04/$0.00+$1.50

Cartilage implants or tissue-engineered constructs experience a relatively low immune response in the knee compared to the rest of the body. Since articular cartilage is avascular, there is no simple way for lymphocytes, antigens, and complement proteins to attack the foreign construct. Mild inflammatory responses do occur, though, and a more biocompatible scaffold is always preferred. Biocompatibility, as well as the material properties of the construct, can be controlled based on what components are selected for the scaffold.

In addition to the material's mechanical properties and biocompatibility, a scaffold should elicit a beneficial response from the actual cells. Cell-substrate interactions play an important role in the attachment, viability, and biological response of the cells once they are seeded onto the scaffold. By using a modified scaffold, cells can be guided onto a desired developmental track.

Growth factors and other bioactive agents are increasingly investigated for their ability to stimulate articular cartilage formation *in vitro* and *in vivo*. The addition of these molecules can significantly improve tissue growth, but their incorporation into the scaffold can be a difficult process. Additionally, the activity of a growth factor is usually on the order of days, which restricts its use *in vivo*.

It is the belief of the authors that the ideal scaffold for tissue engineering articular cartilage is obtained by combining bioactive molecules, such as adhesion proteins, peptides, and growth factors, with a mechanically sound scaffold material that has the proper viscoelastic properties, strength, and degradation characteristics. This review will highlight the materials that are most commonly used today for tissue engineering cartilage. Table 21.1 lists representative researchers and their corresponding scaffolds, including any modifications made to the materials using bioactive molecules. A few novel polymers will also be discussed based on their promise as scaffold materials. Surface modification and the incorporation of growth factors will be discussed as an integral part of scaffold design.

21.2 Scaffold Materials

The base scaffold material is the main component when designing a tissue engineering implant. It should fulfill three main requirements: have an interconnected network that allows efficient diffusion of nutrients and room for tissue growth; be biocompatible and bioresorbable, with degradation characteristics that match the rate of new tissue formation; and allow for the attachment, proliferation, and differentiation of chondrocytes that are seeded onto its surface. The last requirement can be fulfilled by using bioactive molecules attached to an inert scaffold, but this option will be discussed later in this review.

Another major concern when making a scaffold is whether it will be used *in vitro* or *in vivo*. If the scaffold is implanted immediately, it must possess the proper mechanical characteristics for the loading environment to retain the implant's shape and partially shield the chondrocytes from the surrounding forces. Injectable scaffold materials have the additional problem of needing to form a mechanically stable implant after entering the body without killing the seeded cells. Typically, injectable materials are photocrosslinked to obtain a high enough stiffness to function under physiological loads, but this process often involves chemicals that are toxic to the cells. Research is ongoing to find a successful approach to this problem.

A cell-seeded scaffold that is cultured *in vitro*, however, does not need extensive structural integrity. Once tissue forms, the engineered construct should have its own mechanical characteristics that do not depend on the partially degraded scaffold. With this approach, the scaffold exists only to support the cells for a period of weeks while new tissue forms. By the time the construct is implanted, the new matrix should be able to function sufficiently under the native loading environment.

Scaffold materials can be sorted into four main categories: natural polymers, synthetic polymers, hydrogels, and composites. There is overlap between the categories, since many natural polymers are hydrogels, and some of those have been used in combination with others to form composite scaffolds. Natural polymers are found in living organisms and can be extracted with relative simplicity. Synthetic polymers are created using chemical processes that are sometimes more complicated, but these polymers are often more conducive to having their material properties changed than natural polymers. Hydrogels can be synthesized, but also occur naturally. They are composed primarily of fluid that significantly swells

TABLE 21.1 Listing of Representative Authors and Their Scaffold Approaches

First Author, Year	Scaffold Material	Protein/Peptide	Growth Factor
Murphy, 2001[2] (*in vitro*)	Alginate		
Mauck, 2000[6] (*in vitro*)	Agarose		
Hunter, 2002[7] (*in vitro*)	Collagen I		
Lee, 2000[8] (*in vitro*)	Collagen II		
Sechriest, 2000[12] (*in vitro*)	Chitosan-GAG		
Silverman, 1999[14] (*in vivo*)	Fibrin glue		
Solchaga, 2000[64] (*in vivo*)	Hyaluronan		
Freed, 1998[29] (*in vitro*)	PGA		
Grande, 1997[28] (*in vitro*)	PLA		
Athanasiou, 1998[20] (review)	PLGA		
Honda, 2000[36] (*in vivo*)	PCL		
Bryant, 2002[49] (*in vitro*)	PEG/PEO		
Suggs, 1999[43] (*in vivo*)	PPF-PEG		
Ameer, 2002[51] (*in vitro*)	Fibrin glue and PLGA		
Marijnissen, 2002[50] (*in vivo*)	Alginate and PLGA		
Bhati, 2001[63] (*in vitro*)	Trimethylene carbonate-PGA	Fibronectin	
Solchaga, 2002[64] (*in vivo*)	Hyaluronan	Fibronectin	
Thomas, 1997[65] (*in vitro*)	Modified quartz (monolayer)	Vitronectin	
Makihira, 1999[66] (*in vitro*)	Plastic (monolayer)	Cartilage matrix protein	
Alsberg, 2001[79] (*in vivo*)	Alginate	RGD (covalent)	
Jo, 2000[69] (*in vitro*)	PPF-PEG	GRGD (covalent)	
Quirk, 2001(*in vitro*)	PLA	RGD (bound to PLL and adsorbed to PLA)	
Carlisle, 2000 (*in vitro*)	PCL and PLLA	RGD (pulsed plasma deposition)	
Eid, 2001[34] (*in vitro*)	PLGA	RGD (adsorption)	
Elisseeff, 2000[47] (*in vitro*)	PEO		TGF-ß (PLGA encapsulated)
Mann, 2001[83] (*in vitro*)	PEG		TGF-ß (tethered)
Athanasiou, 1997[24] (*in vivo*)	PLGA		TGF-ß (physically entrapped)
Toolan, 1996 (*in vitro*)	Collagen I		FGF (soluble)

the polymer network to form a biphasic construct. Composite scaffolds combine two or more materials into one scaffold to take advantage of special characteristics intrinsic to each substance.

New biomaterials are synthesized constantly, but extensive chemical and physical characterization has to be conducted before a material can be used with living cells. The materials summarized in this section have been well characterized and used in experiments involving living cells. Not all have been used with chondrocytes, but their biocompatibility has been proven using other cell types. However, different cells often prefer different materials, and what might work for endothelial cells might not work for chondrocytes. This section summarizes materials that have been used for many tissue engineering applications, so the functional cell type is indicated along with any results.

22.2.1 Natural Polymers

The preference for using natural materials for a scaffold is the belief that many biological materials elicit little or no immune response. Among the natural materials used in cartilage engineering are alginate, agarose, chitosan, fibrin glue, type I and II collagen, and hyaluronic acid-based materials. Each material has its specific advantages, but results vary widely depending on the additional culturing conditions.

Alginate is a polysaccharide extracted from algae and is used to encapsulate cells within the scaffold rather than having them attach to the surface. Encapsulation maintains a chondrocyte's rounded morphology, allowing the redifferentiation of a cell that has been cultured in monolayer.[2] Besides the ability to encapsulate cells, the main advantage to using alginate is its biocompatibility, as reviewed by Hutmacher.[3] For successful use *in vivo*, alginate has to be carefully purified using either filtration, precipitation, or extraction. Alginate grafts have major disadvantages as well. They do not degrade rapidly *in vivo*, which can cause problems as new tissue starts to grow. Long-term implants are not possible because the scaffold loses its functionality within a year.[3] Unlike synthetic polymers, its degradation characteristics cannot be tailored to fit a set timeline.

Agarose is also a polysaccharide but is derived from seaweed and exhibits a temperature-sensitive solubility in water that is used to encapsulate cells.[3] Like alginate, it is biocompatible and provides a three-dimensional environment that helps maintain the chondrocyte's phenotype during culture. Agarose also has degradation properties similar to alginate, thus not allowing control of the scaffold's lifetime in culture. It does not degrade rapidly enough for many *in vitro* experiments. However, several studies have used agarose as a scaffold material when stimulating chondrocytes with direct compression.[4,5] Agarose transmits the applied mechanical forces to the chondrocytes, which stimulates the cells to produce more extracellular matrix proteins than static controls.[6]

One of the most common natural scaffold materials is collagen, specifically type I collagen. Collagen is an extracellular matrix protein that is the major component in connective tissues. It has been studied intensely because of its abundant presence in native tissues. Of course, it has to be purified like most other natural materials to make it less antigenic before it is seeded with chondrocytes. Studies using type I collagen scaffolds in conjunction with direct compression[7] or cross-linked proteoglycans[8,9] showed better results than controls. However, type I collagen scaffolds alone resulted in the dedifferentiation of seeded chondrocytes.[3] Conversely, the use of type II collagen scaffolds helps retain the cells' phenotypes,[10] but fabricating type II collagen scaffolds is a much more difficult and expensive process.

Chitin and chitosan, which are often derived from crab shells, are semicrystalline polymers that have a high degree of biocompatibility *in vivo*, as reviewed by Hutmacher.[3] The molecular structure of chitosan is similar to many glycosaminoglycans (GAGs), which may give it the ability to have interactions with growth factors and adhesion proteins.[3] The degradation characteristics of chitosan are controlled by the degree of deacetylation within the polymer. Unlike alginate and agarose, scaffolds fabricated from chitosan can degrade rapidly *in vivo* depending on the polymer's deacetylation.[3] Researchers can vary the degree of deacetylation to produce a scaffold that degrades over a period of months instead of years so that new tissue can fill the scaffold's space. The porosity can also be controlled, which affects the scaffold's overall strength and elasticity.[11] Studies based on chitosan scaffolds have been conducted with promising results. Sechriest and associates[12] cross-linked chondroitin sulfate with chitosan to form a scaffold that promotes the chondrocytic phenotype when bovine articular chondrocytes were seeded onto it. Endothelial and smooth muscle cell attachment and growth were seen on a dextran sulfate–chitosan composite, heparin-chitosan composite, and chitosan material alone, but a GAG-chitosan composite inhibited attachment and growth.[13] These results indicate that the inclusion of specific proteoglycans in chitosan scaffolds can dramatically change the overall characteristics of the scaffold. As with other biomaterials, chondrocyte response on chitosan has not been well characterized. However, the response of other cell types shows that it could be a beneficial material for articular cartilage engineering.

Fibrin glue has also been used as a carrier for cells. It is often used in conjunction with other scaffold materials, which will be discussed later in Section 21.2.4, "Composite Scaffolds." Fibrin glue is made by mixing fibrinogen with thrombin and allowing it to solidify. This material is advantageous because it is completely biodegradable and can be injected. However, injectable carriers like fibrin glue have little mechanical strength, which is a problem when used in articular cartilage engineering. Researchers have studied chondrocytes in fibrin glue[14] alone and with alginate[15,16] or collagen.[17] Biochemical results did not show a dramatic difference from other scaffold materials.

Hyaluronan (HA) or hyaluronic acid is a polysaccharide that has been used for cartilage engineering applications. HA is a natural material that lubricates articulating joints. It can be cross-linked to form a scaffold that can then be seeded with chondrocytes. One of the main advantages to using HA is that it is also injectable. As with fibrin glue, it can be used in irregularly shaped defects, and implantation is minimally invasive. However, the potential of using hyaluronan as a solid, porous scaffold has also been investigated. Grigolo and associates[18] used a HA-derivative as a prefabricated scaffold *in vivo* and found histological results to be better than controls. Another *in vivo* experiment by Solchaga and associates[19] found that cross-linked HA sponges produced better histological results and integration with the host tissue than benzylated HA, which was, in turn, better than untreated defects.

21.2.2 Synthetic Polymers

Synthetic scaffold materials are man-made polymers that can be fabricated in a laboratory. Unlike natural polymers, synthetics have the advantage of being flexible in varying their physical and chemical properties. The mechanical and degradation characteristics of a polymer can be altered depending on the chemical composition of the macromolecule. This allows researchers the ability to design a scaffold that degrades over a set period, while still retaining a portion of its strength.

The most prevalent synthetic polymers for scaffolding are polyglycolides, polylactides, and their copolymers.[20-25] These polymers can be fabricated as porous scaffolds or nonwoven meshes and felts. Poly-glycolic acid (PGA), probably the most common synthetic polymer used in cartilage engineering, is an alpha polyester that degrades by hydrolytic scission. Total degradation, defined as time to complete mass loss, usually occurs in 4 to 12 months, which is short in comparison to other polyesters used as implants.[26] Its degradation products are naturally resorbed into the body, making it useful as a biocompatible material for many medical applications. PGA has a tensile strength of 57 MPa and a modulus of 6.5 GPa,[26] but these properties do not translate directly to the scaffold stiffness because the material is formed into a mesh or felt instead of a solid structure. PGA has been used extensively as a suture material when copolymerized with polylactic acid (PLA) and also as a tissue engineering scaffold material. It can be fabricated as a porous scaffold through a salt-leaching process that controls the porosity and interconnectivity of the pores. More commonly, PGA is used as a mesh or felt for cartilage engineering purposes. Since PGA is often extruded into thin polymer strands (~13 μm in diameter),[27] it must be molded into nonwoven mesh discs to be used as a scaffold. This provides a highly porous environment in which cells can be seeded. However, the structure of the scaffold prevents its immediate use in loading-bearing environments. Tissue would have to fill much of the void space to give the construct sufficient mechanical integrity. In articular cartilage engineering studies, Grande and associates[28] found that PGA promoted proteoglycan synthesis to a greater extent than PGA/PLA copolymers or collagen matrices. Freed and associates[27,29,30] have also used PGA scaffolds extensively in their research, obtaining good extracellular matrix production along with predictable polymer degradation.

Polylactic acid is another alpha polyester used extensively in the medical field and, as with PGA, has been approved by the FDA for implantation in humans. In general, PLA degrades slower than PGA. Total degradation time for PLA ranges from 12 months to over 2 years.[31] Alone, PLA can have a tensile strength between 11.4 and 72 GPa and a modulus ranging from 0.6 to 4 GPa, depending on which isomer is used in the polymer.[26] PLA exists in two stereoisometric forms, which gives rise to four different types of PLA: poly(D-lactide), poly(L-lactide), poly(D, L-lactide), and poly(meso-lactide).[32] Poly(D,L-lactide) is an amorphous polymer that is used primarily for drug delivery. However, the D and L monomers form semicrystalline polymers, the materials used primarily in cartilage engineering. Like PGA, PLA is used primarily as a nonwoven mesh for tissue engineering applications, although many researchers have investigated porous PLA scaffolds for their application in orthopedics. When observing cell attachment, Ishaug-Riley and associates[33] found that fewer chondrocytes attached to PLLA than to PGA initially, but both surfaces allowed extensive proliferation of the cells, giving similar total cell numbers at confluence.

Polylactic-co-glycolic acid (PLGA) is a copolymer that is composed of varying ratios of PGA and PLA. The material properties of the copolymer can be controlled depending on the ratio of each monomer present in the macromolecule. For example, a 75/25 ratio of PLA/PGA has a degradation time of 4 to 5 months, while a 50/50 ratio of the monomers has a total degradation time of only 1 to 2 months.[31] The modulus of elasticity of these copolymers stays relatively constant at 2 GPa with no major variation due to the monomer ratio.[31] Again, this value is the tensile modulus measured for the solid material, not a scaffold, which would be considerably less stiff. The biocompatibility of PLGA has been proven in numerous clinical trials using it as an implant in large and small animal models.[24,34] Like both PGA and PLA, the copolymer can be fabricated as a nonwoven mesh or felt when used as a cartilage engineering scaffold, as well as a highly porous, solid scaffold. The interconnectivity of the pores, pore size, and void fraction can all be adjusted during the fabrication process to give the construct the proper architecture to function successfully as a tissue engineering scaffold.[35]

Another synthetic polymer that has been used in cartilage engineering is polycaprolactone (PCL). Its degradation and strength characteristics fit well for orthopedic applications, and it also has good biocompatibility. PCL has a tensile strength between 19 and 27 MPa and a modulus of 0.34 GPa[26] and is most commonly formed into a porous scaffold through a salt-leaching process. Like other polyesters, PCL degrades through hydrolytic scission, but it can take as long as 24 months to totally degrade the material.[31] Because of its resistance to rapid hydrolysis, PCL is often copolymerized with other materials to produce the desired degradation characteristics.[33] Honda and associates[36] used poly (L-lactide-epsilon-caprolactone) as a biodegradable sponge that was implanted into nude mice, and after 4 weeks histology data showed the formation of cartilage-like structures in the construct.

A newer trend in synthetic polymers is to control and restrict the attachment of cells and proteins on the scaffold. Polyethylene glycol (PEG), also known as polyethylene oxide (PEO), is a polymer that resists the adsorbance of proteins and cells onto its structure because it is very hydrophilic. By using PEG in a copolymer, researchers can take advantage of this property and control the cell attachment characteristics of the scaffold. The primary reason for using PEG is to enhance the biocompatibility of the copolymer.[37] With increased hydrophilicity, antibodies and other proteins find it difficult to attach to the construct, thereby lessening any immune response. PEG alone has a compressive modulus ranging from 200 to 500 kPa, with the higher modulus corresponding to a higher molecular weight.[38] PEG is versatile in its ability to be copolymerized. Work has been done with PEG-PLA constructs,[39] PEG-poly(propylene fumarate),[37,40-44] PEG dimethacrylate,[45] and lactide-based PEG networks.[45] These copolymers often have better degradation characteristics than PEG alone, while still retaining good biocompatibility. PEG-PPF samples have been found to lose 40 to 60% of their mass in 1 week,[41] whereas PEG does not degrade at all over that duration.[44] For articular cartilage engineering, significant degradation of the scaffold is necessary to provide room for new tissue formation. Oftentimes, copolymerization is the only viable solution when working with specific polymers.

21.2.3 Hydrogels

Hydrogels are a subclass of natural and synthetic polymers that are characterized by being composed mainly of fluid and having a network of polymer chains that allow the macroscopic construct to swell significantly when placed in a polar, liquid solution. Alginate, agarose, and fibrin glue are all natural hydrogels, and many PEG-based polymers are classified as synthetic hydrogels. As stated before, the major characteristic of this subclass of polymers is their ability to swell significantly in water. Hydrogels can have up to 99% water by volume while still retaining their shape. This highly hydrated composition is reminiscent of native articular cartilage, both having a large liquid phase that permeates a solid phase, composed of either polymer or extracellular matrix.

Hydrogels are used in cartilage engineering to encapsulate cells and growth factors in a polymer network (Figure 21.1).[47] This process effectively immobilizes the cells and encourages differentiation in chondrocytes by forcing them to retain a rounded shape. Growth factors that have been encapsulated are present throughout the scaffold, removing any complications that might be present due to concentration gradients in the media. By encapsulating the cells in a polymer matrix, researchers aim to replicate the mechanotransduction present in native cartilage. Meshes and felts do not transmit external loads to the cells in the same way as hydrogels because stress exists only along the fibers if nothing is present in the void spaces. However, hydrogels exert a controlled compressive force on the encapsulated cells that is similar to physiological conditions.[4]

Experiments focusing on the effect of direct compression on chondrocytes most often use agarose or a similar hydrogel.[6,48] The reason for this is twofold. First, dynamic compression is usually conducted at

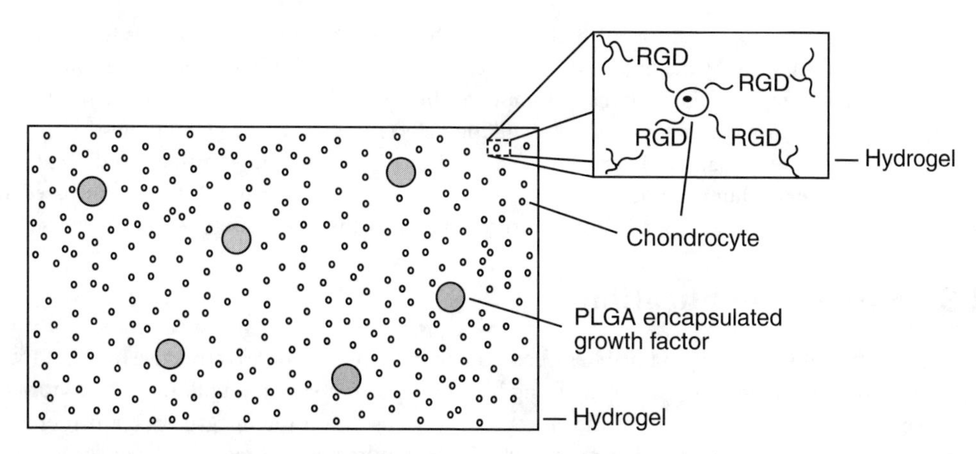

FIGURE 21.1 This is one possible approach to bioactive scaffold design. The base polymer is a hydrogel with RGD covalently attached. PLGA-encapsulated growth factors are dispersed throughout the scaffold. Chondrocytes retain their spherical shape within the hydrogel and are stimulated by the peptides and growth factors.

frequencies of approximately 1 Hz.[1] At this speed, the scaffold material must have sufficient elasticity and recovery from compressive deformation to stay in contact with the loading platen. Hydrogels can easily be fabricated to have this property, whereas a fibrous mesh cannot. Second, as discussed before, the mechanotransduction through a gel may be more similar to native cartilage than other scaffold architectures. Since the overall goal is cartilage regeneration, researchers want to replicate the native loading environment as closely as possible.

Hydrogels are being tested by many researchers for their use in both *in vitro* and *in vivo* cartilage engineering applications.[15,37,41,42,47,49,50] In addition to their suitability for mechanical stimulation studies, hydrogels are ideal as injectable scaffolds because their mass is composed primarily of water.[43] However, major problems still exist when encapsulating cells in a three-dimensional hydrogel. Almost all cross-linking agents are cytotoxic at the levels needed to produce a sufficiently stiff synthetic scaffold. In addition, none of the natural hydrogels have sufficient stiffness to function immediately *in vivo*. The encapsulation process has to be mild enough to have high viability while still producing the necessary mechanical properties. For *in vitro* experiments in general, studies suggest that fibrous, mesh scaffolds support chondrogenesis to a greater degree than hydrogels, indicating that hydrogels might not be the best scaffold material for articular cartilage engineering *in vitro*.[1]

21.2.4 Composite Scaffolds

Composite scaffolds consist of two or more of the previously discussed materials used together to produce a better scaffold. For example, Ameer and associates[51] encapsulated chondrocytes in fibrin glue, which was subsequently used to fill the void volumes of PLGA meshes. This approach produced 2.6 times more GAG (wet weight composition) after 4 weeks than PLGA alone. The authors hypothesized that the fibrin network more effectively retains the GAG within the construct by resisting diffusion out of the construct. However, there was no difference between the amount of collagen in the composite and the PLGA scaffolds.

Marijnissen and associates[52] studied two different composite scaffolds. Cells seeded in alginate were combined with either PLGA or demineralized bone matrix (DBM) and then implanted in nude mice for 8 weeks. Results showed that the PLGA-alginate composite produced type II collagen while the DBM-alginate composite did not. This shows that the type of material used can have an impact on the type of products secreted by the cells. Scaffold materials should be carefully selected based on the tissue that is to be grown. For example, articular cartilage constructs should contain little or no type I collagen, while meniscal cartilage should have mostly type I collagen. Therefore, to achieve articular cartilage regeneration, materials that stimulate type I collagen and not type II collagen should be avoided.

Fibers, either of the same or different bulk material, have also been used in composite scaffolds to improve structural support. Slivka and associates[53] reinforced PLGA with PGA fibers. The compressive modulus and yield strength of the material was improved by up to 20% using this method. Carbon fibers have also been used with satisfactory results for filling defects *in vivo.* Kus and associates[54] implanted carbon fiber scaffolds in human knee defects and had a 71% success rate, while Brittberg and associates[55] used carbon fiber to fill human knee defects and had an 83% success rate. Both studies based the effectiveness of the procedure on qualitative measures of pain at the defect site after several years.

21.3 Surface Modification

The surface of a scaffold can be modified in several ways to make it more or less attractive to cells. Protein coating, peptide attachment, and micropatterning have been used in various applications to control the attachment of cells on a surface. All of these procedures are based on the integrin-receptor properties that exist between cells and extracellular matrix proteins. Chondrocytes express specific integrins, many of which are present on other types of cells.[56] These integrins attach to a corresponding protein, effectively adhering the cell to whatever the protein is adsorbed onto. Studies have shown that $\alpha_1\beta_1$, $\alpha_2\beta_1$, $\alpha_5\beta_1$, $\alpha_V\beta_5$, $\alpha_V\beta_3$, and $\alpha_3\beta_1$ are all integrins that exist on chondrocytes, the latter two being more predominant in the superficial zone of articular cartilage than in the deep zone.[57,58] Modifying biomaterials to take advantage of these integrins allows researchers the ability to control cellular attachment to a scaffold.

21.3.1 Protein Coating

Protein coating is a common method for changing the attachment characteristics of a surface. By using a scaffold material that is hydrophobic, proteins can be readily adsorbed to the surface. The type of coating can affect what cell types attach, along with changing the construct's biocompatibility. The most common adhesion-promoting proteins that are present in the body are collagen, thrombospondin, osteopontin, bone sialoprotein, fibronectin, vitronectin, fibrinogen, von Willebrand factor, laminin, entactin, and tenascin.[56,59] A protein is chosen for surface coating depending on the target cell's integrin receptors. Chondrocytes, based on the integrins present, can attach to collagen, laminin, fibronectin, vitronectin, fibrinogen, bone sialoprotein, thrombospondin, and von Willebrand factor.[60] These extracellular matrix molecules convey mechanical and chemical stimuli in native tissue. Tissue engineered constructs should be able to replicate this function, using either supplemental or naturally secreted proteins. Collagen and fibronectin are the most common proteins used for cartilage applications. The reasoning is that if a scaffold is coated with a specific protein, then only cells that express the corresponding integrin can attach to the surface.

Collagen has been discussed previously as a scaffold material. It is used primarily as the main component of the scaffold and not as a coating. However, monolayer studies have shown that chondrocytes readily attach to collagen surfaces as in native tissue.[61] When type II collagen fragments are introduced to a chondrocyte-on-collagen culture, cell attachment is inhibited, indicating the binding of cell integrins to the fragments rather than the surface.[62] Collagen is much more effective as a matrix material than a coating, so the number of studies on this application is limited.

Extracellular matrix proteins promote the haptotactic and chemotactic motility of chondrocytes, which can be used to increase the migration of cells into a scaffold.[58] Bhati and associates[63] found that cell ingrowth and attachment was increased when a polymer scaffold was coated with fibronectin. The best results came when a coated scaffold was seeded and cultured in a spinner flask, but even under static conditions cell attachment was greater for the coated scaffolds. Solchaga and associates[64] used a hyaluronan scaffold coated with fibronectin as an implant in rabbits and observed total tissue ingrowth into the plug.

Vitronectin has also been studied as a scaffold coating, although focus has been on the attachment of bone-derived cells rather than chondrocytes. Thomas and associates[65] found that vitronectin, not fibronectin, was the protein that controlled osteoblast attachment and spreading. Media without fibronectin had no effect on cell attachment, but media without vitronectin greatly reduced attachment and spreading. Whether this effect holds for chondrocytes has yet to be determined.

A molecule that has not been studied extensively but holds promise as a coating material is cartilage matrix protein (CMP). As reviewed by Makihira and associates,[66] CMP is a noncollagenous protein that is expressed almost exclusively in cartilage. It binds to aggrecan and type II collagen and has been found to involve the $\alpha_1\beta_1$ integrin during chondrocyte adhesion. Makihira and associates[66] studied the adhesion and spreading of chondrocytes on a CMP-coated dish. CMP enhanced both attachment and spreading on the surface, and there was an even more dramatic increase when type II collagen was added to the media. Makihira and associates propose that CMP would be more appropriate in cartilage applications than other proteins because it is specific to chondrocytes.

Protein adsorbance can be varied depending on the type of base material for the scaffold. Unless the protein is cross-linked to the surface, which would likely reduce its effectiveness, it will eventually disassociate from the scaffold. The more hydrophobic the material, the stronger the attachment of the protein, so most base scaffold materials for coating applications are very hydrophobic. For two-dimensional surfaces, the protein adsorbance can be controlled using self-assembled monolayers. The surface chemistry can be varied to produce hydrophobic and hydrophilic regions, which will change the protein adsorbance to the surface.[67] For most three-dimensional applications, the only way to modulate surface adsorbance is to choose an appropriate base material for the scaffold.

For some applications, only two dimensions are needed. As far as cartilage engineering is concerned, a functional scaffold has to be three-dimensional. However, many preliminary experiments are done in monolayer. If the concept of protein coating is taken further, then cell patterns can be made on a material's surface. Areas of the material can be coated while others are left blank. If the underlying material does not promote attachment of cells by itself, then the cells will only attach to the areas that have the protein. This concept can be implemented using full proteins, but more often short peptide sequences are used instead.

21.3.2 Peptide Attachment

Peptides are short amino acid sequences derived from large, adhesion proteins. The reason cells attach to a protein-coated surface is because of amino acid recognition sequences located in the protein structure. Researchers have determined which sequences are recognized by cells and use that knowledge to create scaffolds incorporating peptide sequences instead of full proteins. The major advantage of this technique is that a peptide can be permanently attached to a material without seriously affecting its function. Proteins on the other hand can lift off from a surface in an unpredictable manner. In general, the attachment and surface properties of a biomaterial can be strictly controlled using peptides instead of full proteins.

A peptide is most often bound to a material using a covalent bond. This securely attaches the sequence to the surface, assuring localized effects due to the peptide. One problem that can occur is a reduction in peptide activity. By attaching the peptide to a linker chain, it can be moved away from the surface of the material and allowed more flexibility in its function.[56] The biomaterials chosen as base scaffolds often have properties that inhibit the adherence of cells and proteins. This forces the attachment characteristics of the material to be totally dependent on the bound peptides. However, the steric hindrance of the base material requires peptides to be far enough away from the surface for binding between cellular integrins and peptides to occur.

Another design parameter is the density of peptides on the material. Increasing the concentration of peptides will increase cellular attachment, but it will also decrease cell motility on the scaffold.[56] A balance between promoting attachment and allowing cell motility has to be found for specific cell types and applications. Migration of cells into a material will not occur if the peptide concentrations are too high. However, a migration response to extracellular matrix proteins can be mediated by clustering integrins on the material.[58] This approach can be useful if an implant wants to encourage the ingrowth of native cells.

The most common peptide sequence used for cell attachment is Arg-Gly-Asp (RGD), which corresponds to a portion of the fibronectin protein.[56] It is present in many species of both plants and animals, which hints at its longevity in biological life.[68] RGD is useful in tissue engineering because it has an almost generic attachment with many integrins. Of the 20 known integrins, 8 to 12 of them recognize the RGD sequence in their ligands.[59] In chondrocytes, RGD binds strongly to $\alpha_5\beta_1$, $\alpha_V\beta_5$, and $\alpha_V\beta_3$ and weakly to $\alpha_3\beta_1$. This corresponds with both the superficial and deep zone chondrocytes present in cartilage.

Many peptides used for tissue engineering incorporate the RGD sequence but are more than three amino acids long. Researchers have used peptide sequences such as G**RGD**,[69] G**RGD**SP,[70] and CGGNGEPRGDTYRAY[71] to utilize the benefits of the RGD sequence. A peptide is chosen based on what protein it is modeled after (the last sequence is from bone sialoprotein) and how it will be attached to the scaffold. For example, a short peptide sequence like GRGD can be used on the end of hydrophilic spacers when modifying a hydrophobic bulk material.[69]

Various attachment peptides have been studied extensively for use in tissue engineering and drug delivery applications. Some of the recognition sequences that have known activities are: KGD ($\alpha_{IIb}\beta_3$), PECAM ($\alpha_V\beta_3$), KQAGDV ($\alpha_{IIb}\beta_3$), LDV ($\alpha_4\beta_1$ and $\alpha_4\beta_7$), YGYYGDALR and FYFDLR ($\alpha_2\beta_1$), and RLD/KRLDGS ($\alpha_V\beta_3$ and $\alpha_M\beta_2$).[59,68,72] Other peptide sequences have been studied, but specific integrin relationships were not found. For chondrocytes, the functional sequences of those listed (not including RGD) are PECAM, YGYYGDALR, FYFDLR, and RLD/KRLDGS with weak binding occurring with KQAGDV and LDV.[59]

The attachment of peptides to a biomaterial can be controlled to form desired patterns on the surface. This process is known as micropatterning and has been used for attachment studies in monolayer.[73-76] The peptides are bound to the surface in such a way as to restrict either a single cell's shape or a community of cells' pattern. Areas that have the peptide will allow integrin binding, while blank areas will not allow cell attachment. If the peptides are cell specific, then different regions will promote attachment for different cells.

Micropatterning is often used to control the shape of a cell by restricting the degree of spreading. A cell's shape governs whether it will grow, die, or differentiate.[76] When a cell spreads more, there is an increase in cell survival and proliferation, but when a cell cannot spread and balls up on a surface, it enters apoptosis and dies. A patterned surface that supports neither growth nor apoptosis will induce the cells to differentiate.[75] A cell at this stage will express proteins and produce extracellular matrix in greater amounts than in either other state. Physically, the spreading is controlled by placing spacer ligands apart at different distances. The cell will spread further if the ligands are spaced apart than if they are grouped in one small clump. If the spacers are too far apart, then the cells will not spread because the focal adhesions cannot be made.

Proliferation is controlled in the same manner. If the peptide concentration is too high, then the cells do not move apart because they are bound too tightly to the surface, leaving little room for cells produced through division. If the peptide concentration is too low, then the cells still cannot migrate because there is no place to form focal adhesions, resulting in overcrowding like before. A balance has to be found to allow sufficient migration of the cells over the entire surface.

Although the majority of peptide studies have been conducted on two-dimensional surfaces, there is evidence suggesting that peptides are also beneficial in three-dimensional scaffolds.[77,78] Alginate that contained the RGD peptide promoted cell adhesion and spreading as well as increased differentiation compared to controls.[79] However, Mann and associates[80,81] found that PEG hydrogels modified with adhesion peptides decreased proliferation throughout the construct and decreased extracellular matrix secretions as well. However, this result could be caused by using too high a concentration of peptides. Future research can investigate this hypothesis. Unlike hydrogels, porous scaffolds have surfaces that can be modified similarly to two-dimensional materials. Research on the benefits of peptides in these situations is limited, but it appears that it would be just as beneficial as in two dimensions.

21.4 Growth Factor Inclusion

Another way that a scaffold can be modified is to include growth factors (GFs). Proteins such as TGF-β, IGF, PDGF, HGF, and FGF all produce an effect on the proliferation and differentiation of chondrocytes. These proteins will likely be required to engineer functional articular cartilage. GFs stimulate cells to secrete extracellular matrix in greater amounts than without them. For example, Bonnassar and associates[82] used IGF-I to increase protein and proteoglycan synthesis in cartilage explants 90 and 120%, respectively. Other experiments confirm the dramatic effect of GFs on extracellular matrix synthesis in explants and cell-seeded constructs.

The results due to GFs make their use a certainty in future cartilage engineering studies. Problems arise, however, when attempting to include GFs in a cartilage scaffold. In *in vitro* experiments, GFs can be added to the media to stimulate the cells, but under *in vivo* conditions GFs must somehow be incorporated into the scaffold for extended effects. The *in vitro* experiments might also benefit from the inclusion of GFs in the scaffold because stimulants would be dispersed evenly throughout the construct, whereas before, diffusion might keep a significant amount of the GFs outside the scaffold.

There are three main methods of GF inclusion: encapsulation, covalent bonding, and in solution. Encapsulation requires the use of a hydrogel as either the entire scaffold or as a GF carrier. This means that the whole construct can be made of the same hydrogel, such as alginate or PEG, or only one component of a composite scaffold is a hydrogel, such as using alginate gel in a PGA felt. Nonhydrogel scaffolds by themselves usually have too high of porosity to effectively retain GFs in the construct, but Athanasiou and associates[24] used physical entrapment to load TGF-β into PLGA scaffolds (65 to 75% porous) and obtained positive results. The most common method of including a GF in a hydrogel is to load it into a microparticle and then encapsulate the microparticle in the hydrogel.[47] The protein is released into the hydrogel in a predictable fashion, thereby stimulating the chondrocytes seeded in the scaffold. Microparticle encapsulation can also be used in fibrous scaffolds as a form of GF delivery.

Covalent bonding is another way to include a GF in a scaffold. Immobilizing proteins often decreases their effectiveness because access to the active regions of the molecule is restricted, but Mann and associates[83] covalently bonded TGF-β1 to PEG and found no decrease in its ability to stimulate the cells. This approach appears to be an effective method for physical inclusion of the GF in the scaffold if the material is not a hydrogel. The difficulty lies in attaching GFs to various base materials while not losing their activity and ability to affect matrix synthesis.

Including GFs in the media solution is the most common and simplest method of stimulation for *in vitro* experiments. This approach obviously would not work for an *in vivo* study. The GF is added in controlled amounts to the media and replaced along with the media. The activity of the GF does not decrease because it is continuously replaced, which is not the case in the other two methods. However, a larger amount of GF is used because of its continuous replenishment, making this approach expensive for use in large, fluid-dominated bioreactors.

Including GFs in the articular cartilage engineering process is undoubtedly a must, but it still remains to be seen which GFs are best for chondrogenesis. Certain GFs might stimulate proliferation, while others promote synthesis of the various extracellular molecules. Blunk and associates[84] found that IGF-I increased GAG fractions, TGF-β1 increased total collagen, and IL-4 minimized the GAG-depleted region on an engineered construct's surface. It is possible that several GFs will be necessary to encourage seeded chondrocytes into producing native levels of extracellular matrix. Whether they are included in solution, encapsulated in a gel, or covalently bonded to a scaffold, growth factors have to be a part of bioactive scaffold design.

21.5 Conclusion

The creation of a bioactive scaffold will increase the chances of producing a functional articular cartilage construct *in vitro* or *in vivo*. By controlling the attachment of cells and stimulating their differentiation, scaffolds can promote the formation of the correct type of tissue in the correct location. Initially, the materials have to be chosen based on the characteristics that are desired. Degradation time, strength, and elasticity are physical properties that can be controlled by using various base materials for the scaffold. To a limited degree, attachment and differentiation can also be affected by the scaffold material. However, the surface properties are more effective when the biomaterial is modified with proteins or peptides. Biocompatibility and cell attachment are two major benefits to altering the surface of the scaffold. Some results also indicate an effect on proliferation and differentiation. To get the most out of the seeded cells, growth factors should be included in the scaffold design. They can be added as a supplement in the media, but incorporating them into the actual scaffold will assure an interaction between the growth factors and the cells. The combinations and permutations available between the different parameters described in this paper leave plenty of room for future research. By using the proper combination of scaffold components, researchers will move closer to the goal of successfully engineering a functional articular cartilage construct.

Acknowledgment

This work was funded in part by NSF-IGERT Grant DGE-0114264.

References

1. Darling, E.M. and Athanasiou, K.A., Articular cartilage bioreactors and bioprocesses, *Tissue Eng.*, manuscript accepted.
2. Murphy, C.L. and Sambanis, A., Effect of oxygen tension and alginate encapsulation on restoration of the differentiated phenotype of passaged chondrocytes, *Tissue Eng.*, 7, 791, 2001.
3. Hutmacher, D.W., Scaffold design and fabrication technologies for engineering tissues — state of the art and future perspectives, *J. Biomater. Sci. Polym. Ed.*, 12, 107, 2001.
4. Saris, D.B., Mukherjee, N., Berglund, L.J., Schultz, F.M., An, K.N., and O'Driscoll, S.W., Dynamic pressure transmission through agarose gels, *Tissue Eng.*, 6, 531, 2000.
5. Elder, S.H., Goldstein, S.A., Kimura, J.H., Soslowsky, L.J., and Spengler, D.M., Chondrocyte differentiation is modulated by frequency and duration of cyclic compressive loading, *Ann. Biomed. Eng.*, 29, 476, 2001.
6. Mauck, R.L., Soltz, M.A., Wang, C.C., Wong, D.D., Chao, P.H., Valhmu, W.B., Hung, C.T., and Ateshian, G.A., Functional tissue engineering of articular cartilage through dynamic loading of chondrocyte-seeded agarose gels, *J. Biomech. Eng.*, 122, 252, 2000.
7. Hunter, C.J., Imler, S.M., Malaviya, P., Nerem, R.M., and Levenston, M.E., Mechanical compression alters gene expression and extracellular matrix synthesis by chondrocytes cultured in collagen I gels, *Biomaterials,* 23, 1249, 2002.
8. Lee, C.R., Breinan, H.A., Nehrer, S., and Spector, M., Articular cartilage chondrocytes in type I and type II collagen-GAG matrices exhibit contractile behavior *in vitro, Tissue Eng.,* 6, 555, 2000.
9. van Susante, J.L.C., Pieper, J., Buma, P., van Kuppevelt, T.H., van Beuningen, H., van Der Kraan, P.M., Veerkamp, J.H., van den Berg, W.B., and Veth, R.P.H., Linkage of chondroitin-sulfate to type I collagen scaffolds stimulates the bioactivity of seeded chondrocytes *in vitro, Biomaterials,* 22, 2359, 2001.
10. Nehrer, S., Breinan, H.A., Ramappa, A., Shortkroff, S., Young, G., Minas, T., Sledge, C.B., Yannas, I.V., and Spector, M., Canine chondrocytes seeded in type I and type II collagen implants investigated *in vitro, J. Biomed. Mater. Res.,* 38, 95, 1997.
11. Madihally, S.V. and Matthew, H.W., Porous chitosan scaffolds for tissue engineering, *Biomaterials,* 20, 1133, 1999.
12. Sechriest, V.F., Miao, Y.J., Niyibizi, C., Westerhausen-Larson, A., Matthew, H.W., Evans, C.H., Fu, F.H., and Suh, J.K., GAG-augmented polysaccharide hydrogel: a novel biocompatible and biodegradable material to support chondrogenesis, *J. Biomed. Mater. Res.,* 49, 534, 2000.

5. Zeltinger, J., Sherwood, J. K., Graham, D.A., Mueller, R., and Griffith, L.G., Effect of pore size and void fraction on cellular adhesion, proliferation, and matrix deposition, *Tissue Eng.*, 7, 557, 2001.
36. Honda, M., Yada, T., Ueda, M., and Kimata, K., Cartilage formation by cultured chondrocytes in a new scaffold made of poly(L-lactide-epsilon-caprolactone) sponge, *J. Oral Maxillofac. Surg.*, 58, 767, 2000.
37. Suggs, L.J., Shive, M.S., Garcia, C.A., Anderson, J.M., and Mikos, A.G., In vitro cytotoxicity and in vivo biocompatibility of poly(propylene fumarate-co-ethylene glycol) hydrogels, *J. Biomed. Mater. Res.*, 46, 22, 1999.
38. Zimmermann, J., Bittner, K., Stark, B., and Mulhaupt, R., Novel hydrogels as supports for *in vitro* cell growth: poly(ethylene glycol)- and gelatine-based (meth)acrylamidopeptide macromonomers, *Biomaterials,* 23, 2127, 2002.
39. Anseth, K.S., Metters, A.T., Bryant, S.J., Martens, P.J., Elisseeff, J.H., and Bowman, C.N., In situ forming degradable networks and their application in tissue engineering and drug delivery, *J. Control Release,* 78, 199, 2002.
40. Fisher, J.P., Vehof, J.W., Dean, D., van der Waerden, J.P., Holland, T.A., Mikos, A.G., and Jansen, J.A., Soft and hard tissue response to photocrosslinked poly(propylene fumarate) scaffolds in a rabbit model, *J. Biomed. Mater. Res.*, 59, 547, 2002.
41. Suggs, L.J., Krishnan, R.S., Garcia, C.A., Peter, S.J., Anderson, J.M., and Mikos, A.G., In vitro and in vivo degradation of poly(propylene fumarate-co-ethylene glycol) hydrogels, *J. Biomed. Mater. Res.*, 42, 312, 1998.
42. Suggs, L.J., Kao, E.Y., Palombo, L.L., Krishnan, R.S., Widmer, M.S., and Mikos, A.G., Preparation and characterization of poly(propylene fumarate-co-ethylene glycol) hydrogels, *J. Biomater. Sci. Polym. Ed.*, 9, 653, 1998.
43. Suggs, L.J. and Mikos, A.G. Development of poly(propylene fumarate-co-ethylene glycol) as an injectable carrier for endothelial cells, *Cell Transplant*, 8, 345, 1999.
44. Temenoff, J.S., Athanasiou, K.A., Lebaron, R.G., and Mikos, A.G., Effect of poly(ethylene glycol) molecular weight on tensile and swelling properties of oligo(poly(ethylene glycol) fumarate) hydrogels for cartilage tissue engineering, *J. Biomed. Mater. Res.*, 59, 429, 2002.
45. Bryant, S.J. and Anseth, K.S., The effects of scaffold thickness on tissue engineered cartilage in photocrosslinked poly(ethylene oxide) hydrogels, *Biomaterials,* 22, 619, 2001.
46. Han, D.K., Park, K.D., Hubbell, J.A., and Kim, Y.H., Surface characteristics and biocompatibility of lactide-based poly(ethylene glycol) scaffolds for tissue engineering, *J. Biomater. Sci. Polym. Ed.*, 9, 667, 1998.
47. Elisseeff, J., McIntosh, W., Anseth, K., Riley, S., Ragan, P., and Langer, R., Photoencapsulation of chondrocytes in poly(ethylene oxide)-based semi-interpenetrating networks, *J. Biomed. Mater. Res.*, 51, 164, 2000.
48. Buschmann, M.D., Gluzband, Y.A., Grodzinsky, A.J., and Hunziker, E.B., Mechanical compression modulates matrix biosynthesis in chondrocyte/agarose culture, *J. Cell Sci.*, 108, 1497, 1995.
49. Bryant, S.J. and Anseth, K.S., Hydrogel properties influence ECM production by chondrocytes photoencapsulated in poly(ethylene glycol) hydrogels, *J. Biomed. Mater. Res.*, 59, 63, 2002.
50. Marijnissen, W.J., van Osch, G.J., Aigner, J., van der Veen, S.W., Hollander, A.P., Verwoerd-Verhoef, H.L., and Verhaar, J.A., Alginate as a chondrocyte-delivery substance in combination with a non-woven scaffold for cartilage tissue engineering, *Biomaterials,* 23, 1511, 2002.
51. Ameer, G.A., Mahmood, T.A., and Langer, R., A biodegradable composite scaffold for cell transplantation, *J. Orthop. Res.*, 20, 16, 2002.
52. Marijnissen, W.J., van Osch, G.J., Aigner, J., Verwoerd-Verhoef, H.L., and Verhaar, J.A., Tissue-engineered cartilage using serially passaged articular chondrocytes. Chondrocytes in alginate, combined in vivo with a synthetic (E210) or biologic biodegradable carrier (DBM), *Biomaterials,* 21, 571, 2000.
53. Slivka, M.A., Leatherbury, N.C., Kieswetter, K., and Niederauer, G.G., Porous, resorbable, fiber-reinforced scaffolds tailored for articular cartilage repair, *Tissue Eng.*, 7, 767, 2001.

13. Chupa, J.M., Foster, A.M., Sumner, S.R., Madihally, S.V., and Matthew, H.W., V
to polysaccharide materials: *in vitro* and *in vivo* evaluations, *Biomaterials,* 21,
14. Silverman, R.P., Passaretti, D., Huang, W., Randolph, M.A., and Yaremchuk, M.J
engineered cartilage using a fibrin glue polymer, *Plast. Reconstr. Surg.*, 103, 1809
15. Almqvist, K.F., Wang, L., Wang, J., Baeten, D., Cornelissen, M., Verdonk, R.,
Verbruggen, G., Culture of chondrocytes in alginate surrounded by fibrin gel: ch
the cells over a period of eight weeks, *Ann. Rheum. Dis.*, 60, 781, 2001.
16. Perka, C., Arnold, U., Spitzer, R.S., and Lindenhayn, K., The use of fibrin beads for
neering and subsequential transplantation, *Tissue Eng.*, 7, 359, 2001.
17. Perka, C., Schultz, O., Lindenhayn, K., Spitzer, R.S., Muschik, M., Sittinger, M., and
G.R., Joint cartilage repair with transplantation of embryonic chondrocytes embedded in
fibrin matrices, *Clin. Exp. Rheumatol.*, 18, 13, 2000.
18. Grigolo, B., Roseti, L., Fiorini, M., Fini, M., Giavaresi, G., Aldini, N.N., Giardino, R., and Fa
A., Transplantation of chondrocytes seeded on a hyaluronan derivative (hyaff-11) into car
defects in rabbits, *Biomaterials,* 22, 2417, 2001.
19. Solchaga, L.A., Yoo, J.U., Lundberg, M., Dennis, J.E., Huibregtse, B.A., Goldberg, V.M., and Cap
A.I., Hyaluronan-based polymers in the treatment of osteochondral defects, *J. Orthop. Res.*,
773, 2000.
20. Athanasiou, K.A., Agrawal, C.M., Barber, F.A., and Burkhart, S.S., Orthopaedic applications for
PLA-PGA biodegradable polymers, *Arthroscopy,* 14, 726, 1998.
21. Athanasiou, K.A., Niederauer, G.G., Agrawal, C.M., and Landsman, A.S., Applications of biodegradable lactides and glycolides in podiatry, *Clin. Podiatr. Med. Surg.*, 12, 475, 1995.
22. Athanasiou, K.A., Singhal, A.R., Agrawal, C.M., and Boyan, B.D., In vitro degradation and release characteristics of biodegradable implants containing trypsin inhibitor, *Clin. Orthop.*, 272, 1995.
23. Athanasiou, K.A., Niederauer, G.G., and Agrawal, C.M., Sterilization, toxicity, biocompatibility and clinical applications of polylactic acid/polyglycolic acid copolymers, *Biomaterials,* 17, 93, 1996.
24. Athanasiou, K.A., Korvick, D., and Schenck, R.C., Biodegradable implants for the treatment of osteochondral defects in a goat model, *Tissue Eng.*, 3, 363, 1997.
25. Vunjak-Novakovic, G. and Freed, L.E., Culture of organized cell communities, *Adv. Drug Deliv. Rev.*, 33, 15, 1998.
26. Daniels, A.U., Chang, M.K., and Andriano, K.P., Mechanical properties of biodegradable polymers and composites proposed for internal fixation of bone, *J. Appl. Biomater.*, 1, 57, 1990.
27. Freed, L.E., Grande, D.A., Lingbin, Z., Emmanual, J., Marquis, J.C., and Langer, R., Joint resurfacing using allograft chondrocytes and synthetic biodegradable polymer scaffolds, *J. Biomed. Mater. Res.*, 28, 891, 1994.
28. Grande, D.A., Halberstadt, C., Naughton, G., Schwartz, R., and Manji, R., Evaluation of matrix scaffolds for tissue engineering of articular cartilage grafts, *J. Biomed. Mater. Res.*, 34, 211, 1997.
29. Freed, L.E., Hollander, A.P., Martin, I., Barry, J.R., Langer, R., and Vunjak-Novakovic, G., Chondrogenesis in a cell-polymer-bioreactor system, *Exp. Cell Res.*, 240, 58, 1998.
30. Freed, L.E., Vunjak-Novakovic, G., and Langer, R., Cultivation of cell-polymer cartilage implants in bioreactors, *J. Cell Biochem.*, 51, 257, 1993.
31. Middleton, J.C. and Tipton, A.J., Synthetic biodegradable polymers as orthopedic devices, *Biomaterials,* 21, 2335, 2000.
32. Hutmacher, D.W., Goh, J. C., and Teoh, S.H., An introduction to biodegradable materials for tissue engineering applications, *Ann. Acad. Med. Singapore,* 30, 183, 2001.
33. Ishaug-Riley, S.L., Okun, L.E., Prado, G., Applegate, M.A., and Ratcliffe, A., Human articular chondrocyte adhesion and proliferation on synthetic biodegradable polymer films, *Biomaterials,* 20, 2245, 1999.
34. Eid, K., Chen, E., Griffith, L., and Glowacki, J., Effect of RGD coating on osteocompatibility of PLGA-polymer disks in a rat tibial wound, *J. Biomed. Mater. Res.*, 57, 224, 2001.

54. Kus, W.M., Gorecki, A., Strzelczyk, P., and Swiader, P., Carbon fiber scaffolds in the surgical treatment of cartilage lesions, *Ann. Transplant.*, 4, 101, 1999.
55. Brittberg, M., Faxen, E., and Peterson, L., Carbon fiber scaffolds in the treatment of early knee osteoarthritis. A prospective 4-year followup of 37 patients, *Clin. Orthop.*, 155, 1994.
56. LeBaron, R.G. and Athanasiou, K.A., Extracellular matrix cell adhesion peptides: functional applications in orthopedic materials, *Tissue Eng.*, 6, 85, 2000.
57. Woods, V.L., Jr., Schreck, P.J., Gesink, D.S., Pacheco, H.O., Amiel, D., Akeson, W.H., and Lotz, M., Integrin expression by human articular chondrocytes, *Arthritis Rheum.*, 37, 537, 1994.
58. Shimizu, M., Minakuchi, K., Kaji, S., and Koga, J., Chondrocyte migration to fibronectin, type I collagen, and type II collagen, *Cell Struct. Funct.*, 22, 309, 1997.
59. Ruoslahti, E., RGD and other recognition sequences for integrins, *Annu. Rev. Cell Dev. Biol.*, 12, 697, 1996.
60. Hubbell, J.A., Matrix effects, in *Principles of Tissue Engineering*, Lanza, R., Langer, R., and Chick, W., Eds., R.G. Landes Company, Austin, 1997.
61. Lee, V., Cao, L., Zhang, Y., Kiani, C., Adams, M.E., and Yang, B.B., The roles of matrix molecules in mediating chondrocyte aggregation, attachment, and spreading, *J. Cell Biochem.*, 79, 322, 2000.
62. Jennings, L., Wu, L., King, K.B., Hammerle, H., Cs-Szabo, G., and Mollenhauer, J., The effects of collagen fragments on the extracellular matrix metabolism of bovine and human chondrocytes, *Connect. Tissue Res.*, 42, 71, 2001.
63. Bhati, R.S., Mukherjee, D.P., McCarthy, K.J., Rogers, S.H., Smith, D.F., and Shalaby, S.W., The growth of chondrocytes into a fibronectin-coated biodegradable scaffold, *J. Biomed. Mater. Res.*, 56, 74, 2001.
64. Solchaga, L.A., Gao, J., Dennis, J.E., Awadallah, A., Lundberg, M., Caplan, A.I., and Goldberg, V.M., Treatment of osteochondral defects with autologous bone marrow in a hyaluronan-based delivery vehicle, *Tissue Eng.*, 8, 333, 2002.
65. Thomas, C.H., McFarland, C.D., Jenkins, M.L., Rezania, A., Steele, J.G., and Healy, K.E., The role of vitronectin in the attachment and spatial distribution of bone-derived cells on materials with patterned surface chemistry, *J. Biomed. Mater. Res.*, 37, 81, 1997.
66. Makihira, S., Yan, W., Ohno, S., Kawamoto, T., Fujimoto, K., Okimura, A., Yoshida, E., Noshiro, M., Hamada, T., and Kato, Y., Enhancement of cell adhesion and spreading by a cartilage-specific noncollagenous protein, cartilage matrix protein (CMP/Matrilin-1), via integrin alpha1beta1, *J. Biol. Chem.*, 274, 11417, 1999.
67. Prime, K.L. and Whitesides, G.M., Self-assembled organic monolayers: model systems for studying adsorption of proteins at surfaces, *Science*, 252, 1164, 1991.
68. Koivunen, E., Wang, B., Dickinson, C.D., and Ruoslahti, E., Peptides in cell adhesion research, *Methods Enzymol.*, 245, 346, 1994.
69. Jo, S., Engel, P.S., and Mikos, A.G., Synthesis of poly(ethylene glycol)-tethered poly(propylene fumarate) and its modification with GRGD peptide, *Polymer*, 41, 7595, 2000.
70. Pierschbacher, M.D. and Ruoslahti, E., Variants of the cell recognition site of fibronectin that retain attachment-promoting activity, *Proc. Natl. Acad. Sci. U.S.A.*, 81, 5985, 1984.
71. Rezania, A., Thomas, C.H., Branger, A.B., Waters, C.M., and Healy, K.E., The detachment strength and morphology of bone cells contacting materials modified with a peptide sequence found within bone sialoprotein, *J. Biomed. Mater. Res.*, 37, 9, 1997.
72. Pasqualini, R., Koivunen, E., and Ruoslahti, E., Peptides in cell adhesion: powerful tools for the study of integrin-ligand interactions, *Braz. J. Med. Biol. Res.*, 29, 1151, 1996.
73. Britland, S., Clark, P., Connolly, P., and Moores, G., Micropatterned substratum adhesiveness: a model for morphogenetic cues controlling cell behavior, *Exp. Cell Res.*, 198, 124, 1992.
74. Lom, B., Healy, K.E., and Hockberger, P.E., A versatile technique for patterning biomolecules onto glass coverslips, *J. Neurosci. Methods*, 50, 385, 1993.
75. Dike, L.E., Chen, C.S., Mrksich, M., Tien, J., Whitesides, G.M., and Ingber, D.E., Geometric control of switching between growth, apoptosis, and differentiation during angiogenesis using micropatterned substrates, *In Vitro Cell Dev. Biol. Anim.*, 35, 441, 1999.

76. Chen, C.S., Mrksich, M., Huang, S., Whitesides, G.M., and Ingber, D.E., Geometric control of cell life and death, *Science*, 276, 1425, 1997.
77. Mann, B.K., Gobin, A.S., Tsai, A.T., Schmedlen, R.H., and West, J.L., Smooth muscle cell growth in photopolymerized hydrogels with cell adhesive and proteolytically degradable domains: synthetic ECM analogs for tissue engineering, *Biomaterials*, 22, 3045, 2001.
78. Gobin, A.S. and West, J.L., Cell migration through defined, synthetic ECM analogs, *FASEB J.*, 16, 751, 2002.
79. Alsberg, E., Anderson, K.W., Albeiruti, A., Franceschi, R.T., and Mooney, D.J., Cell-interactive alginate hydrogels for bone tissue engineering, *J. Dent. Res.*, 80, 2025, 2001.
80. Mann, B.K. and West, J. L. Cell adhesion peptides alter smooth muscle cell adhesion, proliferation, migration, and matrix protein synthesis on modified surfaces and in polymer scaffolds, *J. Biomed. Mater. Res.*, 60, 86, 2002.
81. Mann, B.K., Tsai, A.T., Scott-Burden, T., and West, J.L., Modification of surfaces with cell adhesion peptides alters extracellular matrix deposition, *Biomaterials*, 20, 2281, 1999.
82. Bonassar, L.J., Grodzinsky, A.J., Frank, E.H., Davila, S.G., Bhaktav, N.R., and Trippel, S.B., The effect of dynamic compression on the response of articular cartilage to insulin-like growth factor-I, *J. Orthop. Res.*, 19, 11, 2001.
83. Mann, B.K., Schmedlen, R.H., and West, J.L., Tethered-TGF-beta increases extracellular matrix production of vascular smooth muscle cells, *Biomaterials*, 22, 439, 2001.
84. Blunk, T., Sieminski, A.L., Gooch, K.J., Courter, D.L., Hollander, A.P., Nahir, A.M., Langer, R., Vunjak-Novakovic, G., and Freed, L.E., Differential effects of growth factors on tissue-engineered cartilage, *Tissue Eng.*, 8, 73, 2002.

V

Interventional Disease Treatment

Contributions of Technology to Direct Disease Treatment

The role of technology in health care certainly goes far beyond the initial diagnosis of disease. It is only basic human nature to desire to fix a problem once it has been identified. Exciting new technologies for the direct treatment of disease have thus been readily accepted.

There is perhaps no direct healthcare interface with a higher need for reliable technology development than the surgical suite. The act of entering the human body for direct manipulation cannot be undertaken without tremendous care. A wide variety of technologies have made surgical procedures more reliable, less traumatic, and shorter in duration. The savings in mortality and morbidity are added to the direct savings from less expensive procedures.

The nature of any surgical procedure requires constant monitoring of the patient during and after the procedure. While reliable monitoring technologies have allowed the surgeon to pay more attention to the procedure itself, human observation is still required. This has resulted in an interesting hybrid of automated devices that provide constant feedback and controllability of anesthetics.

Advances in materials know-how have led to the development of fantastic technologies that allow for the minimally invasive treatment of a variety of diseases. The ability to design miniature devices that are deployed via small catheters has revolutionized patient care. Procedures that once took hours of highly invasive surgery and required weeks of recovery are now being replaced with nearly outpatient-delivered procedures. The pharmaceutical industry has been quick to adapt many of the technologies presented in other sections of this book to develop new medicines. New chemical pathways to attack disease are being identified and applied with astonishing results.

The continued development of treatment technologies will provide tremendous benefits for patients in terms of improved safety, shorter hospital stay, improved post-procedure care, and faster recovery; while at the same time healthcare providers will enjoy the benefits of increased efficiency, reliability, and speed.

This section includes the following chapters:

22

Anesthesia/Monitoring Devices

Spencer Kee
M.D. Anderson Cancer Center

CONTENTS

22.1 Technical Background

The conduct of safe anesthesia relies upon adequate monitoring of the patient. This is crucial as the patient is unable to communicate when under general anesthesia. Vital parameters such as pulse rate and blood pressure are affected by the patient's condition, the surgery being performed and anesthesia agents. The minimum standard for monitoring during anesthesia care has been defined by the American Society of Anesthesiologists initially in 1986 then amended in 1998.[1]

The first standard of anesthesia monitoring is the mandatory presence of qualified anesthesia personnel to supervise the care of the patient. The next minimum standard involves the monitoring of the patient's oxygenation, ventilation, circulation and body temperature. Each monitoring system will be considered in turn and then ancillary monitoring will be dealt with in detail.

22.1.1 Oxygenation

Adequate oxygen concentration in the inspired gases and in the blood is to be monitored and suitable alarms enabled to warn of hypoxia or hypoxemia. We will consider measurement of oxygen in both gases and its saturation in the blood in turn.

Oxygen concentration in inspired gases can be measured in a variety of ways.

22.1.1.1 Oxygen Analysis with Other Gases

Mass spectrometry. (See Figure 22.1.) The principle behind this monitor is that each component of the gaseous mixture can be separated by its unique mass/charge ratio.[2] An electron beam ionizes the mixture of gases after the mixture has been subjected to a molecular sieve. This beam strips off electrons from the molecules and renders a variable positive charge to the molecules. The electron beam also splits off atomic particles and this helps to differentiate nitrous oxide and carbon dioxide as these two molecules have the same molecular weight (mol wt = 44). The mass/charge ratio of the molecule will influence its behavior in a magnetic and an electrostatic field that are at right angles to each other. The positively charged ion is accelerated toward a negatively charged plate and as it is accelerating, the magnetic field will influence its trajectory according to the mass of the ion. Ion collectors placed in specific positions record the quantity of each mass/charge combination and this is proportional to the total mixture. Thus,

0-8493-1140-3/04/$0.00+$1.50

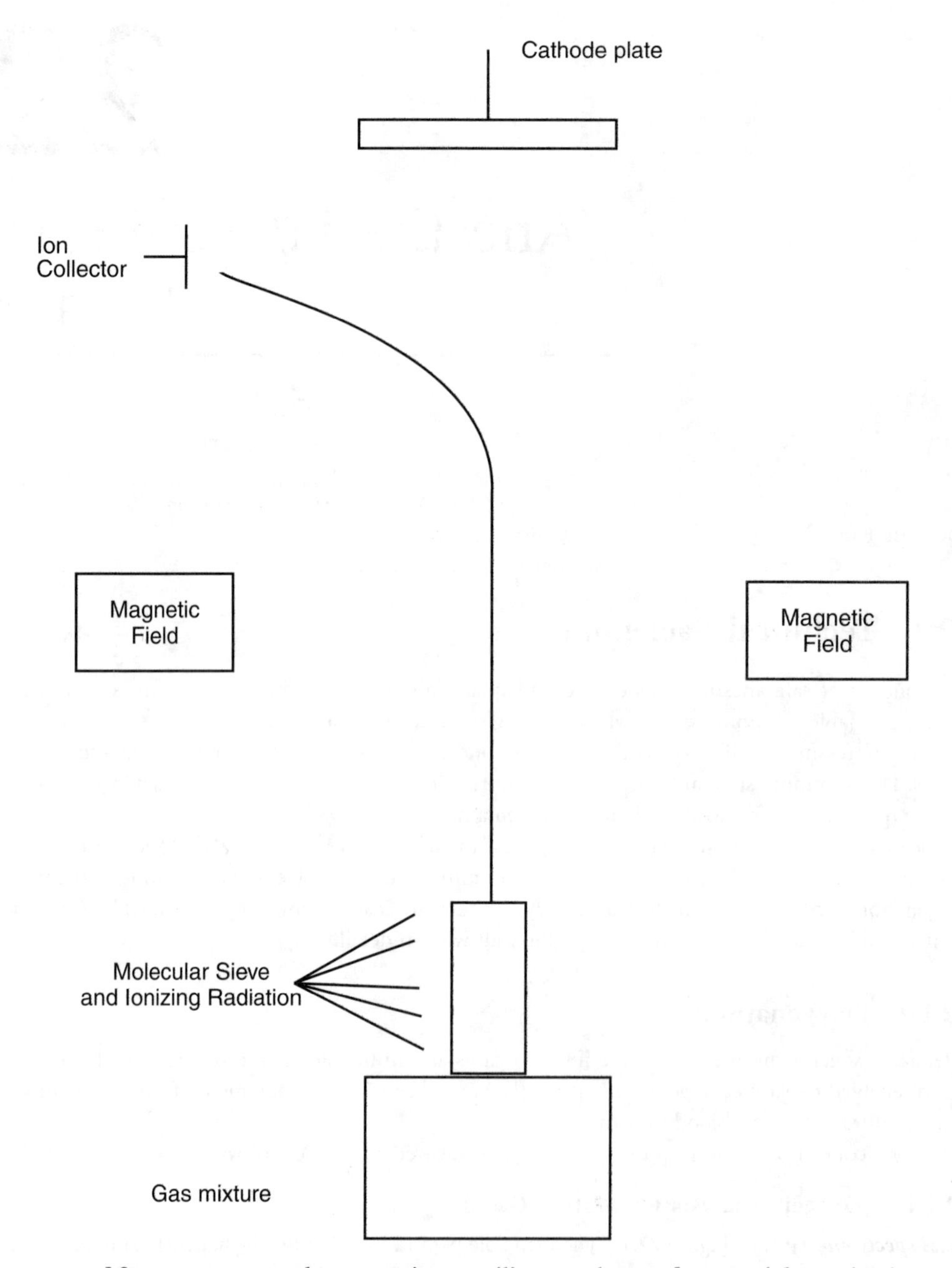

FIGURE 22.1 Mass spectrometer demonstrating curvilinear pathway of gas particles under the influence of electrostatic and magnetic fields.

the concentration of each component can be determined. This is very accurate and has the additional advantage of being able to analyze all the component concentrations of the inspired/exhaled gases. Since the molecular weight of carbon dioxide and nitrous oxide are the same, the mass spectrometer will determine the total quantity of all molecules having a molecular weight of 44. Thus another principle must be invoked to determine the relative amounts of each. The electron beam will also render a fixed proportion of carbon monoxide and nitric oxide from each of the parent compounds. Thus analysis of the amounts of carbon monoxide and nitric oxide will be able to determine the relative amounts of each of the parent compounds that were present. However, there can be a significant delay in obtaining the information as the analyzer is often centralized in an operating suite consisting of a number of operating rooms. This means that each anesthesia machine must wait in line for its gas sample to be analyzed, and the delay is dependent on how many machines are multiplexed into one analyzer and the physical distance between the anesthesia machine and the analyzer, as the sample of gases must travel from anesthesia machine to analyzer. The cost of purchasing and maintaining this analyzer and the lack of immediacy of the information has been a clinical obstacle in the installation of this mode of analyzer. Newer versions are less bulky but are still more expensive than alternative analyzers.

Quadrapole mass spectrometer. The principle is the same as above. However, instead of a magnetic field used to deflect mass/charge combinations into ion detectors, the four poles utilize radio frequency and electric fields to select out specific mass/charge combinations to collide with the ion collector. This reduces the number of ion collectors needed to one, and the field and radio frequency combinations across the poles determine which component of the gas is measured. The poles undergo different combinations to select out specific components. The collected ions are proportional to their concentrations.

Raman spectroscopy. The principle depends on Raman scattering. When photons collide with molecules, they may be scattered without loss of energy; this is called Rayleigh scattering. The colliding photons may also impart some energy to the molecule with resultant lower energy photon being re-emitted (Raman scattering). The quanta of energy absorbed by the molecule is dependent on the molecular weight and structure of the molecule. Thus, when an argon laser is fired at a 488-mm wavelength through the gaseous mixture, spectroscopy of scattered light will reveal the component parts of the mixture. The peaks of each lowered wavelength will correspond to the individual concentration of that component.[3]

22.1.1.2 Measurement of Oxygen Partial Pressure by Itself

Paramagnetic oxygen analyzer. The principle uses the paramagnetic property of oxygen to deduce the partial pressure of oxygen. Oxygen molecules are attracted to a magnetic field and this property is paramagnetic. Nitrogen has the opposite property of being diamagnetic, which means that it is repelled by a magnetic field. A dumbbell construction using two spheres filled with nitrogen is suspended in a magnetic field. If any oxygen molecules are present in the gaseous mixture, they will tend to occupy the center of the field and thus displace the nitrogen-filled spheres. The displacement of the spheres is proportional to the number of molecules of oxygen and thus its partial pressure. A mirror mounted on the suspending wire helps to measure the displacement tendency. A restoring current is applied to the coil to keep the spheres in the zero position. The restoring current works from an electric feedback relay to keep a beam of light reflected off the mirror at the zero position. Therefore the restoring current is proportional to the oxygen concentration. This is very accurate and has a fast rate of response and thus can analyze inhaled and exhaled oxygen concentrations.[4]

Fuel cell (galvanic) oxygen analyzer. This is a fuel cell that generates a current that is directly proportional to the exposed oxygen partial pressure. Like a chemical battery, the components of the fuel cell get exhausted faster when exposed to higher concentrations of oxygen. The generation of current is proportional to the oxygen available to react with the component parts of the electrodes. An oxygen-permeable membrane separates the electrolyte gel from the gas sample. As oxygen diffuses into the electrolyte solution, it will react with the electrodes to generate a current. Calibration of the fuel cell is essential for proper performance. The response time for this type of analyzer is relatively slow so it should only be positioned in the inhalation limb of the anesthesia circuit; however, there is no warm-up time for this analyzer.[5]

Polarographic (Clark electrode) oxygen analyzer. This differs from a galvanic analyzer in that an external power source must be used to provide energy for the reaction. Both the galvanic and the polarographic analyzer have electrodes, electrolytic gels and oxygen-permeable membranes. However, the response time for the polarographic analyzer is much faster due to the external power source. This analyzer takes a few minutes to warm up and must also be calibrated for optimal performance.

22.1.1.3 Blood Oxygenation

The principle monitor for the measurement of this parameter is pulse oximetry. Oximetry utilizes the fact that different species of hemoglobin have different absorption spectra, particularly hemoglobin and oxyhemoglobin. By choosing different wavelengths of light to transilluminate the tissue, the total amount of hemoglobin and the relative amount of oxyhemoglobin can be derived. Modern pulse oximeters use two or more light-emitting diodes with one photo diode acting as a sensing transducer. A variable fluctuation is essential in determining the absorption of the wavelength by the hemoglobin moiety, as all tissues will absorb some of each wavelength. Therefore, the fluctuating portion of the absorbed light will refer to the arterial hemoglobin portion of the blood, as the venous and capillary hemoglobin will be relatively constant. The fluctuating portion of the absorption spectrum will be seen in all frequencies that are absorbed by hemoglobin. Pulse oximeters will not work in patients who are on cardiopulmonary bypass because the blood flow through the tissues is constant rather than intermittent like a pulse. It is this pulsating element of the absorption spectrum that allows the determination of the amount of total hemoglobin that is present in the tissue. Once an estimate of the total hemoglobin is made, it becomes a matter of ratio adjustment to derive the saturation of that hemoglobin. The ratio of the fluctuating parts of both wavelengths is applied to an internal algorithm that derives the arteriolar oximetry. If we define the following conditions, we will be able to derive an equation for that ratio (R).

AC660 = fluctuating absorption at 660 nm wavelength
DC660 = background absorption at 660 nm wavelength
AC940 = fluctuating absorption at 940 nm wavelength
DC940 = background absorption at 940 nm wavelength

$$R = \frac{AC660/DC660}{AC940/DC940}$$

The value R is then applied to a "look-up table" that has a pulse oximeter saturation derived from healthy human volunteers. For example if R = 1, then the saturation will be 85%. The accuracy of the system is between 1 and 2%.[6]

Error correction is designed into pulse oximeters by increasing the light emitted when a poor quality signal is received at the photo diode receiver, by longer averaging periods to reduce motion artifacts, by correcting for the ambient light received at the photo diode and by ensuring a closed fit between tissue and photo diode. However, there are a few caveats. Pitfalls in pulse oximetry occur when there is the presence of greater than 5% of other species of hemoglobin such as carboxyhemoglobin, methemoglobin and sickle cell hemoglobinemia. The machine will "read" carboxyhemoglobin as oxyhemoglobin and will thus over-read the true saturation.[7] Methemoglobinemia will falsely lower the perceived saturation readout and if the true saturation should drop, the presence of methemoglobinemia will "mask" the desaturation so the readout remains unchanged.[8] The presence of injected dyes will cause artifacts, as the dyes will absorb some of the wavelengths employed. Methylene blue and, to a lesser extent, indocyanine green cause a perceived drop in saturation readout when there has been no change.[9,10] The pulse oximeter also becomes inaccurate in low cardiac output states such as shock, heart failure and hypothermia.[11] When the probe is positioned incorrectly, the light from the light source to the photo diode may go through the tissues at a grazing incidence. This incidental light will effectively decrease the "signal-to-noise" ratio so that real changes in saturation are masked. This effect is known as the "penumbra" effect and can be addressed by correct repositioning of the probe.[12] Pulse oximeters are also subject to interference with electrocautery devices and mechanical factors such as blood pressure cuffs and motion artifacts. The newer generation of pulse oximeters use adaptive digital filtering such as pioneered by Masimo Incorporated, which reduces motion artifact and adjusts for venous blood pulsation.[13]

22.1.2 Ventilation

All cases should have the ability to ensure adequate ventilation of the patient. Monitors are divided into two broad categories: capnography and ventilator alarms.

22.1.2.1 Capnography

This provides a trace of the carbon dioxide content within each respiratory cycle. Carbon dioxide can be detected by mass spectrometry or Raman analysis, and both of these methods have been discussed above (see oxygen analyzer). However the majority of capnographs rely on infrared absorption. Carbon dioxide, like nitrous oxide and water vapor, has the property of absorbing infrared radiation. Selection of a specific wavelength (4.3 μm) will lessen the collateral absorption effect. Nitrous oxide will absorb infrared at 4.5 μm thus the use of highly specific filters makes this a nonissue. However, nitrous oxide will affect the infrared absorption of carbon dioxide by a phenomenon called collision broadening where the spectral absorption peaks of a gas (carbon dioxide) are broadened by the presence/collision of another gas (nitrous oxide).[14] This can be corrected for if the concentration of nitrous oxide is known. If nitrous oxide is present at 70%, then the perceived carbon dioxide readout must be corrected by a factor of 0.90, and similarly if nitrous oxide is present at 50%, then the carbon dioxide readout needs a correction factor of 0.94 to render the true carbon dioxide concentration.[15] Of the infrared absorption analyzers, there are two types of capnographs: sidestream and mainstream.

Sidestream capnographs continuously aspirate a sample of the respiratory gases and analyze the carbon dioxide content of that sample. Setting the wrong aspiration rate, leaks within the sampling system, water vapor condensation causing blockages and dust particles all are sources of error. Water traps are designed to prevent the entry of liquids into the measuring chamber as liquids have a high infrared absorbance. After the gases have been analyzed, the waste gases may be returned to the anesthesia gas circuit on the exhalation side before the soda-lime canister.

Mainstream capnographs will analyze the whole of the respiratory gases at one point in the anesthesia circuit. The measuring chamber (cuvette) is placed as close as possible to the endotracheal tube. The analyzer uses infrared absorbance to detect carbon dioxide. The chamber is heated to 40°C to prevent liquid condensation of the water vapor present in exhaled gases. The chamber is heavy and needs to be supported away from the patient's face as it may cause burns or cause pressure ulceration. Particulate matter such as mucus or saliva from the airway will cause errors by absorbing infrared if they enter the cuvette. However, the response time of this type of analyzer is much faster than with the sidestream capnographs, mass spectrometers or Raman analyzers. There are also no issues about sampling rate flow time, blockages in the aspirating tubing or leaks or malfunction of the aspirating pump which are all present in the other types of capnographs. All capnographs must be calibrated periodically to prevent equipment drift.

22.1.2.2 Ventilator Alarms

These can be either of two types. Pressure threshold alarms are designed to detect ventilator or anesthesia circuit disconnections. Volumes of exhaled gases can be monitored for adequacy of ventilation during cases where an endotracheal tube is in place.

Ventilator disconnection alarms are pressure gauges that have a set threshold limit that must be exceeded once every 15 to 20 sec. The monitor is a modified manometer that transduces the airway pressure energy to mechanical energy (the needle movement in the gauge) or an electrical output seen on a monitor display. A triggered relay with a time-out function is activated whenever this alarm is switched on. Some alarms allow the user to set the threshold pressure that must be exceeded before monitor declares a ventilator disconnection. This type of alarm will still function in the presence of a small leak, but large leaks in the anesthesia circuit will prevent the threshold pressure from being exceeded. Typical setting of the threshold pressure should be between 3 to 5 cm water pressure below the peak inspiratory airway pressure. This type of monitor is usually incorporated into the ventilator design as a safety feature and is activated as soon as the ventilator is cycled. This alarm cannot determine a disconnection without a ventilator cycling positive pressure within the anesthesia circuit. The capnograph can also be used as a disconnection type alarm but it will only function as such when the disconnection is between the sampling point in the circuit and the patient's airway. If the anesthesia circuit is disconnected between the sampling point and the anesthesia circuit, and the patient is breathing spontaneously, there will be a continuous capnograph waveform despite the disconnection.

Volume monitors are usually based on the principle of a rotameter. This is a vane/turbine being rotated in a flow of gas They tend to underestimate the volume recorded at very low tidal volumes and overestimate large tidal volumes. This is because of inertia in its moving parts. An optical counter will determine how many times the vanes are turned and thus the patient's tidal volume can be calculated. Other ways of measuring gas volumes are Fleisch pneumotachography, screen-type pneumotachography and vortex-type pneumotachography, with hot wire anemometer and with ultrasonic flow meter. Fleisch pneumotachographs consist of a bundle of capillary tubes placed parallel with the airflow. The flow within the capillary tubes is laminar and thus the pressure drop across the capillary tubes is linearly related to gas flow.[16] Screen-type pneumotachographs are much lighter and less bulky than the Fleisch type and measure a pressure drop across the screen mesh. The pressure drop is nonlinear as the flow across the mesh is turbulent (flow across orifices). The characteristics of the mesh are very sensitive to deposition of moisture or debris across the mesh and so their performance suffers. Vortex-type pneumotachographs are usually incorporated into ventilators. An ultrasonic beam is disrupted by vortices that are generated when laminar flow is broken up by struts placed across the tube. The formation of vortices is related to the velocity and thus the flow. Hot-wire anemometers pass a current along a conductor to maintain the conductor at constant temperature. When gases flow across the wire, heat is lost and more current is needed to restore the set temperature. However, the presence of mucus and droplets affect the heating characteristics of the wire. Ultrasonic flow meters are mounted coaxially and measure the change in speed in a wave that is pulsed parallel to the direction of flow.[17]

22.1.3 Circulation

The basic parameters that are monitored for the circulatory system are heart rate and blood pressure. Heart rate measurement can be done by pulse oximetry (see above) or by electrocardiogram.

22.1.3.1 The Electrocardiogram

The electrocardiogram (EKG) is a measure of the electrical activity of the heart and does not equate to an output from the heart. However, it is a simple and noninvasive monitor to apply in the OR. Standard lead II is used to monitor the rhythm of the heart as the p wave is best seen in this lead. A modified lead V5 is used whenever the anesthesiologist/anesthetist feels that the patient is at risk from ischemia as this lead displays lateral wall ischemia by ST segment depression/elevation. The monitor counts the heart rate by identifying the R wave in the QRS complex and measures the R–R interval between adjacent R waves to derive the heart rate. Because there is natural beat-to-beat variability in the heart rate, there is usually an averaging of the heart rate over the last 5 to 15 sec. Modern telemetry devices will have a moving average filter that places more weight on recent changes in rate. Thus, the averaging interval is variable depending on new changes in the rate measured. Errors arise from multiple sources: improper electrode placement, poor electrical conduction across the skin due to dehydrated conducting gel, poor cable integrity to conduct the evoked potential to the monitor, noncardiac muscle activity that also generate electrical potentials, electrocautery instruments that generate radio frequency waves, 60 Hz interference from fluid warmers, inappropriate signal gain, inappropriate R wave signal threshold, displacement of one or several electrodes.

22.1.3.2 Blood Pressure

Blood pressure can be monitored by two different methods: using noninvasive and invasive blood pressure monitors.

Noninvasive blood pressure measurement methods can be manual or automated. The correct size cuff and position of the pneumatic bladder are both pivotal in obtaining reliable readings. The correct width of cuff should be 20% greater than the diameter of the arm and the pneumatic bladder must be positioned so that the artery is in the center of the bladder. The cuff should be applied to have a snug fit to the limb and the bladder must be deflated. Manual cuff blood pressure can use a variety of pulse detection probes from stethoscopes, Doppler ultrasound, arterial wall motion changes by ultrasound, oscillotonometry or oscillometry. Automated machines depend on the principle of oscillometry. Here, the cuff pressure is inflated above the systolic pressure and slowly deflated in an incremental stepwise manner. At each step of deflation, the pressure is stabilized and small fluctuations in the occluding pressure are measured. These small fluctuations are the result of a partial column of blood passing under the occluding cuff; their oscillations vary with the occluding cuff pressure. Variables such as systolic, mean and diastolic blood pressures may be derived from the oscillations. Peak oscillations correlate closely with the mean arterial pressure. The systolic and diastolic pressures are extrapolated from the peak oscillations. The systolic pressure is usually set when the oscillations are between 25 and 50% of the peak oscillation as the pulsations are increasing in size. This derived systolic pressure has less accuracy than the mean arterial pressure when compared to direct arterial blood pressure measurement. Finally, the diastolic pressure is derived from about 80% decay from the peak oscillation and has less correlation to the true diastolic pressure. Each manufacturer has its own propriety algorithm to determine the mean, systolic and diastolic pressures. As a general rule, automatic blood pressure machines tend to under-read the systolic and over-read the diastolic blood pressure compared to arterial line pressure readings.[18-20] Errors are seen when the wrong cuff is selected, in the presence of a small leak in the pneumatic system, and when there is partial obstruction to pneumatic system, movement artifacts by the patient or by a surgeon and muscle tremors from shivering. Problems caused by noninvasive blood pressure machines including bruising from the cuff, nerve palsies from ischemia induced by cuff pressures, limb edema, thrombophlebitis and even compartment syndrome.

Invasive blood pressure monitors depend on the placement of an arterial line and measuring the pressure wave. Unlike the noninvasive system, this gives continual beat-by-beat information of the blood pressure. This system is more costly and has the potential for more complications and requires more technical skill to initiate and maintain; it is considered the "gold standard" for measuring blood pressure. The waveform can display information about the regularity of the pulse, small but significant variations of the blood pressure with changes in respiration and the status of the circulating volume. The pressure transducer converts mechanical energy to electrical energy. The majority of these use a strain gauge principle. A wire or silicone crystal is stretched over a dome and, as the pressure within the dome rises, the resistance of the wire/silicone crystal changes. This resistance is arranged in a Wheatstone bridge circuit so that the voltage output is proportional to the pressure applied to the diaphragm. There are now disposable transducers with a simple calibration method to zero the transducer to atmospheric pressure. The arterial cannula/pressure tubing/ transducer complex is capable of resonating due to the reverberation of the pressure wave within the complex. The natural frequency of the complex and its damping coefficient are important determinants to whether the system will overshoot or undershoot the true systolic blood pressure. One way to measure this at the patient interface is to perform a fast flush test. After several fast flushes, the flush artifact is examined. The distance between two adjacent peaks or troughs should be constant and represents the natural frequency of the system. It is calculated by the paper speed (mm/sec) divided by the horizontal distance between two flush artifacts (mm) to give a frequency (f/sec = f Hz). The higher the frequency value, the less likely the whole system will reverberate. Systems with a natural frequency of less than 7 Hz are unsatisfactory. Examining the flush artifact and measuring the vertical heights of two successive waves will derive the damping coefficient. The ratio of these two successive vertical heights will render an amplitude ratio. This ratio should be between 0.05 and 0.10 as this will equate with a damping coefficient of 0.6 to 0.7 which would be ideal for a pressure transducer system. Errors can be in multiple areas: improper selection of arterial cannula, partial kinking of the cannula as it enters the skin, partial obstruction to the artery that the cannula is measuring (e.g., the blood pressure cuff, poor patient positioning on the table so that the artery to the limb is partially obstructed), incorrect compliant pressure tubing connecting arterial cannula to transducer, air bubbles within the cannula or pressure tubing or transducer, incorrect transducer height in relation to the heart, incorrect calibration of the transducer, overdamping and underdamping of the pressure wave. Clinical studies show that most systems are underdamped and therefore overestimate the systolic blood pressure.[22,23]

22.1.4 Temperature

There are two types of body temperatures recorded. They are peripheral temperatures and body core temperatures. Body core temperatures reflect core blood and core organ temperature. They are taken at the following sites and require placement of specialized probes: nasopharynx, tympanic membrane, circulating blood in the pulmonary artery, distal third of the esophagus, bladder and rectum. Peripheral temperatures can be recorded from forehead, nose, armpit, groin and peripheral limbs. The core temperature is a reflection of the body's ability to maintain an isothermic environment in the face of challenges in the operating room, e.g., cool environments, cold intravenous fluids, heat loss from opened body cavities and vasodilating medication. The core-peripheral temperature is a reflection of the peripheral cooling of the body and a measure of vasodilatation of the epidermal vasculature. There are various technologies used in temperature measurement. These consist of thermistors, thermocouples, infrared readers for tympanic membrane and thermometers. Thermistors are semiconductors whose resistance decreases in a predictable manner with increasing temperature. Thermocouples are two dissimilar metals joined in a circuit; when one junction has a temperature different from the other, a potential difference is generated. Infrared tympanic membrane scanners are unreliable as they are dependent on good reproducible techniques and an unobstructed external auditory canal. Thermistors in pulmonary artery catheters, esophageal probes and urinary Foley catheters remain the most reliable way to measure core temperature. All these probes are disposable but are they are invasive. Temperature probes placed on the skin are also thermistors and will help determine core-peripheral temperature gradient, but are subject to the environmental conditions at the site. The operating room environment is invariably hypothermic, the majority of anesthetic agents cause vasodilatation encouraging the loss of heat from the body to the environment. Finally patients under general anesthesia reduce their activity to basal metabolic rate that impairs their ability to maintain core temperature. It is common for the core temperature to fall by 0.5 to 1.5°C within the first 30 min of general anesthesia. Hyperthermia is also a relatively late sign of a peculiar disease triggered by some anesthesia agents in susceptible individuals. Malignant hyperthermia appears to be a genetic defect in calcium metabolism in skeletal muscles, and prompt recognition of this disorder is essential to ensure a favorable outcome.

22.2 Signal Processing

Through digital signal processing, information from unrelated sources can be assembled into one place and displayed in a central location where the anesthesiologist reads the screen. The digital signal processors have the capability to display information in various formats such as numerical data, warning and alert information or information to be displayed in continuous real-time waveform and trend information. These processors allow the data to be displayed in their own channels in a clear and concise way without interference from adjacent channels, and yet still allow the user to customize the display to their personal preference. Signal processors also store data in a contemporaneous manner and this can be downloaded and viewed at a more convenient time. Clinical data in the form of trend information is sometimes just as crucial as the absolute values displayed and the ability to capture and store this information is important to signal processors. Signal processors are pivotal in incorporating all the available information from discrete modular parameters into one main display and a possible secondary display unit. They convert all the data to digital format and are able to manipulate the data to reduce the "noise" level by adaptive filtering, Fourier transformation, signal acquisition to partially recover a degraded signal by modeling the signal distortions due to data acquisition and sampling, use of filters at high-pass, low-pass, and band-pass, and notch filters to select out "noise."

References

1. American Society of Anesthesiologists, Standards for Basic Intraoperative Monitoring, adopted October 6, 1986; amended October 18, 1989; effective January 1, 1990.
2. Gillbe, C.E., Heneghan, C.P., and Branthwaite, M.A., Respiratory mass spectrometry during general anaesthesia, *Br. J. Anaesth.*, 53(1), 103–109, 1981.

3. VanWagenen, R.A., Westenskow, D.R., Benner, R.E., Gregonis, D.E., and Coleman, D.L., Dedicated monitoring of anesthetic and respiratory gases by Raman scattering, *J. Clin. Monit.*, 2(4), 215–222, 1986.
4. Hill, R.W., Determination of oxygen consumption by use of the paramagnetic oxygen analyzer, *J. Appl. Physiol.*, 33(2), 261–263, 1972.
5. Torda, T.A. and Grant, G.C., Test of a fuel cell oxygen analyzer, *Br. J. Anaesth.*, 44(10), 1108–1112, 1972.
6. Chaudhary, B.A. and Burki, N.K., Ear oximetry in clinical practice, *Am. Rev. Respir. Dis.*, 117(1), 173–175, 1978.
7. Barker, S.J. and Tremper, K.K., The effect of carbon monoxide inhalation on pulse oximetry and transcutaneous PO2, *Anesthesiology*, 66(5), 677–679, 1987.
8. Barker, S.J., Tremper, K.K., and Hyatt, J., Effects of methemoglobinemia on pulse oximetry and mixed venous oximetry, *Anesthesiology*, 70(1), 112–117, 1989.
9. Scheller, M.S., Unger, R.J., and Kelner, M.J., Effects of intravenously administered dyes on pulse oximetry readings, *Anesthesiology*, 65(5), 550–552, 1986.
10. Kessler, M.R., Eide, T., Humayun, B., and Poppers, P.J., Spurious pulse oximeter desaturation with methylene blue injection, *Anesthesiology*, 65(4), 435–436, 1986.
11. Lawson, D., Norley, I., Korbon, G., Loeb, R., and Ellis, J., Blood flow limits and pulse oximeter signal detection, *Anesthesiology*, 67(4), 599–603, 1987.
12. Barker, S.J., Hyatt, J., Shah, N.K., and Kao, Y.J., The effect of sensor malpositioning on pulse oximeter accuracy during hypoxemia, *Anesthesiology*, 79(2), 248–254, 1993.
13. Bohnhorst, B., Peter, C.S., and Poets, C.F., Pulse oximeters' reliability in detecting hypoxemia and bradycardia: comparison between a conventional and two new generation oximeters, *Crit. Care Med.*, 28(5), 1565–1568, 2000.
14. Raemer, D.B. and Calalang, I., Accuracy of end-tidal carbon dioxide tension analyzer, *J. Clin. Monit.*, 7, 19–20, 1991.
15. Kennell, E.M., Andrews, R.W., and Wollman, H., Correction factors for nitrous oxide in the infrared analysis of carbon dioxide, *Anesthesiology*, 39, 441–443, 1973.
16. von der Hardt, H. and Zywietz, C.H., Reliability in pneumotachographic measurements, *Respiration*, 33(6), 416–424, 1976.
17. Blumenfeld, W., Turney, S.Z., and Denman, R.J., A coaxial ultrasonic pneumotachometer, *Med. Biol. Eng.*, 13(6), 855–860, 1975.
18. Carroll, G.C., Blood pressure monitoring (review), *Crit. Care Clin.*, 4(3), 411–434, 1988.
19. Davis, R.F., Clinical comparison of automated auscultatory and oscillometric and catheter-transducer measurements of arterial pressure, *J. Clin. Monit.*, 1(2), 114–119, 1985.
20. Forster, F.K. and Turney, D., Oscillometric determination of diastolic, mean and systolic blood pressure — a numerical model, *J. Biomech. Eng.*, 108(4), 359–364, 1986.
21. Kleinman, B., Powell, S., Kumar, P., and Gardner, R.M., The fast flush test measures the dynamic response of the entire blood pressure monitoring system, *Anesthesiology*, 77(6), 1215–1220, 1992.
22. Schwid, H.A., Frequency response evaluation of radial artery catheter-manometer systems: sinusoidal frequency analysis versus flush method, *J. Clin. Monit.*, 4(3), 181–185, 1988.
23. Hipkins, S.F., Rutten, A.J., and Runciman, W.B., Experimental analysis of catheter-manometer systems *in vitro* and *in vivo*, *Anesthesiology*, 71(6), 893–906, 1989.

23

Intraoperative Neurophysiological Monitoring

Carla S. Hatten
Premier Neurodiagnostic Services

George Zouridakis
University of Houston

CONTENTS

23.1 Introduction

During the past several years, refined surgical techniques and better equipment for life support have dramatically improved the outcome of many complex surgical procedures.[1] At the same time, in an attempt to minimize neurological sequelae from these complicated procedures, an enormous effort was made to develop intraoperative monitoring (IOM) procedures that could provide accurate information on the functional integrity of the nervous system of an anesthetized patient.

Early applications of IOM were limited to only a few tests, such as somatosensory-evoked potentials (EPs) in the late seventies to monitor spinal cord function during surgery for scoliosis,[2,3] and the recording of facial muscle activity in cases requiring facial nerve dissection.[4] Later on, auditory brainstem responses were employed in operations for acoustic tumors[5,6] with the intention to preserve hearing and vestibular nerve functions. Today, a variety of complicated neurophysiological tests specifically developed for intraoperative use cover a wide range of applications in neurological, orthopedic, and vascular surgery, and they are gradually becoming part of standard medical practice.

In general, two consequences of surgical intervention can compromise the functional integrity of the nervous system and lead to postoperative neurological deficits, ischemia, and mechanical injury. These insults are typically manifested as changes in the morphology, amplitude, or frequency content of electrophysiological signals. Thus, continuous monitoring of these waveforms provides an objective way to detect and quantify changes in brain, spinal cord, or peripheral nerve function early enough so that

0-8493-1140-3/04/$0.00+$1.50

actions can be taken to reverse the effects of an insult, prevent permanent injury, and restore normal function. Additionally, given that IOM is delivered continuously throughout a procedure, it can be used to assess the efficacy of a corrective action, and the overall effectiveness of surgical intervention. IOM has also been effective in localizing specific neuronal structures that cannot be easily identified solely on anatomical grounds, such as peripheral nerves and the sensorimotor cortical strip.

23.2 Overview

23.2.1 Types of Tests

IOM employs recordings of both spontaneous and evoked activity. The scalp-recorded electroencephalogram (EEG) can be used to monitor cerebral function during neurological or vascular surgery, while activity recorded directly from the exposed cortex can be used to map the margins of epileptogenic tissue and identify the cortical areas involved with certain normal brain functions such as speech.

Evoked activity is obtained through external stimulation of a neural pathway. Common sensory stimuli include electrical shocks, clicking sounds, and flashes of light, which result in the familiar somatosensory, auditory, and visual EPs, respectively. Similarly, electrical or magnetic stimulation of motor pathways gives rise to the so-called motor EPs. Evoked responses usually are very small compared to the ongoing activity, and averaging of a large number of single-trial responses is necessary to obtain clear waveforms. In certain cases, however, individual stimuli result in large responses, and averaging is not needed. For example, an electrical stimulus delivered to a spinal nerve root results in a well-defined high-amplitude muscle response known as triggered electromyographic (EMG) activity.

Evoked responses can be recorded from the brain, the spinal cord, a peripheral nerve, or a muscle, depending on the site of stimulation. During surgery, the type of test to be used and the sites of recording and stimulation are chosen on a case-by-case basis, depending on what structures are at risk in the context of a particular procedure. Unfortunately, there is no single monitoring procedure that can be used in all circumstances. On the contrary, very often it is necessary to administer multiple tests simultaneously, in order to maximize the sensitivity of IOM.

This chapter provides an overview of the various techniques and equipment for neurophysiological monitoring and the rationale for their intraoperative use, as well as the main principles on which they are based. The various IOM tests and the surgical procedures that employ them can be found elsewhere.[7]

23.2.2 Affecting Factors

Electrophysiological monitoring in the operating room poses several specific challenges. The two major risks, ischemia and mechanical insult, will typically result in a reduction in the amplitude, an increase in the latency, and an overall change in the morphology of waveforms. Although there are no exact values of amplitude or latency changes that absolutely predict neurological outcome,[8] for each test there are recommended values that can be used as a "rule of thumb" for warning the surgical team.

However, a plethora of additional factors can result in drastic changes in the waveforms just like ischemia and mechanical injury. These include changes in blood pressure, body temperature, and most importantly anesthesia regime; nearly all anesthetic agents affect cerebral blood flow, perfusion, and metabolic rate. Moreover, extraneous biological noise, such as heart and muscle activity, electrical noise, like the omnipresent 60-Hz interference, and equipment failure will contribute to the difficulty in interpreting the recordings correctly and reduce the ability of differentiating artifactual from true changes due to surgery.

Familiarity with all these factors and careful observation of the context in which signal changes occur — namely, surgical maneuvers like tissue retraction and instrumentation placement, bolus injection of drugs, and a decrease in blood pressure — as well as communication with the surgeon and the anesthesiologist is necessary for proper interpretation of changes in the neurophysiological signals. We have previously presented a detailed description of the effects of anesthetic agents and other perisurgical factors on all neurophysiological recordings currently used intraoperatively.[7]

23.2.3 Usefulness

The merits of IOM have been extensively reported in the literature from different institutions worldwide and for a variety of types of procedures, including spine surgery,[9,10] neurovascular cases,[11,12] cranial nerve operations,[13-16] and cases involving peripheral auditory structures and brainstem pathways.[17] IOM has made brain retraction, which is required for adequate exposure in many intracranial procedures, a much less common source of morbidity,[4] and has therefore allowed for overall safer operations.[18]

Continuous feedback regarding neurological function provides the medical team with additional reassurance and allows the surgeons to carry out the operation in an optimal way[14] attempting, for instance, more aggressive maneuvers that otherwise they would not risk attempting.[10] Also, certain high-risk patients previously regarded as inoperable can now be considered as candidates for surgery.

Intuitively, then, the cost-effectiveness of IOM would seem obvious, since it can decrease the risk of permanent postoperative neurological deficit and often the time it takes to perform an operation. Moreover, with regard to economic terms, even when the cost of suffering is not included, it has been estimated that IOM is clinically cost effective as the risk of postoperative complications approaches 1%.[10]

23.2.4 Personnel

Guidelines for proper IOM have been set forth by the American Electroencephalographic Society[8] and include recommendations for equipment, personnel, and documentation. The American Clinical Neurophysiology Society has also published guidelines for EEG and EPs. According to these guidelines, personnel should have a board registration and a minimum of 5 years experience in EEG and EPs, with a minimum of 1 to 2 years of EEG and EP monitoring in the operating room. Selection of proper personnel is critical, as the experience of the monitoring team is the primary predictor of neurological complications; the rate of postoperative deficits in teams with the least experience was found to be twice as high compared to the most experienced teams.[10]

Typically, a clinical neurophysiologist or a physician is the leader of a monitoring team and supervises several operating rooms, while a technologist is available in each room at all times and can place electrodes, set up equipment, and monitor the case during the less critical phases of an operation. This is similar to how anesthesia teams are organized in many hospitals. The current Health Care Financing Administration guidelines state that monitoring may also be performed by a technologist with on-line real-time contact with a physician. Insurance carriers generally adopt and apply these requirements.

All personnel involved with monitoring should be able to interpret the recordings and communicate the findings in a way that the surgeons find useful. This implies that at least the leader of the IOM team should have a strong background in neurophysiology and anatomy, as well as knowledge about the specific surgical operation being performed.

23.2.5 Equipment

When IOM first began, machines typically had two or, in extremely rare cases, four channels, and thousands of responses were needed to arrive at recognizable averaged waveforms. To accomplish monitoring of more than one structure the technologist was required to crawl under the operating table to switch wires around. Printing waveforms generally took the whole next workday to recall from floppy discs and print via a plotter. Times have really changed. Memory and speed of computers has dramatically increased, making monitoring faster and offering a broader range of simultaneous monitoring procedures. Today's multimodality machines can have as many as 32 recording channels and can monitor several structures simultaneously. Clear responses can be obtained with a smaller number of trials, which means that waveforms can be updated more frequently, and thus neural pathways monitored more accurately.

Most modern systems consist of a portable, self-contained, computer-controlled apparatus that has the capacity to perform stimulation, recording, data processing, display, storage, printing, and teleconferencing. The choice of equipment for IOM is very important and should allow for simultaneous multimodality recordings. For example, to meet the needs of specific brain operations, it should be possible to monitor auditory and somatosensory EPs simultaneously. Or, in cases involving placement of instrumentation in the lumbar spine where the nerve roots, and not the spinal cord, are mostly at risk, the equipment should allow simultaneous monitoring of EPs and free-running EMG, since the EMG provides instantaneous and specific information on root insult that would be missed if recordings of only EPs were monitored. The capability of multiple stimulation sites is also desirable for monitoring primary and secondary nerve structures at risk. For instance, following lumbar spine procedures where the patient has been prone with arms extended for several hours, postoperative ulnar nerve palsies are not uncommon, and can be prevented by monitoring responses from both the median (primary site) and ulnar nerves (secondary site). The case is the same for peroneal palsies, when the leg has been poorly padded and compressed for hours.

However, equipment should also be easy to use and flexible to allow fast interpretation of the results. An example of latest generation equipment (model Endeavor, Nicolet Biomedical, Madison, WI) is shown in Figure 23.1.

23.3 Neurophysiological Recordings: Spontaneous Activity

Several structures in the body that are part of either the nervous or the muscular system can generate spontaneous bioelectrical activity that can be recorded externally. The most common generators are neurons in the brain that produce activity recorded on the scalp as the electroencephalogram (EEG), and muscles that, when contracting, give rise to signals captured in an electromyogram (EMG).

23.3.1 Electroencephalogram

Clinical Use — Intraoperatively EEG is commonly used for monitoring cerebral function during carotid endarterectomy, aneurysm clipping, repair of arteriovenous malformation, and balloon angioplasty, as it can reliably detect blood flow changes within 30 sec from the onset of an insult.

Recording Procedure — Intraoperative EEG recordings are typically performed using digital equipment. The preferred type of recording electrodes are hypodermic sterile needles because they are easy to use and maintain a stable impedance over a long period of time.[19] Depending on the constraints imposed by the surgical field, proper IOM requires between 8 and 16 electrodes, that are placed symmetrically on the two hemispheres, following an anteroposterior bipolar montage. Continuous comparison of activity on the hemisphere involved with surgery with the activity on the homotopic unaffected side allows detection of EEG changes in the anterior, posterior, left, or right quadrant, independently.

Because of the need to monitor beta activity, high-frequency filters are set at least to 30 Hz, while low-frequency filtering of 1 Hz is usually adequate, along with standard sensitivities of 5, 7, or 10 mV/mm. On-line visual inspection of the amplitude, frequency content, and symmetry of the EEG traces and computerized techniques, such as compressed spectral array, can clearly visualize the evolution in time of the EEG characteristics, and aid in the interpretation of the recordings.

Interpretation — The most important requirement for interpreting intraoperative EEG is knowledge of the effects of anesthesia depth. Upon induction of anesthesia, the EEG shows widespread slowing (theta and high delta activity) and, at the same time, buildup of fast (beta) activity. Thus, the normal background EEG under typical levels of anesthesia contains a mixture of slow and fast frequencies.

Any changes in the normal pattern during surgery can be due to either ischemia or to perisurgical factors, including depth of anesthesia, body temperature, and administration of a bolus injection of

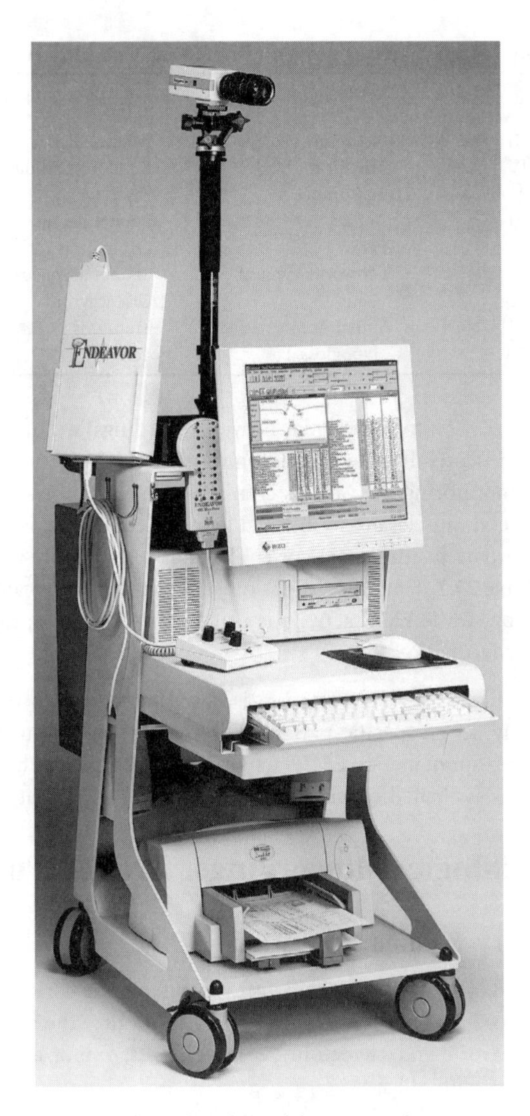

FIGURE 23.1 Example of a modern 32-channel multimodality system for IOM.

drugs. Ischemia of the cerebral cortex typically results in a sudden, localized reduction or total loss of high frequencies, often followed by the appearance of high amplitude slow waves in the delta band. Long intervals of cortical ischemia will produce a further decrease in both the amplitude and frequency, until EEG silence is reached.[20]

Unfortunately, several anesthetic agents may have similar effects on the EEG. In general, EEG changes due to ischemia are abrupt and localized, while changes from perisurgical factors are relatively slow and generalized. Successful differentiation of EEG changes can be achieved by correlating the observed EEG changes with surgical maneuvers, anesthesia regime, blood pressure, oxygen level, heart rate, body temperature, and administration of drugs.

23.3.2 Electromyogram

Clinical Use — EMG is the recording of the electrical activity of a muscle. EMG monitoring is used to identify and protect cranial nerves and spinal nerve roots from injury during surgical manipulation. Spine surgery, pedicle screw placement, selective rhizotomy, and posterior fossa surgery are good candidates for EMG monitoring.

TABLE 23.1 Muscles Typically Used for Monitoring Cranial Nerves

Cranial Nerve	Nerve Name	Muscle Monitored
III	Oculomotor	Inferior Rectus
IV	Trochlear	Superior Oblique
V	Trigeminal	Masseter
VI	Abducens	Lateral Rectus
VII	Facial	Orbicularis Oris and Oculi
IX	Glossopharyngeal	Stylopharyngeus
X	Vagus	Cricothyroid
XI	Spinal Accessory	Trapezius
XII	Hypoglossal	Tongue

Recording Procedure — When monitoring cranial nerves, recordings are mostly monopolar and EMG needles are typically placed ipsilaterally into muscles innervated by the nerve at risk. Table 23.1 summarizes the muscles used for monitoring the various cranial nerves. For monitoring spinal roots, both the ipsilateral and the contralateral muscles are monitored simultaneously, because of anatomical variations in innervation and reflex events in the spinal cord. The muscles typically used for monitoring spinal roots are summarized in Table 23.2. Thus, recordings must be bipolar. For localization of a nerve, a sterile probe is used for stimulation, while EMG activity is usually displayed on a monitor and also sent to a speaker to provide auditory feedback.[19]

Interpretation — Intraoperative EMG interpretation is based primarily on the presence or absence of muscle activity and partially on its specific pattern. Direct electrical stimulation of a nerve can help localize the neural structure. Spontaneous EMG activity does not assure the integrity of a peripheral nerve. However, triggered EMG elicited consistently can reassure the integrity of the distal nerve.

23.4 Neurophysiological Recordings: Evoked Potentials

23.4.1 Somatosensory Evoked Potentials (SEPs)

Clinical Use — SEPs are used intraoperatively to detect ischemia in the cortex or spinal cord, to monitor the integrity of the spinal cord and peripheral nerves, and to localize the sensorimotor cortex.[21] Spine and neurovascular surgery, carotid endarterectomy, aortic cross-clamping, and localization of sensorimotor cortex can be monitored with SEPs.

TABLE 23.2 Muscles Typically Used for Monitoring Cervical, Lumbar, and Sacral Nerve Roots

Area	Nerve Root	Muscle Monitored
Cervical	C_3	Trapezius
	C_4	Trapezius
	C_5	Deltoid
	C_6	Biceps
	C_7	Triceps
	C_8	Flexor Carpi Ulnaris
Lumbar	L_1	Sartorius, Iliopsoas
	L_2	Rectus Femoris, Vastus Lateralis
	L_3	Rectus Femoris, Vastus Lateralis
	L_4	Tibialis Anterior, Rectus Femoris
	L_5	Tibialis Anterior, Biceps Femoris
Sacral	S_1	Biceps Femoris
	S_2	Gastrocnemius, Biceps Femoris
	S_3	Anal Sphincter
	S_4	Anal Sphincter

Recording Procedure — SEPs are recorded on the scalp after electrical stimulation of a peripheral nerve. To reduce the effect of nonspecific EEG background activity, a large number of single responses must be averaged to increase the signal-to-noise ratio. The median nerve at the wrist is the most common stimulation site for upper extremity monitoring, while the posterior tibial nerve at the ankle is most commonly used for monitoring the lower extremity. Other sites that can be utilized include the ulnar and peroneal nerves, respectively. Recordings are obtained with needle electrodes placed on the scalp and on the cervical spine. Additional electrodes can be placed at the Erb's point for upper extremity SEP recordings, and over the posterior fossa behind the knee for lower extremity recordings. Thus, typical recordings include a cortical, a subcortical, and a peripheral response obtained after stimulation of the left and right sides of the body independently.[21]

Interpretation — Establishing a reproducible baseline prior to any surgical manipulation is important. Baselines should be of familiar morphology, consistent with the clinical picture of the patient, and should contain clear components. Normative values for the responses from various recording sites can be found in the literature.[7] During surgery, interpretation is based on detection of reliable and significant changes compared to the baselines. A change is reliable if it is repeatable at least twice in a row, and significant if its amplitude has decreased by at least 50% or its latency has increased by at least 10%. Anesthetics can alter the evoked responses significantly.

23.4.2 Brainstem Auditory Evoked Responses (BAERs)

Clinical Use — BAERs are used to monitor the function of the entire auditory pathway, including the acoustic nerve, brain stem, and cerebral cortex.[22] Surgery for acoustic tumors, and procedures involving the cerebellopontine angle and the posterior fossa commonly use monitoring of BAERs.

Recording Procedure — BAERs are elicited by auditory stimulation usually with clicks delivered separately in each ear. Stimuli are delivered at a high rate, e.g., 11 Hz, a frequency that does not coincide with the 60-Hz electrical noise. Best responses are obtained from electrodes near the ears (A1, A2) referenced to the vertex (Cz).

Interpretation — Typically, BAERs consist of seven clear waves or peaks (indicated as peaks I to VII), all occurring within the first 10 msec after stimulus onset. Each peak presumably has a specific origin along the auditory pathway, mainly ipsilateral to the stimulated ear. Important parameters to monitor include peak amplitude of waves I, III, and V, latency of wave V, and the interpeak latencies I–III and I–V. Wave V is the most reliably seen wave, particularly in patients with hearing impairment or undergoing surgery. A shift in latency of 1 msec or a drop in amplitude of 50% could be significant and should be reported to the surgeon.

23.4.3 Visual Evoked Potentials (VEPs)

Clinical Use — VEPs can be used to assess the functional integrity of the visual pathway, including the optic nerves, chiasm, optic tracts, and the occipital visual cortex. VEPs are most useful in cases involving the retro-orbital and parasellar regions.[20,23,24] However, their full clinical utility has not yet been determined.

Recording Procedure — A typical montage includes two recording channels, each involving one hemisphere. Visual stimulation is given by red light-emitting diodes (LEDs). Low- and high-frequency filters are set to 1 and 100 Hz, respectively. The stimulus has a duration of 5 msec and a rate between 1 and 5 Hz.

Interpretation — Typically three negative (N1, N2, N3) and three positive (P1, P2, P3) peaks are seen. Interpretation criteria are based on changes that affect the overall morphology, latency, and symmetry of the P1-N2-P2 complex between left and right eye stimulation.[20] However, because of the great variability of flash VEPs, the only reliable change is the complete disappearance of a component.

23.4.4 Motor Evoked Potentials (MEPs)

Clinical Use — SEP monitoring can assess the integrity of primarily sensory tracts, while MEPs are used to protect the motor tracts in the spinal cord.

Recording Procedure — MEPs are elicited by either electrical or magnetic stimulation of the motor cortex or the spinal cord. Electrical stimulation is more common and results in reliable MEPs that can be recorded from either a limb muscle or a peripheral nerve, and they are known as myogenic and neurogenic MEPs. However, optimal use of this technique has yet to be determined.[7]

Interpretation — While the latency of myogenic MEPs is very consistent, their morphology and amplitude can vary wildly. Therefore, intraoperative interpretation is based only on the presence or absence of a response. On the other hand, neurogenic MEPs show more reliable morphology, amplitude, and latency. The most sensitive criterion for intraoperative interpretation is based only on amplitude changes.

23.5 Application Examples

The following paragraphs show some examples in which IOM was shown capable of detecting changes in the functional status of neuronal structures or insults which may have resulted in permanent neurological damage if they had been unnoticed.

23.5.1 EEG Burst Suppression

The effect of depth of anesthesia on the EEG is shown in the example of Figure 23.2, where two channels of frontocentral (F7-C3) and cetro-occipital (C3-O1) activity are seen. Several minutes after induction, a generalized pattern of activity is seen on the entire left hemisphere (left panel), whereas at deeper stages, bursts of activity are followed by segments of EEG suppression (right panel).

23.5.2 Ischemia

Surgery for disc disease performed following an anterior approach is associated with a high risk for vascular complications (e.g., ischemia), due to the close proximity of the areas of interest to major blood vessels.[25] The standard recordings in these cases are SEPs to posterior tibial nerve, with a peripheral, cervical, and cortical response, as shown in Figure 23.3. Temporary occlusion of the abdominal aorta, or one of the vessels that supplies the legs, such as the iliac artery, would cause a partial or complete loss of all responses (including the peripheral ones) ipsilateral to the side of the occluded artery. This situation is shown in Figure 23.3, where inadvertent occlusion of the iliac artery resulted in an increase in the latency and decrease in the amplitude of the responses to posterior tibial nerve stimulation compared to the baselines recorded in the beginning of the operation. The particular components affected are the PF recorded in the posterior fossa behind

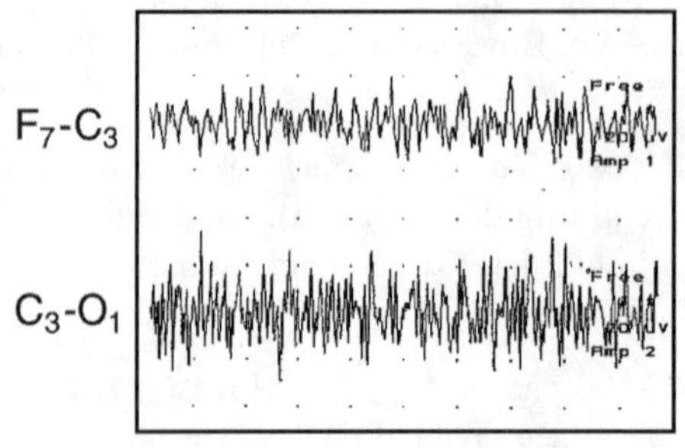

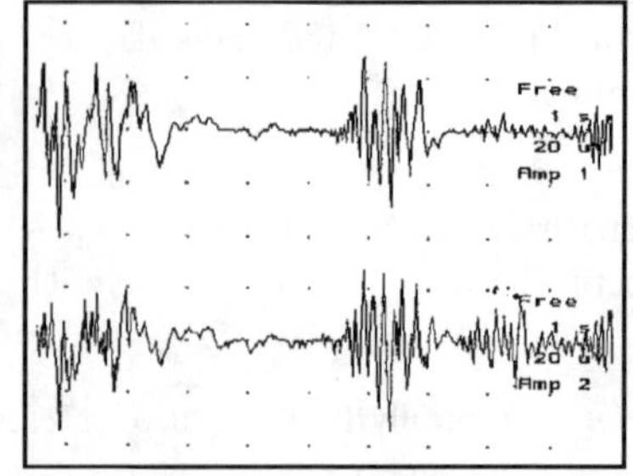

FIGURE 23.2 Example showing the effects of anesthesia depth on the EEG. At typical depths, continuous activity is observed (left) and then at deeper stages, bursts of activity are followed by burst suppression (right).

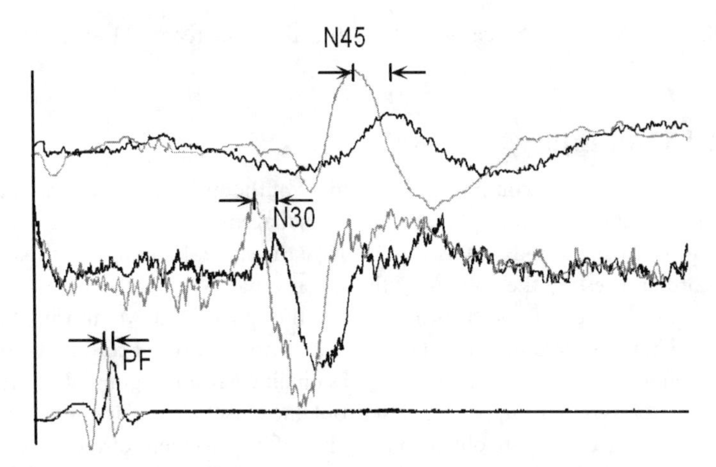

FIGURE 23.3 SEPs obtained after inadvertent occlusion of the iliac artery. Increased latency and decreased amplitude is seen in all responses (dark traces) to posterior tibial nerve stimulation. Gray traces correspond to the baselines.

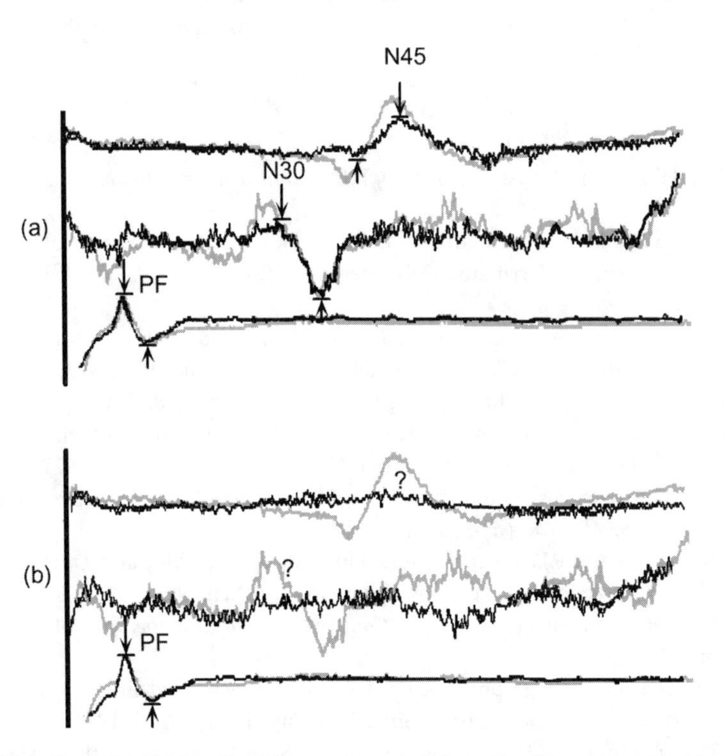

FIGURE 23.4 SEPs indicating cord injury. Baselines are shown in lighter color. The responses in (a) were obtained just before placement of instrumentation, while the ones in (b) were obtain after. The cortical (N45) and cervical responses (N30) disappeared just after placement of instrumentation, while the peripheral response (PF) remained unchanged.

the knee, the N30 recorded at cervical level two, and the N45 recorded at a contralateral central scalp location.

23.5.3 Spinal Cord Injury

During surgery for spinal fracture, compression or damage of the spinal cord by bone and disc fragments that enter the spinal canal is a common threat. Surgical management in these cases requires fusion with instrumentation, whereby metal rods are used to stabilize the spine. In addition, it may be necessary to decompress the cord and restore the volume of the spinal canal. A variety of complications can occur during these operations, including mechanical injury to the spinal cord. Monitoring SEPs to posterior tibial nerve stimulation is standard practice in these cases.[21b] An example of cord injury due to misplaced instrumentation is shown in Figure 23.4. Baseline SEPs obtained at the beginning of the case are shown in lighter color. The responses in the upper panel were obtained just before placement of instrumentation, while the ones in the lower panel were obtained after. Just after placement of the instrumentation, both the cortical (N45) and cervical (N30) responses disappeared, while the peripheral response (PF) obtained from the popliteal fossa remained unchanged.

23.6 Conclusions

Several factors contribute to successful IOM, including knowledge about the neuroanatomical structures that generate the signals under study and their function, understanding of the effects of surgical and perisurgical factors on the recordings, properly trained personnel and adoption of the established guidelines, ability to recognize and troubleshoot equipment failures, and finally integration of the monitoring personnel into the surgical and anesthesia teams. Only then can intraoperative monitoring be used as a safe, very useful, clinically valid, and cost-effective procedure that can improve the outcome of a variety of surgical procedures.

References

1. Albert, T.J., Balderston, R.A., and Northup, B.E., *Surgical Approaches to the Spine*, W.B. Saunders, Philadelphia, 1997.
2. Engler, G.L., Spielholz, N.J., Bernhard, W.N., Danziger, F., Merkin, H., and Wolff, T., Somatosensory evoked potentials during Harrington instrumentation for scoliosis, *J. Bone Joint Surg.*, 60, 528–532, 1978.
3. Nash, C.L., Lorig, R.A., Schatzinger, L.A., and Brown, R.H., Spinal cord monitoring during operative treatment of the spine, *Clin. Orthop. Related Res.*, 126, 100–105, 1977.
4. Delgado, T.E., Bucheit, W.A., Rosenholtz, H.R., and Chrissian, S., Intraoperative monitoring of facial muscle evoked responses obtained by intracranial stimulation of the facial nerve: a more accurate technique for facial nerve dissection, *Neurosurgery*, 4, 418–421, 1979.
5. Daspit, C.P., Raudzens, P.A., and Shetter, A.G., Monitoring of intraoperative auditory brain stem responses, *Otolaryngol. Head Neck Surg.*, 90, 108–116, 1982.
6. Grundy, B.L., Jannetta, P.J., Procopio, P.T., Lina, A., Boston, J.R., and Doyle, E., Intraoperative monitoring of brain-stem auditory evoked potentials, *J. Neurosurg.*, 57, 674–681, 1982.
7. Zouridakis, G. and Papanicolaou, A.C., *A Concise Guide to Intraoperative Monitoring*, CRC Press, Boca Raton, FL, 2001.
8. American Electroencephalographic Society, Guideline eleven: guidelines for intraoperative monitoring of sensory evoked potentials, *J. Clin. Neurophysiol.*, 11, 77–87, 1994.
9. Keith, R.W., Stambough, J.L., and Awender, S.H., Somatosensory cortical evoked potentials: a review of 100 cases of intraoperative spinal surgery monitoring, *J. Spinal Disorders*, 3, 220–226, 1990.

10. Nuwer, M.R., Dawson, E.G., Carlson, L.G., Kanim, L.E., and Sherman, J.E., Somatosensory evoked potential spinal cord monitoring reduces neurologic deficits after scoliosis surgery: results of a large multicenter survey, *Electroencephalogr. Clin. Neurophysiol.*, 96, 6–11, 1995.
11. Matsui, Y., Goh, K., Shiiya, N., Murashita, T., Miyama, M., Ohba, J., Gohda, T., Sakuma, M., Yasuda, K., and Tanabe, T., Clinical application of evoked spinal cord potentials elicited by direct stimulation of the cord during temporary occlusion of the thoracic aorta, *J. Thoracic Cardiovasc. Surg.*, 107, 1519–1527, 1994.
12. North, R.B., Drenger, B., Beattie, C., McPherson, R.W., Parker, S., Reitz, B.A., and Williams, G.M., Monitoring of spinal cord stimulation evoked potentials during thoracoabdominal aneurysm surgery, *Neurosurgery*, 28, 325–330, 1991.
13. Kartush, J.M. and Lundy, L.B., Facial nerve outcome in acoustic neuroma surgery, *Otolaryngol. Clin. North Am.*, 25, 623–647, 1992.
14. Møller, A.R., Intraoperative neurophysiologic monitoring of cranial nerves, in *Neurosurgical Topics Book 13, Surgery of Cranial Nerves of the Posterior Fossa*, Barrow, D.L., Ed., American Association of Neurological Surgeons, Park Ridge, IL, 1993.
15. Sekiya, T., Hatayama, T., Iwabuchi, T., and Maeda, S., Intraoperative recordings of evoked extraocular muscle activities to monitor ocular motor nerve function, *Neurosurgery*, 32, 227–235, 1993.
16. Yingling, C.D. and Gardi, J.N., Intraoperative monitoring of facial and cochlear nerves during acoustic neuroma surgery, *Otolaryngol. Clin. North Am.*, 25, 413–448, 1992.
17. Markand, O.N., Brainstem auditory evoked potentials, *J. Clin. Neurophysiol.*, 11, 319–342, 1994.
18. Schepens, M.A., Boezeman, E.H., Hamerlijnck, R.P., ter Beek, H., and Vermeulen, F.E., Somatosensory evoked potentials during exclusion and reperfusion of critical aortic segments in thoracoabdominal aortic aneurysm surgery, *J. Cardiac Surg.*, 9, 692–702, 1994.
19. Zouridakis, G., Papanicolaou, A.C., and Simos, P.G., Intraoperative neurophysiological monitoring. III. Analysis of spontaneous activity, *J. Clin. Eng.*, 23, 223–231, 1998.
20. Freye, E., *Cerebral Monitoring in the Operating Room and the Intensive Care Unit*, Kluwer Academic Publ., Dordrecht, The Netherlands, 1990.
21. Zouridakis, G., Papanicolaou, A.C., and Simos, P.G., Intraoperative neurophysiological monitoring. IV. Analysis of evoked activity, *J. Clin. Eng.*, 24, 309–319, 1999.

21b. Zouridakis, G., Papanicolaou, A.C., and Simos, P.G., Intraoperative neurophysiological monitoring. V. Surgery for spinal disorders, *J. Clin. Eng.*, 24, 372–379, 1999.

22. Zouridakis, G., Papanicolaou, A.C., and Simos, P.G., Intraoperative neurophysiological monitoring. VI. Cranial surgery, *J. Clin. Eng.*, 25, 54–64, 2000.
23. Møller, A.R., Neurophysiologic monitoring: cranial neurosurgery, in *Intraoperative Neuroprotection*, Andrews, R.J., Ed., Williams & Wilkins, Baltimore, 1996, 20.
24. Strauss, C., Fahlbusch, R., Nimsky, C., and Cedzich, C., Monitoring visual evoked potentials during para- and suprasellar procedures, in *Intraoperative Monitoring Techniques in Neurosurgery*, Loftus, C.M. and Traynelis, V.C., Eds., McGraw-Hill, New York, 1994.
25. Prior, P., The rationale and utility of neurophysiological investigations in clinical monitoring for brain and spinal cord ischemia during surgery and intensive care, *Comp. Meth. Prog. Biomed.*, 51, 13–27, 1996.

24

Technical Considerations in the Construction of Vascular Anastomoses

Mark A. Grevious
University of Illinois at Chicago

Francis Loth
University of Illinois at Chicago

Steven A. Jones
Louisiana Tech University

Nurullah Arslan
Fatih University

Michael A. Curi
University of Chicago

Lewis B. Schwartz
University of Chicago

Hisham S. Bassiouny
University of Chicago

CONTENTS

24.1 Introduction

Over the past several years, great strides have been made with respect to the way many surgeons construct vascular anastomoses. The word "anastomosis" comes from a Greek word meaning *outlet* and also comes from the Latin root word *anastomoun* which means *to furnish with a mouth.* The definition of anastomosis is the surgical connection of separate or severed tubular hollow organs to form a continuous channel, as between two parts of an artery or a vein. Vascular anastomoses of some kind are used in many of the surgical subspecialties. Vascular surgeons perform procedures such as arterial to venous bypass grafts for hemodialysis, and arterial bypass grafts for arterial insufficiency. Cardiac surgeons perform coronary artery bypass grafting as a means to revascularize the heart. They use autologous saphenous vein grafts and bypass blood directly from the aorta to the major vessels of the heart (e.g., left anterior descending, and the circumflex artery). Other fields in which vascular and microvascular anastomoses are used include otolaryngology, plastic surgery, neurosurgery, and pediatric surgery. The field of transplantation surgery routinely utilizes the concept of anastomoses. The organs harvested from the cadaver must include vessels that are long enough to be anastomosed to the recipient vessels. Additionally, it is important to realize that other structures such as the common bile duct in liver transplantation, the small bowel in small

0-8493-1140-3/04/$0.00+$1.50

bowel transplantation, and the ureters in renal transplantation are tubular structures which require coaptation via suture anastomosis.

The person credited with the first vascular anastomosis was J.B. Murphy in 1897. However, it was Alexis Carrel who developed a method of vessel triangulation to allow consistent and reproducible success with vascular anastomoses.[1] Carrel began the study of experimental vascular suture in the laboratory of Mariel Soulier in France, but was unable to pass the requisite clinical examinations and continue training. He became disillusioned with European medical training, traveled briefly to Montreal, and then secured a position within the University of Chicago Department of Physiology under the direction of Dr. George Stuart. Along with another of Stuart's young pupils, Charles Claude Guthrie, Carrel began an intensive study on the feasibility of experimental blood vessel surgery. Using fine silk suture and meticulous technique, Carrel and Guthrie successfully created a variety of vascular anastomoses and reconstructions, including the first-ever vein grafts, termed "biterminal venous transplantation." He was awarded the Nobel Prize in 1912 for his work on the suturing of vessels and transplantation of organs.

Most vascular anastomoses, such as the ones performed by cardiac and vascular surgeons, are performed under direct vision or, more commonly, loupe magnification. In addition to the well-publicized endovascular surgical techniques, (i.e., angioplasty, endovascular stent placement, and aneurysm repair) endoscopic vascular anastomoses, endoscopic vascular repair, and endoscopic vascular reconstruction can be performed. Furthermore, with the advent of the operating microscope, vascular anastomoses of vessels as small as 1 mm can be performed.

The history of microsurgery begins with Jules Jacobsen, a vascular surgeon from the University of Vermont, who in 1960 first reported suturing vessels together that were less than 1.5 mm in diameter. The father of microsurgery, however, is Harry Buncke. He is credited with performing the first two successful replantation procedures on laboratory animals.[2] He performed replantation of a rabbit ear and in 1966 he reported performing free tissue transfer of a monkey great toe to its hand.[3]

The purpose of this section is to provide insight on some of the current techniques used to construct vascular anastomoses. Although there have been many advances in construction of vascular anastomoses, the principles that were outlined by Alexis Carrel in his Nobel Prize Address in 1912 remain the same (i.e., aseptic technique, delicate handling of the tissue, and meticulous attention to detail). The basic techniques of three different types of anastomoses (rectus abdominis free tissue transfer, infrainguinal bypass, and arteriovenous graft) will also be discussed. This chapter will also discuss the importance of hemodynamics in graft patency and describe the basic fluid dynamics present within infrainguinal bypasses and arteriovenous grafts.

24.2 Materials

Monofilament sutures are the suture of choice when constructing macrovascular anastomoses or microvascular anastomoses. Braided suture tends to cause a significant amount of friction when passed through the vessel wall. Because both nylon suture and polypropylene suture are monofilament sutures, they do not cause this problem. Nylon monofilament is often employed when performing microvascular anastomoses. Polypropylene suture is often used when performing procedures such as coronary bypass grafting, arteriovenous (AV) fistulas, or AV Grafts. Additionally, PTFE (polytetrafluoroethylene) suture may be used when performing vascular procedures that require the use of a prosthetic vascular conduit made of PTFE. Polypropylene is a vinyl polymer, and is similar to polyethylene. Synthetic grafts are used widely in vascular reconstructive surgery, but their long-term patency is limited. The most widely used prosthetic materials for vascular grafts are PTFE and Dacron.

24.2.1 PTFE

Poly(tetrafluoroethylene) is prepared via suspension polymerization. It was later discovered that PTFE could be altered by stretching. This material was noted to be very strong and could be used for many things including clothing and prosthetic vascular conduits.[4]

24.2.2 Dacron

This type of graft is used for abdominal aortic aneurysm surgery and for aorto-iliac occlusive disease among many other uses. Dacron grafts are made in either knitted or woven form. Woven grafts have smaller pores and do not leak as much blood. Some Dacron grafts have recently been manufactured coated with protein (collagen/albumin) to reduce the blood loss and with antibiotics to prevent graft infection.

24.3 Anastomoses

One of the more important concepts is to have adequate flow into and out of a vessel. Obstruction and disturbance of flow dynamics proximal or distal to an anastomosis may cause undesirable effects whether the anastomosis is for a vascular conduit or tissue that will be transferred or transplanted. Prior to performing the anastomosis, proximal and distal control of the vessels is necessary with either vessel loops or vessel clamps of the appropriate size. There is not one specific way to perform an anastomosis. There are several different methods to perform a running anastomosis and an interrupted anastomosis depending on surgeon preference. However, the surgeon should adhere to a meticulous nontraumatic technique when handling the vessels. Two principal types of anastomoses are performed: either end-to-end or end-to-side.

24.3.1 End-to-End

End-to-end anastomoses can be performed using an interrupted technique, or a running technique. Interrupted end-to-end anastomoses are performed by first approximating the vessels via two opposing sutures. Additional sutures may be placed to construct a triangulated pattern as described by Alexis Carrel, or four sutures may be placed equidistant from one another. Once these sutures are placed, the surgical assistant places slight tension on two of the sutures, and the surgeon places additional sutures to bisect the distance between the sutures until adequate coaptation of the vessels is completed. The surgeon must make sure that the intimal layers from each vessel end are in direct contact. Meticulous surgical technique is required. The vessel ends must be relatively similar in diameter. If there is a size discrepancy, the smaller vessel may be beveled slightly to make the diameter larger. When performing microsurgical anastomoses, the adventitia is stripped, and the intima is inspected for injury. If a running technique is performed, the same core sutures are used, but the vessels are approximated in a running fashion.

24.3.2 End-to-Side

End-to-side anastomoses can also be performed using an interrupted or a running technique. An example is an infrainguinal arterial bypass with prosthetic PTFE graft. Adequate proximal and distal control must be obtained. The recipient artery (side artery) is prepared by performing an arteriotomy (small cut in the vessel along the longitudinal axis the recipient artery is made) (Figure 24.1). The first sutures to be placed are at the heel of the anastomosis. Once this is done, one end of a double-armed suture (suture with a needle on each end) is passed inside out at the apex of the arteriotomy site and the other needle is passed from inside to out of the PTFE graft. A separate double-armed suture is placed adjacent to the first suture in the same manner. The two sutures are tied down and then the vessels are brought together with one suture for the near side of the artery and the other suture for the far side of the artery. It is best to perform the far side first because that is usually the most difficult part of the anastomosis. For an interrupted technique, one suture is placed at the heel and one at the toe. The distance between the sutures is bisected until the anastomosis is complete.

24.4 Surgical Applications

Vascular anastomoses are necessary in a variety of surgical procedures, and the basic techniques of rectus abdominis free tissue transfer, infrainguinal bypass, and arteriovenous graft are described here.

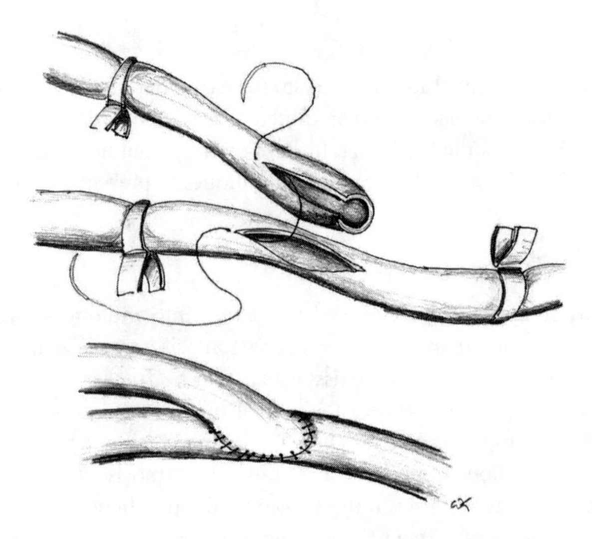

FIGURE 24.1 Sketch of an end-to-side anastomosis.

24.4.1 Rectus Abdominis Free Tissue Transfer

Patients who have large soft tissue defects from trauma or from wounds created surgically following extirpation of various types of tumors require coverage with well-vascularized tissue. Plastic surgeons have developed many methods to solve these very difficult problems. One method that is commonly employed for large soft tissue defects on the lower extremity, for example, is the transfer of the rectus abdominis muscle either as a muscle flap or as a muscle flap with the overlying skin attached (myocutaneous flap). The rectus abdominis muscle is classified as a Mathis-Nahai Type III flap, which means that it has a vascular arterial supply that comes from two dominant sources. The two dominant vascular arteries are the superior epigastric artery, a branch from the internal thoracic artery and the deep inferior epigastric artery (DIEA), a branch of the external iliac artery.

If the recipient site for the muscle flap is the lower extremity, the vessels of the lower extremity are identified and prepared prior to harvesting of the muscle. Large defects of the leg may involve injury to one or more of the major arteries in that region. The artery and a suitable vein are prepared with tenotomy scissors under loupe magnification first, followed by stripping of the adventitia under the operating microscope. A medium-sized branch of one of the major arteries (e.g., anterior tibial artery, peroneal artery, or the posterior tibial artery in the lower leg) is identified and sacrificed, then this can be used as the recipient artery for an end-to-end anastomosis with the DIEA. An adequately sized vein is used for an end-to-end anastomosis with the vein of the flap. If there are no vessels of adequate caliber, then the artery and its accompanying vein can be used as the recipient vessels in an end-to-side fashion. Proximal and distal control of the artery and vein are obtained with either small vascular clips or with small vessel loops. If a myocutaneous flap is to be harvested, then an elliptical vertical skin paddle over the rectus muscle is sketched over the muscle. This vertical skin paddle is incised around the markings and the subcutaneous tissue is dissected down to the anterior rectus sheath. The width of the elliptical skin paddle must be small enough to ensure that the donor site will be able to be closed primarily (bring skin edges together). The muscle is identified under the rectus sheath, and the muscle along with the skin paddle is harvested. The vascular contributions to the muscle from the superior epigastric artery and vein and the intercostal neurovascular bundles are ligated and divided. The vascular pedicle on which the muscle is harvested is the deep inferior epigastric artery. This vascular pedicle is dissected to its origin at the external iliac artery. Once this is performed, all soft tissue attachments of the muscle to the anterior and posterior rectus sheath are divided, taking care not to injure the vascular pedicle. At this point, the flap is being perfused only by the DIEA and its accompanying vein.

The operating microscope is placed in position at the leg where the vessels have been previously prepared. Some surgeons give systemic heparin at this point. The artery and vein are ligated at the origin of the vessels, and the tissue is brought down to the leg and the microsurgical anastomosis is performed. The anastomoses are performed meticulously, but with steady progress to decrease ischemia time. The anastomoses are performed using 8-0 or 9-0 nylon suture. It is the surgeon's preference on which vessel to suture first. Some surgeons prefer to perform the arterial anastomosis first to decrease ischemia time. Once the arterial anastomosis is performed, the venous blood is allowed to flow out of the flap for a short while. The vein is then clamped and the venous anastomosis is performed. Other surgeons prefer to perform the venous anastomosis first, then immediately perform the arterial anastomosis because the surgeon does not want the flap to experience any venous congestion that may occur following re-establishment of arterial flow to the flap. Once the anastomosis is completed, the muscle is then inset around the entire circumference of the wound with absorbable suture. If the flap is a muscle flap only, then a split thickness skin graft is harvested and placed directly over the muscle and secured with absorbable suture. A posterior mold plaster splint is placed on the lower extremity for the period of about a week to decrease any excess motion around the surgical site.

24.4.2 Infrainguinal Bypass

Patients with long-segment femoropopliteal occlusive disease are best treated with bypass originating from the groin. The major groin artery is the common femoral artery. The arterial inflow can originate from either the common femoral, the origin of the superficial femoral artery, or the profunda femoris artery. Preoperative evaluation includes assessment of medical risk, with use of myocardial stress testing to identify coronary disease. A general anesthetic is usually used; however, in some cases a regional block may be performed. Bypass to the popliteal artery above the knee may be performed using either the patient's own vein (autologous vein) or PTFE with acceptable results. Prosthetic bypass to arteries below the knee have a much lower overall patency rate, and thus these distal bypass procedures are best accomplished using autologous vein.

The patient is placed supine on the operating table and the leg is prepared from the lower abdomen to the ankle. The leg is externally rotated and supported behind the knee. A patient that has occluded superficial femoral and proximal popliteal arteries will require femoro-posterior tibial artery grafting. If the entire saphenous vein is available, then the *in situ* technique is preferable.

An incision is made in the groin over the saphenofemoral junction and the proximal saphenous vein is exposed. The entire length of the saphenous vein is exposed on its anterior surface. Visualization and protection of the vein is of utmost importance and one should not hesitate to connect multiple incisions if exposure is impaired. The proximal saphenous vein is dissected to its junction to the common femoral vein, and branches are ligated and divided. The saphenofemoral junction is fully mobilized and exposed. The adjacent common femoral artery is exposed, and control of the femoral, superficial femoral, and profunda femoris arteries secured.

After exposure and control of posterior tibial artery and distal portion of the saphenous vein in the calf, the patient is systemically heparinized. A vascular clamp is placed on the femoral vein at the saphenofemoral junction and the saphenous vein amputated. The defect in the common femoral vein is repaired with polypropylene monofilament suture. The saphenous vein is opened proximally to expose the highest venous value. Using loupe magnification, both leaflets of the superior saphenous valve are surgically removed under direct vision. Vascular clamps are applied to the femoral bifurcation, and a longitudinal arteriotomy is made in the common femoral artery. The proximal portion of the vein is anastomosed to the femoral artery using continuous 5-0 or 6-0 monofilament suture.

After completion of the proximal anastomosis, the clamps are removed and flow is established in the proximal portion of the saphenous vein. Flow stops at the first competent valve; this can usually be identified by the distention of the proximal vein and the collapse of the distal vein. Through large-sized distal side branches, a special valve-cutting device (called a valvulotome) is introduced and passed proximally through the closed valves. The vein valves are bicuspid; the plane of closure of the valves is parallel to the skin. Flow of arterial blood through the proximal anastomosis closes the valve cusps; this is essential for valve lysis. The valvulotome passes through the cusp in a plane parallel to the skin (parallel to the plane of valve closure) and is then rotated 90° anteriorly. The valvulotome is withdrawn and the tip is transluminally visualized on the anterior wall of the vein. When a valve is engaged, resistance will be felt. The valvulotome is withdrawn and a sudden release or pop is felt as the cusp is cut. The valvulotome is then again advanced in a plane parallel to the skin, past the location of the cut anterior leaflet, rotated 90° posteriorly, and withdrawn to cut the posterior leaflet. After cutting both valves, cusps are rendered incompetent allowing for unimpeded antegrade flow. Thus prepared, the vein graft is cannulated through its distal cut end; successful valve lysis is confirmed by a strong pulsatile stream of blood from the distal end of the vein.

The posterior tibial target artery is again located. The vein is controlled proximally. The distal end of the vein is spatulated and sutured end to side to the posterior tibial artery using continuous 6-0 or 7-0 monofilament suture. The anastomosis is completed and flow is established to the distal posterior tibial artery. After flow is established, all remaining side branches and fistulas are ligated leaving a continuous unbranched bypass conduit. Localization of these fistulas can be facilitated by the use of intraoperative hand-held continuous-wave Doppler ultrasound. Arteriography confirms wide patency of the reconstruction.

24.4.3 Arteriovenous Grafts for Hemodialysis

Construction of AV grafts for hemodialysis is one of the more commonly performed vascular surgery procedures in the United States. The procedure that is associated with the best long-term patency for hemodialysis is construction of an AV fistula. AV fistulas are surgically created arterial to venous connections for hemodialysis. One method of performing these fistulas is to construct an anastomosis between the cephalic vein and the radial artery at the wrist. However, this type of surgery can only be performed if the patient has an adequate caliber and quality of vein to be used. A prosthetic vascular conduit is used when the patient does not have suitable vein available. The AV grafts for hemodialysis are usually placed on the nondominant arm and can be placed on the upper or lower extremities. The upper extremity is most often used first, either in the forearm area or the upper arm. The arm is prepped and draped sterilely. An incision is made in the arm to achieve access to the brachial artery and to identify a large caliber vein in the cubital fossa (e.g., profunda cubitalis). If an AV graft procedure is to be performed, the PTFE graft is tunneled subcutaneously toward the wrist. A separate counter-incision is made 5 to 10 cm proximal to the distal wrist crease. The distal end of the PTFE graft is then brought out through this incision, and then tunneled back toward the proximal incision forming a loop on the anterior surface of the forearm. The distal incision is then closed. An end-to-side anastomosis of both the artery and the vein is performed using 5-0 or 6-0 prolene suture. Care is taken to ensure that little to no air is introduced into the vessels once blood flow through the AV graft is established. The wounds are closed over the graft anastomoses.

24.5 Patency

The surgeon concentrates on constructing a vascular anastomosis that will accommodate the required blood flow to the tissue or organ. After surgery, however, the concern shifts to how long the vessel will remain patent, and a great deal of research has been done to try and understand what causes the failure of grafts. In a recent study at the University of Chicago hospitals, patients were followed to determine patency rates following placement of 568 infrainguinal grafts. Vein grafts showed significantly better patency compared with PTFE grafts (Figure 24.2). Only limited differences were observed for different points of the distal anastomosis for femoral bypass grafts (Figure 24.3).

Hemodynamics has been shown to play an important role in chronic graft failure. However, the short-term effects of the anastomotic geometry are not so important. In an acute study, Blaisdell et al.,[5] reported that graft diameter and angle of attachment do not in themselves affect blood flow in arteries or arterial

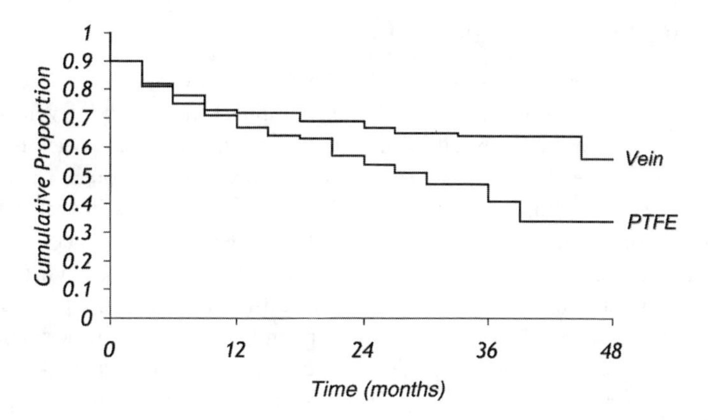

FIGURE 24.2 Cumulative proportion of vascular grafts remaining patent with synthetic (PTFE-215 grafts) and autologous (vein-349 grafts).

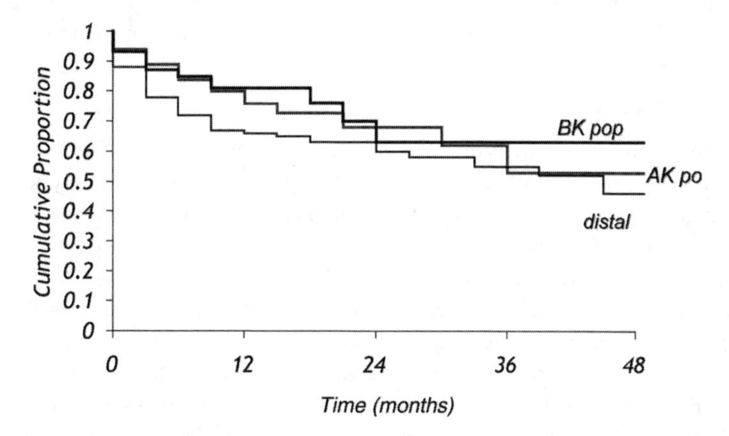

FIGURE 24.3 Cumulative proportion of vascular grafts remaining patent for femoral bypass grafts to different points of the distal anastomosis. These include: popliteal artery above the knee (AK pop-167 grafts), popliteal artery below the knee (BK pop-61 grafts), and anterior tibial artery, peroneal artery, etc. (distal-333 grafts).

substitutes. In general, there is significant concern about how the anastomostic geometry and graft hemodynamics affect patency rates. A detailed description of the hemodynamics of vein grafts and its relationship to patency is given by Skelly et al.[6] and is briefly described here.

24.5.1 Blood Flow (ml/sec)

Transit-time ultrasound devices have made intraoperative measurement of blood flow much easier. While the correlation is weak, infrainguinal vein grafts with high mean flow enjoy higher patency rates;[7,8] however, extended patency with low mean flow is often observed clinically. While low sensitivity and specificity of individual measurements limit its ability to guide therapy, patency curves for high flow grafts do exceed low flow grafts by about 20%.[9,10] For these reasons, routine clinical measurement of mean blood flow has not gained popularity. Stimulated mean blood flow >140 ml/min has predictive value for graft patency, but only when using univariate analysis and ignoring more specific measures of conduit and/or outflow bed resistance.[9,10] The poor correlation between mean blood flow and graft patency might well be expected since it only considers the mean components within the pulsatile waveform. Mean blood flow is primarily dependent on the state of the peripheral outflow bed. This can be demonstrated by a transient 100% increase in mean flow after a single dose of papaverine. An intraoperative measurement of mean blood flow is basically a measure of outflow resistance since skeletal muscle outflow is almost entirely governed by arteriolar tone.

24.5.2 Outflow Resistance (dynes/cm^5)

Outflow resistance (R) is a frequently studied and somewhat controversial variable of bypass grafting. This outflow can be estimated anatomically using the angiographic runoff score,[11,12] which has advantages, as it is quantifiable preoperatively. The results using this method, however, have been mixed, and positive correlations with patency, when found, have been only on the order of 20 to 30%. Thus, the conclusions of the SVS/ISCVS Ad Hoc Committee on Reporting Standards appear valid in that "[the angiographic runoff score] has not correlated well with the patency of infrainguinal vein grafts (where patency rates are usually good despite compromised runoff)."[13] Outflow can also be measured indirectly using a pulse-generated runoff.[14-17] A more direct method of estimating runoff is to compute R of the completed vascular reconstruction as the ratio of measured pressure and flow ($R = P/Q$). A relationship between outflow resistance and graft patency using this technique has been documented by several groups, including our own.[10,14,15,18-20] However, R has a fairly low specificity and sensitivity as a predictor of patency. The difference in patency between high R ($>50 \times 10^3$ dynes/cm^5) and low R ($<50 \times 10^3$ dynes/cm^5) grafts is only about 20%. In addition, long-term patency in a high R circuit (such as a popliteal-to-dorsalis pedis bypass) can routinely be achieved given adequate inflow and a high-quality autologous conduit. Thus, R is not very useful for selecting or excluding patients for revascularization.

24.5.3 Diameter (cm)

The most basic dimensions of a graft, its diameter and length, give a measure of the "resistive" properties of the conduit that is independent of the outflow bed. Based on steady or pulsatile equation of the flow through a straight graft, the effect of radius (fourth power) and length (first power) are important. The relationship between internal diameter and patency has not been well studied despite this seemingly obvious connection. An early report by Bernhard et al. suggested 4.0 mm as the smallest acceptable diameter for successful infrainguinal vein grafting.[21] Later, LiCalzi and Stansel showed veins as small as 3.5 mm achieved patency similar to larger conduits.[22] Sanders et al.[23] conducted a canine study to examine the importance of diameter. They concluded that the diameter of a prosthesis should approximate or be 2 mm larger than that of the outflow vessel, depending on the runoff, the location of the graft, and the recipient's exercise potential. Lastly, a study of factors influencing the development of vein graft stenoses[24] concluded that the only factor significantly predictive of stenosis was a minimum graft diameter <3.5 mm.[25] The lack of studies examining vein graft diameter is likely due to the difficulty of its precise measurement. Measurements are often inaccurate because of the variation in vessel wall thickness and degree of taper. It is not unusual for even relatively short vein segments to taper by 25% especially at points of confluence.[26] In addition, measurements of internal diameter using intraoperative angiography suffer greatly from magnification and parallax artifact.

24.5.4 Wall Shear Stress (dynes/cm^2)

Estimation of wall shear stress (WSS) in human vein grafts is quite complex. Based on the Poiseuille flow, WSS is $4\,\mu Q/\pi r^3$, where μ = blood viscosity, Q = mean flow, and r = internal radius. While this equation neglects the pulsatile nature of the flow, there are also problems with neglecting vessel taper and the measurement of the internal radius. Even with an assumed value of the vessel radius as uniform and rigid, vein grafts tend to vary only modestly with respect to diameter (3 to 6 mm) but widely with respect to mean outflow resistance (10 to 300×10^3 dynes/cm^5). Therefore, the primary determinant of the mean WSS is ultimately outflow resistance or volume flowrate.

The effect of WSS on the artery wall has been an important research topic during the last decade, and several investigators have demonstrated that the artery wall responds to prolonged changes in WSS by undergoing a significant degree of remodeling. Kamiya and Togawa[27] used a dog model to demonstrate that the carotid artery alters its diameter in response to changes in flow rate so as to maintain the mean WSS at approximately 15 dynes/cm^2. Changes in diameter in response to decreased flow in the rabbit carotid were shown to be dependent upon the presence of an intact endothelium

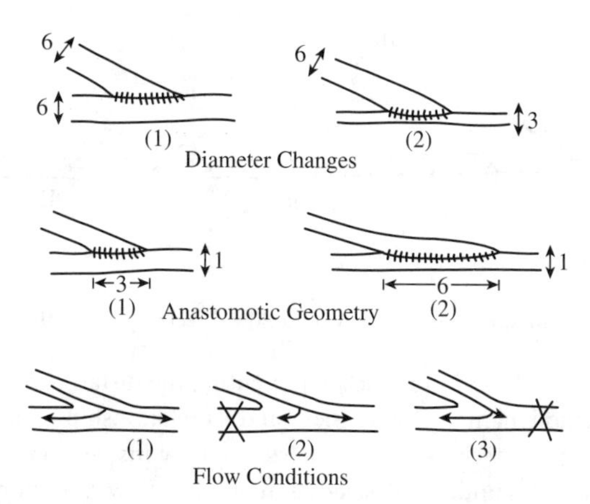

FIGURE 24.4 Variations in graft diameter, geometry, and flow conditions

by Langille and O'Donnell.[28] Zarins et al.[29] have shown that the artery lumen in cynomolgus monkeys, when subjected to up to ten-fold increases in blood flow, increased in diameter over a period of months until a mean WSS of 15 dynes/cm^2 was restored. Thus, there is considerable evidence that WSS is one mechanism which regulates artery lumen diameter, and intimal thickening is characteristic of the remodeling process. Of particular relevance is the evidence that intimal thickening occurs in localized regions where the WSS is low in magnitude and/or oscillates in direction during the cardiac cycle.[30] Thus, vascular geometries such as bifurcations and anastomoses, which create localized zones with such WSS behavior may be more prone to intimal thickening.

24.5.5 Importance of Geometry on Graft Hemodynamics

The vascular graft geometry is, to some extent, determined by the vascular surgeon and can vary in several ways (i.e., ratio of graft-to-artery diameter, graft angle, and hood length), as shown in Figure 24.4. Figure 24.5 shows the graft geometry at the midplane and the nomenclature employed. There are also considerable variations in blood flow waveforms between subjects, both in shape and time-averaged values, for the inlet as well as the proximal and distal outlet segments (POS and DOS). Blood flow in the POS is possible because the bypass graft is typically constructed distal to patent collateral vessels as shown in Figure 24.6. The ratio of POS:DOS flow will have a major influence on the velocity and WSS behavior. Autologous conduits vary greatly in diameter, thus the significant size mismatch between the host and graft vessels. The anastomostic geometry can also vary with respect to hood length, which is controlled by the surgeon. These variations in geometry and flow conditions make the hemodynamics inside an end-to-side anastomosis difficult to predict, and significantly different from the more commonly studied flow bifurcations such as the carotid, left coronary and aortic bifurcations.[31]

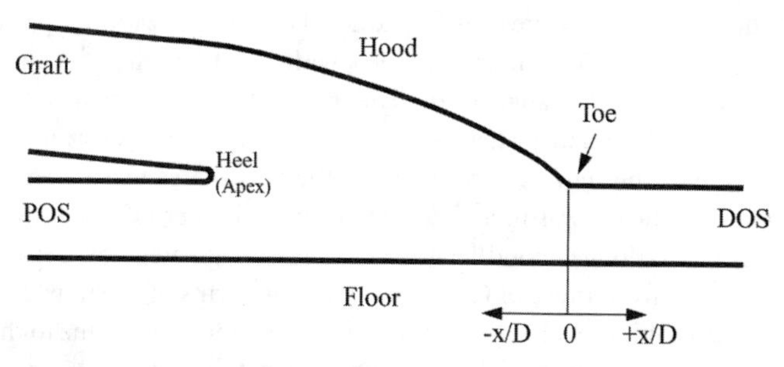

FIGURE 24.5 Nomenclature for an end-to-side anastomosis. (From Loth, F. et al., *J. Biomech. Eng.*, 124, 44, 2002. With permission.)

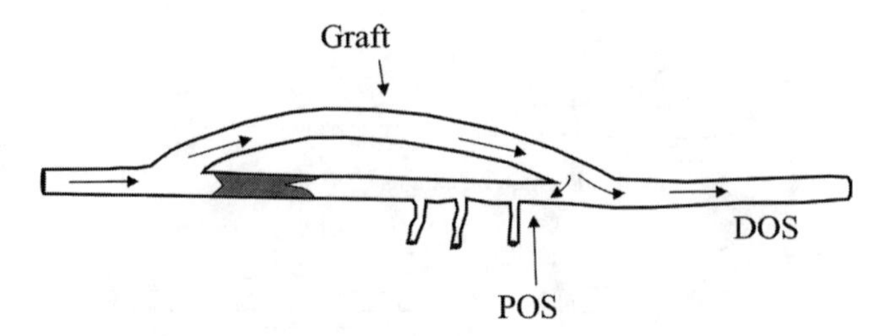

FIGURE 24.6 Sketch of an end-to-side anastomosis with a flow directed proximally and distally.

Several studies have employed *in vitro* models representing the distal segment of end-to-side anastomoses to investigate the hemodynamics environment and its relationship with graft failure. Ojha et al.[32] employed a photochromic tracer technique to visualize the flow inside a 45° graft model to determine the axial velocity and WSS profiles under both steady and pulsatile flow conditions with the POS occluded. The Plexiglas model represents an anastomosis with equal graft and artery diameters and a hood length of 1.4 diameters. The results demonstrate the types of flow structures that exist inside end-to-side vascular graft under this configuration and serve as an excellent reference for further studies employing models with different geometries and flow conditions.

Shu and Hwang[33] conducted an *in vitro* study of an end-to-side graft using flow visualization and LDA under pulsatile flow conditions. They used an elastic transparent flow model to simulate the venous anastomosis of arteriovenous hemodialysis angioaccess loop grafts based on silicone rubber casts obtained from grafts of this type implanted in dogs. Arterial bypass grafts are similar in geometry although the flow rates and Reynolds numbers are significantly lower than those employed in this arteriovenous graft study. Both the different flow conditions and the differences between vein and artery suggest that intimal hyperplasia in hemodialysis grafts and arterial bypass grafts should be considered as two distinctly different phenomena.[34] Nonetheless, this study demonstrates the type of flow field to be expected in arterial bypass grafts under high blood flow conditions such as during exercise or with a distal arteriovenous fistula.

The effect of the different parameters on the flow field inside arterial bypass grafts under steady flow conditions has been investigated by several researchers. These flow and geometric parameters include Reynolds number, POS:DOS flow ratio, graft angle, hood length, and ratio of graft-to-artery diameter. Steady flow experiments by Keynton et al.[35] using a laser Doppler anemometer (LDA) examined the effects of graft angle on the local velocity field inside *in vitro* end-to-side graft models with the POS occluded. The three models examined had graft angles of 30°, 45°, and 60° with equal graft-to-artery diameters. They found circumferential motion to be greatest for the 60° model and least for the 30° model.

The effect of outlet flow conditions, POS to DOS flow ratio and Reynolds number on the flow phenomena was investigated by Crawshaw et al.[36] and White et al.[37] Using a clear plastic model with inlet graft angles of 15° and 45°, Crawshaw et al.[36] demonstrated that the formation of separation regions under steady flow conditions is minimized by a small graft angle and occlusion of the POS. Flow separation near the toe of the anastomotic hood occurred in the 15° model under conditions of POS flow less than that in the 45° model. White et al.[37] conducted flow visualization experiments under steady and pulsatile flow conditions for two vein graft models with hood lengths of 4 and 8 diameters, equal graft and artery diameters, and a graft angle of 0°. These models were constructed as scaled-up models from plastic casts of the *in vivo* geometry. They demonstrated separation occurring along the lateral walls of the sinus at the junction of the vein and artery due to the lateral area expansion created by the sinus. Separation on the hood near the toe was more likely to occur for higher POS flows, and there was a clear tendency for the model with a longer hood length to experience greater flow separation on the hood. Their results differ somewhat from those of Crawshaw et al.[36] in terms of the flow division at which they occurred and, as discussed by White et al.,[37] these differences are undoubtedly due to the specific geometry studied. Flow studies on a simplified model consisting of two tubes connected at an angle give good insight into the types of flow behavior inside the distal segment of end-to-side grafts. However, the presence and location of flow features (separation, stagnation point) may differ from that of the *in vivo* case due to geometric differences.

The ratio of graft-to-artery diameter can also significantly affect the location of flow features. Crawshaw et al.[36] also used a realistic geometry constructed by grafting a 10-mm knitted Dacron graft end to side to a 6-mm PTFE main channel at 45°. Comparing this model to the plastic model with straight tubes, they found similar separation zones to occur in the model of Dacron-PTFE anastomosis, despite the discrepancy in size between the graft inlet diameters; however, details about the position and flow division at which they occurred are not provided. The ratio of graft-to-artery diameter can greatly affect the WSS distribution since WSS is related to the reciprocal of the radius cubed. Binns et al.[38] conducted a study on the effect of WSS on vascular healing in which PTFE grafts with internal diameters of 3, 6, and 8 mm were inserted end to end in the femoral and carotid arteries of ten mongrel dogs. They found lower WSS produced greater amounts of pseudointimal thickening within PTFE grafts and neointimal thickening at their anastomoses. Conversely, the higher WSS from small-diameter grafts was associated with poor graft patency. This suggests that, based on the WSS, an optimal diameter may exist for maximum patency. The optimal diameter is not known at this time; however, grafts of diameter smaller than the host vessel are not commonly employed due to the increased resistance of the smaller grafts.

24.5.6 Arterial Bypass Graft Hemodynamics

We have reported on the fluid dynamics within an end-to-side graft geometry using an upscaled model.[39,40] Some of the results of those studies will be summarized here. The model geometry was based on a vinyl polysiloxane cast taken from an acute PTFE canine ilio-femoral graft that was representative of the 12 anastomoses constructed in a set of preliminary canine studies (anastomosis is shown in Figure 24.7). This geometry is also representative of PTFE femoral-popliteal bypass grafts commonly employed in humans. The *in vitro* model of this cast was scaled up in diameter nine times. This scaling parameter was selected such that standard tubing (50.8 and 31.75 mm) could be used for the inlet and exits of the model and to provide good spatial resolution in the LDA measurements. Dynamic similarity between the original graft and the scaled-up model was ensured by maintaining physiologic Reynolds numbers and POS:DOS flow ratios. Based on internal dimensions, the graft to artery diameter ratio was 1.6 to 1, representing an *in vivo* graft lumen diameter of 5.6 mm and an artery lumen diameter of 3.5 mm (*external* diameter measurements for the graft and artery are 6 and 4 mm, respectively, with a graft-to-artery diameter ratio of 1.5). The graft branching angle was 5°, while the hood length to host artery diameter was 5:1 based on lumen measurements (approximately 4.5:1 based on external dimensions). Proximal and distal to the anastomosis, the artery and graft diameters were modeled to be constant in size.

The graft model incorporated several important features. First, the model geometry was defined such that the three-dimensional boundaries were described analytically in order to facilitate numerical solutions for this geometry.[40] Second, the model was idealized to be symmetric about the plane of the anastomosis, which reduced the total measurements needed to describe the flow and allowed the main flow features to be more clearly observed. Last, the model was constructed from Sylgard elastomer (Dow Corning) with a wall thickness of 2 cm or greater, which provided an optically clear and essentially rigid model. The dimensions of the plastic cast as a function of position along the host vessel were measured from images obtained from a high-resolution GE 9800 computerized tomography (CT) scanner at Grady

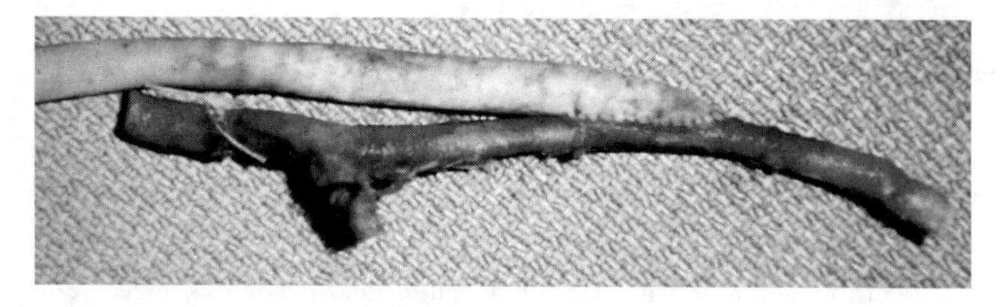

FIGURE 24.7 Photograph of an end-to-side anastomosis.

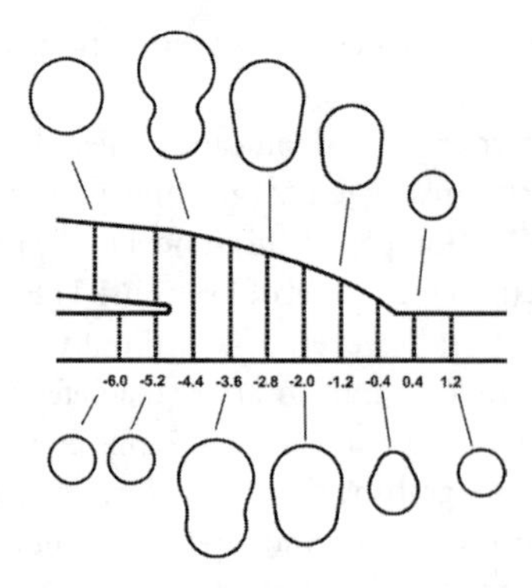

FIGURE 24.8 Cross-sectional view of an end-to-side anastomosis. (From Loth, F. et al., *J. Biomech. Eng.*, 124, 44, 2002. With permission.)

Memorial Hospital in Atlanta, Georgia. Each image represented the cross-sectional shape of the plastic cast at sections 1.5 mm apart in the axial direction of the host vessel, although the CT scanner had a boundary detection program that caused the cross-sectional profile to appear smoother than the true profile. The resulting cross-sectional geometry of the end-to-side configuration is shown in Figure 24.8.

A variety of flow conditions can exist for the fluid exiting the graft. However, it is common in clinical experience — and in the canine studies upon which this particular geometry was based — for the majority of the flow to exit the anastomosis in the distal direction and for a portion to exit proximally to supply small arterial branches in the proximal segment. Thus, the flow division into the DOS and POS is a very influential boundary condition. The *in vivo* canine studies indicated that the POS:DOS flow ratio immediately after surgery was typically between 20:80 and 30:70. The LDA measurements were conducted with the division of flow set at 20:80 for a Reynolds number of 208 based on the host artery diameter. (*Note:* The Reynolds number based on the graft inlet diameter is 130.) This corresponded to an *in vivo* mean flow rate value of 1.9 ml/sec which is typical of that found in our canine ilio-femoral anastomoses. The Reynolds number for this study was based on the host artery diameter and *not* on the graft diameter (thus, $Re = 4\rho Q_{Graft}/\pi D_A \mu$, where *in vivo* values are: $Q_{Graft} = 1.9$ cm^3/sec, $D_A = 0.35$ cm, $\mu = 0.035$ g/sec/cm, and $\rho = 1.05$ g/cm^3).

The experimental setup was such that either steady or pulsatile flow could be generated and the velocity measurements were conducted using laser Doppler anemometry. The WSS values were obtained from the product of the velocity gradient at the wall and the viscosity of the fluid. The velocity gradient was estimated as the slope of a linear least squares fit of three velocity measurements near the wall. Details of the steady flow experimental setup are given by Loth et al.[39]

Velocity measurements at the midplane of the anastomosis are displayed as two-dimensional vectors in Figure 24.9. The zero reference position is located at the toe of the graft. The graft velocity profile at

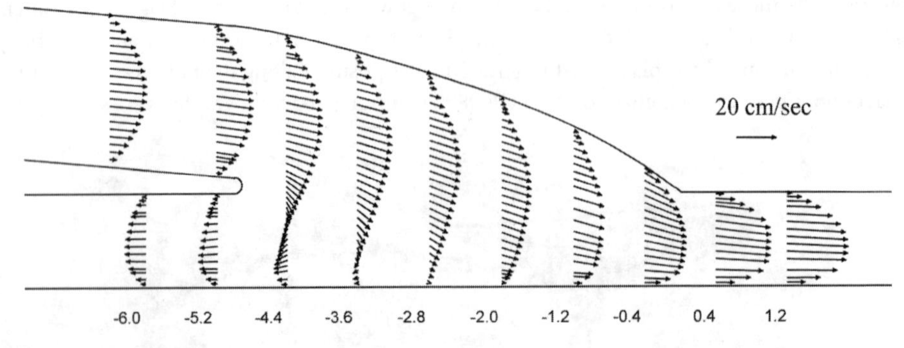

FIGURE 24.9 Velocity distribution at the midplane of an end-to-side anastomosis under steady flow conditions. (From Loth, F. et al., *J. Biomech. Eng.*, 119, 187, 1997. With permission.)

position –6.6 is parabolic in shape (Poiseuille flow) while at position –5.2, just upstream from the anastomosis, the velocity profile is slightly skewed toward the heel. The amount of skewing was examined for POS:DOS flow ratios of 50:50 and 0:100 and found to increase with increasing POS flow. The flow from the graft into the anastomosis has some similarities to flow in a sudden expansion. Specifically, the peak velocity maintains its magnitude as the flow moves distally into the anastomosis, and the velocity gradient along the hood at the midplane decreases as the flow moves distally in the graft until position –2.0 is reached. Distal to position –2.0, the decreasing cross-sectional area of the anastomosis causes the velocity gradient to increase along the hood until the flow exits through the DOS.

The velocity profiles in the DOS entrance are blunt with high velocity gradients near the wall. As the flow moves from positions 0.4 to 1.2 in the DOS, the velocity profile becomes less blunt and the peak velocity increases from 23 to 25 cm/sec. This increase in peak velocity is an entrance flow effect and is also observed in the POS where the peak velocity increases in magnitude from –7.6 to –8.4 cm/sec from positions –5.2 to –6.0. Velocity profiles are skewed toward the floor in both the POS and DOS. It is interesting to note that, throughout the midplane, the measured velocities have a component that is directed toward the floor of the graft.

The flow field changes significantly under pulsatile flow conditions although the main features shown in the steady flow field are still present throughout most of the cardiac cycle. The pulsatile flow waveform is shown in Figure 24.10. On average, the flow split remained at 20:80. The mean and peak Reynolds numbers were 850 and 222, respectively. Figure 24.11 shows the WSS trace at each measurement location inside the graft. The time averaged (mean), maximum, and minimum values of the WSS over the cycle are given in Table 24.1. The WSS values measured inside the vascular graft model are generally lower than the values that exist inside a normal healthy artery except at the inlet to and inside the DOS on the floor side (traces V, W, and X) where the mean for trace V was double that of trace Z. Traces A and K at the graft entrance are approximately one quarter in magnitude of trace Z. This was expected since shear varies with the inverse of the radius cubed in straight tubes and the ratio of graft diameter to host artery diameter is 1.6 to 1 (i.e., $1.6^{-3} = 0.244$). Note that the shapes of traces A and K are very similar to that of the flow waveform.

After entering the anastomosis, flow impinges on the floor forming a stagnation point where flow splits to exit through the DOS or POS. The sign of the WSS indicates direction with positive WSS directed

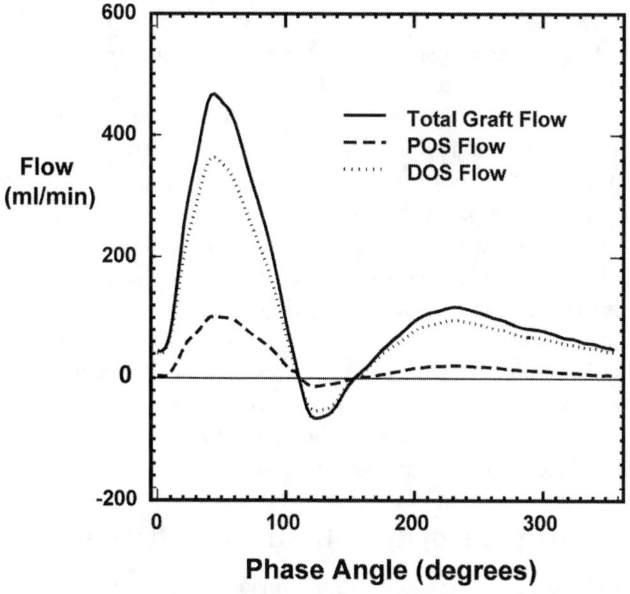

FIGURE 24.10 Example flow waveform of a femoral to popliteal bypass graft. (From Loth, F. et al., *J. Biomech. Eng.*, 124, 44, 2002. With permission.)

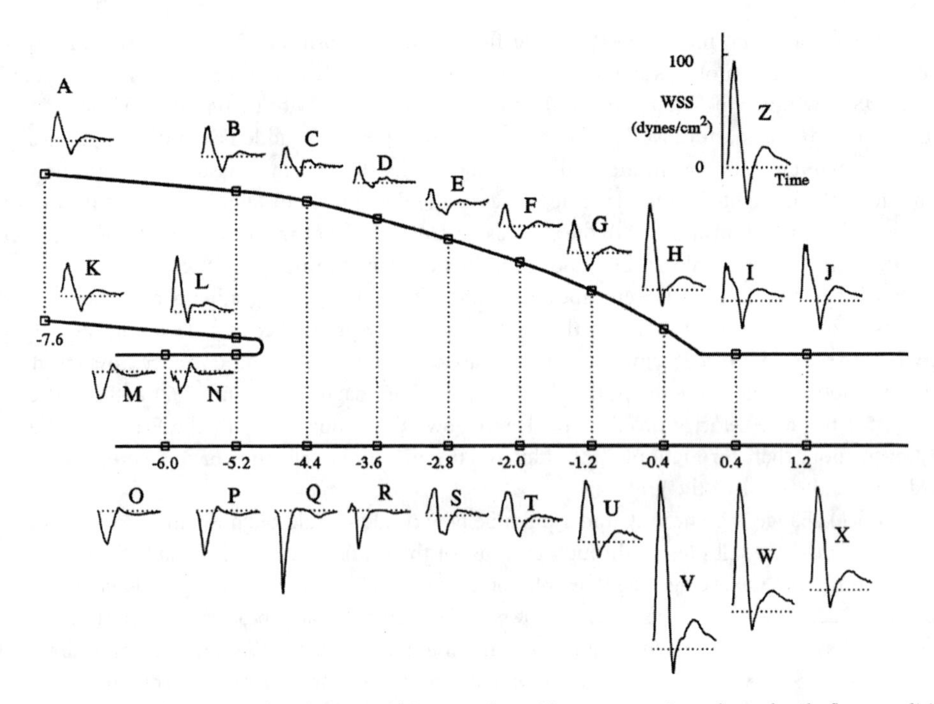

FIGURE 24.11 Wall shear stress distribution within an end-to-side anastomosis under pulsatile flow conditions.

distally and negative WSS directed proximally. The WSS traces on the floor near the stagnation point demonstrate how quickly the WSS environment can change significantly in a short distance (traces R, S, and T). The minimum mean WSS along the floor was located slightly proximal to the midway point of the anastomosis at position –2.8 (see trace S).

Along the hood, the mean WSS also decreases to a minimum near the midway point of the anastomosis at position –2.8 (trace E). At this position, near wall reverse flow during the cardiac cycle occurs earliest and was reversed for the longest period (between phase angles 66° and 174°). On the hood near the entrance to the DOS, WSS increases greatly due to the reduction in cross-sectional area (see trace H). Inside the DOS, the mean WSS decreases just distal to the toe as flow was skewed toward the floor.

Proximal to position –3.6 on the floor and inside the POS, WSS traces follow the inverse of the flow waveform trace as flow moves retrograde in the POS. WSS values are again low inside the POS with slightly higher values found on the floor side as expected since velocity profiles were skewed toward the floor inside the POS throughout most of the cycle.

Quantitative and concurrent experiments were carried out to determine the correlation between intimal hyperplastic thickening (IHT) *in vivo* and the distribution of hemodynamic WSS *in vitro* for this end-to-side anastomosis model.[39] The spatial distribution of IHT and the reciprocal of mean WSS were correlated ($r = 0.525$, $p < 0.01$). However, this correlation was only present for positions located on the PTFE graft itself. The data indicate that IHT is most evident at the suture line and along the juxta anastamotic PTFE graft hood, in contrast to the native artery. The conclusion from this study was that the relationship between IHT development and hemodynamics is significantly affected by multiple biological and mechanical factors (i.e., hemodynamics, surgical injury, and the presence of PTFE).

24.5.7 Arteriovenous Hemodialysis Graft Hemodynamics

An AV graft is constructed from an artery to a vein to provide an access site for hemodialysis patients. By bypassing the high resistance vessels (arterioles and capillaries), high flow rates can be achieved that are necessary for efficient hemodialysis (Figure 24.12). A synthetic graft material, polytetrafluoroethylene (PTFE), is often used for these grafts. More than half of the AV grafts fail and require surgical reconstruction

TABLE 24.1 Mean, Maximum and Minimum Values of Wall Shear Stress Inside the Anastomosis

Location	Position (x/D)	Mean	Maximum	Minimum
		Hood Side		
A	−7.4	3.7	25.6	−11.8
B	−5.2	3.2	27.1	−13.8
C	−4.4	3.1	17.7	−8.4
D	−3.6	2.4	14.8	−4.3
E	−2.8	1.4	13.5	−8.7
F	−2	1.2	18.9	−10.4
G	−1.2	2.7	28.7	−15.9
H	−0.4	14.6	75.6	−14.1
I	0.4	7.1	33.2	−24.8
J	1.2	9.8	50	−24.8
		Heel-Graft Side		
K	−7.4	4.3	28.9	−13.3
L	−5.2	8.8	49.5	−9.3
		Heel-POS Side		
M	−6	−4.6	23.5	−6.6
N	−5.2	−3	18.9	−7.4
		Floor Side		
O	−6	−5.9	29.3	−3.1
P	−5.2	−6.6	38.5	−3.7
Q	−4.4	−8.6	73.1	−1.6
R	−3.6	−3.9	33.6	−5.9
S	−2.8	1.6	23.4	−16.6
T	−2	3.9	25.1	−13.8
U	−1.2	11.1	53.6	−13.2
V	−0.4	32.4	146.8	−21.5
W	0.4	24.3	112	−16
X	1.2	20.8	90.5	−15
		Theory in Artery*		
Z	—	16.3	94.1	−32.4

* A theoretical solution of WSS values[45] for the present waveform inside a straight tube of diameter equal to that of the artery is given for comparison.

within 3 years.[41] The majority of these graft failures are caused by occlusive venous anastomotic intimal hyperplasia (VAIH) which is a stenosis or narrowing of the vein downstream of the graft. The stenoses are predominately located near and just downstream of the venous anastomosis. Biomechanical forces in the AV graft are unique with generally high wall shear stress (WSS) acting on the vein with a region of flow separation and pressure fluctuations that vibrate the vein wall and surrounding tissue. In an AV graft canine animal model, Fillinger et al.[42,43] measured the level of vibration in the tissue surrounding the venous anastomosis and found that this level had a strong correlation with VAIH ($r = 0.92$, $p < 0.001$). However, since WSS was not examined in this study, it remains unclear if the distribution of WSS also plays a role in the development of VAIH.

Further experimental studies using laser Doppler anemometry were conducted using the model described previously to examine the steady flow environment within an AV graft[44] and are briefly described here. All results are presented scaled to *in vivo* values. The experimental setup was such that 90% of the flow returning to the venous side was from the graft. The Reynolds number was 2275, which is approximately 10 times the value used in the vascular graft study. The time-averaged mean velocity vectors are shown in Figure 24.13. The mean velocity profile at the inlet was blunt (not parabolic) since flow at this

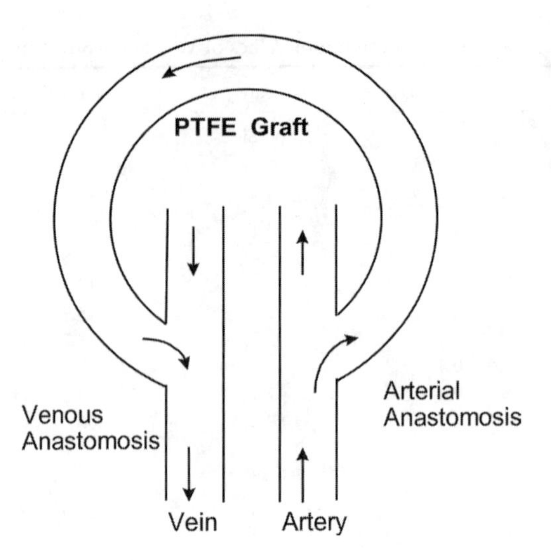

FIGURE 24.12 Schematic arteriovenous bypass graft.

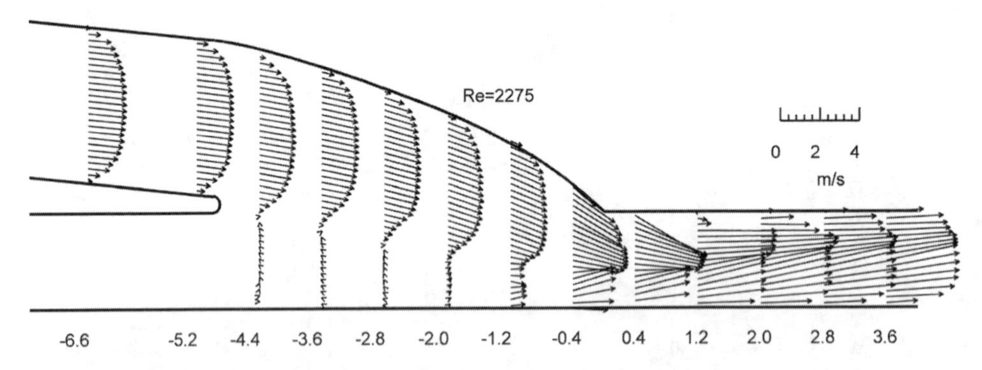

FIGURE 24.13 Velocity distribution at the midplane of an end-to-side anastomosis under steady flow conditions representative of that present in an arteriovenous graft (Re = 2275).

Reynolds number is transitional. The velocity profiles stay blunt inside the anastomosis and a recirculation cell forms on the floor side of the graft. A stagnation point is formed between position –2.8 and –2.0. Flow appears to be separated somewhere between positions 0.4 and 1.2. The distribution of turbulent fluctuations is shown in Figure 24.14 as the root mean square of the velocity component parallel to the floor of the graft. Turbulent intensities are greater near the wall throughout the model with the exception of the recirculation zone near the floor. The highest turbulent intensities and Reynolds stresses were found on the toe side of proximal venous segment between positions 1.2 and 3.6 (0.55 m/sec and 1263 dynes/cm^2, respectively).

These results indicate three types of flow regimes: (1) stagnation point flow on the floor within the recirculation cell, (2) separated flow just downstream to the toe inside the PVS, and (3) increased turbulence intensity and Reynolds stresses downstream of the toe extending more than three diameters inside the PVS. Localized regions of low WSS present within regimes 1 and 2 may be significant in the development of intimal hyperplasia. The increased turbulence downstream of the toe within the PVS corresponds to the location of high tissue vibration and intimal hyperplasia found by Fillinger et al.[42]

Despite the advancements in our understanding of the failure of vascular anastomoses, research in this area is still necessary. The technical aspects of constructing anastomoses are still evolving. While there are no recent major advances with respect to graft material, companies are continually developing and testing new prefabricated grafts products. Numerical simulation techniques now allow researchers to better understand the hemodynamic environment of both prosthetic and autologous vascular conduits.

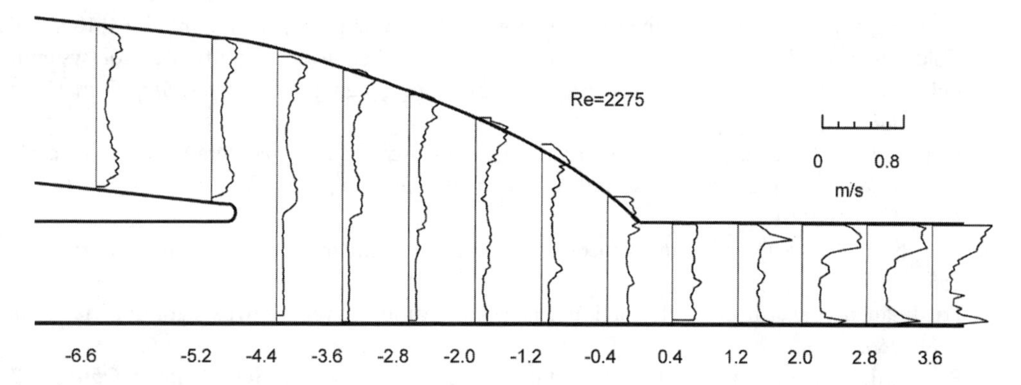

FIGURE 24.14 Root mean square of the axial component of velocity that demonstrates the fluctuations present in this weakly turbulent flow.

However, use of this fluid dynamic information in the prediction of patency or graft design still remains a challenge.

References

1. Brieger, G.H., The development of surgery, in *Textbook of Surgery. The Biological Basis of Modern Surgical Practice*, Sabiston, D.C., Ed., W.B. Saunders, Philadelphia, 1991.
2. Buncke, H.J., Jr. and Schulz, W.P., Total ear reimplantation in the rabbit utilizing microminiature vascular anastomoses, *Br. J. Plast. Surg.*, 19, 15, 1966.
3. Buncke, H.J., Jr., Buncke, C.M., and Schulz, W.P., Immediate Nicoladoni procedure in the Rhesus monkey, or hallux-to-hand transplantation, utilizing microminiature vascular anastomoses, *Br. J. Plast. Surg.*, 19, 332, 1966.
4. Moneta, G.L. and Porter, J.M., Arterial substitutes, in *Textbook of Surgery. The Biological Basis of Modern Surgical Practice*, Sabiston, D.C., Ed., W.B. Saunders, Philadelphia, 1991.
5. Blaisdell, F., Steele, M., and Allen, R., Management of acute lower extremity arterial ischaemia due to embolism and thrombosis, *Surgery*, 84, 822, 1978.
6. Skelly, C.L. et al., The hemodynamics of vein grafts: measurement and meaning, *Ann. Vasc. Surg.*, 15, 110, 2001.
7. Casha, A. et al., Infrainguinal saphenous vein graft aneurysm and aortic aneurysm, *Eur. J. Vasc. Endovasc. Surg.*, 12, 380, 1996.
8. Davidson, E. and DePalma, R., Atherosclerotic aneurysm occurring in an autogenous vein graft, *Am. J. Surg.*, 124, 112, 1972.
9. Peer, R. and Upson, J., Aneursmal dilatation in saphenous vein bypass grafts, *J. Cardiovasc. Surg.*, 31, 668, 1990.
10. Desoutter, P. et al., Anevrysme developpe au niveau d'un pontage femoro-poplite par greffon veineux ex-situ datant de dixs ans, *Presse Med.*, 25, 1039, 1996.
11. Wight, J. et al., Asymptomatic large coronary artery saphenous vein bypass graft aneurysm: a case report and review of the literature, *Am. Heart J.*, 133, 454, 1997.
12. Alexander, J. and Liu, Y.-C., Atherosclerotic aneurysm formation in an in situ saphenous vein graft, *J. Vasc. Surg.*, 20, 660, 1994.
13. Ascer, E. et al., Intraoperative outflow resistance as a predictor of late patency of femoropopliteal and infrapopliteal arterial bypasses, *J. Vasc. Surg.*, 5, 820, 1987.
14. Teja, K., Dillingham, R., and Mentzer, R., Saphenous vein aneurysms after aortocoronary bypass grafting: postoperative interval and hyperlipidemia as determining factors, *Am. Heart J.*, 113, 1527, 1987.
15. Dzavik, V., Lemay, M., and Chan, K.-L., Echocardiographic diagnosis of an aortocoronary venous bypass graft aneurysm, *Am. Heart J.*, 118, 619, 1989.

16. Liang, B. et al., Atherosclerotic aneurysms of aortocornary vein grafts, *Am. J. Cardiol.*, 61, 185, 1988.
17. Goldfarb A. et al., Massive aneurysmal dilatation of saphenous vein grafts used for systemic-pulmonary artery shunts: a role for magnetic resonance imaging in diagnosis, *Am. Heart J.*, 116, 870, 1988.
18. Frapier, J. et al., Aneurysm of a saphenous vein aorto-coronary bypass graft. Report of a case presenting with a presternal mass and review of the literature, *Ann. Chir. Chir. Thorac. Cardio-Vasc.*, 45, 657, 1991.
19. Murphy, J. et al., Rupture of an aortocoronary saphenous vein graft aneurysm, *Am. J. Cardiol.*, 58, 555, 1986.
20. Friedman, S. et al., Aneurysm formation: a late complication of venous bypass grafting, *Am. Heart J.*, 89, 366, 1975.
21. Bernhard, V. et al., Bypass grafting to distal arteries for limb salvage, *Surg. Gynecol. Obstet.*, 135, 219, 1972.
22. LiCalzi, L.K. and Stansel, H.C., The closure index: prediction of long-term patency of femoropopliteal vein grafts, *Surgery*, 91, 413, 1982.
23. Sanders, R.J. et al., The significance of graft diameter, *Surgery*, 88, 856, 1980.
24. Idu, M.M. et al., Factors influencing the development of vein-graft stenosis and their significance for clinical management, *Eur. J. Vasc. Endovasc. Surg.*, 17, 15, 1999.
25. Ferreira, A.C. et al., Saphenous vein graft aneurysm presenting as a large mediastinal mass compressing the right atrium, *Am. J. Cardiol.*, 79, 706, 1997.
26. Ennis, B. et al., Charactrization of a saphenous vein graft aneurysm by intravascular ultrasound and computerized three-dimensional reconstruction, *Catheterization Cardiovasc. Diagn.*, 24, 328, 1993.
27. Kamiya, A. and Togawa, T., Adaptive regulation of wall shear stress to flow change in the canine carotid artery, *Am. J. Physiol.*, 239, H14, 1980.
28. Langille, L. and O'Donnell, F., Reductions in arterial diameter produced by chronic decreases in blood flow are endothelium-dependent, *Science*, 231, 405, 1986.
29. Zarins, C.K. et al., Shear stress regulation of artery lumen diameter in experimental atherogenesis, *J. Vasc. Surg.*, 5, 413, 1987.
30. Ku, D.N. et al., Pulsatile flow and atherosclerosis in the human carotid bifurcation: positive correlation between plaque location and low and oscillating shear stress, *Arteriosclerosis*, 5, 293, 1985.
31. Giddens, D.P., Tongdar, D.T., and Loth, F., Fluid mechanics of arterial bifurcations in, *Biological Flows*, Jaffrin, M.Y. and Caro, C., Eds., Plenum Press, New York, 1995.
32. Ojha, M. et al., Steady and pulsatile flow in an end-to-side arterial anastomosis model, *J. Vasc. Surg.*, 12, 747, 1990.
33. Shu, M.C.S. and Hwang, N.H.C., Haemodynamics of angioaccess venous anastomoses, *J. Biomed. Eng.*, 13, 103, 1991.
34. Glagov, S. et al., Hemodynamic effects and tissue reactions at graft to vein anastomosis for vascular access, in *Vascular Access for Hemodialysis-II*, Sommer, B.G. and Henry, M.L., Eds., W. L. Gore & Associates, Inc. and Precept Press, Inc., Chicago, IL, 1991.
35. Keynton, R.S., Rittgers, S.E., and Shu, M.C.S., The effect of angle and flow rate upon hemodynamics in distal vascular graft anastomoses: an in vitro model study, *J. Biomech. Eng.*, 113, 458, 1991.
36. Crawshaw, H.M. et al., Flow disturbance at the distal end-to-side anastomosis, *Arch. Surg.*, 115, 1280, 1980.
37. White, S.S. et al., Hemodynamic patterns in two flow models of end-to-side vascular graft anastomoses: effects of pulsatility, flow division, Reynolds number and hood length, *J. Biomech. Eng.*, 115, 104, 1993.
38. Binns, R.L. et al., Optimal graft diameter: effect of wall shear stress on vascular healing, *J. Vasc. Surg.*,10, 326, 1989.
39. Loth, F. et al., Relative contribution of wall shear stress and injury in experimental intimal thickening at PTFE end-to-side arterial anastomoses, *J. Biomech. Eng.*, 124, 44, 2002.

40. Loth, F. et al., Measurements of velocity and wall shear stress inside a PTFE vascular graft model under steady flow conditions, *J. Biomech. Eng.*, 119, 187, 1997.
41. Hodges, T.C. et al., Longitudinal comparison of dialysis access methods: risk factors for failure, *J. Vasc. Surg.*, 26, 1009, 1997.
42. Fillinger, M.F., Kerns, D.B., and Schwartz, R.A., Hemodynamics and intimal hyperplasia, in *Vascular Access for Hemodialysis-II*, Sommer, B.G. and Henry, M.L., Eds., W. L. Gore & Associates, Inc., and Precept Press, Inc., Chicago, IL, 1991.
43. Fillinger, M.F. et al., Graft geometry and venous intimal-medial hyperplasia in arteriovenous loop grafts, *J. Vasc. Surg.*, 11, 556, 1990.
44. Arslan, N., Experimental characterization of transitional unsteady flow inside a graft-to-vein junction, Ph.D. Dissertation in MIE, University of Illinois at Chicago, 1999.
45. Womersley, J.R., An elastic tube theory of pulse transmission and oscillatory flow in mammalian arteries, Wright Air Development Center, Technical Report WADC-TR 56-614, 1957.

25

Minimally Invasive Cardiovascular Technologies

James E. Moore, Jr.
Florida International University

Marc Jalisi
Florida International University

Michael R. Moreno
Florida International University

Eric Crumpler
Florida International University

CONTENTS

25.1 Introduction

Cardiovascular disease remains the most common cause of death in western countries despite considerable advances in treatment strategies. In the 20th century, technologies such as the heart/lung bypass machine were developed to enable surgeons to operate on virtually any part of the system, including the heart itself. While these procedures have saved countless lives, they suffer from relatively high mortality and morbidity rates due to their invasiveness. The procedures often take several hours in the surgical suite, followed by several days to weeks of recovery in intensive care wards. The cost to the patient and/or their insurance carrier for these procedures exceeds $30,000. Many of the most severely diseased patients were excluded from surgery because of the danger associated with the procedure itself.

An effort began in the 1960s to move toward less invasive procedures to treat cardiovascular disease states. Advances in materials science, imaging, and pharmaceuticals have led to a wide variety of devices to treat such pathologies such as occlusive atherosclerotic plaques, heart valve deficiencies, aneurysms, and deep venous thrombosis. These procedures are less traumatic to the patient, require fewer hospital resources, and shorten recovery times. In most cases, a small entry point is established in the femoral artery, located near the groin. Catheters are inserted and led up to the disease location. The patient can be under general or local anesthesia. This is advantageous in neural procedures, in which the patient can be asked certain questions or to perform certain tasks to monitor neural function. Once the procedure is completed, the entry point is closed, and the patient is sent to recovery. In many cases, the patient goes home within days to resume normal activities. The cost of such procedures is approximately one third less than the equivalent surgical procedure, although this savings varies considerably (Hltaky et al., 1997). As the long-term performance of these devices is improved, the savings over surgical procedures will continue to increase.

The move toward less invasive procedures has occurred in parallel with an overall trend of increasing numbers of total cardiovascular procedures. From 1979 to 1999, the total number of cardiovascular

0-8493-1140-3/04/$0.00+$1.50

operations and procedures rose 413%. In 1999, there were approximately 571,000 coronary artery bypass graft (CABG) procedures performed in the U.S. In that same year, an estimated 601,000 percutaneous transluminal coronary angioplasty (PTCA) procedures were performed. This was the first year that PTCA procedures outnumbered CABG procedures. The number of PTCA procedures increased by 285% from 1987 to 1999, compared to 135% over the same period for CABG (American Heart Association, 2001).

The purpose of this section is to describe some of the technologies that have emerged for minimally invasive treatment of cardiovascular pathologies. It is important to recognize that new devices are being developed constantly. However, a sufficient ground level of these devices has emerged that demonstrates the feasibility of the minimally invasive approach. These exciting technologies are increasing in application because both clinicians and patients recognize their potential benefits.

25.2 Angioplasty

Percutaneous transluminal angioplasty (PTA) involves the deployment of a small balloon inside a blocked vessel using a catheter. The PTA procedure begins by introducing a delivery sheath into a superficial artery, such as the femoral artery. A guidewire is then pushed up to the disease site using a guiding catheter. Guidewires are typically less than 0.4 mm in diameter, and serve as the delivery vehicle for the remainder of the devices to be delivered to the diseased vessel. The guiding catheter is withdrawn so that the PTA balloon catheter, stent delivery catheter, or other device can be guided to the disease site. The balloon is then inflated to widen the blockage (Figure 25.1). PTA is the most common therapeutical intervention worldwide. It was developed in response to the need for a less invasive, less traumatic treatment for patients who could not tolerate open surgical bypass. It is hoped that the vessel remains open when the balloon is removed, although this is not always the case. If the vessel is not permanently deformed by the balloon inflation, it will simply return to its previous blocked state (elastic recoil). Even if the artery remains open initially, it may occlude weeks or months later due to tissue proliferation. This process, termed *restenosis*, occurs in approximately 40% of patients (Fleisch and Meier, 1999). The history of PTA can be traced back to the pioneering work of Charles Dotter in the 1960s.

It is believed that angioplasty enlarges the lumen through permanent deformation of the plaque and healthy artery. Postmortem inspection of arteries treated with PTA reveals fracture of the plaque near its thinnest margin (Zarins et al., 1982). Balloon inflation can also provoke damage to the healthy artery structure, including disruption of the internal and/or external elastic laminae. The risk of restenosis increases with greater arterial injury because of the increase in hyperplasia, a natural response to injury.

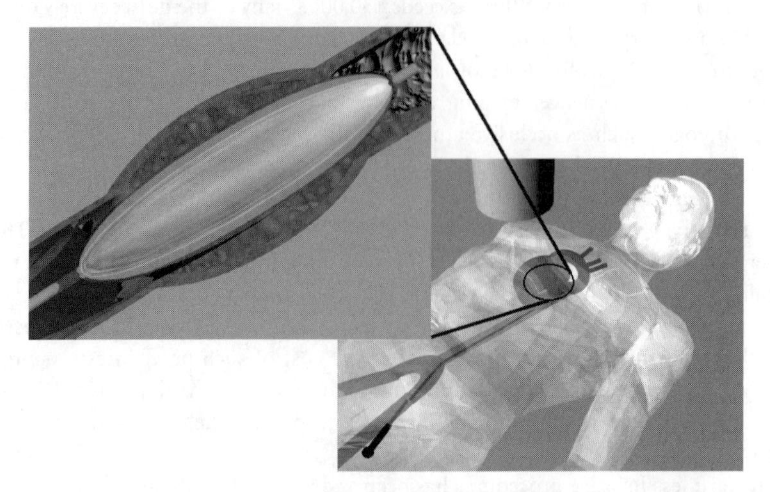

FIGURE 25.1 Illustration of a percutaneous transluminal angioplasty (PTA) procedure. Entry into the systemic arterial circulation is gained via the femoral artery in the groin. A small diameter catheter is threaded to the blockage site with the aid of fluoroscopy, and the balloon is inflated to spread open the artery lumen.

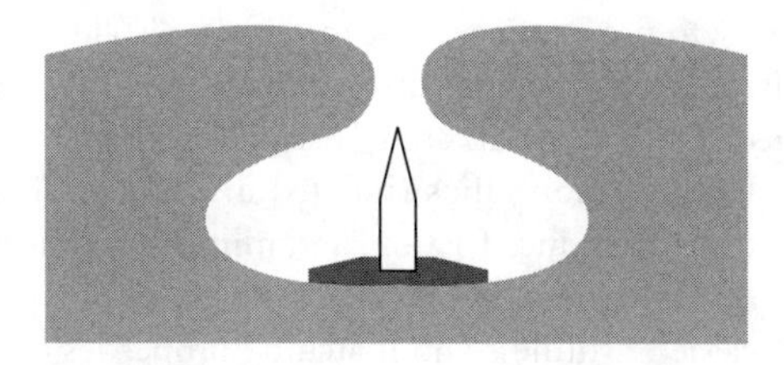

FIGURE 25.2 Angioplasty cutting balloon detail. Radially protruding blades are placed on the exterior surface of the balloon. These blades are contained within the folds of the undeployed balloon as shown. Once the balloon is in place, the blades push into the plaque, promoting fracture to facilitate expansion of the lumen.

Realizing that plaque fracture is key to permanent lumen expansion, cutting balloon catheters have been developed that include radially protruding blades that cut into the plaque as the balloon is inflated (Figure 25.2).

Important design considerations for guidewires include the ability to deliver it to the vessel reliably and quickly while minimizing the trauma to the vessel wall. While the trauma to the vessel wall can be lessened by coating the guidewire with low friction materials such as Teflon, the stiffness of the guidewire will primarily determine the degree of injury. The main considerations in this trade-off are the column strength, which depends on diameter to the fourth power. The guidewire should move precisely when pushed without buckling, but at the same time be able to negotiate tortuous vessels with ease. It is often desirable to have a guidewire that is relatively stiff along most of its length, but which has a more flexible end to avoid vessel trauma and dissection. Core to tip guidewires are often designed using step tapered metallic core and a 3-cm-long flat, soft shapeable atraumatic tip welded/soldered to the tapered distal core. When the design is not core to tip, the intermediate or tapered section is connected to the shaft by glued hypo-tube and a 3-cm-long flat, soft shapeable atraumatic tip welded/soldered to the tapered distal core. The 3-cm tip is often covered by a radio-opaque coil for improved visibility in fluoroscopy as well as bending flexibility. Materials used for guidewire core designs are often from high modulus, high resistance and chemically reactive biocompatible materials and SS304V (vacuum remelt for improved purity and homogeneity stainless steel), Cr-Co alloys (i.e., MP35N, Elgiloy, L605, etc.), and superelastic Ni-Ti (Nitinol). Other than Nitinol, these materials need to be stress relieved and hardened by precipitation or age-hardening heat treatment process for improved kink resistance.

Once a suitable guidewire has been delivered to the diseased vessel, the PTA balloon catheter is placed concentrically over the guidewire and pushed directly to the blockage. These balloons come in a range of sizes, from small coronary artery sizes (2 to 4 mm) to large diameter balloons for peripheral vessels (15 to 20 mm). Balloons are typically designed to expand to a specified diameter at a deployment pressure of approximately 10 atm, with very little further expansion at higher pressures. This allows the operator to predetermine the final expanded diameter. A variety of complex balloon shapes can be fabricated from polyethylene to completely fill various body cavities. Other balloon materials are low- and high-density polyethylene, polyvinyl chloride (PVC), and nylon. However, when lower precision balloons are desired, elastomeric balloons are used that conform to the lumen shape as they expand. There are numerous balloon shapes such as conical balloon, spherical balloon, dog bone balloon, conical/square long balloon, stepped balloon, offset balloon, etc., which could be fabricated/formed in different diameters and lengths. A specific shaped balloon may be used depending upon anatomical site, the requirements of the treatment process, or both. Platinum or gold marker bands are attached at each end of the balloon for distinctive tip radiopacity. This allows the operator to position the balloon precisely prior to inflation.

Important design considerations for balloon catheters extend beyond their ability to expand the lumen of the diseased vessel. The trackability of a catheter refers to its ability to track through tortuous vessels, or how easily the catheter follows over the guidewire through a tortuous vessel. Obviously this is a function of catheter sliding friction force (frictional resistance between the guidewire, catheter, and vessel wall), constructing elements/materials, and geometrical configurations (shaft diameter and length, column strength, lateral flexibility). Small diameter catheters have greater flexibility, but lack column strength. This makes it necessary to use stronger shaft materials, distal tapering and/or reinforcing with braids, coils, or stiffening wires. The crossability of a catheter refers to the ability of its distal end to traverse the lesion to be treated. Thus, the goals are to design low-profile catheters with small diameter distal tips, and balloons with high inflation ratios (inflated to deflated diameters). These strategies are augmented with polymeric coatings to reduce friction, and minimizing the amount of adhesive used for balloon-catheter attachment. The adhesion spots create relatively stiff sections that impede crossability. Finally, gradual transitions in catheter stiffness and matching properties of catheters to guidewires help to optimize crossability.

In many cases, clinicians determine that some of the atherosclerotic plaque must be removed to increase the long-term chances for an open lumen. This process is referred to as "debulking." There are a variety of technologies developed for this purpose, but the degree of success has been limited. Despite considerable development work in the 1980s and 1990s, laser angioplasty has never enjoyed widespread clinical use. This procedure uses high laser energy to vaporize plaque by breaking molecular bonds. The guidewire is positioned across target coronary lesion, and the laser catheter is activated and advanced slowly through the lesion. In a laser balloon angioplasty device used in coronary angioplasty, the laser is mounted inside the balloon and transmits light through the balloon walls. Mechanical atherectomy catheters aim to physically destroy and remove, rather than displace, the plaque material. The design of this type of device requires pulverization and vacuum aspiration of material to prevent thromboembolic events. In a subset of these devices, directional coronary atherectomy, a catheter/cutter is pushed against arterial plaque. A related application of such technologies is the removal of thrombus from bypass and AV fistula grafts (thrombectomy).

25.3 Stents

First described in the modern era by Dotter (1969), stents were designed to improve upon the limited success of balloon angioplasty for the treatment of occlusive vascular disease. A stent is a tubular scaffold that is expanded inside the artery in order to prop open the lumen. Dotter attempted placement of plastic stents in canine politeal arteries that thrombosed after 24 h. Later animal studies using both stainless steel coil stents and nitinol coils were tried successfully (Dotter et al., 1983). The first human use of stents occurred in 1986 (Sigwart et al., 1987).

The variety of stent designs conceived or developed is staggering. A search of the U.S. Patent and Trademark Office database in late 2002 revealed more than 4500 patents including the term "stent." While not all of these patents were for medical devices, it is interesting to note that approximately half of these patents were applied for in the year 2000 or later. Most stents can be classified as either balloon-expandable or self-expanding. Balloon-expandable stents are mounted over an angioplasty balloon, delivered to the diseased vessel site, and expanded through inflation of the balloon. The stent is permanently or plastically deformed to the desired diameter, and the balloon is removed (Figure 25.3). Balloon-expandable stents are often made of 316 stainless steel or other non-corrosive, stiff alloy metals (e.g., Tantalum, or Cr-Co super alloys Elgiloy, MP35N, and L605). Self-expanding stents are produced at the desired final diameter, and spring-loaded into a much smaller catheter (Figure 25.4). Once the stent is delivered to the diseased vessel, the catheter sheath is withdrawn, and the stent expands elastically outward into the artery. The need for a high degree of elastic deformation requires that self-expanding stents be made of more elastic materials such as Nitinol, a nickel-titanium alloy with shape memory capability (Duerig et al., 2000). Nitinol can be strained approximately 8% and remain elastic if processed correctly, compared to less than 0.5% for stainless steel. Its shape memory properties have also been exploited in the design of stents. Polymer stents are also under development (Tsuji et al., 2001). The ability of a polymer stent to degrade safely once the artery has remodeled is desirable, but much development work remains to be done for this process to be dependable.

The key parameters in stent design are numerous, and in some cases conflicting (Table 25.1). The first important issue is that the material be biocompatible, since it will be exposed directly to the blood stream. In order to be deployed in small narrowings, a high expansion ratio (deployed diameter/crimped

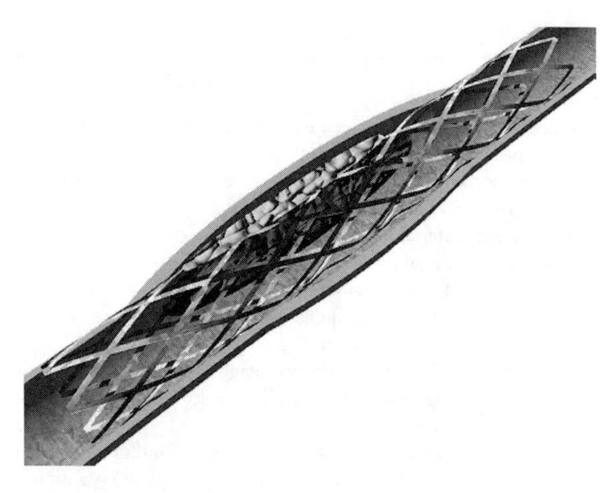

FIGURE 25.3 Illustration of a balloon expanded stent deployed inside a stenotic artery. The atherosclerotic plaque material is displaced and held outward by the more rigid stent structure.

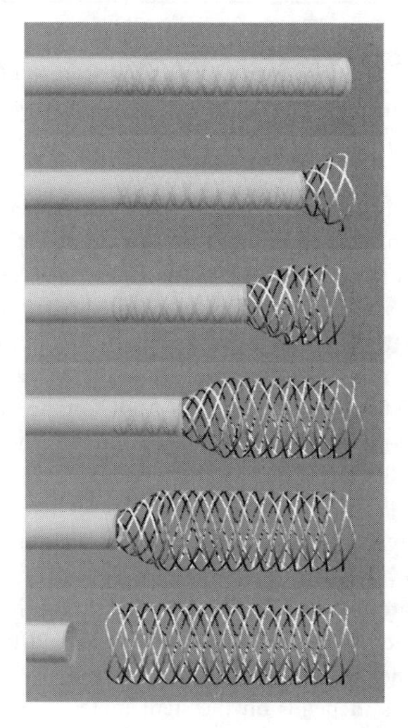

FIGURE 25.4 Illustration of a self-expanding stent being deployed. The sheath is withdrawn, releasing the spring-loaded stent to its full diameter.

diameter) is required. The crimped diameter of the stent is often referred to as its profile, which should be as low as possible. Deploying the stent often requires navigating tortuous vessels or entering branches with an acute angle. Thus, the stent must have good longitudinal flexibility. The above considerations generally require a minimum amount of material in the makeup of the stent. Propping open the previously blocked passage while remaining in place following deployment requires a high degree of radial strength. Accurate positioning of the stent requires that it be sufficiently radiopaque. These two considerations generally require a high amount of material in the stent, thus there must be a trade-off in the design process. The expansion of the stent from the crimped to the deployed state must result in as little axial foreshortening as possible, or it will be difficult to predict the final position of the stent.

TABLE 25.1 Design Considerations for Vascular Stents

Characteristic	Comment
Outward radial force	Necessary to prop open artery. Excessive radial force can injure artery wall and promote hyperplasia over time.
Material	Must be biocompatible and non-corrosive. Typical: SS316, Co/Cr Alloys, Nitinol, Polymers.
Radiopacity	Depends on material properties and total mass present. More radiopaque markers or coatings of different material may be added to stent.
MRI artifacts	Depends on material properties.
Profile	Diameter of catheter containing crimped stent. Must be as low as possible.
Expansion ratio	Ratio of deployed to crimped diameter. Higher is better.
Expansion mode	Typically balloon or self-expanding.
Foreshortening	Ratio of deployed length to crimped length. Should be 1 for accurate placement.
Longitudinal flexibility	Necessary to navigate tortuous arteries. Deployment in curved arteries should not injure wall at ends of stent.
Surface treatment	Highly polished and passivated to reduce thrombus and inflammation.
Surface coating	Polymers with embedded anti-inflammatory drugs show promise.
Manufacturing method	Typically laser-machined from tube stock. Also knitted mesh and coils. Thermal treatments may be necessary.
Fatigue resistance	Must be able to withstand at least 10 years of cyclic fatigue.

Other considerations include the ability to retrieve the stent in case of mal deployment, and minimal interference with CT and MRI imaging. The delivery system must work well with the particular stent design, and must hold the stent in place in a way that does not injure or snag on the artery wall as it is guided to the disease site.

Perhaps the most important design characteristic for stents is that they do not provoke the development of a new blockage either acutely through thrombosis or later on due to hyperplasia. Unfortunately, there is little direct information on how stent design affects these processes. The reaction of the body to a stent implanted in an artery is a multistage process (Edelman and Rogers, 1998). First, the exposure of the subendothelium and the stent material to the blood stream initiates thrombus formation (Figure 25.5). This process, which takes place within minutes/hours, includes an aggregation of platelets, fibrin, and erythrocytes. The degree of platelet adhesion depends not only on the surface characteristics of the stent, but also on the strut configuration. Areas of flow stagnation, which depend heavily on strut design, influence the degree of platelet adhesion (Robaina et al., 2002). Areas that are subjected to intermittent flow stagnation and low wall shear stress showed greater platelet accumulation in their *in vitro* experiments. The second stage of the reaction to the stent is inflammation. The peak of this process occurs approximately 4 to 14 days following stent implantation. Deposits of surface adherent and tissue infiltrating monocytes can be seen around stent struts, demonstrating the degree to which the struts are injuring the wall. These monocytes release cytokines, mitogens, and tissue growth factors that further increase neointimal formation. The third stage is the proliferation of vascular smooth muscle cells in the media and neointima. This process depends on the stent material, as well as the stress placed on the artery wall by the stent. The final stage of arterial adaptation is remodeling. One can think of this phase as the artery's attempt to reach a new homeostatic state in the presence of the persistent injury caused by the stent. The final thickness of the neointima depends heavily on the degree to which the stent injures the artery wall, as indicated by the disruption of the internal and external elastic laminae (Rogers and Edelman, 1995).

Acute thrombosis was a common cause of failure for stenting procedures in the early 1990s, but advances in stenting technology and aggressive antiplatelet drug regimens have reduced these failures to nearly negligible levels. The deployment of a stent with or without balloon inflation substantially denudes the endothelial layer of the artery, which normally provides perfect antithrombotic protection. The complete re-establishment of the endothelial layer takes weeks to months, leaving a considerable time gap for clinically significant thrombosis to form. The potential for thrombus is enhanced by the fact that the stent itself is a foreign material that provokes platelet attachment and buildup. Electrochemical surface

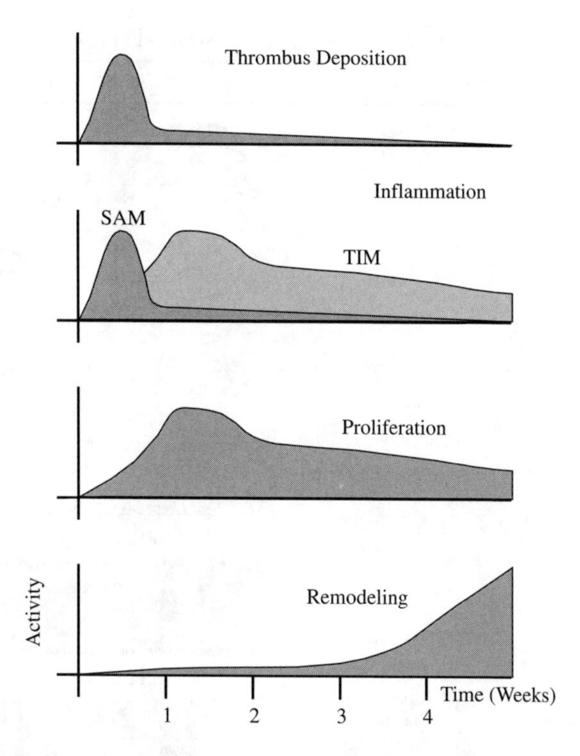

FIGURE 25.5 Response of the artery wall to the presence of a stent. The process begins with thrombus deposition, followed quickly by inflammation. Surface adherent monocytes (SAMs) respond to the injury presented by the stent, then enter the wall as tissue infiltrating monocytes (TIMs). Cellular proliferation (mainly smooth muscle) provides additional tissue to shore up stress concentrations in the artery wall. Finally, the remodeling stage takes place in which the artery attempts to redefine a new homeostatic state. (Adapted from Edelman and Rogers, 1998.)

treatments have reduced the risk associated with the stent itself. However, the use of systemic antiplatelet drugs has played a more dominant role in reducing acute stent thrombosis. Aspirin enjoys widespread use as an anticoagulant. Its use as an adjunct to stent deployment is limited because it inhibits only one of the many pathways to platelet activation. Currently, daily usage of aspirin is recommended for all persons at risk of circulatory disorders, including stent patients. Ticlopidine, another platelet activation inhibitor, can be effective when used in conjunction with aspirin, but suffers from a number of undesirable side effects. Clopidogrel, like Ticlopidine, inhibits platelet activation, but has fewer side effects. Heparin is commonly used during stent procedures, but not afterward. Much recent success has resulted from the use of glycoprotein IIb/IIIa inhibitors such as Abciximab. Activated platelets secrete GP IIb/IIIa in order to bind fibrinogen and von Willebrand factor, which encourage binding with other platelets. Abciximab is administered prior to and during the interventional procedure.

The growth of tissue into the stented region can cause a new blockage, a process called in-stent restenosis. This process is responsible for the clinical failure of 20 to 30% of stenting procedures within 6 months following implantation. Among the factors that influence the risk for restenosis is stent design. In a clinical study of more than 4500 coronary stent implantations (Kastrati et al., 2001), it was shown that restenosis rates for different stent designs vary from 20 to 50% (Table 25.2). The exact relationship between stent design and the development of intimal hyperplasia is not well understood. It is generally thought that the percent area covered by the stent and the mechanical mismatch between the stent and artery wall are important factors. The characteristics of the original atherosclerotic plaque also play an important role.

The problem of restenosis is being addressed by coating stents with polymers in which drugs have been embedded. The polymers provide a stable matrix into which drugs are uniformly distributed and

TABLE 25.2 Restenosis Rates of Different Stent Designs Implanted in Human Coronary Arteries*

Stent	Restenosis rate	Design (strut thickness)
Guidant Multi-Link	20.0%	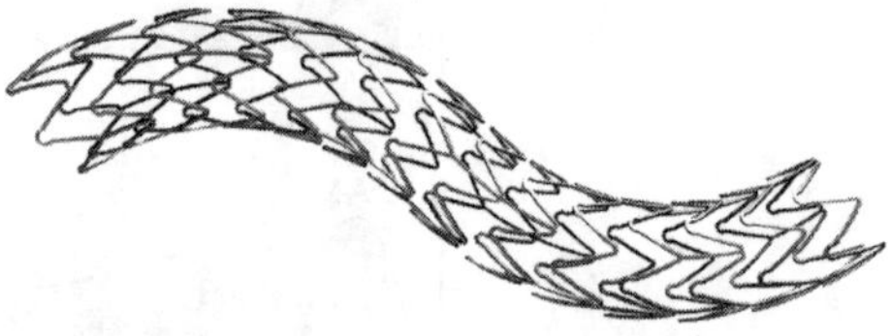 (0.14 mm thick × 0.10 mm wide)
Jomed Jostent	25.8%	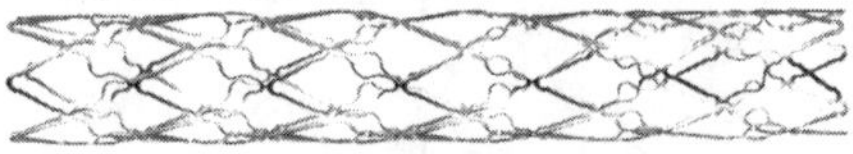 (0.09 mm × 0.09 mm)
J&J Palmaz-Schatz	29.0%	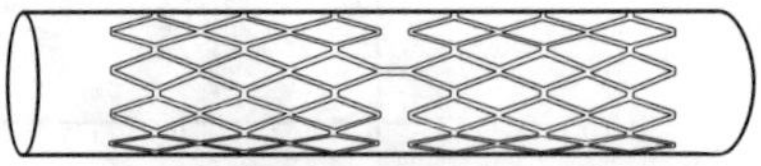 (0.15 mm × 0.15 mm)
PURA-A	30.9%	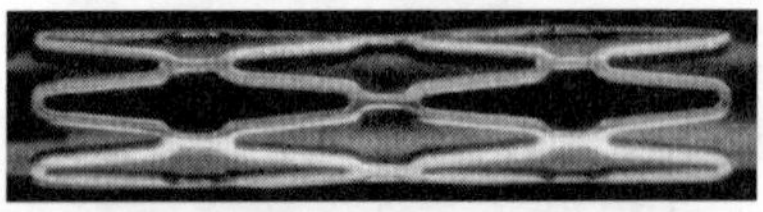 (0.12 mm × 0.12 mm)
Inflow Steel	37.3%	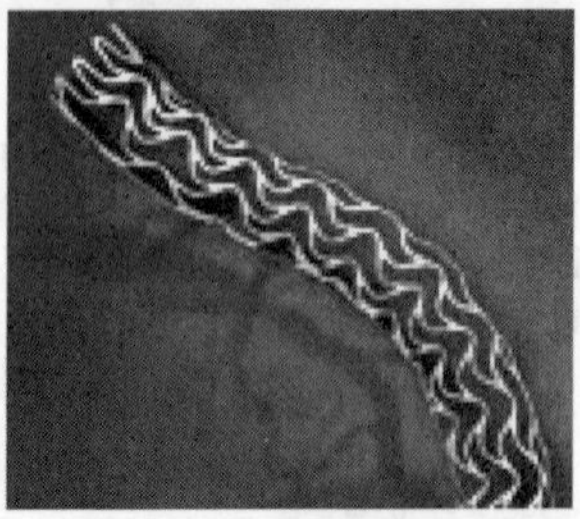 (0.075 mm × 0.075 mm)
NIR	37.8%	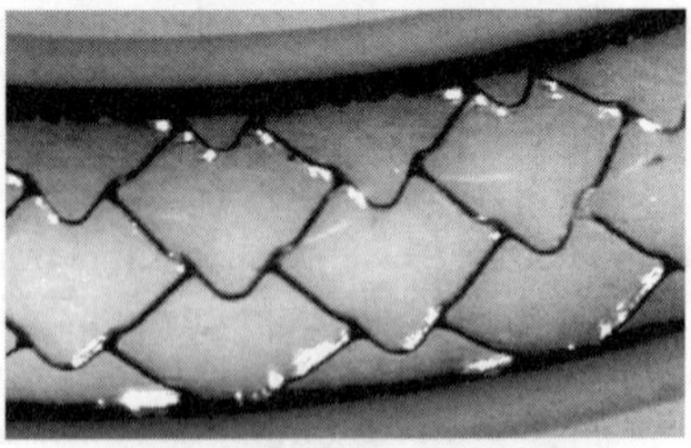 (0.1 mm × 0.1 mm)
Inflow gold	50.3%	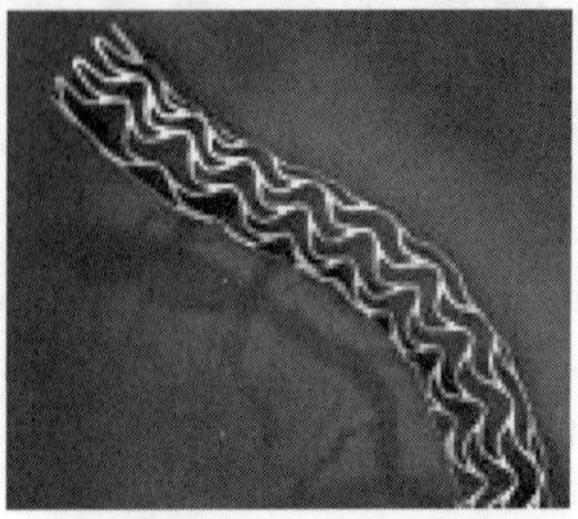 (0.075 mm × 0.075 mm)

* All stents included in this study are laser machined from 316L stainless steel, and balloon expanded. The Inflow gold stent is coated with gold to improve radiopacity.

Adapted from Kastrati et al., 2001.

released over a specific period of time, typically days to weeks (Uhrich et al., 1999). Although most stent-coating technology is closely guarded, several coating techniques have been described. The most common polymer coating that is often applied to the surface of the stent struts uses nonerodable and nonbiodegradable methacrylate and/or ethylene base copolymers. The other biodegradable and non-biodegradable polymers often employed include nylon, polyurethane, silicone, polyethylene terphthalate, polyglycolic acid/polylactic acid (PLGA), polycaprolactone, polyhydroxybutyrate valerate, poly(n-butyl methacrylate), polyorthoester, poly(ethylene-co-vinyl acetate), and polyethyleneoxide/polybutylene terephthalate (Uhrich et al., 1999). One important factor in the choice of polymers is the adherence of the polymer to the stent. With deployment, mechanical stress/strain may have a tendency to delaminate the coating or cause uneven drug distribution (Hwang et al., 2001). Other factors involve uniform distribution of the drug for expected efficacy. One of the first examples of coated stents involved heparin (Hirsh, 1991), which reduces platelet adhesion. Heparin coating of stents is an attractive method because of its anticoagulant properties and inhibitory effects on mesenchynmal cell growth and differentiation (Hirsh, 1991; Clowes and Karnovsky, 1977). A number of materials have been evaluated (*in vitro* and *in vivo*) as potential thrombo-resistant stent coatings such as hydrogels and polyurethanes. However, the endpoint-attached heparin surface proved to be significantly superior to other models (Serruys et al., 1994; Ragosta et al., 1999; Clowes and Karnovsky, 1977). While antithrombogenic compounds (heparin) and minimally thrombogenic compounds (phosphorycholine) have been integrated into polymers, novel approaches based on anti-inflammatory or antiproliferation agents are being evaluated. Two of the more promising pharmaceutical drugs suitable for coating include Paclitaxel (Taxol), including taxane analogues and Rapamycin (Sirolimus). Paclitaxel, previously used as an anticancer agent that reduces cellular proliferation, migration and signal transduction, has demonstrated *in vitro* and *in vivo* success, and is currently being evaluated in human clinical trials. Early clinical trial data show that stents coated with this drug have demonstrated reduced restenosis rates (Grube and Büllesfeld, 2002). Early clinical studies of stents coated with Sirolimus showed near zero restenosis rates (Degertekin et al., 2002). This drug has been systemically applied to patients for the prophylactic prevention of renal transplant rejection (Poon et al., 2002). Sirolimus is a natural microlide immunosuppressant that inhibits vascular smooth muscle cell proliferation through blocking the cellular transition from the G1 to the S phase (Gallo et al., 1999). This proliferation is prevented when Sirolimus (or Rapamycin) binds to its cytosolic receptor, FKBP12, and blocks the activation of T cells, the lymphocytes responsible for cell-mediated immunity. Through this mechanism, Sirolimus also prevents smooth muscle cell migration, thus interrupting the cascade of cellular activity leading to neointimal hyperplasia causing restenosis (Sousa et al., 2001). Widespread clinical use of these devices over time will reveal if these exciting new devices really solve the problem of restenosis.

25.4 Aneurysm Treatment

The development of PTA and stenting led clinicians to explore other conditions that might be treated with adaptations of these technologies. In 1991, Juan Parodi treated a patient with an abdominal aortic aneurysm (AAA) with a balloon expandable stent to which a vascular graft had been attached (Parodi et al., 1991). This stent graft, or endograft, was deployed via a percutaneous catheter approach. The idea was to seal the aneurysm from arterial pressure and reduce the risk of its rupture (Figure 25.6). AAAs, the 13th leading cause of death in the U.S., manifest as a local ballooning of the aortic wall that forms 1 to 2 cm distal to the renal arteries. The aneurysm often extends into the iliac arteries. The large radius and reduced wall thickness in the aneurysm make it prone to rupture, often a fatal event.

Since Parodi's initial clinical experience, there have been numerous endografts developed for AAA treatment. There are at least 15 designs currently in development or already in clinical use. The important design considerations include the ability to remain sealed against healthy portions of the artery wall proximal and distal to the aneurysm, ability to clot off the porous graft material, and minimal delivery profile. It is also important to recognize that aneurysm geometry is highly individual. The device must be prepared to treat a wide variety of vessel diameters, lengths, and degrees of tortuosity. Although

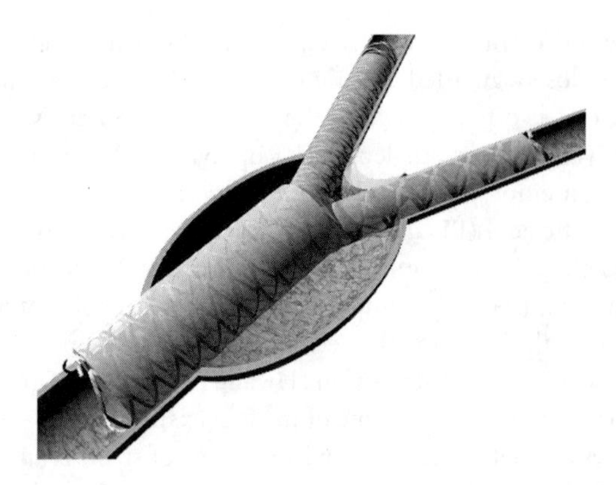

FIGURE 25.6 Illustration of an endograft deployed to seal off an abdominal aortic aneurysm (AAA). The graft material clots off, sealing the aneurysm from being subjected to arterial pressure, and reducing the risk of rupture.

Parodi's initial design was a single tube, the extension of many aneurysms into the iliac arteries required adaptation to bifurcated designs. A typical approach is to deploy the main body and one leg of the endograft via one femoral artery, then deploy the other leg of the endograft via the contralateral femoral artery. It is also possible to extend a single tapered graft into one iliac artery, then implant a femoral cross-over graft surgically to supply the contralateral side. The contralateral side must then be sealed using an iliac occluder plug. Regardless of the particular design, the ability to make a reliable seal between the endograft components is crucial. Both balloon expanded and self-expanding stents have been used to make endografts. In some designs, the stents extend the whole length of the endograft, while in others short stents are included only at the proximal and distal attachment regions (Figure 25.7). The proximal attachment site is particularly worrisome because the aneurysm may extend proximally to the level of the renal arteries. The length of "healthy neck" in the aorta between the renal arteries and the beginning of the aneurysm is an important criterion in determining patient eligibility for this treatment. This has led endograft designers to devise ways of securing endografts above the renal arteries without blocking their outflow. The graft material is typically PTFE or Dacron, and is attached to the graft material with sutures or other means.

The clinical experience with endografts has demonstrated mixed success. While this technology has offered hope to AAA patients too sick for surgical intervention, unanticipated device failures have stopped endografts from enjoying widespread clinical use. The failures of endografting have been classified into four different categories (Table 25.3). Type I failures are leaks that occur at the proximal or distal attachment sites. Type II failures occur when the aneurysm sac receives pressurization from communicating circulation,

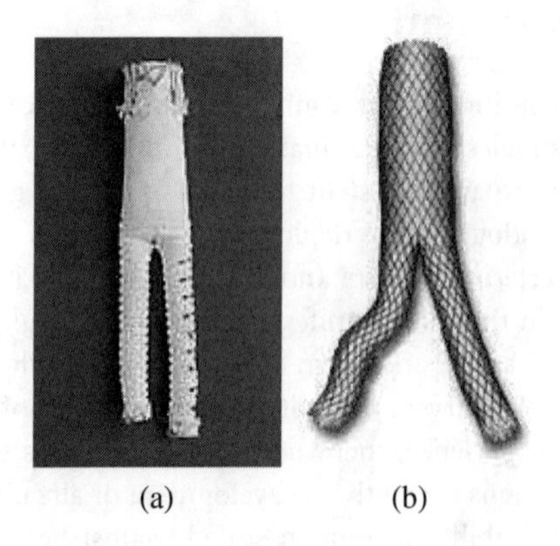

FIGURE 25.7 Illustrations of two endografts used to treat abdominal aortic aneurysms. The Guidant Ancure device (a) is an "unspported" design in which stents are placed at the proximal and distal ends, but not the middle portion. The Medtronic Aneurx device (b) is a fully supported device in which the stents run the entire length.

TABLE 25.3 Failure Classifications for AAA Endografts

Endoleak Type	Description
I	Attachment site leak
IA	Proximal end of graft
IB	Distal end of graft
IC	Iliac occluder (plug)
II	Branch leaks from communicating arteries
IIA	One branch inlet only
IIB	Complex, flow-through, or multiple branches
III	Graft defect
IIIA	Junctional leak or modular disconnection
IIIB	Fabric disruption (hole)
IV	Graft porosity

typically from arteries that connect to the inferior mesenteric artery. Type III failures are seen when leaks occur at endograft component junctions, or there is some other breach in the structural integrity of the middle portion of the endograft. Type IV failures include sac pressurization due to continued graft material porosity. The occurrence of these different failures depends on endograft design and patient-specific conditions (van Marrewijk et al., 2002). Type I and III failures can be treated with the deployment of additional endograft components. In many cases, sleeves of bare or graft-coated stents are inserted over the trouble area. There is considerable controversy concerning the treatment of Type II endoleaks. Coil embolization can be performed at the time of endograft implantation or later, but access to these often small communicating arteries is difficult. Many clinicians prefer to monitor these cases for changes in aneurysm morphology rather than actively treat the endoleaks. As a last resort, the patient can undergo conversion to surgical treatment, in which an artificial graft is sewn in place of the diseased aorta. Endograft design is evolving to minimize the risk of failure, but progress is impeded by lack of knowledge concerning the truly physiologic mechanical conditions to which endografts are subjected. In addition to tortuous geometries and cycling pressures, which are included in FDA required device testing, endografts are subjected to complex hemodynamic forces (Liffman et al., 2001). Changes in vessel geometry that occur during normal physiologic movement such as hip flexion may be important as well, but these changes are not well understood at present.

Minimally invasive devices have also been developed to treat aneurysm forming in the cerebral circulation. Ruptures of cerebral aneurysms eventually kill approximately half of those afflicted. It is desirable in this case to form a thrombus inside the aneurysm so that the structural weakness is sealed off and eventually covered with neointima. This can be accomplished with the catheter-based deployment of a thin, metallic wire. Once a sufficient length of the "coil" has been deployed into the aneurysm, an electric charge is applied to the end of the catheter, breaking it off from the catheter. Platinum is often used for the wire material (Byrne et al., 1999; Uda et al., 1998). The placement of a stent across the neck of the aneurysm is also a treatment option. In this case, the blood flow in the aneurysm is slowed by the stent mesh, causing thrombus to form (Lieber and Gounis, 2002). The stent mesh also aids in forming neointima.

25.5 Embolic Filters

There are a variety of clinical situations in which embolic material shedding from a plaque, thrombosis, or intervention site need to be trapped and prevented from reaching distal tissues. If emboli from a deep vein thrombosis reach the heart or lungs, the results can be deadly. Deep vein thrombosis can result from extended periods in which the legs are kept stationary, such as postoperative situations. Emboli can also result from clinical interventions to treat occlusive atherosclerotic plaques. Balloon angioplasty and stenting provoke plaque fracture, thus the possibility that pieces will break off and lodge downstream in a smaller artery. This is a particular concern for carotid stenting, where emboli can cause serious brain

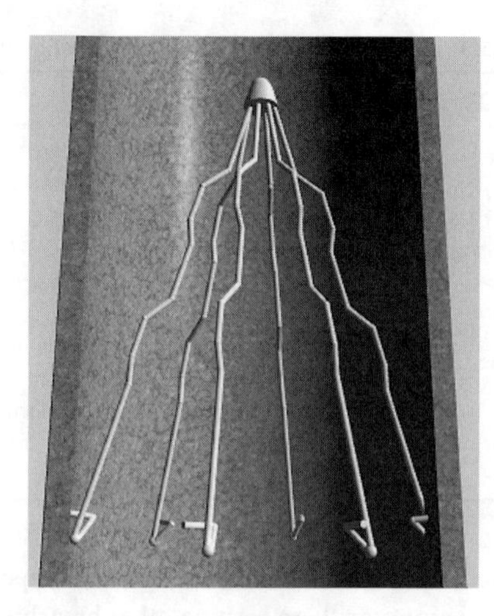

FIGURE 25.8 Illustration of the Greenfield vena cava filter. This device is deployed percutaneously to prevent emboli from deep vein thrombi from reaching the heart and pulmonary circulation.

ischemia (Sievert and Rabe, 2002). Emboli may also result during the treatment of stenoses in saphenous vein coronary bypass grafts (Morales and Heuser, 2002).

Emboli from deep vein thrombosis are responsible for an estimated 200,000 deaths per year in the U.S. (Zwaan et al., 1995). Vena cava filters deployed via a catheter approach have been in use since the 1960s to prevent emboli from reaching the pulmonary circulation. The most common current design is the Greenfield filter (Figure 25.8). It is thought that the filter captures larger emboli in its middle section, then these emboli get broken down by the body's natural thrombolysis process (Greenfield and Proctor, 2000). Competing designs have emerged recently that feature different capture basket designs and deployment schemes. Problems with permanent filters include vena cava thrombus rates of up to 19% (Ferris et al., 1993). More recent designs have emerged that can be withdrawn, dissolved, or converted to simple stents once the danger of emboli is thought to have subsided (Stecker et al., 2001). Testing of all filter designs *in vitro* with artificial emboli have reported trapping rates ranging from 22 to 98%, depending on filter design and flow conditions (Lorch et al., 1998).

Another class of temporary embolic protection devices has emerged to augment endovascular treatments, so-called distal protection devices. Because they remain in place only as long as the intervention itself, designs for distal protection devices ranges from total occlusion balloons to basket-like porous membranes (Figure 25.9).

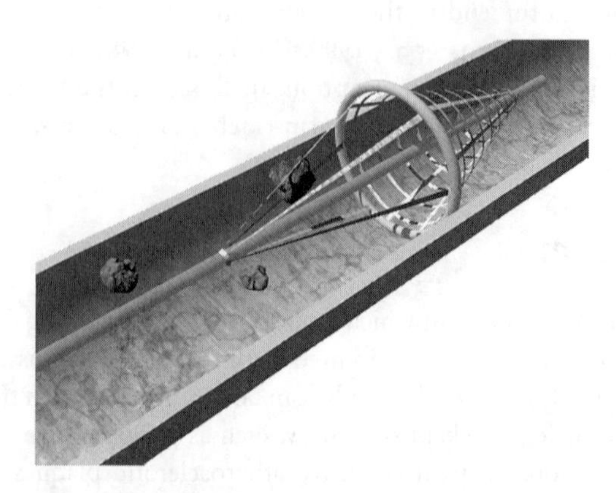

FIGURE 25.9 Illustration of a distal protection device deployed in an artery. Emboli from a procedure being performed proximal to the device are captured, then removed when the device is recaptured into the catheter.

25.6 Cardiac Ablation Catheters

Minimally invasive arrhythmia surgery has renewed interest in the treatment of atrial fibrillation and other cardiac abnormalities due to the developments in catheter-based ablation (Keane, 2002; Bella et al., 2001; Lustgarden et al., 1999). This technology involves the production of scar tissue in areas of the myocardium that exhibit irregular electrical activity. Techniques ranging from the traditional radiofrequency-based to laser-enhanced approaches have simplified surgical treatment and avoided several of the drawbacks of surgery. Although the current standard in catheter ablation is radiofrequency, it has its limitations. Radiofrequency-based catheter ablation has a relatively safe record, producing precisely defined lesions. Long-term outcomes have shown to be effective in a wide population of patients (Bella et al., 2001). However, the energy required to produce these lesions can cause endocardial disruption. This is often due to the primary requirement of continuous contact between the electrode and the endocardium during ablation. Alternatively, other ablation techniques have been employed, including cryogenic, and thermal ablation (microwave-, infrared-, and laser-based) approaches that are undergoing preclinical and clinical evaluation. The first method, cryoablation, has been deemed safe in the treatment of cardiac arrhythmias. Recently, cryoablation has been used specifically in the percutaneous transvascular mapping and ablation of arrhythmias (Lustgarden et al., 1999; Keane et al., 1999). Some of the potential advantages of cryoablation with regards to radiofrequency ablation include a stable adhesion of the cryothermal catheter to the endocardium throughout the process, reduced incidence of endocardial thrombus formation at the site of cryoablation, and freedom from electrical interference by intracardiac echo imaging during ablation. The latter effect is often seen during radiofrequency ablation. The second method, microwave ablation, uses electromagnetic radiation rather than radiofrequencies. Because of this, microwave does not require a contact dependency, unlike radiofrequency- or cryo-based ablation (Maessen et al., 2002; Williams et al., 2002). Recently, microwave ablation has been used as an intra-operative tool in the surgical maze procedure and evaluated as an alternative for radiofrequency epicardial ablation in minimally invasive access surgery (Knaut et al., 2001; Benussi et al., 2002). Finally, in order to apply a highly focused beam of energy, laser ablation is being evaluated. Early studies in the use of laser ablation met with significant difficulties. Lesions created through the use of high-energy pulsed lasing (Nd-YAG, i.e., infrared wavelength) carried a risk of crater formation (Lee et al., 1985). This risk was addressed by the use of a higher frequency laser, argon (630 nm) vs. Nd-YAG (1064 nm), which reduced the creation of craters (Sakena et al., 1989). These results were encouraging for the potential application of laser ablation. This application of the continuous lower energy diode laser facilitates the ability to heat and create controlled and precisely located lesions uniformly. To this end, the ability to focus a narrow beam will enhance refined lesions through more versatile devices. The introduction of alternative ablation techniques may overcome some of the limitations of conventional radiofrequency ablation and the overall ability to decrease the risk of endocardial disruption. Finally, we may see more preclinical and eventually clinical applications of the thermal-based ablation techniques with the expectation of increased overall efficacy of cardiac ablation. The favorable safety profiles, in early results, ensure ablation as a technique in future cardiac arrhythmia management.

References

American Heart Association, 2002 Heart and Stroke Statistical Update, Dallas, 2001.

Bella, P.D., De Ponti, R., Uriarte, J.A.S., Tondo, C., Klersy, C., Carbucicchio, C., Storti, C., Riva, S., and Longobardi, M., Catheter ablation and antiarrhymic drugs for haemodynamically tolerated post-infarction ventricular tachycardia, *Eur. Heart J.*, 23, 414–424, 2001.

Benussi, S., Nascimbene, S., Agricola, E., Calori, G., Calvi, S., Caldarola, A., Oppizzi, M., Casati, V., Pappone, C., and Alfieri, O., Surgical ablation of atrial fibrillation using the epicardial radiofrequency approach: mid-term results and risk analysis, *Ann. Thorac. Surg.*, 74, 1050–1057, 2002.

Byrne, J.V., Sohn, M.J., Molyneux, A.J., and Chir, B., Five-year experience in using coil embolization for ruptured intracranial aneurysms: outcomes and incidence of late rebleeding, *J. Neurosurg.*, 90(4), 656–663, 1999.

Clowes, A.W. and Karnovsky, M.J., Suppression by heparin of smooth muscle cell proliferation in injured arteries, *Nature*, 265, 625–626, 1977.

Degertekin, M., Regar, E., Tanabe, K., Lee, C.H., and Serruys, P.W., Sirolimus eluting stent in the treatment of atherosclerosis coronary artery disease, *Minerva Cardioangiol.*, 50(5), 405–418, 2002.

Dotter, C.T., Transluminally-placed coilspring endarterial tube grafts: long term patency in canine popliteal artery, *Invest. Radiol.*, 4, 329–332, 1969.

Dotter, C.T., Buschman, R.W., McKinney, M.K., and Rösch, J., Transluminal expandable nitinol coil stent grafting: preliminary report, *Radiology*, 147, 259–260, 1983.

Duerig, T.W., Tolomeo, D.E., and Wholey, M., An overview of superelastic stent design, *Min. Invas. Ther. Allied Technol.*, 9(3/4), 235–246, 2000.

Edelman, E.R. and Rogers, C., Pathobiologic responses to stenting, *Am. J. Cardiol.*, 81, 4E–6E, 1998.

Ferris, E.J., McCowan, T.C., Carver, D.K., and MacFarland, D.J., Percutaneous inferior vena cava filters: follow-up of seven designs in 320 patients, *Radiology*, 188, 851–856, 1993.

Fleisch, M. and Meier, B., Management and outcome of stents in 1998: long-term outcome, *Cardiol. Rev.*, 7, 215–218, 1999.

Gallo, R., Padurean, A., and Jayaramon, T., Inhibition of intimal thickening after balloon angioplasty in porcine coronary arteries by targeting regulators of the cell cycle, *Circulation*, 99, 2164–2170, 1999.

Greenfield, L.J. and Proctor, M.C., The percutaneous greenfield filter: outcomes and practice patterns, *J. Vasc. Surg.*, 32(5), 888–893, 2000.

Grube, E. and Büllesfeld, L., Initial experience with Paclitaxel-coated stents, *J. Interven. Cardiol.*, 15, 471–476, 2002.

Hirsh, J., Heparin, *N. Engl. J. Med.*, 324, 1565–1574, 1991.

Hlatky, M.A. et al., Medical care costs and quality of life after randomization to coronary angioplasty or coronary by-pass surgery, *N. Engl. J. Med.*, 336(2), 92–99, 1997.

Hwang, C., Wu, D., and Edelman, E., Physiological transport forces govern drug distribution for stent-based delivery, *Circulation*, 104, 600–605, 2001.

Kastrati, A., Mehilli, J., Dirsschinger, J., et al., Restenosis after coronary placement of various stent types, *Am. J. Cardiol.*, 877, 34–39, 2001.

Keane, D., New catheter ablation techniques for the treatment of cardiac arrhythmias, *Cardiac ElectroPhy. Rev.*, 6, 341–348, 2002.

Keane, D., Zhou, L., Houghtaling, C., Aretez, T., McGovern, B., Garan, H., and Ruskin, J., Percutaneous cryothermal catheter ablation for the creation of linear atrial lesions, *Pace*, 22(II), 587, 1999.

Knaut, M., Tugtekin, M., Spitzer, S.G., Karolyi, L., Boehme, H., and Schueler, S., Curative treatment of chronic atrial fibrillation in patients with simultaneous cardiosurgical diseases with intraoperative microwave ablation, *JACC*, 109A(abstr), 2001.

Lee, B.I., Gottdiener, J.S., Fletcher, R.D., Rodriguez, E.R., and Ferrans, V.J., Transcatheter ablation: comparison between laser photoablation and electrode shock ablation in the dog, *Circulation*, 71, 579–586, 1985.

Lieber, B.B. and Gounis, M.J., The physics of endoluminal stenting in the treatment of cerebrovascular aneurysms, *Neurol. Res.*, 24(Suppl. 1), S33–42, 2002.

Liffman, K., Lawrence-Brown, M., Semmens, J.B., Bui, A., Rudman, M., and Hartley, D., Analytical modeling and numerical simulation of forces in an endoluminal graft, *J. Endovasc. Ther.*, 8, 358–371, 2001.

Lorch, H., Zwaan, M., Kulke, C., and Weiss, H.D., In vitro studies of temporary vena cava filters, *Cardiovasc. Interv. Radiol.*, 21, 146–150, 1998.

Lustgarden, D., Keane, D., and Ruskin, J., Cryothermal catheter ablation: mechanism of tissue injury and clinical results, *Prog. Cardiovasc. Dis.*, 41, 481–498, 1999.

Maessen, J.G., Nijis, J.F.M.A., Smeets, J.L.R.M., Vainer, J., and Mochtar, B., Beating-heart treatment of atrial fibrillation with microwave ablation, *Ann. Thorac. Surg.*, 74, S1307–1311, 2002.

Morales, P.A. and Heuser, R.R., Embolic protection devices, *J. Interven. Cardiol.*, 15, 485–490, 2002.

Palmaz, J.C., Richter, G.M., Noldge, G., Kauffmann, G.W., and Wenz, W., Intraluminal Palmaz stent implantation. The first clinical case report on a balloon-expanded vascular prosthesis (in German), *Radiologe*, 27(12), 560–5633, 1987.

Palmaz, J.C., Kopp, D.T., and Hayashi, H., Normal and stenotic renal arteries: experimental balloon-expandable intraluminal stenting, *Radiology*, 164, 705, 1987a.

Poon, M., Badimon, J.J., and Fuster, V., Overcoming restenosis with sirolimus: from alphabet soup to clinical reality, *Lancet*, 359, 619–622, 2002.

Ragosta, M., Karve, M., Brezynski, D., et al., Effectiveness of heparin in preventing thrombin generation and thrombin activity in patients undergoing coronary intervention, *Am. Heart J.*, 137, 250–257, 1999.

Sakena, S., Gielchinsky, J.S., and Tullo, N.G., Argon laser ablation of malignant ventricular tachycardia associated with coronary artery disease, *Am. J. Cardiol.*, 64, 1298–1304, 1989.

Serruys, P.Q., de Jaegere, P., Kiemeneij, F., Macaya, C., Rutsch, W., Heyndrickx, G., Emanuelsson, H., Marco, J., Legrand, V., Materne, P., Belardi, J., Sigart, U., Colombo, A., Goy, J.J., van den Heuvel, P., Delcan, J., and Morel, M., for the BENESTENT Study Group, A comparison of balloon expandable stent implantation with balloon angioplasty in patients with coronary artery disease, *N. Engl. J. Med.*, 331, 489–495, 1994.

Sievert, H. and Rabe, K., Role of distal protection during carotid stenting, *J. Interven. Cardiol.*, 15, 499–504, 2002.

Sigwart, U., Puel, J., Mirkovitch, V., Joffre, F., and Kappenberger, L., Intravascular stents to prevent occlusion and restenosis after transluminal angioplasty, *N. Engl. J. Med.*, 316, 701–706, 1987.

Sousa, J.E., Costa, M.A., Abizaid, A.C., et al., Sustained suppression of neointimal proliferation by Sirolimus-eluting stents. One-year angiographic and intravascular ultrasound follow up, *Circulation*, 104, 2007–2011, 2001.

Stecker, M.S., Barnhart, W.H., and Lang, E.V., Evaluation of a spiral nitinol temporary inferior vena caval filter, *Acad. Radiol.*, 8(6), 484–493, 2001.

Tsuji, T., Tamai, H., Igaki, K., Kyo, E., Kosuga, K., Hata, T., Okada, M., Nakamura, T., Komori, H., Motohara, S., and Uehata, H., Biodegradable polymeric stents, *Curr. Interv. Cardiol. Rep.*, 3(1), 10–17, 2001.

Uda, K., Goto, K., Ogata, N., Izumi, N., Nagata, S., and Matsuno, H., Embolization of cerebral aneurysms using Guglielmi detachable coils — problems and treatment plans in the acute stage after subarachnoid hemorrhage and long-term efficiency, *Neurol. Med. Chir. (Tokyo)*, 38(3), 143–152, 1998.

Uhrich, K., Cannizzaro, S.M., Langer, R.S., and Shakesheff, K.M., Polymeric systems for controlled drug release, *Chem. Rev.*, 99, 3181–3198, 1999.

van Marrewijk, C., Buth, J., Harris, P.L., Norgren, L., Nevelsteen, A., and Wyatt, M.G., Significance of endoleaks after endovascular repair of abdominal aortic aneurysms: the EUROSTAR experience, *J. Vasc. Surg.*, 35(3), 461–473, 2002.

Williams, M.R., Knaut, M., Berube, D., and Oz, M.C., Application of microwave energy in cardiac tissue ablation: from *in vitro* analyses to clinical use, *Ann. Thorac. Surg.*, 74, 1500–1505, 2002.

Zarins, C.K., Lu, C.T., Gewertz, B.L., Lyon, R.T., Rush, D.S., and Glagov, S., Arterial disruption and remodeling following balloon dilatation, *Surgery*, 92(6), 1086–1095, 1982.

Zwaan, M., Kagel, C., Marienhoff, N., Weiss, H.D., Grimm, W., Eberhard, I., and Schweider, G., Erste Erfahrungen mit temporaren vena cava filtern, *Fortschr. Rontgenstr.*, 163, 74–79, 1995.

26

Stereotactic Procedures

CONTENTS

Michael D. Weil
Sirius Medicine, LLC

26.1 Introduction

Stereotaxy employs minimally invasive techniques to precisely locate a target within the body. This requires rendering the internal target and organs relative to an external reference in three-dimensional space. A system of coordinates links the defined exterior and the viewed internal anatomy. The imaging can be performed with diagnostic x-rays, magnetic resonance imaging, or ultrasound. The external reference can be a frame attached to the patient, or marked points on the patient's surface anatomy.

Stereotactic systems can be used to diagnose or treat. Diagnostic procedures can be performed on small lesions with greater precision than conventional biopsy. Diagnostic accuracy is thereby improved. Therapy using stereotaxy can be done with surgery or radiation. The methods permit approach to inaccessible regions of the body with minimal disruption of the intervening tissues. As a result, there is less potential for morbidity and less discomfort for the patient.

Stereotactic procedures are employed in a wide range of applications, from basic scientific research to common clinical problems.[1] The research includes neurologic monitoring[2,3] and gene therapy. The clinical spectrum of usage ranges from cancer diagnosis and treatment to the evaluation and treatment of movement disorders.

26.2 Methods

It is necessary to measure and define the three-dimensional volume around a target (Figure 26.1). An external frame is attached to the patient or, alternatively, prominent surface anatomy is marked ("frameless"). The target and body are next imaged along with the external reference points. The important structures in the space are outlined. The distances of the anatomy relative to the reference frame can then be measured (Figure 26.22). An orthogonal coordinate system (x-, y-, and z-axis) is delineated according to these measurements. The points of interest, outside and inside the patient, are then known by their position in the three-dimensional stereotactic space and given coordinates relative to the refer-

0-8493-1140-3/04/$0.00+$1.50

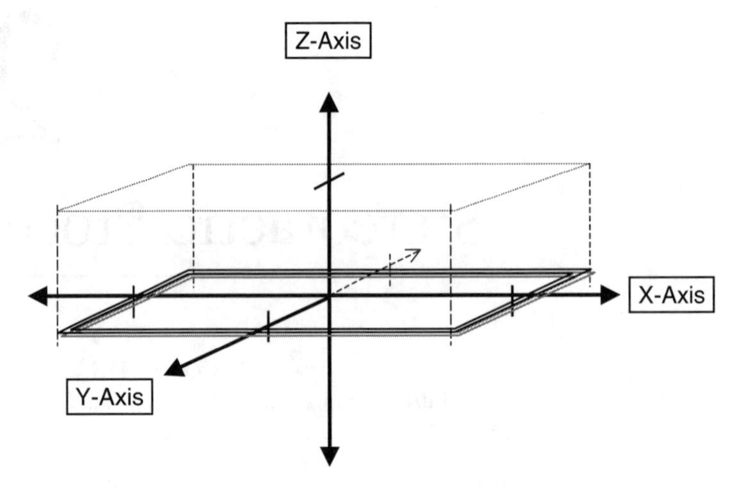

FIGURE 26.1 Stereotactic space is defined relative to a fixed, external reference plane. The coordinate system, x-, y-, and z-axis, is measured in millimeters from the reference plane to define a stereotactic volume (dotted lines). The volumes of the target and normal surrounding structures within the region are defined and localized to these coordinates by planning software.

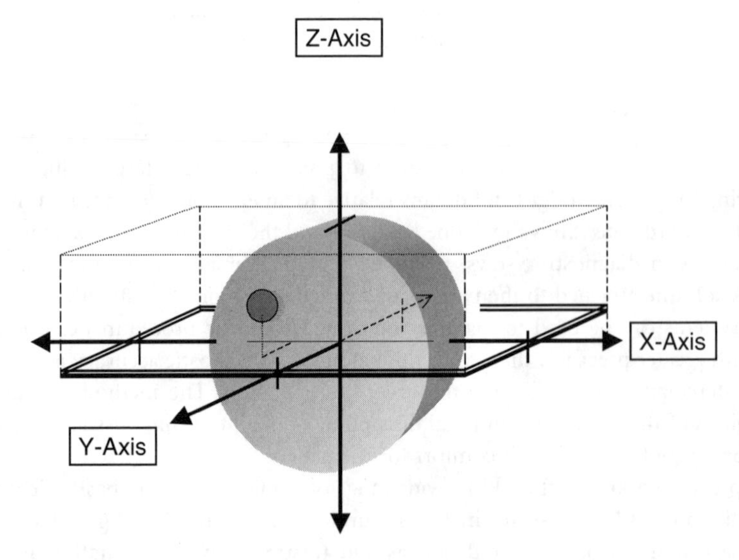

FIGURE 26.2 The stereotactic volume characterizes the anatomy (cylinder) and the target (dark circle). Distances from the reference markers are established by obtaining an image of the lesion within the frame or other orientation points. The coordinates of the lesion at depth can then be targeted from an access point on the surface.

ence. Though the target is unseen by the clinician, it can be readily located and approached by starting at a known point on the patient's surface and proceeding to the coordinates of the target (Figure 26.3).

26.2.1 Frame or Frameless

The methods require an image of the internal structures to be correlated to an accessible external reference. The orientation can be done within a frame to define the borders and coordinates of stereotactic space. Various commercial frames are on the market and most commonly used for neurosurgical procedures. The frame is secured to the patient, often by screws to the bony anatomy, which is then secured to the immobilization mechanism. The images of the patient within the frame can next be scanned into various software.[4] The program can then be used to locate the anatomy based on the distance from the frame.

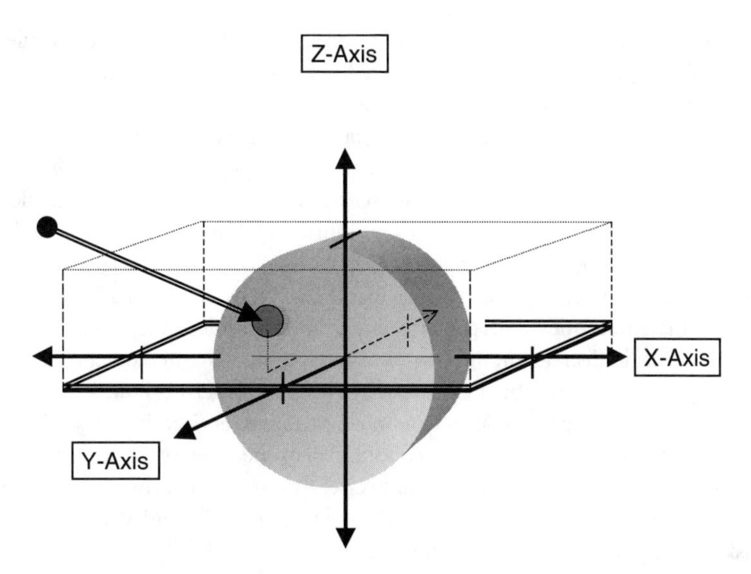

FIGURE 26.3 Trajectory of an instrument or beam is designed through an accessible point on the patient's surface to the coordinates of the target. The coordinates of the surface, interior anatomy, and the target are relative to the frame, or skin markers. Planning software navigates the path (double-lined arrow) and can guide the procedure.

Sophisticated planning systems can then design trajectories of approach for surgery or radiation. The same techniques can be performed by marking the surface anatomy with points (fiducials) that will be visible to the clinician and on the image. Thus, stereotaxy can be performed without the frame as well. The surface is delineated with skin markers,[5] or natural anatomical projections. Various frameless systems are commercially available and are very precise.[6]

Whether the intent of the procedure is biopsy or ablation, the operator must have a mechanism to guide the instrument to the target. In the case of radiosurgery,[7] it is reasonably uncomplicated to aim the beam at the coordinates of the target because the stereotactic frame is attached to the treatment table. The patient lying on the treatment table is aligned with lasers in the room via the frame's coordinate system so that the isocenter of the beam intersects the location of the target. On the other hand, when the lesion is approached with an instrument in the surgeon's hand, a navigation arrangement is needed to know where the needle or scalpel is relative to the target. So-called neuronavigation is accomplished with room sensors that track the instruments.[8] The registration process of the fiducials is critical to the accuracy of these neuronavigation systems. The accuracy of the guidance system is similar whether a frameless or frame-based reference system is employed.[9]

26.3 Clinical Applications

26.3.1 Movement Disorders

Tremor suppression can be accomplished with stimulation, which is as effective as coagulation but with less adverse effects, and the possibility of bilateral operations. Thalamotomy may remain an option in selected patients.[10] By using stereotaxy with MRI and electrophysiology, it is possible to record[11] and stimulate single neuron activity deep within the brain. Electrodes placed at suitable locations can be stimulated with high frequency to treat tremor of different origins.[12] Targets include the ventral intermediate (VIM) region of the thalamus, the subthalamic nucleus (STN), and the medial pallidum (Gpi). Improvement of tremor, rigidity, and akinesia translates into less medication and its associated dyskinesia. In Parkinson's disease,[13] the STN has become the preferred site of stimulation in carefully selected patients, often with the use of ventriculography to improve the accuracy of the stereotactic coordinates.

Stereotactic intracerebral EEG stimulations and recordings can be used to study epilepsy along with other modalities.[14] By mapping somatosensory-evoked potentials via stereotactically placed intracortical electrodes it is possible to study complex projections.[15] The use of standard stereotactic atlases can be expanded with software adapted to compare individuals to averaged anatomy.[16]

Stereotactic surgical techniques can safely reach and ablate deep structures in the brain such as the thalamus. Ventral intermediate (VIM) thalamotomies have been used to treat medically intractable essential tremor,[17] with a 60% success rate and low morbidity. Tremor in multiple sclerosis has been reported to respond to stereotactic surgery of the thalamus, zona incerta and subthalamic nuclei.[18] Stereotactic surgery has been performed with reasonable outcomes in some Parkinson's patients as well. Ventrolateral (VL) thalamotomies and posteroventral (PV) pallidotomies can improve dyskinesias, though without a significant decrease in the levodopa dose.[19] Following stereotactic pallidotomy, patients with Parkinson's disease have been noted to have improvement in perception.[20]

Involuntary, abnormal head movements and pain characterize cervical dystonia. The mechanisms are poorly understood but complex forms of the condition have been reported to respond to stereotactic surgery with bilateral pallidotomy or globus pallidus deep brain stimulation.[21] Unresponsive Tourette's syndrome has been treated with stereotactic surgical zona incerta (ZI) and VL thalamotomy.[22] There is a significant risk of complications with bilateral surgery.

26.3.2 Mass Lesions

Orientation in an operative field in the brain ordinarily requires adequate exposure so the surgeon can identify familiar structures. Image-guided and computer-assisted navigation systems can display accurate spatial information directly from patient images.[23] This data permits delineation of normal anatomy and pathologic lesions with much less manipulation. Therefore, the technique readily lends itself to brain biopsy[24] and drainage of abscesses.[25] Alternatively, the technique can be used with endoscopy. Neuronavigation has been successfully incorporated into surgery for brain and spine masses with improvement in the postoperative course.[8] Computer-assisted guidance has been reported to be of use in transsphenoidal parasellar surgery.[27]

Radiosurgery offers great promise and many advantages over conventional techniques.[28] However, to date there have been no randomized clinical trials to confirm the early hopeful data.[29] Radiosurgical beams, i.e., radiation that is highly conformal to the target, can be delivered to a selected point in a stereotactic volume by several methods. Specially outfitted linear accelerators and the Gamma Knife (multiple cobalt sources) deliver photons. While several specialty centers can treat with protons, there is a huge disadvantage in cost of the protons. Modern accelerators rigged with micro-, multileaf collimation can deliver conformal radiation that is comparable to protons.[30] In rare situations, when a lesion is too intimately involved with a critical structure protons may give a better dose distribution. Intensity modulation along with these dynamic micro-, multileaf collimators can significantly decrease the impact of x-ray beams overshooting the target with unintended consequences.[31]

Delivery of fractionated radiation with stereotactic setups, i.e., fractionated stereotactic radiotherapy, improves reproducibility of multiple treatments,[32] and may be appropriate in selected circumstances.[33,34]

Radiosurgery is playing an increasingly important role in the management of brain metastases when the primary disease is controlled.[35] The role of whole brain radiotherapy with its significant morbidity is challenged by radiosurgery.[36,37]

26.3.3 Vascular Malformations

Endovascular embolization, stereotactic radiosurgery, and microsurgery can be used alone or in combination to effectively treat arteriovenous malformations (AVM) of the brain.[38] Results with stereotactic radiosurgery for the treatment of benign intracranial mass lesions such as AVM[39] have been very good in terms of toxicity and local control. Only 5% of the patients have been reported to suffer adverse symptoms, with a 71% obliteration rate at 2 years. AVMs can reappear after total occlusion with radiosurgery on occasion, particularly in pediatric patients.[40] After being declared cured, 10 of 48 patients had clinical symptoms from AVMs. Radiosurgical procedures for AVMs can be repeated with acceptable risk.[41] Control decreases for bigger lesions. In the case of large AVMs (>3 cm diameter), there was a greater complication rate and significantly less chance of obliteration.[42] The majority of long-term complications after radiosurgery for AVM[43] were associated with radiation injury to the brain. Minimal sequelae after radiosurgery and no history of bleeding resulted in significantly less symptoms. Other vascular pathology, such as cerebral cavernous malformations are presently treated with microsurgical techniques rather than radiosurgery.[44]

26.3.4 Palliation

Posteromedial thalamotomy with stereotactic navigation under MR guidance has been used to successfully relieve intractable pain.[45] Radiosurgery is more effective for idiopathic trigeminal neuralgia[46] than for tumor-related facial pain. Radiosurgery produced control in ≥70% of patients treated for trigeminal neuralgia.[47]

Insertion of Ommaya reservoirs for intrathecal chemotherapy in difficult technical scenarios is facilitated by stereotactic techniques.[48]

26.3.5 Breast

Mammography and biopsy of suspicious lesions can be readily performed with stereotactic methods,[49] where the breast and lesion can be viewed in three-dimensional. Surgical excisional biopsy of nonpalpable suspicious breast lesions are more invasive, and likely more costly than stereotactic large-core needle biopsy.[50] Stereotaxy can be employed for breast biopsy in place of wire localization for nonpalpable abnormalities on mammogram.[51] The procedure is accurate[52] with less surgical trauma. Stereotactic biopsy avoided a surgical procedure in nearly half of the patients in this study. Amorphous calcifications on mammogram remain a diagnostic dilemma. Additionally, there is still risk of false-negative exams,[53] which might be lessened with improved procedures.[54-56] It is expected to be the biopsy technique of choice in the near future for lesions discovered by mammogram.

26.4 Complications

The use of stereotactic navigation is not totally without risk. Seizures can be induced by brain procedures.[24] Bleeding can occur at a biopsy site requiring craniotomy.[57] Tumor seeding along a stereotactic biopsy tract, though rare, has been reported.[58,59] In addition, there have been reports of surgical instruments transferring the infectious agents of variant Creuztfeldt-Jakob disease, though blood-borne agents portend the greatest risk of clinically significant contamination.[60]

It is less difficult to radiate after surgery than vice versa. In a survey of a small group of acoustic neuroma patients retreated with microsurgery after radiosurgery the results were not good.[61] This is likely the result of the technical hurdles from scarring following high dose delivered to a small region.

26.5 New Directions

It may be possible in the near future to perform real-time tissue identification during stereotactic brain biopsies and functional neurosurgery.[62] Cannulas containing microsensors can discriminate cancer from benign tissue via optical scattering spectroscopy *in vivo*. Stereotactic biopsy of parasitic brain lesions; e.g., neurocysticercosis, has been considered the standard of care. However, serodiagnosis might become a reasonable alternative as access to the biopsy techniques is not available in many areas.[63]

Stereotactic methods are commonly employed for brain research, such as electrode placement,[64] or creating precise lesions.[65] Models for tissue transplant into the brain with stereotactic guidance have also been reported,[66] along with early clinical data.[67] Characterization of neuroanatomy is possible by delivering neurotropic viruses into specific regions of the brain with stereotactic guidance.[68] Direct injection of gene therapy into gliomas may be performed routinely with stereotaxy as the efficiency of the vectors is improved.[69]

The impact of precision treatment is often difficult to document initially. Mapping of complex three-dimensional dose distributions of stereotactic radiation treatment can be achieved with polymer gel dosimetry,[70,71] or with radiochromic film.[72]

26.6 Discussion

Stereotactic neurosurgery has been practiced for the past half century.[73] Since its inception, the field has expanded to epilepsy, movement disorders, radiosurgery, frameless techniques, and applied to other sites such as spine and breast. The treatment of Parkinson's disease, for instance, has progressed from open surgical techniques in the 1950s to recording and stimulation with deeply implanted electrodes.[74] These advances were possible with the accuracy of locating the lesions under stereotactic guidance.

The methodology of stereotaxis and image guidance dramatically reduce the potential for harming the patient with invasive procedures in critical areas. However, improved therapeutic modalities will dramatically enhance the impact of these less-invasive delivery systems. Progress in viral vectors for gene therapy,[75] or combinations of treatments could offer the next opportunity for growth of the field of stereotaxy and image-guided navigation.

References

1. Ohye, C., The idea of stereotaxy toward minimally invasive neurosurgery, *Stereotact. Funct. Neurosurg.*, 74(3-4), 185–193, 2000.
2. Stefani, A. et al., Subdyskinetic apomorphine responses in globus pallidus and subthalamus of parkinsonian patients: lack of clear evidence for the 'indirect pathway,' *Clin. Neurophysiol.*, 113(1), 91–100, 2002.
3. Hua, S.E. et al., Microelectrode studies of normal organization and plasticity of human somatosensory thalamus, *J. Clin. Neurophysiol.*, 17(6), 559–574, 2000.
4. Slavin, K.V., Anderson, G.J., and Burchiel, K.J., Comparison of three techniques for calculation of target coordinates in functional stereotactic procedures, *Stereotact. Funct. Neurosurg.*, 72(2-4), 192–195, 1999.
5. Wolfsberger, S. et al., Anatomical landmarks for image registration in frameless stereotactic neuronavigation, *Neurosurg. Rev.*, 25(1-2), 68–72, 2002.
6. Benardete, E.A., Leonard, M.A., and Weiner, H.L., Comparison of frameless stereotactic systems: accuracy, precision, and applications, *Neurosurgery*, 49(6), 1409–1415; discussion 1415–1416, 2001.
7. Chang, S.D. and Adler, J.R., Jr., Current status and optimal use of radiosurgery, *Oncology (Huntingt).*, 15(2), 209–216; discussion 219–221, 2001.
8. Haberland, N. et al., Neuronavigation in surgery of intracranial and spinal tumors, *J. Cancer Res. Clin. Oncol.*, 126(9), 529–541, 2000.
9. Steinmeier, R. et al., Factors influencing the application accuracy of neuronavigation systems, *Stereotact. Funct. Neurosurg.*, 75(4), 188–202, 2000.
10. Speelman, J.D. et al., Stereotactic neurosurgery for tremor, *Mov. Disord.*, 17(Suppl. 3), S84–S88, 2002.
11. Benazzouz, A. et al., Intraoperative microrecordings of the subthalamic nucleus in Parkinson's disease, *Mov. Disord.*, 17(Suppl. 3), S145–S149, 2002.
12. Benabid, A.L. et al., Deep brain stimulation of the corpus luysi (subthalamic nucleus) and other targets in Parkinson's disease. Extension to new indications such as dystonia and epilepsy, *J. Neurol.*, 248(Suppl. 3), III37–III47, 2001.
13. Benabid, A.L. et al., Deep brain stimulation of the subthalamic nucleus for Parkinson's disease: methodologic aspects and clinical criteria, *Neurology*, 55(12), S40–S44, 2000.

14. Baciu, M. et al., Functional MRI assessment of the hemispheric predominance for language in epileptic patients using a simple rhyme detection task, *Epileptic Disord.*, 3(3), 117–124, 2001.
15. Barba, C. et al., Stereotactic recordings of median nerve somatosensory-evoked potentials in the human pre-supplementary motor area, *Eur. J. Neurosci.*, 13(2), 347–356, 2001.
16. Berks, G., Pohl, G., and Keyserlingk, D.G., Three-dimensional-VIEWER: an atlas-based system for individual and statistical investigations of the human brain, *Methods Inf. Med.*, 40(3), 170–177, 2001.
17. Akbostanci, M.C., Slavin, K.V., and Burchiel, K.J., Stereotactic ventral intermedial thalamotomy for the treatment of essential tremor: results of a series of 37 patients, *Stereotact. Funct. Neurosurg.*, 72(2-4), 174–177, 1999.
18. Alusi, S.H. et al., Stereotactic lesional surgery for the treatment of tremor in multiple sclerosis: a prospective case-controlled study, *Brain*, 124(Pt. 8), 1576–1589, 2001.
19. Aguiar, P.M. et al., Motor performance after posteroventral pallidotomy and VIM-thalamotomy in Parkinson's disease: a 1-year follow-up study, *Arq. Neuropsiquiatr.*, 58(3B), 830–835, 2000.
20. Barrett, A.M. et al., Seeing trees but not the forest: limited perception of large configurations in PD, *Neurology*, 56(6), 724–729, 2001.
21. Adler, C.H. and Kumar, R., Pharmacological and surgical options for the treatment of cervical dystonia, *Neurology*, 55(12), S9–S14, 2000.
22. Babel, T.B., Warnke, P.C., and Ostertag, C.B., Immediate and long term outcome after infrathalamic and thalamic lesioning for intractable Tourette's syndrome, *J. Neurol. Neurosurg. Psychiatry*, 70(5), 666–671, 2001.
23. Suess, O. et al., Intracranial image-guided neurosurgery: experience with a new electromagnetic navigation system, *Acta Neurochir. (Wien)*, 143(9), 927–934, 2001.
24. Yu, X. et al., Stereotactic biopsy for intracranial space-occupying lesions: clinical analysis of 550 cases, *Stereotact. Funct. Neurosurg.*, 75(2-3), 103–108, 2000.
25. Strowitzki, M., Schwerdtfeger, K., and Steudel, W.I., Ultrasound-guided aspiration of brain abscesses through a single burr hole, *Minim. Invasive Neurosurg.*, 44(3), 135–140, 2001.
26. Gumprecht, H., Trost, H.A., and Lumenta, C.B., Neuroendoscopy combined with frameless neuronavigation, *Br. J. Neurosurg.*, 14(2), 129–131, 2000.
27. Kacker, A. et al., Transphenoidal surgery utilizing computer-assisted stereotactic guidance, *Rhinology*, 39(4), 207–210, 2001.
28. Weil, M.D., Advances in stereotactic radiosurgery for brain neoplasms, *Curr. Neurol. Neurosci. Rep.*, 1(3), 233–237, 2001.
29. Haines, S.J., Moving targets and ghosts of the past: outcome measurement in brain tumour therapy, *J. Clin. Neurosci.*, 9(2), 109–112, 2002.
30. Baumert, B.G. et al., A comparison of dose distributions of proton and photon beams in stereotactic conformal radiotherapy of brain lesions, *Int. J. Radiat. Oncol. Biol. Phys.*, 49(5), 1439–1449, 2001.
31. Benedict, S.H. et al., Intensity-modulated stereotactic radiosurgery using dynamic micro-multileaf collimation, *Int. J. Radiat. Oncol. Biol. Phys.*, 50(3), 751–758, 2001.
32. Alheit, H. et al., Patient position reproducibility in fractionated stereotactically guided conformal radiotherapy using the BrainLab mask system, *Strahlenther Onkol.*, 177(5), 264–268, 2001.
33. Andrews, D.W. et al., Stereotactic radiosurgery and fractionated stereotactic radiotherapy for the treatment of acoustic schwannomas: comparative observations of 125 patients treated at one institution, *Int. J. Radiat. Oncol. Biol. Phys.*, 50(5), 1265–1278, 2001.
34. Aoyama, H. et al., Treatment outcome of single or hypofractionated single-isocentric stereotactic irradiation (STI) using a linear accelerator for intracranial arteriovenous malformation, *Radiother. Oncol.*, 59(3), 323–328, 2001.
35. Arnold, S.M. and Patchell, R.A., Diagnosis and management of brain metastases, *Hematol. Oncol. Clin. North Am.*, 15(6), 1085–1107, vii, 2001.
36. Weil, M.D., Stereotactic radiosurgery for brain tumors, *Hematol. Oncol. Clin. North Am.*, 15(6), 1017–1026, 2001.

37. Chen, J.C. et al., Stereotactic radiosurgery in the treatment of metastatic disease to the brain, *Neurosurgery*, 47(2), 268–279; discussion 279–281, 2000.
38. Fleetwood, I.G. and Steinberg, G.K., Arteriovenous malformations, *Lancet*, 359(9309), 863–73, 2002.
39. Flickinger, J.C., Kondziolka, D., and Lunsford, L.D., Radiosurgery of benign lesions, *Semin. Radiat. Oncol.*, 5(3), 220–224, 1995.
40. Lindqvist, M. et al., Angiographic long-term follow-up data for arteriovenous malformations previously proven to be obliterated after gamma knife radiosurgery, *Neurosurgery*, 46(4), 803–808; discussion 809-810, 2000.
41. Maesawa, S. et al., Repeated radiosurgery for incompletely obliterated arteriovenous malformations, *J. Neurosurg.*, 92(6), 961–970, 2000.
42. Miyawaki, L. et al., Five year results of LINAC radiosurgery for arteriovenous malformations: outcome for large AVMS, *Int. J. Radiat. Oncol. Biol. Phys.*, 44(5), 1089–1106, 1999.
43. Flickinger, J.C. et al., A multi-institutional analysis of complication outcomes after arteriovenous malformation radiosurgery, *Int. J. Radiat. Oncol. Biol. Phys.*, 44(1), 67–74, 1999.
44. Bertalanffy, H. et al., Cerebral cavernomas in the adult. Review of the literature and analysis of 72 surgically treated patients, *Neurosurg. Rev.*, 25(1-2), 1–53; discussion 54–55, 2002.
45. Balas, I.I. et al. [In Process Citation], *Rev. Neurol.*, 31(6), 531–533, 2000.
46. Chang, J.W. et al., The effects of stereotactic radiosurgery on secondary facial pain, *Stereotact. Funct. Neurosurg.*, 72(Suppl. 1), 29–37, 1999.
47. Pollock, B.E. et al., The Mayo Clinic gamma knife experience: indications and initial results [see comments], *Mayo Clin. Proc.*, 74(1), 5–13, 1999.
48. Al-Anazi, A. and Bernstein, M., Modified stereotactic insertion of the Ommaya reservoir. Technical note, *J. Neurosurg.*, 92(6), 1050–1052, 2000.
49. Bagnall, M.J. et al., Predicting invasion in mammographically detected microcalcification, *Clin. Radiol.*, 56(10), 828–832, 2001.
50. Buijs-van der Woude, T. et al., Cost comparison between stereotactic large-core-needle biopsy versus surgical excision biopsy in The Netherlands, *Eur. J. Cancer*, 37(14), 1736–1745, 2001.
51. Carr, J.J. et al., Stereotactic localization of breast lesions: how it works and methods to improve accuracy, *Radiographics*, 21(2), 463–473, 2001.
52. Berg, W.A. et al., Biopsy of amorphous breast calcifications: pathologic outcome and yield at stereotactic biopsy, *Radiology*, 221(2), 495–503, 2001.
53. Adler, D.D. et al., Follow-up of benign results of stereotactic core breast biopsy, *Acad. Radiol.*, 7(4), 248–253, 2000.
54. Bergaz, F. et al., Clip placement facilitating the approach to breast lesions, *Eur. Radiol.*, 12(2), 471–474, 2002.
55. Atallah, N. et al., Stereotaxic excisional biopsy of non-palpable breast lesions by the ABBI (Advanced Breast Biopsy Instrumentation) technique. Advantages. Disadvantages. Indications. Apropos of 67 cases, *J. Med. Liban*, 48(2), 70–76, 2000.
56. Ancona, A., Caiffa, L., and Fazio, V., Digital stereotactic breast microbiopsy with the mammotome: study of 122 cases, *Radiol. Med. (Torino)*, 101(5), 341–347, 2001.
57. Daszkiewicz, P., [In Process Citation]. *Neurol. Neurochir. Pol.*, 35(5), 899–905, 2001.
58. Aichholzer, M. et al., Epidural metastasis of a glioblastoma after stereotactic biopsy: case report, *Minim. Invasive Neurosurg.*, 44(3), 175–177, 2001.
59. Steinmetz, M.P. et al., Metastatic seeding of the stereotactic biopsy tract in glioblastoma multiforme: case report and review of the literature, *J. Neurooncol.*, 55(3), 167–171, 2001.
60. Brown, P., The risk of blood-borne Creutzfeldt-Jakob disease, *Dev. Biol. Stand.*, 102, 53–59, 2000.
61. Battista, R.A. and Wiet, R.J., Stereotactic radiosurgery for acoustic neuromas: a survey of the American Neurotology Society, *Am. J. Otol.*, 21(3), 371–381, 2000.
62. Andrews, R. et al., Multimodality stereotactic brain tissue identification: the NASA smart probe project, *Stereotact. Funct. Neurosurg.*, 73(1-4), 1–8, 1999.

63. Bedi, S., Prasad, A., and Anand, K.S., Neurocysticercal serodiagnosis — updated, *J. Indian Med. Assoc.*, 99(2), 96, 98–99, 2001.
64. Akaike, K. et al., Regional accumulation of 14C-zonisamide in rat brain during kainic acid-induced limbic seizures, *Can. J. Neurol. Sci.*, 28(4), 341–345, 2001.
65. Bechmann, I. et al., Reactive astrocytes upregulate Fas (CD95) and Fas ligand (CD95L) expression but do not undergo programmed cell death during the course of anterograde degeneration, *Glia*, 32(1), 25–41, 2000.
66. Barami, K. et al., Transplantation of human fetal brain cells into ischemic lesions of adult gerbil hippocampus, *J. Neurosurg.*, 95(2), 308–315, 2001.
67. Hauser, R.A. et al., Bilateral human fetal striatal transplantation in Huntington's disease, *Neurology*, 58(5), 687–695, 2002.
68. Janson, C.G. and During, M.J., Viral vectors as part of an integrated functional genomics program, *Genomics*, 78(1-2), 3–6, 2001.
69. Alavi, J.B. and Eck, S.L., Gene therapy for high grade gliomas, *Expert Opin. Biol. Ther.*, 1(2), 239–252, 2001.
70. Berg, A., Ertl, A., and Moser, E., High-resolution polymer gel dosimetry by parameter selective MR-microimaging on a whole body scanner at 3T, *Med. Phys.*, 28(5), 833–843, 2001.
71. Audet, C. et al., CT gel dosimetry technique: comparison of a planned and measured three-dimensional stereotactic dose volume, *J. Appl. Clin. Med. Phys.*, 3(2), 110–118, 2002.
72. Bazioglou, M. and Kalef-Ezra, J., Dosimetry with radiochromic films: a document scanner technique, neutron response, applications, *Appl. Radiat. Isot.*, 55(3), 339–345, 2001.
73. Gildenberg, P.L., History of the American Society for Stereotactic and Functional Neurosurgery, *Stereotact. Funct. Neurosurg.*, 72(2-4), 77–81, 1999.
74. Gillingham, J., Forty-five years of stereotactic surgery for Parkinson's disease: a review, *Stereotact. Funct. Neurosurg.*, 74(3-4), 95–98, 2000.
75. Lee, E.J., Thimmapaya, B., and Jameson, J.L., Stereotactic injection of adenoviral vectors that target gene expression to specific pituitary cell types: implications for gene therapy, *Neurosurgery*, 46(6), 1461–1468; discussion 1468–1469, 2000.

VI

Ambulatory Adaptations

Use of Technology To Bring Care Outside the Hospital

The following chapter is included in this section:

27

Ambulatory Applications for Monitoring Physiological Parameters

Carolyn B. Yucha
University of Florida

Pei-Shan Tsai
Taipei Medical University

Kristine S. Calderon
University of South Carolina

CONTENTS

27.1 Introduction

Over the past two decades, manufacturers of medical equipment have been struggling to keep pace with the demand for reliable, lightweight, and easy-to-operate medical devices for home and ambulatory use. The frequency with which new and improved devices have been coming to market makes it difficult to keep abreast of current technological advances.

A number of factors have led to this rapidly expanding development of biotechnological instruments for ambulatory use. First, throughout the last two decades, complex financial issues and trends have dramatically reshaped the healthcare industry. In the year 2000, healthcare costs rose 6.9% to $1.3 trillion as Americans spent more on prescription drugs and hospital care. Health care costs are expected to continue to grow at a rate of 7.3% annually over the next 10 years.[1] Government regulations forced a change in third-party reimbursement mechanisms from a retrospective to a prospective payment system.[2] The effect on hospitals was profound, creating an urgent need to control costs. To meet this demand for cost containment, providers have had to reduce patient length of stay in the hospital markedly and to rely on outpatient services rather than hospitalization in many situations. For example, insurance companies are no longer willing to pay for patients to be admitted to the hospital so they can be observed for signs of premature labor or cardiac arrhythmias. The movement of health care

0-8493-1140-3/04/$0.00+$1.50

from the hospital to the outpatient setting has required the development of systems to monitor patients' conditions in the community.

Second, the advancement of biotechnology has allowed for the development of instruments that are easily operable with minimal training. In addition, the miniaturization of components has enabled the creation of lightweight instruments that can be easily worn on a patient's body.

Third, health care researchers and providers are realizing that measurements made in the clinic setting may not accurately represent the patient's average pattern or state. For example, blood pressure measurements taken for a patient who is seated in a familiar clinical setting tend to be lower than those gathered during the normal workday.[3]

Finally, many physiological variables display a circadian rhythm. Cardiovascular indices, such as blood pressure, heart rate, and cardiac output, vary over a 24-h period.[4] For example, nocturnal blood pressure may show a decrease of up to 50 mmHg over daytime measurements, and heart rate may differ by up to 25 beats per minute from day to night. In addition, these cardiovascular rhythms interact and together may trigger a cardiovascular catastrophe, such as a myocardial infarction, sudden cardiac arrest, or stroke, with the highest risk occurring during the first 6 h after awakening and arising. Understanding a patient's fluctuations in cardiovascular indices and being aware of any increases in risk due to rhythmic interactions are crucial components for making accurate health assessments and developing a protective plan of care.

Taken together, these factors have promoted the development of monitoring systems for ambulatory use, which are differentiated from systems that are used in the home. Home systems tend to constrain movement by virtue of their size. Thus, they tend to be more useful for measuring parameters that do not change appreciably over the course of a day or do not depend upon what type of activity is being performed. For example, pelvic floor muscle strength can be measured in the home.[5] It would be impractical, however, for an ambulatory measurement system to be developed in this case as there is no utility in measuring pelvic floor muscle strength over a 24-h period. There are also home systems for the measurement of blood glucose and cholesterol and more recently for the performance of coagulation studies, including prothrombin time, activated partial thromboplastin time, and activated clotting time.[6,7] Though some manufacturers do refer to these systems as "ambulatory," they are not capable of monitoring blood levels as the person goes about normal daily activities.

This chapter focuses on systems that allow for the monitoring of physiological variables (e.g., blood pressure, heart rate) while the person is going about his or her normal daily activities. The requirements for an ambulatory system are that the instrument be easily operated by the patient, be small enough to be carried, and be able to store the data for subsequent downloading and on-line data analysis. Such devices fall into two major categories: specialized and integrated. The first group includes devices with highly specialized sensors and algorithms, such as instruments used to measure thoracic impedance. Because of the complex data collection and analysis involved, these instruments tend to be task specific. On the other hand, there are an increasing number of instruments that can be used to collect many different types of physiological data simultaneously. Typically, these instruments collect anywhere from 1 to 16 parameters and store the data with or without mathematical manipulation. For example, one device can measure skin temperature and/or skin conductance as an indication of hot flashes in menopausal women. These instruments can also be used for more novel applications. For example, White et al. used a combined system to determine the characteristic patterns of tremor, sweating, skin temperature, and locomotor activity in persons undergoing alcohol withdrawal.[8]

Many of the devices described in this chapter are used for research purposes and have not been approved by the FDA. Others are commonly used for clinical care and therefore require FDA approval. FDA's Center for Devices and Radiological Health is responsible for ensuring the safety and effectiveness of medical devices. Their Web site (http://www.fda.gov/cdrh/databases.html) provides up-to-date information about the status of the approval process for new systems. The website also contains a listing of medical devices in commercial distribution by both domestic and foreign manufacturers.

Many developers of these instruments adhere voluntarily to industry standards in their manufacture. The Association for the Advancement of Medical Instrumentation (AAMI) is one of the primary sources of such standards, the details of which are provided on the organization's website (http://www.aami.org). Of the AAMI standards, those specified for ambulatory electrocardiographs and for electronic or automated sphygmomanometers, in particular, are relevant to the information covered in this chapter. The AAMI standard for ambulatory electrocardiographs establishes minimum safety and performance requirements for long-term electrocardiographic monitoring devices (ECGs), also commonly called ambulatory electrocardiographs (AECGs). These devices are intended for use in the analysis of rhythm and of relevant morphology of cardiac complexes. The standard covers the parts of the devices that are directly involved in (1) obtaining a signal from the surface of a patient's body; (2) amplifying and transmitting the signal to recording and display devices; (3) recording and displaying the signal; and (4) providing summaries of rhythms, conduction disturbances, and displacements of the ST segment. The AAMI standard for electronic or automated sphygmomanometers establishes safety and performance requirements for electronic and electromechanical measurement devices that are used with an occluding cuff for the indirect determination of blood pressure. Included within the scope of this standard are devices that sense or display pulsations, flow, or sounds in connection with the electronic measurement, display, or recording of blood pressure. These devices might or might not have an automatic cuff-inflation system.

This chapter is organized into two parts: The first section takes a body systems approach, describing the parameters that can be monitored using ambulatory instruments for each system and providing examples of relevant specialized instruments. The second section focuses on integrated instruments. Though current manufacturers and contact information are provided for the instruments mentioned, this chapter is intended to be used primarily as a general guide to the kinds of ambulatory applications that are available. Because the technological marketplace is a rapidly changing environment, readers are advised to confirm specific manufacturer information when necessary. No prices are provided here as these vary widely with rapidly changing technology and depend on the components needed for specific applications.

27.2 Systems Approach to Ambulatory Applications

This section is organized according to body systems. It describes the parameters that can be monitored using ambulatory instruments for each system and provides examples of relevant specialized instruments.

27.2.1 Cardiovscular System

27.2.1.1 Ambulatory Electrocardiography (AECG) Monitor

27.2.1.1.1 Purpose

An ambulatory electrocardiography (AECG) monitor, also known as a Holter monitor, is a device used for continuous monitoring of the electrical activity of a patient's heart muscle for 24 h or longer. The purpose of Holter monitoring is to detect abnormal electrical activity in the heart that may occur randomly or only under certain circumstances, such as during sleep or periods of physical activity or stress. This information, in turn, may help to identify a previously undetected heart condition, such as cardiac arrhythmia, or ischemia.

27.2.1.1.2 Description

Electrodes are affixed to the surface of the skin at specific points of the patient's chest, using adhesive patches with gel that conducts electrical impulses. The electrodes are connected to the AECG recorder, which is typically worn over the patient's shoulder or attached to a belt around the patient's waist. Current AECG equipment is capable of detecting and analyzing arrhythmias and ST-segment deviation. Some systems also provide more sophisticated analyses of R-R intervals, QRS-T morphology including late potentials, Q-T dispersion, and T-wave alternans.

There are two categories of AECG recorders, continuous recorders and intermittent recorders. Continuous recorders are typically used for investigating symptoms or ECG events during a 24- to 48-h period. The intermittent recorders may be used for weeks to months to provide intermittent recordings of events that occur infrequently. Two types of intermittent recorders are available. A loop recorder is worn continuously, but stores only a brief period of ECG recording when the patient activates the event marker at the time of experiencing a symptom. Another type of intermittent device is the event recorder, which is attached by the patient and activated after the onset of symptoms.

Most recorders utilize five or seven electrodes attached to the chest, which record the signals from two or three bipolar leads onto two or three channels. The most common bipolar lead configuration is comprised of a chest modified V5 (CM_5), a chest modified V3 (CM_3), and a modified inferior lead. Routine identification of ischemic ST-segment deviation requires only two leads. An additional inverse Nehb J lead, in which the positive electrode is placed on the left posterior axillary line, may enhance the ability to detect ischemia. Some systems can record a true 12-lead ECG, whereas others derive a 12-lead ECG from 3-lead data through the use of an algorithm.

Most playback systems use generic computer hardware platforms running proprietary software protocols for data analysis and report generation. Some systems allow for facsimile, modem, network, and internet integration. The computer algorithm is usually capable of identifying ischemia. Accurate diagnosis of arrhythmia morphology and ischemic episodes, however, requires the analysis of an experienced technician or physician.

27.2.1.1.3 Applications

Patients with symptoms related to cardiac arrhythmias (e.g., syncope, palpitation) may benefit from an AECG evaluation. AECG is also useful for assessing anti-arrhythmic drug response and pacemaker and implanted cardioverter/defibrillator function.

27.2.1.1.4 Models

A variety of models with different features (format for recording, storage capacity, playback systems, etc.) manufactured by different companies are available; see Table 27.1.

27.2.1.2 Ambulatory Impedance Cardiogram (AICG) Monitoring

27.2.1.2.1 Purpose

Impedance cardiogram (ICG) provides assessment of a number of indices of cardiac function, including heart rate (HR), stroke volume (SV), pre-ejection period (PEP; an indicator of myocardial contractility), left ventricular ejection time (LVET), and the Heather index (HI; an index of myocardial contractility). Cardiac output (CO) is derived from the HR and SV measurements using the formula $CO = HR * SV$. ICG may also be used in conjunction with a blood pressure monitor to assess total peripheral resistance (TPR) using the formula $TPR = CO \div MAP$, where MAP is mean arterial pressure. Unlike conventional hemodynamic monitoring, which requires the insertion by a physician of a pulmonary artery catheter, ICG monitoring is a safe, noninvasive, and unobtrusive technique.

Ambulatory ICG enables the measurement of cardiac and hemodynamic indices for up to 24 h or more as persons go about their normal daily routines.

27.2.1.2.2 Description

ICG measures the total impedance, or resistance to the flow of electricity, in the thorax. Impedance is represented by the symbol Z and is measured in ohms. Average thoracic impedance, or Zo, is the base impedance and reflects the total fluid status of the thorax. Alternating current is passed along the thorax and recordings are made of impedance changes that occur in synchrony with ejection of blood into the aorta. These data are then used to determine HR, PEP, and LEVT and, in conjunction with an algorithm, to estimate SV.

Typically, an ambulatory ICG device consists of a small plastic container that holds the impedance cardiograph, a small microprocessor, and a battery. Current and recording electrodes connected to the ICG device are attached to the surface of the neck and chest. The current electrodes deliver alternating current generated by the ICG device and the recording electrodes record the average thoracic impedance and the rate of change in impedance during each ventricular ejection.

TABLE 27.1 Ambulatory Electrocardiography (AECG) Monitors

Manufacturer	Model
Del Mar Medical Systems, LLC 1621 Alton Parkway Irvine, CA 92606-4878 Phone: (800) 854-0481 www.delmarmedical.com	Impresario Holter system DartScan Holter analysis system (Model DS-90/DSDI) AccuPlus Holter analysis system (Model 363) Stratascan Holter analysis system (Model 563) Recorders: OmniCorder, DigiCorder, FlashCorder, PacerCorder, Sentinel II, & Aria
TransMedEx, LLC 150 Broadhollow Road, 2nd floor Melville, NY 11747 www.transmedex.com	Digitrak Plus HolterNet Internet Communications (Centralized Holter analysis)
Welch Allyn Phone: (800) 535-6663 www.welchallyn.com/medical/support/contact/	MT-200 Holter System (Model 01420-300) MT-200 Conversion Kit (Model 01420-200) MT-100 (Model 08238-0000)
Scan Tech Medical, LLC 212 Dove Ridge Rd. Columbia, SC 29223 Phone: (877) 722-6800 or (803) 699-1303 www.scantecchmedical.com	Star2000 VX3 Holter System Star2000 Holter System
Forest Medical, LLC 6700 Old Collamer Road Syracuse, NY 13057-1118 Phone: (800) 844-2037 or (315) 434-9000 Fax: (315) 432-8064 www.forestmedical.com	Trillium 3000 Holter System
Reynolds Medical, Inc. 220 Wood Road Braintree, MA 02184 Phone: (877) NEW-HOLTER or (919) 861-0021 Fax: (919) 783-9942 www.reynoldsmedical.com	Pathfinder Holter System Recorders: Tracker, Sherpa, & LifecardCF
Midmark Corporation 60 Vista Drive P.O. Box 286 Versailles, OH 45380–9310 www.midmark.com	IQMark 7700 Holter System IQMark 8800 Holter System

27.2.1.2.3 Applications

Ambulatory ICG is commonly used in psychophysiological research to examine cardiovascular responses to a wide range of stressors in real-life situations or to semistructured naturalistic stressors (public speaking, exams). The ambulatory ICG can also be used for assessing cardiac performance in ambulatory patients for clinical diagnosis or treatment evaluation.

27.2.1.2.4 Models

Currently there are two ambulatory ICG devices available on the market, VU-AMS and AIM. The VU-AMS is considered a valid device for the measurement of PEP, LVET, and inter-beat interval.[9] Correlations between the response of the ambulatory and the standard laboratory devices are high except for SV and CO during exercise, which the VU-AMS tends to overestimate. The AIM yields measures of HR, PEP, LVET, and SV that are comparable to those obtained by using the reference Minnesota 304B system.[10] All between-instrument correlations are greater than 0.87. (See Table 27.2 for a list of ambulatory impedance cardiogram monitors.)

TABLE 27.2 Ambulatory Impedance Cardiogram (Aicg) Monitors

Manufacturer	Model
Vrije Universiteit, Division for Instrumentation of the Department of Psychophysiology de Boechorstsaat 1, Room K1E-29 1081 BT Amsterdam, The Netherlands Phone: +31(20) 444-8822 Fax: +31(20) 444-8832 www.psy.vu.nl/vu-ams	VU-AMS
Bio-Impedance Technology, Inc. 88 VilCom Campus, Suite 165 Chapel Hill, NC Fax: (919) 960-6864 www.microtronics-bit.com	AIM-8

27.2.1.3 Continuous Radionuclide Ventricular Function Monitoring

27.2.1.3.1 Purpose

A continuous radionuclide ventricular function monitor allows for ambulatory monitoring of left ventricular function using a portable nuclear detector (probe).

27.2.1.3.2 Description

The first available ambulatory detector system, called Vest, was equipped with a cadmium telluride detector. The present version uses a sodium iodide (NaI) probe that has been validated in several clinical studies. The Vest system records radionuclide emissions from the left ventricle and transfers the data to a computer. The newest version, the Generation II Vest, is comprised of a NaI crystal detector mounted on a vest garment. It provides synchronized electrocardiography and ambulatory ejection fraction measurements.

27.2.1.3.3 Applications

This device is used for diagnosis and treatment evaluation in patients with coronary artery disease. It can be used to assess cardiac function during exercise and to assess left ventricular functional reserve in patients with hypertrophic cardiomyography.

27.2.1.3.4 Model

The Generation II Vest is the only model currently available (Table 27.3).

27.2.1.4 Ambulatory Blood Pressure Monitoring

27.2.1.4.1 Purpose

Conventional clinic blood pressure (BP) measurements are often poor representations of an individual's average or true BP. BP changes throughout the day and is influenced by various stimuli. It is altered by activity, posture, location (e.g., home, work), food and fluid intake, psychological state, and concomitant medication. Ambulatory blood pressure monitors (ABPMs) can be programmed

TABLE 27.3 Continuous Radionuclide Ventricular Function Monitor

Manufacturer	Model
Capintec, Inc. 6 Arrow Road Ransey, NJ 07446 Phone: (800) 631-3826 or (201) 825-9500 Fax: (201) 825-4829 E-mail: Getinfo@capintec.com	Generation II Vest

to take readings every 15 to 30 min throughout the day and night while patients go about their normal daily activities.

27.2.1.4.2 Description

A variety of reliable, convenient, easy to use, and accurate monitors are commercially available. The typical, fully automatic device for ABPM is battery driven and consists of an arm cuff that can be programmed to inflate automatically throughout a 24- to 48-h period. Readings are stored in a controller/recorder carried on a shoulder strap or belt for subsequent downloading to a personal computer for analysis.

ABPM devices use either auscultatory or oscillometric methods to determine BP. In the auscultatory method, Korotkoff sounds are detected by one or two piezoelectric microphones positioned under the cuff. In the oscillometric method, oscillations are transmitted from the brachial artery to the cuff. The oscillometric instruments detect SBP and mean arterial pressure (MAP) and use an algorithm to calculate DBP. A small air compressor or gas cylinder contained in the controller/recorder inflates the arm cuff. These devices are about the size of a Walkman, weigh a pound or less, and operate quietly.

Typically, the patient keeps a detailed diary with information about physical and mental activity, meals, sleep, medication, and other life events throughout the measurement period to assist in interpretation of the BP data. The validity of the BP data is first analyzed by computer then reviewed by the health care professional, who takes the patient's activity diary into consideration.

27.2.1.4.3 Applications

The Joint National Committee on Prevention, Detection, Evaluation, and Treatment of High Blood Pressure[3] recommends that ABPM be used in patients with suspected "white coat hypertension," those with apparent drug resistance, those exhibiting hypotensive symptoms while taking antihypertensive medications, those with episodic hypertension, and those with autonomic dysfunction.

27.2.1.4.4 Models

A variety of models with different features manufactured by different companies are available. A representative sample is shown in Table 27.4.

27.2.1.5 Heart Rate Monitoring

27.2.1.5.1 Purpose

Heart rate monitoring is an important component of cardiovascular fitness assessment, training programs, and research. Some ambulatory heart rate monitors measure the electrical activity of the heart, which reflects the number of heart contractions per minute. Other monitors on the market rely on plethysmography (photoreflectance), which uses light reflectance to measure the mechanical pulse of blood flow through the capillaries, and then converts those data into a beat-per-minute readout.

27.2.1.5.2 Description

For ambulatory electrical heart rate monitoring, a sealed transmitter containing electrodes is fastened to the chest with an elastic belt. The transmitter detects the voltage differential on the skin during every heartbeat and sends a continuous signal to a wrist receiver via wireless transmission using an electromagnetic field. Most manufacturers use molded construction to make the circuitry of the wrist receivers, making them waterproof and comfortable to wear. For ambulatory plethysmography, or photoreflectance monitoring, a sensor is usually attached to the finger with an elastic band or to the earlobe with a clip. The receiver stores the pulse blood flow, and the data can then be downloaded into a data acquisition system.

27.2.1.5.3 Applications

Ambulatory heart rate monitoring may be used as part of a program to improve cardiovascular fitness, to identify a physiological marker to stress reactivity, and to monitor changes in heart rate related to any cardiovascular disease or condition.

TABLE 27.4 Ambulatory Blood Pressure Monitors

Manufacturer	Model
Welch Allyn Medical Products 4341 State Street Road P.O. Box 220 Skaneateles Falls, NY 13153-0220 Phone: (800) 535-6663 or (315) 685-4100 Fax: (315) 685-3361 www.welchallyn.com	Quiet Trak™ ABPM Model 5100-11
Spacelabs Medical, Inc. 15220 N.E. 40th Street P.O. Box 97013 Redmond, WA 98073-9713 Phone: (425) 882-3700 Fax: (425) 885-4877 www.spacelabs.com	SL-90202 Ultralite SL-90207 Spacelabs' Model 90121-1 Report Management System
A&D Instruments Ltd. Corporate Headquarters 3-23-14 Higashi-Ikebukuro Toshima-ku Tokyo 170-0013, Japan Phone: +81 (3) 5391-6123 Fax: +81 (3) 5391-6128 www.aandd.co.jp	TM-2421/2021 TM-2430
Koven Technology, Inc. 12125 Woodcrest Executive Drive, Suite 220 St. Louis, MO 63141 Phone: (314) 542-2102/(800) 521-8342 Fax: (314) 542-6020 www.koven.com	Nissei DS-250

27.2.1.5.4 Models

A number of devices are available to measure heart rate alone; see Table 27.5. Heart rate may also be measured concurrently with other physiological measures. These integrated systems are described in Section 27.3.

27.2.1.6 Ambulatory Skin Temperature Monitoring

27.2.1.6.1 Purpose

The purpose of skin temperature monitoring is to measure the amount of peripheral blood flow or the relaxation of the arteriolar smooth muscle. Temperatures above 90°F, or 32°C, indicate good peripheral blood flow, presumably due to relaxation of the arteriolar smooth muscle.

27.2.1.6.2 Description

Skin temperature monitoring is usually done via a resistor sensor, known as a thermistor, which is attached to the skin, normally with breathable tape. Changes in skin temperature alter the electrical resistance of the thermistor, resulting in a voltage differential that is recorded and stored for later downloading. Thermistors are usually affixed on the pads of the fingers or on the arm, chest, thigh, and calf. Mean peripheral temperature can be calculated using various sites of placement.

27.2.1.6.3 Applications

Skin temperature monitoring can be used for training people to promote vasodilation or peripheral blood flow. Patients with high blood pressure, migraine headaches, or Raynaud's disease may benefit from temperature training. It can also be used to assess vascular responses to stress.

TABLE 27.5 Ambulatory Heart Rate Monitors

Manufacturer	Model
Polar Electro Inc. 370 Crossways Park Drive Woodbury, NY 11797 Phone: (516) 364-0400 or (800) 227-1314 Fax: (516) 364-5454 www.polarusa.com E-mail: customer.service.usa@polar.fi	Beginner: Beat A-1, Tempo, A-3 Intermediate: Pacer NV, M21, M52, M71ti, A-5 Advanced: S-210, S-410, S-510, S610, ProtrainerXT Competitive: S-210, S-410, S-510, S-610, S-710, S-810
Reebok International Ltd. 1895 J. W. Foster Boulevard Canton, MA 02021 Phone: (866) 725-9666 www.reebokdirect.com	Beginner: Active Trainer Intermediate: Active Trainer Advanced: Fitness Trainer Competitive: Fitness and Precision Trainer
Cardiosport U.K. www.cardiosport.com/uk/index.asp	Beginner: Go Intermediate: Limit Plus, Auto Zone Advanced: Nash Bar, Advanced Competitive: Excel Sport PC, Excel Sport PC and PC Interface
Sensor Dynamics, Inc. 4568 Enterprise Street Fremont, CA 94538 Phone: (510) 623-1459 www.sensordynamics.com E-mail: lseng@sensordynamics.com	All models are entry level: Sensor Dynamics Cardio Pacer, Sensor Dynamics Gemini, Sensor Dynamics Cardio Champ, Sensor Dynamics Phoenix, Sensor Dynamics ProSport II, Sensor Dynamic Hawk
Freestyle 5855 Olivas Park Drive Ventura, CA 93003 www.freestyleusa.com E-mail: product@freestyleusa.com	Beginner: ECG1 – ECG2 Intermediate: ECG2 – ECG3 Advanced: ECG3 – ECG4 Competitive: ECG5
FitSense Technology 21 Boston Road P.O. Box 730 Southborough, MA 01772 Phone: (508) 303-8811 Fax: (508) 357-7990 www.fitsense.com E-mail: info@fitsense.com	All levels: FS-1 Pro
LifeSource by A&D Medical 1555 McCandless Drive Milpitas, CA 95035 Phone: (408) 263-5333 Fax: (408) 263-0119 www.lifesourceonline.com E-mail: support@lifesourceonline.com	Beginner: LifeSource XC100 Intermediate: LifeSource XC200 All Levels: LifeSource XC300
Acumen Inc. 101A Executive Drive, Suite 200 Sterling, VA 20166 USA Phone: (800) 852-7823 Fax: (703) 904-0218 www.acumeninc.com E-mail: acumen@acumeninc.com	Beginner: Basix, Basix ES Intermediate: Excel, Excel ES All Levels: Basix Plus, Basix Plus ES, TZ-Max 50, TX-Max 100, Eon 101, Eon 102, Eon 201, Eon 202

TABLE 27.6 Skin Temperature Monitors

Manufacturer	Model
Ambulatory Monitoring, Inc 731 Saw Mill River Road Ardsley, NY 10502-0609 Phone: (800) 341-0066 Fax: (914) 693-6604 E-mail: info@ambulatory-monitoring.com www.ambulatory-monitoring.com	The Puck – Temperature Telemetry Skin model

27.2.1.6.4 Models

A number of devices are available to measure skin temperature alone; see Table 27.6. Skin temperature may also be measured concurrently with other physiological measures. These integrated systems are described in Section 27.3.

27.2.2 Cerebral/Nervous

27.2.2.1 Ambulatory Electroencephalography (AEEG) Monitoring

27.2.2.1.1 Purpose

Ambulatory electroencephalography (AEEG) monitoring allows for the recording of brain wave activity outside the EEG laboratory.

27.2.2.1.2 Description

Ambulatory recording of EEG requires a multichannel portable recorder and a signal amplifier. Typically, the AEEG unit is battery operated and equipped with a microprocessor for data storage. Recorded signals may be stored and downloaded for later reviewing and computer-aided analysis or may be viewed directly in real-time. EEG electrodes are affixed to the patient's scalp. The electrodes are connected to the recording unit. The recording unit is usually carried in a backpack that can be worn by the patient. During ambulatory recording, the electrode gel may need to be reapplied beneath the electrodes by the patient or caregiver.

27.2.2.1.3 Applications

AEEG is used in clinical practice to (1) confirm a clinical diagnosis of epilepsy, (2) identify interictal epileptiform activity, (3) document seizures of which the patient is unaware, (4) evaluate response to therapy, (5) evaluate suspected pseudoseizures, and (6) evaluate syncope. It can also be used to evaluate nocturnal or sleep-related events.

27.2.2.1.4 Models

A number of ambulatory EEG monitors are available (Table 27.7).

27.2.2.2 Ambulatory Skin Conductance Monitoring

27.2.2.2.1 Purpose

Changes in the skin's ability to conduct electricity are known as electrodermal activity (EDA). Skin conductance monitoring is one method of measuring EDA and involves measuring the ability of the skin to conduct electricity. Skin conductance monitoring detects the ability of the skin to conduct current, which changes in accordance with sweating.

27.2.2.2.2 Description

EDA results from activation of eccrine sweat glands, which are controlled by the sympathetic division of the autonomic nervous system. To measure EDA, a small electrical current is passed through the skin. Skin conductance activity (SCA), or the ability to conduct the current, and skin resistance activity (SRA), or the ability to resist the flow of current, can then be measured. Skin conductance activity is composed

TABLE 27.7 Ambulatory Electroencephalography (AEEG) Monitors

Manufacturer	Model
Grass Telefactor Astro-Med Industrial Park 600 East Greenwich Avenue West Warwick, RI 02893 Phone: (877) 472-7779 or (401) 828-4000 Fax: (401) 822-2430 www.grass-telefactor.com	H2O Recorder
Lifelines Ltd. 7 Clarendon Court Over Wallop, N. Stockbridge Hants, S020 8HU, U.K. Phone: +44 1264 78226 Fax: +44 1264 782088 www.llines.com	Trackit Ambulatory Recorder
Otivus AB Box 513 Enhagsslingan 5 SE-183 25 Täby, Sweden Phone: +46 84646 4500 Fax: +46 8446 4519 www.ortivus.com	Biosaca Ambulatory Recorder
Cadwell Laboratories, Inc. 909 Kellogg Street Kennewick, WA 99336 Phone: (800) 245-3001 or (509) 735-6481 Fax: (509) 783-6503 www.cadwell.com	Easy II EEG System
XLTEK 2568 Bristol Circle Oakville, Ontario Canada L6H 5S1 Phone: (800) 387-7516 or (905) 829-5300 Fax: (905) 829-5304 www.xltek.com	XL TEK Mobee XLTEK Epilepsy/EEG
Flaga hf. Vesturhlid 7 105 Reykjavik, Iceland Phone: +354 510-2000 Fax: +354 510-2010 www.flaga.is	Embla

of skin conductance level (SCL) and skin conductance response (SCR). SCL is the baseline or tonic measure; SCR is the phasic response to stressful situations or events. In skin conductance monitoring two electrodes are placed in close proximity to one another, usually on the chest or on two fingers. A small current is passed from one electrode to the other, allowing for the measurement of skin conductivity. Data are collected and stored for later downloading.

27.2.2.2.3 Applications

Skin conductance is used to monitor stress arousal and hot flashes (as during menopause).

27.2.2.2.4 Models

A number of devices are available to measure skin conductance, usually concurrently with other physiological variables. These are described in Section 27.3.

27.2.2.3 Ambulatory Activity Monitoring

27.2.2.3.1 Purpose

An activity recorder is a small device that measures movement. The monitor can be worn around the wrist (wristwatch style), around the ankle, or on the waist with a belt-clip. Some units can be inserted into a jacket or pouch for animal research.

27.2.2.3.2 Description

Typically the activity monitor contains an accelerometer, which measures acceleration. Acceleration measurements are converted into units of movement intensity and frequency. All activity monitors contain a microprocessor and on-board memory so that the data can be downloaded to either a microcomputer or a PC for off-line processing and display. Some units combine the measurement of activity with simultaneous recording of light exposure (i.e., ambient illumination) and also include other analog measuring devices such as thermistors (see skin temperature monitoring), providing multidimensional ambulatory monitoring. The combination of activity monitor and illumination detector provides information on the rest and activity cycles.

27.2.2.3.3 Applications

The ambulatory activity monitor has applications in many fields of science and medicine for assessment of pathological states with movement-related components, including sleep quality and patterns, geriatric inactivity, hyperactivity (e.g., ADHD), neurological conditions, and cancer-related fatigue or chronic fatigue syndrome. It is useful in monitoring and assessing effects of drugs on the central nervous system. It can also be used in biological and behavioral studies related to activity and chronobiology.

27.2.2.3.4 Models

A variety of models with different features (memory, size, recording models, displays, etc.) are available (Table 27.8).

27.2.3 Orthopedic System

27.2.3.1 Continuous Step Activity Monitoring

27.2.3.1.1 Purpose

An ambulatory step activity monitor continuously records the amount and intensity of an individual's activity within short time intervals over a long period of time. It detects and counts steps for a wide variety of gait styles.

27.2.3.1.2 Description

Typically the device is a small, battery-operated step counter that attaches to a person's ankle with a strap. It contains an accelerometer and an electronic filter to reject extraneous signals.

27.2.3.1.3 Applications

This device is useful in many areas of research and clinical practice where objective data describing an individual's ambulatory function are needed. It can be used in persons with and without gait abnormalities. It is particularly useful for step counting in mobility-impaired subjects (e.g., amputee with prosthetics or neuropathic diabetic).

27.2.3.1.4 Models (Table 27.9)

One device to measure step activity is shown in Table 27.9.

TABLE 27.8 Ambulatory Activity Monitors

Manufacturer	Model
Ambulatory Monitoring, Inc. 731 Saw Mill River Road Ardsley, NY 10502-0609 Phone: (800) 341-0066 Fax: (914) 693-6604 www.ambulatory-monitoring.com	Mini-Motionlogger Micro Mini-Motionlogger Basic Mini-Motionlogger Tri-Mode Basic Mini-Motionlogger Ultra Mini-Motionlogger Actillumes multi-channel data collection Sleep Watch-L and -S Octagonal Basic Sleep Watch Octagonal Sleep Watch and -L Octagonal Sleep Watch version 2.00 Octagonal Ballistogran Sleep Watch
Gaehwiler Electronics, Hombrechtikon, Switzerland (No contact information available)	Actigraph
Innovations in Ambulatory Recording 1055 Taylor Avenue, Suite 300 Baltimore, MD Phone: (410) 296-7723 Fax: (410) 321-0643 www.biotrainer.com	ActiTrac DigiTrac
Stayhealthy, Inc. 222 East Huntington Drive Suite 213 Monrovia, CA 91016 Phone: (800) 321-1218 ext. 28 www.stayhealthy.com	RT3 Triaxial Research Tracker
Mini Mitter Co., Inc. 20300 Empire Avenue, Bldg. B-3 Bend, OR 97701 Phone: (800) 685-2999 or (514) 322-7272 Fax: (541) 322-7277 www.camntech.co.uk	Actiwatch and Actiwatch Plus Actiwatch-L Actiwatch-L Plus Actiwatch-T and Actiwatch-TS Actiwatch-Alert Actiwatch-Score Actiwatch-Neurologica

TABLE 27.9 Continuous Step Activity Monitors

Manufacturer	Model
Prosthetics Research Study 675 South Lane St., Suite 100 Seattle, WA 98104-2942 Phone: (206) 903-8136 Fax: (206) 903-8141 www.pre-research.org	StepWatch Gait Activity Monitor

27.2.4 Muscular System

27.2.4.1 Ambulatory Electromyography (EMG)

27.2.4.1.1 Purpose

When the body performs any activity, the muscles produce an electrical current that is proportional to the level of that activity. Electromyography (EMG) monitoring measures microvolts of electrical current within a muscle or muscle group. The greater the microvolt value, the greater is the electrical current or activity within the given muscle or muscle group.

27.2.4.1.2 Description

There are two basic methods of EMG measurements: intramuscular EMG and surface EMG. The former involves placement of a needle into the relevant muscle and is regularly used in the diagnosis of neuromuscular disorders. The latter involves detection of electrical activity within a muscle by placing electrodes onto the skin directly above the muscle (or muscle group) concerned. This noninvasive technique is therefore a relatively quick and simple method for taking a measurement. Surface EMG is the method used with ambulatory devices. EMG ambulatory monitors include a data collection unit (generally the size of a deck of cards) and sensors. The sensors are applied to the skin using adhesive patches and information is transmitted from the sensors to the data collection unit.

27.2.4.1.3 Applications

EMG has potential applications in all fields of human activity. It was first used as a clinical tool in the field of neurophysiology to study motor unit responses. More recently, physical medicine and rehabilitation as well as industrial medicine and sports research have been the primary fields to make use of EMG.

Ambulatory EMG monitoring allows the collection of objective data to use for diagnosis or research in place of largely subjective descriptions of musculoskeletal aches or injuries. More specifically, EMG monitoring can be used to measure (in order to minimize) the level and nature of force(s) exerted during any work activity; to diagnose the level of musculoskeletal strains or injuries and then to monitor progress during rehabilitation; to measure the level of force, strength or fatigue during a sporting movement or activity; to measure the level of force or stress during any activity for selection and/or investigation purposes; and to measure the level of muscular strain experience by a patient in order to determine the best possible remedy.

27.2.4.1.4 Models (Table 27.10)

A variety of EMG monitors are listed in Table 27.10. Muscle activity may also be measured concurrently with other physiological measures. These integrated systems are described in Section 27.3.

27.2.5 Respiratory System

27.2.5.1 Ambulatory Respiratory Rate Monitoring

27.2.5.1.1 Purpose

Respiration rates are usually expressed as breaths per minute and measured using a respiratory belt (described below). In addition to the respiratory belt, respiration instruments usually include a plethysmography device, which measures the heart rate pattern or respiratory effort tracing (described below).

27.2.5.1.2 Description

A respiratory belt containing a strain gauge (stretch sensor) is positioned around the sternum (to detect thoracic movement) or around the lower ribcage (to detect diaphragmatic movement). With each inspiration, the belt is stretched; with each expiration, the belt relaxes. Plethysmographs (as described previously in the section on heart rate monitoring) usually come in the form of small sensors attached to a finger to collect heart rate pattern or respiratory effort tracing. Data from both devices are collected and stored within a small data collection box for later downloading.

27.2.5.1.3 Applications

Respiration rates may be monitored for the purpose of treating respiration-related disorders and retraining for relaxation breathing. For instance, respiratory rates range from 12 to 14 breaths per minute in

TABLE 27.10 Ambulatory Electromyography (EMG)

Manufacturer	Model
Mega Electronics Ltd. Savilahdentie 6 P.O. Box 1750 70211 Kuopio Finland Phone: +358 (0)17 581-7700 Fax: +358 (0)17 580-0978 E-mail: info@meltd.fi www.meltd.fi	ME3000P2 — 2 channels EMG system (raw/averaged EMG), 1 MB memory ME3000P4 — 4 channels EMG system (raw/averaged EMG), 1–8 MB memory ME3000P8 — 8 channels EMG system (raw/averaged EMG), 1–32 MB memory
Thought Technology, Inc. 2180 Belgrave Avenue Montreal, Quebec Canada 4A 2L8 Phone: (800) 361-3651 or (514) 489-8251 Fax: (514) 489-8255 www.thoughttechnology.com	MyoTrac MyoTrac 2 MyoTrac 3 (pelvic floor) MyoTrac 3G (pelvic floor advanced) ProComp/Biograph — 8 channels
Chattanooga Group A division of Encore Medical Corporation 4717 Adams Road Hixson, TN 37343 Phone: (800) 592-7329 www.chattgroup.com/	EMG Retrainer — 2 channels EMG Retrainer IR

healthy adults under resting conditions. Patients with anxiety disorders or asthma, for example, may have rates as high as 15 to 18 breaths per minute. In addition, respiratory rates can increase significantly during stress and physical exercise in healthy patients or subjects. These increases may be accompanied by an increase or decrease in depth of respiration. Therefore, respiration can be retrained based on monitored breathing rates. During deep relaxation, breathing rates can be slowed to as low as four breaths per minute.

27.2.5.1.4 Models

Anderson and Frank developed a portable device containing a microprocessor that analyzes the output of Respitrace bands via the internet while the subject is wearing the monitor, to retrieve respiratory rate and depth (in units of conductance change) for each breath.[11] They developed this instrument for research purposes, and it is still undergoing reliability testing. A number of devices available to measure respiratory rate are listed in Table 27.11. Respiration may also be measured concurrently with other physiological measures. These integrated systems are described in Section 27.3.

27.2.5.2 Ambulatory Cough Frequency Monitoring

27.2.5.2.1 Purpose

Cough frequency has been measured by recording coughing events with a microphone placed in close contact with a patient's chest or throat. Number and intensity of sounds are used to quantify coughing severity and frequency.

27.2.5.2.2 Description

A portable device developed by Hsu et al.[12] simultaneously records cough sounds and electromyograms of the lower respiratory muscles, including the diaphragm, in order to measure coughing events occurring over a 24-h period. This device uses a 6-vV, battery-operated, solid-state, multiple-channel custom digital logger fitted with a 2-Mb random access memory (Brompton cough recording system, London, U.K.). A unidirectional microphone (Knowles type BL1670, Knowles Electronics Co., W. Sussex, U.K.) attached to the chest wall with double-sided adhesive rings to face the skin transmits the audio signal. Surface

TABLE 27.11 Ambulatory Respiratory Rate Monitors

Manufacturer	Model
Flaga Vesturhlid 7 105 Reykjavik Iceland Phone: (354) 510-2000 Fax: (354) 510-2010 www.flaga.is E-mail: sales@flaga.is	Embletta PDS XactTrace: Respiratory Inductive Plethysmograph (RIP) and sensor
Non-Invasive Monitoring Systems, Inc. 1840 West Avenue Miami Beach, FL 33139 Phone: (305) 534-3694 Fax: (305) 534-9368 E-mail: nims@respitrace.com	*Respitrace 200* *Respitrace 204* — 2 channels of advanced inductive plethysmography and 4 channels of isolated analog to digital conversion *Respitrace 408* — 4 channels of inductive plethysmography and 8 analog inputs

electrodes are used to transmit the electromyogram (EMG) signals (see the EMG section above, for information about ambulatory EMG devices).

27.2.5.2.3 Applications

This type of monitoring can be used to examine cough frequency and diurnal variation for patients who experience chronic cough, asthma patients, and patients who have a predominant symptom of chronic cough with no determined presentation.

27.2.5.2.4 Models

Researchers from Brompton Hospital in London, U.K., developed the Brompton cough recording system for research purposes. To our knowledge, there are no commercially available cough monitors. More advanced unidirectional microphones are available from Emkay Innovative Products, a division of Knowles Electronics Co. for use in development of new recording systems.

Emkay Innovative Products
1151 Maplewood Drive
Itasca, IL 60143
Phone: (630) 250-5930
Fax: (630) 250-5932
E-mail: emkayinfo@emkayproducts.com

27.2.5.3 Ambulatory Hemoglobin Oxygen Saturation Monitoring

27.2.5.3.1 Purpose

The purpose of these monitors is to measure hemoglobin oxygen saturation (SpO_2) noninvasively.

27.2.5.3.2 Description

Pulse oximetry is the measurement of hemoglobin oxygen saturation in the peripheral circulatory system. A sensor is attached to an extremity or an earlobe using adhesive or a clip apparatus. The sensor consists of an emitter that sends red and infrared light through the site to the recessed photodetector. The recessing of the photodetector protects against ambient light and provides "shock absorption" for stabilization during motion. The photodetector measures the differential optical density of the red and infrared light as it is projected through the vascular bed and calculates a ratio of the optical densities. Using the optical density ratios, the device calculates and stores the arterial oxygen saturation (SpO_2) values. While widely used in critical care units, conventional oximetry has been less reliable with conscious, moving patients (e.g., shivering, waving). Measurement of oxygen saturation is particularly challenging due to the effect of movement on local venous blood flow. Recently, signal extraction technology has been coupled with four unique algorithms to deal with movement artifact in pulse oximetry (Masimo SET® Pulse Oximetry). This advance has allowed for the development of ambulatory hemoglobin oxygen saturation monitoring.

27.2.5.3.3 Applications

This type of monitoring is used to evaluate the adequacy of oxygenation and/or the effectiveness of long-term oxygen supplementation in patients with hypoxemia (low oxygen in the blood).

27.2.5.3.4 Models

An ambulatory system called Micropaq™ is made by Welch Allyn Monitoring. In addition to SpO_2, this system also monitors heart rate and ECG. More information about this system can be found in Section 27.3.

27.2.5.4 Ambulatory Pollutant Gases Exposure Monitoring

27.2.5.4.1 Purpose

Pollutant gas monitoring is usually done by measuring levels of carbon monoxide and nitrogen dioxide in the environment surrounding the wearer.

27.2.5.4.2 Description

The levels of carbon monoxide and nitrogen dioxide in the air surrounding the wearer can be monitored using electrochemical gas sensors (City Technology Ltd). These sensors can be calibrated with concentrations of bottled "calibration" gas.

27.2.5.4.3 Applications

This type of monitoring is primarily used to gain insight into the wearer's environment and therefore to help identify sources of pollution.

27.2.5.4.4 Model

An ambulatory system for measuring exposure to pollutant gases was developed by Petley et al.[13] This system also monitors bladder pressure, core body temperature, and skin temperature and is described in Section 27.3.

27.2.6 Reproductive System

27.2.6.1 Ambulatory Uterine Contraction Monitoring

27.2.6.1.1 Purpose

The purpose of home uterine activity monitors (HUAMs) is to detect uterine activity (contractions).

27.2.6.1.2 Description

Monitoring of uterine activity requires a pressure sensor (tacodynamometer), which is held against the abdomen by a belt, and a recording/storage device that is carried by a belt or hung from the shoulder. In clinical practice, the patient typically records uterine activity for q h, twice daily, while performing routine activities. The stored data are then transmitted via telephone to a practitioner's office, where a receiving device prints out the data. The recording of uterine activity by external sensors is comparable to the recording of this activity using an internal uterine pressure catheter, considered to be the gold standard of uterine activity detection.[14]

27.2.6.1.3 Applications

These devices are used for early detection of premature labor in women with high risk of preterm labor. They have not been shown to be useful for screening in normal pregnancy.[15] These devices have also been used in research studies to define the profile of 24-h uterine activity in normal pregnancy.[16]

27.2.6.1.4 Models

Some uterine contraction monitors are shown in Table 27.12.

TABLE 27.12 Ambulatory Uterine Contraction Monitors

Manufacturer	Model
Spacelabs Medical, Inc. 15220 N.E. 40th Street P.O. Box 97013 Redmond, WA 98073-9713 Phone: (425) 882-3700 Fax: (425) 885-4877 www.spacelabs.com	MOM™ Maternal Obstetrical Monitor AMS-02-6701 Antepartum Fetal Monitor — uterine activity and single fetal heart rate AMS-02-6702 Antepartum Fetal Monitor — uterine activity and twin fetal heart rate

27.2.7 Urinary Monitoring

27.2.7.1 Ambulatory Bladder Pressure Monitoring

Petley et al.[13] described a research instrument used to measure bladder pressure. In this system, a pressure sensor located in the bladder detects changes in both detrusor and intra-abdominal pressure. A second pressure sensor located in the vagina or rectum also detects intra-abdominal pressure changes. The true detrusor pressure can then be calculated by subtracting the intra-abdominal pressure from the pressure sensed in the bladder.

Although there are some aspects of routine urodynamic testing for which a frequency response of up to 60 Hz may be thought essential, the restricted nature of the information commonly extracted from the ambulatory pressure data is such that a sample rate of 3 Hz is more than adequate. Using two channels of 8-bit acquisition resolution and a sample rate of 3 Hz allows a recording period of approximately 3 h before the device's memory is full, which is sufficient for most persons evaluated by this technique. This system is not widely used in research or clinical practice.

27.3 Integrated Physiological Data Recorders

The integrated data recorders described in this section are used to collect many different types of physiological data simultaneously. As such they do not fit well into the systems approach used above. Typically, these instruments collect anywhere from 1 to 16 parameters and store the data with no mathematical manipulation. The applications for these instruments depend upon which physiological parameters are being measured (see Section 27.2 for descriptions of applications based on physiological systems). The integrated physiological data recorders are listed below alphabetically according to device.

27.3.1 Device: Biolog® Series

27.3.1.1 Purpose

Three types of ambulatory data recorders known as the Biolog® are available: models 3991, 3992, and 3993. These are used to monitor and record a wide range of signals: ECG, heart rate via photoplethysmography, interbeat interval, heart sounds, electrooculogram, muscle activity (EMG), EEG, respiration, oxygen partial pressure (pO_2), carbon dioxide partial pressure (pCO_2), pressure, temperature, and skin conductance. Data are downloaded to a personal computer. The manufacturer will customize each device according to the customer's specifications for gain, frequency response, data reduction, sample rate, and other criteria.

27.3.1.2 Description

There are three Biolog models in the series with different capabilities. Model 3991 records up to 3 channels and is lightest in weight (8 oz — 1.3 × 2.8 × 5 in.). Model 3992 records up to 7 channels and weighs 20 oz (1.5 × 5 × 7 in.) and model 3993 records up to 14 channels and weighs 50 oz (2.8 × 6 × 8 in.). Data are displayed on a small LCD screen and stored for later downloading. Data can then be viewed, printed, moved to the clipboard, or converted into channel-specific ASCII data files.

27.3.1.3 Manufacturer

U.F.I.
545 Main, C-2
Morro Bay, CA 93442
Phone: (805) 772-1203
Fax: (805) 772-5056
www.ufiservingscience.com

27.3.2 Device: The FlexComp Infiniti™

27.3.2.1 Purpose

The FlexComp is a multimodality, 8-channel system designed for monitoring EMG, EEG, EKG, skin conductance, temperature, heart rate, blood volume pulse, respiration, force, range of motion, and voltage.

27.3.2.2 Description

The FlexComp consists of a lightweight (6.6 oz) encoder and a variety of sensors. It allows the collection of 10 channels at 2000 samples per second. Multiple encoders can be combined to monitor up to 40 channels. Sensors are available for EEG, EMG, SC, BVP, EKG, respiration, temperature, voltage, range of motion, and force. There is a removable compact flash memory up to the maximum available (currently 1 Gb) that provides enough storage to monitor all 10 channels for several days. The memory module can be removed and plugged into a PC to download the raw data. Alternatively, the PC can receive the data via a fiberoptic USB connection or a telemetry compact flash module, which allows data to be beamed more than 100 feet. The FlexComp is similar to the Procomp, described in Section 27.3.6.

27.3.2.3 Manufacturer

Thought Technology
2180 Belgrave Avenue
Montreal, Quebec
Canada, 4A 2L8
Phone: (800) 361-3651 or (514) 489-8251
Fax: (514) 489-8255
www.thoughttechnology.com

27.3.3 Device: The Logger

27.3.3.1 Purpose

The logger is an ambulatory device that was developed for research purposes. It can measure bladder pressure, pollution in the surrounding air, core body temperature, and/or skin temperature.

27.3.3.2 Description

The logger consists of two circuit boards that fit into a case that can be attached to the subject's waist. Two Mallinckrodt transducers are used to measure bladder pressure, and the system is calibrated using a column of water. Data are sent from the transducers to the circuit boards for data storage.

The logger can also be used to monitor the levels of carbon monoxide and nitrogen dioxide in the surrounding air using electrochemical gas sensors (City Technology Ltd). The sensors are calibrated with known concentrations of bottled "calibration" gas. In addition, temperature (National Instruments LM35CZ) and humidity (Mercator RHU-217–5AT) can also be monitored.

Core body temperature can be measured using a tympanic membrane, Type T thermocouple inserted into the external auditory canal. Mean peripheral temperature can be calculated from measurements of skin temperature using thermistors (Yellow Springs Instrument Co, 4000 series compatible) placed on the arm, chest, thigh, and calf.

Data acquired by the system can either be stored to memory as raw data or processed first and then stored. The system is equipped with electrically erasable programmable read only memory (EEPROM), which retains data in the event of power failure. Both hardware and software data protection are offered.

27.3.3.3 Manufacturer

This system was developed for research purposes by Petley, Clitheroe, Clewlow, Deakin, and Chauhan and is not commercially available.[13]

27.3.4 Device: Micropaq™

27.3.4.1 Purpose

Micropaq detects, displays, and stores heart rate, ECG, and oxygen saturation. It can be used alone or can be connected via FlexNet, Welch Allyn's new wireless network, to the Acuity Central Station where the data can be displayed and analyzed.

27.3.4.2 Description

The Micropaq is a small (7.2 × 3.5 × 1.6 in.), lightweight (17 oz with battery), wearable vital signs monitor. Its battery lasts up to 25 h. The display is a backlit LCD that can show two ECG leads at a time, leads I, II, III, AVR, AVF, or V, along with heart rate, SpO_2 numerics, and a pulse bar. Its visual and audible alarms function even when the device is out of telemetry range.

27.3.4.3 Contact Information

Welch Allyn Monitoring
8500 S.W. Creekside Place
Beaverton, Oregon 97008-7107
Phone: (503) 530-7500
Customer Service Phone: (800) 289-2501
Fax: (503) 526-4200
www.monitoring.welchallyn.com

27.3.5 Device: Mini Logger Series 2000

27.3.5.1 Purpose

The Mini Logger Series 2000 is a wearable medical device (120 × 65 × 22 mm) used for obtaining physiological data while the patient or subject pursues his or her normal activity schedule.

27.3.5.2 Description

The Mini Logger Series 2000 is a compact data logger that is capable of monitoring up to five channels of physiological data simultaneously. It can be used to monitor heart rate parameters, such as interbeat interval (IBI) and beats per minute, which is important for determining a subject's heart rate variability (HRV). It can also be used to measure other parameters, such as body temperature and gross motor activity. For all monitored parameters, this device captures the exact timing of physiological changes to allow the clinician or researcher to determine the relationships among, for example, temperature fluctuations, activity patterns, and increase/decrease in heart rate associated with exercise, sleep patterns, shift work, fatigue, etc.

The Mini Logger is equipped with jacks to be used for plugging in the activity and/or temperature sensors worn by the subject or patient. For heart rate monitoring, the subject wears the Polar chest band around his or her chest. Stored data are later downloaded from the Mini Logger through a communications interface, which runs between the serial port of the device and the serial port of a PC-compatible computer that has the Mini Log 2000 software installed.

27.3.5.3 Contact Information

Mini Mitter Co., Inc.
20300 Empire Avenue, Bldg. B-3
Bend, OR 97701
www.minimitter.com

27.3.6 Device: ProComp Infiniti™

27.3.6.1 Purpose

ProComp is a multimodality, 8-channel system designed for monitoring EMG, EEG, EKG, skin conductance, temperature, heart rate, blood volume pulse, respiration, force, range of motion, and voltage.

27.3.6.2 Description

The ProComp consists of a lightweight (6.6 oz) encoder and a variety of sensors. It allows the collection of two channels of 2000 samples per second and six channels of 256 samples per second. There is a removable compact flash memory up to the maximum available (currently 1 Gb), which provides enough storage to monitor all eight channels for several days. The memory module can be removed and plugged into a PC to download the raw data. Alternatively, the PC can receive the data via a fiberoptic USB connection or a telemetry compact flash module, which allows data to be beamed more than 100 ft. The Procomp is similar to the FlexComp, described in Section 27.3.2.

27.3.6.3 Contact Information

Thought Technology
2180 Belgrave Avenue
Montreal, Quebec
Canada, 4A 2L8
Phone: (800) 361-3651 or (514) 489-8251
Fax: (514) 489-8255
www.thoughttechnology.com

27.3.7 Device: Vitaport System

27.3.7.1 Purpose

Vitaport's 18-channel polysomnography/ECG module was designed for full polysomnographic or cardiorespiratory recording. Sensors are available to measures hemoglobin saturation (SpO_2), heart rate, respiration, airflow, ECG, EEG, EOG, EMG, body position, body movement, pressure, or temperature.

27.3.7.2 Description

The Vitaport contains two piezo-resistive accelero-sensors that allow data collection of high resolution posture and movement over 24 h. The polysomnography (PSG) module offers differential diagnosis of apnea and sleep. It contains a full oxygen saturation measurement unit and magnetic coils for monitoring of respiratory excursions. The module can also process sounds of snoring and contains smart sensors for the combined monitoring of body position and movement, as well as a bridge amplifier for measuring esophagus pressure or temperature, and monitors for measuring the ECG and the heart rate. There are five amplifiers for the EEG, EOG, and EMG to be used either for determining quality of sleep (in terms of restless legs) or for performing a full three-lead ECG. External devices, such as a pCO_2 monitor or a CPAP device, can be attached to the auxiliary input if required.

In combination with the recorder base unit, the total weight of the Vitaport is around 700 g, thus enabling the device to be worn on the body. The device allows for 20-channel (including marker and battery channels) polysomnographic recording in the lab, at home under telemetric supervision, or in ambulatory situations. It also can be used in combination with an 8-channel universal (or a 16-channel EEG/Poly) module if more channels are required.

27.3.7.3 Manufacturer

TEMEC Instruments B.V
Spekhofstraat 2
NL-6466 LZ KERKRADE
The Netherlands
Phone: +31 45-5428888
Fax: +31 45-5428584
E-mail: sales@temec.com

References

1. Heffler, S. et al., Health spending projections for 2001–2011, *Health Affairs,* 21(2), 207, 2002.
2. McNeal, G.J., High-tech home care: an expanding critical care frontier, *Crit. Care Nurse,* 16(5), 51, 1996.
3. National High Blood Pressure Education Program (NHBPEP), Sixth Report of the Joint National Committee on the Prevention, Detection, Evaluation and Treatment of High Blood Pressure (JNC VI), NIH Publication No. 98–4080, 1997. Available on-line: http://www.nhlbi.nih.gov/nhlbi/cardio/hbp/prof/hbinfhc.htm.
4. Bridges, E.J. and Woods, S.L., Cardiovascular chronobiology: do you know what time it is? *Prog. Cardiovasc. Nurs.,* 16(2), 65, 2001.
5. Kerschan-Schindl, L. et al., Reliability of pelvic floor muscle strength measurement in elderly incontinent women, *Neurourol. Urodynam.*, 21(1), 42, 2002.
6. Cosmi, B. et al., Accuracy of a portable prothrombin monitor (Coagucheck) in patients on chronic oral anticoagulant therapy: a prospective multicenter study, *Throm. Res.,* 100(4), 279, 2000.
7. Cosmi, B. et al., Assessment of patient capability to self-adjust oral anticoagulant dose: a prospective multicenter study on home use of portable prothrombin time monitor (Coagucheck), *Haematologica,* 85(8), 826, 2000.
8. White, J. M. et al., Twenty-four hour ambulatory monitoring of tremor, sweating, skin temperature, and locomotor activity in the alcohol withdrawal syndrome, *Clin. Autonomic Res.,* 4, 15, 1994.
9. Willemsen, G.H.M. et al. Ambulatory monitoring of the impedance cardiogram, *Psychophysiology,* 33, 184, 1996.
10. Sherwood, A., McFetridge, J., and Hutchenson, J.S., Ambulatory impedance cardiography: a feasibility study, *J. Appl. Physiol.*, 85(6), 2365, 1998.
11. Anderson, D.E. and Frank, L.B., A microprocessor system for ambulatory monitoring of respiration, *J. Ambul. Monitor.*, 3, 11, 1990.
12. Hsu, J.Y. et al., Coughing frequency in patients with persistent cough: assessment using a 24-hour ambulatory recorder, *Eur. Respir. J.*, 7, 1246, 1994.
13. Petley, G.W. et al., Development and application of a general purpose ambulatory monitor, *Med. Eng. Phys.*, 20(1), 33, 1998.
14. Dickinson, J.E. et al., A validation study of home uterine activity monitoring technology in western Australia, *Aust. N.S. J. Obstet. Gynecol.,* 37(1), 39, 1997.
15. Moore, T.R. et al. and the Uterine Activity in Pregnancy Working Group, Diurnal and gestation patterns of uterine activity in normal human pregnancy, *Obstet. Gynecol.*, 83, 517, 1994.
16. U.S. Preventive Services Task Force, *Guide to Clinical Preventive Services,* 2nd ed., U.S. Department of Health and Human Services, Office of Disease Prevention and Health Promotion, Washington, D.C., 1996.

Bibliography

ACC/AHA Task Force on Practice Guidelines, ACC/AHA guidelines for ambulatory electrocardiography, *J. Am. Coll. Cardiol.*, 34(3), 912, 1999.

American Electroencephalographic Society, AEEGS guidelines for long-term monitoring for epilepsy, *J. Clin. Neurophysiol.*, 11(1), 88, 1994.

Aytaclar, S. et al., Association between hyperactivity and executive cognitive functioning in childhood and substance use in early adolescence, *J. Am. Acad. Child Adolescent Psychiatry,* 38, 172, 1998.

Beall, C.M. et al., Percent of oxygen saturation of arterial hemoglobin among Bolivian Aymara at 3,900–4,000 m., *Am. J. Phys. Anthropol.*, 108(1), 41, 1999.

Berger, A.M., Patterns of fatigue and activity and rest during adjuvant breast cancer chemotherapy, *Oncol. Nursing Forum*, 25(1), 51, 1998.

Ceolim, M.F. and Luiz, M.B., Sleep/wake cycle and physical activity in healthy elderly people, *Sleep Res. Online,* 3(3), 87, 2000.

Coleman, K.L. et al., Step activity monitor: long-term, continuous recording of ambulatory function, *J. Rehabil. Res. Dev.*, 36(1), 8, 1999.

Dobkin, P.L. and Pihl, R.O., Measurement of psychological and heart-rate reactivity to stress in the real world, *Psychother. Psychosom.*, 58, 208, 1992.

Fahrenberg, J. and Myrteck, M., *Progress in Ambulatory Assessment*, Hogrefe & Huber Publishers, Seattle, WA, 2001.

Gilliam, F., Kuzniecky, R., and Faught, E., Ambulatory EEG monitoring, *J. Clin. Neurophysiol.*, 16(2), 111, 1999.

Jean-Louis, G. et al., Sleep detection with an accelerometer actigraph: comparisons with polysomnography, *Physiol. Behav.*, 72, 21, 2001.

Jensen, L.A., Onyskiw, J. E., and Prasad, N.G.N., Meta-analysis of arterial oxygen saturation monitoring by pulse oximetry in adults, *Heart Lung*, 27(6), 387, 1998.

Kubicek, W.G. et al., The Minnesota impedance cardiography — theory and applications, *Biomed. Eng.*, 9, 410, 1974.

Leary, A.C. et al., Physical activity level is an independent predictor of the diurnal variation in blood pressure, *J. Hypertension,* 18, 405, 2000.

O'Brien, E., Atkins, N., and Staessen, J., State of the market: a review of ambulatory blood pressure monitoring devices, *Hypertension,* 26, 835, 1995.

Okeie, K. et al., Left ventricular systolic dysfunction during exercise and dobutamine stress in patients with hypertrophic cardiomyopathy, *J. Am. Coll. Cardiol.*, 36(3), 856, 2000.

Pilling, J. and Cutaia, M., Ambulatory oximetry monitoring in patients with severe COPD — a preliminary study, *CHEST,* 116(2), 314, 1999.

Rabito, C.A. et al., Noninvasive, real-time monitoring of renal function — the ambulatory renal monitor, *J. Nuclear Med.*, 34(2), 199, 1993.

Smith, D.G. et al., Step activity monitor: long-term continuous recording of ambulatory function, *Clin. Orthoped. Relat. Res.*, 361, 29, 1999.

Stern, R.M., Ray, W.J., and Quigley, K.S., *Psychophysiol. Rec.,* Oxford University Press, Oxford, 2001.

Webster, J. B. et al., Transducer design and placement for activity recording, *Med. Biol. Eng. Comput.*, 20, 741, 1982.

Wilhelm, F.H. and Walton, T.R., Trusting computerized data reduction too much: a critique of Anderson's ambulatory respiratory monitor, *Bio. Psych.*, 49, 215, 1998.

Ku, Y.E. et al., Physiologic and functional responses of MS patients to body cooling, *Am. J. Phys. Med. Rehabil.*, 79, 427, 2000.

Yucha, C.B., Ambulatory blood pressure monitoring: measurement implications for research, *J. Nursing Measure.*, 9(1), 49, 2001.

VII

Recovery

This section includes the following chapters:

28

Neural Prostheses for Movement Restoration

Dejan B. Popović
Aalborg University

CONTENTS

28.1 Introduction

A neural prosthesis is an assistive system that replaces or augments a function that was lost or diminished because of the injury or disease of the nervous system. The method most frequently applied in neural prostheses (NP) is the external electrical activation of the appropriate impaired sensory-motor systems, that is, use of functional electrical stimulation (FES). FES elicits desired neural activation by delivering the controlled amount of electrical charge patterned as bursts of electrical charge pulses. In principle, it is possible to apply a time varying magnetic field, thereby inducing electrical currents within the selected parts of the neural pathways; however, this technique is not yet efficient enough for functional activation of sensory-motor systems. A detailed presentation of most aspects of neural prosthesis can be found in Popović and Sinkjær (2000).

Figure 28.1 shows the principle of FES-based neural prosthesis. After an injury or disease (e.g., stroke, spinal cord injury, Parkinson's disease) of the central nervous system (CNS) or peripheral lesion some sensory-motor systems will be intact, yet other structures will be paralyzed or paretic. A lesion leads to paralysis with the muscles still being innervated, but sometimes also to denervation of muscles. The innervated muscles are often activated in an unpredicted manner, but they are not controllable volitionally. These muscles are the best candidates for the effective neural prosthesis application. In parallel, many sensory pathways preserve their connections to the CNS, yet their activity does not reach the appropriate centers within the CNS. NP can also restore some elements of the sensory systems. In other words, NP should be considered as a bypass of the damaged sensory-motor systems.

0-8493-1140-3/04/$0.00+$1.50

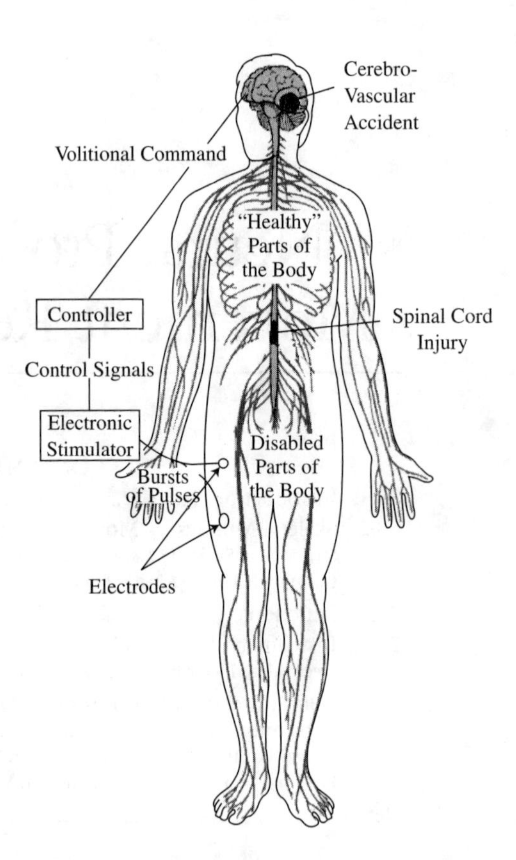

FIGURE 28.1 General schema of the operation of a motor neural prosthesis (NP). Components of the NP are controller, electronic stimulator, sensory feedback (not shown), and electrodes. NP acts as a bypass for the diminished or missing transmission of neural signals from and to the central nervous system.

28.2 Skeletal Muscles — Movement Actuators

The motor system of the human is comprised of three interrelated anatomical systems: the skeletal system, the muscle system, which supplies the power to move the skeleton; and the nervous system, which directs and regulates the activity of the muscles. Man uses about 350 pairs of skeletal muscles of many shapes and sizes that are situated across more than 300 joints, being attached to bones via tendons. A shortening and broadening of the muscle, which brings the muscle ends closer to each other, ultimately changing the angle at the joint across which it acts, produce movement.

Muscle has four well-developed characteristic properties: contractility, irritability, distensibility, and elasticity. The contractility is the capacity of muscle to produce force between its ends; relaxation is the opposite of contraction being entirely passive. Relaxation and contraction progress from zero to maximal values over a finite time. Irritability is the ability of muscle tissue to respond to stimulation. The muscle is the second most highly irritable tissue in the human body, being exceeded in this capacity only by neural tissue. The muscles are distensible; thus, they can be lengthened or stretched by an external force. The stretching force can be the pull of an antagonistic muscle, of gravity, or of a force exerted by an opponent. Distensibility is a reversible process and the muscle suffers no harm so long as it is not stretched in excess of its physiological limits. Unless a muscle has been over stretched, it will recoil from a distended length due to elasticity. Distensibility and elasticity oppose each other, yet they assure that contractions will be smooth and that the muscle is not injured by a sudden strong change in either stretch or contraction.

There are two types of skeletal muscles, distinguishable by speed of contraction and endurance. The designations of "dark" and "pale" muscles have become synonymous with slow and fast contraction, respectively. In addition to a slower contraction/relaxation cycle, dark muscles have lower thresholds, tetanize at lower frequencies, fatigue less rapidly, and are more sensitive to stretch than the faster pale muscles. Most human striated muscles contain both types of fibers, but in differing proportions. The preponderantly slow-fibered muscles are the antigravity muscles, adapted for continuous body support. The predominantly fast-fibered muscles are phasic muscles, which produce quick postural changes and fine skilled movements.

28.2.1 Structure of Skeletal Muscles

A skeletal muscle is composed of two types of structural components: active contractile elements and inert compliant materials. The contractile elements are contained within the muscle fibers. Each muscle is composed of many muscle fibers (a medium-sized muscle containing approximately 1 million fibers). The fibers vary in length from a few millimeters to more than 40 cm, and their width is between 1 and 150 μm. About 85% of the mass of a muscle consists of the muscle fibers, while the remaining 15% is composed largely of connective tissues, which contain variable proportions of collagen, reticular, and elastic fibers. The connective tissues provide an arrangement of simple, spring-like elements (elastic components of the muscle), which exist both in series and in parallel with the contractile elements. A connective tissue sheath, the epimysium, surrounds the muscle and sends septa (the perimysia) into the muscle to envelop bundles of muscle fibers. Larger bundles may be subdivided into several smaller bundles.

28.2.2 Activation of Skeletal Muscles

The muscle activation is linked to activity of neural cells. The essential function of a nerve cell is to transmit excitation to other cells, and it is achieved by releasing a chemical transmitter substance at its synaptic terminal. A number of different kinds of stimuli may excite neurons. The normal stimulus for synaptic neurons is the action upon their membranes of chemical transmitters released by other neurons. Stimulation of receptor neurons is normally provided by chemical, thermal, mechanical, and electromagnetic energies. In a few instances, rare among the vertebrates, a neuron is stimulated by direct electrical stimulation from another neuron.

As the action potential travels along the fiber surface, it consists of a wave of negativity followed by an area of gradually recovering positivity. While an area is in its reversed (active) state, it is absolutely refractory and cannot be restimulated. During recovery, the membrane is relatively refractory, a state that lasts many times longer than the absolute refractory period. Intense or sustained stimuli may restimulate the original site during repolarization. During the relative refractory period both the amplitude and velocity of the neural spike are altered, reflecting changed conditions in the fiber. In some neurons the latter portion of the downward course of the spike is considerably less rapid than its rise. During this period of 12 to 80 msec, the membrane is hyperexcitable or supernormal, hence more easily restimulated.

Neurons normally carry trains of impulses. In general, natural stimuli are of sufficient duration to reactivate the membrane after the absolute refractory period. A single electric shock may produce a single action potential, but only because its duration does not outlast the refractory period of the fiber. The stronger the stimulus, the earlier it will reexcite, and the shorter will be the time span between impulses, hence, the greater the frequency.

Because each action potential is followed by an absolute refractory period, action potentials cannot summate, but remain separate and discrete. The neurons do not conduct impulses at rates as high as the absolute refractory periods would suggest. A fiber with spikes lasting about 0.4 msec might be expected to conduct impulses at a frequency of 2500/sec, but its upper limit will be closer to 1000/sec. Conduction frequencies rarely approximate their possible maxima. Motoneurons usually conduct at frequencies of 20 to 40 (rarely as high as 50) impulses per second although, at the start of a maximum contraction, rates greater than 100 Hz have been recorded. Upper-limit frequencies for sensory neurons normally lie between 100 and 200 impulses per second, although auditory neurons may conduct between 800 and

1000 impulses per second. Information is conveyed by the presence or absence of an action potential, as well as by the frequency of action potentials.

Velocity of conduction depends not only on myelination but also, more importantly, on the diameter of the fiber. It can be fairly accurately said that the conduction velocity is proportional to the diameter of the axon, and is in the range of 50 m/sec. The largest motor and sensory nerve fibers (diameters about 20 μm) have conduction velocities up to 120 m/sec. In small unmyelinated fibers, the velocities are from 0.7 to 2 m/sec. Large fibers have lower stimulus thresholds compared with small fibers.

Nerve fibers are classified into three major groups, A, B, and C, on the basis of conduction velocities. Group C contains the unmyelinated postganglionic fibers and group B the small myelinated preganglionic fibers of the autonomic nervous system. Group A includes the large, rapidly conducting myelinated somatic fibers. Group A has been further divided into four subgroups: α, β, γ, and δ, based on the velocity and diameter.

Nerves enter the muscle near the main arterial branch and divide to distribute both motor and sensory fibers to the muscle bundles. Motor fibers fall into two categories: large fibers (alpha subdivision of Group A) and smaller fibers (gamma subdivision of Group A). Each large alpha motorneuron, with its cell body lying in the ventral horn of the spinal cord, supplies a number of muscle fibers by successive bifurcation of its axis cylinder. One motorneuron and all of the muscle fibers that are innervated with the axon terminals constitute a motor unit. The number of muscle fibers per motor unit varies considerably with both the size of the muscle and the type of its function. Small muscles and muscles concerned with fine gradations of contraction have necessarily smaller motor units than larger bulky muscles whose job is the maintenance of strong contraction.

The excitation of a muscle (contraction) is accomplished by the nervous system: nerve impulses arriving at the neuromuscular junction cause the release of a transmitter substance, which diffuses across the junction and chemically excites the muscle fiber. Action potentials travel along the fiber membrane at a speed of 1 to 3 m/sec and initiate the events that lead to shortening of the contractile elements of the myofibrils and the consequent production of force in the muscle.

Muscle fibers are incapable of lengthening themselves actively.

28.2.3 Contractile Force

The force developed by a contracting muscle is influenced by a number of factors such as the characteristics of the stimulus, the length of the muscle both at the time of stimulation and during the contraction, and the speed at which the muscle is contracting.

Most of what has been learned about muscle has been derived from studies using stimulation by electrical pulses. When a single pulse is applied directly to a motorneuron, the corresponding muscle fiber will respond in an all-or-none fashion. Increasing the intensity of the pulse will not increase the magnitude of the fiber's response. It is important to mention here that the all-or-none response of the muscle fiber is determined by the all-or-none character of its excitation and not by any all-or-none limitations inherent in the contractile mechanism itself. When a single adequate pulse is applied to a whole muscle, the muscle will respond with a quick contraction, followed immediately by relaxation. Such a response is called a twitch. Its magnitude will vary with the number of muscle fibers, which respond to the stimulus, and this will vary directly with the intensity of the pulse up to a finite maximal intensity.

The twitch is an indication of force development by the muscle. After a short latent period, the force becomes evident and rises to a peak, then declines over a slightly longer time course to zero. The time course of the development of force in the twitch is influenced by the interaction of the contractile components of the muscle fibrils with the elastic components of the muscle.

A single electrical pulse must have a certain minimal intensity to be effective. This minimal level is an inverse measure of the irritability of the tissue; the smaller the minimal intensity, the greater the irritability. The minimal effective intensity is designated the threshold or minimal stimulus. These terms refer to the weakest stimulus, which will evoke a barely perceptible response. Subthreshold and subliminal refer to

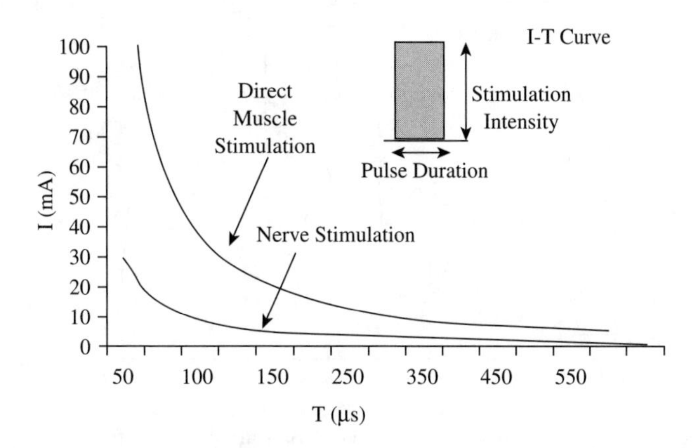

FIGURE 28.2 The intensity (I)–duration (T) curve. Two curves are presented for direct stimulation of the muscle, and stimulation of the muscle via its neural supply. The amount of charge (product of the pulse amplitude and pulse duration) is much higher for the direct muscle stimulation compared with the activation when the neural pathways are stimulated. The upper limb of the I-T curve indicates that a very strong stimulus must be applied for at least the minimal duration, and the minimal pulse intensity is required to activate muscle (lower limb). The minimal current required for stimulation is termed the *reobasis,* and the duration that is required to elicit activation when the stimulation pulse has the intensity twice greater than the reobasis is *the* chronaxia.

a stimulus of inadequate intensity. As the intensity of the single pulse is increased above the minimum, the contractile force in the muscle increases progressively as a result of the activation of more and more muscle fibers. Finally, the intensity is reached that evokes the maximal response of which the muscle is capable. Presumably all fibers are then active. The weakest stimulus intensity that evokes maximal contraction is called the maximal stimulus.

A weak but adequate pulse with a rapid rate of rise from zero to its preset intensity will evoke a stronger contraction than a pulse of the same intensity with a slower rise. A minimal rate is required even for an intense stimulus. If intensity rises too gradually, there will be no response at all; the stimulus is then ineffectual. For any stimulus of adequate intensity, the more abruptly it is applied the greater will be the response it evokes within the limits of the muscle's capacity. The greater the intensity, the less rapidly it needs rise to produce a given level of response.

The relationship of intensity and duration of single current pulses in the production of a barely perceptible contraction is presented in the intensity-duration curve (Figure 28.2). For all points (I-T) right and above the intensity-duration curve the contraction will occurs, yet there will be no contraction if the (I-T) point is left and below the I-T curve.

If a stimulus of constant intensity and duration is applied at various rates of rise, effectiveness will be directly related to the rate. The more abruptly the stimulus is applied, the greater the response of the muscle will be. As the rate decreases, the response will diminish until ultimately, regardless of intensity, the stimulus becomes ineffectual. The decreased effectiveness of a constant intensity at long duration and/or low rate of rise are designated adaptation or accommodation. Many tissues other than muscle adapt to a gradual or persistent stimulus.

If an adequate stimulus is applied to a muscle fiber repeatedly at a rate rapid enough for each succeeding stimulus to reactivate the contractile elements before the previous force has completely subsided, successive responses summate, each building upon the previous one until a maximal level is achieved. If stimulation is continued, the contraction peak is maintained at this level. Such a response is known as tetanus or tetanic contraction. Ultimately, fatigue will cause the peak level to decline progressively. When stimulation ceases, contraction terminates, and the fiber relaxes, the force subsiding quickly to zero. If the repetitive stimulation is too prolonged, however, contracture will result, and relaxation will be significantly slowed as compared with normal. Unlike rigor, contracture is reversible.

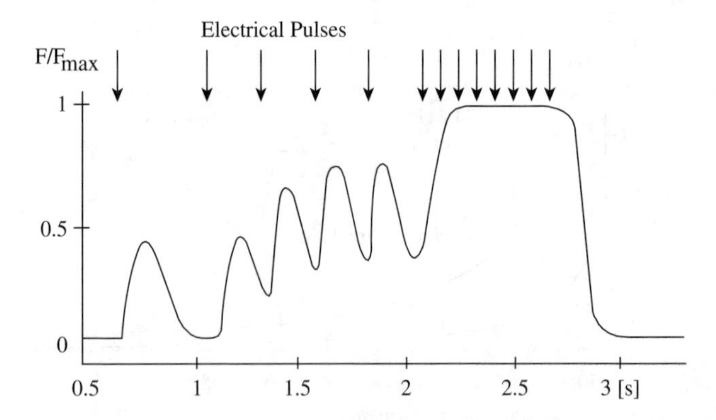

FIGURE 28.3 The effect of the repetition rate (frequency) of stimulation on the force developed in isometric conditions. The first applied stimulus is a single pulse resulting in a muscle twitch; second, 4 pulses per second results with increasing, yet pulsating force; and finally 20 pulses per second results with nonpulsatile (fused) muscle contraction. If the repetition rate is further increased, the force will reach the maximum level (tetanus). The contraction that results with the smooth, time-constant force can be generated with the repetition rate of 20 pulses per second in most human skeletal muscles.

The frequency of stimulation, usually expressed as number of pulses per second or Hertz, determines both the shape and the magnitude of a tetanic contraction traced on a myograph by an excised muscle. When pulses are delivered within an interval that places successive stimuli during the relaxation phase of the preceding response, the contraction approaches a tremor. With a period between pulses short enough to allow for restimulation during the contraction phase, the force becomes smooth (fused contraction) and eventually reaches tetanus. The force developed in response to repetitive pulses is greater than that evoked by a single pulse of the same magnitude (Figure 28.3).

In many muscles, if twitch responses to single pulses are recorded before and immediately after a period of tetanic stimulation, the post-tetanic twitch shows an increase in magnitude and a steeper rise of force than the pre-tetanic control. This phenomenon is known as post-tetanic potentiation (Figure 28.4). The effect occurs whether its motor nerve stimulates the muscle directly or indirectly. Potentiation

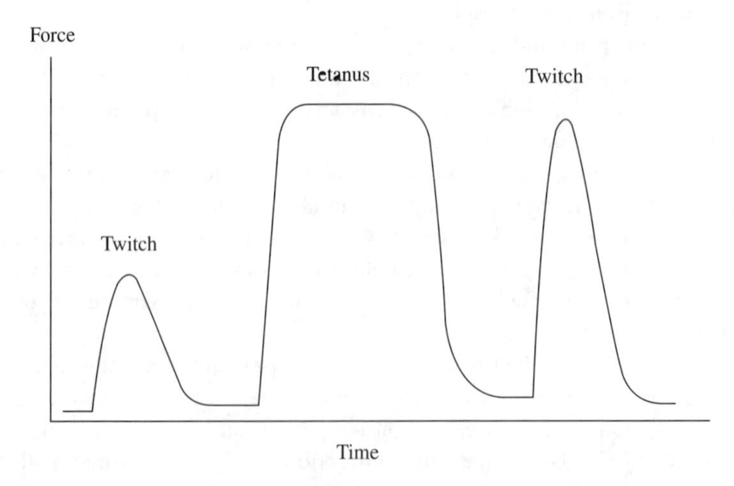

FIGURE 28.4 The diagram demonstrating post-tetanic potentiation. The muscle force (twitch) generated by an isolated singe pulse is smaller compared with a force (tetanus) generated by high frequency stimulation (>50 Hz). The twitch response after the tetanus is much bigger than the twitch response prior to tetanus. This phenomenon suggests that the stimulation by so-called doublets (two pulses applied shortly one after the other) and n-lets (series of n pulses) can be very effective for generating high forces.

is maximal shortly after the repetitive stimulation and then decays exponentially at a rate that is dependent on both the frequency of pulses and the number delivered in the train. Short trains produce potentiation without any alteration of the twitch duration, but longer trains result in lengthening of the contraction time and of the half-relaxation time (the time required for force to drop to 50% of its peak value).

The most obvious property of the muscle is its capacity to develop force against resistance. The length of the muscle at the time of activation markedly affects its ability to develop force and to perform external work. When a muscle contracts, the contractile material itself shortens, but whether the whole muscle shortens or not depends on the relation of the internal force developed by the muscle to the external force exerted by the resistance or load.

Three types of muscle contraction are distinguished according to the length change, induced by the relationship of internal and external forces: isometric, isotonic, and isokinetic. Isometric contraction refers to the case where no change of length occurs, isotonic to the case where the force is kept constant, and isokinetic when the velocity of shortening is kept constant.

The initial length of a muscle, that is, its length at the time of stimulation, influences the magnitude of its contractile response to a given stimulus. A stretched muscle contracts more forcefully than when it is unstretched at the time of activation. This is true whether the contraction is isometric, isotonic, or isokinetic. Within physiological limits, the greater the initial length, the greater the force capability of the muscle will be. Parallel-fibered muscles exert maximal total force at lengths only slightly greater than rest length. Muscles with other fiber arrangements have maxima at somewhat greater relative stretch. In general, optimal length is close to the maximal body length of the muscle, that is, the greatest length that the muscle can attain in the normal living body. This is about 1.2 to 1.3 times the rest length of the muscle. Force capability is less at short and long lengths. Therefore, a muscle can exert the greatest force or sustain the heaviest load when the body position is such as to bring it to its optimal length. In isotonic contractions the increased force and longer length permit greater shortening; hence, more work can be done or, alternatively, the same work can be done at lower energy cost.

The relationship of force to muscle length may be presented graphically in the form of a force-length curve, in which force in an isolated muscle are plotted against a series of muscle lengths from less than to greater than the resting length (Figure 28.5). Both the passive elastic force (Curve 1) exerted by the elastic components in the passively stretched muscle and the total force (Curve 2) exerted by the actively contracting muscle are plotted.

Most isolated unloaded muscles normally shorten by about 50% or less of their rest length. The absolute amount by which any muscle can shorten depends upon the length and arrangement of its fibers, the greatest shortening occurring in the long parallel-fiber muscles such as the *Biceps m.* and *Sartorius m.*

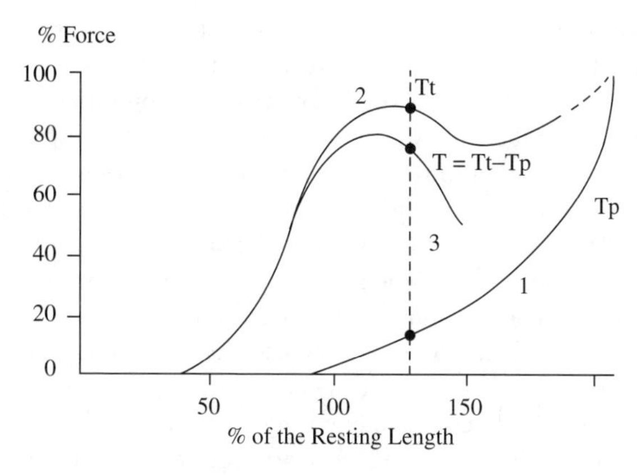

FIGURE 28.5 Force vs. length curve for an isolated muscle. (1) Passive elastic tension, (2) total force, and (3) force obtained by subtracting of passive force from total force. This curves suggests that the muscle force depends on the position of the joint. Maximum force can be generated at muscle lengths that are shorter than the relaxed length of the muscle (this length varies from muscle to muscle).

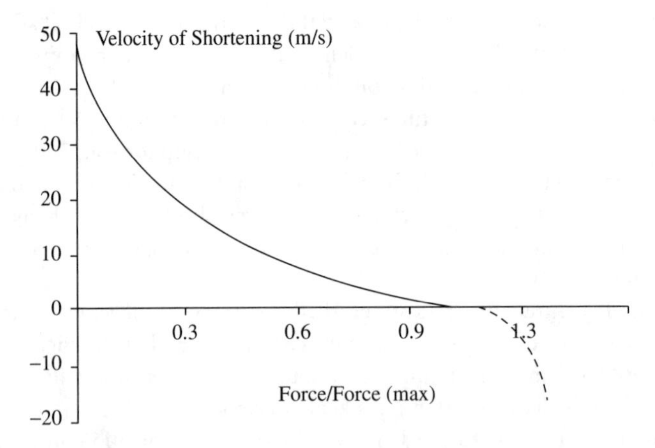

FIGURE 28.6 Relationship among the normalized muscle force and velocity of contraction. Negative velocity relates to eccentric contraction, while the positive to active contraction. The faster the shortening, the smaller is the force, and vice versa. See text for details.

In intact muscle, the structure of joints, the resistance of antagonists, and any load that opposes the muscle further limit shortening. When shortening against resistance, speed varies inversely with the load. Therefore, in isotonic contraction the less the resistance, the more nearly maximal the rate of shortening. When a muscle is required to shorten more rapidly against the same load, less force is produced than when it shortens more slowly.

In concentric contraction the relationship is evidenced by the decrease in velocity as the load is increased. Shortening velocity is maximal with zero load and reflects the intrinsic shortening speed of the contractile material. Velocity reaches zero with a load too great for the muscle to lift; contraction is then isometric and maximal force can be produced. When more muscle fibers are activated than are needed to overcome the load, the excess force is converted into increasing velocity and therefore greater distance of movement.

In eccentric contraction, values for shortening velocity become negative, and the muscle's ability to sustain force increases with increased speed of lengthening, but not to the extent that might be expected from extrapolation of the shortening curve (Figure 28.6).

28.2.4 Muscle Function

Motor skill and all forms of movement result from the interaction of muscular force, gravity, and any other external forces, which impinge on skeletal levers. The muscles rarely act singly; rather, groups of muscles interact in many ways so that the desired movement is accomplished. This interaction may take many different forms so that a muscle may serve in a number of different capacities, depending on the movement. Whenever a muscle causes movement by shortening, it is functioning as a mover or agonist. If the observed muscle makes the major contribution to the movement, that muscle is named as the prime mover. Other muscles crossing the same joint on the same aspect, but which are smaller or which are shown electromyographically to make a lesser contribution to the movement under consideration, are identified as secondary or assistant movers or agonists. The muscles whose action are opposite to and so may oppose that of a prime mover are called antagonists. This does not mean that an antagonist, as the name implies, always exerts force against the prime mover; electromyography has demonstrated conclusively an absence of electrical activity in opposing muscles.

Synergistic action has been defined as cooperative action of two or more muscles in the production of a desired movement. A synergist, then, may be regarded as a muscle that cooperates with the prime mover so as to enhance the movement. Synergic interaction may take many forms and variations as discussed below. Two muscles acting together to produce a movement, which neither could produce alone, may be classed as conjoint synergists. Dorsiflexion of the foot at the ankle is an example. The movement is produced by the combined action of the *Tibialis Anterior m.* and the *Extensor Digitorum Longus m.* The *Tibialis anterior m.* alone would produce a combination of dorsiflexion and inversion, while shortening of the *Extensor Digitorum Longus m.* alone would produce toe extension, dorsiflexion, and eversion. Acting together, the muscles produce a movement of pure dorsiflexion. Another example occurs in lateral deviation of the hand at the wrist; e.g., ulnar deviation results from the simultaneous action of the *Flexor Carpi Ulnaris m.* and the *Extensor Carpi Ulnaris m.*

The *sine qua non* of an effective coordinate movement involves greater stabilization of the more proximal joints so that the distal segments move effectively. The greater the amount of force to be exerted by the open end of a kinematic chain (whether it is the peripheral end of an upper or of a lower extremity), the greater the amount of stabilizing force that is needed at the proximal links.

When a joint is voluntarily fixed rather than stabilized, there is, in addition to immobilization, a rigidity or stiffness resulting from the strong isometric contraction of all muscles crossing that joint. These muscles will forcefully resist all external efforts to move that joint. As fixation can be very tiring, it is seldom used and rarely useful. From the above discussion one should recognize the difference between stabilization and fixation of joints. As stated, fixation denotes a rigidity or stiffness in opposition to all movement, whereas stabilization implies only firmness. Economy of movement involves the use of minimal stabilizing synergy and no fixation of joints.

A muscle crossing two or more joints has certain characteristics, capabilities, and limitations when compared with those muscles that cross only one joint. When a muscle crosses more than one joint, it creates force moments at each of the joints crossed whenever it generates force. The moments of force it exerts at any given instant depend on two factors: the instantaneous length of the moment arm at each joint and the corresponding amount of force that the muscle is exerting. The joint with the longest moment arm, and hence with the greatest moment of force, is normally the one at which the multiactuator muscle will produce or regulate the most action. For example, the *Hamstrings m.* has the moment arm at the hip at least 50% longer than the one at the knee; thus, it contributes more to knee flexion then to hip extension.

28.3 Functional Electrical Stimulation Principles

The literature dealing with electrical stimulation frequently uses terms other than FES, such as neuromuscular stimulation (NMS) and functional neuromuscular stimulation (FNS), aiming to precisely describe the structures that are activated by electrical stimulation. The term FES is used throughout this chapter.

FES systems aim to achieve sensory-motor integration; thereby a better function of humans with paralysis or paresis. FES activates motoneurons or reflex pathways by stimulating efferent or afferent nerve fibers, respectively.

FES can be delivered using monopolar or bipolar configuration. In the bipolar configuration two electrodes are positioned in the vicinity of the muscle that should be stimulated. In the monopolar configuration active electrodes (cathodes) are positioned in the vicinity of the structures to be stimulated, while a single common electrode (anode) is positioned distant to the stimulated structure, yet somewhere along the neural pathway to the CNS.

FES delivers trains of the electrical charge pulses, mimicking to an extent the natural flow of excitation signals generated by the CNS in nonimpaired structures. FES operation can be modeled with a relatively simple electric circuit: generator, electrodes, and tissue. The tissue is an ionic conductor with an impedance of about 10 to 100 Ω, and electrodes are capacitive conductors whose electrical properties depend on many variables, but their impedance is from 500 Ω to 5 kΩ, and they induce a phase shift of about 10 to 30°. The generator can work as a current or voltage regulated device.

The amplitude and duration of stimulus pulses, output impedance of the generator, and impedance of electrodes determine the electrical charge that will be delivered to neuromuscular structure. Stimulators are usually referred to as constant-current or constant-voltage devices. High-output impedance devices will deliver the desired current to the tissue, regardless of the changes in electrode properties up to the

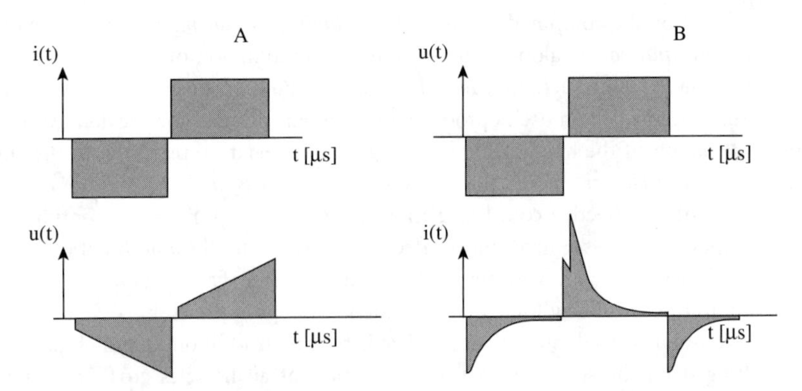

FIGURE 28.7 The stimulator output shape of pulses. (A) Current-regulated stimulation; (B) voltage-regulated stimulation. The top panels show the output of the stimulator; the bottom shows the current and voltage applied to the tissue. Note that the current-regulated output ensures that the amount of charge is controlled. The exponential drop of the current with the voltage-regulated stimulator depends on the impedance (capacitance) of the electrode/tissue interface. If the capacitance is large, the exponential drop will be very fast resulting with almost no charge transferred to the tissues.

voltage capacity available. These constant-current stimulators should be correctly termed current-regulated stimulators.

The electrical charge delivered to the stimulated structure depends on the impedance of electrodes to tissue interface when the stimulators that have a low-output impedance, or so-called constant-voltage or voltage-regulated devices, are applied. This is the reason to use the current-regulated electronic stimulator so that the consequences of typical impedance changes can be ignored. Figure 28.7 shows the patterns of the voltage and current for the current-regulated and (A) voltage-regulated (B) stimulators. Since the electrode-skin interface has electro-capacitive properties, the voltage regulates the stimulation results with uncontrolled electrical current (Figure 28.7); thus, although the voltage may be substantial, the actual charge delivered to the tissue may be very small. This may result in pain, yet very weak or no muscle contraction. In contrast, current-regulated stimulators precisely control the charge delivered to the tissue (Figure 28.7). The issue that has to be considered is that the current-regulated stimulator may cause tissue damage if the surface of the electrode is too small.

The stimulus waveform selected for the excitation process must take into consideration the desired physiological effect (action potential generation), potential damage to the tissue, and potential degradation of the electrode. The process is discussed in detail by Mortimer and collaborators (Mortimer, 1981; Scheiner et al., 1990; McCreery et al., 1995). The waveform selected is generally rectangular. A nonrectangular pulse could be utilized, but the rise time must be sufficiently fast so that the nerve membrane does not accommodate and fails to open its channels. The stimulus waveform may be unidirectional (monophasic) or bidirectional (biphasic) as shown in Figure 28.8.

Biphasic stimulus is recommended for several reasons. Surface stimulation is more comfortable with biphasic than monophasic stimulation. For implanted electrodes, the potential for damage to the tissue will be lessened with the biphasic stimulus. Tissue damage is significantly related to the pH change at the electrode tissue interface. At the cathode, the pH may increase due to the production of OH^-, while at the anode the environment will become more acidic (Scheiner et al., 1990). While some buffering capacity for pH changes exists in the tissue, the changes with monophasic stimulation are greater than those with biphasic stimulation. Although reactions at the electrodes are not completely reversed with the biphasic stimulation, this stimulus allows significantly greater charge injection before tissue damage is encountered (Mortimer, 1981).

The shape of the secondary pulse is also important. Conceptually, one would like the electrode reactions to be totally reversible, suggesting a rapid current reversal in the secondary phase. With the metallic conductors presently used, the electrode reactions are not completely reversed. The biphasic pulse limits

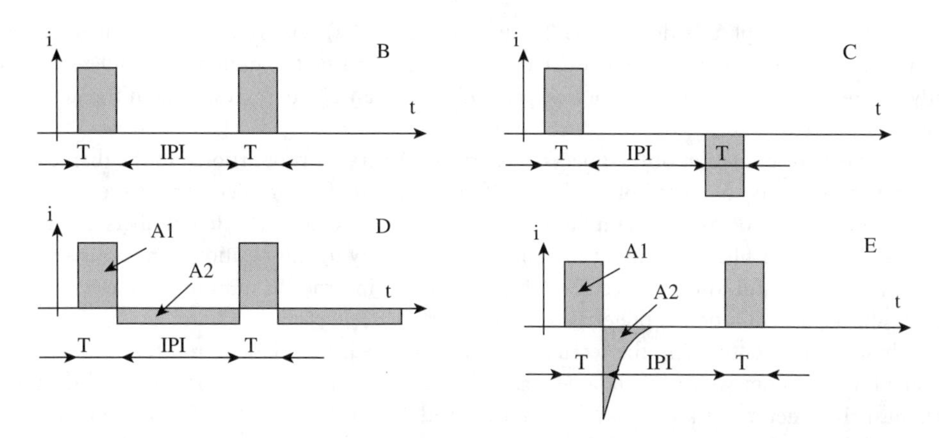

FIGURE 28.8 The pattern of stimulation pulses. (B) Monophasic constant current; (C) biphasic constant current; (D) biphasic balanced constant current; (E) biphasic compensated constant current. The size of area A2 (electrical charge) has to be at least 80% of the size of the area A1 for safe subcutaneous stimulation (minimal tissue damage and electrode corrosion). T is the pulse duration, IPI is the interpulse interval, and the height of a shaded square is the amplitude of the pulse (current intensity).

the extent of irreversibility of the reactions. Balanced charge stimuli are generally used in which equal charge is delivered in each half-cycle. Some degree of imbalance may be allowed, but this issue is still being studied.

Both electrodes receive a pulse of each polarity (Figure 28.8). By convention, the electrode that receives the negative stimulus pulse first is called the cathode. During the cathodic phase (assuming a monopolar configuration) the charge is delivered first to the active (working) electrode, which is near the depolarization site. This is important in order to minimize the risk of possible tissue damage. The anodic pulse is then applied after a short interphase delay following the cathodic pulse.

This second pulse will allow the action potential to fully develop on the nerve since immediate current reversal may stop the firing of a nerve fiber, which is just at its threshold. This prevents the electrode potential developed on the working electrode from corroding due to the application of excessive anodic potentials. The cathodic pulse does not contribute to the corrosion of the electrode. For example, using non-noble i.m. electrodes, the cathodic amplitude may be 20 to 40 times greater than the anodic phase.

The surface area of the electrode is important in defining the safety of the stimulation. The geometric surface area may be many times less than the real surface area, depending upon the surface structure of the stimulating electrodes. Large surface areas will diffuse the current and may not affect the excitation desired. A small surface area may result in a high charge density and current density. When selecting an electrode, one must know these values in order to assess the safety of the stimulation. Although absolute safe levels of stimulation have not been established for all electrode types and all stimulus waveforms, the values presented by Grill and Mortimer (2000) provide the investigator with estimated safe levels for neural stimulation. With i.m. electrodes, safe stimulation is demonstrated at a charge density of 2.0 μC/mm^2 in the cathodic phase using balanced biphasic monopolar stimulation with a current-regulated stimulus with a capacitively coupled recharge phase (Grill and Mortimer, 2000).

Either amplitude modulation (AM) or pulse width (duration) modulation (PWM) may govern the level of recruitment. A comparison of the method of recruitment modulation to be selected should include consideration of recruitment linearity, charge injected (for safety reasons), and ease of implementation and control of the circuitry that generates the stimulus pulses. This comparison has been made for intramuscular (i.m.) electrodes. The results showed that, in consideration of recruitment, the differences between AM and PWM were small. PWM utilized a slightly lower charge density than AM to evoke a response of equal magnitude, a result that has been theoretically confirmed. Since timing circuits (i.e., regulating pulse width) can be easily constructed and controlled with a resolution of 1 μsec or less, many designers of stimulator use this technique.

As shown in the amplitude-duration (I-T) curve (Figure 28.2) relatively short stimulus rectangular pulses result in the muscle nerve being excited. Much larger charge is required to stimulate the muscle directly. Therefore, FES utilizes short pulses, generally less than 200 μsec, resulting in the activation of the nerve.

The threshold for excitation of the fibers of a peripheral nerve is proportional to the diameter of the fiber. Since the nerve is composed of a mixture of afferent and efferent fibers with a spectrum of fiber diameters, short pulses of constant amplitude will excite large afferent and efferent fibers. Longer pulses may also excite smaller fibers, including afferents normally carrying information of noxious stimuli, and therefore may be painful to the subject. For this reason and in order to minimize the electrical charge injection, short pulse duration is preferred.

In a physiological contraction, the recruitment order is fixed; slow, fatigue-resistant motor units are active at a lower voluntary effort than larger, fast, fatigable units. In an electrically induced recruitment, the recruitment order is not known *a priori*, but depends upon the variables of position and geometry as well as fiber size. An inverse order of electrically induced recruitment is typical when applying FES; the largest fibers are being easily excited, compared with small fibers. This implies that the recruitment has to be considered at all times in order to provide controlled and graded externally induced activation. The recruitment of nerve fibers with increasing stimulus pulse amplitude or duration is nonlinear as shown in Figure 28.9. For this reason, a linear increase of muscle output force cannot be achieved by a linear change in the input. The selection of the most effective parameter for regulation of recruitment has been studied by many (e.g., Bajzek and Jaeger, 1987; Baratta et al., 1989; Baratta and Solomonow, 1990; Crago et al., 1974, 1980; Popović et al., 1991).

The second mechanism affecting the overall force developed by the muscle is temporal summation. Stimulus pulses applied in rapid succession to the nerve will produce a mechanically additive effect of the twitch response. At low frequencies the response is unfused, and variations of the muscle force are noticeable. As the mechanical responses sum with increasing frequency, the force variability ceases, and the force increases (Figure 28.10).

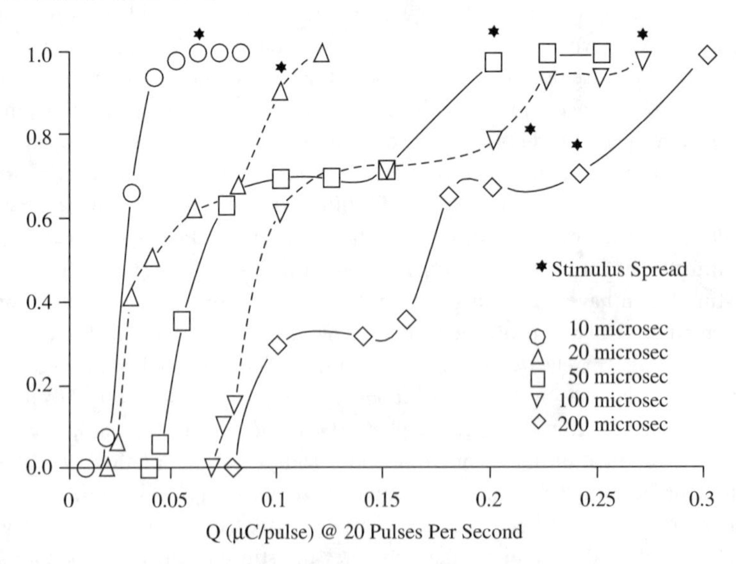

FIGURE 28.9 An example of a so-called recruitment curve, that is, the relation between the stimulation strength and the force. This example shows the recordings of the force developed in *Medial Gastrocnemius m.* of a cat when the stimulation strength was varied. Intramuscular electrodes were used in this experiment. Shorter pulses required less charge to elicit a force, but the recruitment range was very steep (narrow range for control of the force). Longer pulses were less effective and produced sharply expressed nonlinear effects (multistep raising of the force). The best-suited stimulation strength can be accomplished by varying the pulse duration between 50 and 150 μs.

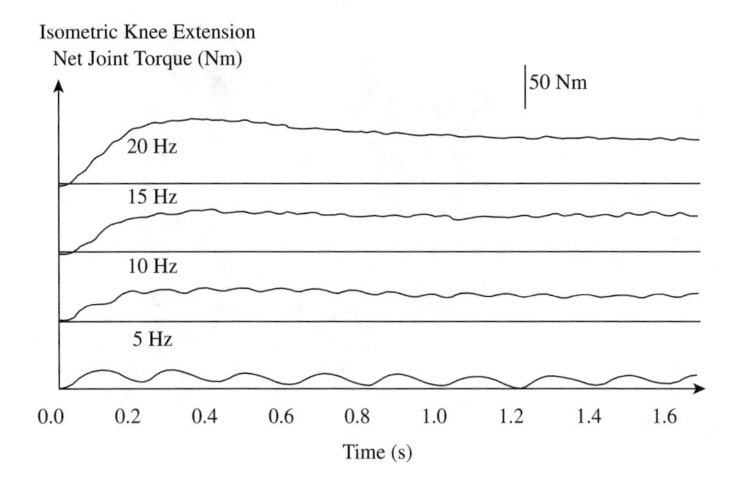

FIGURE 28.10 The schema of the change of the externally elicited force vs. the stimulation frequency. The presented example is from measurements of the isometric knee extension net joint torque in a paraplegic subject (spinal cord injury at the level T8) elicited by stimulating *Quadriceps m.* with surface electrodes. The stimulation parameters were pulse duration T = 300 μsec and current intensity I = 100 mA.

The frequency at which the mechanical responses produced are sufficiently smooth is known as fusion frequency. At this frequency sufficient smoothness of muscle force is expected. The point at which fusion is achieved depends upon the speed of contraction of the activated muscle fibers, and therefore ultimately upon the level of recruitment. In most human upper extremity muscles, the fusion occurs at less then 20 Hz. Increasing the stimulus frequency above the fusion frequency to the level of tetanus results in a further increase in force. Up to 40 or 50% of the maximum muscle force may be regulated by temporal summation from fusion to tetanus. Temporal summation leads to temporal modulation being inversely proportional with the frequency (f) of stimulation. In order to grade the force, the muscle temporal modulation of the interpulse interval (IPI = 1/f) or a combination of recruitment and temporal modulation can be selected.

28.4 Instrumentation for FES

A functional diagram of the FES system (Figure 28.11) shows the main components of a neural prosthesis: (1) electrodes, (2) stimulator, (3) sensors, (4) command interface, and (5) controller.

28.4.1 Electrodes

Surface electrodes (e.g., Bowman and Baker, 1985) are placed on the skin surface over the area where the stimulus is to be delivered. McNeal and Baker (1988) and McNeal and Reswick (1976) defined the criteria for surface electrodes: low impedance and even distribution of current, flexibility to maintain

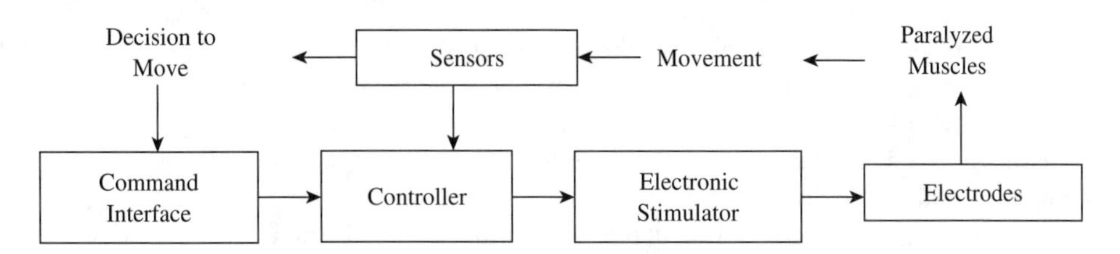

FIGURE 28.11 Components for an FES system: command interface, control system, controller, electronic stimulator, electrodes, and sensors. Decision to move is at the voluntary level of the user. The arrow from sensors to the decision to move indicates possible biofeedback.

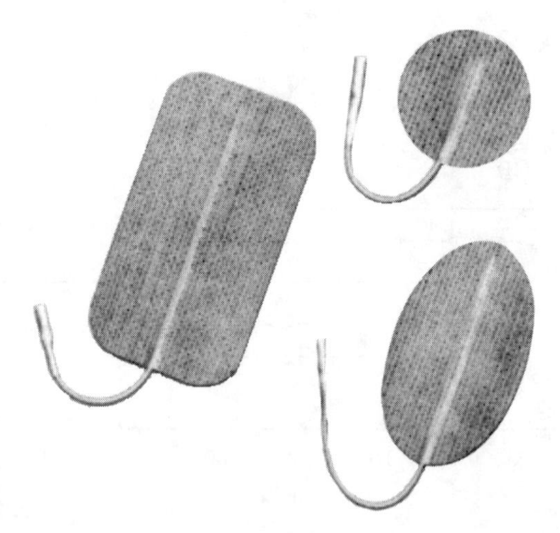

FIGURE 28.12 An example of surface electrodes made as multilayer structure. These electrodes can be used in the same subject for several times during a period of about 2 weeks. The electrodes can be moisturized for better contact if they start drying up; this will decrease the impedance (capacitance). The bottom (skin side) layer is a polymer with strong adhesive properties that sticks to the skin, the middle is a conductive layer (metal) connected with the lead, and the top (external) layer is the isolating material. The construction provides an interface with the evenly distributed current density over the surface of the electrode. The electrodes are flexible and manufactures in different sizes (e.g., small circular electrodes D = 2.5 cm, small square electrodes a = 4 cm, big rectangular electrodes a × b = 8 cm × 12 cm).

good skin contact, ease of application and removal, and suitable mounting for days without irritation of the skin. A surface electrode has three elements: the conductor, the interfacial layer, and the adhesive. The earliest electrodes used metal plates for the conductor, gel- or saline-saturated fabric for the interfacial layer, and tape or circumferential bands for maintaining position. Substantial improvements of these electrodes have been directed toward resolving some of the problems, such as drying of the conductor, difficulties in application, and maintaining position and good electrical contact of the entire electrode surface, especially on the skin surfaces with a large radius of curvature (back and abdomen). Usage of conductive polymer and conductive adhesives proved to be effective for clinical and home usage. Surface electrodes for most applications have a rather large surface area of 5 cm^2 or more (Figure 28.12).

The stimulus parameters required for activation by using surface electrodes depend on the stimulus waveform, the surface area, electrode materials, placement, skin impedance, and other factors. Typically, for the rectangular pulsatile waveform frequently used, threshold values are 30 mA or greater for a pulse width of 100 to 300 μsec. Stimulus pulses shorter than the 50 μsec cause a stronger, unpleasant sensation (pain), and thus are not used. The frequency of stimulation depends on the application but it is typically between 16 and 50 pulses per second.

The primary limitation encountered with surface electrodes is that small muscles generally cannot be selectively activated, and deep muscle cannot be activated without first exciting muscles that are more superficial. Furthermore, fine gradation of force can be difficult because relative movement between the electrode and muscle will alter the stimulation-force relationship. Physical movement of the electrode can cause such movement, from length changes in the muscle induced by the contraction process, or from internal change in the nerve-electrode geometry during isometric contraction. The pain is definitely a limiting factor in applying surface electrodes in subjects with preserved sensory and diminished motor functions.

Subcutaneous (s.c.) electrodes can be divided into those in which the electrode is secured to the muscle exciting the motorneurons, and those that contact the nerve that contains the motoneurons. The advantages of s.c. electrodes vs. surface electrodes are better selectivity, repeatable excitation, and permanent positioning. The sensation to the users is much more comfortable because the electrodes are placed away from the pain receptors, and the current amplitude is much lower. The potential disadvantage of implanted electrode is the damage that can result from improper design and implantation (e.g., irreversible deleterious effects to the neural tissue, physical failure of an electrode requiring an invasive revision procedure).

The mechanisms of failure of s.c. electrodes may be separated into three categories: physiological, biological, or physical (Mortimer, 1981; Scheiner et al., 1990). The biological failures include those mechanically induced at surgical installation, excess encapsulation, infection or rejection, and those induced with stimulation (Mortimer, 1981). The physical failures are those of the conductor, such as electrochemical degradation or mechanical failures (breakage), and of the insulator. Categorization of electrode failure requires, if possible, identification of the failure mechanisms to at least this level (Scheiner et al., 1990; Smith et al., 1994).

Subcutaneous electrodes that are secured to the muscle include two types: the i.m. electrode (Bowman and Erickson, 1985; Handa et al., 1989a; Smith et al., 1994), which can be injected using a hypodermic needle either nonsurgically through the closed skin or through an open incision, and the epimysial electrode (Grandjean and Mortimer, 1986), which is fixed to the muscle surface and must be placed surgically. The i.m. electrode is a helical coil fabricated from a multiple-strand wire (Figure 28.13). Such a configuration provides a structure that is able to sustain multiple flexions without fracture. Generally, non-noble alloys are employed (e.g., type 316L stainless steel) and wire insulation is Teflon. A hook formed at the end of the coil keeps the electrode from being pressed out of the needle during insertion and assists in securing the electrode when the needle is withdrawn (Figure 28.13).

The i.m. electrode is used as the cathode electrode in a monopolar configuration with a surface electrode as the indifferent (anode) electrode. The i.m. electrode is implanted, using the hypodermic needle as the carrier, into a site near a motor point of the target muscle. Stimulation applied through the needle shaft assists in identifying the position of the needle tip. Positioning of the electrode within an individual muscle can be achieved in 80% of the injections by an experienced investigator, although the absolute position will vary somewhat from one injection to the next in the same muscle.

Placement of multiple i.m. electrodes within a single muscle enables one to employ sequential stimulation techniques on rather small muscles, since the extent of recruitment can be quite focused and restricted.

Electrodes are either inserted directly through the skin with the needle (the target muscle is near the skin interface), or implanted and tunneled subcutaneously (the target muscles extend distances of 15 cm from the skin interface). Intramuscular electrodes generally elicit a maximal muscular contraction with a 20-mA, 200-μsec stimulus. This is on the order of 10% of the stimulus charge required by surface electrodes. The impedance of the i.m. electrode is typically 300 Ω, but the entire load impedance of tissue and surface anode may be as high as 1.5 kΩ. The probability of functional operation of i.m. electrodes in the upper extremity is 80% after one year. Of the failures, one third are physical failures. In the case of a fracture, the broken segment will remain in place and the external segment will be withdrawn. Two thirds of failures are due to an altered physiological response, believed to be caused by a physical

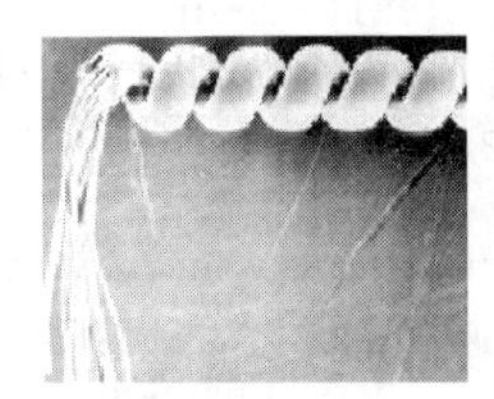
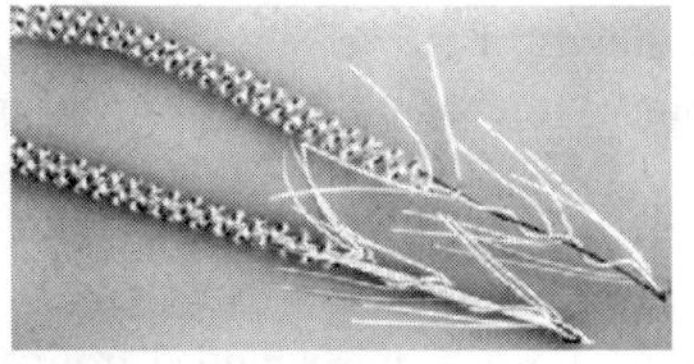

FIGURE 28.13 Two different types of i.m. electrodes. The left panel shows an electrode made of multistranded stainless steel and Teflon insulated. The electrode is coiled, and the tip of electrode is bared from the insulation. The right panel shows the Peterson-type electrodes with the core (surgical thread) for minimizing the breakage of the electrodes. The multistranded Teflon-insulated stainless steel wire is rapped around the core. The tip of the electrode shows the wires when the insulation was taken off.

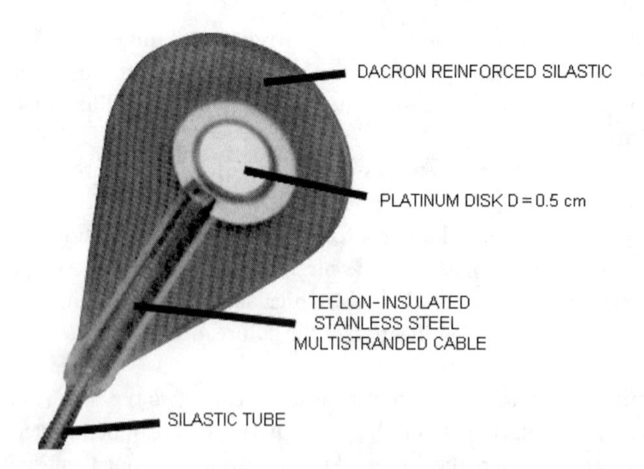

FIGURE 28.14 An example of the epimysial electrode. The electrode is made out of platinum (disk with the diameter of 0.5 cm) that is welded to the stainless steel wire. The stainless steel wire is Teflon insulated and pulled through a silastic tube filled with silastic, thereby eliminating air bubbles in the tube. The electrode is surgically positioned at the surface of the muscle and sutured to the fascia by using the Dacron-reinforced silastic material surrounding the metal contact.

displacement of the electrode, and present modifications on electrode design are under way to correct both problems.

The primary disadvantage of percutaneous electrodes is the maintenance of the skin interface, yet reports show that only few infections occurred in implantation of over 2000 electrodes, some implanted for more than 5 years (Peckham, 1988). Granulomas at the skin interface are infrequent, but they are treated with local cauterization. The advantage of percutaneous (i.m.) electrodes over surface electrodes is that they provide a means of eliciting focused, repeatable responses over time with a nonsurgical technique.

The epimysial electrode (e.g., Grandjean and Mortimer, 1986) is a disk-shaped metal with a reinforced polymer for shielding the surface away from the muscle and for suturing to the muscle (Figure 28.14). The electrode is surgically placed on the muscle near the motor point. The conductive surface of the disk is 3 mm in diameter. In contrast to the i.m. electrode where the placement is surgical and small size is not so essential, the lead may have a more mechanical redundancy than the i.m. lead.

The impedance and physiologic characteristics of stimulation over this electrode are also similar to the i.m. electrode. That is, the recruitment is nonlinear with either pulse-amplitude or pulse-width modulation and may be approximated by piecewise linear segments. The recruitment may also be length dependent, meaning that the force output changes with muscle length due to changes in the electrode to nerve coupling. This is in addition to the length-tension properties of the muscle.

Another type of surgically placed electrodes are nerve electrodes. Nerve electrodes have the potential for producing the most desired physiological response (Sweeney and Mortimer, 1986; Naples et al., 1988; Rutten et al., 1991; Sweeney et al., 1990; Loeb and Peck, 1996). The electrode must be designed with an appreciation for the sensitivity of the nerve to mechanical trauma, manifest by swelling, its longitudinal mobility during muscle movement, and the necessity of maintaining a constant orientation between the nerve fibers and the electrode.

The nerve electrodes are characterized by their placement relative to the nerve: encircling or intraneural. Cuff electrodes encircle the nerve; they have either a tube or a spiral configuration (Figure 28.15). The latter is a loose, open helix, which is wrapped around the nerve in a monopolar configuration. Cuff electrodes come in a variety of configurations; they all have a longitudinal opening to allow installation on the nerve without damaging it. The cuff is formed of a polymer (usually silicone rubber or recently polyamide), sometimes reinforced with Dacron. The electrodes within the cuff are made out of metal, usually being circumferential around the inner surface of the cuff. A self-wrapping cuff (Naples et al., 1988) uses the same materials, yet it is self-sized, thus eliminating the problem of selecting the appropriate

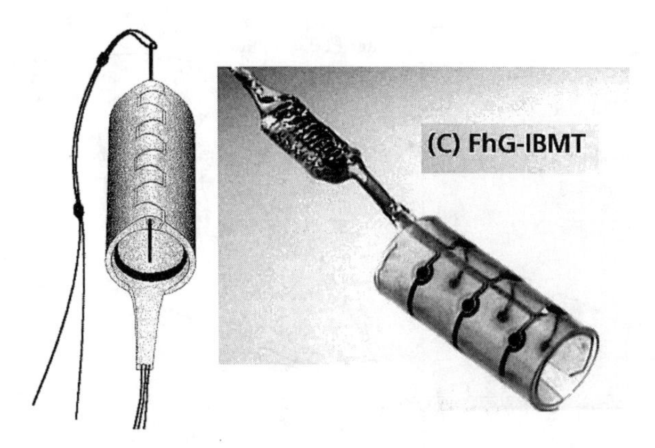

FIGURE 28.15 The sketch representation of the cuff (around the nerve) electrodes (left) and the newly designed 12-contact circular cuff electrode (with a longitudinal slit) for selective stimulation with a four-channel stimulator. In order to minimize contamination of the neural signal from the surrounding biological signals the electrodes must fit tightly around the nerve and be well closed. An electrode can be closed with the flap covering the longitudinal slip, and kept in position by means of the surgical threads around the cuff (right side), and it can be closed by using a "zipper" method where the ends of the cuff have little holes and the plastic baton can be pulled through the holes. (Left side) The novel self-wrapping polyamide multipolar electrode for selective recording/stimulation of the whole nerve (C). (Courtesy of T. Stieglitz, Fraunhofer Institute, St Ingbert, Germany, 2000.)

size. Both cuff and spiral electrode configurations may be used in various monopolar, bipolar, or tripolar configurations (Sweeney and Mortimer, 1986; Naples et al., 1988).

With the choice of the proper geometric relationship between the nerve and electrode and the configuration, it is possible to restrict the direction of current flow and generate action potentials that propagate unidirectionally along the nerve. Encircling cuff electrodes typically require one tenth the charge required with muscle (i.m. or epimysial) electrodes, with maximal responses elicited with stimulus amplitudes on the order of 2 mA and pulse widths of 300 μsec. The recruitment gain is often higher compared with the i.m. electrodes, and similar nonlinearities are encountered.

Today the design of new cuff electrodes is oriented toward selective stimulation, that is, possible steered stimulation of various fascicles within the same large nerve (Sweeney et al., 1995; Veraart et al., 1993). Figure 28.15 shows the multipolar cuff electrode for selective stimulation of nerves. Experiments have been done with a tripolar electrode (12 contacts) and monopolar (4 contacts) cuff electrodes and a four-channel stimulator (Figure 28.16). It has been shown that by using "intelligent" control it is possible to stimulate several muscles by activating corresponding fascicles within a sciatic nerve of a cat (Qi et al., 1999) and peripheral nerve of humans (Popović and Sinkjær, 2000).

Intraneural electrodes utilize a conductor that invades the epineurium. Many studies have been done with intraneural electrodes. There is sufficient evidence that maximal contraction is elicited at stimulation levels an order of magnitude lower than with nerve cuff electrodes (200 μA, pulse duration 300 μsec). The variations of such a design would be a valuable clinical tool, yet the connectors, fixation, and neural damage are still not resolved to allow clinical usage.

In order to maximize the usage of the preserved neural networks after the injury of CNS it could be effective to stimulate higher CNS structures, rather than to directly activate the last-order motoneurons. There is evidence in humans that the neural circuitry of the spinal cord is capable of generating complex behaviors with coordinated muscle activity (Dimitrijević, 1998). This method is currently receiving more attention (Mushahwar and Horch, 1997, 2000). Clinical applications in the motor system include stimulation of the sacral anterior roots for bladder function (Brindley et al., 1986; Davis et al., 1997; Rushton, 1990). The behaviors that can be mediated by the isolated spinal cord include reaching-like limb movements (Lemay and Grill, 1999), standing, and walking (Barbeau et al., 1999). Spinal circuits can be activated by epidural and intraspinal electrical stimulation (Veraart et al., 1993). Two methods are equally appealing: intraspinal microstimulation enables direct activation

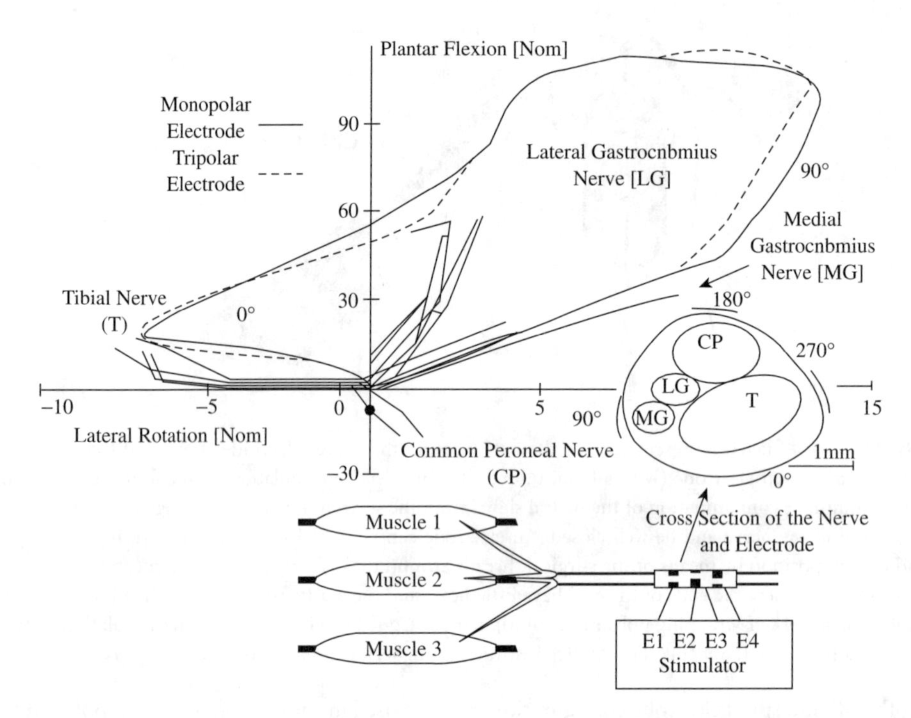

FIGURE 28.16 Selective activation of four fascicles with a four-polar cuff electrode positioned around the sciatic nerve of a cat. Appropriate voltages applied to four polls result with desired activation; thus, a single cuff and four-channel stimulator can control the activity of several muscles.

of spinal neurons, and afferent input makes synaptic contacts on spinal neurons, and thus also could be used for stimulation of CNS.

A new interface to stimulate spinal cord neurons has been developed: microwires finer than a human hair have been tested in animal experiments (Mushahwar and Horch, 1997). The microwires were implanted in the spinal cord of animals (Figure 28.17). The implants caused no pain or discomfort,

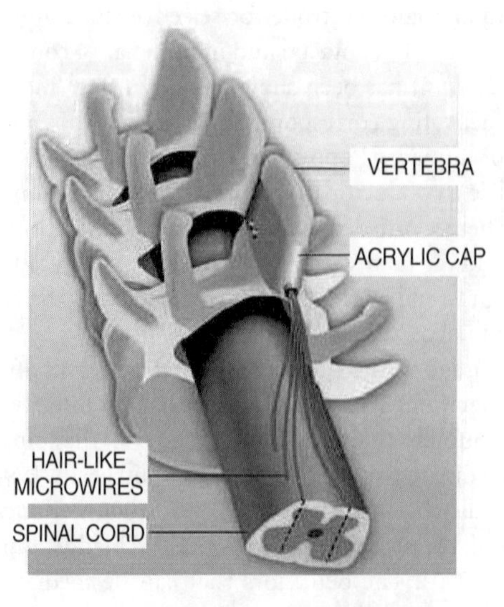

FIGURE 28.17 The schema of using very fine metal wires to directly microstimulate the spinal cord, thereby activating movement. See text for further explanation. (Courtesy of Prof. Dr. Arthur Prochazka, University of Alberta, Edmonton, Canada, 2000.)

and the motor activity remained normal, indicating that the wires had not damaged the spinal cord. When trains of electrical micropulses were delivered through the microwires, the stimuli were not perceived, yet strong coordinated limb movements were produced, sufficient to support body weight. This indicates that spinal cord microstimulation could generate useful movement in people with paraplegia or tetraplegia.

28.4.2 Electronic Stimulators

An electronic stimulator for FES application has to be a self-contained device with a low power consumption, small, light, and must have the simplest possible user interface (Bijak et al., 1999; Brindley et al., 1978; Buckett et al., 1988; Donaldson, 1986; Ilić et al., 1994; James et al., 1991; Minzly et al., 1993; Smith et al., 1987; Thrope et al., 1985; Bogataj et al., 1989). The stimulator should be programmable, and the programming should be done wireless, although using wires is acceptable. The stimulator needs a set-up mode; mode of programming when communicating with the host computer. Once the programming is finished, the stimulator should be turned to the autonomous mode.

An electronic stimulator must have the following elements: power source or communication link to a remote unit that delivers energy for operation, DC/DC converter, output stage that generates current-regulated or voltage-regulated pulses, and the controller that defines the shape, intensity, and frequency of pulses (Ilić et al., 1994). The DC/DC is a system that generates the needed high voltage for stimulation. In some cases the required voltage must be as high as 300 V, yet in others it is within 10 V. The output stages are parts that secure that the pulse applied will be effective, yet not harmful.

Implantable stimulators for FES may be separated into single- or multichannel devices. Single-channel implants, which have been fabricated, are all radio frequency powered and controlled devices (Figure 28.18). They use relatively few discrete components and have a receiving antenna, which is integrated into the circuitry. The packaging materials are epoxy or glass-ceramic. The most common single-channel configuration is one in which lead wires are used to place the electrode away from the site of the receiver

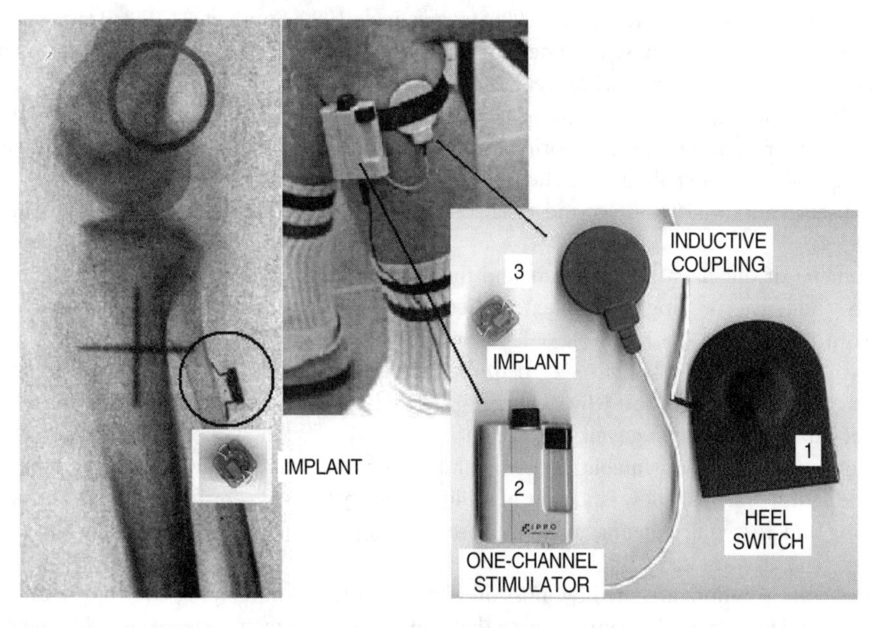

FIGURE 28.18 The single-channel implantable system for correcting foot-drop. Left panel shows the xerogram showing the implant in place. Right panel shows the shoe insole-based heel-switch (1) for triggering of the stimulation (heel-off), external stimulator (2) powered by one AA battery and connected to the RF transmission coil, and the implant (3). The middle panel shows the transmitting coil and stimulator positioned on the patient. The wire going down from the stimulator connects to the heel-switch.

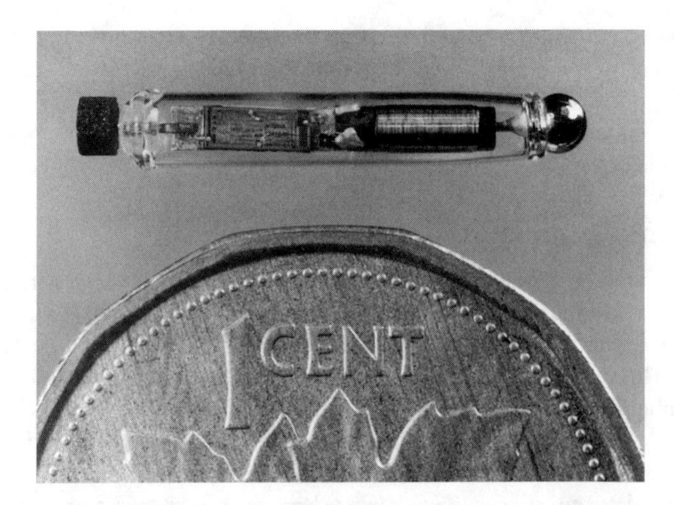

FIGURE 28.19 BION — the microstimulator with anodized Tantalum (left) and Iridium surface-activated ball (right) electrodes. The electronic circuitry is hermetically sealed with glass beads in the glass capillary tube (length 13 mm, diameter 2 mm). (Courtesy of Prof. Dr. Gerald E. Loeb, University of Southern California, Los Angeles, 1996.)

unit. Avery and Medtronics employed this design for neuromuscular applications in commercially available devices many years ago.

Alternatively, the electrodes may be an integral part of the packaging of the circuitry, allowing the entire device to be placed adjacent to the nerve such as it is in the Ljubljana-designed implantable foot-drop system (Strojnik et al., 1987).

Two alternative schemes have been considered for multimuscle excitation. It is possible, in principle, to use several one-channel units that are controlled from one controller (Cameron et al., 1997; Strojnik et al., 1987), or to use a single implantable stimulator that will connect with multiple electrodes (Holle et al., 1984; Thoma et al., 1978; Rushton, 1990; Strojnik et al., 1990; Smith et al., 1996; Davis et al., 1997).

The single channel devices have been developed originally for foot-drop correction and implanted in many subjects with positive experience, yet the development was continued in a different direction, i.e., toward multichannel stimulators (Strojnik et al., 1990, 1993). The wireless single-channel stimulator has been developed for extensive use in restoring motor functions, and up to now animal experiments show great promises (Cameron et al., 1997). The BION, single channel wireless stimulator is sealed with glass beads and uses an anodized Tantalum and surface activated Iridium electrodes to minimize tissue damage (Figure 28.19).

The diameter of the glass tube is 2 mm, and the length of the whole device is 13 mm. The BION is powered by inductive coupling from an external coil at 2 MHz. A total of 256 units can be driven from a single control based on the Motorola 68HC11 microcomputer. The pulse width control is from 3 to 258 sec with the increment of only 1 sec, the pulse amplitude control from 0.2 to 30 mA in two ranges of 15 linear steps. The stimulator delivers charge-balanced monophasic pulses, allowing for selection of a square of exponential discharge tail.

The problem with all implantable devices without batteries, which require a lot of power to drive sensory and motor systems, is low efficiency of radio frequency transmission. In order to transmit energy, the emitting and receiving antenna must be close and aligned; this is very difficult if a stimulator is injected into a deep muscle.

The alternative solution, accepted by most other research teams developing electronic stimulators, is a miniature, implantable, multichannel device that will excite as many muscles as needed. The difficulty is that such a stimulator will be remote from the stimulation points; therefore, connectors and leads have to be used between the stimulator and stimulation points.

The use of long leads should be eliminated after the technique of selective nerve stimulation, including potential stimulation of the spinal cord directly, or spinal roots is perfected. The experiments conducted

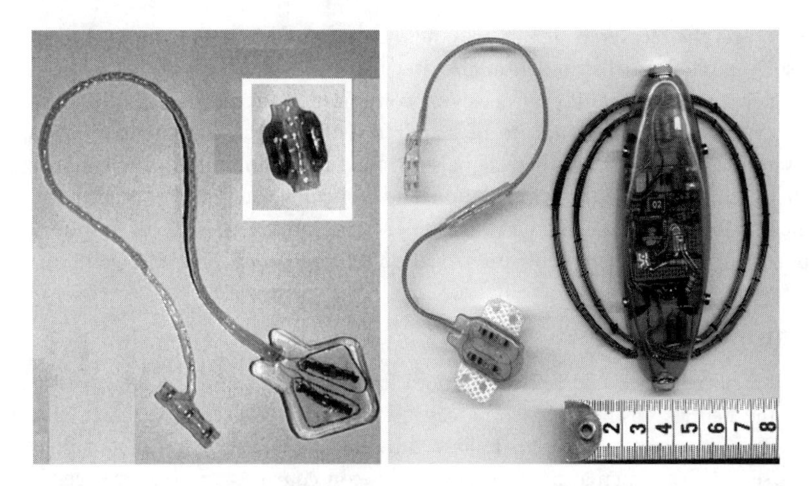

FIGURE 28.20 Two types of fully implantable cuff-electrode-based stimulators under development. Stimulators include the multipolar neural interface and electronic circuitry for energy and control signals communication. (Courtesy of Dr. Morten Haugland, Aalborg University, Denmark, 2002.)

at Aalborg University with the two-channel fully implanted RF-driven stimulators (Haugland et al., 1999) integrated in the cuff electrode (Figure 28.20) suggest that this is a viable technique. Selective activation of different muscle groups has been achieved in a sitting and walking subject.

The stimulation-telemetry system described by Smith et al. (1998) is an example of state-of-the-art technology (Figure 28.29). The device can be configured with the following functions: (1) up to 32 independent channels of stimulation for activation of muscles (or sensory feedback), with independent control of stimulus pulse interval, pulse duration, pulse amplitude, interphase delay (for biphasic stimulus waveform), and recharge phase duration (for biphasic stimulus waveform); (2) up to eight independent telemetry channels for sensors, with independent control of sampling rate and pulse powering parameters of the sensor (power amplitude and duration); (3) up to eight independent telemetry channels for processed (rectified and integrated) signals measured from muscles or nerves (EMG or ENG), with independent control of the sampling rate and provisions for stimulus artifact blanking and processing control; (4) up to eight independent telemetry channels for unprocessed MES channels, with independent control of sampling rate; and (5) up to eight independent telemetry channels for system functions, providing control or sampling of internal system parameters, such as internal voltage levels.

Due to overall timing constraints, implant circuit size, implant capsule size, number of lead wires, circuit and sensor power consumption, and external control and processing requirements, it is not practical to realize a single device having the maximal capabilities outlined above. However, the intent of the stimulator-telemeter system is to provide the means of realizing an optimal implantable device having all the necessary circuitry and packaging to meet the anticipated clinical applications, without requiring design or engineering effort beyond that of fabricating the device itself. For example, a basic upper extremity application would require, minimally, eight channels of stimulation for providing palmar and lateral grasp and sensory feedback, along with one joint angle transducer as a command control source.

The stimulation-telemetry implant device comprises an electronic circuit that is hermetically sealed in a titanium capsule with feedthroughs. A single internal radio frequency (RF) coil provides transcutaneous reception of power and bidirectional communication. The lead wires connected to the feed-through holes extend to the stimulating electrodes, to the implanted sensors, or to the recording electrodes. The later two connections are used as control input. The circuit capsule, coil, and lead wire exits are conformably coated in epoxy and silicone elastomer to provide physical support for the feedthroughs and RF coil, and stress relief to the leads making it suitable for long-term implantation.

The functional elements required to realize the system include the following: (1) an RF receiver for recovering power and functional commands transmitted from an external control unit; (2) control logic circuitry to interpret the recovered signals, execute the command function, and to supervise functional circuit blocks; (3) multichannel stimulation circuitry for generating the stimulus pulses that are sent to the stimulating electrodes; (4) multichannel signal conditioning circuitry which provides amplification, filtering, and processing for the signals to be acquired (MES and sensor signals); (5) data acquisition circuitry for sampling and digitizing these signals; (6) modulation circuitry for telemetring the acquired data through the RF link; (7) power regulation and switching circuitry for selectively powering the included functional blocks of the circuitry, as needed, to minimize power consumption of the device; and (8) system control circuitry to allow interrogation or configuration of the operation of the device.

28.4.3 Sensors

Sensors for NP applications should provide to both the system and the user information regarding the conditions of the neural prosthesis. In some cases, it is not obvious that the user does need instant information (e.g., if automatic execution follows the desired trajectory), yet if anything unexpected is happening, the sensory warning may prevent catastrophic consequences. Sensors are needed in FES systems for the command interface (e.g., activating the neural prosthesis, changing the mode of operation).

The sensory system to be used should provide information of various kinds, such as the contact force or pressure over the area of contact (grasping, standing, and walking), the position of the joints (prehension, reaching, standing, and walking), and perhaps the activity of the muscle. The dynamic range, resolution, and frequency response of sensors must be determined upon the application. For example, force sensors for walking and standing must withstand several times body weight under dynamic loading and joint position sensors must allow unrestrained movement over the entire range of motion of the joint (Figure 28.21).

The constraints imposed on the sensors for FES systems are significant; they must be cosmetically acceptable and easy to mount, they should be self-contained, have low power consumption, and must provide adequate information. In most available FES systems sensors are placed externally. The sensor positioned at the surface of the body is not a suitable solution for many situations (e.g., an external-force sensor on the digits of the hand requires donning and needs a cable to communicate with the control box, and it should work in variable temperature conditions and hazardous environment). The alternative is to use implanted sensors. They have to meet the same performance specifications while functioning in a more hostile environment. These sensors should communicate with the remote control box, and the device must be powered via radio frequency (RF) link. The ultimate solution is to use available sensor in the organism; to record from nerves and muscles and process the information in a real-time useful signal. This solution requires the ability to interface without the nerves and interpret the signals they are supplying to the central nervous system.

28.4.3.1 Artificial Sensors for Neural Prostheses

In order to control the position of the extremity, it is of interest to know the joint angles and joint angular velocities, and if in contact with the environment, the contact forces. The most commonly used sensors for measuring joint angles are potentiometers. However, joint angle can be effectively measured with optocouplers, optical fibers, strain gages, Hall-effect transducers, and magneto-transistors as well as many other transducers.

The field-effect transistor (FET) is a micro-miniature electronic device in which the current amplification depends on the applied voltages. In principle, the FET transistor has three zones, source, gate, and drain; the width of the gate determines the gain of the transistor. The arrays of FET devices mounted on specially designed support rely on the change of the gate width provoked by force. This device is able to measure microstrains and displacements in parallel with measuring of finite displacements. A single FET could record small displacements; multiple devices built in a single semiconductor support are convenient for measuring bigger displacements.

The piezoresistive sensors are very frequently used in recording of displacements, forces, and pressures. The most frequently used sensors are strain gauges, yet they are often unsuitable for neuroprosthetics

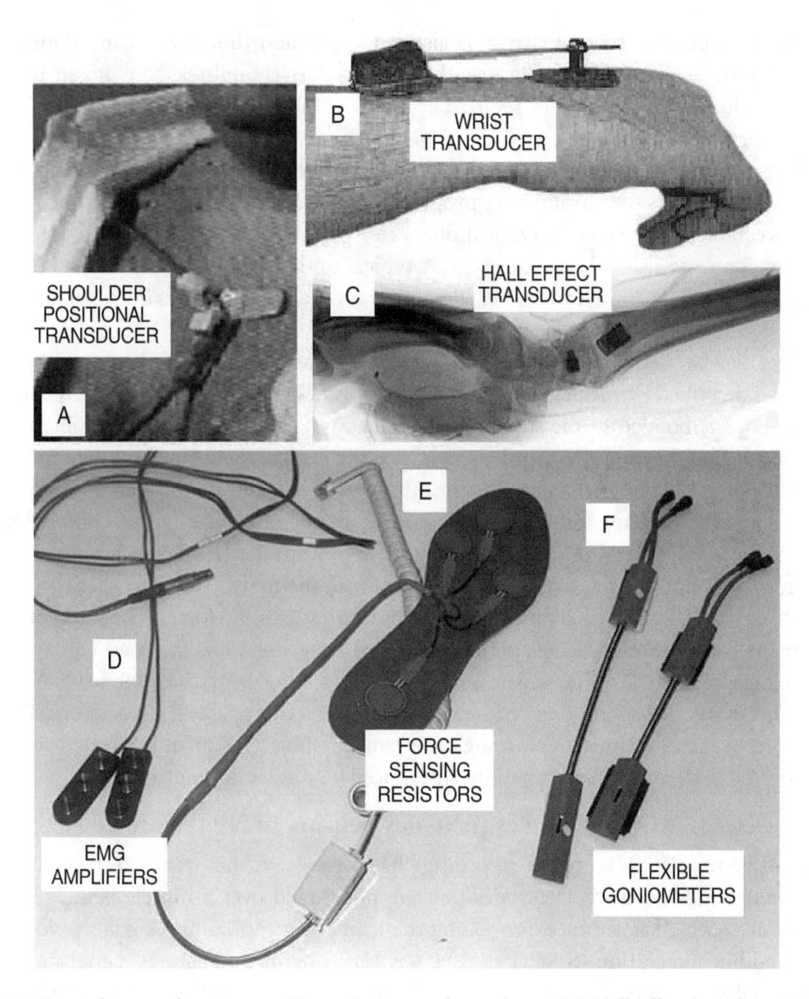

FIGURE 28.21 Several types of sensors used in various neural prostheses. (A) Hall-effect-based position transducer for volitional generation of commands; (B) wrist position sensor for measuring wrist movement; (C) implantable version of the Hall-effect transducer for measuring wrist movement; (D) EMG electrodes and preamplifier for EMG feedback; (E) force sensing resistors built into an insole for measuring the ground reaction forces and pressures; (F) flexible goniometers (Penny and Giles, Blackwood, U.K.) for measuring joint angles. The later three are used in sampled data feedback and closed loop control schema.

because of the size, power consumption, and temperature variability. The use of polymer elastomer is effective for recordings of the forces and pressures. The elastomers can be stretched or compressed appreciably, but they return to their original shapes after the stress is removed. The elastomers are made conductive by impregnating them with metal powders or carbon black. The electrical conductivity of elastomers using metal fillers is good, but elastomers exhibit nonuniformly large hysteresis, and poor tensile and compression properties. Moreover, it was found that the hardness of the rubber couldn't be made independent of the metallic loading for a given conductivity (Webster, 1988). Maalej and Webster (1988) have investigated the Interlink manufactured Force Sensing Resistors (FSRs) based on elastomer material. With the instrumentation capable of dealing with the hysteresis and nonlinearity, the sensor was suggested as a valuable asset for neuroprosthetics.

It is possible to use piezoelectric sensors in NP. The high level of piezoelectricity was obtained by polyvinylidene fluoride-based polymers. Polyvinylidene fluoride (PVF2) became a popular sensor (Dario et al., 1983). PVF2 films mechanically appear the same as a thin sheet of plastic. These films are flexible and durable. Their flexibility allows them to be manufactured in large thin sheets or complex shapes, depending on the application. The material is also very light and thin. PVF2 can be manufactured in thickness ranging from 6 to 2000 μm because the film is relatively unbreakable. It can be stretched up to 14% before yielding (Hausler et al., 1980). The PVF2 is highly temperature sensitive because of its pyroelectric properties.

Optical fibers can be used for measurements of displacements. The compactness, sensing ability, relative durability, and light-ray conducting properties make optical fibers good candidates for the use as miniature, wearable tactile sensors. Optical fibers can withstand tensions of up to 690 kPa. They are noise and corrosion resistant and very compact. A typical optic fiber sensor bundle is 1.3 to 3.2 mm in diameter and composed of individual fiber elements, each with an approximate diameter of 75 μm (Coulombe, 1984).

Optocouplers may be used in many different devices for measurements of force, pressure, and displacement. A load cell described by Maalej and Webster (1988) is designed for forces between 0 and 50 N. The light-emitting diode is bonded to the support in such a way that it is only partly visible from the phototransistor mounted at the same U shaped frame. Once the frame is loaded, then it bends; the amount of light falling to the phototransistor changes, and the output voltage at the phototransistor is highly correlated to the force loading the U-shape frame. The nonlinearity of such a device can be compensated with the adequate electronic circuitry, and the measurements are reproducible. The device has small hysteresis, the random error is small, and the thermal drift is only minimal; the drawback is low spatial resolution.

The capacitive changes can be used for measurements of pressures and forces. The series of multielement capacitive sensors was fabricated using specially designed capacitor films that had contacts at each end (Seow, 1988; Crago et al., 1986). The sensor is an array of 8×8 fields. Each of the fields has the capacity of only 5 pF. The small capacity imposes series problems coming from parasite capacitance. The sensor was designed for force feedback control in grasping of tetraplegic subjects with an implanted system.

The use of optical gyroscopes has been recently introduced for measuring joint angles and angular velocities.

28.4.3.2 Muscles (EMG) and Nerves (ENG) as Sensors in NP (Figure 28.22)

Signals that can be used for NP are the recordings from a muscle, that is, an electromyogram (EMG). The signals are recorded by using electrodes that are positioned over a muscle being able to generate EMG (Frigo et al., 2000). The simplest processing that can produce a control signal is the amplification, rectification, and bin-integration (Saxena et al., 1995). The obtained integrated signal can be compared with the preset value (threshold), and the results applied as a switch within a state machine (Saxena et al., 1995). A comparator with hysteresis works well enough eliminating the on-off bouncing because of the nonvoluntary variation of the processed EMG signal.

A multithreshold comparator can also be used (Figure 28.23, bottom), allowing the user to control in steps the selected function (e.g., strength of the grasp). The clinical results favor the simple, single-threshold systems because of the difficulties in tuning of the internal components, variability of EMG recordings, and even more because of the lack of feedback about the strength of the grip.

Scott et al. (1996) suggested the use of EMG recordings from *sternocleidomastoid m.* (SCM) to control a FES system for hand control of tetraplegic individuals. Surface electrodes were applied over the SCM muscles to record the EMG. The recording system includes a circuitry that is capable of blanking the stimulation artifacts (Knaflitz and Merletti, 1988). The control could be described as a three-state machine: (1) strong flexion of the SCM opens the hand, (2) weaker flexion closes the hand, and (3) no flexion (below the selected threshold) locks the grasp. This is to say that three levels of EMG recordings trigger the controller to activate the following programs: (1) increase the stimulation of the muscles that are contributing to the opening of the hand, (2) increase the stimulation of the muscles that are contributing to the closing of the hand, and (3) keep the activation of the muscles at the selected level. A laboratory version of the myoelectric control of a grasping system has been developed by the ParaCare group at the University of Zurich, Switzerland (Popović et al., 2000). The system controls grasping based on: (1) analogue EMG control that uses recordings from the deltoid muscle of the ipsilateral arm, and (2) discrete EMG control (i.e., digitally processed EMG based on the coded series of integrated, rectified, and compared with a threshold signal).

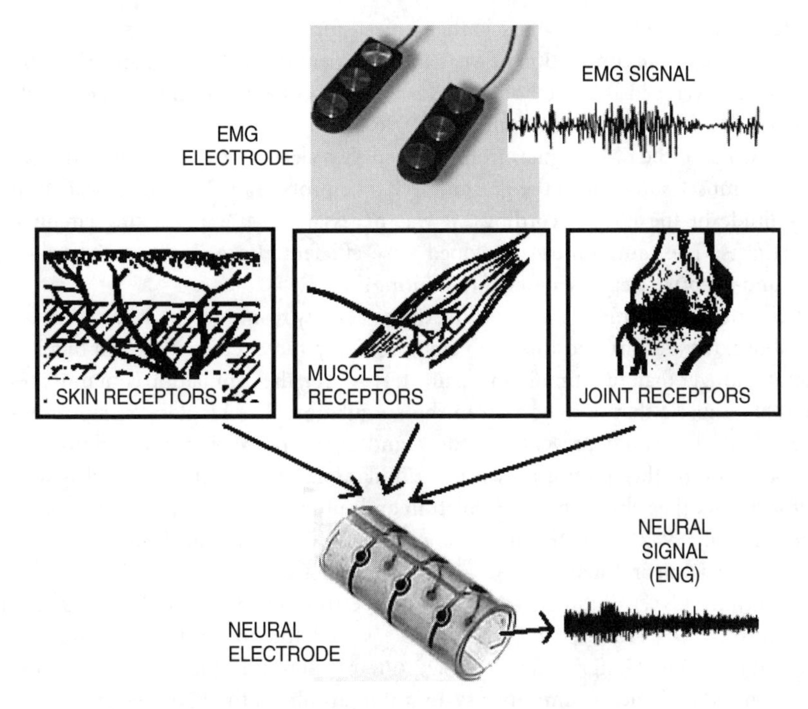

FIGURE 28.22 The principle of using natural sensors in neural prostheses. Most of the receptors (skin, muscle, joint) generate signals, although they are not connected to the appropriate centers in the CNS. These signals can be recorded with the adequate neural and muscle interface and used within implantable neural prostheses.

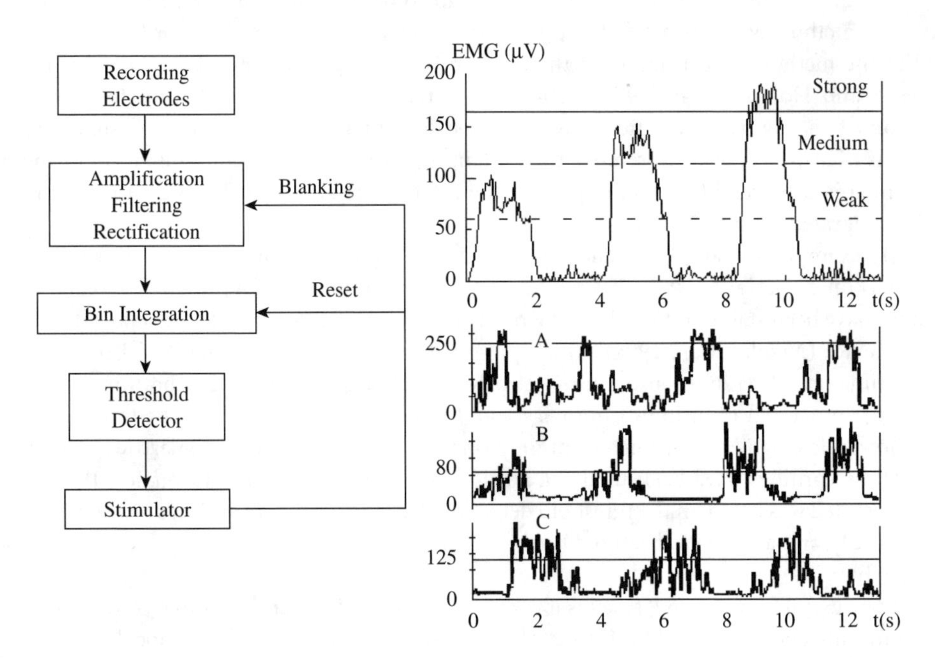

FIGURE 28.23 The flow-chart diagram of processing of EMG signals for a grasping neural prosthesis (left). The recordings (right panels) are from the wrist extensor in three tetraplegics (bottom panel: A, B, and C) during their contraction of the wrist extensors (the finger flexors were stimulated at 20 Hz). The right top panel shows the possible grading of the output based on three-threshold state control method. (Based on Saxena et al., 1995.)

It is possible to stimulate the same muscle that is used for control (Vossius et al., 1987). The aim of this method is to enhance the contraction of weak muscles. Sennels et al. (1997) and Thorsen et al. (1998, 1999) have further developed this method, and some therapeutic application of electrical stimulation benefit greatly (Francisco et al., 1998; Glanz et al., 1996).

Hart et al. (1998) used the EMG signals from three surface electrodes (bipolar recordings) placed over the wrist extensor muscles to control the grasping NP. The proportional signals were determined based upon the amplitude of the EMG recordings. It was necessary to use a blanking circuit to minimize stimulation artifacts. The same group developed very efficient processing techniques: adaptive time constant filter and adaptive step size (slow rate limiting) filter.

One of the common problems in the recording of the activity from muscles is the stimulation artifact. As described above, the way around this problem is to apply the circuitry that will blank the response for a period that is longer than the stimulation artifact. However, the stimulation contaminates the natural signals even at the muscle that is remote from the stimulation. The blanking circuitry is sufficient to eliminate the effects that could prevent recording and signal processing, yet additional filtering can improve the canceling of the noise imposed by stimulation. One possible method is to estimate the artifact waveform from the subthreshold stimulation and subtract it from the sub-threshold stimulation response (McGill et al., 1982). Adaptive noise canceling (ANC) can be much more effectively achieved by means of an artificial neural network.

Electroneurogram (ENG) obtained from a cuff electrode (Hoffer and Loeb, 1980; Stein et al., 1975; Hoffer et al., 1995; Hoffer, 1988) is a viable signal for NP (Haugland and Sinkjær, 1995; Upshaw and Sinkjær, 1998; Haugland et al., 1999; Inmann, 2001). In the current implants at Aalborg University, Denmark a telemetric amplifier system that amplifies the ENG recorded from a tripolar nerve cuff electrode and transmits it from the implanted amplifier through the skin to an external control unit was demonstrated to work good enough in both walking and grasping NP. The output is raw ENG, bandpass filtered from 800 Hz to 8000 Hz. The implant is powered by radiofrequency induction and will operate for a coil-to-coil separation up to 30 mm. Input-referred noise is not more than 1 μV (r.m.s.). The device is small enough to be implanted in the extremities of human adults. The method used for artifact suppression in nerve cuff electrode recordings is intimately related to the method for extraction of the envelope of the signal as described above for the EMG (Haugland and Hoffer, 1994a, 1994b) and is essentially based on rectification followed by the integration of the signal during noise-free periods (bin-integration). Initially, the signal from the amplifier is high-pass filtered to remove the remaining EMG and noise contamination of the nerve signal, which is still present even after passing the filter in the amplifier. The signal is then rectified and bin-integrated (Figure 28.24).

An early example of using EMG and ENG for NP in animal demonstrated the feasibility of this approach (Popović et al., 1993). Several cats have been implanted for up to 3.5 years, and the recordings have been stable and reliable. The recordings have been processed with a portable, battery-powered device (Nikolić et al., 1994), which provided amplification, filtering, and BIN integration; thus real-time use of natural sensors for control was facilitated. Figure 28.25 (bottom panel) shows 10 sec of the processed recordings from nerves and muscles in a walking cat. The top panel (Figure 28.25) shows the original recordings from only one stride (indicated with the arrow in the bottom panel). The recordings have been used for a rule-based controller. The information that could be reliably extracted was based on the threshold detection. Since two nerve recordings have been captured simultaneously, and a separate threshold level was adopted for each nerve, four pieces of information were available.

It might be useful for future NP systems if control signals could be derived from recordings of afferent activity (Yoshida and Horch, 1996). Riso et al. (2000) used a rabbit ankle as a model for the human ankle. They characterized the responses evoked in a pair of complementary mixed nerves (the tibial and peroneal components of the sciatic nerve) that carry muscle afferents from the main ankle extensor and ankle flexor muscles. Simultaneous recordings were obtained using tripolar cuffs installed around the two nerves (Figure 28.26).

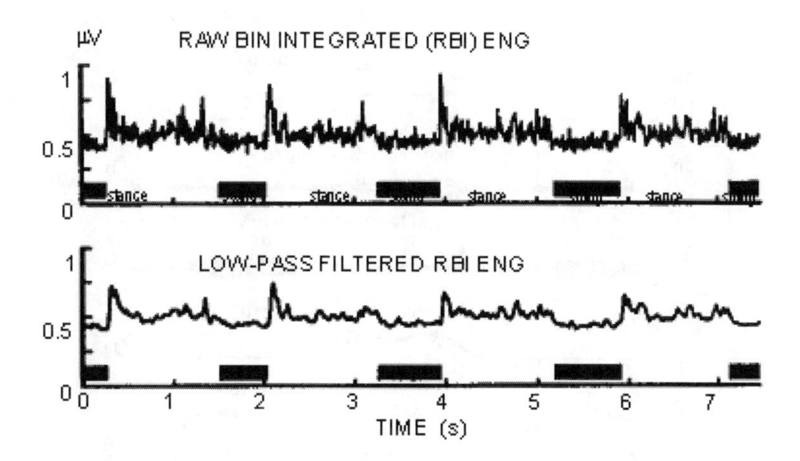

FIGURE 28.24 The processed recordings from a cuff-electrode at the sural nerve of a walking human. Four consecutive steps are presented: rectified bin integrated (RBI) electroneurogram (ENG) at the top, and the same signal low-pass filtered (bottom). Black bars are the timings recorded by a heel-switch positioned in the shoe during walking.

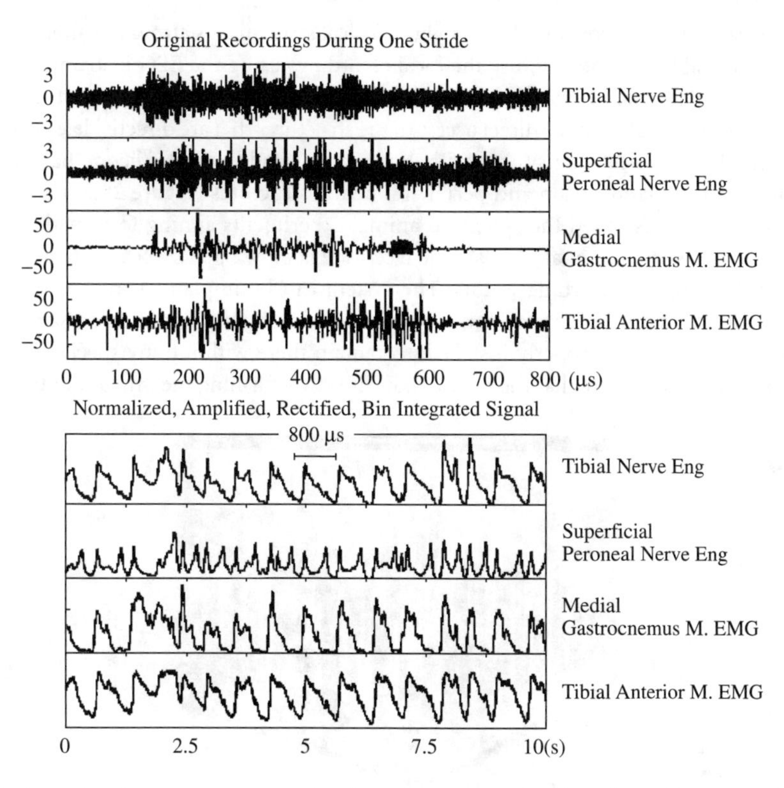

FIGURE 28.25 Raw signal from one stride and real-time processed recordings from 10 sec from the Tibial (TI) n, Superficial Peroneal (SP) n, *Medial Gastrocnemius* (MG) m, and *Tibialis Anterior* (TA) m in a cat walking on a powered treadmill. The recordings were used for rule-based control of FES-supported walking. Both EMG and ENG signals (natural sensors) were used for control. The cuff and epimysial electrodes were implanted in cats for a period longer than 3 years; the recordings were stable throughout the experiments. (Adapted from Popović et al., 1993, © IEEE.)

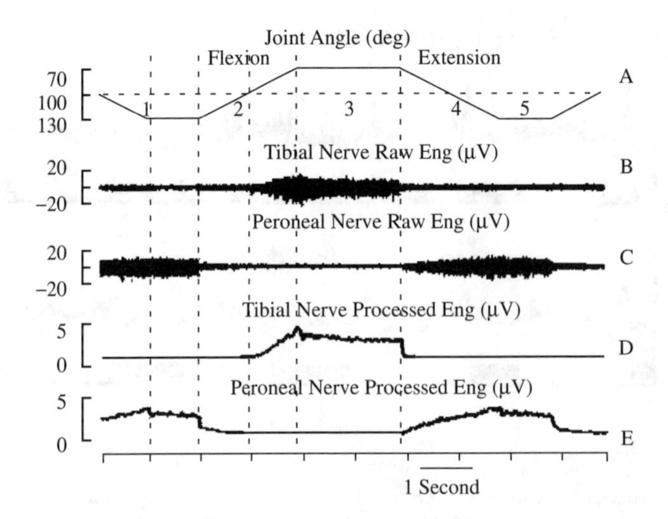

FIGURE 28.26 Joint angle and nerve activity recorded from the tibial and peroneal nerves in a rabbit during passive ankle movement over a range of 60°. The nerve activities before processing are in B and C, while D and E are the rectified and integrated signals using a moving window average. (Adapted from Riso et al., 2000, © IEEE.)

28.4.3.3 Recording from the Cortex — Brain Interface

Recently, the possible use of recordings from higher cortical structures is attracting attention from many researchers. One possible method is to use the focal recordings using the EEG instrumentation (McFarland et al., 1998; Wolpaw et al., 1998; Vaughan et al., 1998). The other rather invasive technique is much more attractive because it will provide direct access to the structures that are directly delegated for sensory-motor functions. A multi-electrode system with 100 needles made out of silicone has been tested for both recording and stimulating brain and peripheral neural structures (Figure 28.27).

Normann and colleagues tested the system in animal experiments aiming to provide a possible tool for visual prostheses (Normann et al., 1999). The electrode is only 2.5 × 2.5 × 2 mm^3 and provides 100 independent stimulation or recording points. The system can be implanted in the cortex by using a special tool, which allows the device to penetrate into the brain or peripheral nerve (Normann, personal communication, 1999) and, if properly installed, to remain there without any special attachment. The longer-term experiments indicate that the neural tissue is slowly pushing the implant out; thus, it is likely

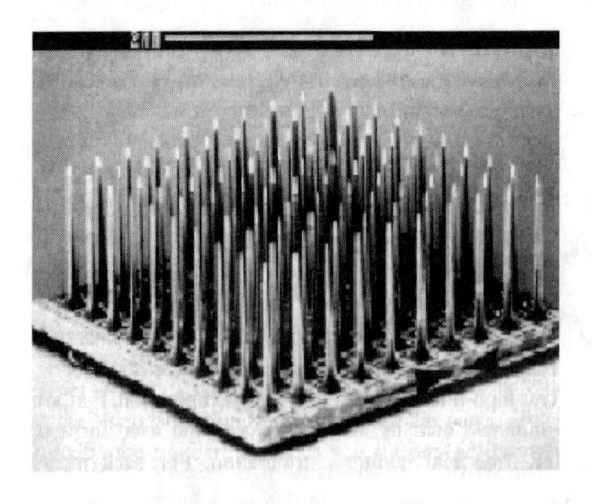

FIGURE 28.27 The 100-electrode array for interfacing the central nervous and peripheral nervous system. The back silicon-based plate is used to host electronic circuitry if necessary. Each of the 100 electrodes that could have various lengths to allow variable penetration into the tissue can be independently controlled. The maximum length of needle electrodes (made out the same silicon bulk) is 2.5 mm. (Courtesy of Dr. Richard Norman, University of Utah, Salt Lake City, 1998.)

that after some time, the electrode will not operate. The same electrode array is currently being tested in peripheral nerves and dorsal ganglion with great promises (Stein, personal communication, 2002).

28.4.4 Controller

A controller for NP is a system that has to be programmable to provide the following functions: (1) use data from analog and analog sensors in real-time for sensory driven feed-forward or closed-loop control, (2) use switches for finite state control, and (3) generate signals that define the shape, amplitude, duration, and repetition rate of impulses to be delivered. Today many stimulation patterns are needed that require sophisticated programming. A controller must produce sufficient number of output signals that accommodate the stimulator number of channels. Today most microcontrollers can do the simple real-time control, yet most are not capable of executing complex model-based control algorithms. Digital signal processors can be used, yet their power consumption is at this stage still questionable for portable, self-contained systems, especially implantable systems.

The controller should communicate with the host computer. This communication today can be easily accomplished by infrared communication, radio frequency transmission, or using USB and serial wire-based communication link. The host computer needs an interface that allows the user to efficiently program the stimulation protocol with regard to number of channels to be used, number and type of sensors and switches that will be applied, timing sequences, and special events. The host computer interface must allow the user to potentially control the pulse amplitude and duration, repetition rate, and rise and fall time of the strength of stimulation.

The control schemes for different applications are explained in the text that follows.

28.5 Neural Prostheses for Restoring Upper and Lower Extremity Functions

During the last 40 years many NPs for restitution of upper and lower extremity functions have been developed, yet only a few have reached the production of even prototype series for clinical studies. The main reason is that the application of motor NP is extremely demanding and that in many cases the pathology does not allow sufficient improvement in function to make a NP effective enough. Many neural prostheses are used for therapeutic purposes. The advancements of technology, better understanding of sensory-motor systems, and greatly improved computer power that facilitates the implementation of much more complex control schema raise great hopes for the future.

28.5.1 Neural Prostheses for Reaching and Grasping

NPs for upper limbs are being developed to establish and augment the independence to the user (Figure 28.28). The target population for many years has been tetraplegics with diminished, yet preserved shoulder and elbow functions who lack wrist control and grasping ability (Triolo et al., 1996).

Controlling the movement of the whole arm has lately received more attention (Crago et al., 1998; Grill and Peckham, 1998; Lemay and Crago, 1997; Popović and Popović, 1998a, 1998b, 2000, 2001; Smith et al., 1996). The feasibility of restoring upper extremity function to individuals with high cervical spinal cord injury (C4 or higher) using FES and/or reconstructive surgery has been evaluated. Externally controlling movement to these individuals is challenging and not very successful for two primary reasons: (1) the number of retained voluntary functions is so low that there is a minimal opportunity to substitute for lost functions or even to use these motions to control external devices; and (2) individuals with C3 or C4 level spinal cord injuries exhibit extensive denervation of the shoulder and elbow muscles, which limits the possibility of using FES to restore movement.

The NP developed by Reberšek and Vodovnik (1973) was one of the first FES systems for grasping. This NP had three stimulation channels (two stimulation electrodes per channel), used to generate the grasping functions by stimulating the finger flexors and extensors, and the thumb flexors. Although this

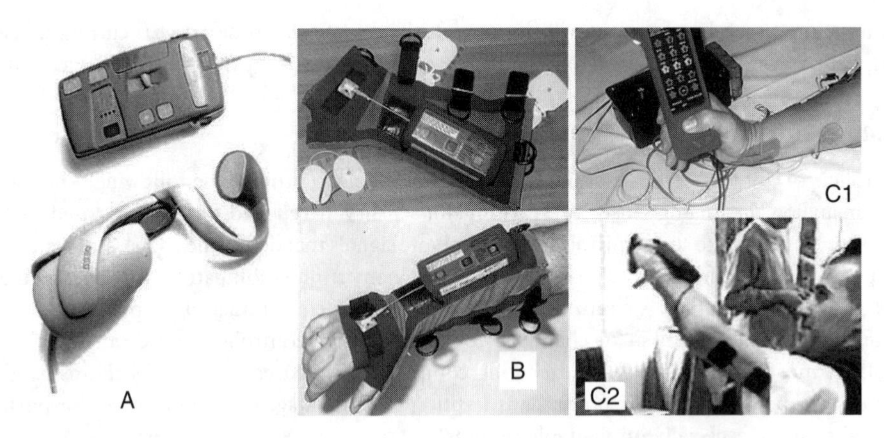

FIGURE 28.28 Three neural prostheses for restoring upper extremity function. (A) Handmaster NMS-1® (Ness, Raanana, Israel) includes a plastic splint that incorporates electrodes for easy and fast mounting; (B) Bionic Glove® (University of Alberta, Edmonton, Canada) that is a garment-based system that incorporates metal contacts with the polymer-based electrodes that have to be positioned on the skin; (C1 and C2) Belgrade Grasping System® (Medicina TS, Belgrade, Yugoslavia) designed for lifelike control of grasping and reaching.

device was developed almost three decades ago, it is one of the rare FES systems that allowed a subject to control the stimulation intensity via different sensory interfaces such as EMG sensor, sliding resistor, and pressure sensor. As a result, the subject was able to select the most appropriate command interface. The main disadvantage of this neuroprosthesis was that donning and doffing times were long, and that the selectivity of stimulation was rather low. A much more complex system with surface electrodes was developed at Ben Gurion University, Israel (Nathan, 1989; Nathan and Ohry, 1990). A voice control was used for driving the twelve bipolar stimulation channels and controlling the elbow, wrist, and hand functions. There was very little practical experience with the system, because of the complexity of tuning it for the needs of potential users. Surface stimulation did not allow control of the small hand and forearm muscles necessary to provide dexterity while grasping. Daily mounting and fitting of the system has been problematic.

There were several modifications of the surface stimulation system, yet in most cases that ended in research laboratories, without being brought to the clinical evaluations. The most advanced among many surface stimulation systems is the Handmaster NMS-1.® The Handmaster is a neuroprosthesis designed for tetraplegic and stroke subjects (Nathan, 1993). There is a maximum of five stimulating electrodes connected to three channels of the stimulator. The Handmaster is controlled with a push button that triggers the hand opening and closing functions. The subject is expected to push the button with the contralateral arm, or alternatively the one mounted in the splint. By pressing the push button, the stimulator turns on and after a short time delay extends the subject's fingers for a short period of time followed by the thumb and finger flexion. The fingers and thumb remain flexed until the subject presses the push button for the second time. The consecutive activation of the push-button generates finger extension that lasts a predefined period of time followed by switching off of the stimulator. Besides the push-button (i.e., the switch) a sliding resistor is provided that allows the subject to regulate the way in which the thumb flexes. This feature helps the subject to adjust the grasp to the size and the shape of the object he/she wants to grasp. In addition, the subject can increase or decrease the grasping force using two additional push buttons.

Tetraplegic subjects in principle can grasp objects by extending a wrist, thereby causing passive finger flexion due to the limited length of the finger flexors. Typically C6-C7 tetraplegic subjects are able to generate this so-called tenodesis grasp. The grasp generated with tenodesis is rather weak. In order to hold an object using tenodesis grasp it is necessary to maintain the wrist extension during the entire duration of the object manipulation, and that is often very difficult or impossible to do. At the University of Alberta, Edmonton, Canada, Prochazka et al. (1997) developed the Bionic Glove,® a neuroprosthesis that enhances the tenodesis grasp. The Bionic Glove applies a position transducer attached to the wrist to detect voluntary wrist flexion and extension. When the patient flexes the wrist, the finger extensors are stimulated causing hand opening. When the patient voluntarily extends the wrist, the finger flexors are stimulated to provide hand closure. A dead-zone (hysteresis) allows movement of the wrist once the "open" or "close" stimulation pattern is activated. The electrical stimulation is provided via three self-adhesive surface stimulation electrodes that are placed over the muscles' motor points, and an anode that is placed proximal to the wrist crease. Each stimulation electrode has a metal stud on its back that is connected to one of four stainless steel meshes placed inside the neoprene glove above the expected electrode positions. The stimulator and the position sensor used by the glove are located on the forearm part of the glove. An easy-to-use interface with three push-buttons on the stimulator is used to set the stimulation parameters and the optional audio feedback that facilitates faster learning. To the best of the authors' knowledge, the Bionic Glove is not commercially available at the moment. The Bionic Glove is currently being modified and its new version named "Tetron" incorporates several grasping strategies. In the clinical evaluation (Popović et al., 1999) it was indicated that the stimulation is beneficial to tetraplegic subjects (therapy effects and orthotic assistance), but that the overall acceptance rate for long-time use is at about 30% of potential users. One of the conclusions was that the control, donning, and doffing should be improved, as well as its cosmetic appearance.

The Belgrade Grasping/Reaching System (BGS®) is a four-channel system (Popović and Popović, 1998a; 1998b) allowing two modalities of grasping: side and palm grasps by generating opposition and control of elbow movement. A preprogrammed sequence is triggered using a switch interface, similar to the Handmaster system. The grasping is separated into three phases: (1) prehension (forming the correct aperture); (2) relaxing (allowing the hand to get good contact with the object); and (3) closing the hand by opposing the palm and the thumb or the side of the index finger and the thumb. The releasing function includes two stages: opening of the hand and resting. It is possible to select the duration of each of the phases of the grasp/release upon the individual characteristics of the subject, as well as his/her preferences. The BGS comprises also a reaching controller. The system uses synergistic control based on mapping of the angular velocities at the shoulder and elbow joints (Popović and Popović, 2001).

The ETHZ-ParaCare® neuroprosthesis was designed recently with the aim to improve grasping and walking functions in SCI and stroke patients (Popović et al., 2001). This four-channel NP is programmable and can be interfaced with many sensors used as feedback or trigger generators. The ETHZ-ParaCare NP provides both palmar and lateral grasps. The controller includes four modalities: proportional EMG, discrete EMG, push button, and sliding resistor strategies. Thus far more than 12 patients have used the system. Four patients used the neuroprosthesis at home in daily living activities. One of the main disadvantages of this system is that it requires between 7 and 10 min to don and doff the system. The system is not yet commercially available. Current efforts are aimed at completing a new generation of the neuroprosthesis that could be used for all FES applications involving surface stimulation electrodes. The ParaCare grasping devices were transferred to Compex Motion Company, Switzerland; the new neuroprosthesis, called Compex Motion® (beta version), became available at the end of 2001.

The likely method to overcome problems of surface electrodes NP for reaching and grasping and reaching, is to use implanted electrode or eventually fully implantable systems. This problem was addressed for more than 20 years in a systematic way in Japan (Handa et al., 1989a; 1998b). Subjects have been implanted with up to 30 percutaneous i.m. electrodes per extremity. These electrodes were connected to a 30-channel device that delivers a preprogrammed sequence of stimulation pulses. The preprogrammed sequence was prepared based on the activity of muscles recorded in able-bodied subjects. The i.m. EMG determined the pattern of muscle activity in able-bodied subjects. This stimulation program in the Sendai Hospital, Japan was most often applied as a therapy, with a plan to design a self-contained orthosis for daily continuous usage.

The most advanced grasping NP follows from more than 20 years of dedicated work by Peckham (Peckham et al., 1980a, 1980b) from the Case Western Reserve University (CWRU), Cleveland, Ohio. A fully implantable stimulation device (Figure 28.29) is approved for human use under the name Freehand system,® distributed by the NeuroControl Corp. of Cleveland, Ohio. The system has an external unit

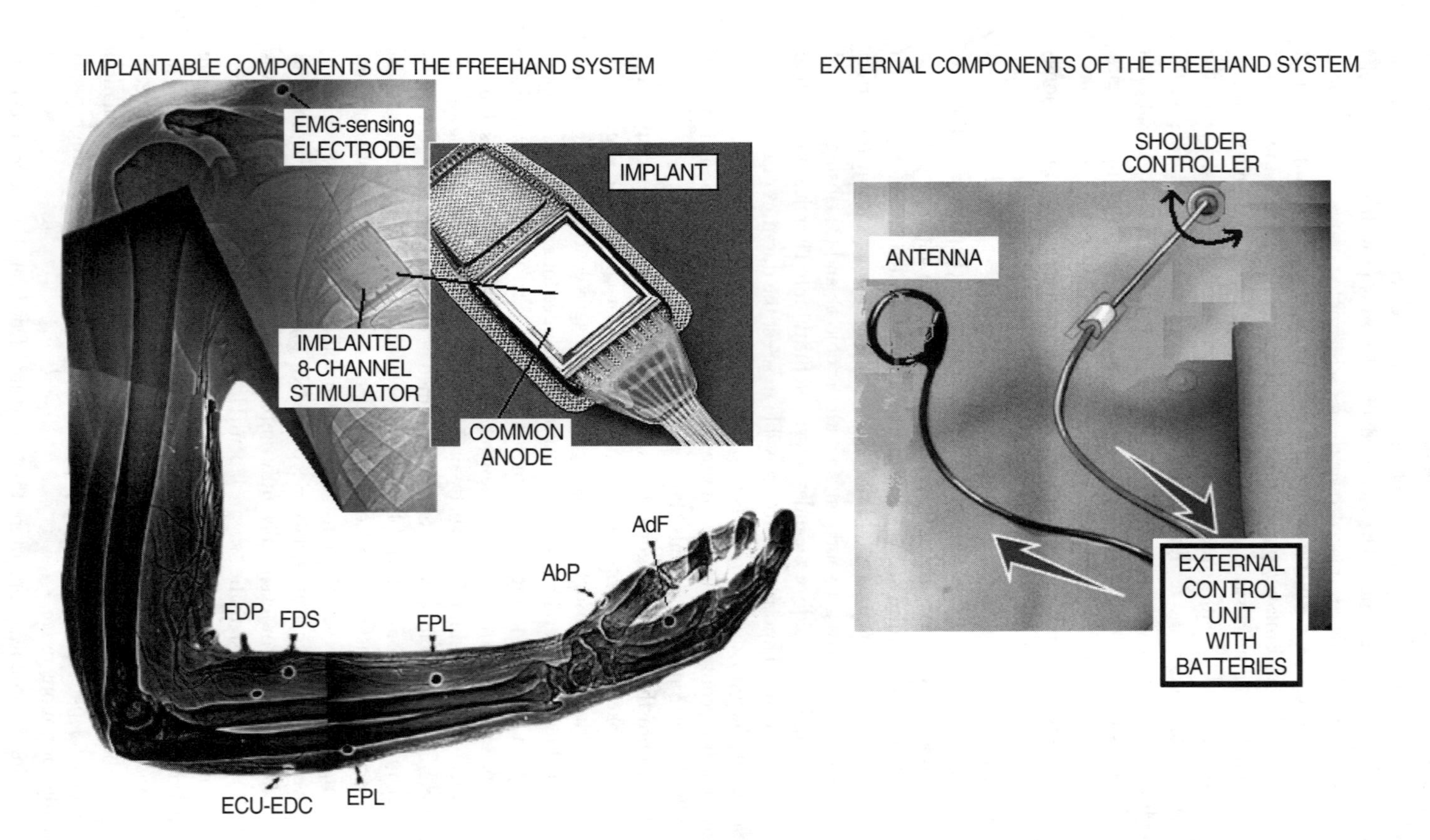

FIGURE 28.29 Drawing of the Freehand System®. The xerogram shows the position of seven stimulating electrodes, cables that were tunneled from the stimulator to the electrodes, and the eight-channel unipolar implanted stimulator. The xerogram also shows the position of one electrode that could be used to record EMG signals and potentially control the grasping system. The right panel indicates the position of the Hall-effect-based transducer used to control opening, closing, and locking the grasp in the desired position. External, microcontroller-based unit generates the control signals that are sent via RF link using the inductive coupling (antenna). The external unit also sends the energy to the implanted unit using the same RF link.

(control box, power source) and an implantable part (remotely powered and controlled stimulator, leads with epimysial electrodes, and a sensory system) (Smith et al., 1987).

The objective of this system is to provide grasp and release for individuals with C5 and C6 level spinal cord injuries. Coordinated electrical stimulation of paralyzed forearm and hand muscles is used to provide lateral (key pinch) and palmar grasp patterns. The subjects obtain proportional control of grasp opening and closing by voluntary movement of either the shoulder or wrist. An external transducer is mounted on the chest to measure the shoulder motion, or on the dorsum of the wrist to measure the wrist flexion/extension. The novel version of the wrist sensor can be implanted (Kilgore et al., 1997; Hart et al., 1998). The control signal is sent to an external control unit, which converts the signal into the appropriate stimulation signals for each electrode. These signals are sent across an inductive link to an implanted stimulator receiver, which generates the stimulus to the appropriate electrode. Seven epimysial electrodes, sewn onto the muscle surface through surgical exposure, are used for muscle excitation. Sensory feedback regarding the control state is provided through an eighth implanted electrode placed in an area of normal sensation.

The electrode leads are tunneled subcutaneously to the implanted stimulator located in the pectoral region. The surgical procedures to enhance both voluntary and stimulated hand functions are often performed in conjunction with the stimulator implantation. More than 250 tetraplegics have received the Freehand® at more than a dozen sites around the world. The subjects have demonstrated the ability to grasp and release objects and to perform activities of daily living more independently when using the neural prosthesis. The subjects utilize the device at home on a regular basis. NeuroControl Corp. of Cleveland, Ohio coordinates the clinical trials. The system is applicable if the following muscles can be stimulated: *Extensor Pollicis Longus m*, *Flexor Pollicis Longus m*, *Adductor Pollicis m*, *Opponens m*, *Flexor Digitorum Profundus m.* and *Superficialis m*, and *Extensor Digitorum Communis m.* A next generation of implantable NP is developed at the CWRU. The implantable stimulator/telemeter extends the capabilities of the existing Freehand stimulator by increasing the number of stimulus channels available. The increased number of stimulus channels allows the following: increased flexibility to control muscles, active extension of the elbow joint, and improved sensory feedback strategies. The system also includes a new implantable transducer for sensing movement of joints such as the wrist or shoulder.

The initial implementation of the advanced stimulator/telemeter provides ten channels of stimulation and one implanted joint angle transducer (Figure 28.29). The stimulator/telemeter unit has been implanted in several individuals. Clinical tests of the implanted joint angle transducer began in 1997. The transducer has been implanted in the wrist, allowing the individual to control grasp opening and closing through voluntary movement of the wrist.

The Freehand system utilizes the individually tuned cocontraction map to provide palmar and lateral grasp. The user voluntarily selects between these two grasps, and controls the prehension proportionally (Peckham and Creasy, 1992). The additional feature of the system is the ability to "lock" the stimulation pattern at any of the preprogrammed combinations. Visual feedback and experience gained through the usage help the subject to perform daily activities (Wijman et al., 1990). The joystick mounted on the contralateral shoulder or some other position at the body controls the preprogrammed sequence of stimulation. The palmar grasp starts from the extended fingers and thumb (one end position of the joystick), followed by the movement of the thumb to opposition and flexing of the fingers (other terminal position of the joystick). The lateral grasp starts from the full extension of the fingers and the thumb, followed by the flexion of the fingers and adduction of the thumb.

A portable version of the hand grasp neuroprosthesis incorporating feedback from natural sensors (Figure 28.30) was developed and used for evaluation of the system performance at the home of a volunteer with tetraplegia (Inmann, 2001). During the evaluation period, the stimulator command signal and the time of usage were stored on a memory card. Additionally, the user's caretaker filled out a form reporting the activity for which the neuroprosthesis was used. The sensory system detects the onset of relative movement of the object and provides for real-time adjustment of the force that prevents the slippage. During the periods of sensory information when there is no slip, the stimulation level is slowly decreasing, thus minimizing the fatigue. Using signals from natural sensors in the skin of the index finger

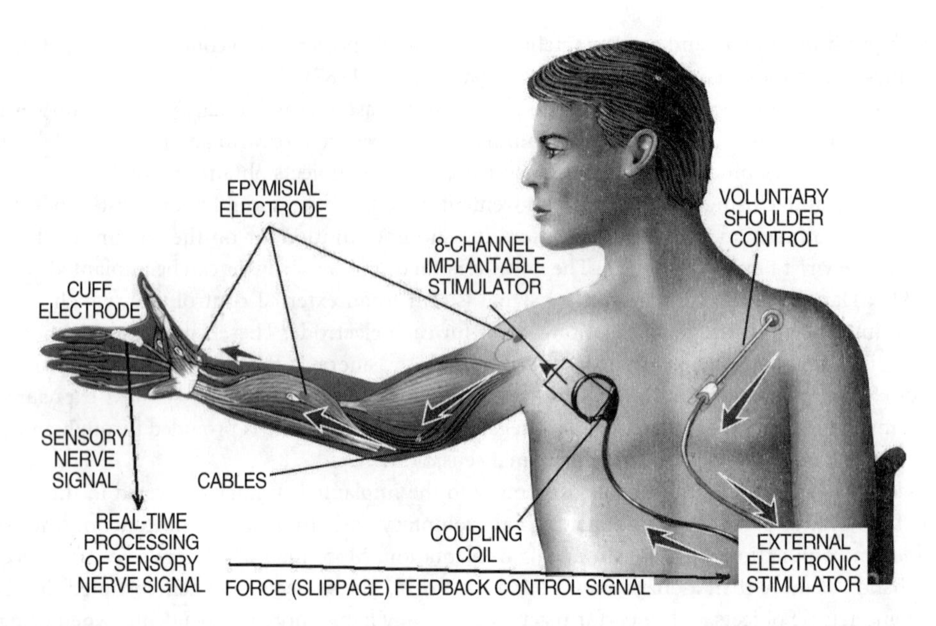

FIGURE 28.30 Drawing of instrumented arm in a tetraplegic subject. Nerve cuff electrodes are positioned at the digital nerve of the index finger in order to record activity from cutaneous mechanoreceptors at the radial aspect of the index finger. Lead wires from the cuff-electrode are routed subcutaneously to a site on the volar forearm where they exit via a small connector. The cuff-electrode is located on a branch of the palmar digital nerve. Signals recorded from the cuff are processed and fed to the control unit. A radiofrequency link is used to provide power for the implanted circuitry. The same subject is instrumented with the Freehand System® described in text and shown in Figure 28.29.

to control automatically the stimulator command signal could reduce the mean lateral pinch force by about 40% compared with using the neuroprosthesis without this feedback signal. Additionally, the control of the neuroprosthesis with push buttons that were mounted permanently on the headrest of the wheelchair, instead of being shoulder controlled was highly accepted by the user (Inmann, 2001). Although the portable system is still a prototype the present system has shown that at least for selected tetraplegics the natural sensory feedback system was superior to the open-loop commercial system that was normally used.

28.5.2 Neural Prostheses for Restoring Standing and Walking

NP started to be used for walking assistance in Ljubljana, Slovenia (e.g., Vodovnik et al., 1967, 1981; Kralj and Bajd, 1989; Bajd et al., 1982, 1983, 1989; Kralj et al., 1980; Gračanin et al., 1967, 1969). The available surface NP systems use various numbers of stimulation channels.

The simplest NP to assist walking, from a technical point, is a single-channel system. This system is only suitable for stroke subjects and a limited group of incomplete spinal cord injured subjects. These individuals can perform limited ambulating with the assistance of the upper extremities without an FES system, although this ambulating may be both modified and/or impaired. The FES in these humans is used to activate a single muscle group. The first demonstrated application of this technique was in stroke subjects (Gračanin et al., 1969), even though the original patent came from Liberson et al. (1961). The stimulation is applied to ankle dorsiflexors so the "foot-drop" can be eliminated.

The Odstock foot-drop stimulator (ODFS, the Department of Medical Physics and Biomedical Engineering, Salisbury District Hospital, Salisbury, Wiltshire, U.K.), the single-channel foot-drop stimulator manufactured by COTAS, Denmark, and MicroFES and FEPA10 peroneal stimulators, Ljubljana, Slovenia are among the few FES systems in clinical use (Figure 28.31). At the time of writing, in excess of 450 people had used the ODFS, more than 3000 COTAS stimulators are sold, and more than 1000 Ljubljana systems have been distributed over more than 20 years.

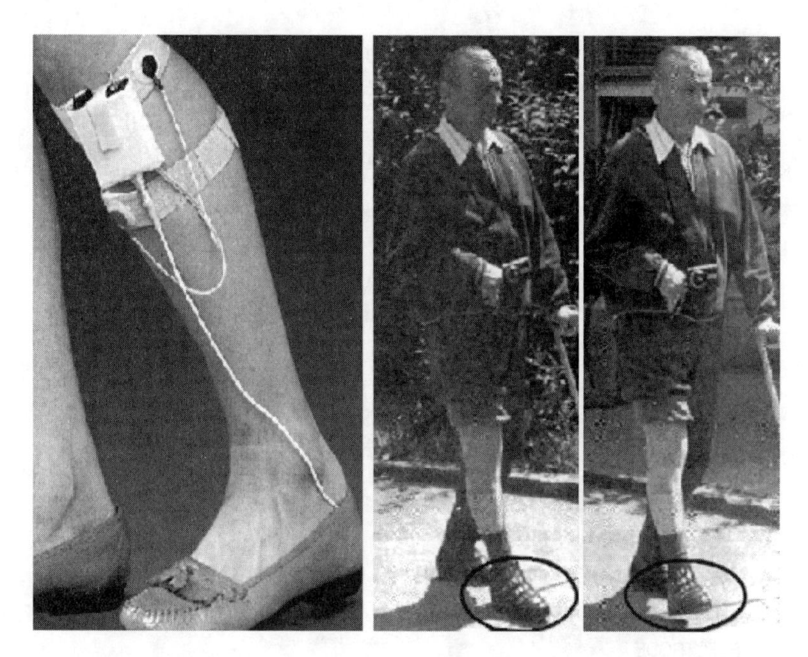

FIGURE 28.31 (Left panel) The KDC 2000A, Cotas, Denmark peroneal stimulator to correct foot-drop problems; (right panel) a hemiplegic subject walking with the stimulator turned off (left) and on (right).

The ODFS is a new technology that follows the work of Liberson et al. (1961). It is a single-channel stimulator providing electrical stimulation to the *Tibialis Anterior m.* or the common peroneal nerve (Granat et al., 1996; Maležič et al., 1984; Stein et al., 1993; Sweeney and Lyons, 1999; Wieler et al., 1999). The stimulation, timed to the gait cycle by using a switch placed in the shoe, causes ankle dorsiflexion with some eversion and/or could elicit a flexor withdrawal reflex (Burridge et al., 1997a, 1997b). The reflex comprises ankle dorsiflexion, hip, and knee flexion, with external rotation of the hip. Adjusting the electrode position and stimulation amplitude may vary the components of the movement. The ODFS stimulator gives an asymmetrical biphasic output of maximum amplitude 80 mA, with a 300-μsec duration of the pulse and the interpulse interval of 40 msec. Stimulation is applied by means of skin-surface electrodes placed, typically, over the common peroneal nerve as it passes over the head of the fibula bone and over the motor point of *Tibialis Anterior m.* The output of the stimulator is normally triggered after heel rises from the ground on the affected side and continues until heel strike occurs. Stimulation can also be triggered by heel strike from the contralateral leg, which is a useful function if heel contact is unreliable on the affected side.

Two stimulation channels; restricting the muscle groups to the *Tibialis Anterior m.* and either the *Hamstrings m.* or *Posterior Tibialis m.*, (calf) muscle groups have been used to correct the foot-drop problem (Taylor, 1997). The stimulation is initiated and terminated using footswitches. A novel programming design allows fine control of timing and parameters of each stimulation channel, yet simple to use by a trained physiotherapist. This follows the application of the Compustim-10B, two-channel, microcontroller-based, neuromuscular stimulator. It was found that stimulating the *Hamstrings m.* and calf muscles (in addition to the *Tibialis Anterior m.*) is most effective.

Stein and colleagues (Dai et al., 1996) have designed an appealing self-contained drop-foot system. The system integrates a single-channel stimulator and a tilt sensor, thus eliminating a foot switch, which was not fully reliable because it easily generated false triggering and malfunctioning. The stimulator has been commercialized, yet the distribution failed to make it a market success.

Medtronic Corp., Minneapolis, MI developed an implantable version of the stimulator with nerve electrodes to deal with foot-drop almost 30 years ago. Waters and colleagues implanted a series of these devices and reported effective and safe operation of the nerve electrodes (no failures), yet Medtronic Co. decided to stop this line of research (McNeal and Bowman, 1985; Waters et al., 1985).

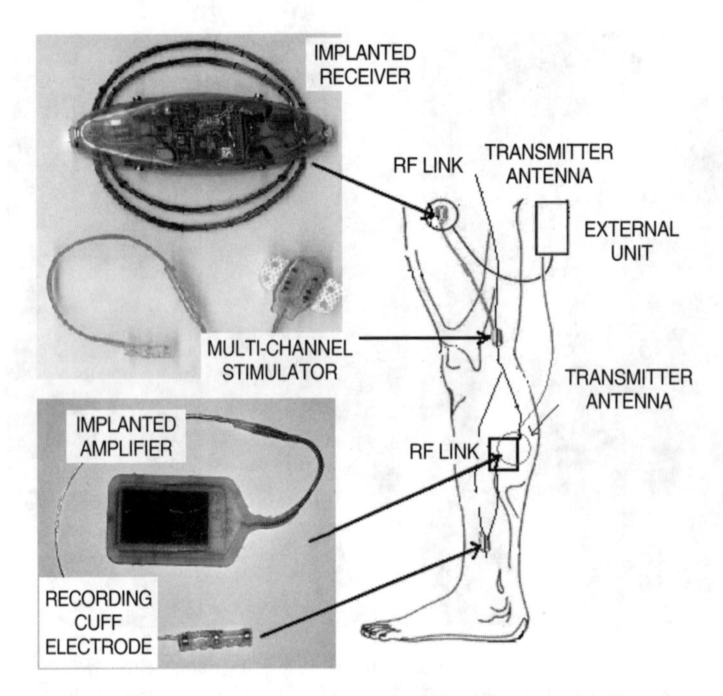

FIGURE 28.32 The new development of the fully implantable system for correcting foot-drop. The neural signal is used (cuff-electrode) for recording of the necessary information for steering of the stimulation; the second cuff is used for selective stimulation of the nerve to allow the appropriate dorsiflexion, controlled inversion/eversion, and internal/external rotation of the foot. The external battery-powered, self-contained unit is providing energy, processing the neural signal based on off-line determined mappings (adaptive logic networks), and delivering control signals for stimulation.

The fully implantable stimulator IPPO (Figure 28.18) has been tested in more than 20 subjects after they had already used the surface stimulation system (Strojnik et al., 1987). The walking pattern did not change with the implanted stimulator compared with the surface electrode based device; however, the ease of application, reproducibility, and cosmetic appearance improved greatly. The implantation is relatively simple, and it is performed in daily surgery.

The dual channel stimulator can be used to correct eversion/inversion of the foot in addition to the dorsiflexion (Hansen, 2001). This new system comprises a cuff-electrode for recording of sensory information from cutaneous receptors. The rationale for implanting a cuff electrode on a cutaneous nerve innervating the foot is to remove the external heel switch used in existing systems for foot-drop correction. Thereby, it is possible to use such systems without footwear and to prepare them to be totally implantable systems. After processing the nerve signal heel contacts can be detected using the afferent nerve signal information alone (Hansen et al., 1998; Kostov et al., 1999) for deciding when the muscle that prevents foot-drop must be stimulated during gait (Figure 28.32).

A multichannel system with a minimum of four channels of FES is required for ambulating of a subject with a complete motor lesion of lower extremities and preserved balance and upper body motor control (Kralj and Bajd, 1989). Appropriate bilateral stimulation of the quadriceps muscles locks the knees during standing (Bajd et al., 1982; Jaeger et al., 1989). Stimulating the common peroneal nerve on the ipsilateral side, while switching off the quadriceps stimulation on that side, produces a flexion of the leg. This flexion, combined with adequate movement of the upper body and use of the upper extremities for support, allows ground clearance and is considered the swing phase of the gait cycle. Hand or foot switches can provide the flexion-extension alternation needed for a slow forward or backward progression (Figure 28.33). Sufficient arm strength must be available to provide balance in parallel bars (clinical application), and with a rolling walker or crutches (daily use of FES).

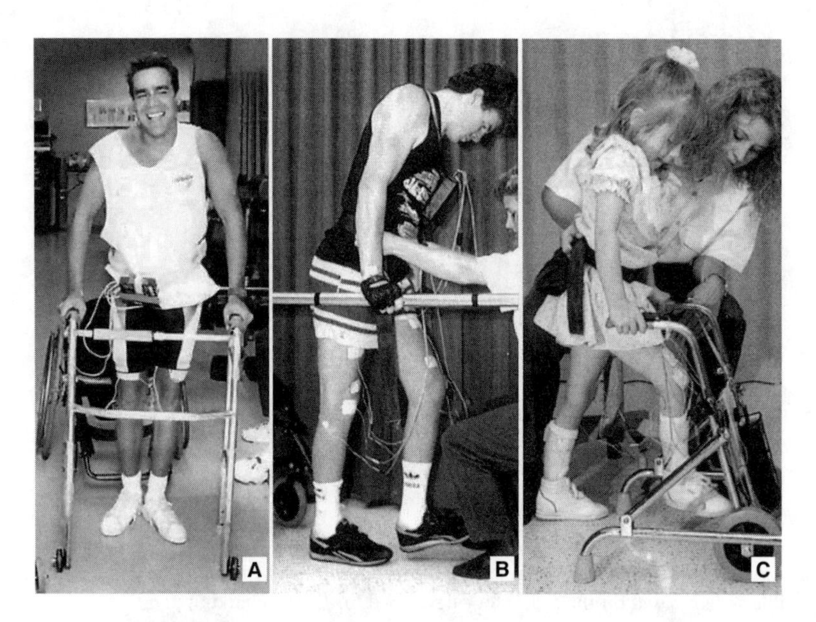

FIGURE 28.33 (A) A paraplegic subject participating at the Miami Project to Cure Paralysis walking study with the Parastep I® system (Sigmedics, Chicago, IL); (B) the use of a six-channel stimulator to restore standing and walking with support over parallel bars, walker, and crutches. Switches are used to trigger the swing phase of the walking; (C) a young girl after a motor vehicle accident caused paraplegia uses the Quadstim® stimulator (Biomech Design, Edmonton, Alberta, Canada) in combination with an ankle-foot orthosis for standing and limited walking.

A dual-channel stimulator Alt-2 (Ljubljana, Slovenia) was developed almost 20 years ago for standing and walking; one stimulator is required per leg. A stimulator comprises three leads for two channels (monopolar stimulation). Stimulating the quadriceps muscle causes extension of the knee and plantar extension; stimulating the peroneal nerve results in a flexion (withdrawal) reflex. A stimulator has a push-button hand-control that switches between the extension (stance phase) and flexion (swing phase) at timings volitionally determined by the user. The system has a safety feature preventing the user from accidentally pressing the flexion function simultaneously in both legs. The switches are mounted in the handles of a walker or crutches and both a wireless and flexible lead connection of switches to the stimulator are available. The use of this assistance for standing and walking has been tested in Ljubljana, Slovenia, in more than 100 subjects over an extended period of time (Kralj and Bajd, 1989), and based on the results, many other rehabilitation research clinics around the world accepted the treatment and built their own similar stimulators (e.g., James et al., 1991). These systems evolved into a commercial product called Parastep-1R (Sigmedics, Chicago, IL), which was approved for home usage in 1994 by the Food and Drug Administration (Graupe and Kohn, 1997; Jacobs et al., 1997; Klose et al., 1997).

Multichannel percutaneous systems for gait restoration with many channels were suggested (Marsolais and Kobetič, 1983, 1987; Kobetič and Marsolais, 1994; Kobetič et al., 1997). The main advantage of these systems is the plausibility to activate many different muscle groups. A preprogrammed stimulation sequence is used for timing and intensity variation of up to 16 channels (Figure 28.34) applied via as many as 64 electrodes. The sequence is cloned from the EMG pattern recorded in able-bodied subjects. Some electrodes are stimulating at very low intensity muscles that are still voluntarily controlled in the abdominal region to provide proprioceptive feedback to the user about the operation of the system. Initially, the method used excluded external bracing, and claimed that FES per se will be adequate, but this method has been changed toward combining the stimulation with some orthotics. Fine-wire i.m. electrodes were positioned by using subdermal needles, and tunneled toward a point where an external connector from several electrodes is attached (externally). These i.m. electrodes serve as the cathodes, positioned close to the motor point of selected muscles. Knee extensors (*Rectus Femoris m*, *Vastus*

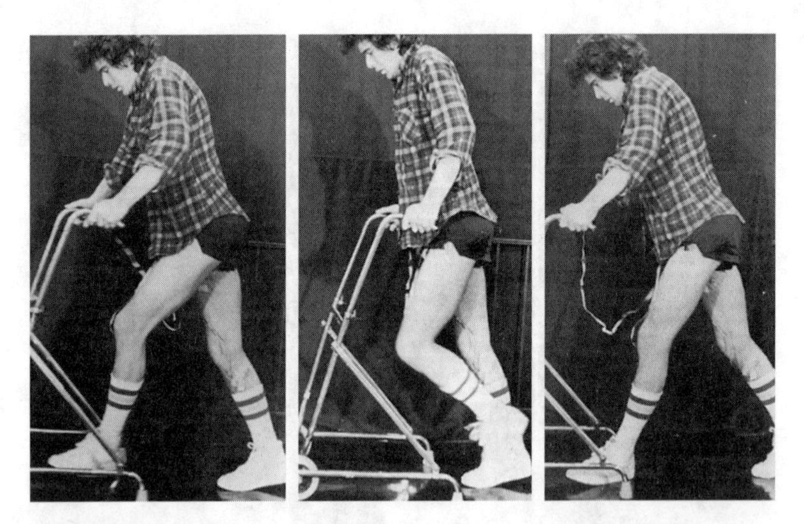

FIGURE 28.34 Paraplegic subject walking with a 16-channel stimulator applied via percutaneous i.m. electrodes. The further development of systems for walking and standing continues with epimysial and i.m. electrodes, yet with a fully implantable system based on the technology developed for the Freehand System®.

Medialis m, Vastus Lateralis m, Vastus Intermedius m), hip flexors (*Sartorius m, Tensor Fasciae Latae m, Gracilis m, Iliopsoas m.*), hip extensors (*Semimembranosus m, Gluteus Maximus m.*), hip abductors (*Gluteus Medius m*), ankle dorsiflexors (*Tibialis Anterior m, Peroneus Longus m*), ankle plantar flexors (*Gastrocnemius Lateralis m, Gastrocnemius Medialis m, Plantaris m, Soleus m*), and paraspinal muscles are selected for activation. A surface electrode has been used as a common anode. Interleaved pulses are delivered with a multichannel, battery-operated, portable stimulator. The hand controller allows the selection of the walking modality. The CWRU system allowed selected humans to walk up to 1.1 m/sec, and walk distances of almost 1000 m. The preprogrammed stimulation sequence included the following walking modes: standing up, sitting down, standing, walking, walking stairs or curb, walking backwards.

Recent projects somewhat changed the initial emphasis of research with implanted systems at the CWRU/Veteran Administration (VA) Center, Cleveland, OH (Kobetič et al., 1999; Sharma et al., 1998). Providing a device to exercise, stand, and maneuver in the vicinity of the wheelchair to individuals with spinal cord injuries (SCIs) through the application of FES is now the primary goal; a system named Freestand, which follows the design of the Freehand, is approved for clinical studies. A single 8-channel CWRU/VA implanted receiver-stimulator (IRS-8) could be used for exercise and standing in individuals with complete motor deficits, and to facilitate walking in selected individuals with partial paralysis. The plan is also to combine both 8- to 16-channel muscle stimulators with a trunk-hip-knee-ankle-foot orthosis with programmable joint locks. The purpose is to provide more immediate mobility to paraplegic individuals and to study functional mobility requirements using the implantable devices currently available.

A different approach to using a multichannel totally implanted FES system (Thoma et al., 1978, 1987) was proposed and tested in a few subjects. This system used a 16-channel implantable stimulator. The electrodes were attached to the epineurium of the selected nerves. Femoral and gluteal nerves were stimulated for hip and knee extension. The so-called "round-about" stimulation was applied in which four electrodes were located around the nerve and stimulated intermittently. This stimulation method was selected to provide physiological-like firing rate to reduce muscle fatigue. The method is finding its extension with the new electrode design that allows selective stimulation of specific fascicles within a nerve.

In 1991 the first 22-channel FES system based on the Nucleus FES22, Cochlear Ltd., Australia, was implanted in a T10-paraplegic male. After a considerable time of training and fitting the program it was possible to achieve sensory feedback-driven standing for about 1 h (Davis et al., 1997). The sensory signals were acquired from the electro-goniometers at the knee joints. Stance stability was assisted with the Andrews' Anterior Floor Reaction Orthosis. The closed-loop control minimizes the time of stimulation; only about 10% of the total standing time are the muscles are externally activated. In 1998, a second T10-paraplegic male was implanted with an updated 22-channel stimulator with telemetry (FES24-A, Neopraxis Pty Ltd, Lane Cove, N.S.W., Australia). Eighteen channels are connected to epineural electrodes on nerves for muscle activation and limb movements thereby allowing exercise and open-loop standing for 30 min. The Praxis FES24-A is a multifunctional stimulator. Ten electrodes are thin, flexible platinum cuffs (Flexi-Cuff), at least twice the diameter of encircled nerve. Eight other electrodes are button-shaped, made of platinum, and placed on the epineurium. Each button has an attached Dacron mesh that is used to suture the electrode to the adjacent connective tissue. The stimulation originates from an external, battery-operated, belt-worn controller (Navigator) microcontroller. The stimulation is delivered via an external RF linked antenna that is magnetically held to the skin by an underlying magnet in the implant. The stimulation parameters are 6.0 to 8.0 mA, with 25- to 500-μsec pulse width and a frequency of up to 60 pulses per second per electrode. The user can select different strategies via a menu-driven protocol based on a simple LCD and keypad interface. A remote RF-linked button is being developed for finger control to complement the keypad. The sensory system comprises two accelerometers and a rate gyroscope.

28.5.2.1 Hybrid Assistive Systems

In order to minimize problems due to the muscle fatigue and to increase the safety, a combination of a mechanical orthosis and FES was suggested. The resulting orthosis is called Hybrid assistive system or Hybrid orthosis (Popović et al., 1989; Tomovič et al., 1995). The support, stability of the joints, and constraint to unwanted motion of the joints are provided by the mechanical component of the orthosis, while FES provides propulsion. Schwirtlich and Popović (1984) suggested a hybrid orthosis that consisted of the self-fitting modular orthosis (SFMO) and surface electrodes FES to provide the knee extension and swing of the leg during walking. A four-channel stimulator was used. The user initiates steps by triggering flexion, and this is followed by sensory-driven knee extensor activity. The SFMO used brakes activated by a micromotor (Schwirtlich and Popović, 1984).

Andrews and Bajd (1984) suggested two variants of hybrid orthoses. One consisted of a combination of a pair of simple plastic splints used to maintain the knee extension and a two-channel stimulator per leg. One channel stimulated gastro-soleus muscles, and the other provided flexor withdrawal response. Since the knee was held in extension, only dorsiflexion of the foot and flexion of the hip were obtained. The other hybrid system comprised the KAFO and two-channel stimulation per leg, The quadriceps and common peroneal nerve were stimulated on each side. The quadriceps stimulation caused knee extension, and the peroneal nerve stimulation produced synergistic flexor response. The mechanical brace incorporated knee joint locks, which were remotely controlled by a solenoid actuator or a Bowden cable.

Andrews and associates (1988) suggested a different way of using the floor reaction orthosis (FOR) in conjunction with FES. This consisted of a rigid ankle foot orthosis, a multichannel stimulator with surface electrodes, body-mounted sensors, a "rule-based" controller, and an electrocutaneous display for supplementary feedback. The finite state controller reacted automatically to destabilize shifts of the ground reaction vector by stimulating appropriate antigravity musculature to brace the leg, The system also featured a control mode to initiate and terminate flexion of the leg during forward progression. A simple mode of supplementary sensory feedback was used during the laboratory standing tests to assist the subject in maintaining the posture.

Solomonow and associates (1989) suggested a hybrid-assistive system that combines FES and reciprocating gait orthosis. The reciprocating gait orthosis was jointly developed by the Louisiana State University Medical Center and Durr-Fillauer Medical Inc. (Douglas et al., 1983). The orthosis includes trunk support, a pelvic assembly, and bilateral knee-ankle-foot-orthosis (KAFO). A rigid pelvic assembly consisting of a pelvic band covering the gluteal and sacral areas bears hip joints. KAFO have posterior offset of the knee joints with drop locks on the lateral sides. The most important feature of the system is the cable coupling of the left and right leg movement. The coupling provides hip joint stability during standing by preventing simultaneous flexion of both hips, yet it allows flexion of one hip and simultaneous extension of the other when a step is taken. The cables can be disengaged to sit down. The FES part of the hybrid system is used for standing up as well as for the swing of the legs. Surface stimulation of *Rectus Femoris m.* and *Hamstrings m* was applied, and the stimulation electrodes were incorporated in a plastic polymer cuff. The electrode cuffs were secured on the thighs with Velcro straps. A four-channel stimulator was worn on a belt. Finger switches were mounted on the handles of the walker. The subject controlled the stimulation himself. Phillips (1989) described a similar system; in addition to the stimulation of *Hamstrings m*, the stimulation of ipsilateral *Gluteus m* was also suggested to improve hip extension of the stance leg, Four two-channel stimulators were used to achieve these functions. The entire bulk of *Quadriceps m.* was stimulated using three-electrode configuration with two channels of one stimulator for each leg, The other two stimulators were used to stimulate *Hamstrings m* and *Gluteus m* on each side.

References

Andrews, B.J. and Bajd, T., Hybrid orthosis for paraplegics, in *Advances in External Control of Human Extremities*, Popović, D.B., Ed., Yugoslav Committee for ETAN (Suppl.), Belgrade, 1984, pp. 55–57.

Andrews, B.J., Baxendale, R.H., Barnett, R., Philips, G.F., Yamazaki, T., Paul, J.P., and Freeman, P.A., Hybrid FES orthosis incorporating closed loop control and sensory feedback, *J. Biomed. Eng.*, 10(2), 189–195, 1988.

Bajd, T. and Bowman, B., Testing and modelling of spasticity, *Biomed. Eng.*, 4, 90–96, 1982.

Bajd, T., Gregorič, M., Vodovnik, L., and Benko, H., Electrical stimulation in treating spasticity resulting from spinal cord injury, *Arch. Phys. Med. Rehabil.*, 66, 515–517, 1985.

Bajd, T., Kralj, A., and Turk, R., Standing-up of a healthy subject and a paraplegic patients, *J. Biomech.*, 15, 1–10, 1982.

Bajd, T., Kralj, A., Turk, R., Benko, H., and Šega, J., The use of a four channel electrical stimulator as an ambulatory aid for paraplegic patients, *Phys. Ther.*, 63, 1116–1120, 1983.

Bajd, T., Kralj, A., Turk, R., Benko, H., and Šega, J., Use of functional electrical stimulation in the rehabilitation of patients with incomplete spinal cord injuries, *J. Biomed. Eng.*, 11, 96–102, 1989.

Bajzek, T.J. and Jaeger, R.J., Characterization and control of muscle response to electrical stimulation, *Ann. Biomed. Eng.*, 15, 485–501, 1987.

Baratta, R. and Solomonow, M., The dynamic response model of nine different skeletal muscles, *IEEE Trans. Biomed. Eng.*, BME-37, 243–251, 1990.

Baratta, R., Zhou, B.H., and Solomonow, M., Frequency response model of skeletal muscle: effect of perturbation level, and control strategy, *Med. Biol. Eng. Comput.*, 27(4), 337–345, 1989.

Barbeau, H., McCrea, D.A., O'Donovan, D.J., Rossignol, S., Grill, W.M., and Lemay, M.A., Tapping into spinal circuits to restore motor function, *Brain Res. Rev.*, 30, 27–51, 1999.

Bijak, M., Sauerman, S., Schmutterer, C., Lanmueller, H., Unger, E., and Mayr, W., A modular PC-based system for easy setup of complex stimulation patterns, Proc 4th Intern. Conf. IFESS, Sendai, 1999, pp. 28–32.

Bogataj, U., Gros, N., Maležič, M., Kelih, B., Kljajić, M., and Aćimović, R., Restoration of gait during two to three weeks of therapy with multichannel electrical stimulation, *Phys. Ther.*, 69(5), 319–327, 1989.

Bowman, B. and Baker, L., Effects of waveform parameters on comfort during transcutaneous neuromuscular electrical stimulation. *Ann. Biomed. Eng.*, 13, 59–74, 1985.

Bowman, R.B. and Erickson, R.C., Acute and chronic implantation of coiled wire intraneural electrodes during cyclical electrical stimulation, *Ann. Biomed. Eng.*, 13, 75–93, 1985.

Brindley, G.S., Polkey, C.E., and Rushton, D.N., Electrical splinting of the knee in paraplegia, *Paraplegia*, 16, 428–435, 1978.

Brodmann, K., Vergleichende Lokalisationslehre der Grosshirnrinde in ibren Prinziplen dargestelit auf Grund des Zellenbaues. Barth, Leipzig, 1909.

Buckett, J.R., Peckham, P.H., Thrope, G.B., Braswell, S.D., and Keith, M.W., A flexible, portable system for neuromuscular stimulation in the paralyzed upper extremity, *IEEE Trans. Biomed. Eng.*, BME-35, 897–904, 1988.

Burridge, J.H., Taylor, P.N., Hagan, S., and Swain, I.D., Experience of clinical use of the Odstock dropped foot stimulator, *Artif. Organs*, 21(3), 254–260, 1997a.

Burridge, J.H., Taylor, P.N., Hagan, S., Wood, D.E., and Swain, I.D., The effects of common peroneal stimulation on the effort and speed of walking: a randomized controlled trial with chronic hemiplegic patients, *Clin. Rehabil.*, 11(3), 201–210, 1997b.

Cameron, T., Loeb, G.E., Peck, R.A., Schulman, J.H., Strojnik, P., and Troyk, P.R., Micromodular implants to provide electrical stimulation of paralyzed muscles and limbs, *IEEE Trans. Biomed. Eng.*, BME-44(9), 781–790, 1997.

Coulombe, R.F., Fiber optic sensors — catching up with the 1980s, *Sensors*, 1(12), 5–11, 1984.

Crago, P.E., Peckham, P.H., Mortimer, J.T., and Van der Meulen, J., The choice of pulse duration for chronic electrical stimulation via surface, nerve and intramuscular electrodes, *Ann. Biomed. Eng.*, 2, 252–264, 1974.

Crago, P.E., Peckham, P.H., and Thrope, G.B., Modulation of muscle force by recruitment during intramuscular stimulation, *IEEE Trans. Biomed. Eng.*, BME-27(12), 679–684, 1980.

Crago, P.E., Chizeck, H.J., Neuman, M.R., and Hambrecht, F.T., Sensors for use with functional neuromuscular stimulation, *IEEE Trans. Biomed. Eng.*, BME-33(2), 256–268, 1986.

Crago, P.E., Memberg, W.D., Usey, M.K., Keith, M.W., Kirsch, R.F., Chapman, G.J., et al., An elbow extension neuroprosthesis for individuals with tetraplegia, *IEEE Trans. Rehabil. Eng.*, TRE-6(1), 1–6, 1998.

Dai, R., Stein, R.B., Andrews, B.J., James, K.B., and Wieler, M., Application of tilt sensors in functional electrical stimulation, *IEEE Trans. Rehabil. Eng.*, TRE-4(2), 63–72, 1996.

Dario, P., Domenici, C., Bardelli, R., DeRossi, D., and Pinotti, P.C., Piezoelectric polymers: new sensor materials for robotic applications, in *Proc. 13th Int. Symp. Indust. Robots,* IEEE Press, Piscataway, NJ, 1983, p. 1434.

Davis, R., Houdayer, T., Andrews, B.J., Emmons, S., and Patrick, J., Paraplegia: prolonged closed-loop standing with implanted nucleus FES-22 stimulator and Andrews' foot-ankle orthosis, *Stereotact. Funct. Neurosurg.*, 69, 281–287, 1997.

Dimitrijević, M.R., Head injuries and restorative neurology, *Scand. J. Rehab. Med. (Suppl.)*, 17, 9–13, 1988.

Donaldson, N., A 24-output implantable stimulator for FES, Proc. 2nd Vienna Int. Workshop Functional Electrostimulation, Vienna, 1986, pp. 197–200.

Douglas, R., Larson, P.F., D'Ambrosia, R., and McCall, R.E., The LSU reciprocating gait orthosis, *Orthopedics*, 6, 34–39, 1983.

Francisco, G., Chae, J., Chawla, H., Kirshblum, S., Zorowitz, R., Lewis, G., and Pang, S., Electromyogram-triggered neuromuscular stimulation for improving the arm function of acute stroke survivors: a randomized pilot study, *Arch. Phys. Med. Rehabil.*, 79(5), 570–575, 1998.

Frigo, C., Ferrarin, M., Frasson, W., Pavan, E., and Thorsen, R., EMG signals detection and processing for on-line control of functional electrical stimulation, *J. Electromyogr. Kinesiol.*, 10(5), 351–360, 2000.

Glanz, M., Klawansky, S., Stason, W., et al., Functional electrostimulation in post stroke rehabilitation: a meta-analysis of the randomized controlled trials, *Arch. Phys. Med. Rehabil.*, 77(6), 549–553, 1996.

Gračanin, F., Kralj, A., and Reberšek, S., Advanced version of the Ljubljana functional electronic peroneal brace with walking rate controlled tetanization, in *Advances in External Control of Human Extremities*, ETAN, 1969, pp. 487–500.

Gračanin, F., Prevec, T., and Trontelj, J., Evaluation of use of functional electronic peroneal brace in hemiparetic patients, in *Advances in External Control of Human Extremities III*, ETAN, 1967, pp. 198–210.

Granat, M.H., Maxwell, D.J., Ferguson, A.C.B., Lees, K.R., and Barbenel, J.C., Peroneal stimulator: evaluation for the correction of spastic drop foot in hemiplegia, *Arch. Phys. Med. Rehabil.*, 77, 19–24, 1996.

Grandjean, P.A. and Mortimer, J.T., Recruitment properties of monopolar and bipolar epimysial electrodes, *Ann. Biomed. Eng.*, 14, 53–66, 1986.

Graupe, D. and Kohn, K.H., Transcutaneous functional neuromuscular stimulation of certain traumatic complete thoracic paraplegics for independent short-distance ambulation, *Neurol. Res.*, 19, 323–333, 1997.

Grill, H.J. and Peckham, P.H., Functional neuromuscular stimulation for combined control of elbow extension and hand grasp in C5 and C6 quadriplegics, *IEEE Trans. Rehab. Eng.*, TRE-6, 190–199, 1998.

Grill, W.M. and Mortimer, J.T., Neural and connective tissue response to long-term implantation of multiple contact nerve cuff electrodes, *J. Biomed. Mater. Res.*, 50(2), 215–226, 2000.

Handa, Y., Hoshimiya, H., Iguchi, Y., and Oda, T., Development of percutaneous intramuscular electrode for multichannel FES system, *IEEE Trans. Biomed. Eng.*, BME-36(7), 705–710, 1989a.

Handa, Y., Ohkubo, K., and Hoshimiya, N., A portable multi-channel functional electrical stimulation (FES) system for restoration of motor function of the paralyzed extremities, *Automedica*, 11(1–3), 221–232, 1989b.

Hansen, M., Machine Learning Techniques for Control of Functional Electrical Stimulation Using Natural Sensors, Ph.D. thesis, Center for Sensory-Motor Interaction, Aalborg University, Aalborg, Denmark, 2001.

Hansen, M., Kostov, A., Haugland, M., and Sinkjær, T., Feature extraction in control of FES using afferent nerve signals in humans, *Can. J. Physiol. Pharmacol.*, 76(2), 1998.

Hart, R.L., Kilgore, K.L., and Peckham, P.H., A comparison between control methods for implanted FES hand-grasp systems, *IEEE Trans. Rehab. Eng.*, TRE-6, 208–218, 1998.

Haugland, M. and Hoffer, J.A., Slip information provided by nerve cuff signals: application in closed-loop control of functional electrical stimulation, *IEEE Trans. Rehab. Eng.*, TRE-2(1), 29–36, 1994a.

Haugland, M. and Hoffer, J.A., Artifact-free sensory nerve signals obtained from cuff electrodes during functional electrical stimulation of nearby muscles, *IEEE Trans. Rehab. Eng.*, TRE-2, 37–39, 1994b.

Haugland, M. and Sinkjær, T., Cutaneous whole nerve recordings used for correction of footdrop in hemiplegic man, *IEEE Trans. Rehab. Eng.*, TRE-3, 307–317, 1995.

Haugland, M., Lickel, A., Haase, J., and Sinkjær, T., Control of FES thumb force using slip information obtained from the cutaneous electroneurogram in quadriplegic man, *IEEE Trans. Rehab. Eng.*, TRE-7(2), 215–227, 1999.

Hausler, E., Lang, H., and Schreiner, F.J., Piezoelectric high polymer foils as physiological mechanic-electric energy converters, in *Proc. IEEE Frontiers Eng. Health Care Conf.*, IEEE Press, Piscataway, NJ, 1980, pp. 333–334.

Hoffer, J.A., Closed Loop, Implant Sensor, Functional Electrical Stimulation System for Partial Restoration of Motor Functions, U.S. Patent No. 4,750,499, 1988.

Hoffer, J.A. and Loeb, G.A., Implantable electrical and mechanical interfaces with nerve and muscle, *Ann. Biomed. Eng.*, 8, 351–360, 1980.

Hoffer, J.A., Stein, R.B., Haugland, K.K., Sinkjær, T., Durfee, W.K., Schwartz, A.B., Loeb, G.E., and Kantor, C., Neural signals for command control and feedback in functional electrical stimulation, *J. Rehabil.*, 33(2), 145–157, 1995.

Holle, J., Frey, M., Gruber, H., Kern, H., Stohr, H., and Thoma, H., Functional electrostimulation of paraplegics: experimental investigations and first clinical experience with an implantable stimulation device, *Orthopaedics*, 7, 1145–1160, 1984.

Ilić, M., Vasiljević, D., and Popović, D.B., A programmable electronic stimulator for FES systems, *IEEE Trans. Rehabil. Eng.*, TRE-2, 234–239, 1994.

Inmann, A., Natural Sensory Feedback for FES Controlled Hand Grasp, Ph.D. thesis, Center for Sensory-Motor Interaction, Aalborg University, Aalborg, Denmark, 2001.

Jacobs, P.L., Nash, M.S., Klose, K.J., Guest, R.S., Needham-Shropshire, B.M., and Green, B.A., Evaluation of a training program for persons with SCI paraplegia using the Parastep 1 ambulation system. II. Effects on physiological responses to peak arm ergometry, *Arch. Phys. Med. Rehab.*, 78(8), 794–798, 1997.

Jaeger, R.J., Yarkony, G.Y., and Smith, R., Standing the spinal cord injured patient by electrical stimulation: refinement of a protocol for clinical use, *IEEE Trans. Biomed. Eng.*, BME-36, 720–728, 1989.

James, K., Waldon, V., Popović, D., and Stein, R., High power four channel stimulator for use in FES systems, Eng. Found. Conf.: Motor Control III — Neuroprostheses, Banff, 1991, p. 25.

Kilgore, K.L., Peckham, P.H., Keith, M.W., Thrope, G.B., Wuolle, K.S., Bryden, A.M., and Hart, R.T., An implanted upper-extremity neuroprosthesis. Follow-up of five patients, *J. Bone Joint Surg. Am.*, 79, 533–541, 1997.

Klose, K.J., Jacobs, P.L., Broton, J.G., Guest, R.S., Needham-Shropshire, B.M., Lebwohl, N., et al., Evaluation of a training program for persons with SCI paraplegia using the Parastep 1 ambulation system. I. Ambulation performance and anthropometric measures, *Arch. Phys. Med. Rehab.*, 78(8), 789–793, 1997.

Knaflitz, M. and Merletti, R., Suppression of stimulation artifacts from myoelectric-evoked potential recordings, *IEEE Trans. Biomed. Eng.*, 35(9), 758–763, 1988.

Kobetič, R. and Marsolais, E.B., Synthesis of paraplegic gait with multichannel functional electrical stimulation, *IEEE Trans. Rehab. Eng.*, TRE-2, 66–79, 1994.

Kobetič, R., Triolo, R.J., and Marsolais, E.B., Muscle selection and walking performance of multichannel FES systems for ambulation in paraplegia, *IEEE Trans. Rehab. Eng.*, TRE-5, 23–29, 1997.

Kobetič, R., Triolo, R.J., Uhlir, J.P., Bieri, C., Wibowo, M., Polando, G., et al., Implanted functional electrical stimulation system for mobility in paraplegia: a follow-up case report, *IEEE Trans. Rehab. Eng.*, TRE-7, 390–398, 1999.

Kostov, A., Hansen, M., Haugland, M., and Sinkjær, T., Adaptive restriction rules provide functional and safe stimulation pattern for foot-drop correction, *Artif. Organs*, 23(5), 443–446, 1999.

Kralj, A. and Bajd, T., *Functional Electrical Stimulation: Standing and Walking after Spinal Cord Injury*, CRC Press, Boca Raton, FL, 1989.

Kralj, A., Bajd, T., and Turk, R., Electrical stimulation providing functional use of paraplegic patient muscles, *Med. Prog. Technol.*, 7, 3–9, 1980.

Lemay, M.A. and Crago, P.E., Closed-loop wrist stabilization in C4 and C5 tetraplegia, *IEEE Trans. Rehab. Eng.*, 5(3), 244–252, 1997.

Lemay, M.A. and Grill, W.M., Spinal force fields in the cat spinal cord (abstract), *Soc. Neurosci.*, 25, 1396, 1999.

Liberson, W.F., Holmquest, H.J., Scott, D., and Dow, A., Functional electrotherapy: stimulation of the peroneal nerve synchronized with the swing phase of the gait in hemiplegic patients, *Arch. Phys. Med. Rehab.*, 42, 101–105, 1961.

Loeb, G.E. and Peck, R.A., Cuff electrodes for chronic stimulation and recording of peripheral nerve activity, *J. Neurosci. Meth.*, 64, 95–103, 1996.

Maalej, N. and Webster, J.G., A miniature electrooptical force transducer, *IEEE Trans. Biomed. Eng.*, BME-35(1), 93–98, 1988.

Maležič, M., Stanič, U., Kljajić, M., Aćimović, R., Krajnik, J., Gros, N., and Stopar, M., Multichannel electrical stimulation of gait in motor disabled patients, *Orthopedics*, 7(7), 1187–1195, 1984.

Marsolais, E.B. and Kobetič, R., Functional walking in paralyzed patients by means of electrical stimulation, *Clin. Orthop.*, 175, 30–36, 1983.

Marsolais, E.B. and Kobetič, R., Functional electrical stimulation for walking in paraplegics, *J. Bone Jt. Surg.*, 69, 728–733, 1987.

McCreery, D.B., Agnew, W.F., Yuen, T.G., and Bullara, L.A., Relationship between stimulus amplitude, stimulus frequency and neural damage during electrical stimulation of sciatic nerve of cat, *Med. Biol. Eng. Comput.*, 33(3), 426–429, 1995.

McFarland, D.J., McCane, L.M., and Wolpaw, J.R., EEG-based communication and control: short-term role of feedback, *IEEE Trans. Rehab. Eng.*, TRE-6(1), 7–11, 1998.

McGill, K.C., Cummins, K.L., Dorfman, L.J., Berlizot, B.B., Leutkemeyer, K., Nishimura, D.G., and Widrow, B., On the nature and elimination of stimulas artifact in nerve signals evoked and recorded using surface electrodes, *IEEE Trans. Biomed. Eng.*, 29(2), 129–137, 1982.

McNeal, D.R. and Baker, L., Effects of joint angle, electrodes and waveform on electrical stimulation of the quadriceps and hamstrings, *Ann. Biomed. Eng.*, 16, 299–310, 1988.

McNeal, D.R. and Bowman, B., Selective activation of muscle using peripheral nerve electrodes, *Med. Biol. Eng. Comp.*, 23(3), 249–253, 1985.

McNeal, D.R. and Reswick, J.B., Control of skeletal muscle by electrical stimulation, *Adv. Biomed. Eng.*, 6, 209–256, 1976.

Minzly, J., Mizrahi, J., Isakov, E., Susak, Z., and Verbeke, M., A computer controlled portable stimulator for paraplegic patients, *J. Biomed. Eng.*, 15, 333–338, 1993.

Mortimer, T., Motor prosthesis, in *Handbook of Physiology* (Sect. 1, Vol. 11, Part 1(5)), Brooks, V.B., Ed., American Physiological Society, Bethesda, MD, 1981, pp. 155–187.

Mushahwar, V.K. and Horch, K.W., Proposed specifications for a lumbar spinal cord electrode array for control of lower extremities in paraplegia, *IEEE Trans. Rehab. Eng.*, TRE-5(3), 237–243, 1997.

Mushahwar, V.K. and Horch, K.W., Muscle recruitment through electrical stimulation of the lumbosacral spinal cord, *IEEE Trans. Rehab. Eng.*, TRE-8(1), 22–28, 2000.

Naples, G.G., Mortimer, J.T., Scheiner, A., and Sweeney, J.D., A spiral nerve cuff electrode for peripheral nerve stimulation, *IEEE Trans. Biomed. Eng.*, BME-35(11), 905–916, 1988.

Nathan, R.H., An FNS-based system for generating upper limb function in the C4 quadriplegic, *Med. Biol. Eng. Comp.*, 27, 549–556, 1989.

Nathan, R.H., Control strategies in FNS systems for the upper extremities, *CRC Press Crit. Rev. Biomed. Eng.*, 21(6), 485–568, 1993.

Nathan, R.H. and Ohry, A., Upper limb functions regained in quadriplegia: a hybrid computerized neuromuscular stimulation system, *Arch. Phys. Med. Rehab.*, 71, 415–421, 1990.

Nikolić, Z.M., Popović, D.B., Stein, R.B., and Kenwell, Z., Instrumentation for ENG and EMG recordings in FES systems, *IEEE Trans. Biomed. Eng.*, BME-41, 703–706, 1994.

Normann, R.A., Maynard, E.M., Rousche, P.J., and Warren, D.J., A neural interface for a cortical vision prosthesis, *Vision Res.*, 39(15), 2577–2587, 1999.

Peckham, P.H., Functional electrical stimulation, in *Encyclopedia of Medical Devices and Instrumentation*, Webster, J.G., Ed., John Wiley, New York, 1988, pp. 1341–1358.

Peckham, P.H. and Creasey, G.H., Neural protheses: clinical applications of functional electrical stimulation in spinal cord injury, *Paraplegia*, 30(2), 96–101, 1992.

Peckham, P.H., Marsolais, E.B., and Mortimer, J.T., Restoration of the key grip and release in the C6 quadriplegic through functional electrical stimulation, *J. Hand Surg.*, 5, 464–469, 1980b.

Peckham, P.H., Mortimer, J.T., and Marsolais, E.B., Controlled prehension and release in the C5 quadriplegic elicited by functional electrical stimulation of the paralyzed forearm muscles, *Ann. Biomed. Eng.*, 8, 369–388, 1980a.

Phillips, C.A., Electrical muscle stimulation in combination with a reciprocating gait orthosis for ambulation by paraplegics, *J. Biomed. Eng.*, 11, 338–344, 1989.

Popović, D.B. and Popović, M.B., Tuning of a nonanalytical hierarchical control system for reaching with FES, *IEEE Trans. Biomed. Eng.*, BME-45(2), 203–212, 1998a.

Popović, D.B. and Popović, M.B., Belgrade grasping system, *J. Electronics (Banja Luka, Bosnia)*, 2, 21–28, 1998b.

Popović, D.B. and Popović, M.B., Control for an elbow neuroprosthesis: cloning biological synergies, *IEEE Med. Biol. Eng. Mag.*, 20(1), 74–81, 2001.

Popović, D.B. and Sinkjær, T., *Control of Movement for the Physically Disabled: Control for Rehabilitation Technology*, Springer, London, 2000.

Popović, D.B., Tomovič, R., and Schwirtlich, L., Hybrid assistive system: neuroprosthesis for motion, *IEEE Trans. Biomed. Eng.*, BME-36(7), 729–738, 1989.

Popović, D.B., Gordon, T., Rafuse, V., and Prochazka, A., Properties of implanted electrodes for functional electrical stimulation, *Ann. Biomed. Eng.*, 19, 303–316, 1991.

Popović, D.B., Stein, R.B., Jovanović, K.L., Rongching, D., Kostov, A., and Armstrong, W.W., Sensory nerve recording for closed-loop control to restore motor functions, *IEEE Trans. Biomed. Eng.*, BME-40, 1024–1031, 1993.

Popović, D.B., Stojanović, A., Pjanović, A., Radosavljević, S., Popović, M.B., Jović, S., and Vulović, D., Clinical evaluation of the bionic glove, *Arch. Phys. Med. Rehab.*, 80(3), 299–304, 1999.

Popović, D.B. and Popović, M.B., Nonanalytical control for assisting reaching in humans with disability, in *Control of Posture and Movement: Neuro-Musculo-Skeletal Interaction and Organization Principles*, Winters, J.M. and Crago, P.E., Eds., Springer-Verlag, New York, 2000, Chap. 39, pp. 535–548.

Popović, M.R., Keller, T., Pappas, I., Dietz, V., and Morari, M., ETHZ-ParaCare grasping and walking neuroprostheses, *IEEE Med. Biol. Eng. Mag.*, 20(1), 82–93, 2001.

Prochazka, A., Gauthier, M., Wieler, M., and Kenwell, Z., The Bionic glove: an electrical stimulator garment that provides controlled grasp and hand opening in quadriplegia, *Arch. Phys. Med. Rehab.*, 78, 608–614, 1997.

Qi, H., Tyler, D.J., and Durand, D.M., Neurofuzzy adaptive controlling of selective stimulation for FES: a case study, *IEEE Trans. Rehab. Eng.*, TRE-7, 183–192, 1999.

Reberšek, S. and Vodovnik, L., Proportionally controlled functional electrical stimulation of hand, *Arch. Phys. Med. Rehab.*, 54, 378–382, 1973.

Riso, R.R., Mosallaie, F.K., Jensen, W., and Sinkjaer, T., Nerve cuff recordings of muscle afferent activity from tibial and peroneal nerves in rabbit during passive ankle motion, *IEEE Trans. Rehab. Eng.*, TRE-8, 244–258, 2000.

Rousche, P.J. and Normann, R.A., Chronic intracortical microstimulation (ICMS) of cat sensory cortex using the Utah Intracortical Electrode Array, *IEEE Trans. Rehab. Eng.*, TRE-7(1), 56–68, 1999.

Rushton, D.N., Choice of nerves roots for multichannel leg controller implant, in *Advances in External Control X*, Popović, D.B., Ed., Nauka, 1990, pp. 99–108.

Rutten, W.L., van Wier, H.J., and Put, J.H., Sensitivity and selectivity of intraneural stimulation using a silicon electrode array, *IEEE Trans. Biomed. Eng.*, 38(2), 192–198, 1991.

Saxena, S., Nikolić, S., and Popović, D.B., An EMG controlled FES system for grasping in tetraplegics, *J. Rehab. Res. Dev.*, 32, 17–23, 1995.

Scheiner, A., Mortimer, J.T., and Roessmann, U., Imbalanced biphasic electrical stimulation: muscle tissue damage, *Ann. Biomed. Eng.*, 18(4), 407–425, 1990.

Schwirtlich, L. and Popović, D.B., Hybrid orthoses for deficient locomotion, in *Advances in External Control of Human Extremities VIII*, Popović, D.B., Ed., ETAN, 1984, pp. 23–32.

Scott, T.R.D., Peckham, P.H., and Kilgore, K.L., Tri-state myoelectric control of bilateral upper extremity neuroprosthesis for tetraplegic individuals, *IEEE Trans. Rehab. Eng.*, TRE-4, 251–263, 1996.

Sennels, S., Biering-Soerensen, F., Anderson, O.T., and Hansen, S.D., Functional neuromuscular stimulation control by surface electromyographic signals produced by volitional activation of the same muscle: adaptive removal of the muscle response from the recorded EMG-signal, *IEEE Trans. Rehab. Eng.*, TRE-5, 195–206, 1997.

Seow, K.C., Capacitive sensors, in *Tactile Sensors for Robotics and Medicine*, Webster, J.G., Ed., John Wiley & Sons, New York, 1988.

Sharma, M., Marsolais, E.B., Polando, G., Triolo, R.J., Davis, J.A., Jr., Bhadra, N., and Uhlir, J.P., Implantation of a 16-channel functional electrical stimulation walking system, *Clin. Orthop.*, 347, 236–242, 1998.

Smith, B.T., Betz, R.R., Mulcahey, M.J., and Triolo, R.J., Reliability of percutaneous intramuscular electrodes for upper extremity functional neuromuscular stimulation in adolescents with C5 tetraplegia, *Arch. Phys. Med. Rehab.*, 75(9), 939–945, 1994.

Smith, B.T., Mulcahey, B.J., and Betz, R.P., Development of an upper extremity FES system for individuals with C4 tetraplegia, *IEEE Trans. Rehab. Eng.*, TRE-4, 264–270, 1996.

Smith, B.T., Peckham, P.H., Keith, M.W., and Roscoe, D.D., An externally powered, multichannel, implantable stimulator for versatile control of paralyzed muscle, *IEEE Trans. Biomed. Eng.*, BME-34(7), 499–508, 1987.

Smith, B.T., Tang, Z., Johnson, M.W., Pourmehdi, S., Gazdik, M.M., Buckett, J.R., and Peckham, P.H., An externally powered multichannel, implantable stimulator-telemeter for control of paralyzed muscles, *IEEE Trans. Biomed. Eng.*, BME-45, 463–475, 1998.

Solomonow, M., Baratta, R., Hirokawa, S., Rightor, N., Walker, W., Beaudette, P., Shoji, H., and D'Ambrosia, R., The RGO generation. II. Muscle stimulation powered orthosis as a practical walking system for thoracic paraplegics, *Orthopedics*, 12(10), 1309–1315, 1989.

Stein, R.B., Bélanger, M., Wheeler, G., Wieler, M., Popović, D.B., Prochazka, A., and Davis, L., Electrical systems for improving locomotion after incomplete spinal cord injury: an assessment, *Arch. Phys. Med. Rehab.*, 74, 954–959, 1993.

Stein, R.B., Charles, D., Davis, L., Jhamandas, J., Mannard, A., and Nichols, T.R., Principles underlying new methods for chronic neural recording, *Can. J. Neurol. Sci.*, 2, 235–244, 1975.

Strojnik, P., Aćimović-Janežič, R., Vavken, E., Simić, V., and Stanič, U., Treatment of drop foot using an implantable peroneal underknee stimulator, *Scand. J. Rehab. Med.*, 19, 37–43, 1987.

Strojnik, P., Schulman, J., Loeb, G., and Troyk, P., Multichannel FES system with distributed microstimulators, in *Proc. Annu. Int. Conf. IEEE EMBS*, IEEE Press, Piscataway, NJ, 1993, pp. 1352–1353.

Strojnik, P., Whitmoyer, D., and Schulman, J., An implantable stimulator for all season, in *Advances in External Control of Human Extremities X*, Popović, D.B., Ed., Nauka, 1990, pp. 335–344.

Sweeney, P.C. and Lyons, G.M., Fuzzy gait event detection in a finite state controlled FES drop foot correction system, *J. Bone Jt. Surg.*, (BR) 81-B, 93–93, 1999.

Sweeney, J.D. and Mortimer, J.T., An asymmetric two electrode cuff for generation of unidirectionally propagated action potentials, *IEEE Trans. Biomed. Eng.*, BME-33, 541–549, 1986.

Sweeney, J.D., Ksienski, D.A., and Mortimer, J.T., A nerve cuff technique for selective excitation of peripheral nerve trunk regions, *IEEE Trans. Biomed. Eng.*, BME-37(7), 706–715, 1990.

Sweeney, J.D., Crawford, N.R., and Brandon, T.A., Neuromuscular stimulation selectivity of multiple-contact nerve cuff electrode arrays, *Med. Biol. Eng. Comp.*, 33, 418–425, 1995.

Taylor, P.N., Ed., *The University of Limerick Drop Foot Stimulator*, The Inst. Phys. Eng. Med., York, England, 1997.

Thoma, H., Holle, J., Moritz, E., and Stöhr, H., Walking after paraplegia — a principle concept, in *Advances in External Control of Human Extremities VI*, ETAN, 1978, pp. 71–84.

Thoma, H., Frey, M., Hole, J., Kern, H., Mayr, W., Schwanda, G., and Stoehr, H., Functional neurostimulation to substitute locomotion in paraplegia patients, in *Artificial Organs*, Andrade, J.D., Ed., VCH Publishers, Weinheim, Germany, 1987, pp. 515–529.

Thorsen, R., Ferrarin, M., Spadone, R., and Frigo, C., An approach using wrist extension as control of FES for restoration of hand function in tetraplegics, in Proc. 6th Vienna Workshop on Functional Electrostimulation, 1998.

Thorsen, R., Ferrarin, M., Spadone, R., and Frigo, C., Functional control of the hand in tetraplegics based on residual synergistic EMG activity, *Artif. Organs*, 23(5), 470–473, 1999.

Thrope, G.B., Peckham, P.H., and Crago, P.E., A computer-controlled multichannel stimulation system for laboratory use in functional neuromuscular stimulation, *IEEE Trans. Biomed. Eng.*, 32(6), 363–370, 1985.

Tomovič, R., Popović, D.B., and Stein, R., *Nonanalytical Methods for Motor Control*, World Scientific Publishing, Singapore, 1995.

Triolo, R., Nathan, R., Handa, Y., Keith, M., Betz, R.R., Carroll, S., and Kantor, C., Challenges to clinical deployment of upper limb neuroprostheses, *J. Rehab. Res. Dev.*, 33(2), 111–122, 1996.

Upshaw, B. and Sinkjær, T., Digital signal processing algorithms for the detection of afferent nerve activity recorded from cuff electrodes, *IEEE Trans. Rehab. Eng.*, TRE-6, 172–181, 1998.

Vaughan, T.M., Miner, L.A., McFarland, D.J., and Wolpaw, J.R., EEG-based communication: analysis of concurrent EMG activity, *Electroencephalogr. Clin. Neurophysiol.*, 107(6), 428–433, 1998.

Veraart, C., Grill, W.M., and Mortimer, J.T,. Selective control of muscle activation with a multipolar nerve cuff electrode, *IEEE Trans. Biomed. Eng.*, BME-40(7), 640–653, 1993.

Vodovnik, L., Bajd, T., Kralj, A., Gračanin, F., and Strojnik, P., Functional electrical stimulation for control of locomotor systems, *CRC Crit. Rev. Bioeng.*, 6, 63–131, 1981.

Vodovnik, L., Crochetiere, W.J., and Reswick, J.B., Control of a skeletal joint by electrical stimulation of antagonists, *Med. Biol. Eng.*, 5, 97–109, 1967.

Vossius, G., Mueschen, U., and Hollander, H.J., Multichannel stimulation of the lower extremities with surface electrodes, in *Advances in External Control of Human Extremities IX*, Popović, D.B., Ed., ETAN, 1987, pp. 193–203.

Waters, R.J., McNeal, D.R., Faloon, W., and Clifford, B., Functional electrical stimulation of the peroneal nerve for hemiplegia, *J. Bone Jt. Surg.*, 67, 792–793, 1985.

Webster, J.G., Ed., *Tactile Sensors for Robotics and Medicine*, John Wiley & Sons, New York, 1988.

Wieler, M., Stein, R.B., Ladouceur, M., Whittaker, M., Smith, A.W., Naaman, S., et al., Multicenter evaluation of electrical stimulation systems for walking, *Arch. Phys. Med. Rehab.*, 80(5), 495–500, 1999.

Wijman, A.C., Stroh, K.C., Van Doren, C.L., Thrope, G.B., Peckham, P.H., and Keith, M.W., Functional evaluation of quadriplegic patients using a hand neuroprosthesis, *Arch. Phys. Med. Rehab.*, 32, 1053–1057, 1990.

Wolpaw, J.R., Ramoser, H., McFarland, D.J., and Pfurtscheller, G., EEG-based communication: improved accuracy by response verification, *IEEE Trans. Rehab. Eng.*, TRE-6(3), 326–333, 1998.

Yoshida, K. and Horch, K., Closed-loop control of ankle position using muscle afferent feedback with functional neuromuscular stimulation, *IEEE Trans. Biomed. Eng.*, 43(2), 167–176, 1996.

29

Pharmaceutical Technical Background on Delivery Methods

Robert S. Litman
Nova Southeastern University

Maria de la Cova

Icel Gonzalez
University of Memphis

Eduardo Lopez

CONTENTS

29.1 Introduction

In the evolution of drug development and manufacturing, drug delivery systems have risen to the forefront in the latest of pharmaceutical advances. There are many new pharmacological entities discovered each year, each with its own unique mechanism of action. Each drug will demonstrate its own pharmacokinetic profile. This profile may be changed by altering the drug delivery system to the target site. In order for a drug to demonstrate its pharmacological activity it must be absorbed, transported to the appropriate tissue or target organ, penetrate to the responding subcellular structure, and elicit a response or change an ongoing process. The drug may be simultaneously or sequentially distributed to a variety of tissues, bound or stored, further metabolized to active or inactive products, and eventually

0-8493-1140-3/04/$0.00+$1.50

excreted from the body. A delivery system that may have an effect upon the absorption, distribution, metabolism, or excretion of a pharmaceutical entity may then affect the potency, half-life, potential for drug interactions, and side-effect profile of that specific entity. Drug delivery systems are developed to enhance the desired pharmacological effect at specific target sites, while reducing the probability of drug interactions and unwanted side effects.

Other reasons for the development of new drug delivery systems include the masking of unpleasant tastes, inability of a patient to swallow a specific dosage form, protecting components from atmospheric degradation, controling the site of drug release, prolonging or delaying the absorption of the drug moiety, improving the drug's physical appearance, and changing the physical surface characteristics of the active ingredients. The following text will present a number of pharmaceutical drug delivery systems used in the treatment of a variety of disease states.

29.2 Central Nervous System: Drug Delivery

29.2.1 Challenges to Delivery: The Blood Brain Barrier

The central nervous system (CNS) consists of the brain and spinal cord. Drug delivery to the brain is challenging because of the blood brain barrier (BBB). The BBB is present in the brain of all vertebrates and is a system that protects the brain from substances in the blood. Because of the presence of the BBB over 98% of new drugs discovered for the CNS do not penetrate the brain following systemic administration.

The BBB is composed of:

1. The continuous endothelium of the capillary wall
2. A relatively thick basal laminal surrounding the external face of the capillary
3. The bulbous feet of the astrocytes that cling to the capillaries

The capillary endothelial cells are almost seamlessly joined all around by tight junctions making them the least permeable capillaries in the entire body. This relative impermeability of the brain capillaries constitutes most of the BBB.[1] In addition, once having traversed this barrier of the capillary endothelial cell, the drug must then penetrate the glial cells that envelop the capillary structure. Cerebral endothelial cells also express ATP-dependent transmemebrane glycoproteins involved in active transport of substances to outside the cell.[2] There are several theories as to what factors affect permeability into the brain. Factors such as lipophilicity, molecular size, polarity, and hydrogen bonding have been studied as methods to predict a drug's penetration capacity into the BBB.[3]

The cerebral spinal fluid (CSF) is a plasma-like fluid that fills the cavities of the CNS and surrounds the CNS externally, protecting the brain and spinal cord. Passage of chemical substances into the CSF is controlled by the blood-CSF barrier. This barrier is created by the ependymal cells of the choroid plexus.[4] The choroid plexus (which is located in the 3rd and 4th ventricles of the brain) has the ability to secrete substances out through an active transport system. Thus, attempts at accessing the brain through the CSF may be unsuccessful due to the protective nature of the choroid plexus. Also, it cannot be inferred that a given drug crosses the BBB just on the basis of its distribution into the CSF.[5]

Access to the CNS can be gained through direct or indirect methods. For drugs with the ability to penetrate the BBB, possible routes of administration are described below as indirect routes of administration. Direct routes of administration are attempts to bypass the BBB and gain access to CNS tissue.

Indirect routes of administration include:

- Intravenous, intraarterial
- Intraperitoneal
- Digestive tract
- Lung
- Skin
- Nasal

- Intramuscular
- Subcutaneous
- Sublingual
- Buccal
- Rectal

29.2.2 Indirect Routes of Administration

As previously described, access to the central nervous system can be achieved through indirect routes of administration, in addition to having to overcome the BBB, such routes of administration are subject to other bodily methods that may decrease or negate the amount of drug that penetrates the brain. For example, the drugs may be subject to being metabolized by the liver, excreted by the kidney, or acted upon by enzymes in the intestine or lung, all of which would result in a decrease in the amount of circulating drug available to the brain. These routes of administration all access the CNS through systemic absorption; in other words, access is gained to the bloodstream, which then attempts to cross the BBB.

Examples of drugs that cross the BBB include clonidine and propranolol, both antihypertensives. Propranolol can be administered via the oral route or i.v. route. Extensive first pass metabolism through the liver makes the oral dose necessarily much higher than the injectable dose. Clonidine is available for administration orally, as a transdermal patch and even for epidural use for intractable pain. Other well-known drugs able to cross the BBB include the opiate analgesics such as morphine, selective serotonin reuptake inhibitors such as Prozac®, and benzodiazepines such as Valium®. These drugs are available in multiple dosage forms ranging from injectable to oral to rectal gels. Fentanyl®, a potent analgesic, is available in transdermal patches and buccal formulations and generally used to treat cancer pain.

Still, the BBB and the blood-CSF barriers remain the largest challenge in developing drugs to effectively treat CNS disorders. Therefore, numerous ways to circumvent these barriers such as direct delivery to the CNS or attempted interruption of the BBB system have been researched.

29.2.3 Direct Routes of Administration

29.2.3.1 Nasal Drug Delivery

The nasal route of administration bypasses the BBB. Common drugs of addiction such as cocaine or amphetamine derivative may rapidly enter the brain by the nasal route. Nasal drug intake appears to be a fast and effective route of administration, suitable for drugs that must act rapidly and are taken in small amounts. Examples include antimigraine drugs such as Imitrex Nasal Spray® and analgesics such as Stadol Nasal Spray®. Unfortunately, frequent use of this route of administration may lead to complications such as mucosal damage that can lead to infections. Also, some patients may lose the ability to smell.

29.2.3.2 Epidural Drug Delivery

Drugs administered into the epidural space in order to reach the spinal cord must traverse the dura mater, arachnoid mater, then enter the CSF to reach the spinal cord gray and white matter. This occurs through simple diffusion. Epidural infusion and anesthesia is a common tool in the U.S. for pain relief from contractions during labor. Pharmacologic means to prevent the redistribution of drug to the systemic circulation or to prolong the drug effect have been used. One such example is the addition of epinephrine to local anesthetics and epidural opioids. The addition of epinephrine has been shown to improve the quality and prolong the duration of epidural anesthesia and analgesia. Other pharmaceutical modifiers of redistribution include preparations that provide slow-release "depot" formulations, encapsulating drugs in liposomes, embedding drugs in biodegradable polymers, or using drugs that are themselves nearly insoluble in aqueous solutions.[6]

29.2.3.3 Intrathecal Drug Delivery

This method involves direct injection into the CSF via a spinal needle or catheter. Drug injection into the CSF results in mixing of the drug product and the CSF which does not occur with epidurally administered drugs. Drugs enter the CSF as a solution, instead of as individual molecules in the case of epidural administration. This causes the density of the solution and the patient's position to be the most important factors with regard to where the drug initially distributes along the spinal cord. The more dense the solution, the more the tendency to move down the spinal column until complete mixture with the CSF makes the solution isobaric. Hydrophobic drugs have poor permeability into the CSF. One way to improve the permeability is to increase their aqueous solubility.

Research into compounds such as cyclodextrins shows that combining drugs, for example sufentanil with cyclodextrin, increases its permeability into the meninges more than twofold *in vitro*. However, it is also possible that when used *in vivo* the redistribution of drugs into unintended sites might occur. Rigorous toxicology trials in animals are still necessary in this area.[6,10]

29.2.3.4 Intracerebroventricular Drug Delivery

Invasive brain drug delivery systems have been the most widely used for circumventing the BBB drug delivery problem. This invasive strategy requires either a crainiotomy by a neurosurgeon or access to the carotid artery by an interventional radiologist. The neurosurgical-based systems include intracerebroventricular (ICV) infusion of drugs or intracerebral implants of biodegradable polymers.[7] Unfortunately, drug penetration following ICV injection is minimal.[5] Also, because of the one-way flow of CSF in the brain following ICV injection, the distribution of drug to both sides of the brain following ICV injection would require the placement of catheters in both lateral ventricles.[5] ICV has been used primarily in three treatment areas: chemotherapy for brain tumors, treatment of infections of the central nervous system,[12] and delivery of analgesics in the setting of intractable pain.[8] In the case of chemotherapy, direct injection into the CNS also avoids significant systemic toxicity by limiting chemotherapy exposure to the CNS.

29.2.3.5 CNS and Drug Targeting

Drug targeting describes a process for attempting site specific delivery of drugs. For drugs needing access to the CNS for their action to be exerted, the need for drug targeting and avoidance of the BBB is an obvious one.

Drug targeting has been classified into three types:[9]

1. Delivery to a discrete organ or tissue
2. Targeting to a specific cell type (e.g., tumor cells vs. normal cells)
3. Delivery to a specific intracellular compartment in the target cells (e.g., lysosomes)

Targeting can be achieved through different methodologies: Biologic agents that are selective to a particular site in the body, preparation of prodrug that becomes active once it reaches the target site, and using a biologically inert macromolecular carrier system that directs a drug to a specific site in the body.

For example, 3.85% carmustine (Gliadel®) impregnated polymers consisting of CPP:SA have shown improved survival in patients with high-grade recurrent gliomas (brain tumor).[7] Carmustine itself crosses the BBB; however, the polymers allow higher tissue levels to be achieved with minimal systemic side effects. The polymer wafers are placed after the surgical removal of the brain tumor itself in the cavity left behind once the tumor is removed.

Drug targeting is a promising field of research to aid in drug delivery to the CNS.

29.3 Cardiovascular System: Drug Delivery

Cardiovascular disease has become an important cause of morbidity and mortality as the population ages. The new millennium holds even greater promise as genetic engineering produces new and even more effective drugs and devices to prevent and treat patients with cardiovascular disease.[53] In this section the latest cardiovascular drug delivery methods will be discussed.

29.3.1 Chronotherapeutics

Chronotherapeutic medications deliver medications in concentrations that vary according to changes in physiologic need.[54,55] In hypertension, chronotherapeutic medications deliver the drug in highest concentrations during the morning period, when blood pressure is the greatest, and in lesser concentrations at nighttime, when blood pressure is the lowest.[54,55] Verapamil, a calcium channel blocker, has been marketed in two formulations that use novel delivery systems to provide chronotherapy: Verelan PM™ (Schwarz Pharma Inc, Milwaukee, WI) and Covera-HS™ (Pharmacia Corp, Peapack, NJ).[54] Verelan PM uses chronotherapeutic oral drug absorption system (CODAS) technology, and Covera-HS uses the controlled-onset, extended-release (COER-24) delivery system.[54] The CODAS delivery system incorporates a 4- to 5-h delay in drug delivery followed by an extended drug release, with a peak concentration occurring approximately 11 h after administration, which is designed for bedtime dosing.[54] Trough concentrations occur approximately 4 h after dosing.[54] "Each capsule contains numerous pellets that consist of an inert core surrounded by active drug and rate-controlling membranes that combine water-soluble and water-insoluble polymers."[54] As the pellets lie in the gastrointestinal tract, water washes over the pellets, slowly dissolving the water-soluble polymer and allowing the drug to diffuse through pores in the coating.[54] The water-insoluble polymer continues to provide a barrier that allows the drug to be dosed every 24 h.[54] For the Covera-HS™ the outermost component of the (COER-24) delivery system is a semipermeable membrane that regulates absorption of water into the tablet.[54] Water is absorbed from the gastrointestinal tract at a fixed rate until the second layer, or delay coat, is reached.[54] The second layer then absorbs water and temporarily prevents the passage of water into the inner core of the tablet.[54] This process delays drug release for approximately 4 to 5 h while the patient is sleeping, when blood pressure is lower.[54] When sufficient moisture has been absorbed, a third layer expands by osmosis, pushing verapamil out of the tablet at a constant rate that adequately controls the patient's blood pressure during the morning hours.[54] Continued absorption of water and ongoing osmotic expansion of the third layer provide for extended release of drug and once-daily dosing.[54]

In conclusion, chronotherapeutic verapamil formulations provide effective 24-h control of blood pressure.[54,55] The delay in drug release avoids problems with excessive blood pressure lowering during sleep and provides blood pressure control in the late morning and early afternoon hours when blood pressure is the highest.[54,55]

29.3.2 Grafts/Stents

Since 1952, when the first vascular prostheses was constructed out of the fabric Vinyon N, many researchers have focused upon the production of an ideal synthetic vascular graft.[56] Restenosis complicates the outcome of most of the interventional cardiovascular procedures for relieving coronary artery obstruction.[57] The pathogenesis of restenosis is incompletely understood, but seems to be due to a number of factors which include: acute fibrin thrombus, platelet binding, smooth muscle proliferation, and inflammation.[57] Thus the search for the ideal graft that will maintain a long patency is still on. Drug-eluting vascular stents with a variety of coatings including fibrin, heparin, and polymers that contain NO donors have been tested with differing outcomes.[58] NO-containing cross-linked polyethylenimine microspheres that release NO with a half-life of 51 h have been applied to vascular grafts to prevent thrombosis and restenosis. The incorporation of the NO to the polymeric matrices has shown powerful antiplatelet activity in cardiovascular grafts.[58] Alternatively, liposomal drug delivery systems bearing arginine-glycine-aspartic acid (RGD) peptides on the surface could emulate the function of fibrinogen in binding GPIIb-IIIa on activated platelets, and therefore represent a means to target liposome-encapsulated anticoagulant or antiplatelet effects to discrete regions of the cardiovascular system.[59] The RGD peptide utilized has demonstrated to inhibit fibrinogen binding to platelets which is one of the factors for restenosis.[59] Due to their relative chemical simplicity, peptides are versatile ligands for use in liposomal drug delivery to molecular targets within the cardiovascular system.[59] Poly(ethylene oxide) (PEO)-grafted phospholipids were shown to dramatically increase liposome survival in the circulation by avoiding rapid reticuloendothelial system uptake.[59] Recently, investigators inserted silastic tubing into the peritoneal cavity of rats and rabbits.[56] "The resulting inflammatory reaction to the silastic covered the tubes with layers of myofibroblasts, collagen matrix, and a monolayer of mesothelial cells. By withdrawing the tubing from the laminar, multicellular remains of the inflammatory response and then everting this biological tube, these investigators discovered synthetic arteries with architecture similar to that of native blood vessels."[56] The mesothelial cells mimicked endothelial cells, the myofibroblasts act as smooth muscle cells lying in a collagen bed, and the entire structure was surrounded by a collagenous adventitia.[56] The vessels also developed structures similar to high-volume myofilaments that are able to respond to pharmacological agonists.[56] In conclusion, the presumably higher patency rates and longer half-lives of tissue-engineered vascular prostheses and the use of liposomes as potentially advantageous targeted drug carriers for such intravascular applications will be the future for the treatment of restenosis.[56,59]

29.4 Orthopedic: Drug Delivery

29.4.1 Metabolic Bone Diseases

The skeletal system is affected by a host of disorders including osteoporosis, osteomalacia, renal osteodystrophy, Paget's disease, osteomyelitis, and numerous others. Osteoporosis, a disorder frequently encountered as bone loss associated with aging in postmenopausal women, is now recognized as a major health issue in the United States. Osteoporosis is defined as a universal, gradual reduction in bone mass to a point where the skeleton is compromised.[14] The majority of current treatments for osteoporosis are limited to antiresorptive therapy that slow bone turnover and loss, rather than building new bone mass. Current therapeutic prophylactic and treatment alternatives for osteoporosis include hormone replacement therapy, calcitonin, bisphosphonates, and selective estrogen receptor modulators.

29.4.1.1 Indirect Routes of Administration

Indirect routes of administration include nasal, transdermal, intravenous (i.v.), oral, and subcutaneous (s.c.).

29.4.1.2 Nasal

Calcitonin is a polypeptide hormone composed of 32 amino acids secreted by the parafollicular cells of the thyroid gland. Although the actions of calcitonin on bone are still not completely understood, it inhibits bone resorption by decreasing the number of osteoclasts and their resorptive activities and limiting osteocytic osteolysis.[15] A synthetic nasal calcitonin formulation is available (Miacalcin®). Calcitonin is also available for s.c. injection.

29.4.1.3 Transdermal

Hormone replacement therapy (i.e., estrogen or estrogen-progestin combinations) has been shown to be beneficial in post-menopausal women at risk for osteoporosis. Women exposed to estrogen therapy for 7 to 10 years have a 50% reduction in the incidence of osteoporotic fractures.[16] Estrogen therapy for osteoporosis is available as oral tablets and transdermal patches. The patch itself is usually composed of three layers: a backing layer, an adhesive layer, and protective release layer.

Transdermal patches generally have one of two different designs of the drug compartment: (1) form-fill and seal design and (2) monolith design. In form-fill and seal design, drug is contained as a liquid or semisolid reservoir in shallow pouches within the backing layer. The monolith design is further subdivided into the peripheral adhesive laminate structure and solid-state laminate structure, in the peripheral adhesive design, the active delivery area is generally much less than the patch size, in the solid state laminate structure, the active delivery area is identical to the size of the patch. Monolith patches are uniform in composition throughout. They can be cut to smaller sizes without compromising their basic delivery function.[16] There are numerous transdermal estrogen patches available ranging from 25 to 100 mcg of delivery per day. Generally, the patches are changed every 72 h; now several weekly patches have been introduced into the market.

29.4.1.4 Intravenous

Bisphosphonates are a class of drugs indicated to treat Paget's disease, hypercalcemia of malignancy, and osteoporosis. They can be given orally and intravenously to humans. Clinical studies of the feasibility of bisphosphonate transdermal delivery and direct delivery to bone via prodrug are being conducted. The i.v. route, though available, is seldom used for the treatment of osteoporosis. This is because large amounts and rapid injection of i.v. bisphosphonates can result in kidney failure.

29.4.1.5 Oral

Bisphosphonates are the mainstay of osteoporosis treatment in the oral setting. The mechanism of action of the bisphosphonates is based on their affinity to bone mineral hydoxyapatite. The bisphosphonates bind strongly to the calcium phosphate crystals and inhibit their growth, aggregation, and dissolution. The biological effects of the bisphosphonates in calcium-related disorders are due to their incorporation in bone enabling direct interaction with osteoclasts and/or osteoblasts.[15] The oral route, as can be imagined, is the most preferred route for chronic drug therapy. The major disadvantage of the clinically utilized bisphosphonates is their poor bioavailability (less than 1%) due to their hydrophilic nature and their side effects of gastrointestinal irritation, in addition, food can further suppress absorption, as much as four- to fivefold. Therefore, these drugs are taken on an empty stomach. Attempts at circumventing the bioavailability issue have included: absorption enhancement through use of EDTA, development of prodrugs that are lipophilic, and prodrugs that would use carrier mediated transport systems.[26] EDTA can improve the absorption of these compounds by directly enhancing intestinal permeability. Unfortunately, EDTA damages the mucosal integrity and cannot be used in humans. The other approaches are still in initial stages of research, none yet available for marketed use in humans.

29.4.1.6 Bone Infections

The term osteomyelitis describes any infection involving bone. Osteomyelitis represents a difficult infection to treat for various reasons. First, it has a tendency to be chronic and recurrent and second, there is a need to deliver high concentrations of antimicrobial agents in the blood to achieve adequate levels in bone.[23] Traditional therapy includes intravenously administered antimicrobials (to avoid issues with bioavailability). Since the classic organisms that infect bone are of a Gram-positive nature, the most frequently used antimicrobials are cephalosporins, extended spectrum penicillins, and vancomycin for resistant species. Three major considerations are critical in managing these infections in bone:

1. Spectrum of activity of agent chosen
2. Ability of antimicrobial to penetrate and reach the site of infection
3. Duration of therapy

29.4.1.7 Direct Routes of Administration

Other treatment options used for treatment of osteomyelitis include the use of ceramic composites as implantable systems. The treatment of osteomyelitis as previously discussed is a complicated process involving surgical removal of dead bone tissue and prolonged systemic antibiotics. Hydroxyapatite cement systems have been developed to deliver drug to the skeletal tissue at therapeutic concentrations without causing systemic toxicity.[18] These hydroxyapatite cement formulations are loaded with antibiotics such as cephalexin and then placed directly at the site of infection or fracture.

Tricalcium phosphate and amino acid antibiotic composite ceramics and PMMA antibiotic-impregnated beads have also been used to treat osteomyelitis with success.[18,19]

29.4.1.8 Drug Targeting

Targeting of bisphosphonate release from bone has been the subject of recent study. This drug delivery system is based on the concept of a site-specific bisphosphonate prodrug. The system, which is used only in animal trials thus far, is called the osteotropic drug delivery system. This approach is based on the chemical adsorption of the prodrug to the mineral component, hydroxyapatite.[20] Also the subject of recent study was the use of the osteotropic drug delivery system to deliver diclofenac (a nonsteroidal anti-inflammatory drug). This study in rats showed that once the prodrug complex was injected into the animals it was predominantly distributed to the skeleton. This study showed hope for this approach for highly potent and nontoxic therapy of diclofenac with less frequent medication administration.[21] Studies of other nonsteroidal anti-inflamatory drugs are also being conducted.[22] Future studies will elucidate if these will be of value in humans.

29.5 Muscular System: Drug Delivery

Muscles of the skeletal system in our body have adapted to contract in order for us to carry out daily functions of motion. Contraction of these muscle fibers is achieved when these cells are stimulated by nerve impulses. Acetylcholine is the neurotransmitter released presynaptically from axon terminals at the neuromuscular junction causing an electrical activation of the skeletal fibers. The interaction of acetylcholine with receptor proteins causes a change in membrane structure that results in the opening of sodium and potassium channels leading to depolarization.[45]

This perfect mechanism of motion is sometimes affected by autoimmune diseases. Myasthenia Gravis is a disease characterized by episodic muscle weakness caused by loss or dysfunction of acetylcholine receptors. Current treatments for myasthenia gravis are limited to relieving the symptoms or immunosuppressing the pathogenesis.[46] Anticholinesterase muscle stimulants such as Neostigmine and Pyridostigmine have been formulated to inhibit the destruction of acetylcholine by cholinesterase, therefore allowing constant stimulation of postsynaptic cells leading to muscle contraction.[46]

Access to the skeletal muscle can be gained through indirect (oral, i.v.) or direct (i.m.) routes. As it can be imagined, oral route is the preferred route for chronic drug therapy; however, the major disadvantage of these agents are the poor bioavailability (<10%). Poor bioavailability requires frequent administration of large doses leading to many gastrointestinal adverse events.[47]

Parenteral routes are also available. These routes of administration are most desirable for treatment when patients have difficulty swallowing or are undergoing a myasthenic crisis.[47] No clinical trials have been done concluding which route of administration is preferred. If the i.v. route is chosen over the i.m., then medication should be infused slowly to be able to look for cholinergic reactions (i.e., bradycardia).[49]

Neostigmine and Pyridostigmine also have other therapeutic indications. Both agents can be used for the reversal of nondepolarizing muscle relaxants.[47] Nondepolarizing muscle relaxants such as Mivacurium, Vecuronium, and Pancuronium are used in adjunct to general anesthesia to facilitate endotracheal intubation or to provide skeletal muscle relaxation during surgery or mechanical ventilation.[47] These agents act by antagonizing acetylcholine by competitively binding to cholinergic site on motor endplate leading to inhibition of skeletal muscle movement.[45] All nondepolarizing neuromuscular blockers are only available in injection form, intravenous use is recommended due to tissue irritation caused by i.m. administration.[50] Duration of action is the only factor that sets a difference between these agents. Currently available short-acting agents include Mivacurium and Cisatricurium, intermediate acting agents are Atracurium, Rocuronium, and Vancuronium, and long-acting agents include Pancuronium and Pipecuronium. Generally, short-acting neuromuscular blockers are preferred since limited complications related to prolonged or excessive blockade are avoided.[47] Numerous reports have described the use of neuromuscular blocking agents to facilitate mechanical ventilation; however, none of these reports have compared neuromuscular blockers to placebo.[50]

Currently, there are other pharmacological agents available that affect the skeletal muscle system. These agents are classified into centrally (i.e., Baclofen, Cyclobenzaprine) or direct acting (i.e., Dantrolene) muscle relaxants.[47] Baclofen is a widely used centrally acting agent for the management of spasticity associated with multiple sclerosis or spinal cord lesion. Baclofen works by inhibiting transmission of reflexes at the spinal cord by hyperpolarization.[51] Baclofen is also available in direct (intrathecal) or indirect (oral) routes of administration, intrathecal administration involves a direct injection into the CSF. This route of administration is indicated for the management of severe spasticity of spinal cord origin for patients who are unresponsive to oral Baclofen therapy or who experience intolerable CNS side effects at effective doses.[51] When used intrathecally, Baclofen is given as single bolus test dose or for chronic use, only in an inplantable pump approved by the FDA specifically for Baclofen administration.[47] Oral route is preferred for the rest of the patients because is convenient and absorption is rapid from the GI tract.

Dantrolene is another muscle relaxant used for the management of spinal cord spasticity, but, as opposed to Baclofen, Dantrolene acts directly on skeletal muscle. This agent works by interfering with the release of calcium ions from the sarcoplasmic reticulum.[52] Dantrolene is administered orally for the management of this condition. A major disadvantage of this route of administration is the slow and incomplete absorption from the GI tract, injections are also available, but this route of administration is reserved for the treatment of malignant hyperthermia.[52]

29.6 Sensory: Drug Delivery

Advances in biopharmaceutical technology have led to sophisticated drug delivery devices that allow drugs to be delivered through the skin and mucous membranes of the mouth. Transdermal drug delivery requires that drug molecules have biphasic solubility.[60] The transdermal drug needs lipid solubility to pass through the first layer of skin, the stratum corneum and aqueous solubility to move through the dermis.[60] The drug must contain high potency, low molecular weight, and insignificant cutaneous metabolism, and the skin must be able to tolerate long-term contact with the drug.[60] Most transdermal drug systems have a rate-controlling membrane that can be a disadvantage because of the slow systemic absorption of the drug.[60] One method used to increase the absorption rate of drugs through the skin is that of iontophoresis.[60] Iontophoresis is defined as "the introduction of ions of soluble salts into the skin or mucosal surfaces of the body by mean of an electric current."[60] Once one activates the current, electrons flow through the skin beneath the electrode being attracted by the oppositely charged electrode on the other side of the skin.[60] The use of ultrasound (sonophoresis), defined as sound of frequency greater than 20 kHz, has also been considered to improve the delivery of transdermal medications.[61] In addition to the elevation of skin temperature, sonophoresis is also reported to induce an increase in pore size and the formation of small gaseous pockets within cells (cavitation), which is thought to be the predominant mechanism by which low-frequency ultrasound promotes skin penetration enhancement and probably accounts for the enhanced transport of polar molecules.[61] Yet another method being considered is electroporation, which uses high-voltage short duration pulses to open up new pathways through the stratum corneum, which is thought to create localized regions of membrane permeabilization by producing aqueous pathways in lipid membrane bilayers.[61,62] In this section different medications and drug delivery devices will be discussed that deal with the sensation of pain.

29.6.1 Ultrasound

In this particular study ultrasound was applied continuously at a frequency of 1 MHz, and at an intensity of 2 W/cm^2 using an ultrasound generator to deliver radiolabeled lidocaine, a local anesthetic, through a piece of stratum corneum.[63] Stratum corneum permeability was enhanced by a factor of about 9 due to ultrasound application, which led to an enhanced diffusion coefficient of most molecules, by a factor ranging from 2.6 to 15 depending on the molecule. [63] Ultrasound is thought to disrupt lipid bilayers thus allowing a higher rate of solute diffusion.[63] On the other hand, ultrasound in some cases enhanced partition coefficient of some solutes by up to 60% and at the same time decreased the partition coefficient of some drugs by 30%.[63] In any case the enhanced diffusion coefficients outweigh the decreases in partition coefficients.[63] In another study ultrasound was used to enhance the permeability of fentanyl, a transdermal opioid agonist, in this experiment ultrasound was applied using a frequency of 20 kHz with the diameter of the ultrasound probe being 1.3 cm^2, pulsed for 1 h or continuously for 10 min.[64] "When ultrasound was used in pulsed mode, the diffusion flux of fentanyl was 35-fold greater than controls; however, diffusion flux calculated 7 h after the end of ultrasound exposure was not significantly different from controls." [64] Microscopic study of the skin after ultrasound revealed no damage to the stratum corneum.[64]

The administration of ultrasound to a transdermal patch might allow self-regulation of pain by the patient. Further studies will be needed to conclude the efficacy and safety of ultrasound in the delivery of transdermal medications.

29.6.2 Iontophoresis/Electroporation

In this study the transdermal delivery of buprenorphine, a synthetic opiate analgesic, was assisted using iontophoresis and/or electroporation.[62] A current of 0.5 mA/cm^2 was applied for 4 h and sampling was continued for 24 h.[62] The amount delivered under anode was much higher than that delivered under cathode due to the fact that buprenorphine has a positive charge at a pH of 4.[62] Electroporation alone was unable to enhance transport of buprenorphine across the skin.[62] On the other hand, electroporation and iontophoresis combined produced a delivery, which was over six times higher than that achieved by electroporation alone and about twice that achieved by iontophoresis alone.[62] In conclusion, the combination of iontophoresis and electroporation may be used in the future to control drug release and to increase drug permeation across the skin.

29.7 Digestive System: Drug Delivery

In general, the digestive system is made up of the stomach, small intestine, and large intestine. The fasting pH of the stomach is about 2 to 6, while in the presence of food the stomach pH is about 1.5 to 2, thus basic drugs are solubilized rapidly in the presence of stomach acid.[65] Stomach emptying is influenced by the food content and osmolality. Food often slows down the gastric emptying time usually allowing an oral medication anywhere from 3 to 6 h to empty out of the stomach.[65] The duodenum, the upper portion of the small intestine, is the optimum site for drug absorption.[65] This is because of the unique anatomy of the duodenum which possess microvilli that provide a large surface area for drugs to passively diffuse through.[65] The ileum, which is the terminal part of the small intestine, also plays a role in the absorption of hydrophobic drugs.[65] On the other hand, the large intestine lacks the microvilli that the small intestine has so it is very limited in drug absorption.[65] In this section new delivery methods to the digestive tract will be discussed.

29.7.1 GI Stents

Expandable metal stents have been approved by the Food and Drug Administration for the treatment of gastrointestinal obstruction due to cancer and could possibly be used in other benign diseases.[66] In the past, plastic stents have been used since they are relatively inexpensive when compared to these new metal stents.[67] In this study by Knyrim et al., where two groups of patients either received plastic or metal stents for esophageal obstruction complications of device placement and functioning were significantly more frequent in the plastic-prosthesis group than in the metal stent group.[67] In addition, metal stents are easier to place and require less dilation than plastic stents, and are less expensive after cost analysis.[67] The major problem with metal stents is tumor ingrowth, but this can be treated by laser ablation, which can be done in an outpatient setting.[67] These gastric stents are made up of different metal alloys and are put in by gastroenterologists.[67] The stents collapse to 3 mm in diameter at placement but can then expand up to 16 mm after positioned in the stricture.[67] These metal stents are used for esophageal carcinoma, in which all other treatment options have failed to produce any relief of dysphagia.[66] Dysphagia is usually relieved in up to 90% of patients who have metal stents placed and in all the patients in the Knyrim et al. trial.[66,67] Esophageal expandable metal stents are also used to treat tracheoesophageal fistulas due to cancer and may increase the survival of the patient, and that is why it is considered the primary treatment option.[66] Stents may also be used in the upper gastrointestinal tract and for cancerous large-bowel obstruction.[66] In the future, biodegradable stents could be used for benign diseases and stents that release chemotherapeutic agents or radiation can also be developed that could cause tumor regression.[66]

29.7.2 Colonic Drug Delivery

There are many different designs of colonic delivery systems and targeting has been achieved in several ways: coating drugs with pH-sensitive polymer, coating drugs with bacterial degradable polymers, using prodrugs, and delivering drugs through bacterial degradable matrixes.[68] The colon-targeted delivery capsule was recently developed at Tanabe Co. Ltd., and was designed by making three different layers along with an organic acid that is used as a pH adjusting agent along with the medication.[68] The three different layers are an enteric-coated layer, a hydrophilic layer, and an acid-soluble layer.[68] Using this system, the drug does not release until at least 5 h without regard to fed or fasted patients.[68] Electrostatic interaction between polyanions and polycation led to the formation of polyelectrolyte complexes (PECs), which can provide a greater barrier to drug release in the upper GIT than either material alone.[69] Thus pectin, a polyanion, and chitosan, a polycation, can be used together to better improve drug delivery to the colon.[69] In this study the optimum ratio of PEC was 10:1 weight ratio of pectin to chitosan.[69] Another study found that the ratio of pectin to chitosan to hydroxypropyl methylcellulose of 3:1:1 also had the potential of colonic selective delivery.[70] The delivery to the colon would ultimately occur when the bacterial enzymes commence to breakdown the pectin and the medication is released.[69,70] In another study using 5-aminosalicylic acid (5-ASA), which is used to treat ulcerative colitis, it was found that using an 80:20 pectin-hydroxypropyl methylcellulose (HPMC) coating mixture provided an intermediate erosion pattern for the colonic delivery of 5-ASA tablets.[71] This is promising to patients who have ulcerative colitis, whose current treatment options include rectally applied foams, suppositories, and enemas.[71]

29.8 Pulmonary: Drug Delivery

Inhalation is one of the oldest modes of drug delivery dating back to the earliest days of medical history. Medications were added to boiling water for patients to inhale.[26] Many advances have come from the renewed interest in this form of drug delivery.

Direct administration using inhalation as a method of drug delivery to the respiratory tract has become well established in the treatment of lung disease. This route has several advantages. Medication is delivered directly to the tracheobronchial tree allowing for rapid and predictable onset of action; the first-pass effect is circumvented; degradation within the gastrointestinal tract is avoided; much lower dosages than by the oral route can be administered with equivalent therapeutic efficacy, minimizing the potential for undesired side effects; and it can be used as an alternative route to avoid potential drug interactions when two or more medications are used concurrently.

For many years theophylline was the gold standard for the treatment of asthma. It is now known that asthma is an inflammatory process best treated on a chronic basis with corticosteroids. Nonetheless, theophylline continues to be used to treat asthma. It is available as an injectable to be administered via i.v. infusion, as controlled-release tablets, and liquid suspensions and rectal suppositories.

Bronchodilators and corticosteroids are the mainstay of treatment for asthma and chronic obstructive pulmonary disease (COPD). Administration via inhalation reduces systemic exposure of these compounds and unwanted systemic side effects. Bronchodilators exert their action by relaxing airway smooth muscle. Numerous compounds are available on the market with varying degrees of duration of action. Some bronchodilators are available for injectable use such as terbutaline, isoproterenol, and epinephrine. Others are available as oral solutions or tablets such as albuterol. Unfortunately, systemic use of these drugs to treat respiratory conditions results in unwanted systemic side effects. These side effects include such conditions as tachycardia; therefore, direct administration into the lungs is desirable.

Corticosteroids affect the inflammation that is present in these airway diseases. Corticosteroids are available for injectable use as intravenous or intramuscular depot injections, as oral solutions and tablets. Again, systemic use of corticosteroids can lead to many undesirable side effects including osteoporosis, hyperglycemia, and electrolyte imbalances.

29.8.1 Indirect Routes of Administration

Indirect routes of administration for agents available to treat the respiratory system include i.v., i.m., oral, and rectal. A discussion of direct methods of administration follows.

29.8.2 Direct Routes of Administration

Direct routes of administration through the mouth and into the lungs can be categorized in the following manner:

1. Nebulizers (ultrasonic or jet)
2. Metered dose inhalers
3. Dry powder inhalers
4. Administration through chest tube into the pleural cavity

The respiratory tract consists of multiple generations of branching airways (pharynx, larynx, trachea, bronchi, bronchioles, and alveoli) that progressively decrease in diameter but increase in number and total surface area. The large surface area of bronchioles and alveoli facilitates the rapid absorption of inhaled drugs.[31]

29.8.2.1 Jet Nebulizers

Jet nebulizers use compressed gas (air or oxygen) from a compressed gas cylinder, hospital air-line, or electrical compressor to convert a liquid into a spray. The aerosol leaving the nebulizer is diluted by atmospheric air and inhaled through a face mask or mouthpiece. The ability of an aerosol to penetrate the respiratory tract is directly related to its efficacy. The most important property to possess that governs penetration and deposition in the respiratory tract is particle size. Particles must be less than 5 μm and preferably less than 2 μm for alveolar deposition.[27] For the most part, drugs are in aqueous solution form when available for nebulization. There are multidose preparations available, but most nebulizer formulations are packaged as sterile, isotonic preservative-free unit doses. Examples include albuterol, n-acetylcysteine, and cromolyn sodium, all drugs used in the treatment of asthma.

29.8.2.2 Ultrasonic Nebulizers

In ultrasonic nebulizers, the energy required to atomize a liquid comes from a piezoelectric crystal, usually a man-made ceramic material, vibrating at high frequency.[31]

Commercially available ultrasonic nebulizers produce aerosol droplets that are often significantly larger than those produced by jet nebulizers. The absence of droplets with size less than 2 μm suggests that such nebulizers may be inappropriate for applications requiring that the drug penetrates to the most peripheral lung regions.[28]

As previously mentioned, most solutions for nebulization are aqueous; however, drugs poorly soluble in water can be formulated as suspensions. For example, Pulmicort Respules® consists of a suspension of the corticosteroid budesonide; in general, ultrasonic nebulizers are less efficient and more variable in delivering suspensions than jet nebulizers.[28] Nebulizers are established devices for the delivery of therapy to the lungs. They have advantages over other systems in the elderly and pediatric population. This advantage stems from the fact that the drug may be inhaled during normal tidal breathing through a mouthpiece or face mask. Other delivery methods require coordination of inhalation and activation of the device, which would be unsuitable for the very elderly or the very young.

29.8.2.3 Metered Dose Inhalers

The metered dose inhaler (MDI) is currently the most widely used inhalation delivery device. This is due to its portability, durability, long shelf life, cost-effectiveness, and relative ease of use. Unlike nebulizers, MDIs require metering and dispensing in coordination with the patient's inspiratory cycle. Therefore, successful lung delivery depends on a patient's ability to operate the inhalation device properly. Current improvements include the use of spacer devices. One of the biggest challenges with MDIs is to reduce the amount of drug that is deposited in the oropharyngeal area instead of the lungs. Spacer devices have the ability to reduce the speed of the emitted aerosol cloud and reduce the deposition of drug in the throat by as much as 45%.[29]

Drugs available for delivery through these devices include β-agonists for smooth muscle relaxation, corticosteroids, and mast cell stabilizers. MDIs available on the market containing these products are numerous. As previously mentioned, all these drugs treat asthma and COPD.

29.8.2.4 Dry Powder Inhalers

Prior to 1987, aerosolized MDIs were delivered via systems that relied on chlorofluorocarbon (CFC) propellant systems. There was a subsequent ban on all nonmedical uses of these CFC products that could deplete the ozone layer. Pharmaceutical manufacturers were encouraged to investigate other propellant systems, in addition to researching new propellants following the ban on CFC, pharmaceutical companies began to develop inhalable drugs in new forms such as dry powders.[30]

There are several different designs for dry powder inhalation devices (DPIDs). One such design is the Spinhaler®, in this device a gelatin capsule filled with drug and excipient is mounted in a rotor upon which are several small fan blades. The capsule is pierced by two small needles by sliding the outer casing of the inhaler relative to the inner casing. When the patient inhales, the capsule rotates rapidly and empties its content.[31] Some devices such as the Diskhaler® make it possible for the patient to know how many doses remain. This is an advantage over the MDI, which does not have this capacity. As with MDI, these devices rely on the patient's inspiratory effort; in frail, elderly patients or small children this can be an issue with adequate drug delivery. The drug formulations for these devices exist as capsules or disks. The majority of the drug formulations again consist of β-agonists, corticosteroids, and mast cell stabilizers. A novel formulation being investigated with these devices is the use of vaccines by inhalation. It is postulated that there is potential for enhanced biological efficacy since pulmonary delivery may produce mucosal immunity superior to that produced by parenteral administration of vaccines. Studies have shown the safety and efficacy of measles vaccine delivered as a liquid aerosol from a nebulizer. A powder formulation of measles vaccine has been formulated for aerosol delivery in feasibility study. Challenges remain such as the development of appropriate delivery technology and reduction in the hygroscopic nature of the formulation.[32]

29.8.2.5 Chest Tube Administration

Malignant pleural effusions are a common complication in advanced malignancy. Metastatic lung and breast cancer account for 75% of the cases.[33] In this procedure a small bore thoracostomy tube is placed under local anesthesia. Then a sclerosing agent is instilled through the tube. Agents that have been used with success include bleomycin, doxycycline, and talc poudrage. The sclerosing agent instillation, if successful, will stop the accumulation of the fluid in the lung.

29.9 Ear, Nose, and Throat: Drug Delivery

29.9.1 The Ear

Diseases of the ear, most commonly infections, are very prevalent in children. Extensive use of antibiotics for this indication has lead to marked antimicrobial resistance. Recently, the American Academy of Otolaryngology convened to set consensus on the treatment of common ear ailments. These included chronic suppurative otitis media, otitis externa, and tympanostomy tube otorrhea. The consensus was that in the absence of systemic infection or serious underlying disease topical antibiotics alone should constitute first line treatment.[34]

29.9.1.1 Indirect Routes of Administration

Indirect routes of administration include oral, i.v., and i.m. antibiotics. Using these routes the antibiotic reaches the systemic blood circulation, which then enters the middle and inner ear.

29.9.1.2 Direct Routes of Administration

Direct administration includes the use of antibiotic and anti-inflammatory ear drops such as Cipro HC Otic Suspension® or Otobiotic Otic® (which contains a mixture of antibiotic and anti-inflammatory). Solutions such as Otocain® contain topical analgesics (benzocaine) to alleviate ear pain.

Novel direct delivery devices being studied in animals include a biodegradable support matrix incorporating a therapeutically releasable amount of antibiotic. This device is then inserted into the middle ear and is capable of drug delivery for 3 months. Progression into human studies may show potential for this device to be used as a source of inner ear drug delivery.[35]

Intratympanic therapy for Meniere's disease has also been studied. Gentamicin solution of 0.5 ml has been injected transtympanically using a tuberculin syringe and a 27-gauge long needle. Patients treated in the study had good response to treatment with over 50% having complete control of their vertigo.[36]

29.1.2 The Nose

Drugs have been administered nasally for both topical and systemic action. Common ailments that affect the nose and are treated with topical therapy include: allergic rhinitis, congestion, and sinusitis. Acute sinusitis is a condition manifesting inflammation and infection, usually of the frontal and maxillary sinuses. Goals of therapy are to improve drainage in the blocked sinuses and resolve the infection. Steam inhalation can cause vasoconstriction and help with drainage as can topical vasocontrictors such as phenylephrine spray.

29.1.2.1 Indirect Routes of Administration

Indirect routes of administration include oral and i.v. use of antibiotics.

29.1.2.2 Direct Routes of Administration

Direct routes of administration include the use of nasal sprays and, for more accurate dosing, mechanical pumps and pressurized aerosol systems. Allergic rhinitis is a condition that is prevalent in our society. Frequently present in patients who also have asthma, it is best treated by nasal corticosteroids. The use of these medications directly to the nasal mucosa avoids exposing the body to systemic levels of corticosteroids and their potential side effects.

One of the simplest and oldest methods of nasal drug delivery is the use of a device to administer solutions via dropper. This system, while cost-effective and easy to manufacture, has the disadvantage of not accurately measuring drugs because of the inability to control the exact volume delivered. Squeezed nasal bottles are mainly used as a delivery device for decongestants, such as Afrin Spray®. They function by pressing the bottle and pushing air inside the bottle through a simple jet, which atomizes a certain volume of fluid. Metered-dose pump sprays (MDPSs) allow for the application of a defined dose with a high dosing accuracy. These systems consist of the container, the pump with the valve, and the actuator.[37] Powder dosage forms are understudy and include inhaled insulin. Although dry powders have advantages over liquid formulations, they are infrequently used in nasal drug delivery. Nasal gels have also been studied as a means of prolonging drug contact with the nasal mucosa. One product is marketed as vitamin B-12 (Nasocobal gel®).

29.1.3 The Throat

Infection of the throat is a common ailment as is cough. Many throat infections are self-limiting and require treatment only with analgesics. Streptococcal throat infections, however, do require antimicrobial treatment because of their potential to damage the heart valves. Treatment for these infections consists of systemic oral antibiotics; the drug of choice is a simple penicillin. Cough is another common ailment that is treated with different medications depending on the cause of the cough. For cough from the common cold and allergic rhinitis, oral antihistamines and decongestants along with ipratropium nasal spray can be used. If the cough is due to COPD, a 2-week trial of oral corticosteroids can be utilized.[38]

Other over-the-counter treatment modalities include liquid sprays that contain topical anesthetics for throat pain, such as Orasept Throat Spray®, or lozenges such as Cepacol®.

A novel treatment in throat disorders involves the use of botulinum toxin to treat spasmodic dysphonias. This condition is a disorder that results in the patient having either a strained or strangled voice or a breathy, whispery voice. The toxin, injected directly into the posterior cricoarytenoid muscle, paralyzing the muscle that is causing the spasm and resulting in relief of the condition.[39]

29.10 Lymphatic System: Drug Delivery

The human body is exposed to a wide variety of diseases of benign and malignant origin. These diseases affect the lymphatic system at the early stages of the process. Cancers, as well as many infections (viral, bacterial, or fungal), spread by lymphatic dissemination.[40] The high prevalence of lymph node involvement in these diseases is not surprising because the primary function of the lymphatic tissue is to provide the body's immune response.

Appropriate diagnosis and treatment of diseases affecting the lymph nodes depend on the availability of drugs that are retained by the lymph nodes. Effective accumulation of drugs into the lymph nodes can be achieved by intralymphatic or interstitial administration.[41] Since there is a high variability of lymphatic networks and drainage routes, systemic administration would always be preferred and currently represents a focus in lymphotropic drug design.[42]

The interstitial space constitutes a significant barrier to the diffusion of macromolecules and particulates and may limit the rate and extent of drainage from site of administration. Macromolecules dissolved in the interstitial fluid are readily drained by lymphatics; therefore, the limiting factor to macromolecular transfer from blood capillary to lymph is capillary permeability. The rate of macromolecule and particle extravasation depends on size and structure. Macromolecules may be transferred in liquid phase, while some proteins are transported by transcytosis-associated receptors. The nature and size of lymphatic vessels vary along the route.[41]

Access routes to the lymph nodes can be accomplished through lymphatic vessels or blood vessels. Drug delivery through the lymphatic vessels is highly efficient; interstitial macromolecules are cleared from the injection site almost exclusively by lymphatics, but do not return to blood capillaries. Direct drug delivery through blood vessels to intranodal tissue is not very effective unless homing receptors are utilized.[40] Different local administration routes have been utilized to deliver diagnostic or therapeutic drugs to the lymph nodes.

For intralymphatic administration, a peripheral lymphatic vessel has to be cannulated by surgical cutdown. This method results in high concentration of drug in the lymph nodes, but it is only limited to draining lymph nodes leading to an uneven drug distribution. This method has been used for x-ray lymphography and CT. Agents used include iodized oils.[41]

Interstitial administration does not require cannulation of a lymphatic vessel, and therefore is easier to perform. Agents can be injected at any accessible anatomical site, where they penetrate from the interstitial space into small lymphatic vessels through intercellular gaps of lymphatic endothelium. The agents are then transported through the network of lymphatic vessels to peripheral lymph nodes. The disadvantage of the interstitial route is that it provides low, unreliable drug delivery to mediastinal and abdominal lymph nodes, which are involved in the majority of carcinomas.[44]

Oral delivery of lipophilic drugs to the lymph nodes is associated with the formation and transport of lipoproteins, which are formed after the adsorption of lipid digestion products. Lymphatic transport of polar drugs after intestinal absorption is lower because of their preferential absorption by blood.

Intra-arterial injections of drugs carrying particulates that are too large to pass through capillary vessels result in high local tissue concentration of the released drugs, which can then diffuse to local lymph nodes. This method is used to chemoembolize tumors rather than to treat metastatic diseases.[41]

In addition to locally administered drugs, there are systemic agents that can be injected intravenously and can accumulate in the lymph nodes by different mechanisms.

Low molecular weight compounds such as gallium citrate accumulates in normal lymphatic tissue and lymphomas; however, because its nonspecific biodistribution, it is not used very often except for imaging of lymphomas, tumor recurrence, or sarcoid imaging. Metalloporphyrins also have been used for selective lymphatic imaging and MRI of human colon carcinoma.[43]

Radiolabeled lymphocytes are another source for clinical use in detecting sites of inflammation and lymphoreticular malignancies. Usually, lymphocytes are incubated with an Indium oxide complex and the resulting labeling efficiency is 50 to 60%.[42]

Homing receptors of lymphocytes are responsible for cell accumulation in lymphatic tissue and inflammations (where homing molecules are also expressed). Because the homing process is highly selective, it is possible that the future availability of vector molecules with specificity to lymphocyte adhesion glycoproteins will allow efficient drug delivery.

Colloidal iron oxide particles have been studied as diagnostic MR contrast agents. It has been found that after i.v. administration, some dextran-coated colloids accumulate in lymph nodes in much higher concentrations than any other particulate.[43]

Lymph nodes are an easy target for drug delivery through intralymphatic or interstitial administration with local concentrations achievable. These administration routes are rarely used because of the unreliable and highly variable delivery to different lymph node groups. Because of these factors, system carriers are being developed for lymph node delivery. The two classes of agents are (1) agents that have long circulation times and are able to extravasate into interstitium and then are cleared by lymphatics (i.e., dextran-covered particles of dextran-based graft copolymers); (2) agents targeting lymph node-specific lymphocyte homing receptors or antigens.[40]

29.11 Reproductive System: Drug Delivery

The female reproductive tract is divided into external and internal genitalia. Parts of the female anatomy include the pelvis, bladder, urethra, and vagina.[72] For reproduction, the human endometrium must receive hormonal signals that prepare it for implantation.[72] When conception does not occur, these signals initiate mechanisms that lead to menses and controlled regeneration of this tissue, and the cycle repeats itself again.[72] In contrast, the male reproductive system is composed of the scrotal sac, testes, genital ducts, accessory glands, and penis.[73] The scrotal sac performs an important role in maintaining the testes at a temperature about 2°C below the temperature of the internal organs so that spermatogenesis can occur.[73] In this section new reproductive system drug delivery methods will be discussed.

29.11.1 Contraceptive Implants

Norplant™ (The Population Council) and Jadelle are the only subdermal implants currently available in the United States, even though there are several more that are currently being used in other countries.[74] Norplant consists of six capsules that release the progestin, levonorgestrel for at least 5 years; after this time there is still 69% of the original steroid load left in the silastic capsules to act as a safety margin for women who don't remove the implants after the recommended 5 years.[74–76] The system consists of six silastic capsules, 34 mm long and 2.4 mm in diameter.[75] Jadelle™ (The Population Council) also uses levonorgestrel just like Norplant.[76] The only difference between the products is that Jadelle uses two silastic rods instead of six capsules, thus making insertion and removal easier for the Jadelle implant.[76] Each Jadelle implant is 4.4 cm long and is composed of a polydimethylsiloxane elastomer covered by silicone rubber tubing.[74] Jadelle is approved by the FDA for 3 years of use, but has been shown to be effective for up to 5 years.[74] The next implant that is currently used in other countries is the Implanon™ (NV Organon, Oss, The Netherlands).[76] Implanon is a single-rod implant that is 4 cm long and 2 mm in diameter.[74] It contains 68 mg of 3-keto-desogestrel (etonogestrel) in an ethylene vinyl acetate (EVA) polymer core surrounded by an EVA membrane with a contraceptive dose maintained for 3 years.[74,75] Its contraceptive efficacy is excellent since there has not been one report of a single pregnancy in over 5000 woman-years of experience with this product.[76] Yet another implant used in other countries is the

Uniplant™. Uniplant is a single silastic 3.5-cm-long, 2.4-mm-diameter capsule containing 55 mg nomegestrol acetate developed as a single 1-year contraceptive implant.[74–76] An alternative approach to resolving the difficulties of implant removal which is considered a minor surgery and usually takes about 20 min, is to eliminate the need for removal altogether.[74–76] Capronor™ is a 40-mm rod containing levonorgestrel in an E-caprolactone polymer.[74] The polymer releases levonorgestrel about ten times faster than silastic and thereby one implant can achieve adequate serum concentrations, instead of normally two implants.[74] The implant is biodegradable and it appears to remain for about 1 year.[74] Another form of biodegradable implants is pellets.[74] These pellets are expected to dissolve within 2 years of application, but are impossible to take out after several months of implantation.[74] In conclusion, some of the advantages of progestin implants are long unattended use, efficacy, no compliance issues, and lower levels of progestin when compared to oral contraceptives.[76] Disadvantages are that minor surgery is required for insertion and removal and there is a high cost associated with the method if early removal is performed.[76]

29.11.2 Contraceptive Patch

Ortho Evra/Evra™ (Janssen Pharmaceutica, NV Belgium) is the only available female contraceptive transdermal patch in the market. The matrix patch which is 20 cm^2 is thin and consists of three layers: an outer protective layer of polyester; a medicated, adhesive middle layer; and a clear, polyester release liner that is removed prior to patch application.[77,78] The patch is designed to deliver 150 μg of norelgestromin and 20 μg of ethinyl estradiol daily to the systemic circulation.[77–79] The patch can be applied to the buttocks, upper outer arm, lower abdomen, or upper torso (excluding the breast).[77] Because the patch is replaced weekly on the same day of the week for 3 consecutive weeks (followed by 1 week patch-free) and the next patch cycle begins on the same day, it makes patient compliance easier when compared with oral contraceptives.[79]

29.11.3 Male Contraceptive

Androgen therapy is predominantly used for replacement in primary hypogonadism but may be used for male contraception.[80] Desogestrel DSG (300 μg daily) and transdermal testosterone (T0) (5 mg daily) patches were given to male patients for 24 weeks.[81] Using this regimen 71% of the patients were azoospermia (no sperm) by the end of week 12.[81] This regimen wasn't as effective as using IM T enanthate.[81] The lower efficacy of the transdermal T is likely to be due to failure of the transdermal T system in maintaining circulating T levels consistently in the required range.[81] In conclusion, the use of desogestrel and IM T enanthate might lead to male contraception in the near future.

References

1. Marieb, E., The central nervous system, in *Human Anatomy & Physiology, 4th ed.*, Fox, D., Ed., Benjamin/Cummings Science Publishing, Menlo Park, CA, 1997, pp. 405–455.
2. Minn, A. et al., Drug metabolism in the brain: benefits and risks, in *The Blood-Brain Barrier and Drug Delivery to the CNS*, Begley, D., Bradbury, M., and Kreuter, J., Eds., Marcel Dekker, New York, 2000, pp. 145–170.
3. Bradbury, M., History and physiology of the blood-brain barrier in relation to delivery of drugs to the brain, in *The Blood-Brain Barrier and Drug Delivery to the CNS*, Begley, D., Bradbury, M., and Kreuter, J., Eds., Marcel Dekker, New York, 2000, pp. 1–8.
4. Madaras-Kelly, K. et al., Central nervous system infections, in *Pharmacotherapy: A Pathophysiologic Approach, 3rd ed.*, Dipiro, J. et al., Eds., Appleton-Lange, Norwalk, CT, 1997, pp. 1971–1993.
5. Partridge, W.M., Invasive brain drug delivery, in *Brain Drug Targeting: The Future of Brain Drug Development*, Cambridge University Press, New York, 2001, pp. 13–35.
6. Bernards, C.M., Epidural and intrathecal drug movement, in *Spinal Drug Delivery*, Yaksh, T., Ed., Elsevier, New York, 1999, pp. 239–252.
7. Haroun, R.I. and Brem, H., Local drug delivery, *Curr. Opin.Oncol.*, 12, 187, 2000.

8. Harbaugh, R.E, Saunders, R.L., and Reeder, R.F., Use of implantable pumps for central nervous system drug infusions to treat neurological disease, *Neurosurgery*, 23, 693, 1988.
9. Kumar, M. and Banker, G., Biological processes and events involved in drug targeting, in *Modern Pharmaceutics*, Vol. 72, Banker, G. and Rhodes, C., Eds., Marcel Dekker, New York, 1996, pp. 613–625.
10. Wallace, M.S., Human spinal drug delivery: methods and technology, in *Spinal Drug Delivery*, Yaksh, T., Ed., Elsevier, New York, 1999, pp. 345–370.
11. Boylan, L. et al., Routes of parenteral administration, in *Modern Pharmaceutics*, Vol. 72, Banker, G. and Rhodes, C., Eds., Marcel Dekker, New York, 1996, pp. 442–447.
12. Scheld, W.M., Drug delivery to the central nervous system: general principles and relevance to therapy for infections of the central nervous system, *Rev. Infect. Dis.*, 11S, 1669, 1989.
13. Bomgaars, L., Blaney, S.M., and Poplack, D.G., Inthrathecal chemotherapy, in *Spinal Drug Delivery*, Yaksh, T., Ed., Elsevier, New York, pp. 503–512.
14. O' Connell, M.B. and Bauwens, S.F., Osteoporosis and osteomalacia, in *Pharmacotherapy: A Pathophysiologic Approach, 3rd ed.*, Dipiro, J. et al., Ed., Appleton-Lange, Norwalk, CT, 1997, pp. 1689–1716.
15. Patton, J.S., Pulmonary delivery of drugs for bone disorders, *Adv. Drug Deliv. Rev.*, 42, 239, 2000.
16. Ramachandran, C. and Fleisher, D., Transdermal delivery of drugs for the treatment of bone diseases, *Adv. Drug Deliv. Rev.*, 42, 197, 2000.
17. Norden, C., Gillespie, W., and Nade, S., Antimicrobial agents and other forms of therapy, in *Infections in Bones and Joints*, Blackwell Scientific, Cambridge, 1994, pp. 119–136.
18. Dash, A. and Cudworth, G., Therapeutic applications of implantable drug delivery systems, *J. Pharmacol. Toxicol. Methods*, 40, 1, 1998.
19. Alonge, T.O. and Fashina, A.N., Ceftriaxone-PMMA beads—a slow release preparation? *Int. J. Clin. Practice*, 54, 353, 2000.
20. Fujisaki, J. et al., Osteotropic drug delivery system (ODDS) based on bisphosphonic prodrug. IV. Effects of osteotropic estradiol on bone mineral density and uterine weight in ovariectomized rats, *J. Drug Targeting*, 4, 129, 1997.
21. Hirabayashi, H. et al., Bone-specific delivery and sustained release of diclofenac, a non-steroidal anti-inflammatory drug, via bisphosphonic prodrug based on the Osteotropic Drug Delivery System, *J. Controlled Release*, 70, 183, 2001.
22. Otsuka, M. and Nakahigashi, Y., A novel skeletal drug delivery system using self-setting calcium phosphate cement. VII. Effect of biological factors on indomethacin release from cement loaded on bovine bone, *J. Pharm. Sci.*, 83, 1569, 1994.
23. Norden, C., Gillespie, W., and Nade, S., Principles of management, in *Infections in Bones and Joints*, Blackwell Scientific, Cambridge, 1994, pp. 115–118.
24. Hosking, D. and Ringe, J., *Treatment of Metabolic Bone Disease Management Strategy and Drug Therapy*, Martin Dunitz, London, 2000.
25. Aviva, E. and Golomb, G., Administration routes and delivery systems of bisphosphonates for the treatment of bone resorption, *Adv. Drug Deliv. Rev.*, 42, 175, 2000.
26. Newman, S.P. and Busse, W.W., Evolution of dry powder inhaler design, formulation, and performance, *Respir. Med.*, 96, 293, 2002.
27. McCallion, O. et al., Jet nebulisers for pulmonary drug delivery, *Int. J. Pharm.*, 130, 1, 1996.
28. Taylor, M. and McCallion, O., Ultrasonic nebulisers for pulmonary drug delivery, *Int. J. Pharm.*, 153, 93, 1997.
29. Keller, M., Innovations and perspectives of metered dose inhalers in pulmonary drug delivery, *Int. J. Pharm.*, 186, 81, 1999.
30. Anderson, P., Delivery options and devices for aerosolized therapeutics, *CHEST*, 120, 89s, 2001.
31. Timsina, M.P. et al., Drug delivery to the respiratory tract using dry powder inhalers, *Int. J. Pharm.*, 101, 1, 1994.

32. LiCalsi, C. et al., A powder formulation of measles vaccine for aerosol delivery, *Vaccine,* 19, 2629, 2001.
33. Diacon, A.H., Prospective randomized comparison of thorascopic talc poudrage under local anesthesia versus bleomycin instillation for pleurodesis in malignant pleural effusions, *Am. J. Respir. Crit. Care Med.*, 162, 1445, 2000.
34. Hannley, M.T., Denney, J.C., and Holzer, S.S., Use of ototopical antibiotics in treating 3 common ear diseases, *Otolaryngology,* 122, 934, 2000.
35. Goycoolea, M.V., Extended middle ear drug delivery. A new concept; a new device, *Acta Otolaryngol.*, 493, 119, 1992.
36. Quaranta, A., Intratympanic therpay for Meniere's disease: effect of administration of low concentration of gentamicin, *Acta Otolaryngol.*, 121, 387, 2001.
37. Kublik, H. and Vidgren, M.T., Nasal delivery systems and their effect on deposition and absorption, *Adv. Drug Deliv. Rev.*, 29, 157, 1998.
38. Irwin, R.S. and Madison, J.M., Primary care: the diagnosis and treatment of cough, *N. Engl. J. Med.*, 343, 1715, 2000.
39. Neuenschwander, M.C. and Prtibitkin, E.A., Botulinum toxin in otolaryngology: a review of its actions and opportunites for use, *ENT-Ear Nose Throat J.*, 79, 799, 2000.
40. Swartz, M.A., The physiology of the lymphatic system, *Adv. Drug Deliv. Rev.*, 50, 3, 2001.
41. Porter, C.J., Transport and absorption of drugs via the lymphatic system, *Adv. Drug Deliv. Rev.*, 50, 1, 2001.
42. Porter, C.J., Lymphatic transport of proteins after subcutaneous injection: implications of animal model selection, *Adv. Drug Deliv. Rev.*, 50, 157, 2001.
43. Swart, P.J., Homing of negatively charged albumins to the lymphatic system: general implications for drug targeting to peripheral tissues and reservoirs, *Biochem. Pharmacol.*, 58, 1425, 1999.
44. Porter, C.J., Intestinal lymphatic drug transport: an update, *Adv. Drug Deliv. Rev.*, 50, 61, 2001.
45. Goodman Gilman, A., Goodman, L.S., and Gilman, A., Drugs acting at synaptic and neuroeffector junctional site, in *Goodman and Gilman's The Pharmacological Basis of Therapeutics,* MacMillan, New York, 1980, chap. 2.
46. Fauci, A.S. et al., Myasthenia gravis and other diseases of the neuromuscular junction, in *Harrison's Principles of Internal Medicine,* McGraw-Hill, New York, 1998, chap. 382.
47. Kastrup, E.K. et al., Central nervous system agents, in *Facts and Comparisons,* Wolters Kluwer, St. Louis, 2002, chap. 7.
48. Madaras-Kelly, K. et al., Central nervous system infections, in *Pharmacotherapy: A Pathophysiologic Approach, 3rd ed.*, Dipiro, J. et al., Ed., Appleton-Lange, Norwalk, CT, 1997, pp. 1971–1993.
49. Briassoulis, G., Continuous neostigmine infusion in post-thymectomy juvenile myasthenic crisis, *J. Child Neurol.*, 15, 747, 2002.
50. Murray, M.J. et al., Clinical practice guidelines for sustained neuromuscular blockade in the adult critically ill patients, *Crit. Care Med.*, 30, 1, 2002.
51. Nielsen, J.F., Baclofen increases the soleus stretch reflex threshold in the early swing phase during walking in spastic Multiple Sclerosis, *Multiple Sclerosis,* 6, 105, 2000.
52. Borasio, G.D., Palliative care in amyotrophic lateral sclerosis, *Neurol Clin.*, 19, 829, 2001.
53. Zaret, B.L., Berliner, R.W., Moser, M., et al., Cardiovascular drugs, in *Yale University School of Medicine Heartbook,* Goetz, D.M., Ed., Hearst Books, New York, 1992, chap. 23.
54. Smith, D.H.G., Pharmacology of cardiovascular chronotherapeutic agents, *Am. J. Hypertension,* 14(9), Suppl. 1, S296, 2001.
55. Smolensky, M.H. and Portaluppi, F., Chronopharmacology and chronotherapy of cardiovascular medications: relevance to prevention and treatment of coronary heart disease, *Am. Heart J.*, 137(4), S14, 1999.
56. Sahil, A.P. and Edelman, E.R., Endothelial cell delivery for cardiovascular therapy, *Adv. Drug Delivery Rev.*, 42(1–2), 139, 2000.

57. Levy, R.J., Labhasetwar, V., Song, C., Lerner, E., et al., Polymeric drug delivery systems for treatment of cardiovascular calcification, arrhythmias, and restenosis, *J. Controlled Release*, 36, 137, 1995.
58. Ignarro, L.J., Napoli, C., and Loscalzo, J., Nitric oxide donors and cardiovascular agents modulating the bioactivity of nitric oxide: an overview, *Circ. Res.*, 90(1), 21, 2002.
59. Lestini, B.J., Sagnella, S.M., Xu, Z., Shive, M.S., et al., Surface modification of liposomes for selective cell targeting in cardiovascular drug delivery, *J. Controlled Release*, 78, 1–3, 235, 2002.
60. Ashburn, M.A. and Rice, L.J., *The Management of Pain, 1st ed.*, Churchill Livingstone, New York, 1998, chap. 11.
61. Naik, A., Yogeshvar, N.K., and Guy, R.H., Transdermal drug delivery: overcoming the skin's barrier function, *Pharm. Sci. Technol. Today*, 3(9), 318, 2000.
62. Bose, S., Ravis, W.R., Lin, Y., Zhang, L., Hofmann, G.A., et al., Electrically-assisted transdermal delivery of buprenorphine, *J. Controlled Release*, 73(2–3), 197, 2001.
63. Mitragotri, S., Effect of therapeutic ultrasound on partition and diffusion coefficients in human stratum corneum, *J. Controlled Release*, 71(1), 23, 2001.
64. Boucaud, A., Machet, L., Arbeille, B., and Machet, M.C., In vitro study of low-frequency ultrasound-enhanced transdermal transport of fentanyl and caffeine across human and hairless rat skin, *Int. J. Pharm.*, 228(1–2), 69, 2001.
65. Shargel, L. and Yu, B.C., *Applied Biopharmaceutics and Pharmacokinetics, 3rd ed.*, Appleton-Lange, Norwalk, CT, 1993, chap. 7.
66. Baron, T.H., Expandable metal stents for the treatment of cancerous obstruction of the gastrointestinal tract, *N. Engl. J. Med.*, 344(22), 1681, 2001.
67. Knyrim, K., Wagner, H.J., Bethge, N., Keymling, M., and Vakil, N.A., Controlled trial of an expansile metal stent for palliation of esophageal obstruction due to inoperable cancer, *N. Engl. J. Med.*, 329, 1302, 1993.
68. Ishibashi, T., Pitcairn, G.R., Yoshino, H., Mizobe, M., et al., Scintigraphic evaluation of a new capsule-type colon specific drug delivery system in healthy volunteers, *J. Pharm. Sci.*, 87(5), 531, 1998.
69. Macleod, G.S., Collett, J.H., and Fell, J.T., The potential use of mixed films of pectin, chitosan, and HPMC for bimodal drug release, *J. Controlled Release*, 58, 303, 1999.
70. Macleod, G.S., Collett, J.H., Fell, J.T., Sharma, H.L., et al., *Int. J. Pharm.*, 187(2), 251, 1999.
71. Turkoglu, M. and Ugurlu, T., In vitro evaluation of pectin-HPMC compression coated 5-aminosalicylic acid tablets for colonic delivery, *Eur. J. Pharm. Biopharm.*, 53(1), 65, 2002.
72. Bernhisel, M.A., Braly, P.S., Branch, W.D., and Bristow, R.E., *Danforth's Obstetrics and Gynecology, 8th ed.*, Lippincott, Williams & Wilkins, Philadelphia, 1999, chap. 3.
73. Pizzorno, J.E., *Textbook of Natural Medicine, 2nd ed.*, Churchill Livingstone, New York, 1999, 1378, 74.
74. Kovalevsky, G. and Barnhart, K., Norplant and other implantable contraceptives, *Clin. Obstet. Gynecol.*, 44(1), 92, 75, 2001.
75. Jordan, A., Toxicology of progestogens of implantable contraceptives for women, *Contraception*, 65(1), 3, 2002.
76. Croxatto, H.B., Progestin implants, *Steriods*, 65, 681, 2000.
77. Audet, M.C., Moreau, M., Koltun, W.D., Waldbaum, A.S., et al., Evaluation of contraceptive efficacy and cycle control of a transdermal contraceptive patch vs an oral contraceptive: a randomized controlled trial, *J.A.M.A.*, 285(18), 2347, 2001.
78. Abhrams, L.S., Skee, D.M., Natarajan, J., Wong, F.A., et al., Pharmacokinetics of norelgestromin and ethinyl estradiol delivered by a contraceptive patch (Ortho Evra/Evra™) under conditions of heat, humidity, and exercise, *J. Clin. Pharmacol.*, 41, 1301, 2001.
79. Dittrich, R., Parker, L., Rosen, J.B., Shangold, G., et al., Transdermal contraception: evaluation of three transdermal norelgestromin/ethinyl estradiol doses in a randomized, multicenter, dose-response study, *Am. J. Obstet. Gynecol.*, 186(1), 15, 2002.
80. Anderson, R.A., Martin, C.W., Kung, A.W., Everington, D., et al., 7Alpha-methyl-19-nortestosterone maintains sexual behavior and mood in hypogonadal men, *J. Clin. Endocrinol. Metab.*, 84(10), 3556, 1999.

81. Hair, W.M., Kitteridge, K., O'Connor, D.B., and Wu, F.C., A novel male contraceptive pill-patch combination: oral desogestrel and transdermal testosterone in the suppression of spermatogenesis in normal men, *J. Clin. Endocrinol. Metab.*, 86(11), 5201, 2001.
82. Danckwerts, M. and Fassihi, A., Implantable controlled release of drug delivery systems: a review, *Drug Dev. Ind. Pharm.*, 17(11), 1465, 1991.
83. Coukell, A.J. and Balfour, J.A., Levonorgestrel subdermal implants. A review of contraceptive efficacy and acceptability, *Drugs*, 55(6), 861, 1998.
84. Van Os, W.A., The intrauterine device and its dynamics, *Adv. Contraception*, 15(2), 119, 1999.

VIII

Alternative and Emerging Techniques

The incorporation of technology in so many areas of patient care has inspired many researchers who strive to develop radically new ideas. New treatment strategies, as well as new applications of existing technologies, have emerged from seemingly limitless imagination. The degree to which these therapies become accepted as commonplace depends on many factors. However, proof of efficacy remains the dominating determinant.

The therapies outlined in these chapters are chosen from a wide range of ideas as case studies in innovation. It would be beyond the scope of this volume to attempt to summarize the domain of alternative and emerging medical technologies. Nevertheless, one can see the promise that technology brings to health care in the applications described below.

The chapters included in this section are:

30

Hyperbaric Oxygen Therapy

Tonja Weed
University of Virginia

Timothy Bill
University of Virginia

Thomas J. Gampper
University of Virginia

CONTENTS

30.1 Introduction

Hyperbaric oxygen (HBO) therapy is the delivery of 100% oxygen at pressures greater than atmospheric, which by convention is considered to be 760 mmHg or 1 atmosphere (atm) at sea level. The therapeutic effects are dependent upon the increase in both pressure and oxygen delivered to tissues. Although the primary oxygen delivery mechanism in humans is hemoglobin, which binds, carries, and delivers up to 4 molecules of oxygen per hemoglobin molecule, a certain amount of oxygen is dissolved freely in plasma. The amount dissolved depends upon the percent of inspired oxygen (F_iO_2), the solubility of oxygen in plasma, and the surrounding pressure. Ambient conditions allow for plasma oxygen concentrations of 0.3 ml/dl. When the inspired oxygen concentration is raised to 100% and the ambient pressure to 3 atm, the amount of dissolved oxygen rises to approximately 6 ml/dl.[1] This equals the volume of oxygen extracted by the human tissues at rest, which means hyperbaric oxygen conditions can theoretically support aerobic metabolism without utilizing the hemoglobin transport mechanism.[1,2]

Hyperbaric therapy was first documented in 1664, when a British physician, Dr. Henshaw, attempted to treat chronic illnesses, such as arthritis, with hypobaric pressure, and acute illnesses, such as fever, with hyperbaric pressures.[3] The discovery of oxygen waited another 100 years until described by Joseph Priestly in 1775.[4] By the 1800s, hyperbaric chambers were in fashion with Europe's wealthy class, despite the scarcity of scientific evidence to support actual medical benefit. It was not until 1917 that Drager described the application of HBO therapy for decompression sickness and it was first clinically applied by Behnke in the 1930s.[5] Then, in 1960, the Dutch cardiac surgeon Boerema published the landmark article, *Life without Blood*, which described an experimental group of pigs

0-8493-1140-3/04/$0.00+$1.50

who underwent serial replacement of their blood with plasma expanders. In a powerful demonstration of the potential of hyperbaric oxygen, these pigs were able to lead active lives without any hemoglobin while maintained at 3 atm of pressurized oxygen.[6] Following this, research interest and clinical applications expanded in a dramatic fashion. In response to this growth, the Undersea Medical Society was founded in 1967 with the mission to evaluate and support only those applications based in scientific methodology. This group continues today as the Undersea and Hyperbaric Medical Society (UHMS) to actively support research and education and publishes a triennial committee review of approved HBO indications.[7]

These published guidelines support the use of hyperbaric oxygen therapy for the conditions of air or gas embolism, decompression sickness, carbon monoxide poisoning, clostridial myositis and myonecrosis (gas gangrene), necrotizing soft tissue infections, refractory osteomyelitis, intracranial abscess, acute blood loss anemia, crush injury, compromised skin grafts and flaps, enhancement of healing in selected problem wounds, complications of radiation therapy, and thermal burns. Other applications include cyanide poisoning, acute traumatic ischemia, sudden hearing loss, acoustic trauma, tinnitus, and selected cases of facial palsy.[8] Conditions under current investigation include stroke, head trauma, cerebral palsy, acute myocardial infarction, chronic Lyme disease, and invasive fungal infections.

Hyperbaric oxygen is delivered in either a mono- or multiplace chamber. The monoplace chamber is usually constructed of a clear acrylic shell that accommodates a single person. The operator remains outside to control chamber pressure and observe the patient for any adverse effects of pressurization and hyperoxygenation. The maximum pressure obtainable in a monoplace unit is 3 atm because of the physical properties of the chamber. Multiplace units have the advantage of accommodating two or more people at a time, including medical staff that can attend to patients and perform therapeutic maneuvers. Patients receive 100% oxygen through either a face mask or head tent, while staff members within the chamber are only subjected to pressurized air (21% oxygen). Multiplace chambers are especially useful in treating decompression sickness and air emboli because they can exceed 6 atm of pressure. Disadvantages of these larger chambers include the high initial cost, large space requirements, and the need to closely monitor staff time in the pressurized environment to avoid decompression sickness.

30.2 Indications and Outcomes for Hyperbaric Oxygen Treatment

30.2.1 Air or Gas Embolism and Decompression Sickness

Air embolism can result from traumatic cardiothoracic or vascular injuries, as well as complicate central venous catheter placement or exchange, hemodialysis, cardiothoracic surgery, and mechanical ventilation. Injury occurs when environmental air is entrained into the vascular system through an injured vessel. It can also occur during uncontrolled scuba diving ascents or mountain climbing ascents above 5500 m (altitude decompression sickness).[9] Damage results from the decrease in solubility that a dissolved gas experiences as the atmospheric pressure, and hence its partial pressure, decreases. When the solubility of the gas in plasma decreases, nitrogen (as in decompression sickness of divers) or oxygen reforms gas bubbles within the circulatory system and tissues faster than the ventilatory system can disperse the excess molecules. Treatment with hyperbaric oxygen reduces bubble size, corrects hypoxia, and provides a controlled return to ambient pressure with effective ventilation.

The symptoms of air embolism may vary from rash to weakness, paralysis, altered mental status, and seizures, with death possible in severe cases. A high level of suspicion based upon the clinical setting is critical for the early diagnosis and treatment of air embolism. Treatment begins with 100% oxygen delivered at 2.5 to 3 atm for 2 to 4 h. The best outcomes are achieved when therapy is initiated within 6 h of symptom onset.[10] Further treatments are given until clinical symptoms resolve or fail to show continued improvement.

30.2.2 Carbon Monoxide and Cyanide Poisoning

Carbon monoxide and cyanide poisoning occur as the products of combustion and fumes are inhaled from an accident or suicide attempt. Injury results from the extreme affinity with which carbon monoxide (CO) binds to hemoglobin. Because it does so at a rate 240 times greater than oxygen, carbon monoxide effectively displaces oxygen and prevents its transportation. In addition, CO shifts the hemoglobin–oxygen dissociation curve to the left, which further decreases the release of oxygen to the tissues. Myoglobin oxygen receptors are affected in a manner similar to those for hemoglobin, which completes the overall effect of profound hypoxia.[11–13] The degree of carbon monoxide poisoning may manifest clinically as mild, moderate, or severe. With mild CO exposure, symptoms can mimic those of influenza, with headaches, dizziness, nausea, and vomiting; moderate cases cause confusion, blurred vision, weakness, tachypnea/tachycardia, or ataxia; and severe exposure results in chest pain, palpitations, electrocardiographic ischemia, dysrhythmias, hypotension, syncope, pulmonary edema, disorientation, seizures, obtundation, coma, and finally death. Neurological presentations may be acute, recurrent after a lucid interval of 1 to 40 days, or delayed (from which only 50% of patients fully recover).[14] Laboratory studies may assist in the diagnosis of carbon monoxide poisoning. Normal values for blood carboxyhemoglobin (COHb) range from 0 to 10%, with the upper range seen in cigarette smokers and city dwellers. Because CO moves to the intracellular environment, however, blood levels of COHb after hours of exposure will not accurately reflect the degree of CO intoxication.

The half-life of hemoglobin-bound carbon monoxide averages 5 h under standard conditions (21% oxygen at 1 atm). This may be shortened to 1.5 h by increasing the percentage of inspired oxygen to 100% via a nonrebreathing mask, and further reduced by hyperbaric oxygen therapy to 23 min.[15] Hyperbaric oxygen treatment in carbon monoxide poisoning is significantly more effective at higher pressures (2.8 to 3.0 atm compared to 2.0 atm) and when started shortly after exposure.[16–19] In one study, HBO reduced mortality from 30.1 to 13.5% when initiated within 6 h of CO exposure. The incidence of delayed neurological presentations was also similarly reduced from 36 to 0.7% when HBO was instituted within 6 h of exposure.[19]

In contrast to carbon monoxide, cyanide produces tissue hypoxia by blocking intracellular oxidative phosphorylation. This is manifested clinically as respiratory depression, metabolic acidosis with increased lactic acid levels, and convulsions. Primary therapy consists of thiosulfate (12.5 mg i.v. for adults and 1.65 mg/kg for children), sodium nitrate (300 mg for adults and 0.33 mg/kg for children), 100% oxygen by mechanical ventilation, and anticonvulsants. In cases of inhalational cyanide poisoning refractory to treatment, HBO therapy should be initiated because of the potential for undiagnosed concomitant carbon monoxide poisoning. In addition, studies have shown that mice survive lethal doses of cyanide when treated with HBO at 2.8 atm.[20,21]

30.2.3 Clostridial Myositis/Myonecrosis and Necrotizing Soft Tissue Infections

Because of their rapidly progressive nature and high mortality rates (up to 30 to 50%), soft tissue infections with gas-forming bacteria (e.g., clostridial myositis/myonecrosis) or involvement of the fascial planes (necrotizing fasciitis) are true surgical emergencies.[22,23] Although i.v. antibiotics and surgical debridement of necrotic tissue is the first line of therapy, HBO has proven beneficial in reducing mortality from 42 to 7% in matched cases of necrotizing fasciitis of the perineum (Fournier's gangrene).[23] In other studies of clostridial soft tissue infections, the rate of amputation was decreased from 50 to 24% when HBO was added to surgical debridement and antibiotic therapy.[24] A 15-year retrospective review of clostridial infection reported similar outcome benefits with the addition of HBO therapy.[25]

The improvement seen with hyperbaric oxygen is achieved via several mechanisms. Areas of localized hypoxia are predisposed to infection because oxygen is needed for neutrophil production of the free radicals necessary to kill bacteria.[26,27] Hyperbaric oxygen, therefore, reverses local hypoxia and promotes neutrophil-mediated phagocytosis.[28] Some anaerobic bacteria, such as *Clostridium perfringens*, also lack the antioxidant enzymes dismutase and catalase that degrade superoxide and hydrogen peroxide. This makes them susceptible to the free radicals produced by neutrophils in the setting of hyperbaric oxygen therapy.[29] HBO also inhibits production of the *Clostridium* alpha-toxin that is responsible for tissue liquefaction, septic shock, hemolytic anemia, disseminated intravascular coagulation, renal failure, and cardiotoxicity.[30,31] In addition, HBO may be bacteriostatic for *Escherichia* and *Pseudomonas*.[32–34] Recommended hyperbaric treatments begin at 2.5 to 3 atm, twice daily for 90 min, and continue based on clinical response.[35]

30.2.4 Intracranial Abscess

Although the literature is scant and limited to case reports, the same mechanisms (enhanced host defenses, direct bactericidal/bacteriostatic effects) that make hyperbaric oxygen therapy beneficial in myonecrosis apply to the treatment of brain abscesses as well. The infectious organisms in these reported cases include *Clostridium* (for which HBO was ineffective) and fungal infections with mucormycosis.[36–40] The hyperbaric protocol consists of twice daily treatments at 2.5 atm for 90 min in advanced cases, with the total number of treatments ranging between 5 and 20.[41,42]

30.2.5 Refractory Osteomyelitis

Standard treatment of osteomyelitis includes surgical debridement of devitalized bone coupled with antibiotics. Intraoperative bone biopsies are obtained for culture to determine the causative organism(s) and select the appropriate antibiotic regimen based on bacterial sensitivities. In some cases, however, debridement and antibiotics are unsuccessful in eradicating the infection because of localized tissue hypoxia. Animal models in infected rabbit tibiae show a decrease in oxygen tension when compared to normal controls (23 and 45 mmHg, respectively). As noted above, decreased oxygen levels impair the bactericidal action of neutrophils. This condition is reversed with the increased oxygen levels achieved during hyperbaric oxygen treatments. Multiple human studies have confirmed the efficacy of HBO in refractory osteomyelitis when combined with secondary surgical debridement and antibiotics, with reports of 70 to 89% disease-free rates.[43–47] One study failed to confirm that these results were nonrandomized, however, and its authors felt that the conservative initial debridement may have contributed to the treatment failures.[48] The current recommended treatment protocol is 2.0 atm for 90 min twice daily for inpatients, daily for outpatients or if the infection is under control, and 2.5 atm if *Pseudomonas* or *E. coli* is the causative organism.[42]

30.2.6 Acute Traumatic Ischemia, Crush Injury, and Reperfusion Injury

Interruption of blood flow deprives dependent tissues of oxygen and nutrients. This results in multiple sequelae that must be recognized to prevent further morbidity. The vascular compromise may be apparent, as in the case of open extremity fractures with loss of pulses, or occult, as with electrical injuries, crush injuries, or compartment syndrome. Compartment syndrome exists when the pressure within an anatomic compartment exceeds the capillary perfusion pressure of 20 mmHg. At that point, nutritive blood flow to tissues ceases. The recognition of vascular compromise is classically described in terms of the 5 P's: *P*ain out of proportion to the clinical situation (the earliest clinical symptom, usually within the first 30 min); *P*aresthesias in the distribution of nerves within the affected compartment; *P*aralysis/weakness of involved muscles; *P*oikilothermia (coolness as compared to other areas); and *P*ulselessness (a very late finding). In addition, compartment syndrome may have the additional "P" of pressure, presenting as tense, shiny skin. The subsequent time course of hypoxic tissues involves functional muscle weakness at 2 to 4 h, decreased capillary integrity and soft tissue edema within 3 h, and irreversible muscle damage with the onset of myoglobinuria in 4 to 6 h. Restoration of perfusion is critical to stop this progression, but with the return of blood flow comes a further increase in tissue edema. This occurs because damaged capillaries allow fluid to leak into the interstitium. Treatment of compartment syndrome includes fasciotomy, which is the release of the fascia enveloping the affected tissues. Fasciotomy can be performed prophylactically at the time of vascular repair in anticipation of complications or definitively to treat an existing compartment syndrome.

Hyperbaric oxygen is used in the setting of ischemia to limit edema, support hypoxic tissues, and limit the extent of reperfusion injury. Edema is limited because hyperoxia causes a reflexive vasoconstriction that slows further extravasation.[49] Tissue oxygenation is supported by diffusion from the hyperoxygenated plasma into the soft tissues, improving neutrophil phagocytic activity and fibroblast proliferation (which is inhibited when oxygen levels are less than 30 mmHg).[50] In a postischemic animal model, adenosine triphosphatase (ATPase), phosphocreatine kinase, and lactate levels from the HBO-treated group were similar to levels in uninjured controls. Despite the restoration of blood flow, the non-HBO treated postischemic group continued to have high lactate levels indicative of ongoing anaerobic metabolism.[51] Other studies have shown that oxygen-free radicals interact with cell membrane lipid layers to produce lipid peroxidation, a reperfusion event that is decreased by HBO.[52–54] Hyperbaric oxygen's greatest protective effect, however, is the inhibition of neutrophil adherence to postcapillary venules.[52,55]

A special category of traumatic ischemia includes amputation of the ear or nose, for which successful salvage has been reported utilizing hyperbaric oxygen.[56,57] In cases where the small caliber of vessels in the amputated tissue precludes microvascular repair, the reattached tissue behaves as a composite graft. Animal studies transferring a composite graft of skin, subcutaneous tissue, and cartilage to the opposite ear demonstrated postoperative HBO therapy to significantly improve graft survival.[58] In experimental studies, grafts require approximately 72 h for neovascularization to occur.[59] Because of their low oxygen levels, ischemic composite grafts are at risk for decreased ATP, increased osmolarity and edema, and further impairment of imbibition and inosculation.[60] HBO stimulates macrophages to secrete angiogenic factors that then increase fibroblastic activity, forming a new fibrous matrix and stimulating inosculation.[61] In fact, capillaries have been shown to grow three times farther into pedicled guinea pig flaps treated with HBO.[62] Evidence also shows that fibroblasts behave as facultative anaerobes and intermittent episodes of hypoxia (as occur between HBO treatments) have a stimulatory effect on collagen synthesis.[63]

The HBO protocol is 2.5 atm for 90 min three times daily in the first 24 h, then twice daily for 2 to 4 days if treating compartment syndrome postfasciotomy, or 5 to 7 days for crush injury or composite graft of amputated tissues.

30.2.7 Compromised Skin Grafts and Flaps

Human clinical studies have shown a beneficial effect of HBO on skin grafts and flaps, especially when compromised or when placed on poorly vascularized tissue beds (90% salvage rate).[64] A prospective, randomized study of 48 consecutive patients receiving skin grafts demonstrated an 84% skin graft survival rate with HBO therapy compared to 62% graft survival without HBO.[65] The mechanisms responsible for flap and graft salvage are those described for acute traumatic injury and reperfusion injury. In flaps with evidence of ischemia, measured oxygen tensions are commonly less than 15 mmHg.[66] This is harmful because fibroblast synthesis, collagen production, and angiogenesis require oxygen tensions of 30 to 40 mmHg.[63] Commonly used protocols include 2 to 2.5 atm for 90 min twice daily tapered to 120 min daily once clinical improvement is sustained.

30.2.8 Complications of Radiation Therapy and Prevention of Osteoradionecrosis

Radiation therapy is widely used for selected tumors as both curative and adjuvant therapy. Though effective against neoplasms, radiation has detrimental effects on adjacent tissues. There are progressive changes in the irradiated arterioles and capillaries, beginning with thickening of the vessel walls, followed by endarteritis and vasculitis, and ending with vessel obliteration. The soft tissues become fibrotic and occasionally painful. The time course for these changes is 6 months to 5 years after the ionizing radiation treatments.[67] This creates a hypoxic and hypocellular zone that exhibits poor wound healing following even minor trauma or surgery. Hyperbaric oxygen therapy addresses this by creating a wound oxygen gradient sufficient to stimulate neoangiogenesis and reverse the effects of radiation.[62,68]

Bone is particularly sensitive to irradiation because its high density results in absorption of a greater proportion of the delivered dosage. Osteoporosis and osteonecrosis are not uncommon late findings months to years after treatment. In head and neck cancer, for example, the mandible is often included in the radiation field. Even procedures as minor as tooth extraction within this zone can precipitously lead to osteoradionecrosis (ORN), osteomyelitis, and pathologic fractures. These are particularly difficult to treat and prove refractory to the conventional therapy of debridement and antibiotics in over half of cases.[69] Hyperbaric oxygen therapy has been successfully applied to these wounds with reported healing rates of up to 93%.[70–73] Prophylactic hyperbaric oxygen has also been shown to be more effective than penicillin in preventing osteoradionecrosis of the mandible in previously irradiated patients, with incidences of 5.4 and 30%, respectively.[71,74] The accepted protocol for ORN prophylaxis in an irradiated mandible is 20 presurgical treatments at 2.4 atm for 90 min followed by another 10 postsurgical treatments.

There are also reports of improvement in soft tissue radiation injury. Women undergoing breast conservation therapy for breast cancer (lumpectomy + radiation) may have late sequelae common to radiation-induced soft tissue changes. Patients treated with hyperbaric oxygen at 2.4 atm for 90 min daily for an average of 25 sessions showed a significant reduction in postirradiation pain, erythema, and edema when compared to untreated controls ($p < 0.001$).[75] Radiation prostatitis is likewise responsive to HBO therapy, typically applied as an extended treatment course consisting of daily 90-min treatments at 2.4 atm for 4 to 8 weeks.[76–78]

30.2.9 Thermal Burns

The beneficial effects of HBO in thermal injury include edema reduction (improved capillary integrity and hyperoxic vasoconstriction), support of marginal tissue in the zone of stasis, and an increased rate of neovascularization. When compared to control patients, burn patients receiving hyperbaric treatments demonstrated a 30% decrease in mortality, a 50% increase in wound healing rate (in TBSA burns of less than 50% the mean healing time was 19.7 days vs. 43.8 days in untreated group), and required 35% less fluid during the initial resuscitative period.[79] In another series, HBO reduced the average hospital length of stay from 73 to 43 days and surgical procedures from 4.2 to 2.4, with an overall cost reduction of 34%.[80] Recommended treatment parameters are 2.0 atm for 90 min three times in the first 24 h postburn, and then twice daily for 5 to 45 treatments depending upon patient response and extent of burn.

30.2.10 Enhanced Healing in Selected Problem Wounds

In addition to wounds in an irradiated field, hyperbaric oxygen therapy may benefit other chronic nonhealing wounds.[81] Diabetic patients with nonhealing lower extremity wounds have benefited from HBO as a part of a comprehensive diabetic wound care program, reducing major amputation rates from 40.5 to 23.5% in one study and similarly in others.[82–85] A later randomized controlled study by the same investigators found similar results with the HBO-treated group demonstrating an increase in transcutaneous oxygen measurements (TCOMs) on the dorsum of the foot.[83] This would seem to indicate that collateral neovascularization of the foot was stimulated by HBO therapy. TCOM studies are often obtained before initiating therapy to predict the possible benefit from HBO intervention.[86,87] One method of testing includes exposure to supplemental normobaric oxygen via a nonrebreathing mask for 10 min. When the resulting transcutaneous oxygen values increase by at least 100 mmHg over the baseline, the patient is likely to benefit from HBO therapy.[88]

The recommended protocol is 2.0 atm for 90 min twice daily if the wound is gangrenous or otherwise daily for 14 days. When improvement is evident, HBO is continued Monday through Friday, with a possible 7-day halt in treatments to monitor whether healing progresses without HBO therapy.

30.2.11 Acute Blood Loss Anemia

The acute loss of a significant portion of the blood volume leads to circulatory collapse. Immediate blood transfusion is not always possible because of technical (blood type incompatibility) or religious beliefs (as in

Jehovah's Witnesses). In these situations, hyperbaric oxygen therapy may be used in the interim until blood type crossmatching is complete or erythropoeisis adequate. As previously noted, there is sufficient oxygen dissolved in plasma under hyperbaric conditions (3 atm and 100% oxygen) to sustain life in the absence of red blood cells.[1,2,6] Multiple reports describe the successful use of HBO in cases of organ dysfunction secondary to acute blood loss.[89,90] Because wide variations exist in the tolerance to anemia, treatment is based upon patient symptoms rather than an arbitrary hemoglobin/hematocrit laboratory value.

30.2.12 Other Possible Applications

Recent research efforts have focused on ischemic injury of the brain and spinal cord. Possible benefits successfully demonstrated in animal models include reducing infarct size by 18%, preventing reperfusion injury as measured by lipid peroxidation products, decreasing paralysis, and protecting neuron viability against both acute and delayed injury.[91,92] The time period from onset of ischemia to intervention with HBO therapy is a variable that is still open to debate, since most of the animal studies provide evidence of efficacy after a short period of ischemia (15 to 40 min), but not after treatment delayed beyond 6 h.[91,92] Another variable that must be clarified is the optimal hyperbaric pressure. One human clinical study of ischemic stroke patients (prospective, double-blinded randomized trial) demonstrated improvement after HBO using some but not all outcome measures. This study used only 1.5 atm of pressure, while the animal studies used 3 atm of pressure (most of the application protocols for HBO utilized 2 to 3 atm of pressured 100% oxygen).[93]

30.2.13 Complications of Hyperbaric Oxygen Therapy

Complications of HBO therapy fall into two major categories: barotrauma and oxygen toxicity. Barotrauma of the ear is the most common complication from treatment, with published reports placing the incidence anywhere from 5 to 82%.[94] This occurs when eustachian tube dysfunction does not allow adequate pressure equalization under hyperbaric conditions. Barotrauma may also affect any air-filled space, including the facial sinuses, where "sinus squeeze" can cause severe pain. Pulmonary barotrauma, however, is the most concerning pressure-related complication of hyperbaric oxygen treatments. Potentially life-threatening pneumothorax or pneumomediastinum may occur. This is more likely in the setting of preexisting pulmonary diseases such as emphysema and COPD.

Oxygen toxicity is dependent upon the partial pressure of inspired oxygen and the duration of exposure. At 3 atm, toxicity occurs after 3 h, but at 4 atm, only 10 to 40 min of exposure are necessary before unwanted side effects occur.[95] The pathophysiology is most likely related to oxygen free-radical mechanisms,[96] although the effects are reversible and clinical protocols avoid these levels. The four most important manifestations of oxygen toxicity are: lowered seizure threshold; diffuse pulmonary alveolar injury; myopia; and increased rate of cataract formation. A history of seizure disorder predisposes patients to oxygen-induced seizures with HBO treatments. This necessitates maintenance of antiepileptic medications within therapeutic levels during the course of treatment.[97] Other factors that lower the seizure threshold can also increase the risk of oxygen-induced seizures, including fever, nicotine, aspirin, and alcohol. At the typical treatment pressure of 2.4 atm, the incidence of HBO-induced seizures is approximately 1/10,000.[98]

There are no reports of pulmonary toxicity in patients with healthy lungs who receive HBO at 1.5 to 2 atm for periods of less than 1 h.[99] Under normobaric conditions, more than 24 h of treatment with 100% oxygen are needed for pulmonary toxicity to occur. This usually first manifests as a reversible reduction in vital capacity from an oxygen-dependent inhibition of surfactant production or from a depletion of natural antioxidants.

Myopia, commonly called near-sightedness, is frequently reported during HBO therapy and averages a change of 3 diopters. This side effect, however, is transitory and reverts to the patient's baseline vision within 6 months of completing therapy.[100] Because there are few antioxidants in the lens, oxidation of lens proteins may result in the formation of aggregates. An increased rate of cataract formation can also occur, especially in patients with preexisting cataracts.[100]

30.3 Summary

Hyperbaric oxygen is an efficacious therapeutic and prophylactic modality for a number of disease processes. Although historically used as a panacea for well-being and health improvement, critical scientific investigation has yielded specific uses that decrease both patient morbidity and mortality. As laboratory and human clinical trials evaluate further applications, hyperbaric oxygen therapy will continue to expand and more patients may hope to benefit from this unique manipulation of the environment.

References

1. Lambertson, C.J. et al., Oxygen toxicity: effects in man of oxygen inhalation at 1 and 3.5 atmospheres upon blood gas transport, cerebral circulation, and cerebral metabolism, *J. Appl. Physiol.*, 5, 471–486, 1953.
2. Kety, S.S. et al., The effects of altered arterial tensions of carbon dioxide and oxygen on cerebral flow and cerebral oxygen consumption of normal young men, *J. Clin Invest.*, 27, 484–492, 1948.
3. Henshaw, N., *A Register for the Air*, In Five Chapters, Samuel Dancer, Dublin, 1664.
4. Priestly, J., Experiments and observations on different kinds of air, in *The Discovery of Oxygen*, Part 1, Vol. 11, The Alembic Club, Edinburgh, 1923; in *Foundations of Anaesthesiology*, Faulconer, A. and Keys, T.C., Eds., Vol. 1, Charles C Thomas, Springfield, IL, 1965, pp. 39–70.
5. Behnke, A.R., The effect of oxygen on man at pressures from 1–4 atmospheres, *Am. J. Physiol.*, 110, 563–570, 1935.
6. Boerema, I., Meyne, N.G., et al., Life without blood, *J. Cardiovasc. Surg.*, 182, 133–146, 1960.
7. Thom, S.R., Hyperbaric oxygen therapy: a committee report. Bethesda, *Undersea Hyperbaric Med.*, 1992.
8. Takahashi, H. and Kobayashi, S., New indications for hyperbaric oxygen therapy and its complication, in *Hyperbaric Oxygen Therapy in Otorhinolaryngology*, Yanagita, N. and Nakashima, T., Eds., S. Karger AG, Basel, Switzerland, 1998, p. 1.
9. Blumen, I.J. et al., Flight physiology: clinical considerations, *Crit. Care Clin.*, 8, 597–618, 1992.
10. Moon, R.E. and Gorman, D.F., Treatment of the decompression disorders, in *The Physiology and Medicine of Diving, 4th ed.*, Bennett, P.B. and Elliot, D.H., Eds., W.B. Saunders, Philadelphia, 1993, pp. 506–541.
11. Wittenberg, B.A. and Wittenberg, J.B., Role of myoglobin in the oxygen supply of red skeletal muscle, *J. Biol. Chem.*, 250, 9038, 1975.
12. Chen, K.C. and McGrath, J.J., Response of the isolated heart to carbon monoxide and nitrogen anoxia, *Toxicol. Appl. Pharmacol.*, 81, 363, 1985.
13. Ginsberg, M.D. et al., Experimental carbon monoxide encephalopathy in the primate. II. Clinical aspects, neuropathology, and physiologic correlation, *Arch. Neurol.*, 30, 209, 1974.
14. Bartlett, R., Carbon monoxide poisoning, in *Clinical Management of Poisoning and Drug Overdose, 2nd ed.*, Haddad, L.M. and Winchester, J.F., Eds., W.B. Saunders, Philadelphia, 1998, pp. 107–120.
15. Myers, R.A.M., Carbon monoxide poisoning, in *Clinical Management of Poisoning and Drug Overdose, 2nd ed.*, Haddad, L.M. and Winchester, J.F., Eds., W.B. Saunders, Philadelphia, 1998, pp. 1139–1152.
16. Raphael, J.C. et al., Trial of normobaric and hyperbaric oxygen for acute carbon monoxide intoxication, *Lancet*, 1, 414, 1989.
17. Myers, R.A.M., Snyder, S.K. et al., Subacute sequelae of carbon monoxide poisoning, *Ann. Emerg. Med.*, 14, 1163, 1985.
18. Thom, S.R. et al., Delayed neurological sequelae following carbon monoxide poisoning, *Ann. Emerg. Med.*, 25, 474, 1995.
19. Goulon, M. et al., Carbon monoxide poisoning and acute anoxia due to breathing coal gas and hydrocarbons, *Ann. Med. Interne (Paris)*, 120, 335, 1969.

20. Ivanov, K.P., The effect of elevated oxygen pressure on animals poisoned with potassium cyanide, *Pharmacol. Toxicol.*, 22, 476–579, 1959.
21. Skene, W.G. et al., Effect of hyperbaric oxygen in cyanide poisoning, in *Proceedings of the 3rd International Congress on Hyperbaric Oxygen*, Brown, I. and Cox, B., Eds., National Academy of Science, NRC, Washington, D.C., 1966, pp. 705–710.
22. Balcerak, R.J., Sisto, J.M., and Bosack, R.C., Cervicofacial necrotizing fasciitis: report of three cases and literature review, *J. Oral Maxillofac. Surg.*, 46, 450, 1988.
23. Hollabaugh, R.S., Dmochowski, R.R., et al., Fournier's Gangrene: therapeutic impact of hyperbaric oxygen, *Plast. Reconstr. Surg.*, 101(1), 94–100, 1998.
24. Hitchcock, C.R., Demello, F.J., and Haglin, J.J., Gangrene infection: new approaches to an old disease, *Surg. Clin. North Am.*, 55, 1403–1410, 1975.
25. Hart, G.B., Lamb, R.C., and Strauss, M.B., Gas gangrene, *J. Trauma*, 23, 991–1000, 1983.
26. Hunt, T.K., The physiology of wound healing, *Ann. Emerg. Med.*, 17, 1265–1273, 1988.
27. Knighton, D.R., Halliday, B., and Hunt, T.K., Oxygen as an antibiotic: a comparison of the effects of inspired oxygen concentration and antibiotic administration on in vivo bacterial clearance, *Arch. Surg.*, 121, 191–195, 1986.
28. Mader, J.T. et al., A mechanism for the amelioration by hyperbaric oxygen of experimental staphylococcal osteomyelitis in rabbits, *J. Infect. Dis.*, 142, 915–922, 1980.
29. Hill, G.B. and Osterhout, S., Experimental effects of hyperbaric oxygen on selected clostridial species. I. In-vitro studies, *J. Infect. Dis.*, 125, 17–25, 1972.
30. van Unnik, A.J.M., Inhibition of toxin production in *Clostridium perfringens in vitro* by hyperbaric oxygen, *Antonie Van Leeuwenhoek*, 31, 181–186, 1965.
31. Kaye, D., Effect of hyperbaric oxygen on Clostridia *in vitro* and *in vivo*, *Proc. Soc. Exp. Biol. Med.*, 124, 360–366, 1967.
32. Boehm, D.E. et al., Oxygen, and toxicity inhibition of amino acid biosynthesis, *Nature*, 262, 418–420, 1976.
33. Brown, O.R., Reversible inhibition of respiration of *Escherichia coli* by hyperoxia, *Microbios*, 5, 7–16, 1972.
34. Park, M.K. et al., Hyperoxia prolongs the aminoglycoside-induced postantibiotic effect in *Pseudomonas aeruginosa*, *Antimicrob. Agents Chemother.*, 35, 691–695, 1991.
35. Scher, R.L., Hyperbaric oxygen therapy for necrotizing cervical infections, in *Hyperbaric Oxygen Therapy in Otorhinolaryngology*, Yanagita, N. and Nakashima, T., Eds., S. Karger AG, Basel, Switzerland, 1998, p. 50.
36. Anand, V.K. et al., Intracranial complications of mucormycosis: an experimental model and clinical review, *Laryngoscope*, 102, 656–662, 1992.
37. Keogh, A.J., Clostridial brain abscess and hyperbaric oxygen, *Postgrad. Med. J.*, 49, 64–66, 1973.
38. Couch, L., Theilen, F., and Mader, J.T., Rhinocerebral Mucormycosis with cerebral extension successfully treated with adjunctive hyperbaric oxygen therapy, *Arch. Otolaryngol. Head Neck Surg.*, 114, 791–794, 1988.
39. Price, J.C. and Stevens, D.L., Hyperbaric oxygen in the treatment of rhinocerebral mucormycosis, *Laryngoscope*, 90, 737–747, 1980.
40. Ferguson, B.J., Mitchell, T.G., Moon, R., et al., Adjunctive hyperbaric oxygen for treatment of rhinocerebral mucormycosis, *Rev. Infect. Dis.*, 10, 551–559, 1988.
41. Pelton, R.W., Peterson, E.A., et al., Successful treatment of Rhino-orbital Mucormycosis without exenteration: the use of multiple treatment modalities, *Ophthalmic Plast. Reconstr. Surg.*, 17(1), 62–66, 2001.
42. Clarke, D., Treatment protocols, in Primary Training in Hyperbaric Medicine, Hyperbaric Medicine Program at Palmetto Richland Memorial Hospital, 2000, pp. 364–374.
43. Mader, J., Brown, G.L., and Gucklan, J.C., A mechanism for the amelioration by hyperbaric oxygen of experimental staphylococcal osteomyelitis in rabbits, *J. Infect. Dis.*, 142(6), 915–922, 1980.

44. Perrins, D.J.D. et al., OHP in the management of chronic osteomyelitis, in *Proceedings of the 3rd International Conference on Hyperbaric Medicine*, Publ. 1404, Brown, I.W. and Cox, B.G., Eds., National Academy of Sciences, Washington, D.C., 1966, pp. 578–584.
45. Morrey, B.F. et al., Hyperbaric oxygen and chronic osteomyelitis, *Clin. Orthopedic Rel. Res.*, 144, 121–127, 1979.
46. Davis, J.C. et al., Chronic non-hematogenous osteomyelitis treated with adjuvant hyperbaric oxygen, *J. Bone Jt. Surg.*, 68-A, 1210–1217, 1986.
47. Depenbusch, F.L., Thompson, R.E., and Hart, G.B., Use of hyperbaric oxygen in the treatment of refractory osteomyelitis: a preliminary report, *J. Trauma*, 12, 807–812, 1972.
48. Easterhai, J., Pisarello, J., et al., Adjunctive hyperbaric oxygen therapy in the treatment of chronic refractory osteomyelitis, *J. Trauma*, 27(7), 763–768, 1987.
49. Strauss, M.B., Hargens, A.R., et al., Reduction of skeletal muscle necrosis using intermittent hyperbaric oxygen in a model compartment syndrome, *J. Bone Jt. Surg.*, 65A, 656–662, 1983.
50. Hunt, T.K., Zederfeldt, B., and Goldstick, T.K., Oxygen and healing, *Am. J. Surg.*, 118, 521–525, 1969.
51. Nylander, G., Lewis, D., et al., Reduction of postischemic edema with hyperbaric oxygen, *Plast. Reconstr. Surg.*, 76, 596–603, 1985.
52. Thom, S., Functional inhibition of leukocytebeta 2 integrins by hyperbaric oxygen in carbon monoxide-mediated brain injury in rats, *Toxicol. Appl. Pharm.*, 123, 248–256, 1993.
53. Zamboni, W.A., Roth, A.C., et al., Morphologic analysis of the microcirculation during reperfusion of ischemic skeletal muscle and the effect of hyperbaric oxygen, *Plast. Reconstr. Surg.*, 91, 1110–1123, 1993.
54. Thom, S.R. and Elbuken, M.E., Oxygen-dependent antagonism of lipid peroxidation, *Free Rad. Biol. Med.*, 10, 413–426, 1991.
55. Zamboni, W.A., Roth, A.C., et al., The effect of acute hyperbaric oxygen therapy on axial pattern skin flap survival when administered during and after total ischemia, *J. Reconstr. Microsurg.*, 5, 343–347, 1989.
56. Nichter, L.S., Morwood, D.T., et al., Expanding the limits of composite grafting: a case report of successful nose replantation assisted by hyperbaric oxygen therapy, *Plast. Reconstr. Surg.*, 87, 337, 1991.
57. Bill, T.J., Hoard, M.A., and Gampper, T.J., Applications of hyperbaric oxygen in otolaryngology head and neck surgery: facial cutaneous flaps, *Otolaryngol. Clin. North Am.*, 34(4), 756–758, 2001.
58. Zhang, F., Cheng, C., et al., Effect of hyperbaric oxygen on survival of the composite ear graft in rats, *Ann. Plast. Surg.*, 41, 530, 1998.
59. McLaughlin, C.R., Composite ear grafts and their blood supply, *Br. J. Plast. Surg.*, 7, 174, 1952.
60. Nylander, G., Nordstrom, H., et al., Metabolic effects of hyperbaric oxygen in post-ischemic muscle, *Plast. Reconstr. Surg.*, 79, 91, 1991.
61. Knighton, T.R., Hunt, T.K., et al., Oxygen tension regulates expression of angiogenesis factor by macrophages, *Science*, 221, 1283, 1983.
62. Manson, P.N., Im, M.J., and Myers, R.A.M., Improved capillaries by hyperbaric oxygen on skin flaps, *Surg. Forum*, 31, 564, 1980.
63. Knighton, T.R., Silver, I.A., and Hunt, T.K., Regulation of wound healing angiogenesis: effect of oxygen gradients and inspired air concentration, *Surgery*, 90, 262, 1981.
64. Bowersox, J.C., Strauss, M.B., and Hart, G.B., Clinical experience with hyperbaric oxygen therapy in the salvage of ischemic skin flaps and grafts, *J. Hyperbaric Med.*, 1, 141, 1986.
65. Perrins, D.J.D., Influence of hyperbaric oxygen on the survival of split skin grafts, *Lancet*, 1, 868, 1967.
66. Sheffield, P.J., Measuring tissue oxygen tension: a review, *Undersea Hyperbaric Med.*, 25, 179, 1998.
67. Heimbach, R.D., Radiation effect on tissue, in *Problem Wounds: The Role of Oxygen*, Davis, J.C. and Hunt, T.K., Eds., Elsevier, New York, 1988, p. 53.

68. Bayati, S., Russell, R.C., and Roth, A.C., Stimulation of angiogenesis to improve the viability of prefabricated flaps, *Plast. Reconstr. Surg.*, 101, 1290, 1998.
69. Tibbles, P.K. and Edelsberg, J.S., Medical progress: hyperbaric oxygen therapy, *N. Engl. J. Med.*, 334(25), 1642–1648, 1996.
70. Hart, G.B. and Mainous, E.G., The treatment of radiation necrosis with hyperbaric oxygen (OHP), *Cancer*, 37, 2580–2585, 1976.
71. Marx, R.E., Radiation injury to tissue, in *Hyperbaric Medicine Practice*, Kindwell, E.P., Ed., Best, Flagstaff, AZ, 1994, pp. 447–503.
72. Marx, R.E. and Ames, J.R., The use of hyperbaric oxygen therapy in bony reconstruction of the irradiated and tissue-deficient patient, *J. Oral Maxillofac. Surg.*, 40, 412–420, 1982.
73. Mainous, E.G. and Boyne, P.J., Hyperbaric oxygen in total rehabilitation of patients with mandibular osteoradionecrosis, *Int. J. Oral Surg.*, 3, 297–301, 1974.
74. Marx, R.E., Johnson, R.P., and Kline, S.N., Prevention of osteoradionecrosis: a randomized prospective clinical trial of hyperbaric oxygen verses penicillin, *J. Am. Dent. Assoc.*, 111, 49–54, 1985.
75. Carl, U.M., Hyperbaric oxygen therapy for late sequelae in women receiving radiation after breast-conserving surgery, *Int. J. Radiat. Oncol. Biol. Phys.*, 49(4), 1029–1031, 2001.
76. Bem, J., Bem, S., and Singh, A., Use of hyperbaric oxygen chamber in the management of radiation-related complications of the anorectal region: report of two cases and review of the literature, *Dis. Colon Rectum*, 43(10), 1435–1438, 2000.
77. Woo, T.C.S., Joseph, D., and Oxer, H., Hyperbaric oxygen treatment for radiation proctitis, *Int. J. Radiat. Oncol. Biol. Phys.*, 38(3), 619–622, 1997.
78. Warren, D.C., Freehan, P., Slade, J.B., and Ciani, P.E., Chronic radiation proctopathy treated with hyperbaric oxygen, *Undersea Hyperbaric Med.*, 24, 181–184, 1997.
79. Hart, G.B., O'Reilly, R.R., et al., Treatment of burns with hyperbaric oxygen, *Surg. Gynecol. Obstetr.*, 139, 693–696, 1974.
80. Cianci, P.E., Williams, C., et al., Adjunctive hyperbaric oxygen in the treatment of thermal burns: an economic analysis, *J. Burn Care Rehab.*, 11(2), 140–143, 1990.
81. Zamboni, W.A., Wong, H.P., et al., Evaluation of hyperbaric oxygen for diabetic wounds: a prospective study, *Undersea Hyperbaric Med.*, 24, 175–179, 1997.
82. Faglia, E., Favales, F., et al., Change in major amputation rate in a center dedicated to diabetic foot care during the 1980s: prognostic determinants for major amputation, *J. Diabetes Complications*, 12, 96–102, 1988.
83. Faglia, E., Favales, F., et al., Adjunctive systemic hyperbaric oxygen therapy in treatment of severe prevalently ischemic diabetic foot ulcer: a randomized study, *Diabetes Care*, 19(2), 1338–1343, 1996.
84. Oriani, G., Meazza, D., et al., Hyperbaric oxygen therapy in diabetic gangrene, *J. Hyperbaric Med.*, 5, 171–175, 1990.
85. Baroni, G. et al., Hyperbaric oxygen in diabetic gangrene treatment, *Diabetes Care*, 110, 81–86, 1987.
86. Harward, T.R.S., Volny, J., et al., Oxygen inhalation-induced transcutaneous PO(2) changes as a predictor of amputation level, *J. Vas. Surg.*, 2, 200–207, 1985.
87. Pecoraro, R.E., Ahroni, J.H., et al., Chronology and determinants of tissue repair in diabetic lower-extremity ulcers, *Diabetes*, 40, 1305–1313, 1991.
88. Grolman, R.E., Transcutaneous oxygen measurements predict a beneficial response to hyperbaric oxygen therapy in patients with non-healing wounds and critical limb ischemia, *Am. Surg.*, 67(11), 1072–1079, 2001.
89. Greensmith, J.E., Hyperbaric oxygen reverses organ dysfunction in severe anemia, *Anesthesiology*, 93(4), 1149–1152, 2000.
90. Hart, G.B., Lennon, P.A., and Strauss, M.B., Hyperbaric oxygen in exceptional acute blood-loss anemia, *J. Hyperbaric Med.*, 2, 205–210, 1987.

91. Sunami, K., Takeda, Y., et al., Hyperbaric oxygen reduces infarct volume in rats by increasing oxygen supply to the ischemic periphery, *Crit. Care Med.*, 28(8), 2831–2836, 2000.
92. Murakami, N., Horinouchi, T., et al., Hyperbaric oxygen therapy given 30 minutes after spinal cord ischemia attenuates selective motor neuron death in rabbits, *Crit. Care Med.*, 29(4), 814–818, 2001.
93. Nighoghossian, N., Trouillas, P., et al., Hyperbaric oxygen in the treatment of acute ischemic stroke: a double-blinded pilot study, *Stroke*, 26(8), 1369–1372, 1995.
94. Ueda, H., Shien, C.W., et al., Otologic complications of hyperbaric oxygen therapy, in *Hyperbaric Oxygen Therapy in Otorhinolaryngology*, Yanagita, N. and Nakashima, T., Eds., S. Karger AG, Basel, Switzerland, 1988, p. 119.
95. Torbati, D. and Torbati, A., Blood glucose as a predictive measure for central nervous system oxygen toxicity on conscious rats, *Undersea Biomed. Res.*, 13, 147, 1986.
96. Frank, L., Summerville, J., et al., Protection from oxygen toxicity with endotoxin: role of the endogenous antioxidant enzymes of the lung, *J. Clin. Invest.*, 65, 1104, 1980.
97. Clark, J.M. and Fisher, A.B., Oxygen toxicity and extension of tolerance to oxygen therapy, in *Hyperbaric Oxygen Therapy*, Davis, J.C. and Hunt, T.K., Eds., Undersea Medical Society, Bethesda, 1977, p. 61.
98. Davis, J.C., Dunn, J.M., and Heimbach, R.D., Hyperbaric medicine: patient selection, treatment procedures, and side effects, in *Problem Wounds: The Role of Oxygen*, Davis, J.C. and Hunt, T.K., Eds., Elsevier, New York, 1988, p. 225.
99. Clark, J.M. and Lambertson, C.J., Rate of development of pulmonary O_2 toxicity in man during O_2 breathing at 2.0 atm absolute, *J. Appl. Physiol.*, 21, 1477, 1971.
100. Palmquist, B.M., Ophthalmological effects of hyperbaric oxygen therapy in the elderly, *Geriatr. Med. Today*, 5, 135, 1986.

31

Image-Guided Thermal Therapy

CONTENTS

Rajiv Chopra
Sunnybrook and Women's College Health Sciences Centre

31.1 Introduction

Thermal therapy refers to the application of heat to treat disease. This therapeutic approach has been applied for over a century, with initial attempts involving the induction of fever to treat patients with advanced cancers. Since then, investigation into the biological basis for the therapeutic effect of heat, and the development of technology to deliver and monitor thermal therapies has improved the sophistication and accuracy of this treatment modality. The past decade has seen the rapid development of a diverse array of technology for heat generation as well as the introduction of novel noninvasive thermometric techniques such as magnetic resonance imaging (MRI). Today, quantitative knowledge of the temperature distribution within a heated volume, coupled with the ability to control the three-dimensional heating pattern makes thermal therapy a promising technique. These developments are generating a growing interest in the application of high temperatures (>60°C) capable of tissue thermal coagulation as a strategy for thermal therapy. The rapid and indiscriminate destruction of tissues exposed to these temperatures places high demands on the ability to monitor the deposition of energy and quantify the extent of thermal damage.

This manuscript provides an overview of the field of image-guided thermal coagulation therapy. The first section covers the physical principles of thermal therapy, including the relevant biological and physiological responses of tissue to heat. The second section discusses the role for image-guidance in thermal therapy, and the various techniques developed for use in conjunction with heating. The third section examines existing methods of delivering heat to a targeted region of tissue with a special emphasis on interstitial thermal therapy, an area of growing application in this field. Throughout this section, examples of clinical applications of thermal coagulation therapy are given.

0-8493-1140-3/04/$0.00+$1.50

31.2 Thermal Therapy

31.2.1 Mechanism of Tissue Destruction

Above 41°C, heat is cytotoxic to cells, and can be used to elicit a therapeutic effect.[1] Two broad categories exist to classify the different thermal therapeutic regimes used. *Hyperthermia* refers to the exposure of tissue to temperatures between 42 and 46°C for time periods ranging from hours to minutes in order to achieve a therapeutic response through cell death. In this regime, the exposure temperature as well as the duration of heating are important parameters determining cell death. The mechanism of cell killing by heat occurs broadly through the inactivation of proteins through heat-induced conformational changes. The location of these proteins and their functional role, however, varies dramatically from the cytoplasmic cell membrane, the cell nucleus, to the cytoskeleton.[2]

Although the application of hyperthermia alone can be used as a therapeutic modality due to its cytotoxic effects, the predominant application of hyperthermia has been in combination with other therapeutic approaches such as radiation therapy. Studies on the sensitivity of cells to heat and radiation have shown that the two modalities work synergistically to produce an enhanced therapeutic effect compared to either modality alone.[3] Current efforts are directed to the development of reliable delivery strategies to ensure adequate simultaneous heating and radiation delivery to a target volume.[4]

The major challenges with the application of hyperthermia have been related to (1) the technical difficulties of maintaining a volume of tissue at an elevated temperature of 42 to 43°C for periods of up to 2 h, and (2) obtaining accurate knowledge of the thermal dose delivered to tissue due to sparse temperature information.[5] The effects of blood perfusion, heat conduction, and poor control over power deposition from energy sources make the application of hyperthermia for deep seated tumors technically difficult.[1]

At temperatures between 55 and 100°C, the therapeutic mechanism is different, and referred to as *thermal coagulation therapy*, or *high temperature thermal therapy*. The goal of thermal coagulation therapy is to elevate temperatures within a targeted volume above the threshold required to produce thermal coagulation. Thermal coagulation is a process that corresponds to irreversible structural and chemical changes within the intra- and extracellular environment of tissue. These effects occur at temperatures above approximately 60°C for a range of tissue types.[6–8] *In vitro* studies of heat induced cell killing indicate that a cell survival of 0.01% is achieved after 5 sec of heating at 57°C.[9]

Although cell death occurs completely and rapidly above the coagulation temperature threshold, there are various regions of distinct structural changes in tissue, and a range of physiological effects, and time-dependent biological responses between 50 and 100°C. If one considers the region of thermal damage produced by an interstitial heat source radiating energy radially, a number of distinct regions can be seen, reviewed by Thomsen,[10] including those presented below.

31.2.1.1 Ablation and Carbonization

This effect is seen in situations where the temperature elevation generated in tissue is in excess of 100°C and occurs very rapidly. Ablation is defined as the physical removal of tissue components, and can be seen as the presence of craters, holes, and defects within a heated region. Carbonization results in the formation of a thin layer of black residue on the surface of thermal lesion resulting from reduction of tissue components to carbon. These biological changes significantly change tissue optical, acoustic, and physical properties, potentially hampering the delivery of energy for heating. The goal of thermal coagulation therapy is to avoid these effects in tissue.

31.2.1.2 Water Vaporization

As temperatures approach and exceed 100°C in a heated volume, water vapor is formed, and steam collects in small pockets forming vacuoles in tissue. The result is a dessication of tissue, with the presence of small vacuoles throughout.

31.2.1.3 Structural Protein Thermal Coagulation

Structural proteins (collagen, elastin) are found in the extracellular matrix and cytoskeleton of all cells. Upon thermal coagulation, a number of distinct changes occur corresponding to the denaturation of these structural proteins. The semicrystalline network of collagen fibers in tissue is disrupted during coagulation, reduced to an amorphous field of denatured protein. The region of thermal coagulation in most tissues can usually be seen visually as lighter in color, and more opaque. Temperatures above 60°C are usually required to observe coagulation in tissue, and the coagulated volume is often referred to as the *thermal lesion*.

31.2.1.4 Vital Enzyme Denaturation

The denaturation process undergone by functional proteins within cells is similar to that of the structural proteins, but occurs at lower temperatures. These lethal effects occur beyond the visible boundary of the thermal lesion, and can be visualized with various staining techniques.

31.2.1.5 Red Thermal Damage Zone

A red zone appears in tissue peripheral to the coagulation boundary in thermal lesions within 30 sec after heating. This region is characterized by damage to the vasculature, and a number of host physiological responses to heat such as hemorrhage, increased blood flow, and/or hemostasis.

Evaluation of the full extent of thermal damage can be made 1 to 5 days after heating, when all cells undergo cell death. The type of necrosis undergone by cells depends on the initial zone they were located in (structural coagulation, red zone, etc.), and includes effects such as coagulative necrosis, ischemic necrosis, and apoptosis. The extent of thermal necrosis seems to be related to the outer boundary of the red thermal damage zone in tissue.[10]

31.2.2 Dosimetry

The rapid tissue response associated with thermal coagulation therapy has attracted interest from the clinical community as a minimally invasive means to treat localized tumors in tissue. However, accurate delivery of this therapy is predicated on quantitative dosimetry. It is critical to understand the cytotoxic effect of temperature on tissue in a quantitative way so that thermal therapies can be associated with a predictable and repeatable therapeutic response. Two descriptions of thermal damage are used currently: thermal dose and a critical temperature threshold. Both descriptions require knowledge of the temperature distribution over time in a target volume. This has been a long-standing limitation of dosimetry in thermal therapy due to the technological limitations of thermometry. Most dosimetry was based on a few point measurements of temperature from embedded thermocouples around the target region. With the advent of noninvasive thermometry, however, the ability to monitor and control thermal treatments and to implement feedback in delivery is possible. Furthermore, the increase in temperature information in the treatment volume enables the refinement of damage predictions. The relationship between thermal dose, temperature, and the different levels of thermal damage is shown conceptually in Figure 31.1.

31.2.2.1 Thermal Dose

In the realm of hyperthermia, both temperature and time are important variables determining cell death. A number of models have been proposed to relate these two parameters into a combined dose based on the logarithmic relationship between temperature and time for an equivalent cytotoxic effect. It has been observed from temperatures ranging from 43 to 57°C that for an increase in temperature by 1°C the time required to achieve a particular level of cell death could be reduced by approximately one half.[11] This type of observation has led to the formulation of a dose model based on empirical observations and thermodynamic assumptions. The model allows for the calculation of equivalent dose at a reference temperature, arbitrarily chosen as 43°C, and is given by:

$$EQ43 = \sum_{t=0}^{t=final} R^{(43-\bar{T})} \Delta t \qquad (31.1)$$

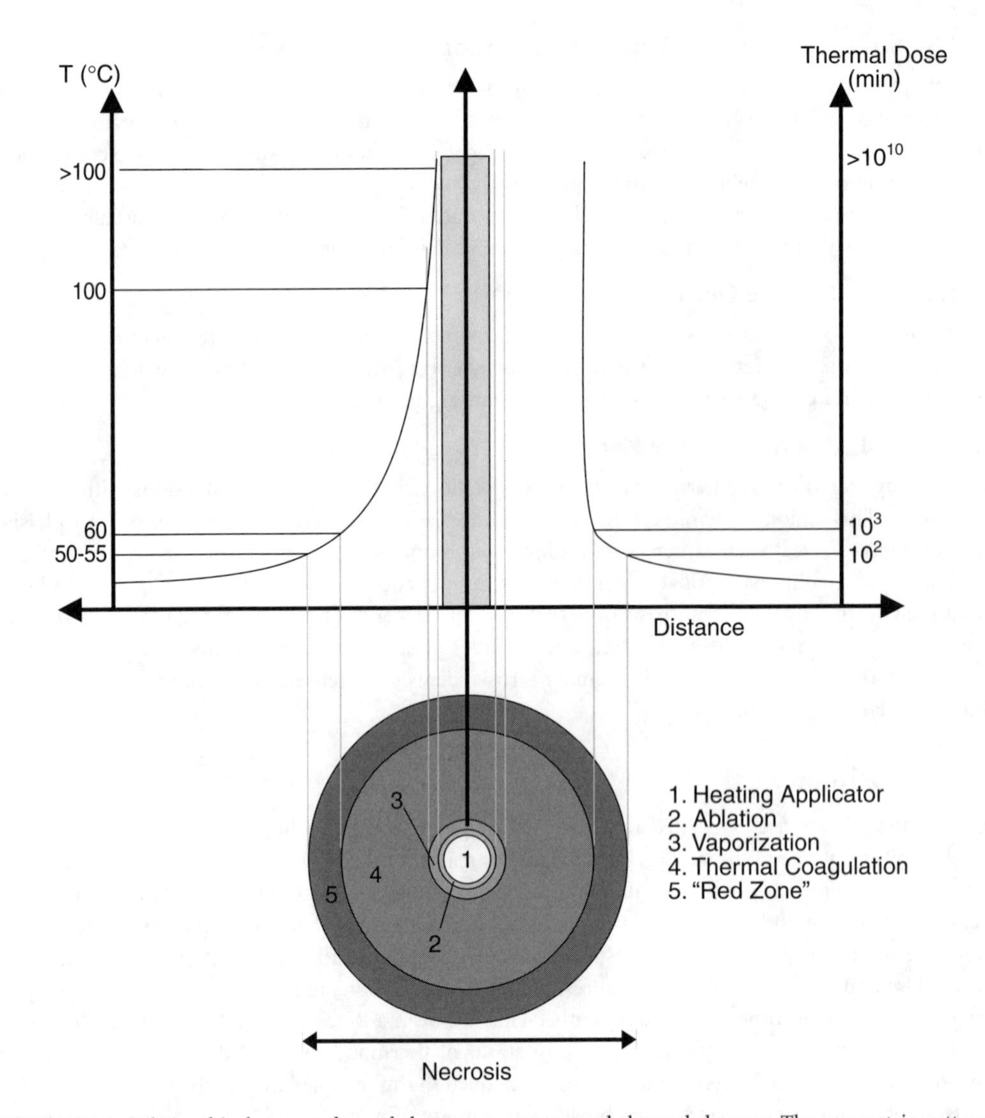

FIGURE 31.1 Relationship between thermal dose, temperature, and thermal damage. The concentric pattern of thermal damage depicted is typical of the thermal lesions produced by interstitial heating applicators. Due to the nature of the thermal dose equation, short exposures at temperatures greater than about 60°C result in very large thermal dose. All of the regions of thermal damage shown in the figure eventually result in necrosed tissue. The extent of the region of thermal coagulation is commonly referred to as the thermal lesion.

where R is a constant equal to 0.25 below 43°C and 0.5 above 43°C, $\overline{T}$ is the average temperature during time Δt, and $EQ43$ is the number of minutes at 43°C required to achieve the equivalent cell kill. This formulation allows many different types of temperature treatment regiments to be standardized into a single unit and compared in terms of cell death. Further corrections have been proposed to account for deviations between observations and predictions below 42.5°C due to the phenomenon of thermotolerance.[11]

31.2.2 Critical Temperature

The thermal dose equation (31.1) has been applied to predict the region of thermal coagulation in high temperature thermal therapy, with the conclusion that about 240 equivalent minutes at 43°C are required to produce a cell survival of 0.01%.[9] Equivalent cell kill can be achieved at 55°C for an exposure time of approximately 5 sec. Above these temperatures, the time required to produce equivalent cell death quickly falls below 1 sec, and measurement or verification of these effects becomes difficult. In thermal coagulation therapy, where exposure times are on the order of minutes and temperature gradients are steep, a number of studies have concluded that the selection of a threshold temperature to describe thermal damage is a sufficient description both *in vitro* and *in vivo*.[6–8] In terms of physical significance, the mechanism of cell death at temperatures above 55°C is of a different nature, relating to the thermal coagulation of proteins,[10] as discussed in Section 31.2.

31.2.3 Heat Conduction

The heating patterns generated in tissue during thermal therapy are influenced by a number of processes including heat conduction, the removal of heat by blood flow, and the deposition of energy from heating applicators. Depending on the nature of the thermal therapy and the anatomy being heated, these processes can have varying influence on the resulting temperature distribution.

Heat conduction depends on the temperature gradients within the heated region and the thermal conductivity of the material, and tends to transport heat to regions of lower temperature. Blood flow tends to remove heat from tissue at a rate that is dependent on the density, size, and flow rate of the vessels, as well as the temperature of the tissue. The elevation of temperatures during heating is determined by the rate of energy deposition from a heating applicator. These effects have been described by Pennes[12] in the Bioheat Transfer Equation (BHTE) given by

$$k\nabla^2 T(r,t) + Q(r,t) - w_b c_b [T(r,t) - T_b(r,t)] = \rho_t c_t \frac{\partial T(r,t)}{\partial t} \tag{31.2}$$

where k is the thermal conductivity of tissue (W/m°C), T(r,t) is the temperature, T_b is the temperature of blood, Q(r,t) is the power deposited by an energy source (W/m^3), w_b is the blood perfusion (kg/m^3·s), c_b is the specific heat capacity of blood (J/kg°C), c_t is the specific heat of tissue, and ρ_t is the density of tissue (kg/m^3). The first term on the left hand side describes the process of heat conduction, and energy deposition is described by the second term. The third term, representing blood perfusion, is an approximation to the actual interaction between tissue and blood, but has been found to be a suitable approximation in the absence of large blood vessels.[5] More sophisticated models based on the actual spatial arrangement of blood vessels have been proposed.[13–15]

The influence of heat loss due to blood flow has a major impact on the outcome of a thermal therapy.[16] For temperature elevations of a few degrees, the vascular network can regulate temperature by increasing the amount of blood flowing through the heated volume. This increase in blood flow can be spatially variable and temperature dependent resulting in the need to compensate the spatial power deposition from heating devices in order to maintain a uniformly heated volume of tissue.[17] This effect has been a major issue for hyperthermia, and places strong emphasis on the ability to measure dynamic temperature distributions during heating for power compensation. If temperatures are increased above the threshold for thermal coagulation, the vessels in the coagulated region are destroyed and flow ceases. This shutting down of flow in coagulated tissue can result in faster rates of heating due to the lack of removal of energy, and must be taken into account to avoid tissue vaporization or ablation.

Another important effect of blood flow related to thermal coagulation therapy is the removal of unwanted heat from normal tissues. In some thermal coagulation therapies, a slight build-up of energy occurs in normal tissues. To avoid thermal damage in these normal tissues, a delay is applied to enable the tissue to return to body temperature through the effects of conduction and blood flow. In these cases a higher value of blood flow can reduce the wait time required.

The role for modeling heat transport in tissues is important for treatment planning in thermal therapies.[18] Knowledge of the effect of blood flow helps predict the power distribution required to achieve a desired temperature distribution.

31.3 Image-Guided Thermal Therapy

Visualization during conventional surgery is incomplete. Anatomical surfaces are exposed visually, but information about surrounding structures, functional information, or tissue characteristics is limited. The result of these limitations is that the localization of targets can be inaccurate, and larger surgical exposures are necessary.[19] Intraoperative imaging can provide information about tissue morphology and function to a surgeon during a procedure, which can potentially reduce invasiveness and improve localization. The introduction of intra-operative imaging information has changed the face of surgery, offering the potential to improve outcomes, reduce uncertainty, and lower morbidity.[20]

Beyond serving as a passive tool offering additional information during surgery, imaging technology can be directly integrated into surgical procedures, guiding the decisions and actions of the surgeon, or in some cases offering novel treatment strategies for procedures. This combination of interventions and imaging technology is known as *image-guided therapy.*

The following subsections describe the various roles for image guidance in thermal coagulation therapy, with special reference to minimally invasive procedures such as interstitial thermal therapy, and image-guidance with magnetic resonance imaging (MRI).

31.3.1 Device Placement

Essential to any image-guided procedure is the ability to visualize a therapeutic device relative to the surrounding anatomy. This capability is met by a wide range of medical imaging technology including ultrasound, magnetic resonance imaging, CT, and x-ray fluoroscopy. In the case of interstitial thermal therapy, correct placement is important to ensure that the boundary of a target volume is within the radial extent of the thermal lesion produced by the applicator.

An important issue when considering image-guided minimally invasive procedures such as interstitial thermal therapy is the compatibility of the interventional device with the imaging technology. Incorrectly chosen materials can interfere with the imaging technology and produce artifacts that reduce the ability to localize the device, or can be undetectable due to a lack of contrast between the device and surrounding tissue.

MRI has the capability to image in multiple planes or three-dimensional which assists in the localization of devices for interventional procedures. Images can also be acquired rapidly (<1 sec) to provide updates of device position during localization. An example of the utility of MRI for device placement is depicted in Figure 31.2, where an interstitial laser fiber was located within a colorectal metastasis in the liver under MR guidance. Most interventional devices are easily distinguished from surrounding tissue in MR

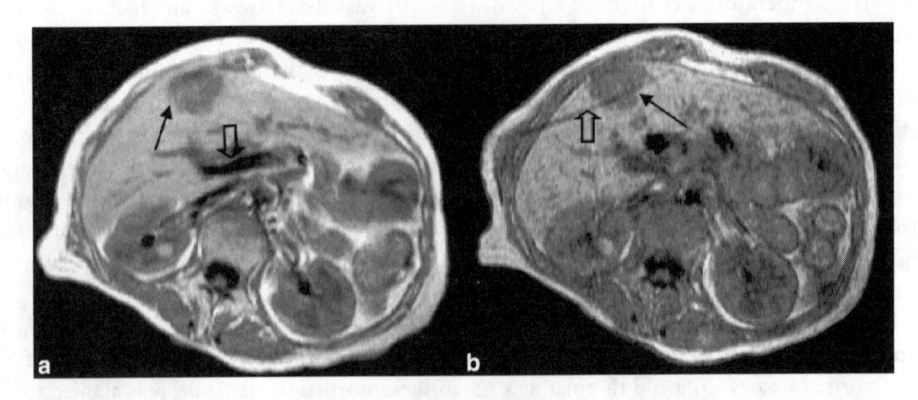

FIGURE 31.2 MRI guidance of an interstitial laser heating applicator for thermal therapy. (a) Axial T_1-weighted image. A catheter, visualized by its susceptibility artifact, has been located in the hepatic artery (open arrow) to occlude blood flow during heating. A subcapsular colorectal metastasis (closed arrow) can also be seen in the image. (b) Axial T_1-weighted image obtained prior to heat delivery shows a laser heating applicator (open arrow) positioned in the lateral third of the metastasis (arrow). (From Wacker, F.K. et al., *J. Magn. Reson. Imaging*, 13, 31, 2001. With permission.)

images, showing up as a signal void due to the absence of water. Incorrectly chosen materials, such as some surgical-grade stainless steel, can present artifacts 5 to 10 times larger than the actual size of the device itself, rendering accurate MRI guidance and localization impossible. Careful selection of materials with a magnetic susceptibility close to that of water is required in order to avoid imaging artifacts that could preclude the use of a device for MRI-guided interventions.[21] The list of available materials is limited to ceramics, plastics, and a few metals, making the design of MRI-compatible equipment and hardware a challenge.

31.3.2 Thermometry

The rate of energy deposition in thermal coagulation therapy is high, and destruction happens within seconds. In addition, all tissues exposed to temperatures sufficient for thermal coagulation are destroyed. A critical component of thermal therapy, therefore, is the monitoring of energy delivery during heating to observe the growth of the thermal lesion, and to reduce damage to normal tissue. This can be accomplished through measurement of the temperature distribution in the target volume during heat delivery.

The requirements of thermometry for thermal coagulation therapy are related to the method of heat application, which can result in large differences in the rate of heating and spatial variation of temperatures. However, general guidelines for the clinical requirements of thermometry techniques are a temperature resolution of about 1°C, a spatial resolution of less than 1 cm, and a temporal resolution of a few seconds.[22]

Traditionally, temperature measurements were performed in the application of hyperthermia through discrete measurements with implanted thermocouples during heating. This form of thermometry results in very high temporal resolution and temperature sensitivity at each of the implanted thermocouples, but suffers from the limited spatial resolution. The entire temperature distribution is usually calculated through interpolation of the point temperature measurements. Errors in the calculated temperature distribution can arise due to the variations caused by blood flow. Increased accuracy can be obtained through the implantation of more thermocouples which undesirably increases the invasiveness of the thermal therapy. However, thermocouples are still used in situations where the temperature at a particular point is required for tissue protection (monitoring the rectal temperature during prostate heating) or in situations where calibration of noninvasive temperature measurements is desired.

Several noninvasive thermometric techniques have been proposed over the past two decades using various imaging modalities including x-ray computed tomography,[23] microwave radiation,[24] ultrasound,[25] and magnetic resonance imaging (MRI).[26] Of these techniques, ultrasound and MR thermometry have seen the furthest development. Ultrasound thermometry is often based on the measurement of time shifts in the RF echo signal.[27] These shifts can be due to temperature-dependent changes in the speed of sound or thermal expansion of the tissue itself.[28] This technique offers very good sensitivity to changes in temperature (0.2°C); however, quantitative application requires knowledge of tissue properties *a priori* and is sensitive to tissue deformation and bulk motion.[29]

The temperature sensitivity of MRI makes it a versatile tool for monitoring the temperature distribution in tissue noninvasively during thermal therapy. Several MR parameters are temperature sensitive including T1,[26] T2,[30] the diffusion coefficient,[31] equilibrium magnetization,[32] and the proton-resonance frequency (PRF).[33] Of these effects, the PRF has seen the most development as a technique for noninvasive MR thermometry due to its linearity with temperature and lack of dependence on tissue type and thermal status.[34] Using this technique at 1.5 Tesla, temperature information can be obtained with millimeter spatial resolution and approximately ± 1°C accuracy in a reasonable imaging time (few seconds), thus meeting the requirements for thermal therapy. Practical implementations of this technique usually measure relative changes in temperature compared to a reference image acquired prior to heating. An example of temperature measurements using the PRF is shown in Figure 31.3. In this experiment, the temperature distribution transverse to an interstitial ultrasound applicator was measured during heating, depicting the shape of the heating pattern. PRF thermometry is sensitive to bulk motion of the object, so care must be taken to

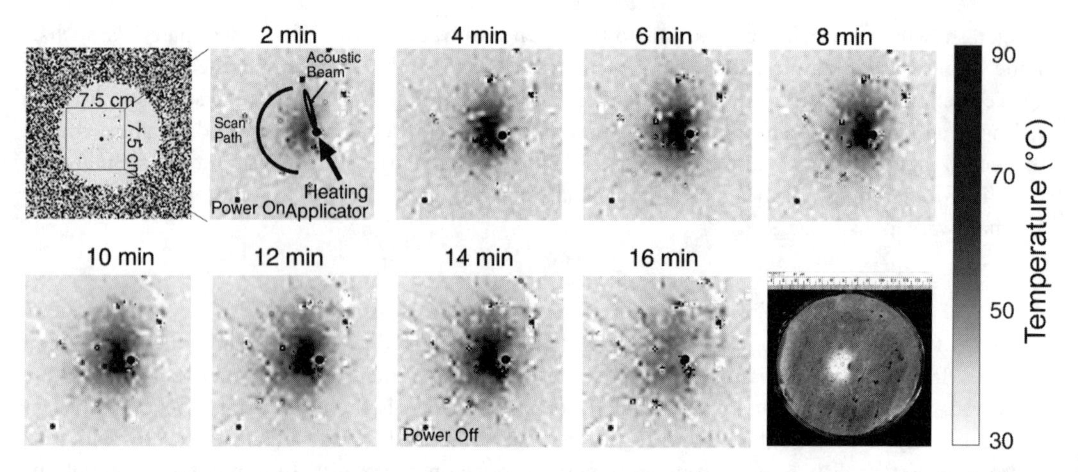

FIGURE 31.3 MR-derived temperature maps during scanned heating with an interstitial ultrasound applicator delivering 7 W of acoustic power, and rotating between 0 and 180°. The location of the heating applicator and the approximate shape of the acoustic beam are superimposed on the second panel. The grayscale is calibrated to temperature. The bottom right panel shows the shape of the thermal lesion generated. (From Chopra, R. et al., *Phys. Med. Biol.*, 46, 3133, 2001. With permission.)

maintain the heated region stationary during a treatment. Spectroscopic imaging techniques are under development to remove the errors associated with phase subtraction for thermometry.[35]

The main difficulties with MR thermometry include the integration of heat delivery technology with standard MRI systems due to the high magnetic fields, and need for non-ferromagnetic equipment. In addition, the PRF shift technique is sensitive to changes in the tissue susceptibility which can arise when interventional devices are placed within the heated region.[36,37] Nonetheless, the ability to measure dynamic temperature distributions noninvasively during thermal therapy makes accurate dosimetry and damage predictions possible.

31.3.3 Assessment of Thermal Damage

The effects of thermal coagulation are immediate, and within a few minutes processes such as tissue swelling and cellular destruction are visible. This feature of thermal therapy is a benefit; the immediate outcome of a treatment can be assessed and, if necessary, certain areas can be reheated to ensure complete coagulation of the targeted volume. Temperature measurements can indicate the size and geometry of the thermal damage region, but a direct imaging method capable of distinguishing the thermal lesion from viable tissue is desirable. A number of imaging modalities have been shown capable of indicating the extent and severity of thermal damage during thermal therapy.

One approach employed to measure thermal damage is the measurement of changes in the vasculature after thermal therapy. The basic idea is that in coagulated tissue, blood flow ceases[9] and the dynamics of contrast enhancement in this region is vastly different. Multiple imaging modalities including MRI,[38] CT,[39] and ultrasound[40] have been shown to exhibit differences in contrast dynamics within the heated region.

Another approach has been to optimize imaging sequences to exploit differences in tissue parameters upon thermal coagulation. Both ultrasound and MRI have been investigated extensively in this area to understand the various changes in tissue parameters with heating.[41–43]

MRI is sensitive to thermal damage, and experiments have shown that most MR parameters, including T1, T2, and the apparent diffusion coefficient (ADC), change upon coagulation.[42,44] Figure 31.4 shows the change in MR signal magnitude with temperature for a range of tissue types. The magnitude and temperature dependence of these changes varies with tissue type, however, the changes are large enough for standard imaging sequences to detect differences between normal and coagulated tissue. Both T1- and T2-weighted imaging sequences are used to detect the varying extent and regions of thermal damage after thermal therapy (Figure 31.5).

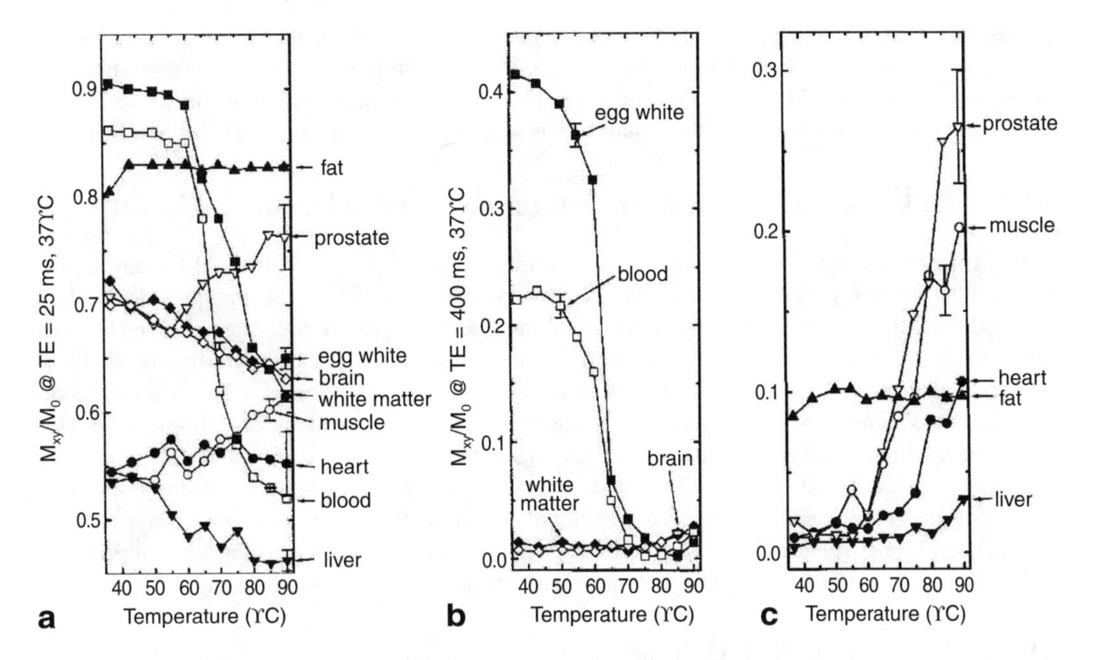

FIGURE 31.4 Plots of normalized T_2-weighted signal at body temperature vs. immersion temperature for a range of tissues and biological materials. (a) Moderate T_2-weighting (TE = 25 ms); (b and c) heavy T_2-weighting (TE = 400 ms). Different relationships are seen among the various tissue types; however, many exhibit rapid changes at temperatures above 60°C. (From Graham, S.J. et al., *Magn. Res. Med.*, 42, 1061, 1999. With permission.)

31.3.4 Summary

Image guidance is essential for the safe and accurate delivery of thermal coagulation therapy. Imaging is required for proper device placement, quantification of the energy delivered, monitoring temperature distributions, and assessing the region of thermal damage. Multiple imaging modalities (MRI, ultrasound, CT) are suitable for one of more of these requirements.

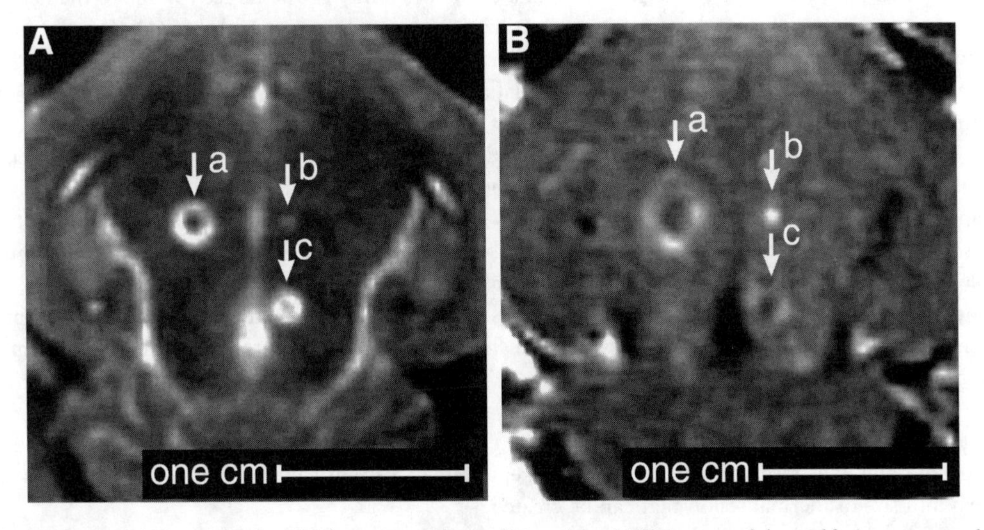

FIGURE 31.5 (A) T_2-weighted and (B) contrast-enhanced T_1-weighted MR images of thermal lesions generated in rabbit brain with a focused ultrasound transducer. Three different power levels were used to create each lesion. In a and c, the thermal lesion consists of a hyperintense rim surrounding a hypointense core. (From Vykhodtseva, N., *Ultrasound Med. Biol.*, 26, 871, 2000. With permission.)

MRI is a promising technology for thermal therapies because of its capability to meet many of the requirements for image-guidance. Current technology offers spatial and temporal resolutions close to clinical needs. The availability of MRI technology for thermal therapy is limited; however, further demonstration of the utility of this technology for image-guided interventions may increase development in this area.[45]

31.4 Delivery Strategies for Image-Guided Thermal Therapy

While the monitoring and assessment tools are an important component of thermal therapy, equally important is the energy source used to deliver heat to a target location. Image guidance provides feedback during thermal therapy enabling the adjustment of heating patterns to ensure adequate treatment; however, this feature is reliant on the capability of delivery technology to control the spatial power deposition in tissue.

The delivery of heat in thermal therapy can be accomplished in three basic ways. External devices can transmit energy through the body to generate heating noninvasively at a target location. Intracavitary devices can be inserted into body cavities such as the esophagus, vagina, and rectum for better access to target volumes otherwise difficult to heat with external energy sources. Finally, interstitial heating involves the delivery of energy from devices inserted directly into or adjacent to the tumor of interest. These techniques are discussed below, with an emphasis on technology for thermal coagulation therapy. The physical principles, heating characteristics, clinical applications, and limitations of each technique are discussed.

31.4.1 Interstitial Heat Delivery

Interstitial heating involves the delivery of energy from devices inserted directly adjacent or into a target volume in tissue. Device placement is achieved by direct penetration through the skin or via body cavities such as the urethra. Heating applicators are usually between 2 and 5 mm in diameter, and are needle or catheter based. Although this technique is invasive, a number of advantages are obtained through the interstitial localization of heating applicators. Devices are located within or adjacent to the target volume of tissue, avoiding the requirement for energy to penetrate through normal tissue. Problems such as skin surface burns, scattering of energy due to intervening tissue layers, or unwanted heating of intervening normal tissue are less prominent in interstitial heating as compared to external heating techniques. The issue of tracking the target volume is greatly simplified because the device moves with the target volume during patient respiration or motion. Finally, due to the proximity of the target volume to the heating applicator, a number of energy sources can be utilized for tissue heating which have short penetration depths, and would be otherwise unsuitable for external heating.

One common limitation with existing interstitial technologies is the lack of control available over the spatial deposition of power. Most heating applicators act approximately as point or line sources of energy, and as a result thermal lesions are usually restricted to spherical or ellipsoidal volumes of tissue. Little adjustment of the heating pattern is possible to account for situations where tumors are not spherical in shape, or the interstitial device is not located exactly at the center of a tumor volume. In anatomy where sensitive normal tissue surrounds a tumor volume, such as the brain or the prostate, this lack of control over the spatial deposition of power can be a critical limitation.

Another characteristic of interstitial technologies is the nature of the temperature distribution produced by heating applicators. The energy deposited in tissue is usually greatest immediately adjacent to the heating applicator resulting in very large temperature increases in this region. It is not uncommon for temperatures capable of ablating, charring, or vaporizing tissue — all of which seriously hamper a treatment — to be generated within a few millimeters of the heating applicator. In order to avoid these effects the power deposited in tissue is usually kept below a certain value, which ultimately limits the maximum size of thermal lesion that can be created.

The following sections briefly describe contemporary interstitial heating technologies for thermal coagulation therapy, from the perspective of their mechanism of operation, heating characteristics, limitations, and areas of application or interest. Table 31.1 serves as a qualitative comparison between the various interstitial heating modalities.

TABLE 31.1 Comparison between Heating Characteristics of Common Interstitial Heating Modalities

	λ	Uniformity of Temperature Distribution	Lesion Size	Control over Spatial Heating Pattern	Comments
RF electrodes	~m	–	++	– –	Limited control over heating pattern Large thermal lesions achieved with cluster or expandable electrodes
Microwave antennae	~cm	–	–	–	Limited control over heating pattern Phased array control possible with multiple antennae Power distribution sensitive to tissue heterogeneities
Laser fibers	~nm	–	–	– –	High absorption can result in tissue vaporization and charring close to applicator Limited control over heating pattern
Ultrasound transducers (cylindrical)	~mm	+ –	+	+	Require acoustic window for application Can be sectored to deliver energy directionally Transducer requires cooling
Ultrasound transducers (planar)	~mm	+	++	++	Collimated beam results in rapid heating of localized volume Requires device rotation to cover large volume Transducer requires cooling Require acoustic window for application

++ = excellent, + = good, + – = average, – = poor, – – = very poor

31.4.1.1 RF Electrodes

Interstitial RF heating is typically performed between 0.3 and 30 MHz. Below about 100 kHz, undesirable stimulation of nerve and muscle fibers occurs, and above 30 MHz resistive heating is no longer the main mechanism of action. The primary mechanism of absorption of electromagnetic energy in tissue in this frequency range is resistive loss from conduction currents.[46] The absorbed power density (SAR, units W/kg) for an electromagnetic wave in a dissipative medium is given by,

$$SAR = \frac{1}{2}\frac{\sigma}{\rho}|\mathbf{E}|^2 \tag{31.3}$$

where σ is the electrical conductivity (S/m), ρ is the density of tissue (kg/m^3), and **E** is the electric field. The SAR drops away rapidly with distance from the heating applicator, thus the primary mechanism for temperature elevation in a target volume is heat conduction. At the lower end of this frequency range (~500 kHz) electrodes are in direct contact with tissue, while at the upper end (~27 MHz) the coupling between the tissue and electrode is capacitive. All techniques require a ground return for current, either implanted in tissue or attached to the skin surface. The large wavelengths associated with RF energy in this frequency range precludes the ability to focus energy to particular locations in tissue.

The conductivity of tissue depends on temperature, frequency, and water content.[47] Electrical current tends to avoid regions with low water content due to a low conductivity. Tissue dessication, which occurs as temperatures approach the vaporization threshold, can result in a decrease in tissue conductivity in the region surrounding the applicator, which in turn adversely affects the penetration of RF energy into tissue. Attempts to increase tissue conductivity with direct saline injection during heating[48] have been implemented. Reduction of tissue temperature adjacent to the applicator through the use of perfusate-cooled electrodes has also been investigated[49] as a means to avoid excessive tissue dessication. Another approach to increase SAR distribution has been to use multiple clusters of RF electrodes[50] or electrodes with expandable electrodes.[51]

Interstitial thermal therapy with RF electrodes has been applied for a variety of neoplasms including primary and metastatic liver tumors, renal cell carcinomas, and breast tumors, reviewed by Gazelle et al.[52] The primary advantage of this technique is the small size of applicators, and the ability to generate thermal lesions with diameters between 3 and 4 cm *in vivo* through the use of expandable electrodes. The technique has seen the furthest development, and arguably the greatest interest for the treatment of isolated primary and secondary liver tumors. Studies investigating the long term survival of patients with unresectable liver tumors who were treated with interstitial RF thermal therapy demonstrated the ability to coagulate tumors with a local recurrence rate of only 2% in 169 treated tumors.[53] Recent long-term studies of over 100 patients undergoing interstitial treatment of colorectal carcinoma metastases in the liver with RF heating applicators have demonstrated survival curves comparable to surgical treatments of similar populations.[54] The main challenge with the application of RF thermal therapy is the strong influence of blood flow on the shape of the generated thermal lesion, witnessed in recent trials for the treatment of renal cell carcinomas.[55]

31.4.1.2 Microwave Antennae

Interstitial microwave applicators typically operate between 300 and 2450 MHz, where the predominant mode of propagation for electromagnetic waves is radiative. Commonly used frequencies of operation are 433, 915, and 2450 MHz with respective wavelengths in muscle tissue of 10, 4.5, and 1.7 cm. These frequencies are based on the permitted ISM (Industrial, Scientific, and Medical) radio frequency transmission bands in Europe and the United States. Tissue absorption in this frequency range occurs primarily due to dielectric losses, and the absorbed power (SAR) is given by the same relationship as in Equation 8.3.[56] Unlike RF energy, the short wavelength at microwave frequencies enables using phased applicators to focus energy within a target volume. However, the main challenges with microwaves are the limited depth of penetration (2 to 3 cm) and the strong reflections at soft tissue interfaces.

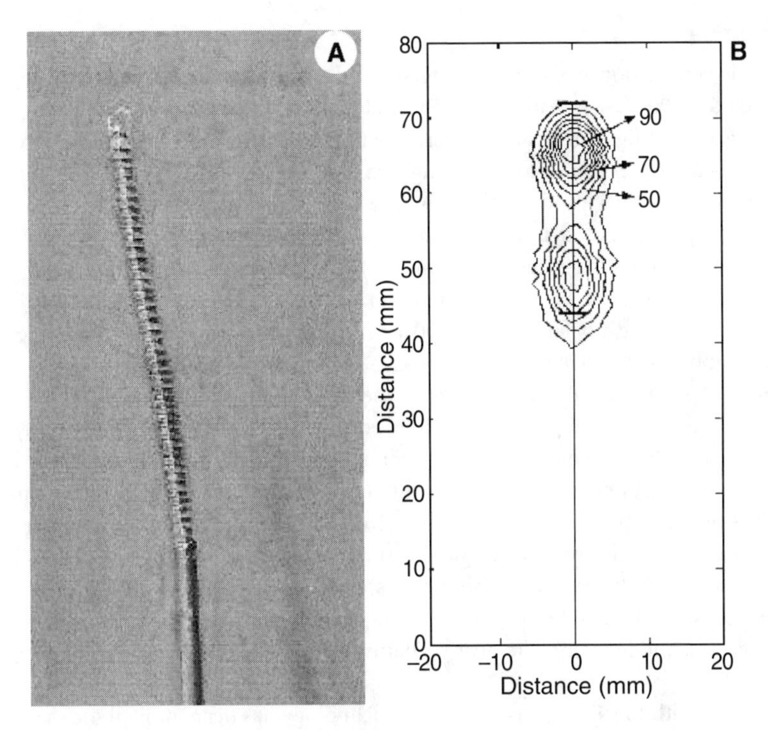

FIGURE 31.6 (A) Helical radiating tip microwave antenna with 3-cm active element and 1.5 mm outer diameter. This device was use in thermal therapy for prostate cancer. (B) SAR contour plot produced by infrared thermography shows the expected pattern of heating. (From Sherar, M.D. et al., *J. Urol.*, 166, 1707, 2001. With permission.)

A number of designs exist for interstitial microwave antennae. The simplest design is called the dipole antenna and consists of a length of semirigid coaxial cable with a section of the outer conductor removed near the end of the cable. The maximum SAR, and consequently heating occurs at the location of this junction point, and drops off on either side.[57] There is a portion of the cable near the tip that does not contribute to heating, making the insertion of the antenna past the target volume necessary. Finally, the SAR pattern is dependent on the insertion depth of the applicator. One feature of this design is that multiple antennae can be phased to produce a maximum power deposition at the geometric center for heating of larger volumes.[58]

A more recent design is the helical coil antenna which consists of a coil of wire wrapped around the exposed inner conductor in the coaxial cable.[59] This design produces an approximately cylindrical heating pattern in the immediate vicinity of the device. The heating pattern produced by this design is not dependent on insertion depth, and has an increased penetration depth compared to that of the simple dipole antenna.[56] Figure 31.6 shows the measured SAR pattern from a helical coil antenna.

The clinical use of interstitial microwave antennae is under investigation with trials underway for the treatment of prostate cancer[60] and hepatocellular carcinoma.[61] Earlier studies have investigated the benefit of interstitial microwave hyperthermia plus radiotherapy for the treatment of glioblastoma multiforme.[62] For the treatment of prostate cancer, multiple antennae are inserted percutaneously into the prostate gland under ultrasound guidance.[60] Results from these studies indicate that temperatures capable of thermal coagulation can be achieved at the within the prostate gland without thermal damage to the rectal wall and urethra. Comparative studies for thermal therapy of hepatic neoplasms indicate that microwave antennae are suitable for thermal therapy of liver tumors; however, the size of thermal lesion produced by these applicators results in the need for multiple insertions, as compared with RF heating.[63] Some of the difficulties associated with the application of microwave heating include sensitivity of the power distribution to tissue heterogeneities, as well as heating of the proximal feed line to the antenna.[64]

31.4.1.3 Laser Fibers

The most common application of lasers for interstitial thermal therapy (LITT) is through the use of infrared light (800 to 1300 nm) transmitted via optical fiber into tissue, first demonstrated by Bown in 1983.[65] The propagation of light in tissue is determined by the scattering and absorption characteristics of tissue. Commonly used lasers used to produce light in this range are the Nd-YAG (Neodymium yttrium aluminium garnet) laser which produces light with a wavelength of 1064 nm, and diode lasers. The optical penetration depth of light, defined as the depth where the percent of collimated light transmitted into tissue is reduced to 37%,[66] reaches a maximum of 7.46 mm in liver tissue between 800 and 1100 nm,[67] justifying the use of these laser wavelengths for interstitial heating. The optical fibers used to transmit light into tissue are no larger then 600 μm in diameter; thus, laser fibers are the smallest interstitial heating applicators currently in use.

A major limitation with laser fibers is the size of thermal lesion that can be generated from a single fiber. Upon tissue coagulation the penetration depth of light decreases by approximately 50% due to a large increase in optical scattering,[67,68] further reducing the optical penetration depth of light. Very high temperatures, capable of charring tissue, are often generated next to the fiber, dropping off rapidly with distance. Thermal conduction plays the major role in the growth of heating patterns due to the rapid drop in absorbed power from the applicator surface. In order to treat clinically relevant tumor volumes, the insertion of multiple fibers is often necessary. Alternative designs of interstitial laser fibers have been investigated to distribute light across a larger area compared with a bare fiber, including diffuser tips, reflectors, and lenses.[69] The heating patterns produced by these various designs is shown in Figure 31.7.

Clinical experience with LITT is growing, and the technology has been applied for the treatment of a number of cancers including isolated hepatic metastases,[70] nasopharyngeal tumors,[71] and breast carcinomas.[72] One of the advantages of LITT is that the light energy does not interfere with most imaging

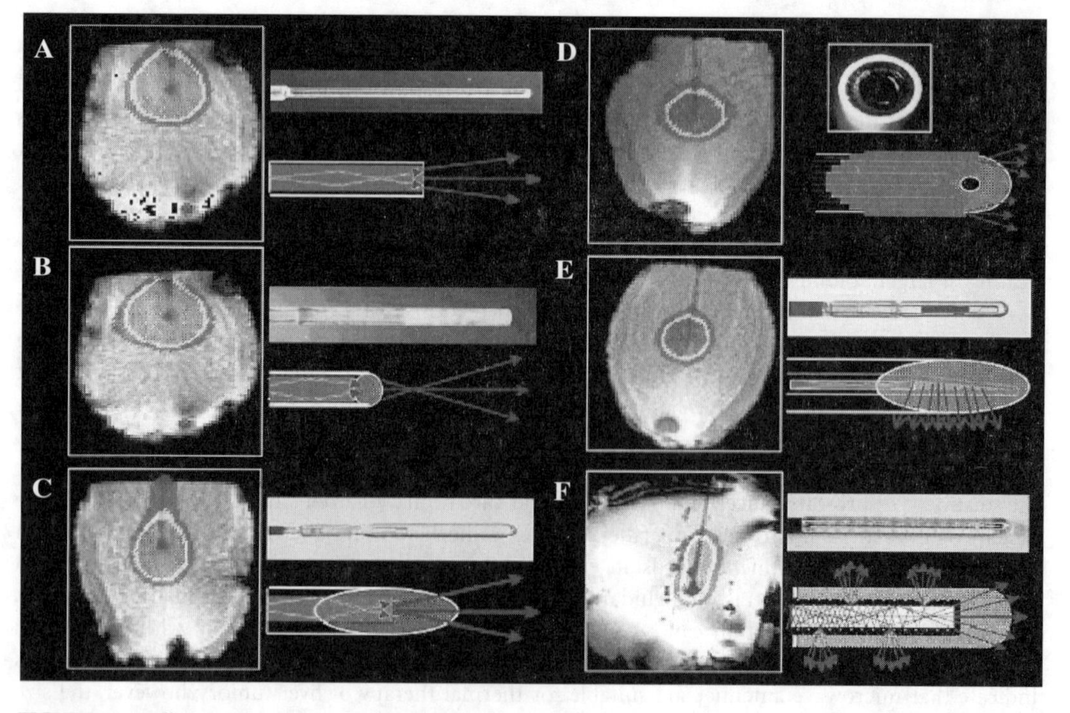

FIGURE 31.7 Illustration, photograph, and heating pattern (measured with MRI) in six different laser fiber configurations. (A) Bare end fiber system; (B) microlens fiber system; (C) microcapsule fiber system; (D) multifiber system; (E) side-firing fiber system; (F) diffuse-projection fiber system. (From Atsumi, H. et al., *Lasers Surg. Med.*, 29, 108, 2001. With permission.)

modalities such as ultrasound or MRI, and integrating these technologies for monitoring and evaluation is a relatively simple task.[73]

31.4.1.4 Ultrasound Transducers

Ultrasound is one of the more recent additions to the list of interstitial technologies, with the first investigations into the feasibility of producing sufficient ultrasound power for interstitial hyperthermia by Hynynen et al.[74] The mechanism of heating for these devices is similar to other ultrasound therapy devices, dependent on the absorption characteristics of tissue and transducer geometry. The frequency range of interstitial ultrasound transducers is typically between 4 and 10 MHz, higher than externally focused transducers for ultrasound therapy due to the proximity of the target region to the transducer. The absorbed power (W/mm^3) in tissue from an ultrasound beam is given by,

$$SAR = \frac{\alpha p_o^2}{\rho c}$$

where α is the absorption coefficient in tissue (Np/m), ρ is the density of tissue (kg/m^3), c is the speed of sound in tissue (m/sec), and p_o is the pressure amplitude at a given point (N/m^2). This expression is valid for any continuous sound field propagating in a medium with zero shear viscosity.[75]

The absorption of ultrasound is primarily due to the macromolecular components of tissue, with a small contribution due to higher order structural organization.[76] With respect to macromolecular contribution, the most important biological molecules appear to be proteins. Tissues high in protein content such collagen (tendon, skin) display the highest values of ultrasonic absorption in the MHz range.[77] The absorption of ultrasound in tissues increases with frequency, and can be described by the relationship,

$$\alpha = \alpha_o f^n$$

where α_o is the absorption of ultrasound at 1 MHz, f is the ultrasound frequency in MHz, and n is the exponent of the frequency dependence. The value of n ranges from 1 to 1.3 for most soft tissues.

The most commonly used design for interstitial ultrasound heat delivery is a multielement array of tubular piezoceramic transducers.[78] These applicators are designed for insertion into standard brachytherapy catheters, or for direct contact with tissue. The tubular transducers produce a cylindrically symmetrical ultrasound wave that propagates into tissue to generate heating, shown in Figure 31.8. This design offers individual control to each transducer element to adjust heating along the axis of the interstitial applicator,[79] and sectored transducers to enable angular directivity of heating.[80]

A more recent design for interstitial ultrasound devices incorporates planar transducers[81–83] with collimated acoustic beams. The absorbed power from a planar transducer is described by,

$$Q \propto e^{-2\mu r}$$

where r is the distance from the surface of the applicator and μ is the ultrasound attenuation coefficient. This expression shows that the main source of power loss is due to the attenuation of ultrasound for this geometry. This design has been shown to generate rapid temperature increases in tissue for the generation of isolated thermal lesions.[82] Theoretical work has investigated the potential for reduced treatment times using this transducer geometry compared to the more conventional cylindrical transducer.[84]

The control over power deposition offered with ultrasound transducers has brought about the potential to adjust the shape of the heating pattern to match the tumor volume, termed *conformal thermal therapy*. The goal of conformal thermal therapy is to deliver sufficient energy to coagulate an entire target volume while reducing the amount of heat delivered to surrounding normal tissues. Control over the three-dimensional shape of the heating pattern can be achieved with interstitial ultrasound devices through the use of multielement configurations[78] (for control along the axis of the device), sectored[80] or planar elements[82] (for angular control), and multifrequency transducers (for control over radial depth of

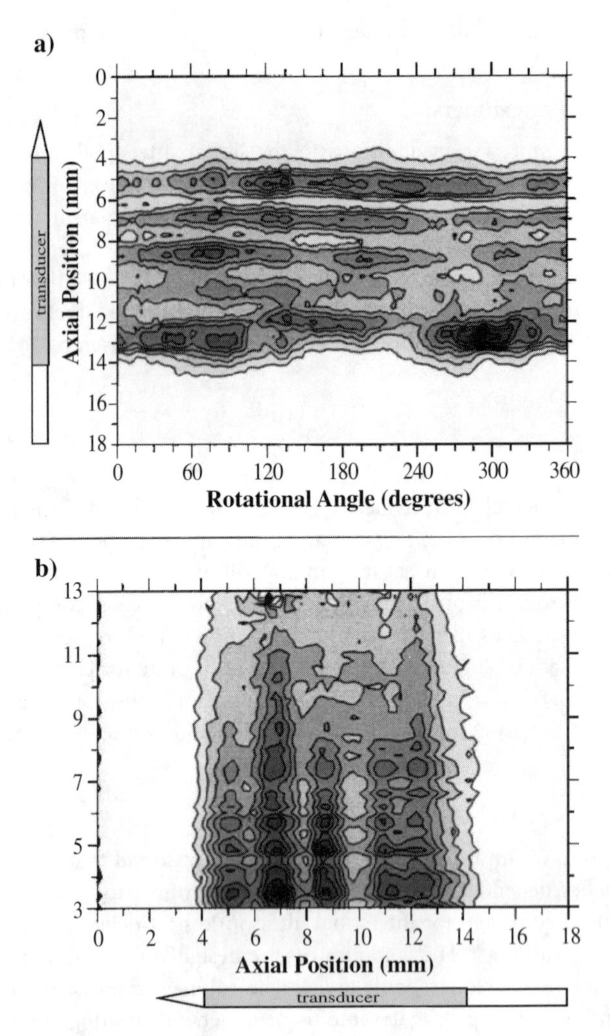

FIGURE 31.8 Acoustic intensity distributions of interstitial US applicator incorporating a 10-mm-long cylindrical transducer (iso-contours at intervals of 10% maximum intensity). (a) Rotational scan around transducer at a radial depth of 8 mm; (b) axial scan along transducer at radial depths of 3 to 13 mm. (The relative position of the US transducer is also shown.) (From Deardorff, D.L. et al., *Med. Phys.*, 28, 104, 2001. With permission.)

heating).[85] Examples of the capability to generate thermal lesions with arbitrary geometry using an interstitial heating applicator with multifrequency planar transducer are shown in Figure 31.9. Important to performing conformal thermal therapy successfully is the incorporation of image guidance into the procedure to provide feedback for continuous monitoring and adjustment of the heating pattern.

The clinical application of interstitial ultrasound heating has been primarily limited to preclinical animal experimentation. Areas of interest are prostate thermal therapy,[78] billiary cancer,[84,86] and cardiac ablation.[81] The major limitation with ultrasound transducers for interstitial heating is the necessity to implement some form of cooling to remove thermal losses in the transducer. In addition, an acoustic window free of air or bone is required in order to heat a volume successfully.

31.4.2 Intracavitary Thermal Therapy

Intracavitary heating applicators are used in situations where a target tumor is accessible via body cavities for energy delivery. By placing the energy source closer to the target volume, tumors in regions inaccessible to energy delivery from external heating applicators can be treated. Inserting devices into body cavities

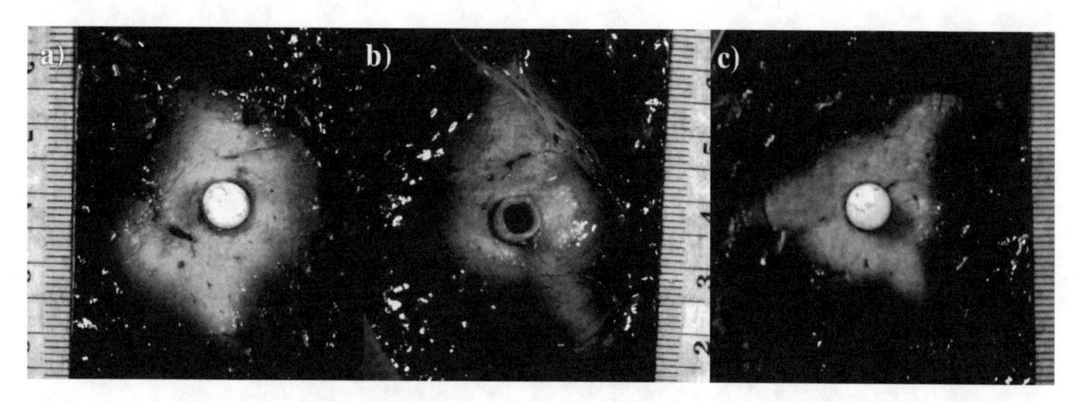

FIGURE 31.9 **(See color insert following page 14-10.)** Examples of conformal thermal therapy with dual-frequency interstitial ultrasound heating applicator. Thermal lesions (shown transverse to the heating applicator) were created by varying the power, frequency, and rate of rotation during heating in excised liver. The ruler scales represent 1-mm increments and the location of the heating applicator is shown by the markers in each panel. Arbitrary thermal lesion geometries are possible with this applicator design.

can also reduce the invasiveness of the procedure relative to interstitial techniques. Commonly used body cavities for intracavitary thermal therapy include the rectum, esophagus, and vagina.

Within this category of heat delivery, a number of energy sources have been applied in the context of hyperthermia including microwave, RF, and ultrasound technology, reviewed by Roos.[87] With respect to temperature coagulation therapy, microwave and ultrasound technology have been developed for intracavitary heating.[88,89] Recent work incorporating MRI guidance with intracavitary ultrasound technology is under development for image-guided thermal coagulation therapy.[90]

31.4.3 Noninvasive Thermal Therapy

The application of noninvasive thermal therapy involves the delivery of energy to a targeted volume of tissue within the body from sources located outside the body. RF, microwave, and ultrasound heating applicators have been applied for both regional and superficial hyperthermia, reviewed by Hand.[91] The unique capability to localize heating to precise volumes of tissue with ultrasound has resulted in its further development for high temperature thermal therapy. Image guidance is a necessity for noninvasive thermal therapies such as high intensity focused ultrasound. In addition to performing thermal dosimetry and evaluation of thermal damage, imaging enables the accurate targeting of energy deposition to the correct region in tissue.

31.4.3.1 MRI-Guided Focused Ultrasound Surgery

MRI-guided focused ultrasound surgery is a technique for the noninvasive treatment of solid tumors[92] that combines the precision of ultrasound power deposition with magnetic resonance imaging for treatment guidance and monitoring. Ultrasound energy is used to destroy a tumor volume without the need for any surgical exposure of the targeted tissue. The entire procedure is performed in an MR imaging environment, providing information to guide, monitor, and evaluate the therapy. The results from this work are encouraging, however, complications that arise due to patient motion, obstructing bone or air, and the sensitivity of intervening tissue have limited the application of this technique to specialized clinical situations.

31.4.3.2 Method of Application

In MRI-guided focused ultrasound therapy, a transducer is located external to the body, coupled to tissue using a water bath or other coupling medium. The transducer produces ultrasound energy which can propagate several centimeters into the body and deposit energy in a well-defined focal volume, shown in Figure 31.10. The ultrasound energy from the transducer is focused to a point within the targeted

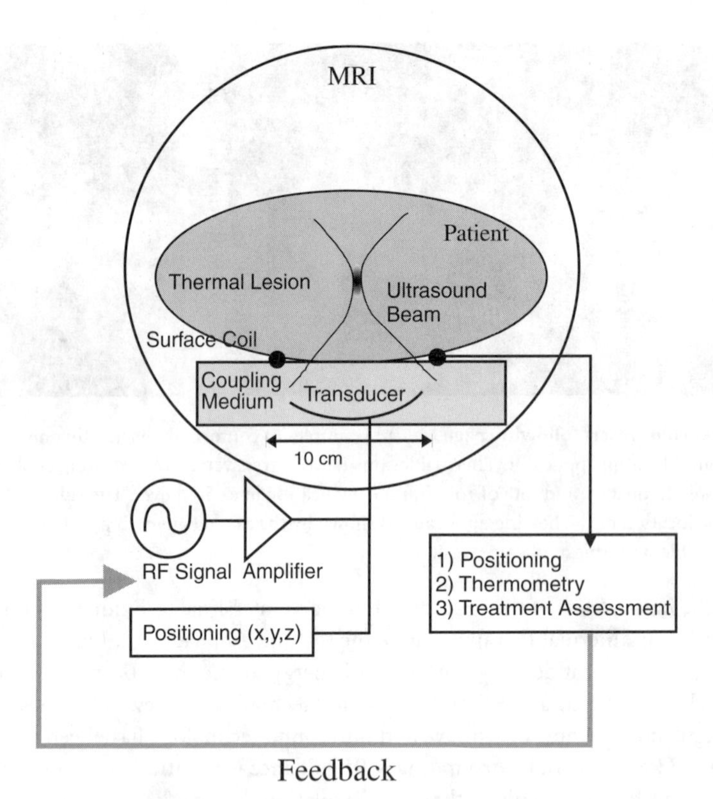

FIGURE 31.10 Concept of MRI-guided focused ultrasound surgery. An ultrasound transducer generates heating at a target location in the patient. MRI is used to target the energy deposition, measure temperature distributions during heating, and assess the thermal lesion generated. This information is used as feedback to adjust the delivery parameters to ensure complete coagulation of the tumor volume.

volume, accomplished with a geometrically focused or phased array transducer. Frequencies between 1 and 2 MHz are used to enable sufficient depth of penetration while maintaining a tight focal volume less than 1 cc.[93] High intensity ultrasound is delivered with the intent of coagulating all tissue within the focal volume of the transducer. Exposure times are approximately 10 sec to achieve thermal coagulation for a spherically focused ultrasound transducer.[6] Following coagulation, the transducer focus is translated to a new location in the tumor volume and the process is repeated until complete coagulation of the tumor is achieved.

MRI is used for monitoring, and guiding the delivery of ultrasound.[94] The location of the ultrasound beam is visualized by depositing a small amount of power resulting in a moderate temperature increase of 3 to 5°C.[95] This change in temperature, localized to the focal volume, can be measured with MR thermometry to reveal the beam location. Based on the knowledge of the size of a thermal lesion created in a single exposure, a number of target locations are prescribed such that successive thermal lesions overlap slightly to create a continuous region of thermal damage.[96] An example of the planning process for treatment of a breast fibroadenoma is shown in Figure 31.11. During heating, MR thermometry is used to monitor the evolution of the temperature generation in tissue, and thermal dosimetry is used to predict the extent of thermal lesion created in a single deposition.[97] After the treatment is complete, the thermal lesion is imaged with MRI to compare with the tumor volume and assess the outcome of the therapy.[98] The appearance of focused ultrasound thermal lesions on MR images is shown in Figure 31.12.

MRI-guided focused ultrasound therapy has been applied for the treatment of localized breast cancer,[99] and high intensity focused ultrasound (HIFU) has been proposed for the treatment of tumors in the bladder,[100] prostate,[101,102] brain,[103] liver, and kidney.[104] Other areas of application for this technique are the treatment of uterine fibroids,[105] glaucoma,[106] the noninvasive removal of fat,[107] and cardiac ablation.[81]

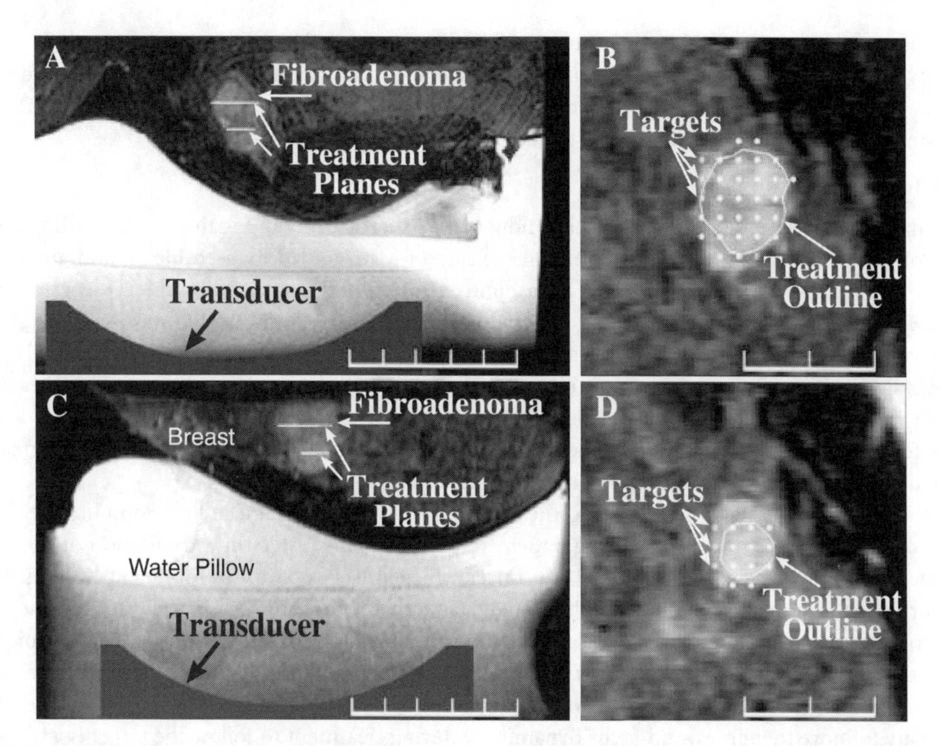

FIGURE 31.11 Treatment planning for MRI-guided focused ultrasound surgery of a breast fiberadenoma. The patient is lying prone with the breast positioned on a water pillow. The imaging sequence used was a fat suppressed T_2-weighted FSE sequence. A and C are transverse sections through the breast showing the tumor, the treatment planes, and the transducer. B and D are coronal sections through the breast showing the prescribed locations for energy deposition from the transducer. (From Hynynen, K. et al., *Radiology*, 219, 176, 2001. With permission.)

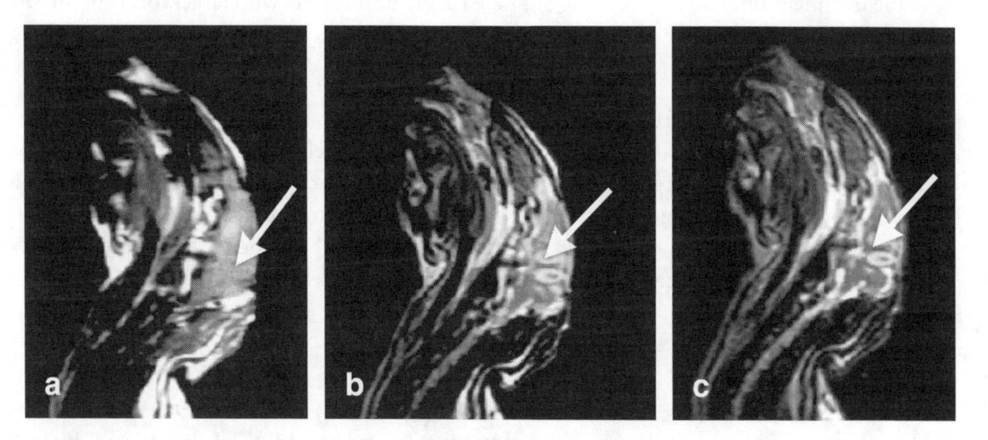

FIGURE 31.12 MR images of thermal lesions created in rabbit brain with a focused ultrasound transducer. (a) T_1-weighted image; (b) T_2-weighted image; (c) FLAIR image. Images were acquired approximately 2 h after delivery. (From Chen, L. et al., *J. Magn. Reson. Imaging*, 10, 146, 1999. With permission.)

Recent results from a number of groups working in the area of high intensity ultrasound thermal therapy have demonstrated that this technique is feasible and that tumors can be coagulated noninvasively.[99,108] Clinical experience with breast tumors has demonstrated that the combination of MRI and ultrasound technology is feasible for the treatment of benign breast fibroadenomas.[99]

31.4.3.3 Limitations

A fundamental requirement for performing noninvasive thermal therapy is the presence of a suitable path for energy to reach the target volume. In the case of MRI-guided focused ultrasound an acoustic window is required. The propagation of ultrasound in soft tissues is affected by the presence of air or bone. The reflection coefficient of these materials is high, and penetration of ultrasound energy to a target volume can be hampered. In the case of bone, reflection and absorption can be problems resulting in excessive heating of the bone-tissue interface.[109] For these reasons, externally focused ultrasound heating is difficult to perform in areas where there may be obstructing bone or air, such as the abdomen, prostate, heart or lungs. In the case of the brain, adjustments to the phase of the ultrasound signal can be made to compensate for the beam disruption due to the skull bone.[110]

Motion of the target volume relative to the ultrasound transducer can also be a complicating factor. Many organs undergo translation during patient respiration. This results in a translation of the target volume relative to the external ultrasound transducer, which must be accounted for during heating. While this correction is not conceptually difficult to understand, there are many technical challenges associated with tracking organ motion. MR thermometry using the proton resonant frequency shift technique is also motion sensitive; thus, large changes in target position preclude the acquisition of reliable temperature information. Some work has been done to correct for motion during thermometry.[111] Furthermore, the ability to move the ultrasound focus dynamically during treatment to follow the target is a technical challenge that has not been tackled to date by any groups. The consequence of target motion is the potential loss of accuracy and control in a thermal treatment.[104]

Finally, the last factor that has limited the application of MRI-guided focused ultrasound is treatment time. Due to the small volume encompassed by the focus of a spherically focused transducer, thermal lesions created in a single insonation are much less than 1 cc. In order to treat a volume with a 3-cm diameter, it would require over 200 lesions to coagulate the complete tumor volume. Fan and Hynynen[112] have looked at this issue in detail and concluded that treatment times greater than 10 h were required to completely coagulate a $3 \times 3 \times 3$ cm^3 tumor volume using a spherically focused transducer. The majority of time is spent waiting for the intervening area to return to body temperature to avoid the buildup of temperatures in normal tissue surrounding the tumor. Considering the fact that MRI is used in conjunction with the ultrasound delivery, treatment times become impractical. Work is being done to reduce the treatment time through the use of phased array transducers with larger focal volumes.[113,114]

31.4.4 Summary

Energy can be delivered to tissue for thermal coagulation therapy through three basic strategies: external, intracavitary, and interstitial heating applicators. Each strategy has characteristics and limitations that make it applicable to particular target volumes within the body. As discussed above, many energy sources can be used to deliver thermal coagulation therapy including RF, microwave, laser, and ultrasound energy. The combination of image-guidance with heat delivery provides feedback for the adjustment of delivery parameters during heating. This capability places requirements on delivery technology for control over the spatial power deposition.

31.5 Conclusions

The field of thermal therapy is evolving rapidly as a deeper understanding of the thermal biology of tissue is obtained, and technology for improved delivery and monitoring of treatments is developed. An increasing number of investigations into the delivery of thermal coagulation therapy have been witnessed in recent years, due to the simple thermal response of tissue at these temperatures, and the large range of temperatures where therapeutic effects are observed (50 to 100°C). The shorter treatment time associated with thermal coagulation therapy is also attractive, especially when compared to conventional hyperthermia.

Imaging technology plays an important role in all aspects of thermal coagulation therapy. The localization of energy deposition to the correct location within a target volume can be achieved with imaging, as well as the capability to monitor the temperature distribution across the heated region. Thermal damage predictions can be made based on the measured temperature distributions, and images of the region of thermal damage can be obtained after the treatment is complete.

MRI has been demonstrated to possess the capability to meet some the clinical needs for monitoring and guiding thermal therapies; however, active investigation into the application of alternative imaging modalities such as ultrasound and CT is ongoing. The potential of imaging technology to provide information for all stages of thermal therapy makes the elimination of surgical exposure of the treatment volume possible. Furthermore, the measurement of the evolution of the spatial heating pattern during treatment provides important information for feedback and active adjustment during heating.

Heat delivery technology for thermal coagulation therapy includes noninvasive, intracavitary, and interstitial heating technologies. Each strategy has various advantages and limitations; however, there is a gradual evolution toward heating technologies that provide the maximum amount of control over the shape of the heating pattern. This development takes full advantage of the information provided by imaging technology as feedback, and enables the adjustment of spatial power distributions to ensure the thermal lesion completely encompasses the tumor volume.

References

1. Engin, K., Biological rationale and clinical experience with hyperthermia, *Control. Clin. Trials*, 17, 316, 1996.
2. Streffer, C., Molecular and cellular mechanisms of hyperthermia, in *Thermoradiotherapy and Thermochemotherapy*, Seegenschmiedt, M.H., Fessenden, P., and Vernon, C.C., Eds., Springer-Verlag, Berlin, 1995.
3. Dewey, W.C. et al., Cell biology of hyperthermia and radiation, in *Radiation Biology in Cancer Research*, Meyn, R.E. and Withers, H.R., Eds., Raven Press, New York, 1980, 589.
4. Moros, E.G., Fan, X., and Straube, W.L., Experimental assessment of power and temperature penetration depth control with a dual frequency ultrasonic system, *Med. Phys.*, 26, 810, 1999.
5. Roemer, R.B., Engineering aspects of hyperthermia therapy, *Annu. Rev. Biomed. Eng.*, 1, 347, 1999.
6. Graham, S.J. et al., Quantifying tissue damage due to focused ultrasound heating observed by MRI, *Magn. Res. Med.*, 41, 321, 1999.
7. Peters, R.D. et al., Magnetic resonance thermometry for predicting thermal damage: an application of interstitial laser coagulation in an in vivo canine prostate model, *Magn. Res. Med.*, 44, 873, 2000.
8. McDannold, N.J. et al., Usefulness of MR imaging-derived thermometry and dosimetry in determining the threshold for tissue damage induced by thermal surgery in rabbits, *Radiology*, 216, 517, 2000.
9. Borrelli, M.J., Time-temperature analysis of cell killing of BHK cells heated at temperatures in the range of 43.5 degrees C to 57.0 degrees C, *Int.J. Radiat. Oncol. Biol. Phys.*, 19, 389, 1990.
10. Thomsen, S., Mapping of thermal injury in biologic tissues using quantitative pathologic techniques, in *Proc. SPIE (Thermal Treatment of Tissue with Image Guidance)*, Ryan, T.P. and Wong, T.Z., Eds., SPIE, San Jose, 1999, 82.
11. Sapareto, S.A. and Dewey, W.C., Thermal dose determination in cancer therapy, *Int. J. Radiat. Oncol. Biol. Phys.*, 10, 787, 1984.
12. Pennes, H.H., Analysis of tissue and arterial blood temperatures in the resting human forearm, *J. Appl. Physiol.*, 1, 93, 1948.

13. Chen, M.M. and Holmes, K.R., Microvascular contributions in tissue heat transfer, *Ann. N. Y. Acad. Sci.*, 335, 137, 1980.
14. Huang, H.W., Chen, Z.P., and Roemer, R.B., A counter current vascular network model of heat transfer in tissues, *J. Biomech. Eng.*, 118, 120, 1996.
15. Kotte, A.N., van Leeuwen, G.M., and Lagendijk, J.J., Modelling the thermal impact of a discrete vessel tree, *Phys. Med. Biol.*, 44, 57, 1999.
16. Kolios, M.C. et al., An investigation of the flow dependence of temperature gradients near large vessels during steady state and transient tissue heating, *Phys. Med. Biol.*, 44, 1479, 1999.
17. Akyurekli, D., Gerig, L.H., and Raaphorst, G.P., Changes in muscle blood flow distribution during hyperthermia, *Int. J. Hyperthermia.*, 13, 481, 1997.
18. Lagendijk, J.J., Hyperthermia treatment planning, *Phys. Med. Biol.*, 45, R61, 2000.
19. Galloway, R.L., The process and development of image-guided procedures, *Annu. Rev. Biomed. Eng.*, 3, 83, 2001.
20. Jolesz, F.A., Image-guided procedures and the operating room of the future, *Radiology*, 204, 601, 1997.
21. Schenck, J.F., The role of magnetic susceptibility in magnetic resonance imaging: MRI magnetic compatibility of the first and second kinds, *Med. Phys.*, 23, 815, 1996.
22. Bolomey, J.C., Le Bihan, D., and Mizushina, S., Recent trends in noninvasive thermal control, in *Thermoradiotherapy and Thermochemotherapy*, Seegenschmiedt, M.H., Fessenden, P., and Vernon, C.C., Eds., Springer, New York, 1995, chap. 16.
23. Fallone, B.G., Moran, P.R., and Podgorsak, E.B., Noninvasive thermometry with a clinical x-ray CT scanner, *Med. Phys.*, 9, 715, 1982.
24. Nguyen, D.D. et al., Simultaneous microwave local heating and microwave thermography. Possible clinical applications, *J. Micro. Power*, 14, 135, 1979.
25. Seip, R. and Ebbini, E., Noninvasive estimation of tissue temperature response to heating fields using diagnostic ultrasound, *IEEE Trans. Biomed. Eng.*, 42, 828, 1995.
26. Parker, D.L. et al., Temperature distribution measurements in two-dimensional NMR imaging, *Med. Phys.*, 10, 321, 1983.
27. Seip, R. and Ebbini, E.S., Noninvasive estimation of tissue temperature response to heating fields using diagnostic ultrasound, *IEEE Trans. Biomed. Eng.*, 42, 828, 1995.
28. Maass-Moreno, R. and Damianou, C.A., Noninvasive temperature estimation in tissue via ultrasound echo-shifts. I. Analytical model, *J. Acoust. Soc. Am.*, 100, 2514, 1996.
29. Ebbini, E. and Simon, C., Temperature imaging using diagnostic ultrasound: methods for guidance and monitoring of thermal treatments of tissue, in *Proc. SPIE (Thermal Treatment of Tissue with Image Guidance)*, Ryan, T.P. and Wong, T.Z., Eds., SPIE, San Jose, 1999, 150.
30. Daniel, B.L., Butts, K., and Block, W.F., Magnetic resonance imaging of frozen tissues: temperature-dependent MR signal characteristics and relevance for MR monitoring of cryosurgery, *Magn. Res. Med.*, 31, 627, 1999.
31. Le Bihan, D., Dalannoy, J., and Levin, R.L., Temperature mapping with MR imaging of molecular diffusion: application to hyperthermia, *Radiology*, 171, 853, 1989.
32. Kamimura, Y. and Amemiya, Y., An NMR technique for noninvasive thermometry using M_o as the temperature-sensitive parameter, *Automedica*, 8, 295, 1987.
33. Ishihara, Y. et al., A precise and fast temperature mapping method using water proton chemical shift, in *Proc SMRM, 11th Annual Meeting*, Berlin, 1992, 4803.
34. Peters, R.D., Hinks, R.S., and Henkelman, R.M., *Ex vivo* tissue-type independence in proton-resonance frequency shift MR thermometry, *Magn. Res. Med.*, 40, 454, 1998.
35. Kuroda, K. et al., Temperature mapping using the water proton chemical shift: self-referenced method with echo-planar spectroscopic imaging, *Magn. Res. Med.*, 43, 220, 2000.
36. Peters, R.D., Hinks, R.S., and Henkelman, R.M., Heat-source orientation and geometry dependence in proton-resonance frequency shift magnetic resonance thermometry, *Magn. Res. Med.*, 41, 909, 1999.

37. De Poorter, J., Noninvasive MRI thermometry with the proton resonance frequency method: study of susceptibility effects, *Magn. Res. Med.*, 34, 359, 1995.
38. Vykhodtseva, N., MRI detection of the thermal effects of focused ultrasound on the brain, *Ultrasound Med. Biol.*, 26, 871, 2000.
39. Purdie, T.G. et al., Dynamic contrast enhanced CT measurement of blood flow during interstitial laser photocoagulation: comparison with an Arrhenius damage model, *Phys. Med. Biol.*, 45, 1115, 2000.
40. Solbiati, L. et al., Radio-frequency ablation of hepatic metastases: postprocedural assessment with a US microbubble contrast agent-early experience, *Radiology*, 211, 643, 1999.
41. Damianou, C.A. et al., Dependence of ultrasonic attenuation and absorption in dog soft tissues on temperature and thermal dose, *J. Acoust. Soc. Am.*, 102, 628, 1997.
42. Graham, S.J. et al., Analysis of changes in MR properties of tissues after heat treatment, *Magn. Res. Med.*, 42, 1061, 1999.
43. Worthington, A.E. and Sherar, M.D., Changes in ultrasound properties of porcine kidney tissue during heating, *Ultrasound Med. Biol.*, 27, 673, 2001.
44. Graham, S.J., Bronskill, M.J., and Henkelman, R.M., Time and temperature dependence of MR parameters during thermal coagulation of ex vivo rabbit muscle, *Magn. Res. Med.*, 39, 198, 1998.
45. Hinks, R.S. et al., MR systems for image-guided therapy, *J. Magn. Res. Imaging*, 8, 19, 1998.
46. Visser, A.G., Kaatee, R.S.J.P., and Levendag, P.C., Radiofrequency techniques for interstitial hyperthermia interstitial and intracavitary thermoradiotherapy, in *Thermoradiotherapy and Thermochemotherapy*, Seegenschmiedt, M.H., Fessenden, P., and Vernon, C.C., Eds., Springer, New York, 1995.
47. Foster, K.R. and Schwan, H.P., Dielectric properties of tissues and biological materials: a critical review, *Crit. Rev. Biomed. Eng.*, 17, 25, 1989.
48. Livraghi, T. et al., Saline-enhanced radiofrequency tissue ablation in the treatment of liver metastases, *Radiology*, 202, 205, 1997.
49. Goldberg, S.N. et al., Radiofrequency tissue ablation: Increased lesion diameter with a perfusion electrode, *Acad. Radiol.*, 3, 636, 1996.
50. Goldberg, S.N. and Gazelle, G.S., Advances in radiofrequency tumor ablation therapy: technical considerations, strategies for increasing coagulation necrosis volume, and preliminary clinical results, in *Proc. SPIE (Surgical Applications of Energy)*, Ryan, T.P. and Katzir, A., Eds., SPIE, San Jose, CA, 1998, 104.
51. Leveen, R.F., Laser hyperthermia and radiofrequency ablation of hepatic lesions. *Semin. Intervent. Rad.*, 14, 313, 1997.
52. Gazelle, G.S. et al., Tumor ablation with radio-frequency energy, *Radiology*, 21, 633, 2000.
53. Curley, S.A., Radiofrequency ablation of unresectable primary and metastatic hepatic malignancies: results in 123 patients, *Ann. Surg.*, 230, 1, 1999.
54. Solbiati, L. et al., Percutaneous radio-frequency ablation of hepatic metastases from colorectal cancer: long-term results in 117 patients, *Radiology*, 221, 159, 2001.
55. Rendon, R.A. et al., The uncertainty of radio frequency treatment of renal cell carcinoma: findings at immediate and delayed nephrectomy, *J. Urol.*, 167, 1587, 2002.
56. Stauffer, P.R., Diederich, C.J., and Seegenschmiedt, M.H., Interstitial heating technologies, in *Thermoradiotherapy and Thermochemotherapy*, Seegenschmiedt, M.H., Fessenden, P., and Vernon, C.C., Eds., Springer, New York, 1995, chap. 13.
57. Zhang, Y. et al., The determination of the electromagnetic field and SAR pattern of an interstitial applicator in a dissipative dielectric medium, *IEEE T. Microw. Theory*, 36, 1438, 1988.
58. Zhang, Y. et al., The calculated and measured temperature distribution of a phased interstitial antenna array, *IEEE T. Microw. Theory*, 38, 69, 1990.
59. Satoh, T. and Stauffer, P.R., Implantable helical coil microwave antenna for interstitial hyperthermia, *Int. J. Hyperthermia*, 4, 497, 1988.

60. Sherar, M.D. et al., Interstitial microwave thermal therapy for prostate cancer: Method of treatment and results of a phase I/II trial, *J. Urol.*, 166, 1707, 2001.
61. Seki, T. et al., Combination therapy with transcatheter arterial chemoembolization and percutaneous microwave coagulation therapy for hepatocellular carcinoma, *Cancer*, 89, 1245, 2000.
62. Sneed, P.K. et al., Survival benefit of hyperthermia in a prospective randomized trial of brachytherapy boost +/– hyperthermia for glioblastoma multiforme, *Int. J. Radiat. Oncol. Biol. Phys.*, 40, 287, 1998.
63. Shibata, T. et al., Small hepatocellular carcinoma: comparison of radio-frequency ablation and percutaneous microwave coagulation therapy, *Radiology*, 223, 331, 2002.
64. Deardorff, D.L., Diederich, C.J., and Nau, W.H., Control of interstitial thermal coagulation: comparative evaluation of microwave and ultrasound applicators, *Med. Phys.*, 28, 104, 2001.
65. Bown, S.G., Phototherapy of tumours, *World J. Surg.*, 7, 700, 1983.
66. Welch, A.J. et al., Definitions and overview of tissue optics, in *Optical-Thermal Response of Laser-Irradiated Tissue*, Welch, A.J. and van Gemert, M.J.C., Eds., Plenum Press, New York, 1995.
67. Ritz, J.P. et al., Optical properties of native and coagulated porcine liver tissue between 400 and 2400 nm, *Lasers Surg. Med.*, 29, 205, 2001.
68. Iizuka, M.N., Sherar, M.D., and Vitkin, I.A., Optical phantom materials for near infrared laser photocoagulation studies, *Lasers Surg. Med.*, 25, 159, 1999.
69. Atsumi, H. et al., Novel laser system and laser irradiation method reduced the risk of carbonization during laser interstitial thermotherapy: assessed by MR temperature measurement, *Lasers Surg. Med.*, 29, 108, 2001.
70. Mack, M.G. et al., Percutaneous MR imaging-guided laser-induced thermotherapy of hepatic metastases, *Abdom. Imag.*, 26, 369, 2001.
71. Vogl, T.J. et al., Recurrent nasopharyngeal tumors: preliminary clinical results with interventional MR imaging — controlled laser-induced thermotherapy, *Radiology*, 196, 725, 1995.
72. Bloom, K.J., Dowlat, K., and Assad, L., Pathologic changes after interstitial laser therapy of infiltrating breast carcinoma, *Am. J. Surg.*, 182, 384, 2001.
73. Vogl, T.J. et al., Interventional MR: interstitial therapy, *Eur. Radiol.*, 9, 1479, 1999.
74. Hynynen, K., The feasibility of interstitial ultrasound hyperthermia, *Med. Phys.*, 19, 979, 1992.
75. Nyborg, W.L., Heat generation by ultrasound in a relaxing medium, *J. Acoust. Soc. Am.*, 70, 310, 1981.
76. Pauly, H. and Schwan, H.P., Mechanism of absorption of ultrasound in liver tissue, *J. Acoust. Soc. Am.*, 50, 692, 1970.
77. Goss, S.A. et al., Dependence of the ultrasonic properties of biological tissue on constituent proteins, *J. Acoust. Soc. Am.*, 67, 1041, 1980.
78. Nau, W.H., Diederich, C.J., and Burdette, E.C., Evaluation of multielement catheter-cooled interstitial ultrasound applicators for high-temperature thermal therapy, *Med. Phys.*, 28, 1525, 2001.
79. Deardorff, D.L. and Diederich, C.J., Axial control of thermal coagulation using a multi-element interstitial ultrasound applicator with internal cooling, *IEEE Trans. Ultrason. Ferroelectr. Freq. Contr.*, 47, 1, 2000.
80. Deardorff, D.L. and Diederich, C.J., Angular directivity of thermal coagulation using air-cooled direct-coupled interstitial ultrasound applicators, *Ultrasound Med. Biol.*, 25, 609, 1999.
81. Zimmer, J.E. et al., The feasibility of using ultrasound for cardiac ablation, *IEEE Trans. Biomed. Eng.*, 42, 891, 1995.
82. Lafon, C. et al., Design and preliminary results of an ultrasound applicator for interstitial thermal coagulation, *Ultrasound Med. Biol.*, 24, 113, 1998.
83. Chopra, R., Bronskill, M.J., and Foster, F.S., Feasibility of linear arrays for interstitial ultrasound thermal therapy, *Med. Phys.*, 27, 1281, 2000.
84. Lafon, C. et al., Theoretical comparison of two interstitial ultrasound applicators designed to induce cylindrical zones of tissue ablation, *Med. Biol. Eng. Comput.*, 37, 298, 1999.

85. Chopra, R. et al., Interstitial ultrasound heating applicator for MR-guided thermal therapy, *Phys. Med. Biol.*, 46, 3133, 2001.
86. Prat, F. et al., Destruction of a bile duct carcinoma by intraductal high intensity ultrasound during ERCP, *Gastrointest. Endosc.*, 53, 797, 2001.
87. Roos, D., Review of intracavitary hyperthermia techniques, in *Interstitial and Intracavitary Thermo-radiotherapy*, Seegenschmiedt, M.H. and Sauer, R., Eds., Springer-Verlag, Berlin, 1993, Chap. 10.
88. Pisa, S. et al., A 915-MHz antenna for microwave thermal ablation treatment: physical design, computer modeling and experimental measurement, *IEEE Trans. Biomed. Eng.*, 48, 599, 2001.
89. Hutchinson, E.B., Buchanan, M.T., and Hynynen, K., Design and optimization of an aperiodic ultrasound phased array for intracavitary prostate thermal therapies, *Med. Phys.*, 23, 767, 1996.
90. Sokka, S.D. and Hynynen, K.H., The feasibility of MRI-guided whole prostate ablation with a linear aperiodic intracavitary ultrasound phased array, *Phys. Med. Biol.*, 45, 3373, 2000.
91. Hand, J.W., Biophysics and technology of electromagnetic hyperthermia, in *Methods of External Hyperthermic Heating*, Gautherie, M., Ed., Springer-Verlag, Berlin, 1990, Chap 1.
92. Hynynen, K. et al., A clinical, noninvasive, MR imaging-monitored ultrasound surgery method, *Radiographics*, 16, 185, 1996.
93. ter Haar, G., Acoustic surgery, *Phys. Today*, 12, 29, 2001.
94. Cline, H.E. et al., MR temperature mapping of focused ultrasound surgery, *Magn. Res. Med.*, 31, 628, 1994.
95. Chung, A.H. et al., Optimization of spoiled gradient-echo phase imaging for in vivo localization of a focused ultrasound beam, *Magn. Res. Med.*, 36, 745, 1996.
96. McDannold, N.J. et al., The use of quantitative temperature images to predict the optimal power for focused ultrasound surgery: in vivo verification in rabbit muscle and brain, *Med. Phys.*, 29, 356, 2002.
97. Chung, A.H., Jolesz, F.A., and Hynynen, K., Thermal dosimetry of a focused ultrasound beam in vivo by magnetic resonance imaging, *Med. Phys.*, 26, 2017, 1999.
98. Vykhodtseva, N. et al., MRI detection of the thermal effects of focused ultrasound on the brain, *Ultrasound Med. Biol.*, 26, 871, 2000.
99. Hynynen, K. et al., MR imaging-guided focused ultrasound surgery of fibroadenomas in the breast: a feasibility study, *Radiology*, 219, 176, 2001.
100. Watkin, N.A. et al., A feasibility study for the noninvasive treatment of superficial bladder tumours with focused ultrasound, *Brit.J. Urol.*, 78, 715, 1996.
101. Bihrle, R. et al., High intensity focused ultrasound for the treatment of benign prostatic hyperplasia: early United States clinical experience, *J. Urol.*, 151, 1271, 1994.
102. Madersbacher, S. et al., Tissue ablation in benighn prostatic hyperplasia with high intensity focused ultrasound, *J. Urol.*, 152, 1956, 1994.
103. Clement, G.T., White, J., and Hynynen, K., Investigation of a large-area phased array for focused ultrasound surgery through the skull, *Phys. Med. Biol.*, 45, 1071, 2000.
104. Daum, D.R. et al., In vivo demonstration of noninvasive thermal surgery of the liver and kidney using an ultrasonic phased array, *Ultrasound Med. Biol.*, 25, 108, 1999.
105. Vaezy, S. et al., Treatment of uterine fibroid tumors in a nude mouse model using high-intensity focused ultrasound, *Am. J. Obstet. Gynecol.*, 183, 6, 2000.
106. Coleman, D.J. et al., Therapeutic ultrasound in the treatment of glaucoma. I. Experimental model, *Ophthalmology*, 92, 339, 1985.
107. Mourad, P.D. and Crum, L.A., A review and examination of ultrasound for lipoplasty, *Clin. Plast. Surg.*, 26, 409, 1999.
108. Visioli, A.G. et al., Preliminary results of a phase I dose escalation clinical trial using focused ultrasound in the treatment of localised tumours, *Eur. J. Ultrasound*, 9, 11, 1999.
109. Lehmann, J.F. et al., Heating produced by ultrasound in bone and soft tissue, *Arch. Phys. Med. Rehab.*, 48, 397, 1967.

110. Clement, G.T. et al., A hemisphere array for noninvasive ultrasound brain therapy and surgery, *Phys. Med. Biol.*, 45, 3707, 2000.
111. de Zwart, J.A. et al., On-line correction and visualization of motion during MRI-controlled hyperthermia, *Magn. Res. Med.*, 45, 128, 2001.
112. Fan, X. and Hynynen, K., Ultrasound surgery using multiple sonications — treatment time considerations, *Ultrasound Med. Biol.*, 22, 471, 1996.
113. Ebbini, E. and Cain, C., Multiple-focus phased array pattern synthesis: optimal driving-signal distributions for hyperthermia cancer therapy, *IEEE Trans. Ultrason. Ferroelectr. Freq. Control*, 35, 561, 1989.
114. Fjield, T., Fan, X., and Hynynen, K., A parametric study of the concentric-ring transducer design for MRI guided ultrasound surgery, *J. Acoust. Soc. Am.*, 100, 1220, 1996.

32

Medical Robotics

Kevin Cleary
Georgetown University Medical Center

Charles C. Nguyen
Catholic University of America

CONTENTS

32.1 Introduction

Medical robotics is an interdisciplinary field that focuses on developing electromechanical devices for clinical applications. The goal of this field is to enable new medical techniques by providing new capabilities to the physician or by providing assistance during surgical procedures. Medical robotics is a relatively young field, as the first recorded medical application occurred in 1985 for a brain biopsy. The field is still emerging. However, medical robotics has tremendous potential for improving the precision and capabilities of physicians when performing surgical procedures and it is believed that the field will continue to grow as improved systems become available.

Although several commercial companies sell medical robots, the total number of robots sold is still very small, and the market will most likely continue to grow slowly. Unlike the area of factory robotics, which grew rapidly during the 1970s and 1980s, medical robotics has not yet gained widespread acceptance. However, the authors feel that the benefits of medical robotics will become increasingly clear, leading to a continued rise in their use in medicine.

This chapter will begin with an introduction to robotics, followed by a historical review of their use in medicine. Clinical applications in several different medical specialties will then be presented. The chapter concludes with a discussion of technology challenges and areas for future research.

32.2 Robotics Review

The word "robot" originated from a 1922 play called "Rossum's Universal Robots (R.U.R.)" by Karel Capek.[1] The play was about a future in which all workers are automatons, who then revolt when they acquire souls.

The initial application of robotics was for handling of nuclear materials during the 1950s. These systems were teleoperated and controlled by a human operator. The first programmable robots were developed

0-8493-1140-3/04/$0.00+$1.50

for industrial applications. The UNIMATE robot was used by General Motors in the early 1960s for stacking hot pieces of metal. The robot could be programmed using a teach pendant to move the system through the desired motions. The robot was hydraulically powered and available with five or six degrees of freedom.

Degrees of freedom (DOF) is a common term in the robotics field and indicates the ability of the robot to position and orient an object in space. To be able to carry out general tasks, a robot must have at least six DOFs: three for translations (such as x, y, and z translations in Cartesian space) and three for rotations (such as rotations about x, y, and z Cartesian axes).

The field of industrial robotics grew rapidly throughout the 1960s and 1970s, when many factories became automated, particularly in the electronics and automotive areas. A trade group, the Robotics Industries Association, was founded in 1974 (www.robotics.org). This group sponsors conferences aimed at industrial applications and publishes a magazine titled *Robotics World*. Their definition of a robot is often quoted, which is "a reprogrammable, multifunctional manipulator designed to move material, parts, tools, or specialized devices through variable programmed motions to perform a variety of tasks." While this definition may seem somewhat narrow, the medical robotics devices we will discuss in this review fall mainly in this category. These robots typically consists of rigid links that allow relative motion from one link to another.[2] Attached to the end of the links is the robot hand, usually referred to as the end-effector. The robot is controlled by a computer system that is used to move the end-effector to any desired point and orientation within its workspace.

On the academic side, robotics became an increasingly popular subject in engineering school and computer science departments in the 1980s. Several of the leading U.S. schools such as Stanford, MIT, and Carnegie Mellon developed robotics groups during this time. Carnegie Mellon formed a Robotics Institute in 1980 and began offering the first Ph.D. in robotics in 1989. While many early students in the field started with the classic text by Richard Paul,[3] several other textbooks began to appear.[2,4,5] International conferences such as the *IEEE International Conference on Robotics and Automation*, which was first held in 1984, began to occur. The *IEEE Transactions on Robotics and Automation* also began publishing in that year, originally as the *Journal of Robotics and Automation.*

In the late 1980s and continuing in the 1990s, the field of robotics began to branch out from factory robotics into other applications such as service robotics and medical robotics. Mobile robotics became a popular topic and medical applications, including surgical robots and robots for rehabilitation, began to appear. In this review of medical robotics, we will focus on robots that play an active role during a surgical intervention. These systems are not meant to replace the physician, but rather to augment the capabilities of the physician. There are other categories of medical robotics, such as robotics for rehabilitation or miniature robots that might be placed inside the body, but these will not be discussed here. The review is not intended to be comprehensive, but rather to give an overview of the field of medical robotics.

Several other medical robotics review articles with a focus on surgical procedures have also been written. Davies[6] describes the history of surgical robotics and gives one classification for the types of robot systems studied by researchers. Taylor[7] discusses several taxonomies for surgical robotics and presents a different classification. Troccaz and Delnondedieu[8] give a historical review and describe passive, semiactive, and active robotic systems. Howe and Matsuoka[9] overview applications in image-based procedures, orthopedic surgery, and neurosurgery, among other specialties. Specialized reviews also exist, such as the article by Caddedu et al.[10] on urology robotics.

32.3 Medical Robotics History

Medical robotics is a relatively new field, with the first recorded medical application of a robot occurring in 1985.[11] Here, the robot was a simple positioning device to orient a needle for biopsy of the brain. A 52-year-old man was put on a CT scanner table and a series of CT images were obtained. The target within the brain was then identified on these images, and a PUMA 560 industrial robot was used to orient a guide tube through which the needle was inserted. Unfortunately, safety issues concerning the operation of the robot in close proximity to people prevented this work from continuing.[6]

About the same time, research groups in Asia, Europe, and the United States began investigating other medical applications of robotics. In Asia, Dohi and colleagues at Tokyo University developed a prototype of a CT-guided needle insertion manipulator.[12] In Europe, a group at Imperial College in London under the direction of Davies began developing a robot for resection of the prostate.[13] At Grenoble University Hospital in France, Benabid, Lavallee, and colleagues started work on neurosurgical applications.[14] In the United States, Taylor and associates at IBM began developing a system for hip implants later known as ROBODOC.[15]

Currently, there are several commercial ventures and a number of research laboratories active in the field of medical robotics. Interest in the topic has grown rapidly in the last few years in particular, and dedicated sessions on medical robotics can now be found at medically related conferences. Early research efforts have led to some commercial products. For example, the work at Grenoble University Hospital led to the NeuroMate robot of Integrated Surgical Systems, as described later.

32.4 Clinical Applications

Robots have been used in a number of clinical applications in medicine as shown in Table 32.1. This table is not exhaustive, but representative research groups and commercial vendors in several areas have been selected to give the reader an overview of the field. The column labeled "Studies" refers to whether human trials, animal studies, cadaver studies, or phantom studies have been done. Each of these areas will be discussed in the following text.

32.4.1 Neurosurgery

As mentioned in the historical review, neurosurgery was the first clinical application of robotics and continues to be a topic of current interest. Neurosurgical stereotactic applications require spatial accuracy and precision targeting to reach the anatomy of interest while minimizing collateral damage. This section presents three neurosurgical robotic systems:

TABLE 32.1 Clinical Application Areas and Representative Robotic Developments

Clinical Area	Country	Institution/Company	System	Studies	Reference
Neurosurgery	Switzerland	Univ. of Lausanne	Minerva	Human	16,17
	US	Integrated Surgical/Grenoble Univ. Hospital	NeuroMate	Human	18
	Japan	Univ. of Tokyo	MRI compatible	Tissue samples	19
Orthopedic	US	Integrated Surgical	ROBODOC	Human	15
	US	Univ. of Tokyo/Hopkins	PAKY/RCM	Phantom	19
	US	Marconi	Kawasaki	Pig	20
	UK	Imperial College	Acrobot	Human	21
Interventional	US	Georgetown/Hopkins	PAKY/RCM	Cadaver	22
	Austria	ARC Seibersdorf Research/ Vienna Univ. Hospital	Custom built	Phantom	23
Urology	UK	Imperial College	Probot	Human	24
	US	Hopkins	PAKY/RCM	Human	25
Maxillofacial	Germany	Charite	SurgiScope	Pig	26
	Germany	Karlsruhe/Heidelberg	RX 90	Pig	27
Radiosurgery	US	Accuray	CyberKnife	Human	28
Ophthalmology	US	Hopkins	Steady-Hand	Phantom	29
Cardiac	US	Intuitive Surgical	da Vinci	Human	30
	US	Computer Motion	Zeus	Human	31
	France	Grenoble	PADyC	Phantom	32

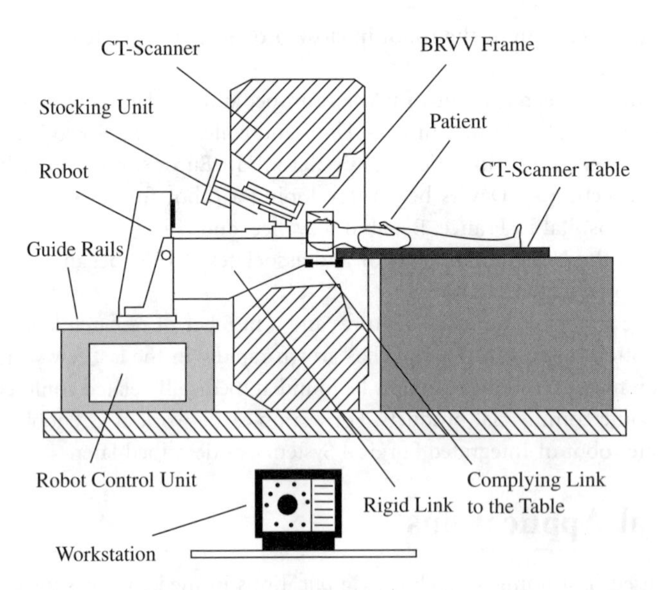

FIGURE 32.1 Minerva components and system overview. (From Burckhart, C.W., Flury, P., and Glauser, D., Stereotactic brain surgery, *IEEE Eng. Med. Biol.*, 14(3), 314–317, 1995. ©1995 IEEE. With permission.)

1. Minerva from the University of Lausanne in Switzerland
2. NeuroMate from Integrated Surgical Systems in the United States
3. An MRI compatible robot developed by Dohi and colleagues in Japan

32.4.1.1 Minerva

One of the earliest robotic systems developed for precise needle placement was the neurosurgical robot Minerva,[16] designed for stereotactic brain biopsy. A special purpose robot was constructed that was designed to work within the CT scanner so that the surgeon could follow the position of the instruments on successive CT scans. This constraint ensured that CT images would be available throughout a procedure, keeping all procedures under the surgeon's supervision and control. A diagram of the system and associated components is shown in Figure 32.1.

The system consists of a five DOF structure with two linear axes (vertical and lateral), two rotary axes (moving in a horizontal and vertical plane), and another linear axis (to move the tool to and from the patient's head).[17] The robot is mounted on a horizontal carrier that moves on rails. A stereotactic frame, the Brown-Roberts-Wells (BRW) reference frame, is attached to the robot gantry and coupled to the motorized CT table by two ball and socket joints arranged in series. The system was used for two operations on patients in September 1993 at the CHUV Hospital in Switzerland, but the project has since been discontinued.

32.4.1.2 NeuroMate

The NeuroMate is a six-axis robot for neurosurgical applications that evolved from work done by Benabid, Lavallee, and colleagues at Grenoble University Hospital in France.[14,18,33] The original system was subsequently redesigned to fulfill specific stereotactic requirements and particular attention was paid to safety issues.[34] The current version (Figure 32.2) is a commercial product that has been licensed by Integrated Surgical Systems (Davis, CA) and is FDA approved.

The system has been used in over 1600 procedures since 1989, covering a range of neurosurgical procedures. The major clinical applications include:

- Tumor biopsies (1100 cases)
- Stereoelectroencephalographic investigations of patients with epilepsy (200 cases)
- Midline stereotactic neurosurgery and functional neurosurgery of the basal ganglia (200 cases)

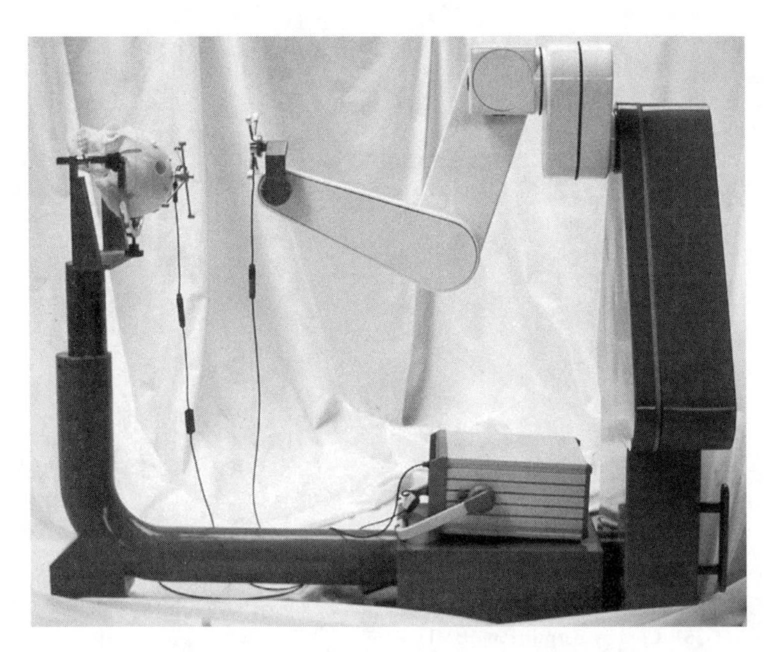

FIGURE 32.2 NeuroMate neurosurgical robot. (Courtesy of Integrated Surgical Systems, Davis, CA.)

A typical clinical procedure consists of an initial data acquisition step, followed by data transfer to the control computer, and then the procedure itself. Data acquisition involves obtaining images of the brain from which path planning from the skin entry point to the target point can be done using a specially developed software program. The images can be in digital form (DSA, CT, or MRI images) or can be digitized (radiographs, for example) using a digitizing table or scanner. Once the path is planned, the images are transferred directly from the planning workstation to the control workstation in the operating room over an Ethernet link.

To carry out the procedure, the robot must know where it is located relative to the patient's anatomy. This is typically done using a calibration cage, which is placed on the end-effector of the robot around the patient's head (Figure 32.3). This cage looks like an open cubic box. The four sides are each implanted with nine x-ray opaque beads, the positions of which have been precisely measured. Two x-rays are taken that show the position of these beads along with the fiducial markers of the patient's frame. This information is used to determine the transformation matrix between the robot and the patient. The defined trajectory is used to command the robot to position a mechanical guide, which is aligned with this trajectory. The robot is then fixed in this position, and the physician uses this guide to introduce the surgical tool such as a drill, probe, or electrode.

32.4.1.3 MRI Compatible Robot

While several robots have been developed for stereotactic neurosurgery, including those mentioned above, almost all of these systems used CT images for guidance. However, many structures in the brain are best visualized using magnetic resonance imaging (MRI). The robotic systems described so far are not suitable for use in an MRI scanner because the strong magnetic fields generated dictate that only nonmagnetic materials can be used. In Japan, in the Mechatronics Laboratory at the University of Tokyo, Dohi, Masamune and colleagues developed an MRI-compatible needle insertion manipulator intended for use in stereotactic neurosurgery.[35] The manipulator frame was manufactured using polyethylene terephthalate (PET) and ultrasonic motors were used for the actuators. Other parts such as bearings, feed screws, and gear that must be strong and precisely fabricated are made of nonmagnetic materials including brass, aluminum, delrin, and ceramics. In phantom tests using watermelons, the robot performed satisfactorily with a positioning error of less than 3.3 mm from the desired target. The unit was small enough at 491 mm in maximum height to fit inside the MRI gantry of 600 mm in diameter.

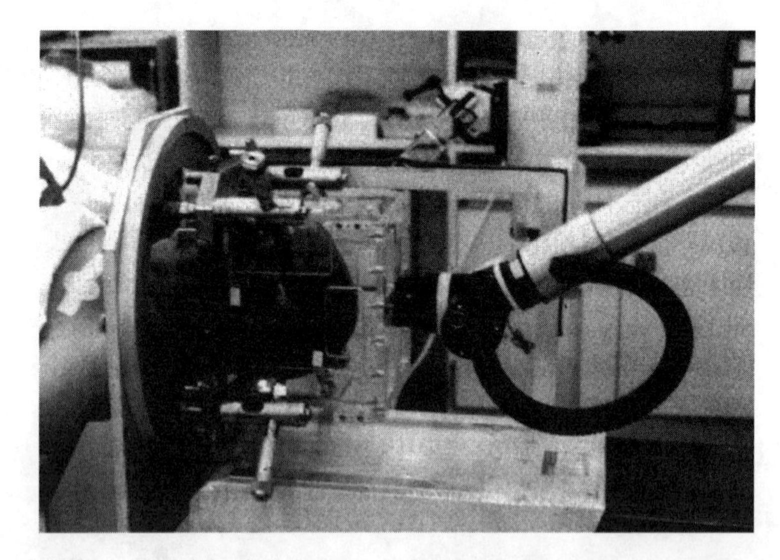

FIGURE 32.3 Calibration cage held by the robot. (From Lavallee, S. et al., Image-guided operating robot: a clinical application in stereotactic neurosurgery, in *Computer-Integrated Surgery*, Taylor, R.H. et al., Eds., MIT Press, Cambridge, 1995, pp. 343–351. Used by permission of MIT Press.)

Rather than retrofitting an industrial robot, Masamune developed a completely new design based on the clinical requirements for safety, MRI compatibility, and compactness. As shown in Figure 32.4, the system includes an X-Y-Z base stage. An arch mechanism is mounted on the base stage along with a linear needle carriage. This isocentric design was adopted for its mechanical safety and simplicity. The system was controlled by a personal computer. The control computer and motor driver boards were remotely located in the MRI control room and connected by shielded cables to the robot.

In a related development, a new MRI compatible robot has been developed to work within the interventional MRI unit at the Brigham and Women's Hospital in Boston, Massachusetts.[36] The interventional MRI has a pair of parallel facing donut-shaped magnets, with an air gap of 560 mm. The robot sits between the magnets and is mounted on at the top of the unit as shown in Figure 32.5. The system is currently undergoing testing. One potential clinical application is needle placement for prostate brachytherapy.

Finally, researchers in Germany have developed an MRI compatible robotic biopsy system, focusing on breast cancer as an initial application. *In vitro* experiments using pig livers in a 1.5-Tesla magnet and 4-mm targets resulted in all eight targets being successfully hit.[37]

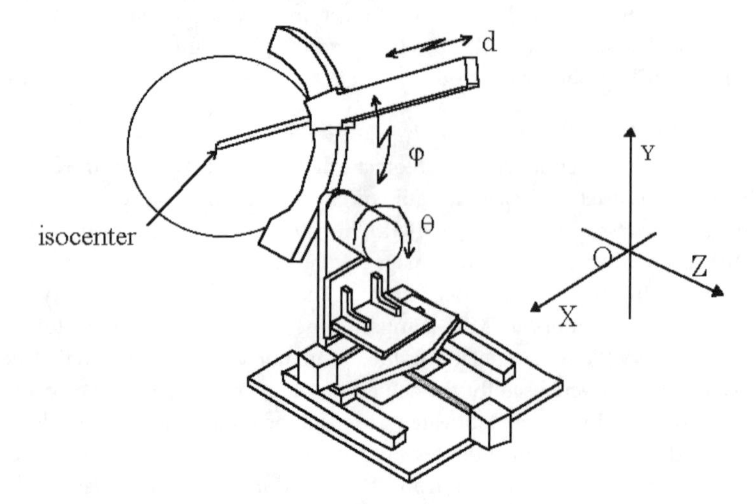

FIGURE 32.4 MRI compatible robot design. (Courtesy of Ken Masamune, Tokyo Denki University, Tokyo, Japan.)

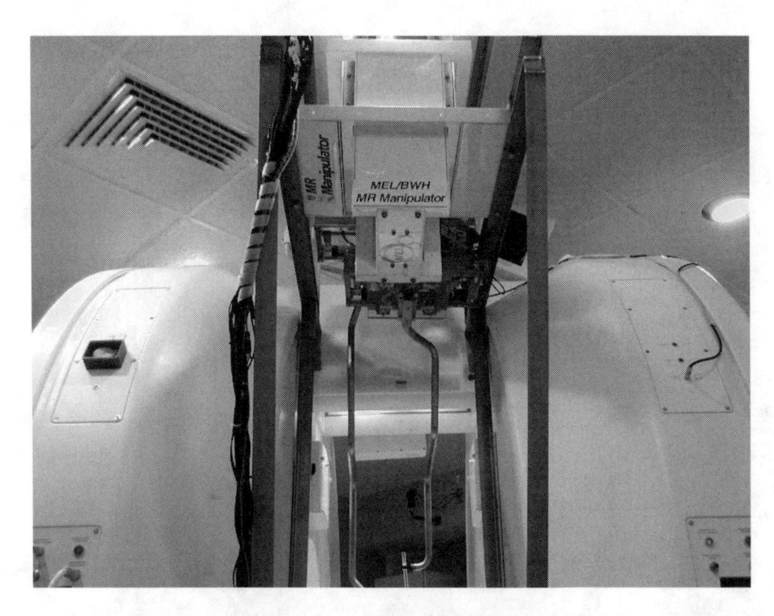

FIGURE 32.5 MRI compatible robot in interventional MRI system. (Courtesy of Kiyoyuki Chinzei, AIST, Tsukuba, Japan, and Ron Kikinis, BWH, Boston, MA.)

32.4.2 Orthopedic

Orthopedics is well suited for robotic assistance due to the rigid nature of bone. Because bone does not deform significantly when it is drilled or cut, it is possible to intraoperatively apply preoperative imaging and planning information more easily than for soft tissues such as the brain or abdominal organs.[38] Orthopedics was also an early adopter of robotics, as the ROBODOC system described next was used to assist surgeons in performing part of a total hip replacement in 1992. The robot was used to mill out the hole for the hip implant. This marked the first use of an active robot for hip surgery.

32.4.2.1 ROBODOC

The ROBODOC system was developed clinically by Integrated Surgical Systems (ISS) for total hip replacement procedures from a prototype created at IBM Research. The system was used in over 1000 cases at a hospital in Frankfurt, Germany from 1994 until 1998.[39] The system consists of three major components: a planning workstation, the robot itself that does the cutting, and the workstation that guides and controls the robot.

A typical hip replacement procedure using ROBODOC is carried out as follows.[40] The procedure starts with the surgeon implanting three locator pins into the hip. These pins are later used as fiducial points for registering the patient anatomy with the robot. A CT scan is then obtained and the CT data is transferred to the planning workstation (ORTHODOC). The surgeon can then choose a suitable implant from a library of possible implants. The surgeon can virtually position the implant on the planning workstation, check different positions, and assess the impact on anteversion, neck length, and stress loading (Figure 32.6). When the planning session is finished, the data is transferred to the computer that controls ROBODOC.

In the operating room, the hip joint is exposed and the robotic system is moved into position to mill out the femoral cavity. The locator pins are used to register the hip joint with the robot. Cutting time is between 20 and 35 min. The surgeon monitors this process by watching a computer screen that that shows the progress of the cutting operation. The robot can also be stopped at any time. When the milling is complete, the robot is removed and the rest of the operation is completed by hand in the conventional manner. A photograph of ROBODOC milling the cavity for the implant is shown in Figure 32.7.

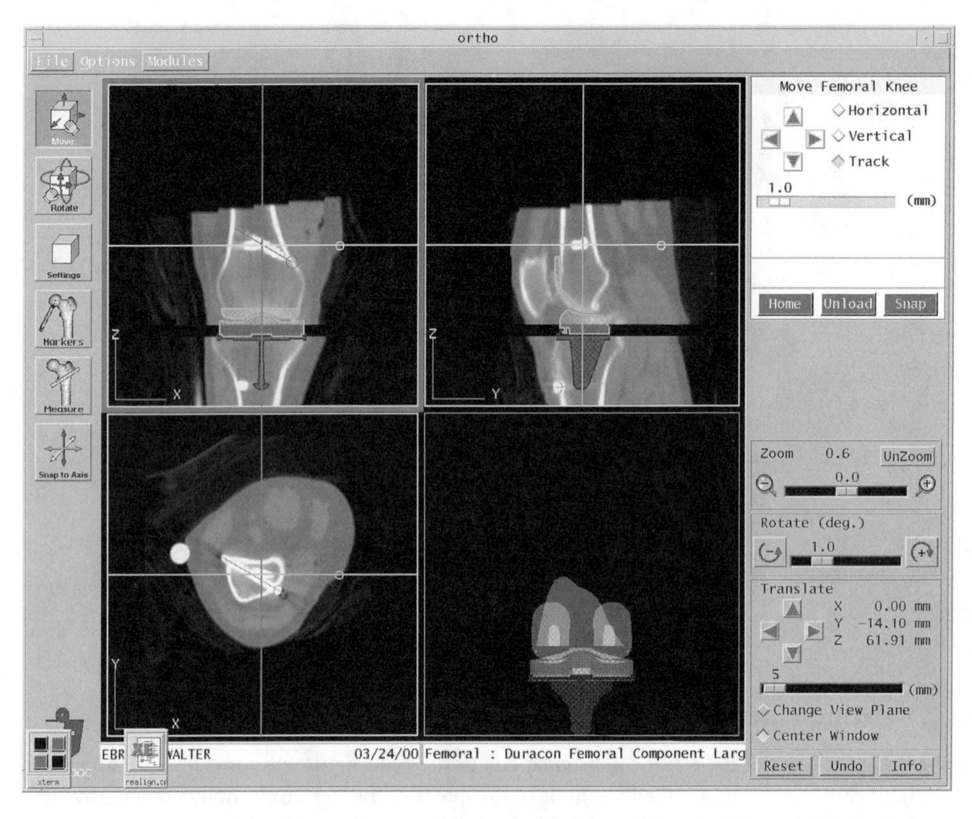

FIGURE 32.6 ORTHODOC planning workstation. (Courtesy of Integrated Surgical Systems, Davis, CA.)

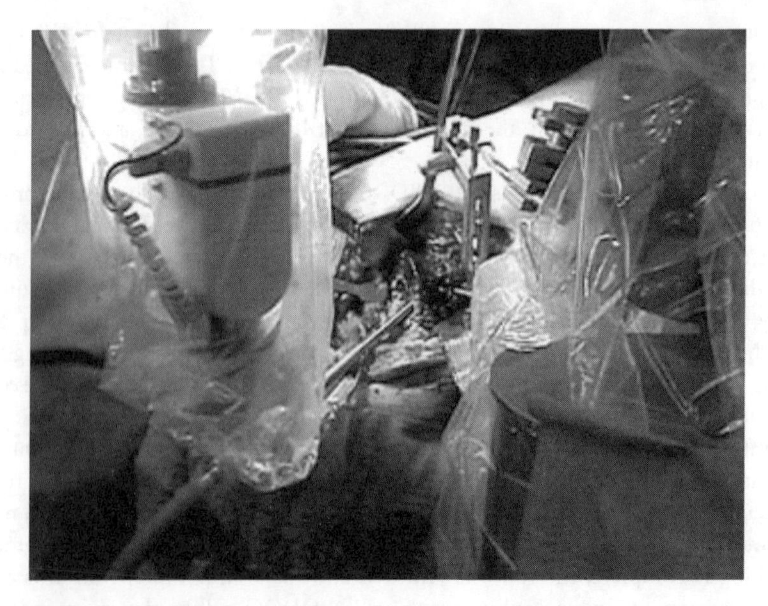

FIGURE 32.7 ROBODOC milling implant cavity for hip replacement surgery. (Courtesy of Integrated Surgical Systems, Davis, CA.)

32.4.2.2 University of Tokyo/Johns Hopkins Collaboration

An integrated robotic system for percutaneous placement of needles under CT guidance was developed by Masamune at the University of Tokyo in collaboration with Johns Hopkins.[19] Single image based co-registration of the PAKY/RCM robot and image space was achieved by stereotactic localization using a miniature version of the BRW head-frame built into the radiolucent needle driver. A phantom study was done with an orientation accuracy of 0.6 degrees and a needle tip to target distance of 1.04 mm. The system is applicable to orthopedic (spine) and many other percutaneous procedures.

32.4.2.3 Marconi Medical Systems

An active robot has been integrated with a CT scanner for interventional procedures by Yanof and colleagues at Marconi Medical Systems.[20] The advantage of this approach is that the coordinate system of the robot can be registered with the coordinate system of the CT during the integration phase. A separate registration step is thus not required for clinical use. Animal experiments using pigs were completed to investigate needle placement in the abdomen. The path was planned based on the CT scans and this information was sent to the robot, which automatically moved to the skin entry point and then oriented and drove the needle.

32.4.2.4 Imperial College

A special purpose robot called Acrobot (for active constraint robot) has been developed for safe use in the operating room for total knee replacement surgery.[21] The surgeon guides the robot using a handle attached to a force sensor attached to the robot tip. The concept is called "active constraint control" and allows for a synergy between the surgeon and the robot. The robot provides geometric accuracy and increases safety by providing motion constraint outside a predefined region. Following two preliminary clinical trials, the first clinical trial was conducted in which the Acrobot was used to register and cut the knee bones.

32.4.3 Interventional

32.4.3.1 Georgetown University/Johns Hopkins Collaboration

At Georgetown University Medical Center, our research group has been focusing on the use of robots for precision placement of instruments in minimally invasive spine procedures.[41,42] This work is a collaboration with the Urology Robotics Laboratory of the Johns Hopkins Medical Institutions and the Computer Integrated Surgical Systems and Technology (CISST) Engineering Research Center at Johns Hopkins University.

Low back pain is a common medical problem, and minimally invasive procedures such as nerve blocks are rapidly growing in popularity as a potential method of treatment. To assist the physician in needle placement during these procedures, we have begun to use a newly developed version of the PAKY/RCM needle driver robot developed at the Urology Robotics Laboratory. Robotic systems such as these have great potential as physician-assist devices for improving the precision of needle placement and enabling the development of the next generation of precision guidance systems for interventional techniques.

The newly developed needle driver robot consists of a three DOF translational stage, a seven DOF passive positioning stage, and a three DOF orientation/driving stage. The robot is mounted on the interventional table and the physician controls the system through a touch screen/joystick interface as shown in Figure 32.8. A cadaver study using the robot to place a 22-gauge needle for nerve and facet blocks has been completed (Figure 32.9).[22] Small metal BB nipple markers (1 mm in diameter) were inserted percutaneously into the paraspinal region of an embalmed cadaver. Six BBs were placed near the nerve root and six BBs near the facet joint. Using the touch screen/joystick interface, the physician controlled the robot to drive the needle toward each target BB. All needles were placed within 3 mm of the target, and the average distance was 1.44 mm ± 0.66 mm (standard deviation).

After the cadaver study was completed, approval was obtained from the Food and Drug Administration (FDA) for a randomized clinical trial of 20 patients for nerve and facet blocks using the robot under an

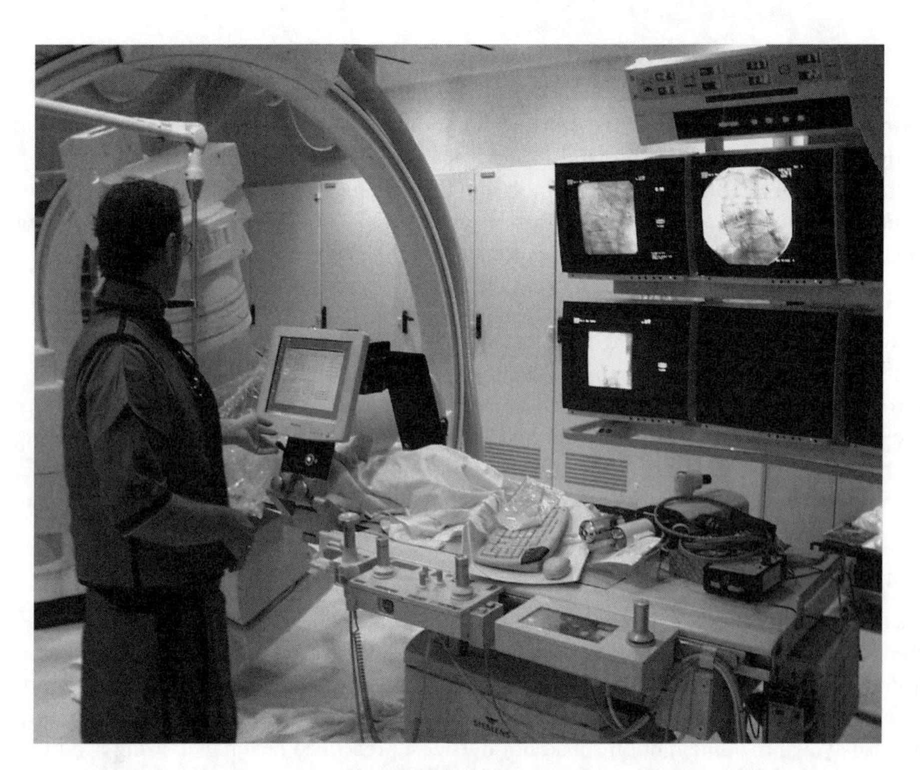

FIGURE 32.8 Needle driver robot cadaver study. Physician uses touch screen/joystick interface to control the robot and monitors the intervention on the fluoroscopy screens.

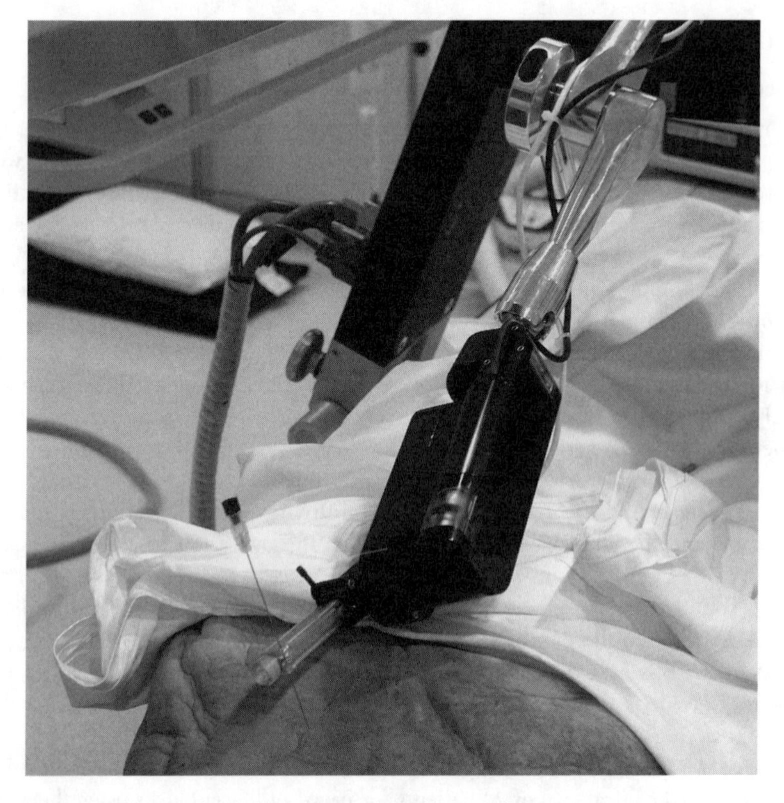

FIGURE 32.9 Close-up of cadaver study showing needle driver and passive positioning arm.

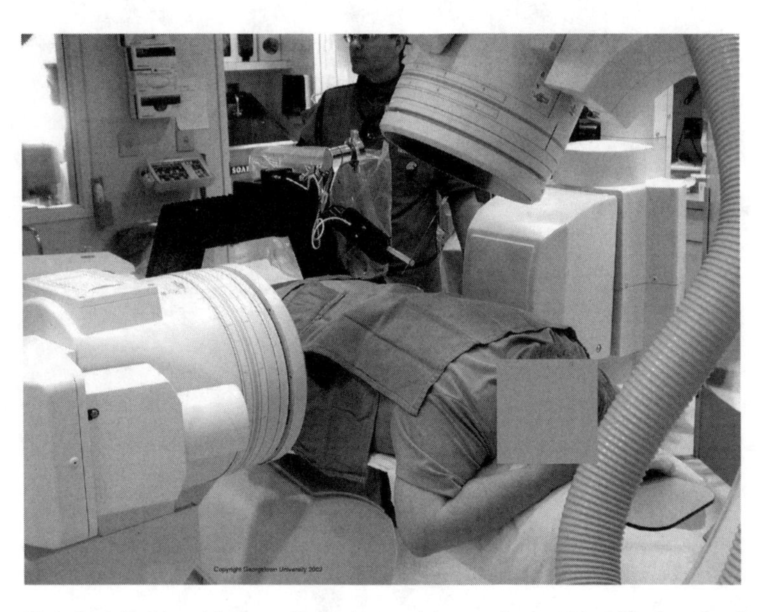

FIGURE 32.10 Clinical trial of joystick-controlled robot to drive needle for spinal block under fluoroscopy.

Investigational Device Exemption (IDE) protocol. This protocol was also approved by the Georgetown Institutional Review Board (IRB) and the U.S. Army Human Subjects Research Review Board. The procedure is done in the standard manner except the robot is used to position, orient, and drive the needle under physician control. A/P fluoroscopy is used to position and orient the needle, and lateral fluoroscopy is used to monitor the depth of insertion. To date, 11 patients have been enrolled and preliminary results show that it is feasible to use the robot for this clinical procedure. A photograph of one of the cases is shown in Figure 32.10.

32.4.3.2 ARC Seibersdorf Research Biopsy Robot

A mobile robotic system to assist interventional radiologists in ultrasound or CT-guided biopsies has been developed by ARC Seibersdorf Research in Austria in cooperation with the Vienna University Hospital.[43] The system includes a four DOF gross positioning system consisting of three linear axes and one rotational axis for initial positioning of the biopsy needle (Figures 32.11 and 32.12). The final pose of the needle is controlled by a three DOF needle positioning stage which includes two DOFs for orienting the needle at any angle, followed by a linear DOF with a stroke of 50 mm for moving the needle along the desired path to the skin entry point. Once the needle is positioned, the physician will then drive the needle to the target point by hand.

The system is controlled by two personal computers (PCs). A Windows 2000-based industrial PC is used for the high-level control of the robot. A Linux-based industrial PC is employed for the user interface and for monitoring of the intervention. The Linux PC includes a video capture card that receives the video input from the ultrasound or CT monitor and displays it on the screen for planning of the biopsy path (Figure 32.13). Once the path has been planned, the robot can then be commanded to move to the desired location and orient the needle.

To register the coordinate system of the robot with that of the ultrasound or CT machine, an optical tracking system (Polaris, Northern Digital, Waterloo, Canada) is used to track the three-dimensional position of all the components. This scheme was tested in a phantom study where peas with a mean diameter of 9.4 mm were embedded within a custom-made gel. The ultrasound transducer was tracked using the Polaris and the path toward each target was placed on the user interface. The robot arm was then commanded to move to the planned insertion point and to orient itself toward the center of the target. A 17-gauge coaxial puncture needle and an 18-gauge biopsy needle were then manually driven toward the center of the target by the radiologist. The goal was successfully achieved for all 20 targets

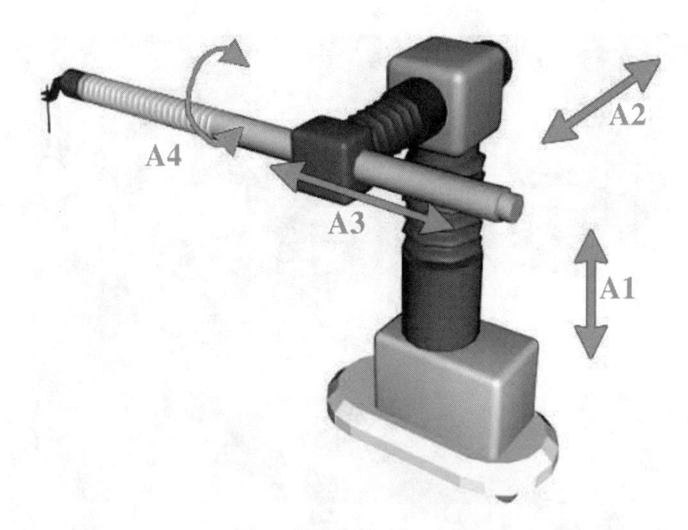

FIGURE 32.11 Degrees of freedom of the gross positioning system. A1–A3 are linear axes and A4 is a rotational motion. (Courtesy of Gernot Kronreif, ARC Seibersdorf Research, Seibersdorf, Austria.)

with only a single needle pass. The average radial distance between the needle tip and the center of the target was 1.9 ± 1.1 mm (standard deviation).

32.4.4 Urology

32.4.4.1 Prostate Resection

One of the pioneering research groups in medical robotics is the Mechantronics in Medicine Laboratory at Imperial College in London. Starting in 1988, the group began developing a robotic system named the *Probot* to aid in transurethral resection of the prostate.[24] While an initial feasibility study was carried out using a standard six-axis PUMA industrial robot, such a system was determined not to be practical for medical

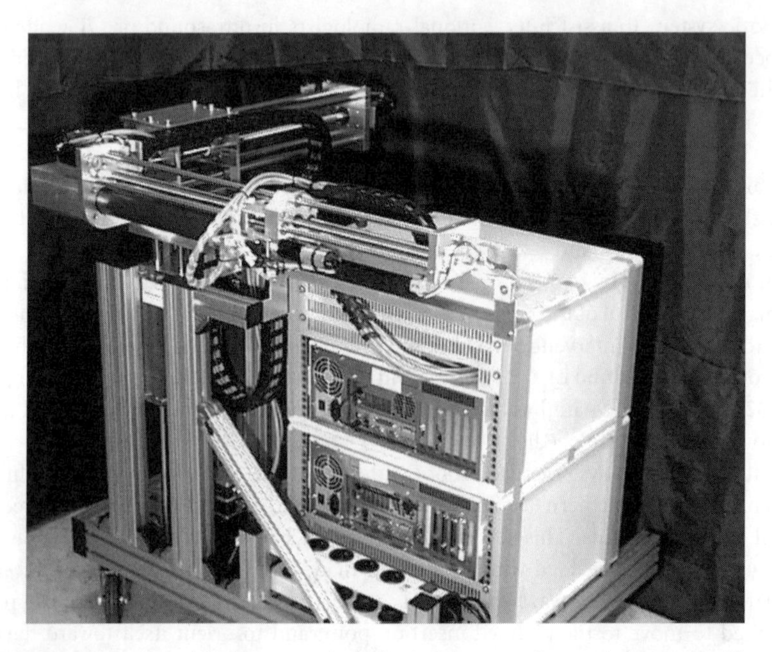

FIGURE 32.12 Prototype gross positioning system includes mobile cart and control electronics. (Courtesy of Gernot Kronreif, ARC Seibersdorf Research, Seibersdorf, Austria.)

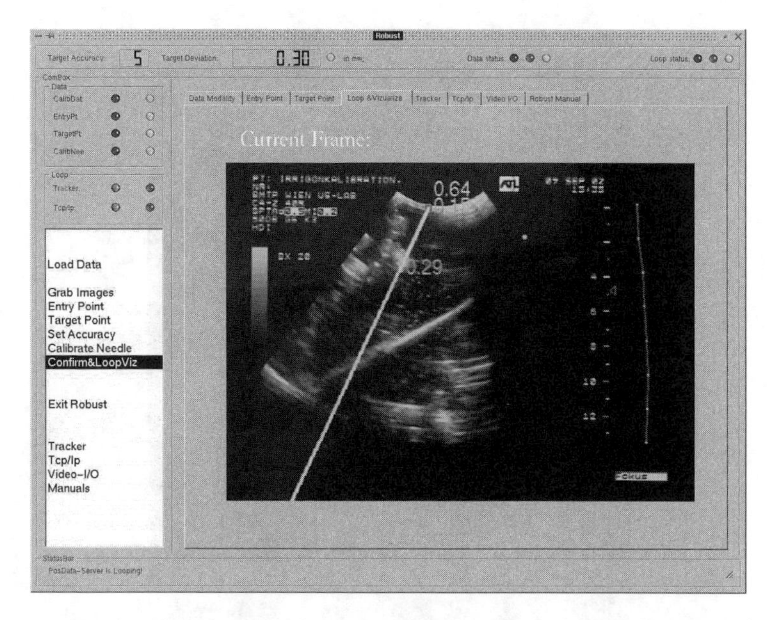

FIGURE 32.13 User interface showing planned and actual biopsy path overlaid with ultrasound scan. (Courtesy of Gernot Kronreif, ARC Seibersdorf Research, Seibersdorf, Austria.)

purposes as these robots are not designed to work in close proximity with humans. Therefore, a special purpose robotic frame was designed to hold the surgical instrument. The first patient was treated in April 1991. This was the first use of a robot to remove substantial quantities of tissue from a human patient.[6]

The robotic frame shown in Figure 32.14 consists of three axes of movement. An additional axis is provided by the resectoscope, which is the surgical instrument used to remove the tissue. The geometry of the system is designed to allow a cavity to be hollowed out from within the prostate and restrict movements outside an allowable range. This restriction provides an additional margin of safety.

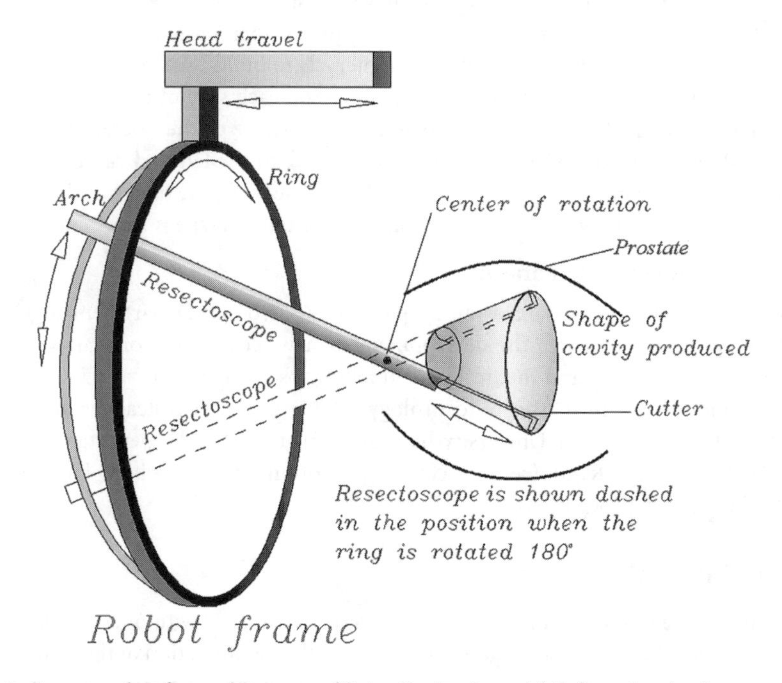

FIGURE 32.14 Prostate robot frame. (Courtesy of Brian Davies, Imperial College, London.)

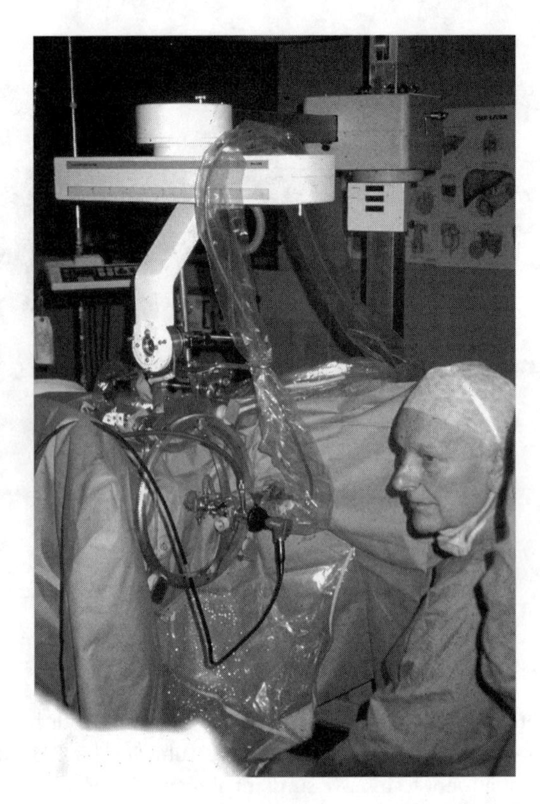

FIGURE 32.15 Probot in clinical use. (Courtesy of Brian Davies, Imperial College, London.)

The clinical application consists of four stages: (1) measurement, (2) imaging, (3) cavity design, and (4) cutting. To begin the procedure, the patient is positioned on the operating table and the Probot is positioned at the bladder neck. The user interface allows the surgeon to view the internal anatomy from a video camera within the resectoscope. An ultrasound probe is then passed down the resectoscope and the robot is set to acquire a series of scans at 5-mm intervals to build up a three-dimensional image of the prostate. The surgeon can then outline the cavity to cut on each slice of the ultrasound image using a light pen. The final step is the actual cutting operation. A picture of the operating room and Probot in clinical use is shown in Figure 32.15. The surgeon is sitting to the left and can observe the progress of the cutting on a video monitor as shown in Figure 32.16. The real-time image of the prostate is at the top left of the monitor and an overlay of the cuts on an ultrasound image is shown at the bottom right.

32.4.4.2 Urology Robotics Laboratory

The Urology Robotics (URobotics) Laboratory, part of the Urology Department at Johns Hopkins Medical Institutions, is dedicated to the development of new technology for urologic surgery.[25] The program combines engineering and medical personnel in close cooperation and is the only academic engineering program devoted exclusively to urology. This group and colleagues at the Engineering Research Center at Johns Hopkins University have developed the PAKY (percutaneous access of the kidney) needle driver[44] and RCM (remote center of motion) robot[45] which has been applied to minimally invasive kidney procedures.

32.4.5 Maxillofacial

Maxillofacial surgery is a branch of surgery that is concerned primarily with operations on the jaws and surrounding soft tissues. Maxillofacial surgery often requires the manipulation of the skull bone including drilling, cutting, shaping, and repositioning operations. Accuracy is at a premium since the shape of the

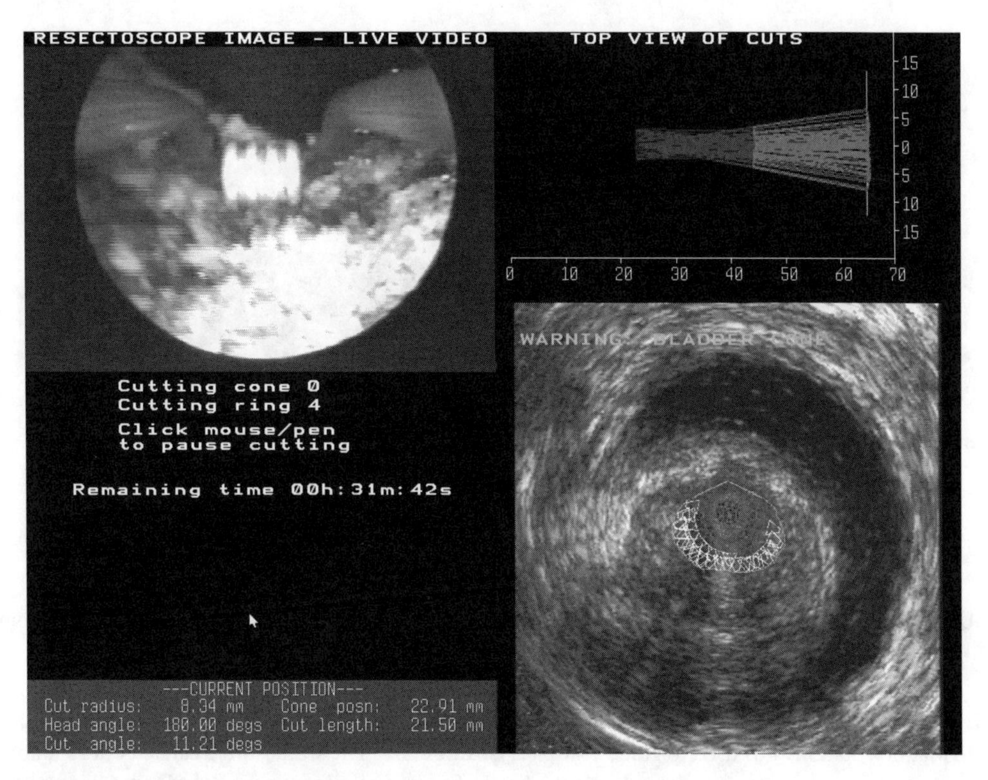

FIGURE 32.16 Video monitor display during procedure. (Courtesy of Brian Davies, Imperial College, London.)

bone and the aesthetic appearance of the skull and face are extremely important to patients. The current procedures are done manually using tools such as pliers, chisels, and electric saws and drills. Maxillofacial surgery may be a good application area for robotics since primarily bony structures are involved and accuracy is at a premium.[26]

For example, the following clinical tasks must be supported by a robot in maxillofacial surgery:[46]

- Guidance for nonflexible catheter implantation (brachytherapy)
- Handling of electric drills, taps, and screwdrivers for fixing bones and implants (anaplastology)
- Handling of electric saw and retractor hooks

32.4.5.1 Experimental Operating Room

For developing an interactive robot system for maxillofacial surgery, an experimental operating room has been set up at the Charite Hospital of Humbolt University in Berlin, Germany as shown in Figure 32.17. This operating room includes a unique robotic system, the SurgiScope. While most robotic systems described in this review are based on a serial kinematic structure in which the links are attached one after the other as in the human arm, at least one company has developed a medical robot based on a parallel kinematic structure. The SurgiScope is a general purpose six DOF robotic device consisting of a fixed base, three parallel links, and a movable end-effector. The system is designed to be fixed on the ceiling and provides a large workspace while not cluttering the operating room floor. The parallel kinematic structure also provides a very stable structure for precision operations. The robot was originally sold by Elekta, but is now being marketed by Jojumarie Intelligente Instrumente in Berlin. The system has been demonstrated in animal studies for placement of the radiation source in brachytherapy.[47]

32.4.5.2 Craniofacial Osteotomy

Another system for maxillofacial surgery has been developed at the Institute of Process Control and Robotics in Karlsruhe, Germany, in cooperation with the Clinic of Craniofacial Surgery at the University

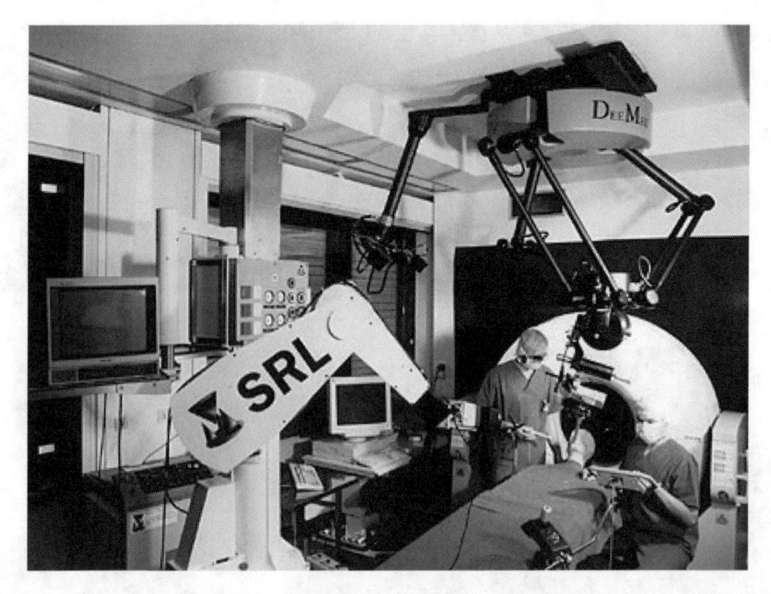

FIGURE 32.17 Surgical robotics laboratory showing parallel robot (ceiling mounted), mobile CT (back of photo), and serial robotics arm (foreground). (Courtesy of Tim Lueth, Charite Berlin.)

of Heidelberg. Animal studies were carried out to perform osteotomies where an RX 90 surgical robot (Orto Maquet, Staubli) was used to guide a surgical cutting saw.[27] The studies were carried out as follows. Twelve titanium screws were implanted into the head of a pig to be used as landmarks. A CT scan with 1.5-mm slice spacing was done, and the resulting images were used to create a surface model for surgical planning. A haptic interface was used to trace the cutting lines on the surface of the skull (Figure 32.18). Once the planning was completed, the robot was registered with the pig in the operating room (Figure 32.19), and the surgeon manually guided the robot arm along the trajectory where his movements

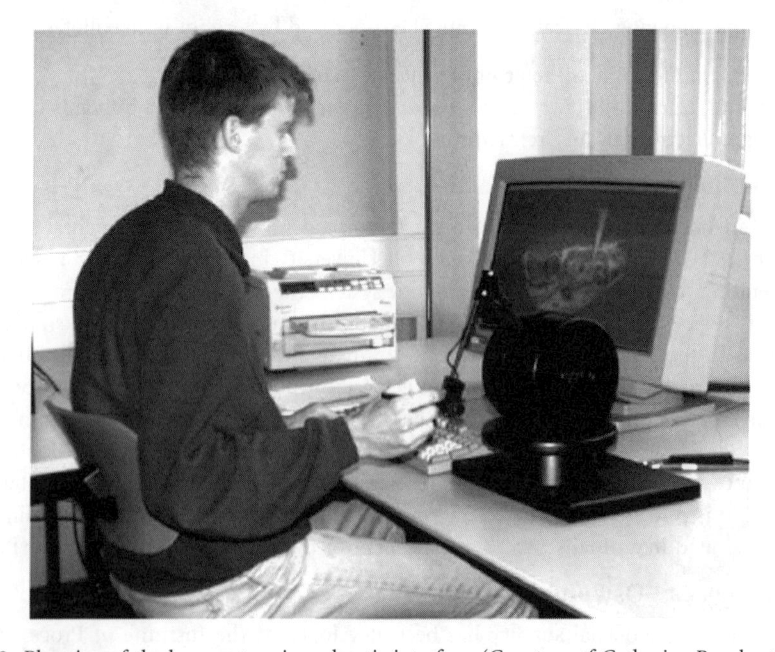

FIGURE 32.18 Planning of the bone cuts using a haptic interface. (Courtesy of Catherina Burghart, University of Karlsruhe, Germany.)

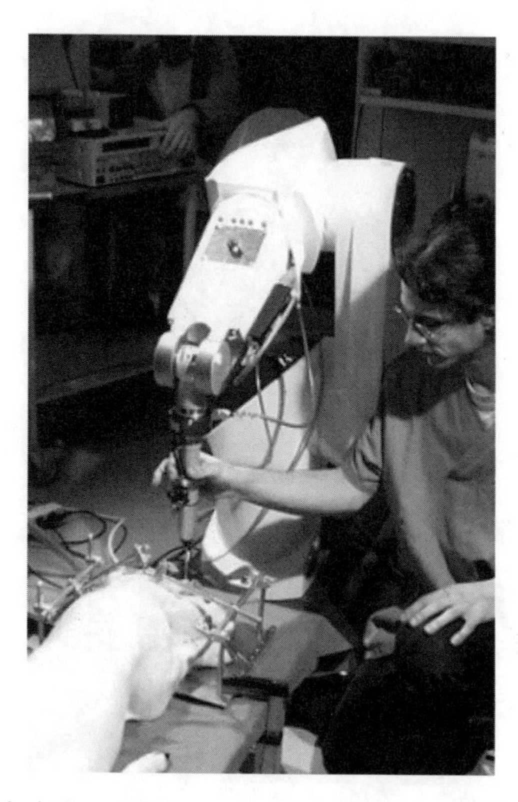

FIGURE 32.19 Registration by force-controlled manual guiding of the robot arm. (Courtesy of Catherina Burghart, University of Karlsruhe, Germany.)

perpendicular to the cutting line were restricted. This system has also been evaluated using sheep for the autonomous milling of a cavity in the skull needed for a customized titanium implant.

32.4.6 Radiosurgery

Radiation is a common means of treatment for tumors. Radiosurgery is the delivery of radiation to a tumor while attempting to spare adjacent normal tissue. In the brain, radiosurgery has typically been carried out using stereotactic frames that are rigidly fixed to the patient's skull. A novel method for precision irradiation called image-guided radiosurgery has been developed by Adler and associates at Stanford University (Stanford, CA).[28] The system consists of a lightweight linear accelerator, a Kuka robot, paired orthogonal x-ray imagers, and a treatment couch as shown in Figure 32.20. During a radiosurgery treatment session, the x-ray imaging system determines the location of the lesion. These coordinates are sent to the robot, which adjusts the pointing of the accelerator beam toward the lesion. The robot arm moves the beam through a series of preset positions to maximize the dose to the lesion while minimizing the dose to the surrounding normal tissue.

32.4.7 Ophthalmology

Many surgical operations on the eye, ear, brain, nerves, and blood vessels require extremely precise positioning and manipulation of surgical instruments. It is not uncommon for a microsurgeon to perform 150 to 200 μm movements during an operation and smaller movements would be desirable.[48] One representative microsurgical application is eye surgery and prototype systems for this purpose have been developed by Das et al.[49] and Hunter et al.[50]

Taylor and colleagues at Johns Hopkins University recently developed a "Steady-Hand" robot for microsurgical augmentation as shown in Figure 32.21.[29] While the initial target application is eye

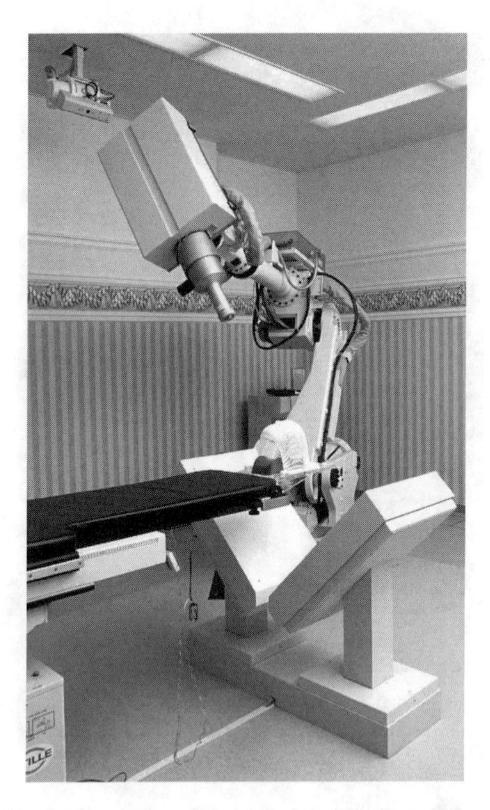

FIGURE 32.20 CyberKnife robotic radiosurgery system. (Courtesy of Accuray, Sunnyvale, CA.)

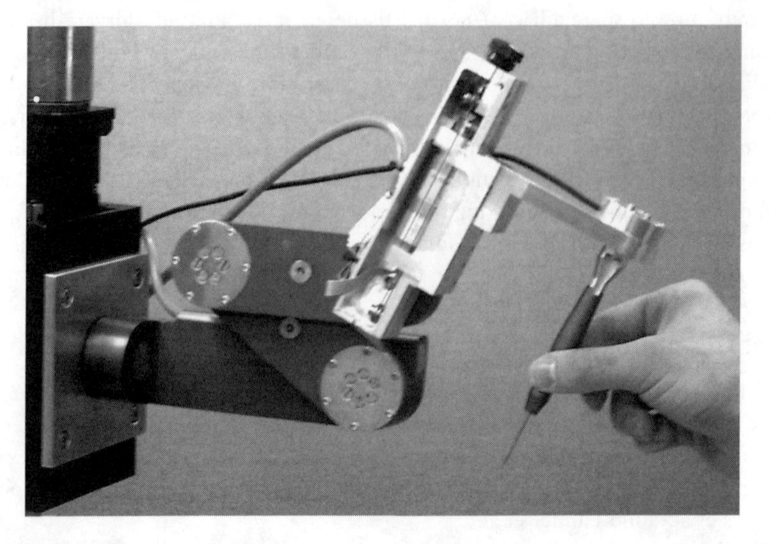

FIGURE 32.21 Steady-Hand robot for microsurgical augmentation. (Courtesy of Russell Taylor, Johns Hopkins University, Baltimore, MD.)

surgery, the system is applicable to numerous clinical specialties. The system consists of four modular subassemblies:

1. An off-the-shelf XYZ translation assembly (only the Z-axis can be seen here)
2. An orientation assembly
3. An end-of-arm motion and guiding assembly including a force/torque sensor
4. Specialized instruments

The major difference between this robotic device and the other robotic systems described in this review is that the Steady-Hand robot is designed to work cooperatively with the physician. In operation, the physician will grasp the tool held by the robot and manipulate the tool with the aid of the robot. The control system of the robot senses the forces exerted by the physician on the tool and by the tool on the environment and responds accordingly. The robot can thus provide smooth, tremor-free, precise positioning and force scaling.

The Steady-Hand robot was employed in a series of experiments to test the ability of a human to position a 10–0 microsurgical needle to 250-, 200-, and 150-μm accuracy.[51] A datum surface was fabricated consisting of two metallic sheets separated by an insulating surface. Three different versions of the experiments were performed: (1) unassisted series (human only); (2) hand-held (human plus Steady-Hand); and (3) autonomous (Steady-Hand was registered to the plates). The use of the Steady-Hand robot was found to significantly improve the ability of the human to position the needle, as success rates improved from 43% unassisted to 79% hand-held for the 150-μm holes (autonomous performance was even better at 96.5%).

32.4.8 Cardiology

Two companies have recently developed master-slave systems for minimally invasive surgery that are aimed at restoring the dexterity that is lost when using traditional laproscopic instruments. The introduction of these systems is a paradigm shift for surgical applications, in that the physician is no longer directly manipulating the surgical tool, but rather controlling the device from a remote interface. While these systems might be used for remote telesurgery in the future, in current practice the master and slave devices are in the same operating room. The initial clinical applications of these systems have been in cardiac surgery, although other applications are beginning to appear as well.

32.4.8.1 Intuitive Surgical: da Vinci

The Intuitive Surgical system (Figure 32.22), called da Vinci, consists of the surgeon's viewing and control console, a control unit, and a three-arm surgical manipulator.[30] The system is designed to combine the freehand movements used in open surgery with the less traumatic methods of minimally invasive surgery. The surgeon sits at the console and sees a high-resolution, three-dimensional image of the surgical field. The surgeon's hands grasp the instrument handles that control the remote endoscopic manipulators and end-effectors. The surgeon's console is shown in Figure 32.22 and a view of the instrument handles along with the remote manipulators is shown in Figure 32.23. The manipulators provide three DOFs (pitch, yaw, and insertion). The end-effector consists of a miniature wrist that adds three more DOFs (pitch, yaw, and roll) and one motion for tool actuation (such as grip). The system allows increased precision by providing motion scaling whereby large motions of the input devices can be scaled down proportionally to produce small motions at the end-effector. Finally, unintended movements caused by tremor, which typically occur with a frequency of 6 to 10 Hz, are filtered by applying a 6-Hz motion filter.[52] Design issues associated with these types of systems are described by Madhani et al.[53]

The da Vinci system had been used to perform over 500 procedures as of October 1999.[30] The system has not only been used for cardiac procedures such as fully endoscopic coronary artery bypass grafts (CABG), but also for a wide variety of other procedures including Nissen fundoplication, cholecystecomy, and lumbar sympathectomy.

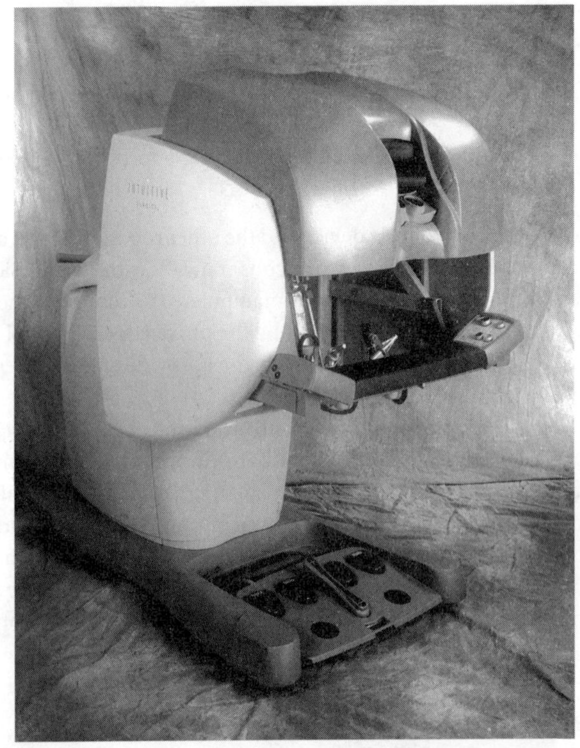

FIGURE 32.22 da Vinci surgeon's console. (Courtesy of Intuitive Surgical, Sunnyvale, CA.)

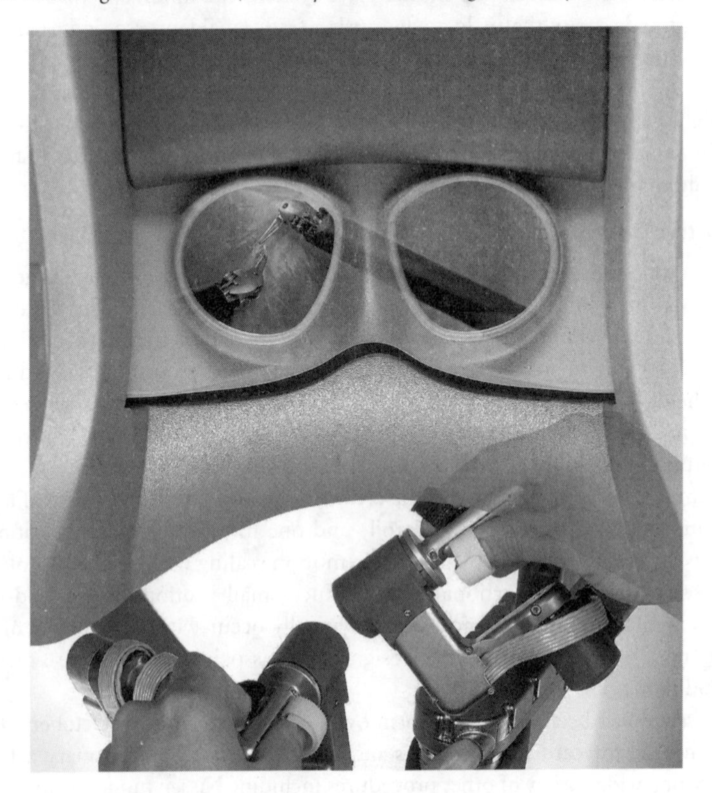

FIGURE 32 23 da Vinci instrument handles and remote manipulators. (Courtesy of Intuitive Surgical, Sunnyvale, CA.)

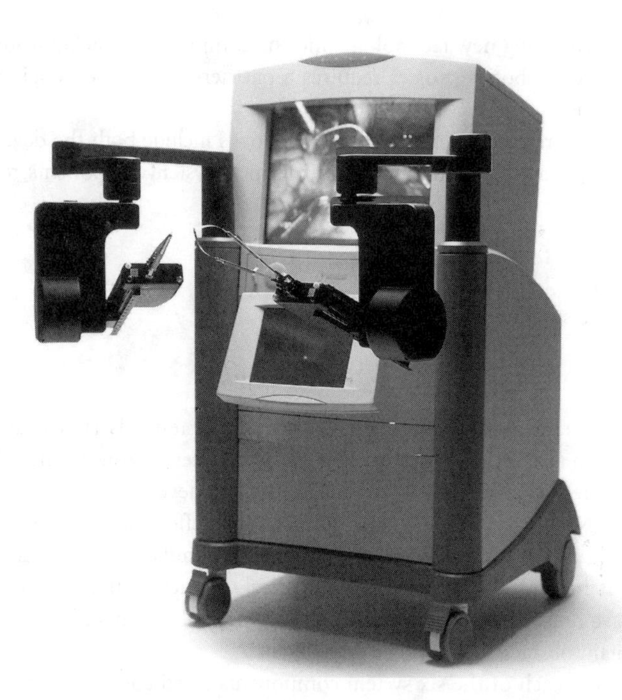

FIGURE 32.24 Zeus surgeon's console. (©2001 Computer Motion, Santa Barbara, CA. Photograph by Bobbi Bennett.)

32.4.8.2 Computer Motion: Zeus

A similar telesurgical system, called Zeus, has been developed by Computer Motion. A picture of the surgeon's console is shown in Figure 32.24. The Zeus slave system consists of three interactive robotic arms (two endoscopic instrument arms and one endoscopic camera arm) which are mounted on the operating room table. However, while the Intuitive Surgical system is a six DOF system (plus grip motion), the Computer Motion system only has four DOFs, and therefore is not as dexterous. Still, the performance of these systems in clinical applications is just beginning to be investigated, and it is difficult to draw conclusions about their efficacy at this point.

The clinical use of the system for endoscopic coronary artery bypass on 25 patients has been described by Boehm et al.[31] This study showed that endoscopic coronary artery bypass on the beating heart is possible, but further development of the technology and techniques is required to minimize the procedure time.

32.4.8.3 Grenoble: Pericardial Puncture

A prototype robot for pericardial puncture has been developed by Troccaz and colleagues at the TIMC/IMAG laboratory of Grenoble University Hospital. The robot is a six DOF SCARA design consisting of a vertical translational axis, three vertical rotational axes, a rotation about a horizontal axis, and a last modular joint which can be a rotational or translational axis. Similar to the Acrobot system for knee replacement surgery described earlier, this robot is designed as a synergistic device that is to be used in cooperation with a human operator. The design of the prototype robot and preliminary experiments are presented in an article by Schneider and Troccaz.[32]

32.5 Technology Challenges/Research Areas

While a number of different clinical areas are being explored as noted in Section 32.4, the field of medical robotics is still in its infancy and we are just at the beginning of this era. Only a handful of commercial companies exist and the number of medical robots sold each year is very small. Part of the reason for this is the difficulty of introducing new technology into the complex medical environment. In addition, the completion of a medical robotics project requires a partnership between engineers and clinicians which is not easy to establish.

Technology challenges and research areas for medical robotics include both the development of system components and the development of systems as a whole. In terms of system components, research is needed in:

1. System architecture
2. Software design
3. Mechanical design
4. Imaging compatible systems
5. User interface
6. Safety issues

For medical robotics systems, the development of application testbeds is critical to move the field forward. These testbeds can also serve to improve the dialog between engineers and clinicians. However, at least in the United States, it is difficult to obtain funding to develop these testbeds. Governmental funding agencies such as NIH or NSF will usually not fund such efforts as they are geared more toward basic research rather than applied research and development. Manufacturers are usually not interested because the environment and investment payback for medical robotics is uncertain. The regulatory issues for medical robotics have not been fully explored, although several systems have been approved by the FDA. These factors remain obstacles to advancing the field.

In the following sections, each of the six system components listed above are briefly discussed.

32.5.1 System Architecture

For medical robotics to evolve as its own field and for the cost and difficulty of developing prototype systems to decrease, the establishment of a system architecture would be an enabling step. The system architecture should emphasize modularity, as noted by Taylor in the design of the Steady-Hand robot, which emphasizes modularity in mechanical design, control system electronics, and software.[29] A modular approach has also been emphasized in the Urology Robotics Laboratory of Stoianovici, where a number of mechanical modules have been developed for precision interventional procedures.[25]

32.5.2 Software Design

The development of a software environment for medical robotics, possibly including an appropriate real-time operating system, is a significant challenge. Many researchers developing medical robotics systems base their software development on commercially available software that may not be suitable for the surgical environment. However, the low cost and widespread availability of these software packages makes their use attractive and there are steps that can be taken (such as watchdog timers, backup systems, and error recovery procedures) to make these systems more reliable. Still, it is believed that along with the system architecture mentioned above, a robust software environment geared to the medical environment would be a substantial contribution. While this software environment would still need to be customized for different surgical procedures, researchers would at least have a starting point for their development work.

32.5.3 Mechanical Design

In addition to better software design, novel mechanical designs are needed to improve the utility of robotics in medical procedures. As noted in the historical review in this paper, the first recorded medical application of a robot was for biopsy of the brain, using a standard PUMA industrial robot. While some other researchers have described the use of industrial robot for medical tasks, it is the belief of these authors and others[54] that special purpose mechanical designs are more appropriate for most applications. In particular, these designs should be safer, as they can be designed specifically for the medical environment and customized for different medical procedures. Novel mechanical designs presented in this review include the Probot[24] and the Steady-Hand robot.[29] However, special purpose designs will not enjoy the same economies of scale as more general designs, and one other solution may be to develop more general purpose medical robots with specialized end-effectors.

32.5.4 Imaging Compatible Systems

With the increasing popularity of image-guided interventions, robotic systems are required that can work within the constraints of various imaging modalities such as CT and MRI. While these systems are for the most part still under the direct control of the physician, in the future they will be increasingly linked to these imaging modalities. In this review, some systems were noted that fall within this category, such as the MRI compatible manipulator of Masamune et al.[35] and the CT integrated robot Minerva.[16]

32.5.5 User Interface

One question that arises in the development of all medical robotics systems concerns the user interface. What is a suitable user interface for a medical robot? Should the robot be given a commanded path or volume and then autonomously carry out the task? Is a joystick or pushbutton interface appropriate? Or would the physician rather manipulate the tool directly with the assistance of the robot? Is force feedback required for a high-fidelity user interface?

These are all questions that require further investigation by the medical robotics community. The answer certainly will vary depending on the medical task for which the robot is designed. It seems that medical robots will at least initially be more accepted by physicians if the physicians feel that they are still in control of the entire procedure.

32.5.6 Safety Issues

Safety is a paramount concern in the application of these systems and must be addressed to move the field forward. Safety issues have been discussed by Davies[54] and Elder and Knight.[55] According to Davies, medical robotics is a completely different application from industrial robotics in that medical robots must operate in cooperation with people to be fully effective. Therefore, appropriate safety levels should be defined and discussed by the community at large. Safety measures that can be taken include the use of redundant sensors, the design of special-purpose robots with capabilities tailored to the task at hand, and the use of fail-safe techniques so that if the robot does fail, it can be removed and the procedure completed by hand. One other safety issue for medical robotics is the need for sterilization and infection control in the operating room and interventional suite.

Davies also presents a hierarchical scheme for the host of tools available to surgeons, ranging from hand-held tools to a fully powered autonomous robot. As the hierarchy moves toward autonomous robots, the surgeon is less and less in control, and more dependent on the mechanical and software systems of the robot. Davies contends that until a consensus is developed on what level of safety is acceptable for what level of autonomy, the medical manufacturers will be slow to develop robotic systems.

While mechanical constraints are one means of assuring safety, programmable constraints, while inherently not as safe, are more flexible. The idea is to dynamically constrain the range of possible motions.[32] Four programming modes can be envisioned: free mode, position mode, trajectory mode, and region mode. As an example, region mode is particularly suited to resection operations such as total knee replacement in that the surgical tool is constrained to remain within a predefined region. This mode could also be valuable in the training of residents and fellows.

32.6 Conclusions

This chapter has reviewed the state of the art in surgical robotics. Several prototype and commercial medical robotics systems were described. Technology challenges and areas for future research were discussed. The use of robots in medicine clearly offers great promise.

We are just in the initial stages of the application of robotics to medicine, and much more work remains to be done. In particular, the development of more testbeds is required for different medical procedures so that more experience can be gained with the technology and how it can be integrated into clinical practice. The issues of cost, safety, and patient outcomes also need to be considered. While there have been some modestly successful commercial medical robots such as ROBODOC and da Vinci, they still are not completely accepted by the medical community.

It may be that the full benefits of robots in medicine will not be realized until more integrated systems are developed, in which the robots are linked to the imaging modalities or to the patient anatomy directly. This link will highlight the potential advantages of robots such as the ability to follow respiratory motion, and enable physicians to successfully complete procedures that can only be imagined today.

Acknowledgments

This is a revised version of an article titled "State of the Art in Surgical Robotics: Clinical Applications and Technology Challenges" that appeared in *Computer Aided Surgery*, Vol. 6, Number 6, 2001, pages 312–328, Copyright © 2002 by Wiley-Liss. The authors would like to thank Wiley for permission to republish this material. The authors would like to thank all their colleagues who generously donated photographs. This work was funded in part by U.S. Army Grants DAMD17–96–2–6004 and DAMD17–99–1–9022. The content of this manuscript does not necessarily reflect the position or policy of the U.S. Government.

References

1. Capek, K., *R.U.R.* (*Rossum's Universal Robots*), Dover Publications, Mineola, NY, 2001.
2. Craig, J.J., *Introduction to Robotics, 2nd ed.*, Addison-Wesley, Reading, PA, 1989.
3. Paul, R.P., *Robot Manipulators: Mathematics, Programming, and Control*, MIT Press, Cambridge, 1981.
4. Fu, K.S., Lee, C.S.G., and Gonzales, R.C., *Robotics: Control, Sensing, Vision & Intelligence*, McGraw-Hill, New York, 1987.
5. Spong, M.W. and Vidyasagar, M., *Robot Dynamics and Control*, Wiley, New York, 1989.
6. Davies, B., A review of robotics in surgery, *Proc. Inst. Mech. Eng. [H]*, 214, 129–140, 2000.
7. Taylor, R.H., Robots as surgical assistants: where we are, wither we are tending, and how to get there, in AIME 97, Genoble, France, 1997, pp. 3–11.
8. Troccaz, J. and Delnondedieu, Y., Robots in surgery, in IARP Workshop on Medical Robots, Vienna, 1996, pp. 161–168.
9. Howe, R.D. and Matsuoka, Y., Robotics for surgery, *Annu. Rev. Biomed. Eng.*, 1, 211–240, 1999.
10. Cadeddu, J.A., Stoianovici, D., and Kavoussi, L.R., Robotic surgery in urology, *Urol. Clin. North Am.*, 25(1), 75–85, 1998.
11. Kwoh, Y.S. et al., A robot with improved absolute positioning accuracy for CT guided stereotactic brain surgery, *IEEE Trans. Biomed. Eng.*, 35(2), 153–160, 1988.
12. Yamauchi, Y. et al., A needle insertion manipulator for x-ray CT image-guided neurosurgery, *Proc. LST*, 5, 814–821, 1993.
13. Davies, B.L. et al., A surgeon robot for prostatectomies, in 5th Int. Conf. on Advanced Robotics (ICAR '91), IEEE, 1991, pp. 871–875.
14. Benabid, A.L. et al., Computer-driven robot for stereotactic surgery connected to CT scan and magnetic resonance imaging. Technological design and preliminary results, *Appl. Neurophysiol.*, 50(1-6), 153–154, 1987.
15. Taylor, R.H. et al., An image-directed robotic system for precise orthopaedic surgery, *IEEE Trans. Robotics Automation*, 10(3), 261–273, 1994.
16. Burckhart, C.W., Flury, P., and Glauser, D., Stereotactic brain surgery, *IEEE Eng. Med. Biol.*, 14(3), 314–317, 1995.

17. Glauser, D. et al., Mechanical concept of the neurosurgical robot Minerva, *Robotica*, 11(6), 567–575, 1993.
18. Lavallee, S. et al., Image-guided operating robot: a clinical application in stereotactic neurosurgery, in *Computer-Integrated Surgery*, Taylor, R.H. et al., Eds., MIT Press, Cambridge, 1995, pp. 343–351.
19. Masamune, K. et al., System for robotically assisted percutaneous procedures with computed tomography guidance, *Comput. Aided Surg.*, 6(6), 370–383, 2001.
20. Yanof, J. et al., CT-integrated robot for interventional procedures: preliminary experiment and computer-human interfaces, *Comput. Aided Surg.*, 6(6), 352–359, 2001.
21. Jakopec, M. et al., The first clinical application of a "hands-on" robotic knee surgery system, *Comput. Aided Surg.*, 6(6), 329–339, 2001.
22. Cleary, K. et al., Robotically assisted nerve and facet blocks: a cadaveric study, *Acad. Radiol.*, 9(7), 821–825, 2002.
23. Kronreif, G., Fürst, M., Kettenbach, J., Figl, M., and Hanel, R., Robotic guidance for percutaneous interventions, *Adv. Robotics*, accepted for publication.
24. Davies, B.L. et al., A clinically applied robot for prostatectomies, in *Computer-Integrated Surgery*, Taylor, R.H. et al., Eds., MIT Press, Cambridge, 1995, pp. 593–601.
25. Stoianovici, D., URobotics — Urology robotics at Johns Hopkins, *Comput. Aided Surg.*, 6(6), 360–369, 2001.
26. Lueth, T.C. et al., A surgical robotic system for maxillofacial surgery, in Proceedings of the 24th Annual Conference of the IEEE Industrial Electronics Society (IECON), 1998, pp. 2470–2475.
27. Burghart, C. et al., Robot assisted craniofacial surgery: first clinical evaluation, in *Computer Assisted Radiology and Surgery*, Elsevier, New York, 1999, 828–833.
28. Adler, J.R., Jr. et al., Image-guided robotic radiosurgery, *Neurosurgery*, 44(6), 1299–1306, 1999; discussion 1306–1307.
29. Taylor, R.H. et al., A steady-hand robotic system for microsurgical augmentation. *Int. J. Robotics Res.*, 18(12), 1201–1210, 1999.
30. Guthart, G.S. and Salisbury, J.J.K., The intuitive telesurgery system: overview and application, in *IEEE International Conference on Robotics and Automation*, 2000, pp. 618–621.
31. Boehm, D.H. et al., Clinical use of a computer-enhanced surgical robotic system for endoscopic coronary artery bypass grafting on the beating heart [In Process Citation], *Thorac. Cardiovasc. Surg.*, 48(4), 198–202, 2000.
32. Schneider, O. and Troccaz, J., A six-degree-of-freedom passive arm with dynamic constraints (PADyC) for cardiac surgery application: preliminary experiments, *Comput. Aided Surg.*, 6(6), 340–351, 2001.
33. Lavallee, S., A new system for computer assisted neurosurgery. in *Proc. 11th IEEE Eng. Med. Biol. Conf.*, 1989, 926–927.
34. Benabid, A.L. et al., Robotic guidance in advanced imaging environments, in *Advanced Neurosurgical Navigation*, E.A. III and Maciunas, R.J., Eds., Thieme Medical Publishers, Inc., New York, 1999, pp. 571–583.
35. Masamune, K. et al., Development of an MRI-compatible needle insertion manipulator for stereotactic neurosurgery, *J. Image Guid. Surg.*, 1(4), 242–248, 1995.
36. Chinzei, K. et al., MR compatible surgical assist robot: system integration and preliminary feasibility study, in *Medical Image Computing and Computer Assisted Intervention*, 2000, pp. 921–930.
37. Kaiser, W.A. et al., Robotic system for biopsy and therapy of breast lesions in a high-field whole-body magnetic resonance tomography unit, *Invest. Radiol.*, 35(8), 513–519, 2000.
38. DiGioia, A.M., What is computer assisted orthopaedic surgery? *Clin. Orthop.*, (354), 2–4, 1998.
39. Borner, M. et al., Experiences with the ROBODOC system in more than 1000 cases, in *Computer Aided Radiology and Surgery*, Elsevier, Amsterdam, 1998, pp. 689–693.
40. Bauer, A., Borner, M., and Lahmer, A., Clinical experience with a medical robotic system for total hip replacement, in *Computer Assisted Orthopedic Surgery*, Nolte, L.P. and Ganz, R., Eds., Hogrefe & Huber, Bern, 1999, pp. 128–133.

41. Cleary, K. et al., Robotics for percutaneous spinal procedures: initial report, in *Computer Assisted Radiology and Surgery (CARS)*, Elsevier, Amsterdam, 2000, pp. 128–133.
42. Cleary, K. et al., Robotically assisted spine needle placement: program plan and cadaver study, in *Computer Based Medical Systems (CBMS) 14th IEEE Int. Symp.*, 2001, pp. 339–342.
43. Kronreif, G. and Fürst, M., Robotic guidance for percutaneous interventions, in *Proc. 11th Int. Workshop on Robotics in Alpe-Adria-Danube Region (RAAD 2002)*, Balatonfüred, Hungary, Budapest Polytechnic, 2002, pp. 277–281.
44. Stoianovici, D. et al., An efficient needle injection technique and radiological guidance method for percutaneous procedures, in *CVRMed-MRCAS*, Troccaz, J., Grimson, E., and Mosges, R., Eds., Springer-Verlag, Grenoble, 1997, pp. 295–298.
45. Stoianovici, D. et al., A modular surgical robotic system for image guided percutaneous procedures, in *MICCAI 98*, Wells, W.M., Colchester, A., and Delp, S., Eds., Springer, Cambridge, MA, 1998, pp. 404–410.
46. Lueth, T. and Bier, J., Robot assisted intervention in surgery, in *Neuronavigation — Neurosurgical and Computer Scientific Aspects*, Gilsbach, J.M. and Stiehl, H.S., Eds., Springer-Verlag, Heidelberg, 1999.
47. Heissler, E. et al., Robot supported insertion of catheters for hyperthermia and brachytherapy, in *Computer Assisted Radiology and Surgery*, Elsevier, Amsterdam, 1998, pp. 660–663.
48. Charles, S., Williams, R.E., and Hamel, B., Design of a surgeon-machine interface for teleoperated microsurgery, in *Proc. Annu. Int. Conf. IEEE Eng. Med. Biol. Soc.*, IEEE, 1989, pp. 883–884.
49. Das, H. et al., Evaluation of a telerobotic system to assist surgeons in microsurgery, *Comput. Aided Surg.*, 4, 15–25, 1999.
50. Hunter, I.W. et al., A teleoperated microsurgical robot and associated virtual environment for eye surgery, *Presence*, 2(4), 265–280, 1993.
51. Kumar, R. et al. Performance of robotic augmentation in microsurgery-scale motions, in *2nd Int. Symp. Medical Image Computing and Computer Assisted Surgery*, 1999, pp. 1108–1115.
52. Falk, V. et al., Quality of computer enhanced totally endoscopic coronary bypass graft anastomosis — comparison to conventional technique, *Eur. J. Cardiothorac. Surg.*, 15(3), 260–264, 1999; discussion 264–265.
53. Madhani, A.J., Niemeyer, G., and J.K.S. Jr., The Black Falcon: a teleoperated surgical instrument for minimally invasive surgery, in *Int. Conf. Intelligent Robots and Systems*, IEEE, Victoria, B.C., Canada, 1998, pp. 936–944.
54. Davies, B.L., A discussion of safety issues for medical robotics, in *Computer-Integrated Surgery*, Taylor, R.H. et al., Eds., MIT Press, Cambridge, 1996, pp. 287–296.
55. Elder, M.C. and Knight, J.C., Specifying user interfaces for safety-critical medical systems, in *Medical Robotics and Computer Assisted Surgery*, Wiley-Liss, Baltimore, MD, 1995, 148–155.

Index

A

C

D

E

F

G

H

I

J

K

L

M

N

O

P

Q

R

S

T

U

V

W

X

Y

Z